Oxford Textbook of
Psychotherapy

Edited by

Glen O. Gabbard

*Brown Foundation Chair of Psychoanalysis and Professor of Psychiatry,
Baylor College of Medicine, Houston, Texas, USA*

Judith S. Beck

*Director, Beck Institute for Cognitive Therapy and Research; Clinical Associate
Professor, University of Pennsylvania, School of Medicine, Philadelphia, Pennsylvania, USA*

and

Jeremy Holmes

*Consultant Psychiatrist/Psychotherapist, Devon NHS Partnership Trust; Visiting Professor
of Psychological Therapies, University of Exeter, and Psychoanalysis Unit,
University College London, London, UK*

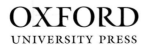

OXFORD
UNIVERSITY PRESS

OXFORD
UNIVERSITY PRESS

Great Clarendon Street, Oxford OX2 6DP

Oxford University Press is a department of the University of Oxford.
It furthers the University's objective of excellence in research, scholarship,
and education by publishing worldwide in

Oxford New York

Auckland Cape Town Dar es Salaam Hong Kong Karachi
Kuala Lumpur Madrid Melbourne Mexico City Nairobi
New Delhi Shanghai Taipei Toronto

With offices in

Argentina Austria Brazil Chile Czech Republic France Greece
Guatemala Hungary Italy Japan Poland Portugal Singapore
South Korea Switzerland Thailand Turkey Ukraine Vietnam

Oxford is a registered trade mark of Oxford University Press
in the UK and in certain other countries

Published in the United States
by Oxford University Press Inc., New York

British Library Cataloguing in Publication Data

Data available

Library of Congress Cataloging in Publication Data

Data available

Typeset by Newgen Imaging Systems (P) Ltd, Chennai, India
Printed in Italy
on acid-free paper by Grafiche Industriali

ISBN 0 19 852064 6   978 0 19 852064 1

10 9 8 7 6 5 4 3 2 1

Contents

Contributors

Gwen Adshead Consultant Psychotherapist, Broadmoor Hospital, Crowthorne, UK
40 Ethics and psychotherapy

Linda B. Andrews Director of Residency Education/Assistant Dean, Menninger Department of Psychiatry, Baylor College of Medicine, Houston, TX, USA
42 Psychotherapy supervision

Mark Aveline Professor, Institute of Lifelong Learning, University of Leicester, Leicester, UK
38 Psychotherapy research

Anthony W. Bateman Visiting Professor, University College London; Consultant Psychiatrist and Psychotherapist, Halliwick Unit, St Ann's Hospital, Barnet, Enfield and Haringey Mental Health Trust, London, UK
24 Borderline personality disorder

Aaron T. Beck Professor, University of Pennsylvania, School of Medicine; President, Beck Institute for Cognitive Therapy and Research, Philadelphia, PA, USA
11 Cognitive-behavior therapy for mood disorders

Judith S. Beck Director, Beck Institute for Cognitive Therapy and Research, Beck Institute, Bala Cynwyd, PA, USA; Clinical Associate Professor of Psychology in Psychiatry and President Elect, Academy of Cognitive Therapy, University of Pennsylvania, Philadelphia, PA, USA

Fred S. Berlin Associate Professor, Department of Psychiatry and Behavioral Sciences, The Johns Hopkins University School of Medicine, Baltimore, MD, USA; Director, National Institute for the Study, Prevention and Treatment of Sexual Trauma
17 Paraphilias

Carlos Blanco New York State Psychiatric Institute, Anxiety Disorders Clinic, New York, NY, USA
3 Interpersonal psychotherapy

Irma J. Bland (deceased) Clinical Professor of Psychiatry, Louisiana State University at New Orleans, New Orleans, LA, USA
36 Cross-Cultural psychotherapy

Sidney Bloch Professor, Department of Psychiatry and Centre for the Study of Health and Society, The University of Melbourne, St Vincent's Hospital, Melbourne, Australia
6 Family therapy

G. R. Bloch-Thorsen Psychiatrist, Rogalund Psychiatric Hospital, Stavanger, Norway
14 Schizophrenia

Louisa M. C. Van Den Bosch Amsterdam Institute for Addiction Research, Psychiatrisch Centrum AMC, Amsterdam, The Netherlands
24 Borderline personality disorder

John W. Burruss Chief of Psychiatry, Ben Taub General Hospital; Assistant Professor, Menninger Department of Psychiatry, Houston, TX, USA
42 Psychotherapy supervision

Fredric N. Busch Assistant Clinical Professor of Psychiatry, Weill Cornell Medical College, Columbia University, New York, NY, USA
13 Anxiety disorders

Veronica Cardenas Doctoral Candidate, Pacific Graduate School of Psychology, Palo Alto, California, USA
5 Cognitive-behavioral group interventions

Sjoerd Colijn Psychotherapist and Cultural Anthropologist; Head, Outpatient Department, Rijngeest Groep, Leiden, The Netherlands
10 Psychotherapy integration

Joan M. Cook University of Pennsylvania, School of Medicine, Philadelphia, PA, USA
32 Psychotherapy with older adults

David W. Coon Associate Professor, Department of Social and Behavioral Sciences, New College of Interdisciplinary Arts and Sciences, Arizona State University, Glendale, AZ, USA
5 Cognitive-behavioral group interventions

Christopher Cordess Emeritus Professor of Forensic Psychiatry, University of Sheffield, Sheffield, UK
22 'Cluster B' antisocial disorders

David Cottrell Professor of Child and Adolescent Psychiatry, Leeds University, Leeds, UK
29 Psychosocial therapies with children

Frank M. Dattilio Clinical Associate Professor of Psychiatry, Department of Psychiatry, Harvard Medical School, Boston, MA, USA
8 Cognitive-behavior therapy with couples

Kate Davidson Consultant Clinical Psychiatrist, Section of Psychological Medicine, University of Glasgow, Glasgow, UK
22 'Cluster B' antisocial disorders

Robert J. DeRubeis Professor and Chair, Department of Psychology, University of Pennsylvania, Philadelphia, PA, USA
2 Cognitive and behavioral therapies

Javier Escobar Chair and Professor of Psychiatry, Robert Wood Johnson Medical School, University of Medicine and Dentistry of New Jersey, Piscataway, USA
20 Psychotherapy of somatoform disorders

Peter J. Fagan Associate Professor of Medical Psychology, Johns Hopkins University School of Medicine, Baltimore, MD, USA
17 Paraphilias

Randy Fingerhut Center for Cognitive Therapy, Department of Psychiatry, University of Pennsylvania, Philadelphia, PA, USA
26 Psychotherapy for avoidant personality disorder

Peter Fonagy Freud Memorial Professor of Psychoanalysis, University College London; Chief Executive, The Anna Freud Centre, London, UK
29 Psychosocial therapies with children

David Fowler Department of Health Policy and Practice, University of East Anglia, Norwich, UK
21 'Cluster A' personality disorders

Arthur Freeman Professor and Chair, Department of Psychology, Philadelphia College of Osteopathic Medicine, Philadelphia, PA, USA
25 Histrionic personality disorder

Sharon Morgillo Freeman Aboite Behavioral Health Sciences, FortWayne, IN, USA
25 Histrionic personality disorder

Peter Fuggle Consultant Clinical Psychologist, Islington Primary Care Trust, London, UK
29 Psychosocial therapies with children

Glen O. Gabbard Brown Foundation Chair of Psychoanalysis, Professor, Department of Psychiatry and Behavioral Sciences, Director, Baylor Psychiatry Clinic, Baylor College of Medicine, Houston, TX, USA
1 Major modalities: psychoanalytic/psychodynamic
28 Psychotherapy of obsessive-compulsive personality disorder

Dolores Gallagher-Thompson Professor of Research, Department of Psychiatry and Behavioral Sciences, Stanford University School of Medicine, Stanford, CA, USA
5 Cognitive-behavioral group interventions
32 Psychotherapy with older adults

Zoë Gillispie Doctoral Candidate, Pacific Graduate School of Psychology, Palo Alto, CA, USA
5 Cognitive-behavioral group interventions

Paul M. Grant Department of Psychology, University of Pennsylvania, Philadelphia, PA, USA
2 Cognitive and behavioral therapies

Jennifer A. Gray Department of Psychology, University of Hawaii, Honolulu, HI, USA
15 Eating disorders

Seth D. Grossman Assistant Dean, Institute for Advanced Studies in Personology and Psychopathology, Coral Gables, FL, USA; Postdoctoral Fellow, Florida International University
23 Psychotherapy for the narcissistic personality disorder

Rex Haigh Consultant Psychiatrist in Psychotherapy, Winterbourne House, Berkshire Healthcare NHS Trust, Reading, UK
21 'Cluster A' personality disorders

Edwin Harari Department of Psychiatry, The University of Melbourne, St Vincent's Hospital, Fitzroy, VIC, Australia
6 Family therapy

Jason Hepple Medical Director, Somerset Partnership NHS and Social Care Trust, BridgeWater, UK
32 Psychotherapy with older adults

Jeremy Holmes Consultant Psychiatrist/Psychotherapist, Devon NHS Partnership Trust; Visiting Professor of Psychological Therapies, University of Exeter, and Psychoanalysis Unit, University College London, London, UK
10 Psychotherapy integration

Michelle Jeffcott Graduate Student, Department of Psychological Sciences, University of Missouri-Columbia, Columbia, MO, USA
18 Sexual disorders

Sigmund Karterud Professor, Department for Personality Psychiatry, Psychiatric Division, Ulleval University Hospital, Oslo, Norway
24 Borderline personality disorder

Jerald Kay Professor and Chair, Department of Psychiatry, Wright State University School of Medicine, Dayton, OH, USA
39 Psychotherapy and medication

Werner Knauss Senior Clinical Psychologist, Heidelberg, Germany
4 Group psychotherapy

Willem Kuyken School of Psychology, University of Exeter, Exeter, UK
11 Cognitive-behavior therapy for mood disorders

Robert L. Leahy Professor, Department of Psychiatry, Weill-Cornell University Medical College, New York Presbyterian Hospital; Director, American Institute for Cognitive Therapy, New York, USA
13 Anxiety disorders

Gregory Lehne Assistant Professor of Psychology, Department of Psychiatry and Behavioral Sciences, Johns Hopkins University School of Medicine, Baltimore, MD, USA
17 Paraphilias

Giovanni Liotti Professor of Cognitive Psychotherapy, School of Cognitive Psychotherapy, Rome, Italy
16 Dissociative disorders

Don R. Lipsitt Clinical Professor of Psychiatry, Harvard Medical School, Boston, MA, USA
20 Psychotherapy of somatoform disorders

James W. Lomax Associate Chairman and Director of Educational Programs, Menninger Department of Psychiatry, Baylor College of Medicine, Houston, TX, USA
42 Psychotherapy supervision

Joseph LoPiccolo Professor of Psychology, Department of Psychological Sciences, University of Missouri-Columbia, Columbia, MO, USA
18 Sexual disorders

B. Martindale Consultant Psychiatrist in Psychotherapy, Early Intervention in Psychosis Service, Monkwearmouth Hospital, Sunderland, UK
14 Schizophrenia

Mary K. McCarthy Assistant Professor of Psychiatry, Harvard Medical School, Department of Psychiatry, Brigham and Women's Hospital, Boston, MA, USA
34 Gender issues in psychotherapy

Lata K. McGinn Ferkauf School of Psychology, Yeshira University, Bronx, NY, USA
13 Anxiety disorders

Delinda Mercer University of Pennsylvania, Philadelphia, PA, USA
19 Individual psychotherapy and counseling for addiction

Barbara L. Milrod Associate Professor of Psychiatry, Weill Medical College of Cornell University, New York, NY, USA
13 Anxiety disorders

Theodore Millon Dean and Scientific Director, Institute for Advanced Studies in Personology and Psychopathology, Coral Gables, FL, USA; Professor Emeritus, University of Miami
23 Psychotherapy for the narcissistic personality disorder

Giuseppe Miti Psychiatrist/Psychotherapist, Department of Mental Health, Forlanini Hospital, Rome, Italy
16 Dissociative disorders

Phil Mollon Head of Adult Psychotherapy and Clinical Psychology Services, Lister Hospital, Stevenage, UK
16 Dissociative disorders

Stirling Moorey Head of Psychotherapy, South London and Maudsley Hospital, London, UK
42 Psychotherapy supervision

Mark Morris Consultant Forensic Psychotherapist, Kneesworth Hospital, Kneesworth, Cambridge, UK
22 'Cluster B' antisocial disorders

Carol C. Nadelson Clinical Professor of Psychiatry, Harvard Medical School, Department of Psychiatry, Brigham and Women's Hospital, Boston, MA, USA
34 Gender issues in psychotherapy

Cory F. Newman Director, Center for Cognitive Therapy, University of Pennsylvania School of Medicine, Philadelphia, PA, USA
26 Psychotherapy for avoidant personality disorder
28 Psychotherapy of obsessive-compulsive personality disorder

Malkah T. Notman Clinical Professor of Psychiatry, Harvard Medical School, Department of Psychiatry, Cambridge Hospital, Cambridge, MA, USA
34 Gender issues in psychotherapy

Helen Odell-Miller Director of Music Therapy; Principal Lecturer in Learning and Teaching, Anglia Polytechnic University, Cambridge, UK; and Head Research Clinical Specialist for Arts Therapies, Cambridge and Peterborough Mental Health Partnership NHS Trust, Cambridge, UK
9 The arts therapies

Glenys Parry Professor of Applied Psychological Therapies, School of Health and Related Research, University of Sheffield, Sheffield, UK
43 Brief and time-limited psychotherapy

J. Christopher Perry Professor of Psychiatry, McGill University, and, Director of Psychotherapy Research, Institute of Community and Family Psychiatry, Sir Mortimer B. Davis Jewish General Hospital, Montreal, Quebec, Canada; Research Affiliate, The Austen Riggs Center, Stockbridge, MA, USA
27 Dependent personality disorder

Sidney H. Phillips Associate Clinical Professor of Psychiatry, Yale University, New Haven, CT, USA
35 Sexual orientation and psychotherapy

Edmond H. Pi Clinical Professor of Psychiatry, David Geffen School of Medicine, University of California at Los Angeles (UCLA), Department of Psychiatry, Harbor-UCLA Medical Center, CA, USA
36 Cross-Cultural psychotherapy

Joan Raphael-Leff Professor, Head of MSc, UCL/Anna Freud Centre, London; Visiting Professor, Centre for Psychoanalytic Studies, University of Essex, Colchester, UK
31 Psychotherapy during the reproductive years

Mark A. Reinecke Northwestern University Medical School, Division of Psychology, Chicago, IL, USA
30 Psychotherapy with adolescents

Justin Richardson Assistant Clinical Professor of Psychiatry, Columbia University College of Physicians and Surgeons, New York, NY, USA
35 Sexual orientation and psychotherapy

Phil Richardson Taristock Clinic, London, UK
12 The psychoanalytic/psychodynamic approach to depressive disorders

Pedro Ruiz Professor and Vice Chair, Department of Psychiatry and Behavioral Sciences, University of Texas Medical Sciences School at Houston, Houston, TX, USA
36 Cross-Cultural psychotherapy

David E. Scharff Co-Director of the International Psychotherapy Institute, Washington, DC, USA
7 Psychodynamic couple therapy

Jill Savege Scharff Co-Director of the International Psychotherapy Institute, Washington, DC, USA
7 Psychodynamic couple therapy

Joy Schaverien Visiting Professor in Art Psychotherapy, University of Sheffield, Sheffield, UK
9 The arts therapies

Stephen R. Shirk Department of Psychology, University of Denver, Denver, CO, USA
30 Psychotherapy with adolescents

Gia Robinson Shurgot Postdoctoral Fellow, Older Adult and Family Center, VA Palo Alto Health Care System and Stanford University School of Medicine, Menlo Park, CA, USA
5 Cognitive-behavioral group interventions

Robert I. Simon Clinical Professor of Psychiatry, Director, Program in Psychiatry and Law, Georgetown University School of Medicine, Washington, DC; Chairman, Department of Psychiatry, Surburban Hospital, Bethesda, MD, USA
41 Clinical–legal issues in psychotherapy

Arietta Slade Professor of Clinical and Developmental Psychology, University College London, London, UK
29 Psychosocial therapies with children

William B. Stiles Professor, Department of Psychology, Miami University, Oxford, OH, USA
38 Psychotherapy research

Julia G. Strand Clinical Psychologist in private practice, Seattle, WA, USA
17 Paraphilias

Bernhard Strauss Professor, Institute of Medical Psychology, Klinikum der Friedrich-Schiller-Universitat, Jena, Germany
38 Psychotherapy research

Mary Target Reader in Psychoanalysis, University College London; Professional Director, The Anna Freud Centre, London, UK
29 Psychosocial therapies with children

David Taylor Medical Director, Tavistock and Portman NHS Trust, London, UK; Training and Supervising Psycho-analyst, British Psycho-Analytical Society
12 The psychoanalytic/psychodynamic approach to depressive disorders

P. M. Trief Professor, Departments of Psychiatry and Medicine, SUNY Upstate Medical University, Syracuse, NY, USA
33 Psychotherapy for medical patients

Rutger Willem Trijsburg Professor of Psychotherapy, Erasmus MC University Medical Center, Department of Medical Psychology and Psychotherapy, Rotterdam; University of Amsterdam, Department of Psychology, Amsterdam, The Netherlands
10 Psychotherapy integration

D. Turkington Senior Lecturer and Consultant Psychiatrist, School of Neurology, Neurosciences and Psychiatry, University of Newcastle-upon-Tyne, Royal Victoria Infirmary, Newcastle-upon-Tyne, UK
14 Schizophrenia

Susan C. Vaughan Assistant Clinical Professor of Psychiatry, Columbia University College of Physicians and Surgeons, New York, NY, USA
35 Sexual orientation and psychotherapy

Kelly M. Vitousek Department of Psychology, University of Hawaii, Honolulu HI, USA
15 Eating disorders

Ed Watkins Clinical Psychology Research Group, University of Exeter, Exeter, UK
11 Cognitive-behavior therapy for mood disorders

Myrna M. Weissman Columbia University, NY State Psychiatric Institute New York, NY, USA
3 Interpersonal psychotherapy

Drew Westen Professor, Department of Psychology and Behavioral Sciences Emory University, Atlanta, GA, USA
37 Implications of research in cognitive neuroscience for psychodynamic psychotherapy

C. A. White Deputy Director, Specialist Psychological Services, NHS Ayrshire and Arran; and Honorary Research Fellow, Faculty of Medicine, University of Glasgow, Scotland, UK
33 Psychotherapy for medical patients

Paul Williams Visiting Professor in Psychoanalysis, Anglia University, Chelmsford, UK
21 'Cluster A' personality disorders

George E. Woody Professor of Psychiatry, University of Pennsylvania, School of Medicine, Philadelphia, PA, USA
19 Individual psychotherapy and counseling for addiction

Paula R. Young Visiting Assistant Professor, Department of Psychology, Northwestern University, Evanston, IL, USA
2 Cognitive and behavioral therapies

Felicity de Zulueta Consulting Psychotherapist, Traumatic Stress Service, Maudsley Hospital, London, UK
36 Cross-Cultural psychotherapy

Introduction

We began the planning of this project with ambitious goals in mind. Above all, we sought to create a textbook that would help psychotherapists treat their patients more effectively. At the same time, we sought to be comprehensive in scope and to provide an evidence base wherever possible to guide the reader. We were aware that most practitioners inhabit a culture of psychotherapeutic pluralism, and we wanted to create a volume where the major psychotherapeutic voices could be heard and valued. We were also aware of a major discrepancy between what typically transpires in academic and training centers and what is actually implemented in the real world of clinical practice. Pure forms of psychotherapy are taught and tested in randomized controlled trials in many universities throughout the world, but most practitioners of psychotherapy in busy practices end up creating their own amalgam of pure and mixed models over time, depending on context and patient need. With this reality in mind, we also wanted to create a text that would encourage an integrated approach to psychotherapy where appropriate.

As if these multiple agendas were not ambitious enough, we also wanted to appeal to a broad market, including students and trainees in psychiatry, psychology, social work, psychotherapeutic counseling, and psychiatric nursing. In addition to trainees, however, we wanted the book to be useable as a reference manual for practicing psychotherapists who might be experienced but nevertheless in need of expert opinion about particular types of psychotherapy or challenges posed by patients with specific problems or issues. Finally, in order to avoid geographical or ideological parochialism, we conceived of the book as an international effort and sought contributions from a multinational panel of experts.

These guiding principles were fundamental to the manner in which we organized the text. We decided to lay the foundation in Section I with chapters describing the major forms of psychotherapy, covering the history, philosophy, and general principles of each of the major therapeutic modalities.

Section II is devoted to the individual psychiatric disorders. Each chapter covers a specific disorder, describing the major theories, evidence base, key practice principles, and guidelines to handle difficult challenges. A practicing psychotherapist who encountered a new patient with bulimia, for example, might wish to consult our book for a refresher on an up-to-date approach to the psychotherapy of eating disorders from a cognitive, psychodynamic, and systemic perspective.

To ensure that each chapter in Section II covered the major theoretical and treatment approaches, we had to devise innovative forms of collaboration. Where, for example, could we find an expert who could write about family, group, and individual therapy for schizophrenia from both a cognitive-behavioral and psychodynamic perspective? We realized that we would have to collect a group of colleagues to function as co-authors. Psychotherapists often think and work in splendid isolation, buttressed mainly by like-minded colleagues, where there is little cross-fertilization across modalities.

Hence at times we had to facilitate an authorial 'shotgun wedding' in which we drew a number of unlikely bedfellows together for the purpose of writing a comprehensive chapter. To avoid theoretical bias, we tried to ensure that the diverse psychotherapeutic strategies were represented in a balanced way in each chapter.

We were pleasantly surprised that in many instances this innovative arrangement had positive results, and the co-authors were admirably collegial. In other instances, we felt it was preferable to opt for two different chapters on the same disorder. For example, we have one chapter on cognitive-behavior therapy for mood disorders and another on psychodynamic therapy for the same diagnostic group.

Next we recognized that the book would be enhanced by a fourth section with chapters focusing on special populations of patients who do not fit neatly into a diagnostically oriented chapter. Psychotherapy varies throughout the lifespan, so we included chapters on children and adolescents, older adults, and the developmental challenges of reproductive and working lives. We have also enlisted authors to write chapters on gender, cultural issues, psychotherapy for medical patients, and the role that sexual orientation plays in psychotherapy.

Our goal to be comprehensive was still not met after we had organized the first section, so we decided to add a sixth and final section that would cover special topics that are highly relevant to most psychotherapists in practice. These include integrating medication with psychotherapy, psychotherapy conducted under time constraints, forensic psychotherapy, ethics, the interface of neuroscience and psychotherapy, and psychotherapy supervision.

With persistence, mutual support, and a possibly exaggerated sense of responsibility, we editors have accomplished much of what we set out to do in the early planning stages. We are pleased with the result and think that a broad audience will benefit from the end product. We owe a special debt of gratitude to Martin Baum and Carol Maxwell at Oxford University Press for keeping us on track and providing moral support when the obstacles seemed overwhelming. We also want to thank Richard Marley for getting the project started and believing that it could be done. We also wish to acknowledge the hard work of each of the authors and their willingness to collaborate with enthusiasm and open-mindedness, even though they were writing with colleagues who spoke a different psychotherapeutic language. In sum, we hope that this volume, comprehensive in scope, integrative in spirit, while respectful of individual psychotherapeutic traditions, will make a useful contribution to a new era of psychotherapy, fit for the challenges and opportunities of mental health care in the twenty-first century.

Glen O. Gabbard
Judith S. Beck
Jeremy Holmes

I

Major modalities

1 Major modalities: psychoanalytic/psychodynamic

Glen O. Gabbard

Introduction

The terms *psychoanalytic* and *psychodynamic* have increasingly been used synonymously in discussions of psychotherapy. Both psychotherapeutic approaches derive from a set of core principles derived from psychoanalysis. Among these principles are transference, countertransference, resistance, the dynamic unconscious, a developmental lens to view adult experience, and psychic determinism. The historical origins of this approach date back to the development of psychoanalysis by Sigmund Freud in the late 1890s and the early 1900s.

Although Freud originally was trained as a neurologist, under the influence of the French neurologist Jean-Martin Charcot, he became intrigued with the mysteries of hysteria. He later collaborated with Josef Breuer on the use of hypnotic suggestion in the treatment of patients suffering from hysteria. In their classical contributions to the subject, Breuer and Freud argued that hysterical patients suffer from 'reminiscences,' suggesting that an unacceptable and repressed idea was responsible for the symptoms of the illness. This understanding led to a therapeutic approach that came to be known as *abreaction*. Freud was initially convinced that bringing a repressed memory of a traumatic event back into the patient's conscious awareness through hypnotic suggestion would produce a catharsis that would result in removal of the patient's symptoms. In other words, the patient would be able to recover and verbalize the feelings that were associated with the original trauma.

Freud soon became frustrated with the use of hypnosis and cathartic abreaction because he learned that this therapeutic approach was often not acceptable and reflected the patient's wish to please the doctor. He also observed that some patients manifested *resistance* to this therapeutic approach. Either they were unable to be hypnotized or incapable of recovering memories that had etiological significance.

In addition, Freud began to recognize that a powerful relationship developed between patient and doctor that had a significant erotic component. One of his patients awoke from a hypnotic trance and threw her arms around Freud's neck. This experience and others led him to develop the concept of *transference*, which referred to the fact that patients displace on to the analyst the feelings, thoughts, and attitudes that were originally linked to parents or other significant figures from the past.

He then modified his technique in such a way that hypnosis was discarded and replaced with the method of *free association*. This technique, involving asking the patient to say whatever comes to mind, is still a cornerstone of technique used by psychoanalysts throughout the world.

Freud went on to immerse himself in the study of dreams, which he viewed as the 'royal road' to the understanding of the unconscious. He recognized that sexualized aspects of childhood life persist into the present and influence adult behavior.

The psychoanalytic approach to psychotherapy has undergone profound transformation since the era of Freud. Each of the core principles retain the remnants of Freudian thinking, however, and much of Freud's edifice remains relevant to our current understanding of patients and the therapeutic strategies used to share that understanding with the patient. While Freud viewed transference and resistance as the essential features of any psychoanalytic approach, today we would expand the fundamental set of concepts to include countertransference, the unconscious, psychic determinism, and a developmental perspective. These basic tenets will be introduced here and elaborated later in the chapter.

Transference

Patients unconsciously relate to the psychotherapist as though the therapist is someone from their past. Although Freud regarded transference as a simple displacement of a past relationship into the present, we now recognize that the therapist's actual characteristics and behavior continuously contribute to the nature of transference (Renik, 1993; Hoffman, 1998). The physical characteristics, way of relating to the patient, gender, and age of the therapist all influence the patient's perception of the therapist. These features trigger neural networks within the patient that contain representations of past figures and revise these 'ghosts' from the past in the present (Westen and Gabbard, 2002a). In addition to the repetitive dimension of transference, the patient also may harbor a longing for a healing or corrective experience to compensate for the problems that occurred in childhood relationships. Hence a longing for a *different* kind of relationship may be inherent in transference.

Resistance

Patients still resist psychotherapy as they did in Freud's day. One of the great discoveries of Freud was that patients may be ambivalent about getting better and unconsciously (or consciously) oppose attempts to help them. Resistance may manifest itself as silence in therapy sessions, as avoidance of difficult topics, or as the forgetting of sessions. In essence, resistance can be viewed as any way that patients defend themselves against changing in the service of preserving their illness as it is. Resistance is no longer viewed as an obstacle to be removed by the therapist. Rather, it is viewed as a revelation about how the patient's past influences current behavior in the relationship with the therapist (Friedman, 1991). If, for example, a male patient experiences his male therapist as critical, he may be reluctant to say much. This reticence may reveal a great deal about his relationship with his father and with other male authority figures. Helping the patient to understand resistance is a central feature of psychodynamic therapy.

Countertransference

Freud wrote very little about countertransference. He originally defined it as the analyst's transference to the patient. He generally regarded it as an interference in the analyst that paralleled transference in the patient. In other words, the analyst would unconsciously view the patient as someone from the past and therefore have difficulty treating the patient. Countertransference is now regarded as an enormously valuable therapeutic tool in psychoanalytic therapy. It is a joint creation that stems in part from the therapist's past but also in part from the patient's internal world.

In other words, patients induce certain feelings in the therapist that provide the therapist with a glimpse of the patient's internal world and what sort of feelings are evoked in other relationships outside of therapy (Gabbard, 1995).

The unconscious

Freud's premise that much of mental life is unconscious has been extensively validated by research in the field of experimental psychology (Westen, 1999). However, psychoanalytic psychotherapists are more likely to refer to unconscious representations or unconscious mental functioning rather than *the unconscious*. The notion of 'the unconscious' as a storage place or reservoir is no longer in keeping with contemporary neuroscience research. We now recognize that memories are stored differently, depending on the type of knowledge being stored. *Declarative* memory involves facts and episodes of one's life, while *procedural* memory involves skills or procedures. Defense mechanisms, for example, are automatic unconscious procedures that regulate affect states. Memories of difficult times in one's life are aspects of declarative knowledge that may be conscious and easily recalled or may be repressed and therefore unconscious. Declarative knowledge is knowledge 'of', whereas procedural knowledge is knowledge 'how' (Westen and Gabbard, 2002b).

In current thinking that integrates psychodynamic and neuroscience data, both procedural and declarative memories can be viewed as either conscious or unconscious (see Figure 1.1). A distinction between *explicit* and *implicit* memory relates to whether knowledge is expressed and/or retrieved with or without conscious awareness. Hence the explicit versus implicit distinction can be understood as equivalent to conscious versus unconscious (Westen and Gabbard, 2000a,b).

Within this model defense mechanisms are primarily in the domain of implicit procedural memory. Suppression, though, one of the few *conscious* defense mechanisms, lies in the realm of explicit procedural memory because it involves the conscious banishment of certain thoughts and/or feelings from one's mind. Implicit declarative knowledge involves repressed ideas and repressed memories of events in one's life and knowledge that involves various kinds of expectations about how others will react in response to what one does. This latter category may be retrievable if one shifts one's attention to it, a category Freud called preconscious. Explicit declarative knowledge consists of facts and events that are fully conscious.

Unconscious aspects of mental functioning may reveal themselves as slips of the tongue, forgetting, or substituting names or words. Nonverbal behavior is also a reflection of unconscious and internalized modes of relating to others. In other words, how the patient relates to the therapist may say a great deal about unconscious representations of self and other within the patient.

Psychic determinism

The principle of psychic determinism asserts that our internal experience, our behaviors, our choice of romantic partners, our career decisions, and even our hobbies are shaped by unconscious forces that are beyond our awareness (Gabbard, 2000a). The psychodynamic therapist approaches a patient with the understanding that any symptom or problem may serve multiple functions. A variety of conflicts from different developmental levels all may converge to form the end result of a behavior or symptom.

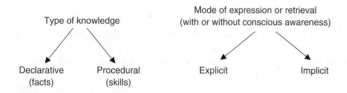

Fig. 1.1 Type of knowledge versus mode of expression. Reprinted from Gabbard, G. O. (2000). *Psychodynamic psychiatry in clinical practice*, 3rd edn, p. 8. Washington, DC: American Psychiatric Press.

A psychoanalytic therapist recognizes that many of the reasons for the patient's difficulties lie outside the patient's awareness, and both therapist and patient must be willing to explore a variety of converging causes.

The developmental perspective

All psychoanalytic thinking is based on a developmental model of behavior. A fundamental assumption is that childhood events shape the adult person. The repetitive patterns of problematic interactions with others stem from intrapsychic issues that are internalized during childhood. In contemporary thinking about the interface between genetics and environment, we know that the genetically based temperament of the child shapes much of the interaction with the parents. In other words, characteristics that are genetically determined evoke specific parental responses, which in turn shape the child's personality (Reiss *et al.*, 1995). Psychoanalytic therapists do not blame parents for their patient's difficulties. They see the patient's difficulties as a complex interaction between the child's characteristics, the parents' characteristics, and the 'fit' between them (Gabbard, 2000a).

Theoretical basis of psychoanalytic/psychodynamic psychotherapy

Ego psychology

During the time that Freud toyed with the idea of cathartic abreaction as his preferred model of healing, he was influenced by the *topographic* model of psychoanalysis. The unconscious mind harbored repressed pathogenic memories. Through the work of psychoanalysis, these memories would become conscious. They would lose their pathogenicity after becoming available to the patient's conscious awareness. The preconscious resided between the conscious and unconscious. The memories residing in the preconscious were available by shifting one's attention and hence were not truly repressed.

As the cathartic abreaction method failed Freud, he developed the tripartite structural model involving, ego, id, and superego. The structural model lends itself to a conflict-based theory that forms the foundation for ego psychology. The id is regarded as the seat of powerful instinctual drives—specifically aggression and sexuality/libido that struggle to emerge into conscious awareness. The superego, which has both conscious and unconscious aspects, is the moral agency that results from the internalization of parents and their value systems. Cultural or social values may also be internalized as part of the superego. The ego itself is partly conscious and partly unconscious, like the superego, and is thought of as the executive organ of the psyche. Conscious aspects of the ego are involved in decision making, perception, calculation, and anticipation of consequences. Among the many unconscious aspects of the ego are most of the defense mechanisms.

Ego psychology is characterized by a view of the intrapsychic world as one in which the three agencies are in constant conflict. Conflict, in turn, produces anxiety, which then results in the activation of a defense mechanism. Symptoms are formed as a result of conflict. The result of the anxiety and defense is a compromise formation. Instinctual drives seek to surface, but the ego and/or superego marshals defensive forces to stop the unacceptable drive from surfacing. The resulting compromise formation contains both the original wish arising from the id and the defense against that wish. Hence compromise gratifies the wish in a disguised and attenuated form. Both neurotic symptoms and character traits can result from these intrapsychic clashes and can be referred to as compromise formations.

Ego psychology de-emphasizes the need to plumb the depths of the unconscious for buried memories. Instead, it focuses on the fact that within the typical defensive operations, one finds the compromises and conflicts that make up the patient's character. A systematic analysis of defenses, as they enter into the treatment in the form of resistances, is a cornerstone of ego-psychological technique. Some common defenses are listed in Table 1.1 and are organized hierarchically from the most immature or pathological defenses to the most healthy or mature.

The developmental model associated with ego psychology involves the epigenetic developmental scheme linked to oral, anal, and phallic libidinal zones. Erik Erikson (1959) described the child's psychosocial crisis that occurred at each developmental phase. In the first month of existence, the infant struggles with basic trust versus basic mistrust while negotiating the oral phase of development. Autonomy versus shame and doubt is typical of the anal phase. Initiative versus guilt characters the phallic-oedipal phase. At about age 3 years and ending somewhere between 6 and 7 is the oedipal phase of developmental where the genitals are the primary source of pleasure. The child wishes to be the exclusive love object of the opposite-sex parent. During this phase the child becomes acutely aware of the triangle of mother, father, and child, having transcended the dyadic mother-child frame of reference in earlier developmental phases. The negative Oedipus complex is often used to describe the child's longing for the same-sex parent, wherein the opposite-sex parent is seen as a rival.

In the positive Oedipus complex, the child wishes to possess the opposite-sex parent exclusively and may harbor murderous wishes toward the same-sex parent. The superego is seen to result from a reluctant resignation

Table 1.1 A hierarchy of defense mechanisms

Defense mechanism	Description
Primitive defenses	
Splitting	Compartmentalizing experiences of self and other such that integration is not possible. When the individual is confronted with the contradictions in behavior, thought, or affect, he/she regards the differences with bland denial or indifference. This defense prevents conflict stemming from the incompatibility of the two polarized aspects of self or other.
Projection	Perceiving and reacting to unacceptable inner impulses and their derivatives as though they were outside the self.
Projective identification	Both an intrapsychic defense mechanism and an interpersonal communication, this phenomenon involves behaving in such a way that subtle interpersonal pressure is placed on another person to take on characteristics of an aspect of the self or an internal object that is projected into that person. The person who is the target of the projection then begins to behave, think, and feel in keeping with what has been projected.
Denial	Avoiding awareness of aspects of external reality that are difficult to face by disregarding sensory data.
Distortion	Significantly altering external reality to meet one's inner wish-fulfilling needs.
Dissociation	Disrupting one's sense of continuity in the areas of identity, memory, consciousness, or perception as a way of retaining an illusion of psychological control in the face of helplessness and loss of control. While similar to splitting, in extreme cases of dissociation, there is alteration of memory of events because of the disconnection of the self from the event.
Idealization	Attributing perfect or near-perfect qualities to others as a way of avoiding anxiety or negative feelings, such as contempt, envy, or anger.
Acting out	Enacting an unconscious wish or fantasy impulsively as a way of avoiding painful affect.
Somatization	Converting emotional pain or other affect states into physical symptoms and focusing one's attention on somatic (rather than intrapsychic) concerns.
Regression	Returning to an earlier phase of development or functioning to avoid the conflicts and tensions associated with one's present level of development.
Higher-level (neurotic) defenses	
Introjection	Internalizing aspects of a significant person as a way of dealing with the loss of that person. One may also introject a hostile or bad object as a way of giving one an illusion of control over the object. Introjection occurs in nondefensive forms as a normal part of development.
Identification	Internalizing the qualities of another person by becoming like the person. While introjection leads to an internalized representation experienced as an 'other,' identification is experienced as part of the self. This, too, can serve nondefensive functions in normal development.
Displacement	Shifting feelings associated with one idea or object to another that resembles the original in some way.
Externalization	Disavowing personal responsibility for a behavior by attributing that responsibility to someone else.
Intellectualization	Using excessive and abstract ideation to avoid difficult feelings.
Isolation of affect	Separating an idea from its associated affect state to avoid emotional turmoil.
Rationalization	Justification of unacceptable attitudes, beliefs, or behaviors, to make them tolerable to one's self.
Sexualization	Endowing an object or behavior with sexual significance to turn a negative experience into an exciting and stimulating one, or to ward off anxieties associated with the object.
Reaction formation	Transforming an unacceptable wish or impulse into its opposite.
Repression	Blocking or expelling unacceptable ideas or impulses from entering consciousness. This defense differs from denial in that the latter is associated with external sensory data, while repression is associated with inner states.
Undoing	Attempting to negate sexual, aggressive, or shameful implications from a previous comment or behavior by elaborating, clarifying, or doing the opposite.
Mature defenses	
Humor	Finding comic and/or ironic elements in difficult situations to reduce unpleasant affect and personal discomfort. This mechanism also allows some distance and objectivity from events so that an individual can reflect on what is happening.
Suppression	Consciously deciding not to attend to a particular feeling, state, or impulse. This defense differs from repression and denial in that it is conscious rather than unconscious.
Ascetism	Attempting to eliminate pleasurable aspects of experience because of internal conflicts produced by that pleasure. This mechanism can be in the service of transcendent or spiritual goals, as in celibacy.
Altruism	Committing oneself to the needs of others over and above one's own needs. Altruistic behavior can be used in the service of narcissistic problems, but can also be the source of great achievements and constructive contributions to society.
Anticipation	Delaying of immediate gratification by planning and thinking about future achievements and accomplishments.
Sublimation	Channeling socially objectionable or internally unacceptable aims into socially acceptable ones.

that it is better to identify with the same-sex parent rather than risk that parent's retaliation in response to incestuous wishes. The male child may fear that father will retaliate in the form of castration, creating castration anxiety. The boy then identifies with the aggressor (father) by deciding to search for a woman like his own mother because he cannot compete with his father.

Freud used the model of male development to understand female psychology. He imagined that a little girl felt like a boy until she discovered the existence of the penis. She then felt inferior and suffered from 'penis envy.' Lack of empirical support for this model of development has led to major rethinking of female developmental experience (Benjamin, 1990; Chodorow, 1996). Current thinking about the construction of gender focuses on the influence of culture, identifications with parents, and internal object relations rather than rigid assumptions about anatomical differences (see Chapter 34, Gender issues in psychotherapy).

Melanie Klein and object relations theory

Object relations theory has become perhaps the predominant theoretical model in contemporary psychoanalytic therapy. The origins of the theory can be linked to the work of Melanie Klein in London in the 1930s and 1940s. Based on her psychoanalytic treatment of children, she developed a theory that emphasized unconscious intrapsychic fantasy and pre-oedipal development.

Klein theorized that the infant began life with a primal anxiety about annihilation. She postulated that to deal with this terror, the ego underwent a splitting process in which the 'badness' or aggression associated with the death instinct was projected into the mother's breast. The child then developed paranoid anxieties about the possibility that the mother would attack the infant. This concern is the primary anxiety of the *paranoid-schizoid position*, an early mode of organizing experience that involves splitting and projection. The good aspects of mother are split off and kept separate from the bad or persecuting aspects so that they will not be contaminated by hate or aggression. In other words, the loving aspects of the mother and the self are kept pure from the contamination of murderous rage and hatred.

The paranoid-schizoid position was proposed as the predominant way that infants organize experiences during the first 6 months. The bad object is projected and then reintrojected throughout this period. The good object may also be projected to keep it safe from 'badness' within the child.

After 6 months, the child begins to integrate the 'bad' mother with the 'good' mother. The child realizes that the mother has both good and bad qualities and starts to integrate the two into a whole object representation of the mother as opposed to a part object of either 'all bad' or 'all good' qualities. This developmental phase is known as the *depressive position*. As part of this developmental epoch, the child has depressive anxiety related to the concern that the child will cause harm to the mother he or she loves. The child may attempt to resolve this depressive anxiety through reparation. In fact, Klein reconceptualized the Oedipus complex as involving the child's effort to address depressive anxieties and guilt through making reparation to those experienced as damaged (Segal, 1964). A child may choose to become a physician, for example, as a way of healing others to repair the damage she imagines she has done to her parents.

Another key component to Klein's theory is the role of envy as a derivative of the death instinct. Envy is a form of hatred directed to the good object rather than the bad object. The envy is partly responsible for the child's perception that he or she has caused damage to the 'good mother' (Klein, 1957). While jealousy involves three persons, envy occurs in a two-person context.

Developmentalists criticize Klein's thinking for attributing complicated forms of cognition and perception to infants in their first several months of life. Her thinking has also been challenged because of her emphasis on the death instinct, a theory that is not endorsed by any other psychoanalytic school of thought and by her tendency to minimize real trauma while emphasizing the child's intrapsychic fantasy life.

Wilford Bion, an analysand of Klein's, was instrumental in moving Kleinian theory away from drives and towards relationships (Bateman and Holmes, 1995). He focused on how the mother serves as a container for the infant's intense affects and 'detoxifies' them through her nurturing so they are taken back by the infant in a more manageable form. This interactional component is considered vital in Bion's model.

While Klein's views were closely linked to Freud's drive theory, the British independent tradition stressed that the infant's drives develop in the context of the mother–infant relationship and therefore must be viewed in that context. Fairbairn (1952) even argued that drives are primarily object seeking in nature rather than tension reducing in the sense of drive theory. A key principle is that relationships are internalized in the early years of life. The object relations building blocks of life involve a representation of self, a representation of the object, and an affect that links the two.

Splitting and projective identification are two of the defense mechanisms most associated with object relations theory (see Table 1.1). Splitting involves the tendency to divide everyone into 'all bad' or 'all good' groups. This polarization of objects involves a corresponding splitting of the self. Hence contradictory presentations of the self may alternate with one another, resulting in a confusing picture both for the patient and for those close to the patient. In a developmental sense, splitting is a defense that occurs *prior to* conflict. As a result, patients who rely on splitting may react with indifference or bland denial when confronted with contradictions in their behavior (Kernberg, 1975).

Projective identification works in tandem with splitting in that object or self-representations that are split off may be placed in others as a way of disavowing them. In projective identification in the psychotherapeutic context, the patient unconsciously projects the self- or object representation into the treater, who then unconsciously identifies with what has been projected. Through interpersonal pressure, the patient coerces a response in the treater that corresponds to what is projected. For example, a 26-year-old female patient with borderline personality disorder had been a victim of physical abuse at the hands of her mother. When she was with her female therapist, she accused the therapist of not listening carefully to what she said. She also accused her therapist of being insensitive toward her. She told her therapist she was convinced that the therapist did not like her and did not want to see her. This behavior in the sessions continued unabated for weeks. Finally, her accusations escalated to the point where the therapist became angry at the constant barrage of accusations, and she told the patient that she was getting fed up with the many distortions that the patient brought to the therapy. She also raised her voice at her patient and exclaimed, 'I can't take your attitude anymore!' Hence through the interpersonal pressure of her behavior, the patient influenced her therapist to conform to the projected bad object. The therapist, in effect, became an attenuated version of the patient's abusive mother. In the ideal therapeutic situation, the projected material is then psychologically processed and modified by the therapist so that what has been projected is transformed by the therapist before it is reintrojected by the patient. This processing generally does not occur in everyday life when patients project certain aspects of themselves into others in the course of their usual contact.

Object relations theory fits well with cognitive neuroscience, in that early self and object representations are etched in specific neural networks as a result of repeated experience with figures in the environment. A central tenet of object relations theory is that the internal representation may not be exactly the same as the external figure on whom the representation is based. Children may exaggerate tendencies in parents, for example, because of their fantasies about the parents. The earliest representations tend to be more polarized and are often referred to as part objects. From the age of 3 to about 6, the part objects and part self-representations are integrated into whole object and whole self-representations and involve both good and bad qualities. When a failure of integration occurs, adult patients may go throughout their lives splitting themselves and others and repeating past object relationships through the mechanism of projective identification.

The independent perspective also was influenced by the thinking of D. W. Winnicott. He stressed the inborn tendency to grow toward self-realization. He felt there was a *true self* whose growth could be either impeded or facilitated by maternal responses (Winnicott, 1965). If the mother, or other caretaking figure, cannot attune herself to the child's authentic self, the child may develop a *false self* designed to please or placate the mothering figure.

Self psychology

Self psychology developed from Heinz Kohut's study of narcissistically disturbed patients who sought analysis (Kohut, 1971, 1977, 1984). Kohut's adult patients were characterized by having a highly vulnerable self-esteem that made them feel easily slighted by friends, colleagues, and romantic partners. He did not view them as suffering from intrapsychic or neurotic conflict. Kohut suggested that these individuals lacked developmentally appropriate empathy by their mothers, creating a *deficit* situation. Individuals with this deficit then go through life attempting to get responses from others that make up for the missing functions within themselves. Kohut called these *selfobject* functions, in that others must perform functions for the patient's self rather than being allowed to behave autonomously.

The selfobject functions tend to fall into three categories, which Kohut viewed as the three kinds of selfobject transferences. The *mirror* transference is an attempt to capture the 'gleam in the mother's eye' in response to phase-appropriate displays of exhibitionism that hearken back to childhood, when the child felt that empathic responses were not forthcoming from the mother. These approving or mirroring responses were viewed by Kohut as essential for the child's development of a cohesive sense of self.

The second form of selfobject transference is the *idealizing* transference, where the patient maintains his or her self-esteem by being in the shadow of an idealized therapist. Basking in the reflected glory of the therapist makes the patient feel whole and worthy.

The third transference is called the twinship or alter-ego transference. This aspect of the self appears as a need to be just like the therapist. The developmental origin is a wish for merger that is gradually transformed into imitative behavior.

Inherent in the self psychological view is the notion that the development and maintenance of self-esteem is equally as important as sexuality and aggression as a motivating factor in human interaction. Moreover, Kohut (1984) felt that separation is a myth that does not reflect our actual need for affirming, empathic responses from others to feel a sense of wholeness throughout life. Eventually, Kohut viewed the self-selfobject connection as responsible for all forms of psychopathology. He viewed oedipal conflicts involving sexuality and aggression as mere 'breakdown products' of developmentally earlier failures involving lack of self or object responses.

Kohut was not clear on a developmental timetable for the difficulties in the sector of the self. However, he suggested that the self begins as fragmented nuclei and only achieves cohesiveness in response to empathic responses from parents. In the absence of those empathic responses, fragmentation of the self occurs, and the child tries to capture the sense of self through seeking out selfobject responses from others.

The self psychological perspective is consonant with the infant observation work of Daniel Stern (1985, 1989). The mothering figure's affirming and validating responses appear to be crucial to the developing infant's sense of self. The child has a sense of self-with-other in response to the caregiver's attunement from very early in infancy. Stern described five discrete senses of self, beginning with the development of a predominantly *body* self from birth to 2 months of age. A *core* sense of self emerges between 2 and 6 months. Between 7 and 9 months, the infant starts to have a greater sense of *subjective* self as intrapsychic states between infant and mother begin to be matched. When the child is approaching the middle of the second year of life, he or she has the capacity to think symbolically and to communicate verbally so a *categorical* or *verbal* sense of self emerges finally. A self with historical continuity, the *narrative* sense of self, arrives between 3 and 5 years of age.

Attachment theory

John Bowlby was responsible for the development of attachment theory, largely in opposition to the existing psychoanalytic theories of his day. Nevertheless, in recent years attachment theory has begun to become integrated with the pluralistic edifice of psychoanalysis. Bowlby (1988) repeatedly emphasized the child's *real* experience and the importance of the external world in the child's healthy development. Borrowing from ethology, attachment behaviors were viewed by Bowlby as not reducible to another drive. An entire system of behaviors on the part of the child serve to optimize proximity to the mother or caregiver (Fonagy, 2001). In contrast to object relations thinking, the motivation of the child is not object seeking. Rather, the goal of the child is to achieve a psychophysiological state related to being in close proximity with the mother or caretaker. Holmes (2001) suggests that the same is true of adults, who, when stressed or threatened, may, if insecurely attached, resort to 'pathological secure base phenomena,' such as substance abuse, deliberate self-harm, or binge eating. These behaviors may re-create a shortcut to the physiological state of the secure base without its relational or psychological components.

The work of Ainsworth *et al.* (1978) was critically important in refining the attachment concept by studying the infant's response to what was called the Strange Situation. In this 20-minute laboratory test, a child is exposed to brief separations from the child's mother. The reaction to these separations led to a classification of children as securely attached, anxious-avoidantly attached, anxious-ambivalent or resistant in the attachment style, or disorganized/disoriented.

Although there is not a one-to-one correlation necessarily between the categories of child attachment and those of adults, attachment theorists have found it clinically useful to think of adult individuals in four somewhat analogous categories of attachment: (1) secure/autonomous individuals who value attachment relationships; (2) insecure/dismissing individuals who deny, devalue, idealize, or denigrate both current and past attachments; (3) preoccupied adults who are overwhelmed or confused by current and past attachment relationships; and (4) disorganized or unresolved individuals who have often suffered neglect or trauma. Compared with other psychoanalytic schools of thought, there is much more rigorous empirical research behind attachment theory. Some of this research demonstrates that expectant parents' mental models of attachment predict subsequent patterns of attachment between mother and infant (Fonagy, 2001). A key concept in attachment theory is *mentalization*, the capacity to understand that one's own behavior and that of others is motivated by internal states, such as thoughts and feelings (Fonagy, 1998). In addition, part of mentalization is an understanding that one's perceptions of others are representations rather than the way reality actually is. The mother's or caregiver's capacity to observe the infant's intentional state and internal world appears to influence the development of secure attachment in the child. The child's secure attachment to the caregiver is highly influential in the child's development of the capacity to mentalize.

Postmodern schools

In recent years a number of theoretical models that emphasize the two-person nature of psychoanalytic treatment have emerged. These various approaches, with labels such as intersubjectivity, relational theory, constructivism, or interpersonal psychoanalysis, all endorse skepticism about any fundamental truth residing in the patient or in the analyst. The truth is co-constructed in the interaction between therapist and patient. They are all postmodernists in outlook in that they doubt the existence of an objective reality 'out there' (Holland, 1983; Leary, 1994; Aron, 1996).

Renik (1993), for example, stresses the irreducible subjectivity of the analyst in the way that the analyst approaches listening and formulating interventions. The treatment situation is intersubjective in that the psychoanalytic therapist can never fully transcend his or her own unconscious motivations for attempting to help the patient. In a similar vein, the postmodernist perspective recognizes that the appearance of the patient's pathology is heavily influenced by the culture, gender, and personal biases of the therapist. The constructivist point of view stresses that we should be hesitant about regarding the patient's transference as a 'distortion,' in t it may be a plausible construct based on the patient's recognition of r aspects of the analyst's behavior (Hoffman, 1983, 1991).

Treatment principles

The principles of technique in psychoanalytic psychotherapy have evolved considerably over the years. The stereotype of the 'blank screen' therapist who is aloof and silent while the patient struggles has misled many to assume that passivity is the hallmark of the psychodynamic therapist. We now practice in a postblank-screen era in which the therapist is actively engaged in the process and recognizes the role of countertransference as much as transference.

The principles of technique vary somewhat according to the therapist's school of thought, but certain themes are universal. Psychodynamic therapists allow their patients to try to articulate the nature of their problems and set goals for what they would like to address in the course of the treatment. Then they invite their patients to say whatever comes to mind as they reflect on the problem. Patients inevitably run into difficulties when they attempt to speak freely to their therapist, and hence resistances to the process become the daily bread and butter of the dynamic therapist's work. As long ago as 1912, Freud made the observation that 'the resistance accompanies the treatment step by step. Every single association, every act of a person under treatment must reckon with the resistance that represents a compromise between the forces that are striving toward recovery and the opposing ones' (p. 103).

A dynamic therapist does not attempt to overcome resistances by insisting that the patient must say what comes to mind. Rather, they strive to understand the meaning of the patient's falling silent or feeling ashamed. In this exploration, dynamic therapists often discover that particular feelings about the therapist are responsible for the resistance. Indeed, transference fantasies about the therapist are a major source of resistance. Patients may wonder if their therapist will be critical of them if they speak their mind. They may also worry that they might hurt the therapist's feelings by saying something negative about the therapy. They may shut down because of concerns that the therapist's motives are other than pure—what if the therapist secretly wants to ridicule them for their foibles? As time goes on in the therapy, more and more of these unconscious concerns are made conscious with the therapist's help, who points out observations of which the patient may not be aware.

The way that the patient resists the process reveals a great deal about the patient's inner world. In 1914, Freud noted that the patient repeats in action what he or she cannot remember and verbalize. Hence the way the patient relates to the therapist—how the patient enters the room, sits in the chair, breaks eye contact with the therapist, and what the patient chooses to call the therapist—all reveal aspects of the patient's internal object relations and unconscious attitudes toward the therapist.

As dynamic therapists begin to understand their patients, they try to enlist them in a collaborative pursuit of common therapeutic goals. This formation of a therapeutic alliance around understanding may be crucial to the success of the therapy. Therapists must help their patients ally themselves with the therapist's task of reflection and understanding. In the optimal situation, patients can observe themselves while also fully participating emotionally in the immediate experience of the therapeutic situation.

Many of the same principles that apply to the patient's optimal attitude also apply to the therapist. Just as patients have transference feelings that are a mixture of the real relationship with the therapist and old relationships from the past, therapists experience countertransference involving the same combination. The *narrow*, or Freudian, view of countertransference was that the analyst's unconscious conflicts about figures in the past are displaced on to the patient in the present. This view has now been superceded by a broader understanding of countertransference. Dynamic psychotherapists think of themselves as containers receiving a variety of projections from the patient. The patient induces certain feelings in the therapist that reflect the patient's internalized relationships. By studying how they feel in response to the patient's projections, therapists start to gain an understanding of how other people feel in relationships with the patient. Therapists must allow themselves to be sufficiently flexible so that they can experience the patient's effort to draw them in to familiar patterns of object relationships. In so doing they are privy to a firsthand experience of the patient's characteristic difficulties with others and can help the patient understand how they are repeating in the present characteristic patterns from the past that are also typical of current relationships.

Terms such as *neutrality*, *abstinence*, and *anonymity* may be misleading in that they can be misconstrued as promoting an aloofness or coldness. These principles of technique have undergone considerable transformation, and all three should now be applied only in a *relative* sense. In other words, therapists are neutral to the extent that they try to remain nonjudgmental about the patient's feelings, wishes, and behaviors in the service of understanding them. Therapists are abstinent in the sense that they do not gratify the patient's every transference wish because they wish to understand it rather than simply indulge it. Therapists certainly provide a good deal of gratification in their warmth and humanity, their laughter in response to a joke, their creation of a holding environment, and their empathic listening (Gabbard, 2000a,b).

Anonymity, especially, has undergone transformation in the way that modern psychodynamic psychotherapists construe the term. Therapists are revealing things about themselves all the time—by the way their office is set up, the way they react to what the patient says, through nonverbal communications such as facial expressions, and by their choice of when to speak versus when to remain silent. They may also self-disclose certain countertransference feelings they are noting within the session in the service of helping patients to understand what they evoke in the therapist and others. Anonymity today is best understood as a form of restraint based on the asymmetry of the therapeutic relationship. Therapists do not talk about their personal problems or their private lives with their families because they are paid a fee or a salary to focus on the *patient's* issues. Too much personal disclosure can burden the patient. The traditional view of anonymity was that the therapist should be like a 'blank screen' so that the therapist's real characteristics would not 'contaminate' the patient's transference. Whatever the therapist does has a continuing impact on the patient's transference so that it is impossible for the therapist to avoid influencing the patient's transference. A spontaneous, natural, warm approach to the patient is much more likely to facilitate a good therapeutic alliance than a remote, silent, aloof posture. We also know that the patient's internal object relations and intrapsychic conflicts will emerge to some degree, regardless of the therapist's behavior.

Spontaneity is certainly a key factor in the therapist's optimal attitude. Psychodynamic therapists allow themselves to be 'sucked in' to the patient's internal world by engaging in the 'dance' that the patient evokes in the consulting room. An example will illustrate one variation of this phenomenon.

> A 30-year-old man came to see his therapist for the first time, and he began by asking him how many patients he had treated. The therapist responded that he did not know the exact number but was curious why the patient asked. In response to this comment, the patient said, 'Oh, I see, you're one of those therapists who turns questions around to the patient so that you never answer anything.' The therapist responded, 'Well, I wouldn't go that far. I do sometimes answer questions if I think it will be useful.' The patient then commented, 'You sound like you're getting defensive now.' The therapist replied, 'No, I don't think I'm being defensive. I'm simply trying to clarify my position.'
>
> At this point the therapist found himself getting irritated by the way he was being challenged by the patient and recognized that he had been drawn in to a particular dance that was typical of this patient, who complained that many of his friends and colleagues found him to be irritating.

In this example the therapist does not hold himself aloof from the patient's influence but rather serves as a container so that he can fully experience what the patient induces in him while also maintaining the capacity to reflect on what is happening between them. As Gabbard and Wilkinson (1994) note: 'The optimal state of mind for therapists is when they can allow themselves to be "sucked in" to the patient's world while retaining the ability to observe it happening in front of their eyes. In such a state, therapists are truly thinking their own thoughts, even though they are under the patient's influence to some extent' (p. 82). This process involves engaging in minor countertransference enactments, in which therapists may feel themselves becoming an object or self-representation within the patient's inner world, followed by a process of working back to thinking one's own thoughts and understanding the enactment in the context of the therapeutic situation.

The dynamic therapist also tracks the affects of the patient. Does anxiety or sadness emerge when the patient's father is discussed? Is there a flash of anger when the patient speaks of demands associated with a sibling's illness? A specific intrapsychic conflict may be heralded by the emergence of affect. Dynamic therapists are equally interested in defenses brought to bear to deal with affect states or drive derivatives. When expression of anger, for example, is stifled by a defensive flight from the subject that evoked the anger, therapists may call attention to the patient's conflict and the defensive strategy used to deal with it (Gray, 1990).

A basic principle of psychoanalytic therapy is *working through*. Calling attention to affect states, defenses, and resistances and understanding their meaning all take time. Freud (1914) noted, 'One must allow the patient time to become more conversant with this resistance with which he has now become acquainted, to *work through* it, to overcome it, by continuing, in defiance of it, the analytic work . . .' (p. 155). The therapist must be prepared to address the same conflicts, the same resistances, and the same transferences as they surface in a variety of different situations, both within the therapeutic relationship and outside the consulting room. Only through repetitive interpretation, observation, and confrontation will the patient finally gain a sense of mastery over a host of haunting internal conflicts and the 'ghosts' responsible for them. Freud (1914) stressed that this working-through process is what distinguishes the psychoanalytic approach from therapies based on suggestion. It also is one of the reasons that dynamic therapy is usually long term or open ended. A significant exception is brief dynamic therapy, but that modality is covered elsewhere in this volume.

Psychodynamic psychotherapy occurs in the context of a frame that assures ethical behavior on the part of the therapist. By adhering to the frame, the enactments occur in an attenuated way that does not threaten harm or exploit the patient. The frame is constituted by a set of professional boundaries that define the limits of a professional relationship and differentiates it from a friendship, a romantic relationship, or a parent–child relationship. Included in these boundaries are the therapist's office, the time frame of 45 or 50 minutes, professional dress and demeanor, limited self-disclosure on the part of the therapist, the acceptance of a fee for a service (or a salary, if publicly funded), confidentiality, and no physical contact. The central point of this asymmetrical relationship is that the therapist's entire focus is on helping the patient with the problems the patient brings to therapy.

Boundaries should not be construed rigidly. Many variations on boundary transgressions occur, some of them benign and even helpful. If a patient falls down entering the office, a therapist may help the patient up. In some cases, therapists may answer personal questions or extend the session. These minor transgressions are referred to as *boundary crossings* (Gutheil and Gabbard, 1998) because they occur in isolation, are attenuated in such a way that no harm is done, and are often explored in the therapy itself. The more egregious boundary transgressions, such as sexual misconduct, are referred to as *boundary violations* because they are exploitative of the patient's vulnerability, may harm the patient, and destroy the viability of the therapy.

The expressive-supportive continuum

Psychodynamic psychotherapy is often referred to as expressive-supportive psychotherapy. This designation reflects the fact that with any one patient, the therapist may be more expressive or exploratory at some times while shifting to a more supportive or suppressive style at another, depending on the patient's needs. Dynamic psychotherapy that is predominantly exploratory or expressive is oriented to analyzing defenses, transference, and intrapsychic conflicts and to making more of the patient's unconscious available to conscious awareness. Supportive or suppressive psychotherapy aims to bolster or strengthen defenses and suppress unconscious conflict. Although psychodynamic psychotherapy as a treatment generally connotes an expressive or exploratory emphasis, supportive interventions are used regularly in such treatments.

The types of interventions that predominate in highly expressive dynamic therapy are interpretation, observation, and confrontation. Interpretations are statements made by the therapist that attempt to explain the patient's thoughts, feelings, behaviors, or symptoms. They link these phenomena to unconscious fantasies, meanings, or childhood origins. An experience that occurs in the therapy that relates to the therapist may be linked to parallel situations outside the consulting room and past situations from long ago. A therapist might use the following transference interpretation to help a patient make unconscious motivations consciously available: 'I wonder if you find it necessary to disagree with any observation I make as a way of defeating the therapy and by implication, triumphing over your dad as well.' Wishes and defenses against those wishes are often the subject of interpretation, and these conflicts can be interpreted as they appear in the transference, childhood memories, and current relationships (Malan, 1976; Gabbard, 2000a).

Observation calls attention to a behavior, the sequence of a comment, a flash of emotion, a pattern within the therapy, or similar phenomena (Gabbard, 2004). Unlike interpretation, observation does not attempt to explain or identify motives. The therapist hopes the observation will lead to a collaborative exploration of meanings. A therapist might say, for example, 'I don't think you're aware of it, but you often grimace when I ask about your mother.'

Confrontation involves an attempt to make the patient face something that he or she is avoiding. While confrontation may have an aggressive connotation, this type of intervention can be delivered gently as well. After a patient's mother died, the therapist noticed that the patient completely avoided the topic of his mother's death. The therapist chose a well-timed moment to point this out: 'I know it's a difficult subject for you, but I don't think you've spoken about your mother a single time since her funeral.' Whereas observation generally focuses on nonverbal communications or patterns that are outside the patient's awareness, confrontations generally target behaviors or topics that are conscious but avoided (Gabbard, 2004).

At the more supportive end of the continuum, therapists may give specific advice to patients on how they should live their lives, how they should decide to behave in a specific situation, or whether they should leave a relationship in which they are involved. Advice giving is unusual in exploratory therapy and sharply distinguishes supportive from expressive therapy. Praise is also used in supportive or suppressive therapy to reinforce certain behaviors or thoughts by approving them. Affirmation is another intervention associated with therapies that are predominantly supportive. In such treatments, therapists make comments such as, 'I don't blame you a bit for feeling the way you do,' or 'you are absolutely right to be angry.' Defenses may be bolstered by such comments as: 'I think you should continue to act kindly to your mother even though you are secretly angry at her.' In this example the therapist reinforced the patient's reaction formation because the patient had a history of getting out of control when expressing anger.

In between the more expressive and supportive interventions are a number of therapist's comments that are used in all dynamic therapies. Empathic validation, particularly associated with self psychological therapists, involves placing oneself in the patient's shoes and attuning oneself to the patient's internal state. This empathic immersion in the patient's inner world helps one to understand feelings, thoughts, or behaviors from the patient's perspective. An example of a comment that is empathically validating is the following: 'I can certainly appreciate why you would feel hurt by your boss's behavior toward you because you had worked hard on the project and expected some recognition.'

Much of psychotherapy involves facilitating the patient's exploration of a particular subject. Hence therapists probably use encouragement to elaborate more than any other intervention. Examples include, 'Please tell me more about that; I'm very interested in it.' Other comments may be more specific: 'At what point in your adolescence did you feel that you really had to leave home?' Sometimes encouragement to elaborate is needed because the patient's communication is confusing: 'Could you please explain to me why you and your previous therapist decided you couldn't work together anymore?'

Clarification is a third intervention that resides in the middle of the expressive-supportive continuum and may take a variety of forms. In dynamic psychotherapy a clarification is often designed to repackage something the patient has said as a way of summarizing key points that the patient is making (Gabbard, 2000a). Clarification may be a way of checking out with the patient if the therapist's understanding is correct. It may also be a way of helping the patient recognize patterns: 'The more I hear you talk, the more I realize that you're basically mad at your mother, your sister, and your girlfriend.' It may also be a way of helping the patient get in touch with specific feelings that are being avoided: 'When you talk about the loss of your boyfriend, I can see that you miss him and are saddened by it even though you'd like to mainly focus on the anger.'

Frequency and transference focus are also a function of the expressive-supportive continuum. Patients who are suited for highly expressive treatment may make greater progress with more than one session per week and more emphasis on transference issues. Patients needing a supportive approach may benefit from sessions less than once per week and avoidance of addressing transference themes.

The goals of psychodynamic psychotherapy are multiple. One basic goal is to expand the patient's awareness of unconscious conflicts, feelings, wishes, fantasies, and motivations. Psychodynamic therapists look for patterns in work or school and in relationships. How do past patterns of relatedness get repeated in the present, both with the therapist and in life outside the consulting room? What recurrent conflicts inhabit the patient in work or school settings? The therapist seeks to formulate interpretations of these unconscious patterns. Another goal is to increase the patient's awareness of problematic attachment patterns so new and different modes of attaching to others are possible.

One of the overall goals of dynamic psychotherapy is to help patients 'live in their own skin' (Gabbard, 1996). Therapists try to help patients understand how they lie to themselves, hide from themselves, and try to project their own conflicts and feelings on to others. From a Kleinian and object relations perspective, therapists interpret how certain aspects of the self have been disavowed and projected on to others so the patient can ultimately take back what has been externalized. Self psychological psychotherapists try to strengthen the patient's self-esteem so that these patients are able to endure slights and narcissistic injuries with greater equanimity.

While most of these goals are more geared to the expressive end of the continuum, patients who have greater deficits may require more supportive strategies with more limited goals. Patients with borderline personality disorder, for example, may need supportive and validating comments to tolerate interpretation (Gabbard, 2000a). They may also need explicit support from the therapist to improve certain ego deficits, such as the capacity for judgment. Therapists may systematically help such patients think through the consequences of their actions to avoid making poor judgments. They may also help them delay impulsive actions by pointing out feelings that trigger the actions. Another goal may be to help the patient deal with internal deficits by providing active soothing or comforting to replace what is missing in the patient's internal world.

Psychodynamic therapists carefully assess each patient to determine whether the emphasis should be predominantly expressive, predominantly supportive, or a mixture of both. Several characteristics suggest that the patient will be responsive to more exploratory approaches. Those patients who are strongly motivated to understand themselves because they are suffering are more suited to an exploratory approach. Other ego strengths auger well for expressive treatment: intact reality testing, good impulse control, a high tolerance for frustration, and a general reflectiveness or psychological mindedness that leads the patient to think about internal motivations for behaviors. Meaningful and enduring interpersonal relationships, above-average intelligence, and a capacity to see parallels between situations in different contexts are also indications for dynamic therapy with an expressive emphasis. Patients who lack these characteristics may require more supportive approaches. In general, a person who is in the throes of a severe life crisis will need support even if ordinarily the person might be suited for a more dynamic approach. Brain-based cognitive dysfunction may also prevent a person from being able to use exploratory therapy. Even patients who are significantly disturbed may benefit from highly expressive

therapy, however, if the therapist is sufficiently skilled to provide support, when necessary, in the areas of the patient's deficits.

Multiple modes of therapeutic action

How does psychodynamic therapy work? Where once upon a time the complete focus was on interpretation of unconscious conflict, almost all psychoanalytic therapists now recognize that there are multiple modes of therapeutic action that vary from patient to patient (Gabbard and Westen, 2003). Fostering insight and the therapeutic relationship itself are probably the primary modes by which change is brought about in psychoanalytic therapy.

Historically, one of the ways that insight has been fostered is to encourage free association. By having the patient say whatever comes to mind, the therapist can demonstrate to the patient how ideas are linked unconsciously through the network of associations. Interpretation is another way to make unconscious wishes, fears, or fantasies more consciously available. The dynamic therapist hopes to instill a way of thinking in the patient's mind so that following termination, the patient continues to do 'self-analytic' or 'self-therapeutic' work to understand anxiety, depression, or conflict as it emerges posttermination period.

Freud (1915) once noted that the analyst pursues a course 'for which there is no model in real life' (p. 166). There is undoubtedly a corrective effect of experiencing a new and different kind of relationship for the patient. When therapists behave differently from what patients expect, the patients must come to grips with the way that they have imposed certain internal expectations on external figures.

Over time the patient internalizes the relationship with the therapist. Soon the internalization process modifies representations that have been present since childhood. Our representations of self and other are etched in neural networks based on childhood experiences (Westen and Gabbard, 2002a,b). These representations are potentials that are activated by situations in external reality that are similar in some way to these internalized self- and object representations. For example, a child who grew up beaten by his father will expect an older male therapist to be violent or critical. When that therapist is calm and caring, the neural network associated with the abusive father and the abused son will gradually be modified in its intensity. While the neural network will not completely disappear, it is weakened because it is now being surpassed by a new neural network involving a representation of an understanding and patient object and a self that feels understood. In keeping with the alteration of representations, the patient also internalizes emotional attitudes of the therapist so that the affect linkage between representations may have a different emotional valence.

Blatt and Auerbach (2001) used the Differentiation-Relatedness Scale to study 40 seriously disturbed treatment-resistant young adults and adolescents. These patients were evaluated at the beginning and end of psychoanalytically oriented inpatient treatment that lasted more than 1 year. Over the course of treatment, internal self- and object representations underwent significant changes. Prior to treatment, these representations were dominated by splitting and polarization, while after treatment, in concert with improved clinical functioning, there were more integrated descriptions of self and others, reflecting a move in the direction of the consolidation of object constancy. Hence the developmental level of mental representations changed significantly with intensive psychoanalytic treatment in an inpatient setting.

Yet another way that the therapeutic relationship may catalyze change is through internalization of the therapist's capacity for mentalization as measured by improved reflective functioning (Fonagy and Target, 1996). Patients who lack the capacity for mentalization related to early attachment problems have difficulty understanding the idea that mental states motivate behavior. Similarly, they have difficulty understanding how the minds of others work. Through the psychotherapeutic relationship, patients may 'find themselves' in the therapist's mind and improve their ability to distinguish representations from external reality. As a result of this improved capacity, patients can then understand both their own mental states and those of others. This capacity may improve in concert with the increased developmental level of internal representations (Blatt and Auerbach, 2001).

The mode of therapeutic action inherent in the therapeutic relationship should not be misconstrued as a simple matter of conscientiously behaving differently than objects from the past (Gabbard and Westen, 2003). To effect change, patients must perceive their therapist as sufficiently similar to the past objects that the core neural networks are activated. Then patients have the opportunity to work through the old representations and affect states that have been problematic to them. The characteristic self-other patterns must come to life in the relationship with the therapist.

In addition to the primary modes of therapeutic action—the fostering of insight and the therapeutic relationship—a variety of secondary strategies are brought to bear in a typical course of psychodynamic therapy (Gabbard and Westen, 2003). Despite the history of eschewing suggestion by psychoanalytic writers, there is little doubt that explicit or implicit suggestions for change accompany most treatments. Problematic beliefs of the patient may be confronted because they are clearly related to behaviors that are self-defeating in one way or another. In addition, therapists may help patients examine conscious methods of decision making or problem solving that create difficulties for them. Even exposure, which is classically associated with behavior therapy, occurs in psychodynamic treatments to some degree. As Fonagy and Target (2000) have emphasized, helping patients to differentiate belief from fact is a form of exposure in that the therapist acknowledges the patient's psychic reality of fear while simultaneously offering an alternative perspective that suggests safety. Moreover, transference anxieties diminish over time in part because of the exposure inherent in the psychotherapeutic situation. For example, patients ultimately realize that their fears of being humiliated or criticized by the therapist are unrealistic as their exposure to the therapist increases.

Some changes undoubtedly occur outside the realm of planned technical interventions. Specific moments of mutual recognition—a tear in the therapist's eye, a shared belly laugh—that are not symbolically represented may have a powerful therapeutic impact (Stern et al., 1998). These changes may occur in the realm of implicit procedural knowledge involving how to feel, think, or behave in a specific relational context.

Two other secondary strategies are worth noting. In recent years, self-disclosure by the therapist in a limited way has become a common intervention. Judicious self-disclosure may promote increased reflective function by helping the patients see that their representation of the therapist is different from the way the therapist actually feels (Gabbard, 2001). Self-disclosures of here-and-now countertransference feelings may also help patients understand the impact they have on others (Gabbard and Wilkinson, 1994). In addition, an affirmation process goes on in most dynamic therapies where patients feel that their point of view is valued and validated. This empathically validating function of the therapist may serve to mitigate longstanding feelings of being disbelieved or dismissed by earlier figures in one's life.

Research findings

Psychoanalysts and psychodynamic therapists have historically been far too complacent about demonstrating the efficacy of their treatments. In some respects, the scarcity of efficacy data based on randomized controlled trials is understandable in light of the unique methodological problems associated with studying long-term psychoanalytic treatment (Gabbard et al., 2002). A long-term follow-up study would be prohibitively expensive as the project would have to persist for 10 years or more to accumulate a large enough sample so that statistically valid analyses would be possible. A suitably matched control group would also be difficult to recruit. Self-selection of treatment is considered important to analysts and analytically oriented therapists because of the motivation necessary to engage in psychodynamic exploration. Patients who are not given the treatments they prefer might well drop out of a randomized, controlled study. Indeed, a substantial number of dropouts would create major problems for a long-term study. Finally, over a period of a decade, uncontrolled variables, such as life events, serious illness,

medication changes, and the comorbidity with Axis I disorders might well effect the meaningfulness of the results (Gunderson and Gabbard, 1999).

The psychodynamic approach has been given credibility by a substantial body of research on brief psychodynamic therapy. In a recent meta-analysis to assess the efficacy of short-term psychodynamic psychotherapy (STPP), (Leichsenring et al., 2004) included only randomized controlled trials that fulfilled rigorous criteria. They found that STTP yielded large and significant effect sizes for social functioning, general psychiatric symptoms, and target problems, and these improvements tended to increase at follow-up. These effect sizes significantly exceeded those of treatment as usual and waiting list control. They also found that there were no differences between STPP and other forms of psychotherapy.

When we examine psychoanalysis and intensive psychoanalytic therapy, we find a small number of outcome studies with the rigor of a randomized controlled design. In the Boston Psychotherapy Study (Stanton et al., 1984), patients with schizophrenia who received supportive therapy were compared with those who were provided with psychoanalytic therapy at a frequency of two or more times a week by experienced psychoanalytically oriented therapists. While certain outcome measures seemed to improve differentially in each group, overall no significant advantage was conferred on patients who were treated with psychoanalytic therapy (Gunderson et al., 1984).

A study of psychoanalytic therapy (three to four sessions per week) for 11 hospitalized diabetic children had profound and lasting effects on their health compared with a comparable sample of diabetic children who received standard medical treatment (Moran et al., 1991). The treatment lasted only 15 weeks, so the study is relevant to intensive psychoanalytic therapy but not to the study of extended psychoanalytic therapy.

Heinicke and Ramsey-Klee (1986) compared intensive psychoanalytic psychotherapy (four times a week) with once-a-week sessions for children with learning difficulties. This randomized controlled trial involved treatments lasting more than a year. The children who were seen once a week showed a greater rate of improvement than those receiving four times weekly sessions. At the time of follow-up, however, the children who had four times weekly sessions showed much greater improvement.

In a more recent study, 38 patients with borderline personality disorder were randomly assigned to a psychoanalytically oriented partial hospital treatment or to standard psychiatric care as a control group (Bateman and Fonagy, 1999). The primary treatments in the partial hospital cell consisted of once weekly individual psychoanalytic psychotherapy and three times weekly group psychoanalytic psychotherapy. The control subjects received no psychotherapy. At the end of treatment at 18 months, the patients who received the psychoanalytically oriented treatment showed significantly more improvements in depressive symptoms, social and interpersonal functioning, need for hospitalization, and suicidal and self-mutilating behavior. These differences were maintained during an 18-month posttreatment follow-up period with assessments every 6 months (Bateman and Fonagy, 2001). Moreover, the treatment group continued to improve during the 18-month follow-up period.

Svartberg et al., (2004) randomly assigned 50 patients with cluster C personality disorders to 40 sessions of either dynamic psychotherapy or cognitive therapy. The full sample of patients showed statistically significant improvement on all measures during treatment and during the 2-year follow-up. Patients who received cognitive therapy did not report significant change in symptom distress after treatment, whereas patients who underwent dynamic therapy treatment did. Two years after the treatment, 54% of the dynamic therapy patients and 42% of the cognitive therapy patients had recovered symptomatically. The researchers concluded that improvement continues after treatment with dynamic psychotherapy.

In Sweden the Stockholm Outcome of Psychoanalysis Psychotherapy Project (Sandell et al., 2000) was able to follow up a large number of patients treated with psychoanalysis and psychoanalytic therapy that was subsidized by national health insurance and provided by private practitioners. This study can best be categorized as a large prepost design. Random assignment was attempted but was unsuccessful. Some patients refused to be assigned, and others who agreed to be assigned did not get the treatment they preferred, so they sought it privately. The patient sample included 756 persons who were subsidized for up to 3 years in psychoanalysis or psychotherapy or on the respective waiting lists for subsidization of those treatments. Complete data for three panel waves were obtained from a group of 331 persons in various phases of long-term psychodynamic psychotherapy and from a group of 74 persons in various phases of psychoanalysis. The psychoanalytic treatments were defined as occurring four to five times a week, while psychotherapy consisted of one to two sessions per week. In measurements of symptomatic outcome using the Symptom Checklist 90, improvement during the 3 years after treatment was positively related to treatment frequency and duration, with patients in psychoanalysis doing better than those in psychoanalytic psychotherapy. This finding may be confounded, however, by the possibility that the psychoanalysts doing once or twice weekly psychotherapy were not conducting their preferred modality. Patients in psychoanalysis continued to improve after termination, a finding not generally noted in outcome studies of other psychotherapies.

Another large prepost study of 763 children who were evaluated and given psychoanalytic treatment at the Anna Freud Centre in London, UK, yielded data that suggested which patients were more likely to benefit from analysis (Target and Fonagy, 1994a,b). Children with phobias appeared to benefit significantly from psychoanalysis, while those with depression did not. Children with severe emotional disorders (three or more Axis I diagnoses) did surprisingly well in psychoanalysis, but they did poorly in once or twice a week psychoanalytic psychotherapy. Children with conduct problems did consistently worse than children with emotional difficulties of equal severity. Children younger than 12 years made more impressive gains with intensive treatment at four to five times per week than with nonintensive treatment at one to three times per week. Adolescents, on the other hand, did not appear to benefit from increased frequency, but the duration of the treatment was correlated with better outcomes. This study nicely illustrates how the findings of research are likely to surprise and inform clinical practitioners.

Several prospective follow-along studies using a prepost design have suggested substantial improvements in patients given psychoanalytic therapies for personality disorders (Stevenson and Meares, 1992; Høglend, 1993; Monsen *et al.*, 1995a,b). Additional data (Stevenson and Meares, 1995) from one of these studies suggest that gains from 1 year of dynamic therapy were maintained at 5-year follow-up. Uncontrolled studies, however, particularly those with relatively small sample sizes and clinical populations whose condition is known to fluctuate wildly, cannot yield data of consequence concerning what type of treatment is likely to be effective for whom.

Conclusions

Psychodynamic psychotherapy is probably the most widely practiced and most well-known form of therapy. Based on psychoanalysis, its unique features include an emphasis on unconscious mental life, systematic attention to transference themes and developmental issues, the exploration of countertransference as an important therapeutic tool, and the working through of resistance, defense, and conflict.

The empirical basis of extended psychoanalytic therapy is far from adequate, but preliminary research is encouraging. Because this form of therapy requires a greater investment of time and money than many other therapies, it should probably be used primarily for conditions that are not likely to respond to brief therapy and/or medication. Patients with complex and longstanding difficulties, especially those firmly entrenched in their character, will probably require open-ended psychoanalytic therapy to make significant gains.

References

Ainsworth, M. D. S., Blehar, M. C., Waters, E., and Wall, S. (1978). *Patterns of attachment: the psychological study of the strange situation*. Hillsdale, NJ: Erlbaum.

Aron, L. (1996). *A meeting of minds: mutuality and psychoanalysis*. Hillsdale, NJ: Analytic Press.

Bateman, A. and Fonagy, P. (1999). The effectiveness of partial hospitalization in the treatment of borderline personality disorder: a randomized controlled trial. *American Journal of Psychiatry*, **156**, 1563–69.

Bateman, A. and Fonagy, P. (2001). Treatment of borderline personality disorder with psychoanalytically oriented partial hospitalization: an 180 month follow-up. *American Journal of Psychiatry*, **158**, 36–42.

Bateman, A. and Holmes, J. (1995). *Introduction to psychoanalysis: contemporary theory and practice*. London: Routledge.

Benjamin, J. (1990). An outline of intersubjectivity: the development of recognition. *Psychoanalytic Psychology*, **7**(Suppl.), 33–46.

Blatt, S. and Auerbach, J. (2001). Mental representation, severe psychopathology, and the therapeutic process. *Journal of the American Psychoanalytic Association*, **49**, 113–59.

Bowlby, J. (1988). *A secure base: clinical applications of attachment theory*. London: Routledge.

Chodorow, N. J. (1996). Theoretical gender and clinical gender: epistemological reflections of the psychology of women. *Journal of the American Psychoanalytic Association*, **44** (Suppl.), 215–38.

Erikson, E. H. (1959). Identity and the life-cycle: selected papers. *Psychological Issues*, **1**, 1–171.

Fairbairn, W. R. D. (1952). *Psychoanalytic studies of the personality*. London: Routledge and Kegan Paul.

Fonagy, P. (1998). An attachment theory approach to treatment of the difficult patient. *Bulletin of the Menninger Clinic*, **62**, 147–69.

Fonagy, P. (2001). *Attachment theory and psychoanalysis*. New York: Other Press.

Fonagy, P. and Target, M. (1996). Playing with reality, I: theory of mind and the normal development of psychic reality. *International Journal of Psycho-Analysis*, **77**, 217–33.

Fonagy, P. and Target, M. (2000). Playing with reality, III: the persistence of dual psychic reality in borderline patients. *International Journal of Psycho-Analysis*, **81**, 853–73.

Freud, S. (1912/1958). The dynamics of transference. In: J. Strachey, trans. and ed. *The standard edition of the complete psychological works of Sigmund Freud*, Vol. 6, pp. 97–108. London: Hogarth Press.

Freud, S. (1914/1958). Remembering, repeating and working-through (further recommendations on the technique of psycho-analysis II). In: J. Strachey, trans. and ed. *The standard edition of the complete psychological works of Sigmund Freud*, Vol. 12, pp. 145–56. London: Hogarth Press.

Freud, S. (1915/1958). Observations on transference-love (further recommendations on the technique of psycho-analysis III). In: J. Strachey, trans. and ed. *The standard edition of the complete psychological works of Sigmund Freud*, Vol. 12, pp. 157–73. London: Hogarth Press.

Friedman, L. (1991). A reading of Freud's papers on technique. *Psychoanalytic Quarterly*, **60**, 564–95.

Gabbard, G. O. (1995). Countertransference: the emerging common ground. *International Journal of Psycho-Analysis*, **76**, 475–85.

Gabbard, G. O. (1996). *Love and hate in the analytic setting*. Northvale, NJ: Jason Aronson.

Gabbard, G. O. (2000a). *Psychodynamic psychiatry in clinical practice*, 3rd edn. Washington, DC: American Psychiatric Press.

Gabbard, G. O. (2000b). Psychoanalysis and psychoanalytic psychotherapy. In: B. J. Sadock and V. A. Sadock, ed. *Comprehensive textbook of psychiatry*, Vol. 2, 7th edn, pp. 2056–80. Philadelphia, PA: Lippincott, Williams and Wilkins.

Gabbard, G. O. (2001). Psychodynamic psychotherapy of borderline personality disorder: a contemporary approach. *Bulletin of the Menninger Clinic*, **65**, 41–57.

Gabbard, G. O. (2004). *Long-term psychodynamic psychotherapy: a basic text*. Arlington, VA: APPI.

Gabbard, G. O. and Westen, D. (2003). Rethinking therapeutic action. *International Journal of Psycho-Analysis*, **84**, 823–41.

Gabbard, G. O. and Wilkinson, S. M. (1994). *Management of countertransference with borderline patients*. Washington, DC: American Psychiatric Press.

Gabbard, G. O., Gunderson, J. G., and Fonagy, P. (2002). The place of psychoanalytic treatments within psychiatry. *Archives of General Psychiatry*, **59**, 505–10.

Gray, P. (1990). The nature of therapeutic action in psychoanalysis. *Journal of the American Psychoanalytic Association*, **38**, 1083–96.

Gunderson, J. G. and Gabbard, G. O. (1999). Making the case for psychoanalytic therapies in the current psychiatric environment. *Journal of the American Psychoanalytic Association*, **47**, 679–703.

Gunderson, J. G., *et al.* (1984). Effects of psychotherapy in schizophrenia, II: comparative outcome of two forms of treatment. *Schizophrenia Bulletin*, **10**, 564–98.

Gutheil, T. H. and Gabbard, G. O. (1998). Misuses and misunderstandings of boundary theory in clinical and regulatory settings. *American Journal of Psychiatry*, **155**, 409–15.

Heinicke, C. M. and Ramsey-Klee, D. M. (1986). Outcome of child psychotherapy as a function of frequency of session. *Journal of the American Academy of Child Psychiatry*, **25**, 247–53.

Hoffman, I. Z. (1983). The patient as interpreter of the analyst's experience. *Contemporary Psychoanalysis*, **19**, 389–422.

Hoffman, I. Z. (1991). Discussion: toward a social constructivist view of the psychoanalytic situation. *Psychoanalytic Dialogues*, **1**, 74–105.

Hoffman, I. Z. (1998). *Ritual and spontaneity in the psychoanalytic process: a dialectical-constructivist view.* Hillsdale, NJ: Analytic Press.

Høglend, P. (1993). Personality disorders and long-term outcome after brief dynamic psychotherapy. *Journal of Personality Disorders*, **7**, 168–81.

Holland, N. N. (1983). Post-modern psychoanalysis. In: I. Hassan and S. Hassan, ed. *Innovation/renovation: new perspectives on the humanities*, pp. 291–309. Madison, WI: University of Wisconsin.

Holmes, J. (2001). *The search for the secure base: attachment theory and psychotherapy.* London: Brunner-Routledge.

Klein, M. (1957). Envy and gratitude. In: *The writings of Melanie Klein*, Vol. 3, pp. 176–235. London: Hogarth Press.

Kernberg, O. F. (1975). *Borderline conditions and pathological narcissism.* New York: Jason Aronson.

Kohut, H. (1971). *The analysis of the self: a systematic approach to the psychoanalytic treatment of narcissistic personality disorders.* New York: International Universities Press.

Kohut, H. (1977). *The restoration of the self.* New York: International Universities Press.

Kohut, H. (1984). *How does analysis cure?* A. Goldberg ed. Chicago, IL: University of Chicago Press.

Leary, K. (1994). Psychoanalytic 'problems' and postmodern 'solutions.' *Psychoanalytic Quarterly*, **63**, 433–65.

Leichsenring, F., Rabung, S., and Leibing, E. (2004). The efficacy of short-term psychodynamic therapy in specific psychiatric disorders: a meta analysis. *Archives of General Psychiatry*, **61**, 1208–16.

Malan, D. H. (1976). *The frontier of brief psychotherapy.* New York: Plenum.

Monsen, J. T., Odland, T., Faugli, A., Daae, E., and Eilertsen, D. E. (1995a). Personality disorders and psychosocial changes after intensive psychotherapy: a prospective follow-up study of an outpatient psychotherapy project, 5 years after end of treatment. *Scandinavian Journal of Psychology*, **36**, 256–68.

Monsen, J. T., Odland, T., Faugli, A., Daae, E., and Eilertsen, D. E. (1995b). Personality disorders: changes and stability after intensive psychotherapy focusing on affect consciousness. *Psychotherapy Research*, **5**, 33–48.

Moran, G., Fonagy, P., Kurtz, A., Bolton, A., and Brook, C. (1991). A controlled study of the psychoanalytic treatment of brittle diabetes. *Journal of the American Academy of Child and Adolescent Psychiatry*, **30**, 926–35.

Reiss, D., *et al.* (1995). Genetic questions for environmental studies: differential parenting and psychopathology in adolescence. *Archives of General Psychiatry*, **52**, 925–36.

Renik, O. (1993). Analytic interaction: conceptualizing technique in light of the analyst's irreducible subjectivity. *Psychoanalytic Quarterly*, **62**, 553–71.

Sandell, R., *et al.* (2000). Varieties of long-term outcome among patients in psychoanalysis and long-term psychotherapy: a review of findings in the Stockholm Outcome of Psychoanalysis and Psychotherapy Project (STOPP). *International Journal of Psycho-Analysis*, **81**, 921–42.

Segal, H. (1964). *An introduction to the work of Melanie Klein.* New York: Basic Books.

Stanton, A. H., Gunderson, J. G., Knapp, P. H., Frank, A. F., Vannicelli, M. L., Schnitzer, R., and Rosenthal, R. (1984). Effects of psychotherapy in schizophrenia, I: design and implementation of a controlled study. *Schizophrenia Bulletin*, **10**, 520–63.

Stern, D. N. (1985). *The interpersonal world of the infant: a view from psychoanalysis and developmental psychology.* New York: Basic Books.

Stern, D. N. (1989). Developmental prerequisites for the sense of a narrated self. In: A. M. Cooper, O. F. Kernberg, and E. S. Person, ed. *Psychoanalysis: toward the second century*, pp. 168–78. Haven, CT: Yale University Press.

Stern, D. N., *et al.* (1998). Non-interpretive mechanisms in psychoanalytic therapy: the 'something more' than interpretation. *International Journal of Psycho-Analysis*, **79**, 903–21.

Stevenson, J. and Meares, R. (1992). An outcome study of psychotherapy for patients with borderline personality disorder. *American Journal of Psychiatry*, **149**, 358–62.

Stevenson, J. and Meares, R. (1995). Borderline patients at 5-year follow-up. Read before the Annual Congress of the Royal Australian-New Zealand College of Psychiatrists, May 6, 1995, Cairns, Australia.

Svartberg, M., Stiles, T., and Seltzer, M. H. (2004). Randomized, controlled trial of the effectiveness of short-term dynamic psychotherapy and cognitive therapy for cluster C personality disorders. *American Journal of Psychiatry*, **161**, 810–17.

Target, M. and Fonagy, P. (1994a). The efficacy of psychoanalysis for children: prediction of outcome in a developmental context. *Journal of the American Academy of Child and Adolescent Psychiatry*, **33**, 1134–44.

Target, M. and Fonagy, P. (1994b). The efficacy of psychoanalysis for children with emotional disorders. *Journal of the American Academy of Child and Adolescent Psychiatry*, **33**, 361–71.

Westen, D. (1999). The scientific status of unconscious processes: is Freud really dead? *Journal of the American Psychoanalytic Association*, **47**, 1061–106.

Westen, D. and Gabbard, G. O. (2002a). Developments in cognitive neuroscience II: implications for theories of transference. *Journal of the American Psychoanalytic Association*, **50**, 99–134.

Westen, D. and Gabbard, G. O. (2002b). Developments in cognitive neuroscience I: conflict, compromise, and connectionism. *Journal of the American Psychoanalytic Association*, **50**, 53–98.

Winnicott, D. W. (1965). *The maturational processes and the facilitating environment: studies in the theory of emotional development.* London: Hogarth Press.

2 Cognitive and behavioral therapies
Paul Grant, Paula R. Young, and Robert J. DeRubeis

Introduction

Cognitive-behavioral therapies represent a class of pragmatic approaches to understanding and treating psychiatric disorders and problems. Although there is much diversity among these treatments, interventions are characteristically problem focused, goal directed, future oriented, time limited, and empirically based. Cognitive-behavioral theories assume that cognitive and emotional processes mediate the acquisition and maintenance of psychopathology. Accordingly, interventions effect change in symptoms, behavior, and functioning via changes in cognition (Dobson and Dozois, 2001). An impressive array of techniques has been developed to help patients learn enduring, portable skills that reduce current distress, improve current functioning, and prevent relapse. An equally impressive research literature supports the application of manual-based, cognitive-behavioral packages to a wide range of disorders.

Behavior therapies are the historical ancestors of cognitive-behavioral therapies. Theoretically allied to Charles Darwin and behaviorists such as Thorndike, Pavlov, Watson, and Skinner, behavior therapies were pioneered in the 1950s by Wolpe and Rachman, among others (Hawton *et al.*, 1989; Craighead *et al.*, 1995). Behavior therapies conceptualize psychopathology in terms of the elementary learning processes of classical and instrumental conditioning (Hawton *et al.*, 1989; Mueser and Leiberman, 1995). Accordingly, the behavior therapist identifies objectively specifiable antecedents and consequences that maintain the maladaptive behavior. Therapy consists in altering environmental contingencies, which leads to change in behavior. Behavioral formulations and interventions are devoid of reference to mediational factors such as thought and cognition, which are inherently unobservable and unreliable (Skinner, 1953; Mueser and Leiberman, 1995).

By the 1970s behavioral therapies had become widely accepted efficacious treatments for a variety of psychological problems (Craighead *et al.*, 1995). However, at this same time, several currents within the field emphasized the role of cognitive factors as mediators of behavioral outcomes: (1) covert behavior such as obsessional thought or observational learning could not be directly addressed by behavioral methods alone; (2) data emanating from the cognitive sciences posed challenges to strictly behavioral models; (3) theorist practitioners such as A. T. Beck, Ellis, and Meichenbaum began calling themselves cognitive-behavioral; and (4) research studies were published demonstrating cognitive-behavioral methods to be equivalent or better than behavioral methods for particular disorders or problems (Dobson and Dozois, 2001; Ingram and Siegle, 2001).

Cognitive-behavioral therapies can be thought to sit on a continuum in terms of how much cognition is included in the formulation: (1) on the one end are behavior therapies that focus upon behavior and environmental determinants in terms of elementary learning theory, and (2) at the other end of the continuum are therapies that formulate therapy purely in cognitive terms, allowing no behavioral intervention at all. Most cognitive-behavioral approaches fall somewhere in between, emphasizing the behavioral and cognitive interventions to differing extents.

Treatment principles

Though the various versions or 'brands' of cognitive-behavioral therapy (CBT) can be distinguished in terms of certain aspects of the client–therapist relationship, the cognitive target for change, the assessment of change, the degree of emphasis placed on the client's self-control, and the degree to which cognitive or behavioral change is the focus (Kendall and Kriss, 1983), treatment principles common to all cognitive-behavioral therapies can be identified.

Cognitive-behavioral interventions are designed to treat specific disorders or problems

The patient's difficulties are operationalized in reliably measurable terms. By making the patient's problems quantifiable in this manner, the therapist introduces objectivity into the therapeutic process (J. S. Beck, 1995). Cognitive-behavioral assessment of a problem can include questionnaires, physiological tests, and behavioral tests that are administered continuously throughout treatment (Blankstein and Segal, 2001). The patient's progress in therapy can then be tracked by objective data that informs treatment decisions. The interventions that cognitive-behavioral therapies deploy are derived theoretically and are consistent with existing models of human learning and cognition (Ingram and Siegle, 2001). The techniques are validated experimentally via group and single-case experimental designs occurring within research and community settings. The utilization of cognitive-behavioral techniques to address problems associated with specific disorders is a direct legacy of behavior therapy (Dobson and Dozois, 2001).

The overarching goal of cognitive-behavioral therapy is to help patients effect desired changes in their lives

Change is conceptualized as a cognitive process, in that thoughts and beliefs mediate changes in behavior (J. S. Beck, 1995). From the patient's perspective, cognitive-behavioral treatment provides an adaptive learning experience that will produce concrete change in domains quite apart from the clinical setting. Importantly, improvement is not contingent on the interpersonal dynamics of the therapeutic relationship, nor does it require insight from the patient as the mechanism of change (Meichenbaum, 1995). Rather, improvement stems directly from change in maladaptive sequences of cognition and behavior.

Cognitive-behavioral therapies are goal oriented

The patient and therapist set explicit goals for the therapy at the outset of treatment. Typically, the patient will desire a reduction in distressing symptoms. The treatment is tailored to the patient's specific set of circumstances, such that any number of problems could be targeted for intervention. Goals such as increasing positive experiences, building coping strategies for future problems, and prevention of relapse are within the purview of cognitive-behavioral therapies. Goal setting focuses the patient's thinking upon gains she can achieve through therapy, and can prompt a discussion of the realistic limits of therapy. For example, the goal of 'never having anxiety again' is unrealistic, as is the goal of 'never being sad again.' Throughout the course of therapy, the patient and therapist can revisit the goals to asses the progress of therapy, revising the goals, if need be, in the face of changing life circumstances.

Cognitive-behavioral intervention occurs over the short term in a time-limited manner

Every attempt is made to effect change rapidly. Many treatment manuals recommend that therapeutic goals be achieved within 12–16 sessions (Chambless et al., 1996). Treatment is based in the present: the therapist and client address current patterns of thinking and behavior with an eye to enabling the patient to anticipate and navigate similar problems in the future. This emphasis upon contemporary problems does not prevent the therapist from taking a detailed client history, nor does it disallow using the past to help conceptualize the patient's problems. However, the action of the therapy resides in current problems and situations (J. S. Beck, 1995).

Cognitive-behavioral therapy is educational

It is axiomatic within cognitive-behavioral approaches that patients are seen as capable of controlling their own thoughts and actions. Therapy, under this assumption, becomes an educative process aimed at helping the patient acquire skills and knowledge that will enable her to function more adaptively. The therapist may instruct the patient throughout treatment: for example, regarding the nature and course of the disorder, as well as the rationale behind specific interventions. Ultimately, the cognitive-behavioral therapist expects the patient to learn which aspects of the process of therapy were most beneficial. And, in the event of an impending recurrence, the patient can use the skills learned in order to limit the severity and duration of symptoms, without needing to reinitiate formal therapy. The educative interaction between the therapist and patient is another factor that sets cognitive-behavioral therapies apart from other schools of therapy (D'Zurilla and Goldfried, 1971; Mahoney, 1974; A. T. Beck et al., 1979; DeRubeis et al., 2001).

Cognitive-behavior therapies attempt to impart to the patient skills that enable more adaptive problem solving

As skill acquisition requires practice, the patient is encouraged to work on a variety of therapeutic tasks outside of the session. The therapist frames these tasks, or homework assignments, as a vital component of treatment that is crucial to its success (J. S. Beck, 1995). The therapist and patient formulate the homework assignments together, customizing each task to the patient's problems and skill set. The therapist clarifies the rationale for each homework assignment and gives specific instructions, allowing the patient to express objections. Whenever possible, the therapist and patient anticipate problems that might hinder completion of the homework task. As homework tasks reinforce and supplement the educational aspects of the therapy, it is important that the patient experience each assignment as a relative success (A. T. Beck et al., 1979; J. S. Beck, 1995).

Cognitive-behavioral therapies emphasize a collaborative relationship between the patient and therapist

The therapist and patient assume an equal share of the responsibility for solving the patient's problems across all therapeutic activity: from setting goals to planning homework assignments to challenging negative cognitions to devising a relapse prevention strategy. The more the therapist and

the patient work together, the greater the learning experience for both. Joint effort not only engenders a cooperative spirit, but also creates a sense of exploration and discovery. These factors enhance motivation and help overcome the many obstacles inherent in psychotherapy (A. T. Beck et al., 1979; J. S. Beck, 1995; DeRubeis et al., 2001).

Cognitive-behavioral therapies require both patient and therapist to take an active role in the moment-by-moment progress of the treatment

Both parties contribute to the therapy in terms of identifying problems and challenging the negative cognitions that mediate negative emotional states and maladaptive behavior (J. S. Beck, 1995). The therapist is active across a variety of tasks: questioning negative thoughts, teaching new skills, educating about the psychological disorder, modeling new behaviors, and planning homework assignments. In a similar vein, the patient is active: monitoring behavior and thought, completing homework assignments, challenging negative thoughts, practicing skills, etc. The active therapist role is one factor that distinguishes cognitive-behavioral treatments from more traditional forms of psychodynamic and psychoanalytic psychotherapy, which prescribe the therapist to follow the patient's lead in session (Meichenbaum, 1995).

Cognitive-behavioral techniques
Goal setting

Collaboratively setting concrete goals with the patient is an important early step that confers several advantages upon the therapeutic process of CBT (Kirk, 1989). First, goal setting helps to clarify the patient's expectations for therapy. Areas of miscommunication or misunderstanding between therapist and patient can be pinpointed and resolved at an early stage within the therapeutic interaction. Additionally, a discussion of goals may enable the patient to formulate a basis for deciding when to continue with and when to discontinue therapy. Goal setting, also, frames the patient's difficulties in terms of change and possibility, which is more hopeful than a framework that emphasizes symptoms, problems, and pain. The process of goal setting can, moreover, serve to reinforce the patient's active role within the therapeutic relationship. CBT is not a passive experience. If the client is going to benefit from treatment, full involvement in the process of therapy is required. Another advantage goal setting bestows upon the therapeutic process is structure. The patient's problems are addressed in a systematic way, and the risk that therapy will become a chaotic series of crisis interventions is reduced. Ultimately, goal setting prepares the patient for discharge, as it explicitly defines the end of therapy as the point when all of the goals are achieved. Therapy can also be terminated if little progress is made towards the goals within an agreed upon timeframe. Thus, goal setting provides a natural means to evaluate the outcome of therapy in terms of the patient's presenting problems.

Cognitive-behavioral assessment

Although most assessment takes place in the initial sessions, the process of assessment continues throughout treatment. Cognitive-behavioral assessment strategies take many forms across four domains: cognition, behavior, emotion, and physiology (Blankstein and Segal, 2001). Each assessment procedure yields specific information about a particular response system. Assessing a problem with multiple techniques produces a more comprehensive identification of the problem, and gives the therapist a better picture of how well the treatment addresses the problem (Kirk, 1989).

Cognitive-behavioral assessment often begins with an initial interview (J. S. Beck, 1995; Blankstein and Segal, 2001). During this interview, the therapist clarifies the patient's problems, formulating the difficulties in manageable units that will encourage the patient to believe that change is possible. Additionally, the assessment process helps the patient learn that variations in the intensity and distress of symptoms are predictable and potentially controllable. The assessment interview also highlights problems that should be prioritized, such as child abuse, suicidality, or problems with serious physical consequences.

The initial interview may be supplemented by a variety of other assessment techniques, including self-report questionnaires, direct observation of behavior, behavioral tests, physiological measures, and self-monitoring. Self-report questionnaires such as the Beck Depression Inventory (BDI-II; A. T. Beck et al., 1996) are easily administered and can be collected periodically throughout the therapy process. Moreover, normative data exist for many self-report questionnaires, which can help to contextualize a patient's score.

A particularly useful assessment technique involves the direct observation of behavior. This can be accomplished through frequency counts, duration of symptoms or behaviors, or observations made during role-plays with the patient. Direct observation of the problem behavior can be repeated during the course of treatment to assess change. Specific behavioral tests also provide direct observation of a wide range of problem behaviors.

Behavioral by-products (e.g., the number of cigarette butts in an ashtray, or the number of hairs pulled out by patients with trichotillomania) are indirect, objective measures that are relatively free from observer bias. While such by-products do not focus on the problem behavior itself, they do provide reliable physical evidence that the behavior has occurred. Patients are easily trained to monitor these by-products as an indication of positive or negative change. While there is accumulating support for the use of physiological measures (Kirk, 1989), they are not routinely used in clinical practice due to the prohibitive cost and availability of measuring equipment. However, less technical measurements can be used effectively, such as self-monitoring of headaches or gastric distress.

Self-monitoring

Self-monitoring is an important assessment tool. The therapist instructs the patient to observe and record her own behavioral and emotional reactions. As these reactions are distributed throughout the patient's daily life, self-monitoring tends to be employed as a homework assignment. The therapist and patient collaboratively select the target of monitoring (e.g., a symptom, behavior, or reaction) based upon the patient's goals and presenting problem list. Self-monitoring serves at least three purposes within a course of CBT: (1) it encourages and effectively trains the patient to observe her own reactions in a more scientific manner; (2) it renders a concrete record of the target symptoms and problems; and (3) new problems can become apparent and targeted for future intervention. Self-monitoring is especially useful in early sessions as a means of assessing the severity or frequency of a particular problem or symptom. However, self-monitoring is equally useful in later sessions as a means of tracking the patient's progress. Examples of self-monitoring include a record of daily activities and corresponding mood; a frequency count of the number of panic attacks per day; a record of the frequency and content of auditory hallucinations; and a food diary in which time, quantity, and type of food eaten are recorded (J. S. Beck, 1995).

Cognitive restructuring

Within the cognitive-behavioral framework, maladaptive thinking is both a symptom and a critical maintenance factor (Meichenbaum, 1995; J. S. Beck, 1995; DeRubeis et al., 2001). Negative automatic thoughts increase negative affect, which in turn increases the likelihood of further negative thought, producing a vicious cycle that tends to maintain dysphoria. It follows from this formulation that patients can overcome their problems by identifying and modifying their negative thoughts.

Within A. T. Beck's formulation (1967; A. T. Beck et al., 1979, 1985), cognitive change depends upon the patient noticing and remembering her own cognition as it occurs. Thus, the patient learns to attend to her own cognitive content as a vehicle for understanding the nature of an emotional episode or disturbance. The heuristic and therapeutic value of the cognitive model lies in its emphasis on the relatively easily accessed mental events that patient can be trained to report (DeRubeis et al., 2001). Once the patient has attended to the content of his or her cognitive reaction, she is then encouraged to view it as a hypothesis, rather than as a manifest fact. Through careful scrutiny and consideration of the belief-hypothesis, the patient gradually alters her perspective. By virtue of changing the relevant belief, change in the emotional reaction and behavior follows. The therapist will characteristically induce cognitive restructuring by asking leading questions that guide the patient to question and alter her faulty cognition (A. T. Beck et al., 1979; Overholser, 1993a,b; J. S. Beck, 1996). This dialogue between patient and therapist is called 'guided discovery' or 'Socratic questioning' (DeRubeis et al., 2001).

Over the course of therapy, the patient will become familiar with the process of evaluating her own thinking, applying it whenever she is confronted with new difficulties. Thus, the ultimate goal of cognitive restructuring is prophylactic: the patient acquires or refines a skill (e.g., to attend to and question her thinking), which she can apply in all domains of her life (Meichenbaum, 1995; J. S. Beck, 1995; DeRubeis et al., 2001). Cognitive restructuring is a central component of specific treatment programs for emotional disorders, personality disorders, eating disorders, and psychotic disorders.

Problem solving

Problem solving is a self-directed process by which a person attempts to identify or discover effective or adaptive solutions for specific problems encountered in everyday life. Initially, the therapist helps the patient identify and define the problems she faces. For each problem, therapist and patient brainstorm potential solutions, evaluate the quality of each solution, and test out the best ones. Problem solving also entails helping the patient identify and overcome difficulties (practical and cognitive) that she might encounter while carrying out the plan. Where testing and evaluation of possible solutions indicates that they are inappropriate, patient and therapist develop either modified or new solutions (D'Zurilla and Goldfried, 1971; D'Zurilla and Nezu, 1980; Hawton and Kirk, 1989).

Problem solving is easily learned and has been applied to a wide range of situations commonly encountered in psychiatric practice: example applications include difficulties associated with mood, anxiety, stress, substance abuse, psychotic symptoms, cancer, and other health problems (D'Zurilla and Nezu, 2001).

Behavioral activation/activity scheduling

The use of activity schedules serves to counteract the patient's loss of motivation, inactivity, and preoccupation with depressive ideas (Lewinsohn, 1974). As inactivity is associated with negative emotional states, the therapist may provide the patient with a schedule to plan activities in advance. By planning the day with the therapist, patients are often able to set meaningful goals. Comparison of the patient's record of the actual activities (compared with what was planned for the day) provides the therapist and patient with objective feedback about his achievements (A. T. Beck et al., 1979). Activities that are scheduled can come from several domains: those that were associated with mastery, pleasure, or good mood, as well as new activities that may be rewarding or informative.

Another tool that the therapist may introduce is 'chunking.' As the patient is likely to perceive some tasks as insurmountably large, the therapist can help the patient to beak (i.e., 'chunk') these larger tasks into smaller, more manageable ones (DeRubeis et al., 2001). The use of 'graded tasks' is a related technique that the therapist may call upon in activity scheduling. Here, the patient first begins to schedule the easier or simpler aspects of larger tasks, before moving on to larger, more difficult tasks (A. T. Beck et al., 1979; J. S. Beck, 1995). Activity scheduling is used to overcome the lethargy and anhedonia of depressed patients, bipolar patients, schizophrenic patients, and eating-disordered patients.

Relapse prevention

Many disorders are characterized by waxing and waning symptomatology. Preparing clients for the possibility that the problem symptoms will return is, accordingly, an important phase of therapy. Central to the relapse prevention model is the distinction between a lapse and a relapse: a lapse is defined as a single isolated emergence of a symptom (e.g., a violation of abstinence), while a relapse is defined as a full-blown return of the pretreatment symptom levels (e.g., addictive behavior) (Marlatt and Gordon, 1995). As a lapse does not inexorably lead to relapse, the therapist and patient can work together to develop skills and strategies to neutralize the lapses that will undoubtedly occur following successful CBT treatment. An equally important application of relapse prevention techniques is to help patients test out whether they have developed realistic expectations of their own ability to cope outside therapy (Young et al., 2003), as unrealistic optimism may be a risk factor for relapse (Alvarez-Conrad et al., 2002).

Relapse prevention consists of four components: (1) identifying high-risk situations; (2) learning coping skills; (3) practicing coping skills; and (4) creating life-style balance. Following the ethos of relapse prevention, the therapist encourages the patient to frame inevitable setbacks as learning experiences within the therapeutic process rather than as personal failures or treatment failures. Therapist and patient anticipate and identify high-risk situations—those which are most likely to trigger relapse—and rehearse coping strategies that can be used in the event that such circumstances occur. Imaginal techniques, importantly, can be employed: the patient vividly imagines a situation that could trigger relapse, applying the coping strategies to see if they effectively neutralize the advancing dysphoria (Ellis and Newman, 1996).

Stress inoculation training within addictions is a specialized application of relapse prevention techniques. Relapse prevention, more generally, has been modified and included as a component of treatments for mood disorders, anxiety disorders, eating disorders, psychotic disorders, and suicidality.

Exposure therapy

Exposure techniques are used to treat fear, anxiety, or other intense negative emotional reactions. The therapist encourages the patient to confront situations that give rise to negative emotion. Typically, the patient will erroneously believe that these circumstances are personally quite dire, and she will actively avoid and escape cues that signal them. Exposure to these feared or avoided situations allows the patient to gather data that are inconsistent with such beliefs. That is to say, she comes to realize that the feared situation is actually safer than she has previously thought. She also learns that avoidance and maladaptive anxiety-neutralizing or 'safety' behaviors, such as ritualizing in obsessive-compulsive disorder (OCD) or taking antianxiety medication, are not required to cope with the anxiety. Exposure can be implemented in vivo or in imaginal mode. In vivo exposure involves actually encountering the feared situation or event, whereas imaginal exposure involves vividly imagining the event as if it were happening in the moment. The newest exposure method is virtual reality, which effectively produces vivid images and sensations of feared objects such as spiders (Garcia-Palacios et al., 2002), as well as feared situations such as airplane flight (Maltby et al., 2002), public speaking (Harris et al., 2002), or the Vietnam War experience (Rothbaum et al., 1999).

When planning exposure therapy, the therapist and patient identify a list of situations that are typically feared or avoided by the patient. The hierarchy should contain representative situations that are important to the treatment goals and the patient's functioning. The situations are then ranked in order of difficulty for the patient. The therapy begins with exposure to one of the easier items on the list, then, in a careful and concerted fashion, the patient and therapist move through the hierarchy until the patient has been exposed to the most difficult item on the list. Cognitive-behavioral applications include exposure to bodily symptoms in panic disorder and OCD, exposure to feared situations in posttraumatic stress disorder (PTSD) and social phobia, exposure to feared objects in specific phobia, exposure to traumatic memories in PTSD, and exposure to worry in generalized anxiety disorder (GAD).

A behavioral experiment (J. S. Beck, 1995) is a therapeutic technique much in the spirit of exposure methods for anxiety; however, it is a more versatile intervention, applying across a range of problems and areas of functioning. The main goal of a behavioral experiment, as with exposure, is to have the patient test out a specific, typically erroneous, belief or thought within a particular situation. When well-designed and carefully executed, such experiments play a pivotal role in the process of cognitive change (Newman et al., 2001). Thus, the depressed patient can, for example, discover the inaccuracy of her belief that exercise is useless or the belief that she won't enjoy a date (J. S. Beck, 1995). Likewise, a patient experiencing command hallucinations can discover the inaccuracy of his belief that the 'voice' is all-powerful or all-knowing (Chadwick et al., 1996).

Effective cognitive-behavioral treatments by disorder

Cognitive and behavioral therapies were pioneered in the late 1950s and 1960s to treat mood and anxiety disorders (Kendall and Kriss, 1983; Meichenbaum, 1995; Dobson and Dozois, 2001). Accordingly, extensive efficacy literature exists that support the success of cognitive-behavioral treatments for major depressive disorder, panic disorder, OCD, social phobia, PTSD, and GAD. Cognitive-behavioral interventions have also been applied successfully to eating disorders, insomnia, substance abuse, paraphilias, and personality disorders. More recently, evidence has accrued indicating cognitive-behavioral treatments are efficacious, in conjunction with medication, for bipolar disorder and schizophrenia.

An exhaustive review is beyond the scope of the present chapter. In the discussion that follows, we briefly sketch the specifics of the effective cognitive-behavioral interventions for each disorder. Readers looking for a more extensive account of the empirical literature supporting the treatments are directed to any one of the publications that have arisen in the context of the empirically validated treatments movement (Roth and Fonagy, 1996; DeRubeis and Crits-Cristoph, 1998; Chambless and Hollon, 1998; Nathan and Gorman, 2002).

Mood disorders

Major depression

More behaviorally oriented approaches theorize that a person becomes depressed when she ceases producing behavior that elicits positive reinforcement (Lewinsohn and Gotlib, 1995). Behavioral interventions, therefore, primarily target daily activities, encouraging the patient to monitor and increase activity frequency. Additional techniques employed include improving social and communication skills, increasing adaptive behaviors, and decreasing negative life events (Craighead et al., 2002b). While less studied than Beck's cognitive therapy, the research that does exist, notably by Jacobson and colleagues, suggests that depressed patients treated with behavior-focused therapy show as much acute improvement as patients treated with a behavior-focused therapy that includes cognitive elements (Jacobson et al., 1996). The equivalence between these treatments was still present at a 2-year follow-up (Gortner et al., 1998).

Beck's CBT (A. T. Beck et al., 1979) conceptualizes depression in terms of cognitive processes (e.g., biases) and products (e.g., thoughts and beliefs) that produce and maintain depression. The therapy is directive and short term, focused upon changing the depressed patient's negative thoughts regarding her self, world, and future. Behavioral methods (e.g., self-monitoring and behavioral activation) dominate early sessions. A shift to cognitively oriented techniques (e.g., cognitive assessment and restructuring) characterizes the mid-treatment sessions. Relapse prevention, finally, is the focal point of late session activity. In the acute reduction of depressive symptoms, CBT is better than a pill-placebo and equivalent to antidepressant medications (Rush et al., 1977; Murphy et al., 1986; Elkin et al., 1989; Hollon et al., 1992). On average, 50–70% of the patients who completed a course of CBT within these trials no longer met Diagnostic and statistical manual of mental disorders (DSM; American Psychiatric Association, 1994) criteria for major depressive disorder (Craighead et al., 2002b). The effectiveness of CBT extends across a wide range of patient severity, including the most severely depressed outpatients (DeRubeis et al., 1999; in press). CBT also appears to prevent depressive relapses at least as effectively as continuous medication (Hollon et al., in press).

McCullough's (2000) cognitive-behavioral analysis system of psychotherapy (CBASP) identifies the root of depression in the impact of behavior and thought upon interpersonal functioning. The patient is encouraged to consider the consequences of her behavior and to utilize social problem solving, among other techniques, to address interpersonal difficulties. In a large outcome study, 12 weeks of CBASP combined with antidepressant medication produces an acute reduction of depressive symptoms in chronically depressed patients that exceeded the reduction that either treatment achieved alone (Keller et al., 2000).

Bipolar disorder

A significant proportion of bipolar patients experience frequent relapses despite adequate medication dosage and compliance. To address this, several manualized cognitive-behavioral treatments have been developed as an adjunct to medications for the treatment of bipolar disorder (Basco and Rush, 1996; Lam et al., 1999; Newman et al., 2002; Scott, 2002). All of these treatments are designed to be administered in conjunction with mood-stabilizing agents. Cognitive aspects of these treatments emphasize negative thinking patterns (e.g., self-statements and dysfunctional beliefs) in the genesis of mood swings. Behavioral aspects focus upon mood fluctuations and vegetative routines (e.g., sleep–wake cycles). The interventions aim to enhance the patient's engagement with the environment via a combination of psychoeducation about the disorder and medication, mood monitoring for episode cues and triggers, as well as the more standard techniques of behavioral activation and cognitive restructuring (Lam et al., 1999; Newman et al., 2002).

When compared with patients treated with mood stabilizers alone, patients treated with combined CBT and mood-stabilizing agents may experience longer latencies between manic episodes (Perry et al., 1999), have fewer hospitalizations (Cochran, 1984), and demonstrate better medication compliance (Lam et al., 2000). In a recent study (Lam et al., 2003), medicated bipolar patients treated with 14 sessions of CBT experience fewer bipolar episodes, fewer days in a bipolar episode, and fewer episode-related admissions across a 12-month period, relative to patients treated with medication alone. The CBT-treated patients also showed higher social functioning, fewer mood symptoms, and less fluctuation in manic symptoms (Lam et al., 2003).

Anxiety disorders

Panic disorder (with and without agoraphobia)

Clark (1996) postulates that panic attacks have a stereotypical phenomenology: first, the patient notices a somatic sensation that is unpleasant (e.g., rapid heart rate); she then begins focusing her attention on internal sensations and potential catastrophic misinterpretation of the sensations (e.g., 'I am going to die'); a vicious cycle ensues in which the patient experiences an escalation of the sense of danger as she interprets her symptoms as pathological, which spurs on the symptoms (e.g., heart races faster, breathing becomes more rapid); finally, despite the patient's every effort, the panic attack intensifies such that the patient believes that it will continue until disaster occurs. Clark's treatment (Clark, 1996) features two behavioral methods: (1) the patient is encouraged to induce the sensations (e.g., hyperventilation) and discover that these sensations do not presage a catastrophe, and (2) patients are encouraged to expose themselves to feared situations that they would otherwise avoid, situations that might lead to panic. However, the cognitive techniques play a more important therapeutic role within the treatment program: (1) developing an idiosyncratic model of panic in terms of the vicious cycle; (2) eliciting and testing maladaptive beliefs with regard to bodily sensations; (3) identifying more adaptive beliefs and evaluating them; and (4) modifying images (e.g., seeing one's own funeral) that spontaneously occur during panic. Craske and colleagues have developed a rather similar treatment that places more emphasis upon the behavioral aspects of the intervention (Craske et al., 2000).

Clark (1996) reports that across five studies between 74% and 95% of patients assigned to cognitive therapy became panic free and maintained this status through the respective follow-up periods (6–15 months). In these trials, CBT outperformed wait-list control, applied relaxation, pharmacotherapy, and exposure therapy. Additionally, Barlow et al. (2000) report evidence that combining medicines with CBT undermines the efficacy of the CBT for panic, as CBT alone produces a more enduring effect (assessed at 12 months) than imipramine or imipramine + CBT.

Obsessive-compulsive disorder

Following the pioneering work of Victor Meyer in 1966, most behavioral and cognitive-behavioral treatments for OCD induce change via exposure and ritual prevention (Franklin and Foa, 2002). Within this behavioral framework, compulsions are conceptualized as safety behaviors (either overt or covert) that reduce the anxiety induced by obsessive ideation. Thus, repeated exposure to obsessional cues when combined with suspension of compulsive rituals should both habituate the anxiety response to obsessional thinking and extinguish the use of the safety behaviors. Treatments for OCD that feature exposure and ritual prevention may also include a cognitive component focused upon preventing relapse. Empirically, treatments that feature exposure and ritual prevention produce better symptom reduction in OCD patients than pill-placebo and anxiety management conditions, and symptom reductions that are equivalent to medication treatments (Franklin and Foa, 2002). The addition of cognitive techniques to exposure and response prevention appears to reduce relapse rates (Hiss et al., 1994).

More cognitively based cognitive-behavioral approaches to OCD theorize that distorted thinking and beliefs support the OCD behavior (Frost and Steketee, 2002). Via Socratic questioning, among other techniques, the therapist helps the patient identify, evaluate, and alter problematic beliefs (Steketee and Barlow, 2002). Whether delivered in 12 sessions or 20 sessions, cognitively focused CBT produces reductions in OCD symptoms that are equivalent—both during active treatment (Van Oppen et al., 1995) and at 1-year follow-up (Cottraux et al., 2001)—to behaviorally focused CBT that emphasizes exposure and ritual prevention. Belief-focused CBT for OCD appears to be especially useful for patients with mental obsessions, and works better as an individualized (i.e., as opposed to group) intervention (Steketee and Barlow, 2002).

Social phobia

Behaviorally oriented models of social phobia emphasize social learning (Hoffman and Barlow, 2002). The socially phobic individual, according to this behavioral formulation, becomes hyperaroused at the prospect of social situations. She learns, moreover, that avoiding and escaping social situations brings a palpable relief in anxiety. However, avoidance and escape behavior have the unintended consequence of maintaining the phobia. Cognitive-behavioral therapists, accordingly, employ exposure methods to habituate anxiety and, thereby, enable the patient to function in the presence of other people (Hoffman and Barlow, 2002). If the patient is deficient in verbal and nonverbal social skills, a social skills training intervention can be included in the treatment (Heimberg and Juster, 1995; Barlow et al., 2002).

Cognitively oriented theorists (Clark and Wells, 1995) propose that social phobia is mediated by maladaptive beliefs about social performance. Specifically, the patient believes that she is apt to behave inappropriately in social situations and that this hapless performance will lead to rejection, loss of status, etc. Preoccupied with negative thoughts about herself and overly concerned with the perceptions others have of her, the social phobic finds social situations noxious and difficult to manage. Cognitive interventions target the negative beliefs about self, attempting to help the patient construct a more accurate image of herself as a social actor (Hoffman and Barlow, 2002).

While exposure and cognitive restructuring produce more improvement in symptoms than a wait-list control group, the combination is better still (Barlow et al., 2002). The combined treatment, delivered in a group context over 12 weeks, also beats a nonspecific therapy and pill-placebo, while demonstrating equal effectiveness with medication that is still present at a 6-month follow-up (Heimberg et al., 1998).

Posttraumatic stress disorder

Behaviorally oriented models propose that avoidance and escape behavior maintain the traumatic response. Exposure—imaginal and/or *in vivo*—is the principal behavioral intervention for PTSD. If imaginal exposure is employed, the patient relives the trauma in imagery, focusing upon key behavioral, emotional, sensory, and cognitive aspects of the experience. For *in-vivo* exposure, patient and therapist construct a hierarchy of feared/avoided situations to be exposed one by one. The goal of exposure is to help the patient master and stop avoiding the cues associated with the traumatic event (Keane and Barlow, 2002). Several studies have shown the efficacy of exposure interventions for PTSD. Foa *et al.* (1991), for example, have demonstrated that rape victims with PTSD treated with exposure—relative to anxiety management, supportive counseling wait-list patients—evidence the fewest PTSD symptoms at a 3.5-month follow-up.

Thrasher *et al.* (1996) postulate that PTSD is maintained by beliefs the patient holds regarding self, the world, the trauma, and the future. Thought identifying, evidence gathering, Socratic questioning, and other standard cognitive therapy techniques are employed in the treatment (A. T. Beck *et al.*, 1979, 1985; J. S. Beck, 1995). Marks *et al.* (1998) report an advantage for PTSD patients treated with 10 sessions of either prolonged exposure or cognitive therapy or the combination of exposure and cognitive restructuring: all three groups demonstrated a greater reduction in symptoms than patients treated with relaxation training; these group differences were still evident at a 6-month follow-up (Marks *et al.*, 1998; Lovell *et al.*, 2001). Thus, while exposure is clearly efficacious, it is not necessary to achieve lasting reduction of PTSD symptoms.

Generalized anxiety disorder

Behavioral approaches propose that anxiety is maintained by avoidance of anxiety producing situations, personal reactions to anxiety, and loss of self-confidence. The interventions often include psychoeducation, applied relaxation, imaginal and *in vivo* exposure, and behavioral activation (Roemer *et al.*, 2002). A. T. Beck *et al.* (1985), on the other hand, argue that anxiety is perpetuated by anxious thoughts and a lack of self-confidence, which can be controlled by helping the patient to recognize anxious thoughts, seeking helpful alternatives, and taking action to test these alternatives. Empirically, several studies find that behavioral and cognitive-behavioral treatments reduce anxiety equally well, as both achieve superior results to wait-list and nonspecific control groups (Barlow *et al.*, 2002). A notable study by Butler *et al.* (1991) found that patients treated with CBT showed less anxiety than patients treated with an exposure-based treatment. CBT has also been found to produce better outcomes for patients with GAD than psychodynamic therapy and benzodiazepines (Roemer *et al.*, 2002).

Specific phobia

The theoretical account of specific phobias is formulated in terms of the elementary learning processes of classical and instrumental conditioning (c.f. for a discussion of this model and further elaborations see Bouton *et al.*, 2001). The phobic stimulus is characterized as a conditioned stimulus (CS) that predicts the coming of an undesirable unconditioned stimulus (US). As situations that are likely to elicit the phobic CS are avoided, and as chance encounters with the phobic stimulus are readily escaped, the CS-US relationship is not allowed to extinguish. Moreover, avoidant and escape behaviors are maintained instrumentally via negative reinforcement (i.e., by avoiding or escaping the situation, the feared undesirable stimulus is not experienced, which increases the likelihood of avoiding and escaping in the future). Behavior treatment for specific phobia entails imaginal and/or *in vivo* exposure to the phobic stimulus (Antony and Barlow, 2002). Barlow *et al.* (2002) report that exposure-based treatments are the treatment of choice, having shown efficacy for animal phobias, fear of heights, fear of flying, and blood-injury phobias. Adding cognitive restructuring to exposure appears to produce better results than exposure alone for patients with dental phobias and patients with claustrophobia (Antony and Barlow, 2002).

Bulimia nervosa (BN)

The cognitive-behavioral model of bulimia centers upon a complex of behavioral and cognitive factors (Fairburn *et al.*, 1993; Fairburn, 1997; Wilson *et al.*, 1997). Both cognitive and behavioral techniques are employed to replace extreme dietary restraint with a normal pattern of eating. Dysfunctional attitudes about body shape, weight, and self are also addressed. Wilson and Fairburn (2002) assert that CBT is the treatment of choice for BN, as it has been found to be more effective than control and nonspecific therapies, equally good or better than other psychotherapies (e.g., interpersonal psychotherapy, supportive therapy, stress management therapy), and equally good or better than pharmacotherapy. A typical result: 50% of the CBT-treated patients stop bingeing and purging, effects that are maintained across 6-month and 1-year follow-up periods (Wilson and Fairburn, 2002). Moreover, the combination of the behavioral and cognitive components of the treatment produces better outcomes than the behavioral components alone.

Binge-eating disorder (BED)

Cognitive-behavioral and strict behavioral weight loss programs have been developed to treat BED. The CBT is based upon the Wilson and Fairburn model for bulimia. Behavioral weight loss introduces caloric restriction, improved nutrition, and increasing physical activity as the method of intervention. Empirically, across medication and psychotherapy trials, a very high placebo response rate is seen in studies. Additionally, CBT and interpersonal therapy appear the same, and only modestly efficacious. Behavioral weight loss program has been less effectively evaluated, though there is evidence that it produces more weight-loss than CBT (Wilson and Fairburn, 2002).

Anorexia nervosa (AN)

Interventions featuring operant conditioning have been implemented with anorexia in inpatient settings. Individualized reinforcers are provided for each 0.5 kg of weight gained. Such programs result in 80% of the AN patients reaching their target weight (Wilson and Fairburn, 2002). Fairburn's (1997) effective cognitive-behavioral model for BN has also been applied to patients with AN. Results thus far are modest: CBT patients are better off than control-treated patients, but still significantly underweight (Channon *et al.*, 1989; Serfaty *et al.*, 1999). Vitousek (2002) discusses current ideas about the application of CBT to anorexia nervosa.

Schizophrenia/schizoaffective disorder

Since the 1960s, several hundred studies have been conducted investigating the impact of behavioral methods (e.g., reinforcement schedules, stimulus control, social modeling, shaping, and fading) upon the full gamut of symptoms and behavior associated with the disorder. Most of these studies utilize A-B-A designs, in which the subject serves as her own control and the active treatment is introduced, and then taken away (Kopelowicz *et al.*, 2002). There is also quite a degree of empirical support for token economy based social learning programs on inpatient wards (Craig *et al.*, 2003). Paul and Lentz (1977), for example, found that a token economy produced changes in symptoms, daily activities, social behavior, and discharge, among other outcomes, as compared with a standard ward.

Social skills training is another behavioral intervention that has an extensive literature. The primary goal of a social skills intervention is to enable individuals with severe mental illness to gain skills that will help them function within their communities (Craig *et al.*, 2003). Typically the intervention is conducted in a group format, with outpatients who are stabilized on medication. The intervention targets the following skills: complying with the use of antipsychotic medication, communicating with mental health professionals, recognizing prodromal signs of relapse, developing a relapse prevention plan, coping with persistent psychotic symptoms, avoiding street drugs and alcohol, and developing leisure skills and conversational skills (Kopelowicz *et al.*, 2002). Empirical evidence supports the idea that social skills programs train skills that are detectable 1-year after the end of treatment. Relapse rates have also been reduced by social skills training relative to medication alone (Hogarty et al., 1986; Craig et al., 2003).

In the UK, several research groups have devised cognitive-behavioral treatment programs to treat the positive symptoms of schizophrenia (Kingdon and Turkington, 1994; Fowler et al., 1995; Chadwick et al., 1996). Delusions, within the cognitive formulation, are beliefs that can be identified, subjected to evidence gathering, and modified. Likewise, distressing auditory hallucinations are percepts about which the patient manifests dysfunctional beliefs (e.g., the voice is omnipotent and powerful) and behavior patterns (e.g., doing what the voice says). Modifications to traditional cognitive-behavioral approaches include a more extensive use of techniques to keep the patient engaged in therapy, flexible use of session structuring (e.g., more or less structure), and a minimally confrontational approach to belief modification (Nelson, 1997).

CBT has demonstrated efficacy for chronic medication-resistant positive symptoms of schizophrenia and schizoaffective disorder (Martindale et al., 2003). Patients receiving CBT adjunctive to medication and case management show a larger reduction in psychotic symptoms than do patients receiving medication and case management alone (Tarrier et al., 1993, 1998, 1999, 2000; Kuipers et al., 1997, 1998; Rector et al., 2003) or patients receiving an active control treatment (Tarrier et al., 1998, 1999, 2000; Pinto et al., 1999; Sensky et al., 2000). Rector et al. (2003) have also found that, relative to routine care, CBT reduces chronic negative symptoms.

CBT has also shown efficacy for the acute symptoms of psychosis. Patients within an acute psychotic episode treated with CBT and routine care improve more rapidly than patients treated with routine care alone or routine care plus active control treatment (Drury et al., 1996a,b; Lewis et al., 2002). CBT also has demonstrated efficacy in the prevention of future psychotic episodes (Drury et al., 1996b; Gumley et al., 2003). Additionally, there is emerging evidence that CBT can delay the onset of the first episode of psychosis, either in conjunction with medicines (McGorry et al., 2002) or without medicines (Morrison et al., 2002). Citing the growing evidence for an effective role of CBT in psychosis (cf., Rector and Beck, 2001), the National Health Service in the UK has recently mandated service providers to include CBT as an option for all individuals being treated for schizophrenia (National Institute of Clinical Excellence, 2002).

Substance abuse

Behavioral approaches for managing substance abuse theorize either from a base of classical or operant conditioning. Cue exposure postulates, in a classical vein, that conditions (e.g., neutral stimuli or CSs) antecedent to drug or alcohol use come, through repeated pairings with drugs or alcohol, to produce conditioned responses that encourage further drinking. The intervention is exposure: the patient experiences the cues without drinking or taking drugs, which, theoretically, extinguishes the Pavlovian spur to use the substances. Within the alcohol abuse literature, cue exposure has been shown to modestly reduce drinking frequency when compared with standard treatments, but has not produced abstinence (Kaddan, 2001).

In contrast to cue exposure, contingency management (CM) is a strict Skinnerian enterprise. Consequences of use (e.g., the feelings that the substance imparts or social factors) are theorized to maintain or reinforce abuse. CM promotes abstinence by introducing a new reinforcement schedule. In methadone clinics, doses of methadone can serve as reinforces for heroin abstinence. However, for cocaine abusers, vouchers exchangeable for valuable goods and services serve to reinforce abstinence behavior. Typically, an escalating schedule of reinforcement is set up such that each specimen of cocaine-free urine is reinforced with a larger reward. CM produces rapid results (e.g., 2 days of abstinence for $100 voucher in 40 of 50 addicts), which are not maintained after CM is stopped (Epstein et al., 2003). CM proves more problematic to apply to alcohol abuse, as it is difficult to verify objectively whether patients have had a drink within the last 24 hours (Kadden, 2001).

Cognitive interventions for substance abuse target beliefs and thoughts as the factors that maintain substance abuse (A. T. Beck et al., 1993). Interventions encourage the abusing patient, first, to identify thoughts, feelings and events that precede and follow each instance of alcohol or drug use. Next, the patient practices resisting and avoiding specific cues associated with using. Additionally, the patient practices alternative strategies for dealing with negative affect and attempts to fill the role of the drug with alternative reinforces (A. T. Beck et al., 1993).

Within the alcohol abuse literature, CBT is called coping skills training. A large number of studies support the efficacy of coping skills training for alcohol abuse (Finney and Moos, 2002). For drug abuse, Carroll and colleagues found that CBT does not reduce acute cocaine abuse at a level that is distinguishable from a clinical management control condition. However, over 6-month and 12-month follow-up periods, CBT-treated cocaine abusers fared substantially better that control subjects, suggesting that the skills imparted by CBT take time to be introduced into daily behavior (Carroll et al., 1994). A recent study finds that adding CBT to CM for cocaine abuse is a promising treatment package: although CBT and CM together perform less well than either treatment alone, at the 12-month follow-up, the patients who received the combined treatment are abstaining from cocaine the most (Epstein et al., 2003).

Somatoform/factitious disorders

For patients suffering hypochondriasis, Clark et al. (1998) have devised a cognitive-behavioral treatment that reduces attention to distressing bodily sensations, corrects misinformation and exaggerated beliefs, and addresses cognitive processes (e.g., selective attention, misattribution, etc.) that maintain disease fears. This CBT package produces better outcomes than no treatment or nonspecific treatments such as relaxation (Clark et al., 1998; Fava et al., 2000). For body dysmorphic disorder, cognitive-behavioral approaches employ an eclectic collection of cognitive and behavioral techniques: patients identify and modify distorted body perceptions, interrupt critical self-thoughts, expose themselves to anxiety provoking situations, and practice response prevention. Group or individual CBT for body dysmorphic disorder is better than no treatment, producing response rates of 50–75% (Simon, 2002). Finally, cognitive-behavioral interventions for somatoform pain include validation that the pain as real, relaxation training, activity scheduling, reinforcement for nonpain behaviors, and cognitive restructuring. Whether implemented as a group or individual intervention, about 30–60% of patients treated with CBT report significant reductions in pain (Simon, 2002).

Personality disorders

Several sophisticated cognitive-behavioral approaches have been developed to address the problems and challenges of personality disorders (A. T. Beck et al., 1990; Linehan, 1993; Young, 1994). It is currently difficult, however, to determine the efficacy of many of these treatments for specific personality disorders, due to a lack of published empirical research (Crits-Cristoph and Barber, 2002). Avoidant personality disorder is one exception to this general trend. In a 10-week study of behaviorally oriented group interventions, Alden (1989) discovered that graded exposure, social skills training, and intimacy focused social skills training conditions all produce better outcomes in patients with avoidant personality disorder than a wait-list group. While improvement was clinically significant, the avoidant patients still tended to fall short of normal functioning. In a further analysis of the data, Alden and colleagues discovered that patient presenting issues moderates the effectiveness of the behavioral treatments; that is, graded exposure worked best for the distrustful and angry patients, while intimacy focused social skills training appeared more effective for the patients who feel beholden to others (Crits-Cristoph and Barber, 2002).

Another empirically supported treatment is Linehan's (1993) dialectical behavior therapy (DBT): a complex cognitive-behavioral treatment for borderline personality disorder that includes group and individual sessions. Group sessions are primarily psychoeducational: teaching interpersonal skills, distress tolerance/reality acceptance, and emotional regulation skills. Individual sessions involve directive problem-solving and supportive techniques. Empirically, DBT produces lower rates of attrition, less parasuicidal behavior, and fewer hospitalizations than treatment as usual (Linehan *et al.*, 1991). DBT also appears to be effective in both outpatient and inpatient settings, and has been found to be superior to a community control group (Koerner and Linehan, 2002).

Limitations and contraindications

It is safe to say that CBT has proved quite versatile, having been successfully applied to a wide spectrum of psychological difficulty. The limits of cognitive therapy have yet to be empirically established. However, several factors may make the cognitive-behavioral approach less effective—in fact, these factors may interfere with the efficacy of *any* psychotherapeutic approach. Low patient motivation, unless appropriately addressed, can impede progress, especially among patients who hold beliefs that they will suffer significant adverse consequences if they comply with treatment. Patients who have positive beliefs about dysfunctional aspects of their disorder likewise need special intervention. Examples include the schizophrenic patient's grandiose delusion (e.g., one who believes he is being persecuted because he is a great deity) and the anorexic patient's social beliefs (e.g., she is superior to others).

Even when motivation is present, the success of cognitive-behavioral methods can be hampered by mental facility. Severely retarded individuals, for example, might not be capable of the reasoning entailed in cognitive restructuring. Self-monitoring might also prove to be too demanding a task for a person with severe intellectual impairment. Behavioral methods may be more appropriate for these individuals than cognitive strategies. Psychopaths (Lykken, 1995) might also have difficulty with certain cognitive interventions; when performing a goal-directed task, they may be less able to attend to peripheral information or to self-regulate, especially under conditions of neutral motivation (Newman *et al.*, 1997).

Finally, cultural differences may impact efficacy if therapists do not tailor the therapy appropriately. Therapists must understand, for example, how these differences may affect the building of a therapeutic alliance and how patients' cultural beliefs affect their thinking and reactions. Different thinking styles and stylistic preferences must often be accommodated for patients to progress.

Future directions

The last 20 years have seen incredible growth in cognitive-behavioral therapies as treatments for psychiatric disorders. What does the future hold? Much current research aims to improve the effectiveness of existing cognitive-behavioral interventions. There is an ongoing attempt, for example, to make cognitive-behavioral interventions more useful in the community (Stirman *et al.*, 2003). Thus, investigators are focusing upon issues of comorbidity and dissemination. Much of the empirical literature that supports cognitive-behavioral interventions for specific disorders has involved screening out a variety of patients with comorbid psychopathology. Newer studies are investigating cognitive-behavioral applications specifically designed for individuals with comorbid diagnoses. An example of this is a current trial being undertaken by Edna Foa and her colleagues that aims to co-jointly treat social phobia and depression (J. D. Huppert, personal communication 2003). Yet another trend involves combining differing treatment modalities. Borkovec, for example, has been piloting a treatment for GAD that combines the best of cognitive-behavioral and interpersonal methods (Roemer *et al.*, 2002). A further example of cross-modality therapeutic synthesis involves the methods of mindfulness mediation, which are being applied to relapse prevention after recovery for depression (Segal *et al.*, 2002) and schizophrenia (D. G. Kingdon, personal communication 2003).

References

Alden, L. E. (1989). Short-term structured treatment for avoidant personality disorder. *Journal of Consulting and Clinical Psychology*, **57**, 756–64.

Alvarez-Conrad, J., Strunk, D. R., Furst, J., and DeRubeis, R. J. (2001). *Mechanisms of relapse prevention in cognitive therapy for depression: investigating schema change and compensatory skills*. Poster session presented at World Congress of the Association of the Advancement of Behavior Therapy, Vancouver.

American Psychiatric Association (1994). *Diagnostic and statistical manual of mental disorders*, 4th edn. Washington, DC: American Psychiatric Association.

Antony, M. M. and Barlow, D. H. (2002). Specific phobias. In: D. H. Barlow, ed. *Anxiety and its disorders: the nature and treatment of anxiety and panic*. New York: Guilford Press.

Barlow, D. H., Gorman, J. M., Shear, M. K., and Woods, S. W. (2000). Cogntive-behavioral therapy, imipramine, or their combination for panic disorder: a randomized controlled trial. *Journal of the American Medical Association*, **283**, 2529–36.

Barlow, D. H., Raffa, S. D., and Cohen, E. M. (2002). Psychosocial treatments for panic disorders, phobias and generalized anxiety disorder. In: P. E. Nathan and J. M. Gorman, ed. *A guide to treatments that work*. New York: Oxford University Press.

Basco, M. R. and Rush, A. J. (1996). *Cognitive-behavioral therapy for bipolar disorder*. New York: Guilford Press.

Beck, A. T. (1967). *Depression: causes and treatment*. Philadelphia, PA: University of Pennsylvania Press.

Beck, A. T., Rush, A. J., Shaw, B. F., and Emery, G. (1979). *Cognitive therapy of depression*. New York: Guilford Press.

Beck, A. T., Emery, G., and Greenberg, R. L. (1985). *Anxiety disorders and phobias: a cognitive perspective*. New York: Basic Books.

Beck, A. T., *et al.* (1990). *Cognitive therapy of personality disorders*. New York: Guilford Press.

Beck, A. T., Wright, F. D., Newman, C. F., and Liese, B. S. (1993). *Cognitive therapy of substance abuse*. New York: Guilford Press.

Beck, A. T., Steer, R. A., and Brown, G. K. (1996). *Manual for the Beck Depression Inventory*, 2nd edn. San Antonio: The Psychological Corporation.

Beck, J. S. (1995). *Cognitive therapy: basics and beyond*. New York: Guilford Press.

Blankstein, K. R. and Segal, Z. V. (2001). Cognitive assessment: issues and methods. In: K. S. Dobson, ed. *Handbook of cognitive-behavioral therapies*. New York: Guilford Press.

Bouton, M. E., Mineka, S., and Barlow, D. H. (2001). A modern learning theory perspective on the etiology of panic disorder. *Psychological Review*, **108**, 4–32.

Butler, G., Fennell, M., Robson, P., and Gelder, M. (1991). Comparison of behavior therapy and cognitive behavior therapy in the treatment of generalized anxiety disorder. *Journal of Consulting and Clinical Psychology*, **59**, 167–75.

Carroll K. M., *et al.* (1994). Psychotherapy and pharmacotherapy for ambulatory cocaine abusers. *Archives of General Psychiatry*, **51**, 177–87.

Chadwick, P., Brichwood, M., and Trower, P. (1996). *Cognitive therapy for delusions, voices and paranoia*. Chichester: John Wiley and Sons Ltd.

Chambless, D. and Hollon, S. D. (1998). Defining empirically supported therapies. *Journal of Consulting and Clinical Psychology*, **66**, 7–18.

Chambless, D., *et al.* (1996). An update on empirically validated therapies. *Clinical Psychologist*, **49**, 5–18.

Channon, S., De Silva, P., Helmsley, D., and Perkins, R. (1989). A controlled trial of cognitive behavioral treatment of anorexia nervosa. *Behaviour Research and Therapy*, **27**, 529–35.

Clark, D. M. (1996). Panic disorder: from theory to therapy. In: P. M. Salkovskis, ed. *Frontiers of cognitive therapy*. New York: Guilford Press.

Clark, D. M. and Wells, A. (1995). A cognitive model of social phobia. In R. G. Heimberg, M. R. Liebowitz, D. A. Hope, and F. R. Schneier, ed. *Social phobia: diagnosis, assessment and treatment*. New York: Guilford Press.

Clark, D. M., *et al.* (1998). Two psychological treatments for hypochondriasis: a randomised controlled trial. *British Journal of Psychiatry*, **173**, 218–25.

Cochran, S. D. (1984). Preventing medical noncompliance in the outpatient treatment of bipolar disorders. *Journal of Consulting and Clinical Psychology*, **52**, 873–8.

Cottraux, J. *et al.* (2001). A randomized controlled trial of cognitive therapy versus intensive behavior therapy in obsessive compulsive disorder. *Psychotherapy and Psychosomatics*, **70**, 288–97.

Craig, T. K. J., Liberman, R. P., Browne, M., Robertson, M. J., and O'Flyn, D. (2003). Psychiatric rehabilitation. In: S. R. Hirsch and D. Weinberger, ed. *Schizophrenia*. Malden, MA: Blackwell Publishing Co.

Craighead, E. W., Craighead, L. W., and Ilardi, S. S. (1995). Behavior therapies in historical perspective. In: B. Bongar and L. E. Beutler, ed. *Comprehensive textbook of psychotherapy: theory and practice*. New York: Oxford University Press.

Craighead, E. W., Miklowitz, D., Frank, E., and Vajk, F. C. (2002b). Psychosocial treatments for bipolar disorder. In: P. E. Nathan and J. M. Gorman, ed. *A guide to treatments that work*. New York: Oxford University Press.

Craske, M. G., Barlow, D. H., and Meadows, E. (2000). *Mastery of your anxiety and panic: therapist guide for anxiety, panic and agoraphobia (MAP-3)*. San Antonio, TX: Graywind/Psychological Corporation.

Crits-Cristoph, P. and Barber, J. P. (2002). Psychological treatments for personality disorders. In: P. E. Nathan and J. M. Gorman, ed. *A guide to treatments that work*. New York: Oxford University Press.

DeRubeis, R. J. (2002). *Cognitive therapy versus antidepressant medications in the treatment of moderate to severe major depressive disorder: response to short-term treatment*. Paper presented at the meeting of the American Psychiatric Association, Philadelphia, PA.

DeRubies, R. J. and Crits-Cristoph, P. (1998). Empirically supported individual and group psychological treatments for adult mental disorders. *Journal of Consulting and Clinical Psychology*, **66**, 37–52.

DeRubeis, R. J., Gelfand, L. A., Tang, T. Z., and Simons, A. (1999). Medications versus cognitive behavioral therapy for severely depressed outpatients: mega-analysis of four randomized comparisons. *American Journal of Psychiatry*, **156**, 1007–13.

DeRubeis, R. J., Tang, T. Z., and Beck, A. T. (2001). Cognitive therapy. In: K. S. Dobson, ed. *Handbook of cognitive-behavioral therapies*. New York: Guilford Press.

Dobson, K. S. and Dozois, D. J. A. (2001). Historical and philosophical bases of the cognitive-behavioral therapies. In: K. S. Dobson, ed. *Handbook of cognitive-behavioral therapies*. New York: Guilford Press.

Drury, V., Birchwood, M., Cochrane, R., and MacMillan, F. (1996a). Cognitive therapy and recovery from acute psychosis: a controlled trial. I. Impact on psychotic symptoms. *British Journal of Psychiatry*, **169**, 593–601.

Drury, V., Birchwood, M., Cochrane, R., and MacMillan, F. (1996b). Cognitive therapy and recovery from acute psychosis: a controlled trial. II. Impact on recovery time. *British Journal of Psychiatry*, **169**, 602–7.

D'Zurilla, T. J. and Goldfried, M. R. (1971). Problem solving and behavior modification. *Journal of Abnormal Psychology*, **78**, 107–26.

D'Zurilla, T. J. and Nezu, A. (1980). A study of the generation of alternatives process in social problem solving. *Cognitive Therapy and Research*, **4**, 73–81.

D'Zurilla, T. J. and Nezu, A. (2001). In: K. S. Dobson, ed. *Handbook of cognitive-behavioral therapies*. New York: Guilford Press.

Elkin, I., *et al.* (1989). National Institute of Mental Health Treatment of Depression Collaborative Research Program: General effectiveness of treatments. *Archives of General Psychiatry*, **46**, 971–82.

Ellis, T. E. and Newman, C. F. (1996). *Choosing to live: how to defeat suicide through cognitive therapy*. Oakland, CA: New Harbinger Publications, Inc.

Epstein, D. H., Hawkins, W. E., Covi, L., Umbricht, A., and Preston, K. L. (2003). Cognitive-behavioral therapy plus contingency management for cocaine use: findings during treatment and across 12-month follow-up. *Psychology of Addictive Behavior*, **17**, 73–82.

Fairburn, C. G. (1997). Eating disorders. In: D. M. Clark and C. G. Fairburn, ed. *The science and practice of cognitive behavior therapy*. Oxford: Oxford University Press.

Fairburn, C. G., Marcus, M. D., and Wilson, G. T. (1993). Cognitive behavioral therapy for binge eating and bulimia nervosa: a comprehensive treatment manual. In: C. G. Fairburn and G. T. Wilson, ed. *Binge eating: nature, assessment, treatment*. New York: Guilford Press.

Fava, G. A., Grandi, S., Rafanelli, C., Fabbri, S., and Cazzaro, M. (2000). Explanatory therapy in hypochondriasis. *Journal of Clinical Psychiatry*, **61**, 317–22.

Finny, J. W. and Moos, R. H. (2002). Psychological treatments for alcohol use disorders. In: P. E. Nathan and J. M. Gorman, ed. *A guide to treatments that work*. New York: Oxford University Press.

Foa, E. B., Rothbaum, B. O., Riggs, D. S., and Murdock, T. B. (1991). Treatment of posttraumatic stress disorder in rape victims: a comparison between cognitive-behavioral procedures and counseling. *Journal of Consulting and Clinical Psychology*, **59**, 714–23.

Fowler, D., Garety, P., and Kuipers, E. (1995). *Cognitive behavior therapy for psychosis: theory and practice*. Chichester: John Wiley and Sons Ltd.

Franklin, M. E. and Foa, E. B. (2002). Cognitive behavioral treatments for obsessive compulsive disorder. In: P. E. Nathan and J. M. Gorman, ed. *A guide to treatments that work*. New York: Oxford University Press.

Frost, R. O. and Steketee, G. (2002). *Cognitive approaches to obsessions and compulsions: theory, assessment, and treatment*. New York: Pergamon Press.

Garcia-Palacios, A., Hoffman, H., Carlin, A., Furness, T. A., Botella, C. (2002). Virtual reality in the treatment of spider phobia: a controlled study. *Behaviour Research and Therapy*, **40**, 983–93.

Gortner, E., Gollan, J. K., Dobson, K. S., and Jacobson, N. S. (1998). Cognitive-behavioral treatment for depression: relapse prevention. *Journal of Consulting and Clinical Psychology*, **66**, 377–84.

Gumley, A., *et al.* (2003). Early intervention for relapse in schizophrenia: results of a 12-month randomized controlled trial of cognitive behavioral therapy. *Psychological Medicine*, **33**, 419–31.

Harris, S. R., Kemmerling, R. L., and North, M. M. (2002). Brief virtual reality therapy for public speaking anxiety. *Cyberpsychology and Behavior*, **5**, 543–50.

Hawton, K. and Kirk, J. (1989). Problem-solving. In: K. Hawton, P. M. Salkovskis, J. Kirk, and D. M. Clark, ed. *Cognitive behaviour therapy for psychiatric problems: a practical guide*. New York: Oxford University Press.

Hawton, K., Salkovskis, P. M., Kirk, J., and Clark, D. M. (1989). The development and principles of cognitive-behavioral treatments. In: K. Hawton, P. M. Salkovskis, J. Kirk, and D. M. Clark, ed. *Cognitive behaviour therapy for psychiatric problems: a practical guide*. New York: Oxford University Press.

Heimberg, R. G. and Juster, H. R. (1995). Cognitive-behavioral treatments: literature review. In: R. C. Heimberg, M. R. Liebowitz, D. A. Hope, and F. R. Schneier, ed. *Social phobia: diagnosis, assessment and treatment*. New York: Guilford Press.

Heimberg, R. G., *et al.* (1998). Cognitive behavioral group therapy vs. phenelzine therapy for social phobia: 12-week outcome. *Archives of General Psychiatry*, **55**, 1133–41.

Hiss, H., Foa, E. B., and Kozak, M. J. (1994). Relapse prevention program for treatment of obsessive-compulsive disorder. *Journal of Consulting and Clinical Psychology*, **62**, 801–8.

Hoffman, S. G. and Barlow, D. H. (2002). Social phobia (social anxiety disorder). In: D. H. Barlow, ed. *Anxiety and its disorders: the nature and treatment of anxiety and panic*. New York: Guilford Press.

Hogarty, G. E., Anderson, C. M., and Reiss, D. J. (1986). Family education, social skills training and maintenance chemotherapy in aftercare treatment of schizophrenia. *Archives of General Psychiatry*, **43**, 633–42.

Hollon, S. D. (2002). *Cognitive therapy versus antidepressant medications in the treatment of moderate to severe depression: prevention of relapse*. Paper presented at the meeting of the American Psychiatric Association, Philadelphia.

Hollon, S. D., *et al.* (1992). Cognitive therapy and pharmacotherapy for depression: singly and in combination. *Archives of General Psychiatry*, **49**, 774–81.

Ingram, R. E. and Siegle, G. J. (2001). Cognition and clinical science. In: K. S. Dobson, ed. *Handbook of cognitive-behavioral therapies*. New York: Guilford Press.

Jacobson, N. S., *et al.* (1996). A component analysis of cognitive-behavioral treatment for depression. *Journal of Consulting and Clinical Psychology*, **64**, 295–304.

Kadden, R. M. (2001). Behavioral and cognitive-behavioral treatments for alcoholism: Research opportunities. *Addictive Behaviors*, **26**, 489–507.

Keane, T. M. and Barlow, D. H. (2002). Posttraumatic stress disorder. In: D. H. Barlow, ed. *Anxiety and its disorders: the nature and treatment of panic and anxiety*. New York: Guilford Press.

Keller, M. B., *et al.* (2000). A comparison of nefazodone, the cognitive behavioral analysis system of psychotherapy, and their combination for the treatment of chronic depression. *New England Journal of Medicine*, **342**, 1462–70.

Kendall, P. C. and Kriss, M. R. (1983). Cognitive-behavioral interventions. In: C. E. Walker, ed. *The handbook of clinical psychology: theory, research and practice*, pp. 770–819. Homewood, IL: Dow Jones-Irwin.

Kingdon, D. G. and Turkington, D. (1994). *Cognitive-behavioral therapy of schizophrenia*. New York: Guilford Press.

Kirk, J. (1989). Cognitive-behavioral assessment. In: K. Hawton, P. M. Salkovskis, J. Kirk, and D. M. Clark, ed. *Cognitive behaviour therapy for psychiatric problems: a practical guide*. New York: Oxford University Press.

Kopelowicz, A., Liberman, R. P., and Zarate, R. (2002). Psychosocial treatments for schizophrenia. In: P. E. Nathan and J. M. Gorman, ed. *A guide to treatments that work*. New York: Oxford University Press.

Koerner, K. and Linehan, M. M. (2002). Dialectical behavior therapy for borderline personality disorder. In: S. G. Hofmann and M. C. Tompson, ed. *Treating chronic and severe mental disorders: a handbook of empirically supported interventions*. New York: Guilford Press.

Kuipers, L., *et al.* (1997). London-East Anglia randomized controlled trial of cognitive-behavior therapy for psychosis. I. Effects of the treatment phase. *British Journal of Psychiatry*, 171, 319–27.

Kuipers, L., *et al.* (1998). London-East Anglia randomized controlled trial of cognitive behavior therapy for psychosis. 3. Follow-up and economic evaluation at 18 months. *British Journal of Psychiatry*, 173, 61–8.

Lam, D. H., Jones, S., Bright, J., and Hayward, P. (1999). *Cognitive therapy for bipolar disorder: a therapists guide to concepts, methods and practice*. Chester, NY: John Wiley and Sons Inc.

Lam, D. H., *et al.* (2000). Cognitive therapy for bipolar illness—a pilot study of relapse prevention *Cognitive Therapy and Research*, 24, 503–20.

Lam, D. H., *et al.* (2003). A randomized controlled study of cognitive therapy for relapse prevention for biploral affective disorder. *Archives of General Psychiatry*, 60, 145–52.

Lewinsohn, P. M. (1974). A behavioral approach to depression. In: R. M. Friedman and M. M. Katz, ed. *The psychology of depression: contemporary theory and research*. New York: John Wiley and Sons Inc.

Lewinsohn, P. M. and Gotlib, I. H. (1995). Behavioral theory and treatment of depression. In: E. E. Becker and W. R. Leber, ed. *Handbook of depression*. New York, Guilford Press.

Lewis, S., *et al.* (2002). Randomised controlled trial of cognitive-behavioural therapy in early schizophrenia: acute-phase outcomes. *British Journal of Psychiatry*, 43, s91–7.

Linehan, M. M. (1993). *Cognitive-behavioral treatment of borderline personality disorder*. New York: Guilford Press.

Linehan, M. M., Hubert, A. E., Suarez, A., Douglas, A., and Heard, H. L. (1991). Cognitive-behavioral treatment of chronically parasuicidical borderline patients. *Archives of General Psychiatry*, 8, 279–92.

Lovell, K., Marks, I. M., Noshirvani, H., Thrasher, S., and Livanou, M. (2001). Do cognitive and exposure treatments improve various PTSD symptoms differently? A randomized controlled trial. *Behavioral and Cognitive Psychotherapy*, 29, 107–12.

Lykken, D. T. (1995). *The antisocial personalities*. Hillsdale, NJ: Erlbaum.

Mahoney, M. J. (1974). *Cognition and behavior modification*. Cambridge, MA: Ballinger.

Maltby, N., Kirsch, I., Mayers, M., and Allen, G. J. (2002). Virtual reality exposure therapy for the treatment of fear of flying: a controlled investigation. *Journal of Consulting and Clinical Psychology*, 70, 1112–18.

Marks, I., Lovell, K., Noshirvani, H., Livanou, M, and Thrasher, S. (1998). Treatment of postraumatic stress disorder by exposure and/or cognitive restructuring. *Archives of General Psychiatry*, 55, 317–25.

Marlatt, G. A. and Gordon, J. R. ed. (1985). *Relapse prevention: maintenance strategies in the treatment of addictive behaviors*. New York: Guilford Press.

Martindale, B. V., Mueser, K. T., Kuipers, E., Sensky, T., and Green, L. (2003). Psychological treatments for schizophrenia. In: S. R. Hirsch and D. Weinberger, ed. *Schizophrenia*. Malden, MA: Blackwell Publishing Co.

McCullough, J. P. (2000). *Treatment of chronic depression: cognitive behavioral analysis system of psychotherapy*. New York: Guilford Press.

McGorry, P. D., *et al.* (2002). Randomized controlled trial of interventions designed to reduce the risk of progression to first-episode psychosis in a clinical sample with subthreshold symptoms. *Archives of General Psychiatry*, 59, 921–8.

Meichenbaum, D. H. (1995). Cognitive-behavioral therapies in historical perspective. In: B. Bongar and L. E. Beutler, ed. *Comprehensive textbook of psychotherapy: theory and practice*. New York: Oxford University Press.

Morrison, A. P., *et al.* (2002). Randomised controlled trial of early detection and cognitive therapy for preventing transition to psychosis in high-risk individuals: study design and interim analysis of transition rate and psychological risk factors. *British Journal of Psychiatry*, 181 (Suppl. 43), s78–84.

Mueser, K. T. and Liberman, R. P. (1995). Behavior therapy in practice. In: B. Bongar and L. E. Beutler, ed. *Comprehensive textbook of psychotherapy: theory and practice*. New York: Oxford University Press.

Nathan, P. E. and Gorman, J. M. (2002). *A guide to treatments that work*. New York: Oxford University Press.

National Institute for Clinical Excellence (2002). *Clinical guideline 1—schizophrenia: Core interventions in the treatment and management of schizophrenia in primary and secondary care* (National Health Service Document N1076). Retrieved April 20, 2003, from http://www.nice.org.uk/pdf/CG1NICEguideline.pdf

Nelson, H. (1997). *Cognitive behavioral therapy with schizophrenia: a practice manual*. Cheltenham: Nelson Thornes Ltd.

Newman, J. P., Schmitt, W. A., and Voss, W. D. (1997). The impact of motivationally neutral cues on psychopathic individuals: assessing the generality of the response modulation hypothesis. *Journal of Abnormal Psychology*, 106, 563–75.

Overholser, J. C. (1993a). Elements of the Socratic method: I. Systematic questioning. *Psychotherapy*, 30, 67–74.

Overholser, J. C. (1993b). Elements of the Socratic method: II. Inductive reasoning. *Psychotherapy*, 30, 75–85.

Paul, G. L. and Lentz, R. J. (1977). *Psychosocial treatment of chronic mental patients: milieu versus social-learning programs*. Cambridge, MA: Harvard University Press.

Perry, A., Tarrier, N., Morriss, R., McCarthy, E., and Limb, K. (1999). Randomized controlled trial of efficacy of teaching patients with bipolar disorder to identify early symptoms of relapse and obtain treatment. *British Medical Journal*, 16, 149–53.

Pinto, A., La Pia, S., Mannella, R., Domenico, G., and DeSimone, L. (1999). Cognitive-behavioral therapy and clozapine for clients with treatment-refractory schizophrenia. *Psychiatric Services*, 50, 901–4.

Rothbaum, B. O., *et al.* (1999). Virtual reality exposure therapy for PTSD Vietnam veterans: a case study. *Journal of Traumatic Stress*, 12, 263–71.

Rector, N. A. and Beck, A. T. (2001). Cognitive behavioral therapy for schizophrenia: an empirical review. *Journal of Nervous and Mental Disease*, 189, 278–87.

Rector, N. A., Seeman, M. V., and Segal, Z. V. (2003). Cognitive therapy for schizophrenia: a preliminary randomized controlled trial. *Schizophrenia Research*, 63, 1–11.

Roemer, L. R., Orsillo, S. M., and Barlow, D. H. (2002). Generalized anxiety disorder. In: D. H. Barlow, ed. *Anxiety and its disorders: the nature and treatment of panic*. New York: Guilford Press.

Roth, A. and Fonagy, P. (1996). *What works for whom?: a critical review of psychotherapy research*. New York: Guilford Press.

Rush, A. J., Beck, A. T., Kovacs, J. M., and Hollon, S. D. (1977). Comparative efficacy of cognitive therapy and pharmacotherapy in the treatment of depressed outpatients. *Cognitive Therapy and Research*, 1, 17–37.

Scott, J. (2002). Cognitive therapy for clients with bipolar disorder. In: A. P. Morrison, ed. *A casebook of cognitive therapy for psychosis*. New York: Taylor and Francis.

Segal, Z. V., Williams, J. M. G., and Teasdale, J. D. (2002). *Mindfulness-based cognitive therapy for depression*. New York: Guilford Press.

Sensky, T., *et al.* (2000). A randomized controlled trial of cognitive-behavioral therapy for persistent symptoms in schizophrenia resistant to medication. *Archives of General Psychiatry*, 57, 165–73.

Serfaty, M. A., Turkington, D., Heap, M., Ledsham, L., and Jolley, E. (1999). Cognitive therapy versus dietary counseling in the outpatient treatment of anorexia nervosa: effects of the treatment phase. *European Eating Disorders Review*, 7, 334–50.

Simon, G. E. (2002). Treatment of somatoform and factitious disorders. In: P. E. Nathan and J. M. Gorman, ed. *A guide to treatments that work*. New York: Oxford University Press.

Skinner, B. F. (1953). *The science of human behavior*. Free Press, New York.

Steketee, G. and Barlow, D. H. (2002). Obsessive-compulsive disorder. In: D. H. Barlow, ed. *Anxiety and its disorders: the nature and treatment of anxiety and panic*. New York: Guilford Press.

Stirman, S. W., *et al.* (2003). Are samples in randomized controlled trials of psychotherapy representative of community outpatients? A new methodology and initial findings. *Journal of Consulting and Clinical Psychology*, **71**(6), 963–72.

Tarrier, N., *et al.* (1993). A trial of two cognitive-behavioral methods of treating drug-resistant residual psychotic symptoms in schizophrenic patients: I outcome. *British Journal of Psychiatry*, **162**, 524–32.

Tarrier, N., *et al.* (1998). Randomised controlled trial of intensive cognitive behavior therapy for patients with chronic schizophrenia. *British Medical Journal*, **317**, 303–7.

Tarrier, N., *et al.* (1999). Durability of the effects of cognitive-behavioral therapy in the treatment of chronic schizophrenia: 12-month follow-up. *British Journal of Psychiatry*, **174**, 500–4.

Tarrier, N., *et al.* (2000). Two-year follow-up of cognitive-behavioral therapy and supportive counseling in the treatment of persistent symptoms in chronic schizophrenia. *Journal of Consulting and Clinical Psychology*, **68**, 917–22.

Thrasher, S. M., Lovell, K., Noshirvani, H., and Livanou, M. (1996). Cognitive restructuring in the treatment of post-traumatic stress disorder: two single cases. *Clinical Psychology and Psychotherapy*, **3**, 137–48.

Van Oppen, P., *et al.* (1995). Cognitive therapy and exposure in vivo in the treatment of obsessive compulsive disorder. *Behavioral Research and Therapy*, **33**, 379–90.

Vitousek, K. (2002). Cognitive behaviour therapy in the treatment of anorexia nervosa. In: C. G. Fairburn and K. D. Brownell, ed. *Eating disorders and obesity: a comprehensive handbook*. New York: Guilford Press.

Wilson, G. T. and Fairburn, C. G. (2002). Treatments for eating disorders. In: P. E. Nathan and J. M. Gorman, ed. *A guide to treatments that work*. New York: Oxford University Press.

Wilson, G. T., Fairburn, C. G., and Agras, W. S. (1997). Cogntive-behavioral therapy for bulimia nervosa. In: D. M. Garner and P. Garfinkel, ed. *Handbook of treatment for eating disorders*. New York: Guilford Press.

Young, J. (1994). *Cognitive therapy for personality disorders: a schema-focused approach*. Sarasota, FL: Professional Resource Press.

Young, P. R., Grant, P., and DeRubeis, R. J. (2003). Some lessons from group supervision of cognitive therapy for depression. *Cognitive and Behavioral Practice*, **10**, 30–40.

3 Interpersonal psychotherapy

Carlos Blanco and Myrna M. Weissman

Introduction

Interpersonal psychotherapy (IPT) was initially developed by the late Gerald Klerman, MD, Myrna Weissman, PhD and colleagues as a time-limited therapy for major depression. Over the last few years, IPT has become increasingly popular among mental health professionals. There are a number of reasons that may partially account for this growing interest in IPT. First, it is easy to teach and to learn. Second, it has been successfully adapted to a number of disorders and to different age and ethnic groups. There is a growing body of literature documenting its efficacy not only in depression, but also in most (although not all) of the disorders for which it has been adapted. Finally, the recent emphasis on evidenced-based medicine has increased the interest in time-limited psychotherapies with proven efficacy.

The idea underlying IPT is simple: psychiatric disorders, although multi-determined in their causes, always take place in a social and interpersonal context: one of the patient's significant relationships is strained, the patient moves to a new location or social role, a loved one dies. The goal of IPT is to achieve symptomatic relief for mental disorders by addressing current interpersonal problems associated with the onset of the disorder. It does not seek to attribute interpersonal problems to personality characteristics or unconscious motivations. Rather, IPT works with the assumption that little can really be said about the patient's personality until the disorder is alleviated.

IPT is continuously evolving, as researchers and clinicians refine its techniques and adapt them to the needs of their patients. In this chapter we present some basic concepts of IPT (see Klerman *et al.*, 1984, for a detailed account of how to conduct IPT, and Weissman *et al.*, 2000, for a comprehensive review of the state of IPT and its adaptations), summarize the data on the efficacy for the disorders for which it has been adapted, describe some of the techniques used in this therapeutic modality and briefly describe some of the potential problems that may arise while conducting IPT.

Theoretical basis of therapy

Theoretical and empirical basis

IPT was initially developed for the treatment of major depressive disorder. While it has since been adapted for treatment of other psychiatric disorders, we are focusing the presentation of its theoretical and empirical basis on the case of depression, consistent with the ideas that led to its creation. However, most of those ideas are readily generalizable to other disorders. IPT is based on three related premises: (1) depression is a medical disorder; (2) depression does not occur in isolation, but in the context of interpersonal relationships and social factors; and (3) the treatment of depression has to be based on empirical data available from any relevant discipline, i.e., epidemiology, phenomenology, neurobiology, and results from clinical trials in diverse populations.

Although the creators of IPT were influenced by a variety of theoretical perspectives, the interpersonal school of thought, founded by Adolf Meyer and Harry Stack Sullivan, was probably the most influential as the theoretical basis for IPT. Meyer's psychobiological approach to understanding psychiatric disorders placed great emphasis on the patient's current psychosocial and interpersonal experiences, in contrast to a psychoanalytic focus on the intrapsychic and the past (Meyer, 1957). Sullivan, who linked clinical psychiatry to other disciplines such as anthropology and social psychology, viewed psychiatry as the scientific study of people and their relationships, rather than the study of the individual in isolation. In Sullivan's interpersonal approach, the unit of observation and therapeutic intervention is the primary social group, the immediate involvement of the patient with the patient's significant others (Sullivan, 1953). IPT's emphasis on interpersonal and social factors in the understanding and treatment of depression also draws on the work of many others clinicians, especially Cohen *et al.* (1954), Fromm-Reichmann (1960), Frank (1973), and Arieti and Bemporad (1978).

The interpersonal approach applied to understanding clinical depression considers three interrelated processes.

1. Symptoms, which are presumed to have biological and psychosocial precipitants.

2. Social and interpersonal relations, such as interaction in social roles with other persons derived from childhood experiences, social reinforcement and personal mastery and competence.

3. Personality problems, which include enduring traits such as low self-esteem or inhibited expression of anger and guilt. Personality patterns can predispose the person to episodes of depression.

IPT attempts to intervene in the first two processes, symptom function and social and interpersonal relations. It does not attempt to modify personality patterns directly. On the other hand, as symptoms lift, it is expected that patients will gain some control over those patterns. Furthermore, mood disorders may mimic personality disorder and resolution of the mood symptoms may result in improvement or resolution of the 'personality disorder'.

IPT intervenes with symptom formation, social adjustment, and interpersonal relations focusing on current problems at conscious and preconscious levels. Typically, those problems include disputes with significant others or relatives, frustrations, anxieties, and wishes as experienced in the interpersonal context. Although the IPT therapist may recognize unconscious factors, they are not directly addressed. The emphasis of IPT is to help the patient change, rather than to understand simply and accept their current unsatisfactory life situation. The influence of past experiences, particularly early childhood experiences, is recognized but the work focuses on the 'here and now', instead of focusing on an attempt to link the past with the present. This focus on the present is very much related to IPT's understanding of depression as a clinical disorder. Following the medical model, etiological factors are taken into account, but the emphasis is on treatment of the current symptoms and improvement of the psychosocial situation. The adoption of the medical model legitimizes the assumption of the 'sick role' on the part of the patient and helps explain the patient's symptoms and decrease the feelings of guilt that are characteristically experienced in depression.

IPT is based not on only on theory, but also on empirical research on the psychosocial aspects of depression. There is evidence to support each of the three key interpersonal problem areas: that people become depressed in the context of complicated bereavement (Maddison and Walker, 1967; Walker *et al.*, 1977), interpersonal disputes (Paykel *et al.*, 1969; Pearlin and Lieberman, 1977) and that interpersonal transitions in the context of life changes can lead to mood symptoms (Overholser and Adams, 1997), particularly in the absence of social supports. Social supports (having close relationships or feeling supported by someone) protect against depression (Brown *et al.*, 1977; Henderson, 1977; Prigerson *et al.*, 1993). Early life events such as the death of a parent (Brown and Harris, 1978) or poor parenting (Parker, 1979) can predispose to depression later in life, particularly when followed by later life stressors. The reverse is also true: once depressed, people have difficulty communicating effectively (Coyne, 1976; Merikangas *et al.*, 1979), as well as generally functioning in their social roles. All this can lead to strained relationships and adverse life events (Weissman *et al.*, 1974; Kendler *et al.*, 1999).

Characteristics of the therapy

The procedures of IPT share many characteristics with other psychotherapeutic approaches. This is not surprising, as most treatment approaches share the goals of helping patients gain a sense of mastery, decrease social isolation and improve satisfaction with their lives. However, IPT differs from other approaches in its overall strategies, some of the techniques used and the aspects it chooses to address (Markowitz *et al.*, 1998):

1. *IPT is time-limited, not long term.* There is substantial evidence that short-term psychotherapy can be efficacious in treating depression in a variety of patients with different demographic characteristics and cultural backgrounds. It is true that short-term therapy might not be efficacious in treating personality disorders. However, that is not the goal of IPT. Furthermore, long-term treatment has the potential for promoting dependence and reinforcing avoidant behavior. Time-limited therapies, on the other hand, are more likely to avoid those adverse effects.

2. *Focused, not open-ended.* Because it is time limited, IPT does not attempt to solve all the problems of the patient's life. Rather, it addresses one or two problem areas of the patient's current functioning. The therapist and the patient agree on the specific focus of the therapy after the initial evaluation sessions. An implicit expectation of IPT is that as patients gain mastery of the problem areas discussed in the sessions, they will be able to address other problems on their own in the future.

3. *Current, not past interpersonal relationships.* Past depressive episodes, significant relationships, friendship patterns, and life experiences are assessed in order to improve the understanding of the patient's world. However, the focus of the treatment is on the patient's symptoms in the present social context, not on the identification of recurrent relationship patterns and their links to childhood experiences.

4. *Interpersonal, not intrapsychic.* In exploring current interpersonal problems with the patient, the IPT therapist may recognize intrapsychic conflicts and mechanisms of defense used by the patient. However, the therapist does not attempt to provide interpretations. Instead, the patient's behavior is explored in terms of interpersonal relations.

5. *Interpersonal, not cognitive-behavioral.* Like cognitive-behavioral therapy (CBT), IPT attempts to change distorted thought patterns that the patient might have. However, unlike CBT, IPT does not attempt to uncover distorted thoughts systematically, nor does it attempt to help the patient to develop alternative thoughts. Rather, the therapist calls attention to those thoughts as they interfere with the interpersonal relationships of the patient. The goal is to change the relationship pattern rather than the associated depressive cognitions, which are recognized as symptoms of depression.

Role of the therapist

The therapist is active, not passive

Consistent with the technique of most time-limited psychotherapies, the IPT therapist is rather active during the sessions, particularly in the initial phase of the therapy. The therapist helps the patient connect feelings with interpersonal behaviors and alerts the patient when the session focuses exclusively on either of these two elements. The therapist also helps the patient discuss progress in the interpersonal problem area, identify potential barriers to improvement and discuss strategies to overcome those barriers. As the therapy progresses, the goal of the therapy becomes not only to solve the current interpersonal problem, but also to help patients learn to solve future problems and pursue their own goals. Thus, the therapist tends to be less active in the later phases of the therapy. For example, the therapist will generally not allow long silences during the session or free associations. If the patient does not talk about the problem area (e.g., role dispute), the therapist will actively ask the patient about episodes of disputes since the last session and help the patient relate the disputes (or their absence) to the mood of the patient.

The therapist is a patient advocate

In IPT the therapist is an explicit ally of the patient. The therapist is nonjudgmental, expresses warmth and positive regard for the patient and congratulates the patient as progress in the problem areas is made. Naturally, this does not imply that the therapist accepts all aspects of the patient, as that would preclude any stimulus for change. Rather, it implies that the therapist works with the patient and for the patient and believes that the patient's problems can be solved. The therapist always tries to have the patient find the solution for the problems discussed in the session. However, the therapist is not afraid to make suggestions or provide direct advice when they seem useful.

The therapeutic relationship is not interpreted as a manifestation of transference

This is a consequence of the medical model of depression adopted by IPT. As the therapist is not neutral but offers an alliance, the patients' expectations of understanding and help are accepted as realistic. Similarly, the relationship between patient and therapist is seen as realistic, and as such not seen as transferential. Naturally, this attitude does not imply that the therapist is not sensitive to the pattern of relationship of the patient, but this pattern is generally not interpreted. Feelings (positive or negative) towards the therapist are left untouched unless they interfere with the progress of the therapy. In that case, the feelings are discussed, as they would be in any other medical or even professional collaboration. However, the focus should remain on the task at hand, namely the resolution of the patient's disorder in the context of the patient's interpersonal relationships outside the therapy and not the exploration of the relationship between the patient and the therapist.

Treatment principles and phases of therapy

Although the number of sessions may vary for different patients (or in different research protocols), IPT is generally conducted in 12–20 sessions, grouped in three phases: evaluation, intermediate, and termination.

The initial phase

The initial sessions, generally three or four, constitute the evaluation phase. They are devoted to defining the disorder in its interpersonal context and the formulation of the interpersonal problem areas. During the initial phase the therapist should accomplish four goals: (1) diagnose the disorder; (2) complete an interpersonal inventory and relate the disorder to the interpersonal context; (3) identify the major interpersonal problem areas; and (4) explain the IPT approach and make a treatment contract that includes the structure and length of the treatment.

During these sessions the patient describes the symptoms and interpersonal situation that led to treatment seeking. The therapist also evaluates the patient's current and past interpersonal relationships, looking for patterns relevant to current relationships. Examining the interactions of these relationships may elucidate the patient's current behavior, expectations, and obstacles to change in the patient's relationship.

In the final phase of the evaluation, the therapist gives the depression a name and provides the patient with the sick role—alleviating the responsibility and sense of guilt for being depressed. The interpersonal problem is then formulated into one of four categories in relation to the onset of symptoms: (1) grief (e.g., death of a loved one); (2) role transition (e.g., marriage, graduation, loss of status); (3) role dispute; and (4) interpersonal deficits (additional problem areas have been suggested for particular age groups or disorders other than depression, see below). If the patient accepts the formulation, an explicit contract is then made with the patient to work on that problem area, with the expectation that improvement in that area will lead to improvement in the depression.

A common difficulty, even for experienced therapists who are treating their first cases with IPT, is to select the focus of treatment. Patients often come with multiple problems, all of which may influence their mood. In those situations it is tempting to suggest that a time-limited treatment is not advisable, or even possible. IPT proposes that it is possible to treat the depression by narrowing the focus to one or two problems. Our experience suggests that patients generally manage the other problems better once their mood improves. Similarly, many 'personality traits' substantially improve or disappear as the depression lifts.

Intermediate sessions: goals and strategies to work on the problems areas

The intermediate phase starts immediately after the treatment contract is set and lasts until the beginning of the termination phase, which typically comprises the last two to three sessions. It is during the intermediate phase that the majority of the therapeutic work is done on the selected interpersonal problem area. During this phase, the problem areas, which were defined in the initial phase, are highlighted and therapist and patient collaborate to find potential solutions for the interpersonal problems. These may require a change in the expectations of the patient or attempts at asserting the patient's wishes in an acceptable way for all the parties involved in the interpersonal situation. There is a continuous emphasis on the connection between the symptoms of the disorder and the interpersonal context.

In our experience, most therapists are skilled at helping the patient establish the connection between the symptoms and the interpersonal context of the patient in the initial phase of therapy. In contrast, when the patient improves therapists appear to forget to point out this connection to the patient. However, it is important to continue to remind the patient of this link. This helps the patient not only understand but also experience the rationale for the therapy. A reminder of the link also rewards patient progress in the problem area, increases patient sensitivity to changes in his or her mood and interpersonal relationships and teaches the patient how to monitor that link to prevent future episodes of the disorder.

Depending on the problem area, the goals and strategies of the intermediate phase may vary:

Grief

From the point of view of IPT, the term grief is reserved for the loss of a loved one. Other losses, such as loss of a job, or the break up of a relationship are categorized as 'role transitions' (see below). Appropriate goals for grief include facilitation of the mourning process and helping the patient reestablish interests and relationships that could substitute for the lost one. The main strategy in the treatment of cases of grief is the reconstruction of the patient's relationship with the deceased, with a particular focus on the events surrounding the death. In those cases, patients have frequently expressed positive feelings about the loved one to their relatives and friends. However, more often than not they have felt guilty about discussing their negative feelings towards the deceased, or feelings of guilt regarding interactions they had soon before the death. As patients discuss those feelings, it becomes easier for them to consider possible ways of becoming involved with others.

Role (or interpersonal) disputes

The goals of treatment in role disputes are: (1) to help identify the dispute, and (2) to make choices about how to address the dispute. The direct approach to the role dispute relies on careful tracking of the sequence of interactions. In this way the patient can make changes in his or her own behavior and expectations that may lead to decreased conflict. Alternatively, after careful consideration the patient may decide that it is preferable to terminate that relationship, in which case part of the therapy will be devoted to assisting the patient in readjusting his or her life after such termination.

Role transition

Issues that are characteristic of role transitions include the mourning of the old role and the restoration of self-esteem by developing a sense of mastery regarding the demands of the new role. As in the previous categories, expression of affect and relating positive and negative feelings to the depressive symptoms are key strategies. Realistic evaluation of what has been lost and what are the opportunities offered by the new role and encouragement for the development of the social support system and new skills necessary to perform the new role are also important in these cases.

Interpersonal deficit

IPT therapists have often used this category when the depressive symptoms could not be easily included under one of the three previous categories. However, some of the new adaptations of IPT for other disorders such as dysthymia and social phobia (or social anxiety disorder) appear to overlap with this category. Patients with interpersonal deficits are encouraged to decrease their social isolation and form new relationships. Exploration of past significant relationships are useful, but, consistent with the focus of IPT on the here and now, it is important to organize work mainly around current relationships or opportunities for new relationships.

Termination

The last two to four sessions constitute the termination phase. The tasks of the termination phase are: (1) explicit discussion of the end of treatment; (2) acknowledgement that the end of treatment is a time of potential grieving and anxiety; and (3) discussion with the patient regarding his or her independent competence. As the goal of IPT is to help the patient cope well without therapy, termination provides an opportunity to internalize strategies.

A certain amount of activity on the part of the therapist is needed here both in terms of helping the patient move from the intermediate to the termination phase and, related to that, helping the patient accept the time-limited nature of the treatment. Although it is openly acknowledged that termination is a time of grieving, the focus of the termination sessions is not the discussion of the feelings towards the therapist. The majority of the work is devoted towards reviewing the gains achieved in the therapy, helping the patient plan how to address other problems that might not have been discussed in the therapy, and helping the patient apply newly learned strategies to possible future situations to minimize the risk of relapse. At the same time, the patient is informed that should a new episode occur, the door is always open to return to therapy, very much the same way that a patient with a new episode of pneumonia would return for a new course of antibiotics.

Treatment techniques and common problems in interpersonal psychotherapy

Most of the techniques used in IPT are common to other psychotherapies, particularly psychodynamic and cognitive therapies. We list them here in order of increasing intrusiveness on the part of the therapist. However, it should be clear that each patient needs a different combination of techniques and that often any of several techniques could be appropriate at particular times of the therapy:

1. Exploratory techniques are geared towards gathering systematic information about the patient's symptoms and presenting problems.

In general, the therapist starts with open-ended questions to allow for nondirective exploration. The therapist may start asking a very general question such as 'where should we start today?' or, in a case of role dispute, say something like 'tell me about your husband'. More direct questioning includes obtaining the interpersonal inventory of the patient, a detailed exploration of the patient's important relationships with significant others.

2. Encouragement of affect encompasses a series of techniques that allow the patient to verbalize painful affects about events or issues that cannot be changed, help the development and constructive expression of new or unacknowledged affects and use the newly gained access to emotional experiences to facilitate growth and change. In a case of grief, the therapist may ask the patient to talk about aspects of the relationship with the dead person that were unpleasant, and how the patient felt on those occasions. The therapist may make supportive remarks such as 'Of course most people would feel angry in that situation', which may allow the patient discuss negative feelings towards the deceased. In a case of role transition, the therapist may encourage the patient to talk about the anxiety generated by the new situation or the demoralization that may follow the failure to meet the demands and expectations of the new role.

3. Clarification is used to make the patient more aware of what has actually been communicated as well as to facilitate the discussion of previously suppressed material. Strategies frequently used for clarification include asking patients to rephrase what they have said, calling attention to the logical extension of a statement by the patient or pointing out the contradiction between statements made by the patient. In a case of role dispute, the patient may say 'I felt there was no point in talking to her any more'. The therapist may then ask 'Did you feel hopeless?' or 'Did you feel angry?', depending on the affect that the therapist suspects predominated in that interaction.

4. Communication analysis is used to examine and identify communication failures in order to help the patient learn to communicate more efficiently and effectively. Communication analysis is most effectively done through a detailed account of important interactions of the patient with a significant other, down to the specific statements made in the interaction. In a case of role dispute with her husband, the patient may feel that she has clearly conveyed why she is angry. Detailed discussion with the therapist may reveal that the reasons for that anger may not have been communicated so clearly, limiting the ability of the husband to cooperate towards a solution. In a case of role transition, the patient may fear criticism from others and be afraid to ask if what was perceived as a criticism was indeed intended as that. Here again, discussion with the therapist may help provide a more realistic view of the interaction.

5. Behavior change techniques are often used in conjunction with communication analysis and their goal is to help the patient consider a wide range of alternative options, and a systematic way of making decisions. Role-playing and modeling can be used to facilitate internalization of these techniques by the patient. In a case of skills deficit, a patient who wants to ask out for lunch a coworker may role-play different possible scenarios with the therapist, and plan how to react to the possible outcomes. An adolescent negotiating a new relationship with her parents may role-play how to ask for more autonomy with assertiveness but without being disrespectful.

6. Use of the therapeutic relationship. In IPT, the patient–therapist relationship is not the primary focus of treatment. Therefore, the use of this technique should be generally limited to instances where the therapist can provide feedback about interpersonal style and behaviors observed in the session and its relation to other interpersonal relationships. In this way, the patient–therapist relationship can be another experimental setting in which to practice new interpersonal skills. In a case of skills deficit, the therapist may encourage the patient to voice any dissatisfaction with the treatment. In a case of role dispute, disagreements between

the patient and the therapist can be used to model how to negotiate divergent point of views without damaging the relationship.

Problems in the treatment with interpersonal psychotherapy

As with any treatment, there are an almost infinite number of problems that can present at different phases of the therapy. We present some common examples here in order to illustrate how an IPT therapist would typically address them, although as always, each case has its own nuances.

The patient substitutes the psychotherapist for friend or family

Patients with poor social support may be tempted to use the therapist as a substitute for these resources. This situation may be chronic or may arise as a result of tendency of patients (especially those with depression) to underestimate their own capabilities to establish interpersonal relationships. To allow the therapeutic relationship to be viewed as a substitute for friends or family is a disservice to the patient. First, because the structure and expectations of friendship is very different than those of therapeutic relationships, topics are likely to be discussed in the sessions that will distract from the focus of the therapy. Equally important, the therapeutic relationship may interfere with the patient's attempts at improving the interpersonal relationships outside the treatment. Finally, it would raise important technical problems for termination, as by design IPT is time limited, while friendships are generally expected to last.

Confronted with this type of problem, the therapist should praise the patient for demonstrating the ability to engage in a close relationship. However, the therapist should also point out how this situation would in reality interfere with the achievement of the patient's goals in the therapy.

The patient misses appointments or is late

In most other therapies, this would be considered a problem in the therapy and probably become a focus of the treatment until it was resolved. In IPT it may be considered a problem related to the disorder itself. The initial approach is to make sure that trivial misunderstandings are clarified or that realistic problems are not responsible, such as difficulty to obtain childcare during the session time. The patient can also be reminded that missed sessions or lateness means less time to work on problems. This uses the pressure of the time limit to motivate the patient and move the therapy forward.

It is also possible that lateness or missed appointments are due to other reasons. The therapist should then try to treat the behavior as an indirect and inefficient communication whether or not the patient is aware of the potentially irritating effects of such behavior. The therapist should ask the patient directly what is getting in the way of arriving on time and, once the reason for lateness is stated, offer to work with the patient to solve that problem. Whenever possible, it is important to point out that the depression may be responsible or at least compound these maladaptive interpersonal behaviors. At the same time, the therapist should try to help the patient discover alternative, more direct methods to get the point across.

The patient is silent or avoids subjects

Some silence occurs in any treatment and in general does not require any intervention. Because the style of the sessions is generally conversational and the therapist is active, silence is rarely a problem. At times it might even be welcome as an expression of the internal work of the patient. If silences become frequent or prolonged, the therapist should assume that the patient is either avoiding recognition of conflicted thoughts or feelings about an issue or would like to bring up something but is concerned about the therapist's reaction.

After reassuring the patient that anything can be discussed during the session, the therapist may begin by asking silent patients what is on their minds or whether there is something they are refraining from discussing. This inquiry usually leads to the discovery of irrational interpersonal fears connected with revealing thoughts and feelings to others. The patient may be afraid of saying something shameful or describing feelings or interactions that may be disapproved by the therapist. In general those concerns should be addressed. However, due to the time limit, it is also important to decide how much time should be reserved for discussion of those topics, as they may distract from the main focus of the therapy.

The patient complains or is uncooperative

As a result of their hopelessness, patients often believe that nothing can help them and that their depression will go on forever. Those feelings may make the patients uncooperative or complain about trivial issues. It is important to instill hope in the patients that the prognosis is good and explain that research suggest that the vast majority of patients improve with treatment. At the same time patients should be made aware of the effects of their behavior on their interpersonal relationships and be provided with alternative ways of handling displeasure. The patients may be encouraged to discuss with others ways of changing the situation or to try to change the relationship that is displeasing them.

In rare cases, patients may completely refuse to discuss the focus of the therapy or decline to participate in the solution of their problems. In those cases, the therapist needs to address the issues directly before the therapy can continue. If the patient refuses to discuss the focus of the therapy, the patient and the therapist need to reconsider whether the selected problem area is the correct one or whether other issues such as hopelessness or shame prevent the patient from discussing the topic. If the patient declines to participate in the solution of the problems, the patient can be asked whether continuing with the current situation (including depression or any other disorder being treated) is a more acceptable alternative, and the impact of that option on the patient's interpersonal relationships.

When the significant other is asked to participate

Although IPT is conceived as an individual treatment (except in the group adaptations discussed below), the patient and the therapist may choose to include significant others in some therapy sessions either to provide information or to obtain information from the relative. In general it is useful to realize that the significant other may feel guilty about the patient's condition and the therapist should initially suspend judgment about the significant others' role in the situation. Naturally, this attitude needs to be balanced with a careful exploration of whether some family members may in fact be contributing the patient's distress. If this is the case, the role of the family member in the patient's difficulty should be acknowledged.

The patient seeks additional, alternative treatment

Exploring alternatives and options in treatment are important themes in IPT. The therapist should maintain an open, nonjudgmental attitude about these activities and they should be discussed in the therapy sessions. It is important to clarify the reasons for the additional treatment and the phase in the therapy where they take place. Additional treatments that are agreed upon during the evaluation phase (e.g., treatment with medication) or that are aimed at addressing very different problems (e.g., smoking cessation) are of less concern. However, treatments that are started during the intermediate or termination phase should immediately alert the therapist to potential dissatisfactions of the patient with the therapy. In those cases, the therapist should help the patient explore the reasons for the need of additional treatment: are there any symptoms left? Is there a lack of hope that the therapy will be able to treat the depression? Does the patient lack the confidence of being able to function autonomously, in the absence of a therapist?

The patient wishes to terminate early

In many cases, early termination cannot be prevented because the assumption of psychotherapy that talking things out should precede action runs counter to the coping styles of many individuals. Patients who express a wish to terminate prematurely should first be asked if they are satisfied with the results of the treatment. This is seldom the case, but provides the patient with an opportunity to express what has been accomplished and what remains for possible future work. In fact, from the interpersonal point of view the wish to terminate treatment can be understood as a role dispute

with the therapist and the patient holding different views of how to resolve it. This view should be made explicit to the patient and attempt to engage the patient in that discussion.

As any dispute, there should be no a priori assumption that one of the parties is right while the other is wrong. Rather, an attempt should be made to clarify the source of the discrepancies and, if possible, to find a solution that is mutually satisfactory. The therapist may ask when the patient started to think about premature termination and what events and interactions led the patient to consider that possibility. This discussion may lead to clarification of the different expectations of the patient and the therapist regarding treatment. It may also expose inefficient modes of communication between patient and therapist. At the end of this discussion there can be an agreement that no further work remains to be done at that time, or the patient may be referred to another psychotherapist or to another form of treatment. If the patient is determined to terminate prematurely, the therapist should communicate, as strongly as possible, that return to therapy is open and would not imply defeat or humiliation.

The patient wants to continue treatment at the end of the therapy

Continuation of treatment is generally discouraged. IPT is time-limited therapy and part of its therapeutic strength may stem from the fact that, by design, it does not allow for unlimited discussion of issues but rather encourages the patient to try to change the situation. On occasion, a change in the circumstances of the patient during the therapy may justify a brief extension of the therapy (Blanco et al., 2001). Another possible exception is when IPT is used for maintenance, where a short-time treatment period would not be sufficient. It is also possible that after finishing IPT, the patient and the therapist agree that other type of treatment are indicated. However, in our experience that is rare. Finally, as previously mentioned, the patient should be reminded that should a relapse of the disorder happen, the patient should seek treatment again, as would be expected in any other medical condition.

Efficacy data

Interpersonal psychotherapy for mood disorders

IPT was initially developed for the acute treatment of major depressive disorder. Similarly to what happens with other medical treatments, over time clinicians and researchers have tried to extend the applicability of IPT for other disorders and for a variety of populations. In this section we present a brief overview of the efficacy data of IPT.

IPT for major depression

The first test of efficacy of IPT as an acute antidepressant treatment was a four-cell, 16-week randomized trial of IPT, amitriptyline (100–200 mg/day), their combination and a nonscheduled control treatment for 81 outpatients with major depression (DiMascio et al., 1979; Weissman et al., 1979). Patients assigned to the control group did not have regular treatment sessions, but could telephone to arrange a session if they experienced sufficient distress. Analyses of the results found all active treatments to be superior to the control condition and the combined treatment to be superior to either active monotherapy. There were no significant differences in efficacy between IPT and amitriptyline, although the therapeutic effects of amitriptyline appeared earlier. On the other hand, IPT and amitriptyline seemed to work preferentially on different symptom clusters: medication appeared to be more effective on the neurovegetative symptoms of depression, while IPT worked mainly on mood, interest, apathy, work, and suicidal ideation (DiMascio et al., 1979).

The efficacy of IPT as an acute treatment for depression was confirmed in the National Institute of Mental Health Treatment of Depression Collaborative Research Program (TDCRP). This study randomly assigned 250 depressed outpatients to 16 weeks of imipramine, IPT, CBT, or placebo. IPT had the lowest attrition rate among the treatments. Because all treatments worked equally well for mildly depressed patients, no overall difference was found among treatments. However, with only severely depressed patients, differences did appear. IPT was similar to imipramine and was superior to placebo. CBT produced an intermediate level of response and was not superior to placebo. A reanalysis of the TDCRP indicated that medication was superior to the psychotherapies, while the psychotherapies were superior to placebo, particularly among the most severe patients (Klein and Ross, 1993).

Follow-up of both the Boston-New Haven and the TDCRP patients suggested that 16 weeks of treatment could induce remission of the acute episode but did not protect against relapse. Based on those results, Frank *et al.* (1989, 1990) compared pharmacotherapy and IPT as prophylaxis for 128 adult outpatients at high risk of relapse. In this study IPT for maintenance (IPT-M) was administered monthly, in contrast with the weekly schedule generally used in the acute treatment. IPT was adapted to focus on the prevention of relapse. The focus of IPT-M was to watch for signs and symptoms of emergent episodes and to develop interpersonal strategies to prevent future episodes. Because the goal of IPT-M was to prevent relapse, it was administered over 3 years as opposed to the usual 12–20 weeks of acute IPT. Owing the longer time frame, therapists and patients were allowed to shift among the four IPT problem areas. The results of the study showed that IPT serves to lengthen the time between episodes in patients not receiving antidepressants. The Frank *et al.* (1989) study is particularly important because it included subjects with multiple episodes of depression and at high risk of relapse, as the placebo cell demonstrated. Reynolds and colleagues (1999) conducted a study with a similar design in 187 geriatric patients, using nortriptyline instead of imipramine. The results of this study showed that all monotherapies were superior to placebo and that combined treatment was superior to IPT-M alone.

Interpersonal psychotherapy in special populations

The rationale for modifying IPT for depressed adolescents (IPT-A) is based on the high prevalence and initial onset of depressive disorders in this population, the recognition of the morbidity and precipitating stressors of depression in adolescents and on the limited data regarding the efficacy of pharmacotherapy in young individuals. Mufson *et al.* (1999) adapted IPT for adolescents with nonpsychotic depression without comorbid substance abuse disorders or conduct disorder. Modifications for adolescents include (1) telephone contact, particularly during the first month, to support engagement in the therapeutic process, and (2) development of an alliance of the therapist with the parents and the school system. This alliance can help the therapist gather information on the patient's behavior and academic performance and to monitor progress. At the same time, the therapist may act as an advocate for the patient, educating parents and teachers on the effects of depression on school performance. To date, there have been two controlled trials of IPT in adolescents (Roselló and Bernal, 1999; Mufson *et al.*, 1999), both of them showing the superiority of IPT-A over controlled waiting-list.

There are also three published trials of IPT in patients with late-life depression. The first two, relatively small studies (Rothblum *et al.*, 1982; Sloane *et al.*, 1985) used the standard IPT approach based on the original manual (Klerman *et al.*, 1984). The latest, a large trial that included a discontinuation treatment design, used a manual developed for maintenance IPT for late-life depression, IPT-LLM (discussed below). The study by Rothblum did not include an IPT-alone cell and, although it suggested that IPT was well tolerated, it could not test its efficacy as a stand-alone treatment. In contrast, the study by Sloane failed to find differences between patients treated with IPT, nortriptyline, and pill-placebo over a treatment period of 6 weeks. In the study by Reynolds all patients received IPT plus nortriptyline in the acute phase, precluding an assessment of IPT as treatment of acute depression in the elderly.

IPT has also been adapted for use with HIV-positive patients and with pregnant and postpartum women. The rationale in both cases is based on the substantial changes that accompany those conditions (although those changes are much less pronounced now for the HIV group than they were

when the therapy was adapted in the late eighties), and the convenience of minimizing the number of medications taken by those individuals. A controlled trial of IPT for HIV-positive individuals, modeled after the TDRCP, indicated that IPT and imipramine plus supportive therapy were both superior to CBT, with supportive therapy a distant but not statistically different third (Markowitz *et al.*, 1999). Regarding postpartum women, O'Hara *et al.* (2000) compared IPT with a waiting-list control group in 120 women with postpartum depression treated for 12 weeks. A significantly greater proportion of women who received IPT recovered from their depressive episode based on Hamilton Depression Rating Scale (HRSD) scores of 6 or lower (37. 5%) and BDI scores of 9 or lower (43.8%) compared with women in the waiting-list group (13.7% and 13.7%, respectively). Women receiving IPT also had significant improvement on the Postpartum Adjustment Questionnaire and the Social Adjustment Scale-Self-Report relative to women in the waiting-list group. In another study (Spinelli and Endicott, 2003) randomized 50 outpatient antepartum women who met DSM-IV criteria for major depressive disorder to IPT or a didactic parenting education program for 16 weeks bilingual. The IPT group showed significant improvement compared with the parenting education control program at termination on the Edinburgh Postnatal Depression Scale, the Beck Depression Inventory, and the Hamilton Depression Rating Scale.

Most recently, Bolton *et al.* (2003) compared group IPT versus usual care for major depressive disorder in rural Uganda. The authors selected 30 villages in two districts of rural Uganda using a random procedure; 15 were then randomly assigned for studying men and 15 for women. In each village, adult men or women believed by themselves and other villagers to have depression-like illness were interviewed using a locally adapted Hopkins Symptom Checklist (SCL-90) and an instrument assessing function. Eight of the 15 male villages and seven of the 15 female villages were randomly assigned to the intervention arm and the remainder to the control arm. The intervention villages received group IPT for depression as weekly 90-minute sessions for 16 weeks, whereas individuals in the other villages received usual care. The authors found a mean reduction in depression severity was 17.47 points in the modified SLC-90 depression score for intervention groups and 3.55 points for controls, a highly significant result.

Interpersonal psychotherapy for other mood disorders

Following the success of IPT in the treatment of major depression, researchers have tested the efficacy of IPT in other mood disorders, namely, dysthymia and bipolar disorder. The motivation to study dysthymia was the general paucity of treatment research in this area and the relatively low (less than 50%) response rate of this disorder to medication treatment. The potential interest in IPT as a treatment for bipolar disorder stems from the manicogenic effects of antidepressant medication.

Although the IPT format for dysthymia (IPT-D) is very similar to the format for major depression, there are some important differences. For instance, IPT-D is usually conducted in 16 weeks, but is not unusual to continue to see the patient monthly for maintenance sessions, a practice that is much less frequent in the treatment of major depression. The problem areas are also often different, with interpersonal deficits being more common in individuals with dysthymia than in patients with major depressive disorder. Consistent with this fact, in most treatments of major depression an acute change in the pattern of the patient's interpersonal relationships can readily be identified. In contrast, the pattern of relationships of the dysthymic patient are generally chronic. As a result, the focus of the therapy is frequently formulated as a 'role transition to health'.

Following promising results from pilot studies at Cornell University Medical College, two large randomized studies are nearing completion. In one of them, Browne *et al.* (2002) at McMaster University in Hamilton, Ontario, randomized 700 overtly dysthymic patients to 12 sessions of IPT, sertraline, or a combination of both over 4 months. Defining response as 40% decrease in the score of the Montgomery-Asberg Depression Rating Scales (MADRS), preliminary results of this study indicate that at 1-year follow-up, 51% of IPT alone subjects responded, compared with 63% in the sertraline and 62% in the combined group. A second study, in Toronto,

Canada, is comparing IPT with the short-term psychodynamic psychotherapy of Luborsky (1984) in the treatment of 72 patients with dysthymia or double depression. Results are not available to date.

Frank *et al.* (2000) have modified IPT for bipolar disorder. This adaptation, called interpersonal and social rhythm therapy (IPSRT) retains the focus on psychosocial factors and the four problem areas characteristic of the original IPT. Moreover, a new component has been added to manage symptoms by regulating social rhythms. The rationale for this new component is that disruption of social rhythms can induce disruptions of biological rhythms, which in turn can trigger the onset of a bipolar episode. Techniques, such as self-monitoring, guided task assignments, and cognitive restructuring, are utilized to regulate the patient's life-style and stabilize social rhythms.

To date, there has been only one study (Frank *et al.*, 1997) of IPSRT as adjunctive treatment to conventional medication clinical treatment of bipolar disorder. Preliminary analysis of this study failed to find differences between the two treatment groups, i.e., in the sample treated to date there was no advantage in treatment outcome for the IPSRT sample. However, the authors found that the IPSRT group showed significantly greater stability in daily routines as treatment proceeded, possibly providing some additional protection against future episodes.

One area that has not been systematically studied to date is the treatment of mood disorders with associated comorbidity, a common presentation in patients seeking treatment. There are three possible reasons for this lack of information. First, although the efficacy of IPT for major depressive disorder has well established, its adaptation for the treatment of other disorders, which should precede its use in comorbid cases, is more recent. Second, from the technical point of view, the focus of IPT in one or two problem areas would, in most cases, force the patient and the therapist select one of the disorders as the focus of treatment, and expect that the comorbid disorder would improve as the result of progress made in the problem area of the main disorder. Third, the emphasis on effectiveness studies is relatively recent. As interest in this type of studies continue, it is likely that IPT researchers will move to include patients with comorbid disorders, who are often excluded from efficacy studies.

Another area where systematic data are lacking is the use of IPT for patients who have failed other treatments for depression. Because IPT tends to be more efficacious in moderate than in severe depression, it will probably not be the treatment of choice in most of those cases as monotherapy. However, studies of a combination of medication plus IPT may help provide empirical evidence for the efficacy of an alternative approach for treatment-resistant cases.

Adaptations of interpersonal psychotherapy for nonmood disorders and innovative formats

Because not only depression, but all psychiatric disorders occur in the context of interpersonal relationships, it is natural to think that IPT may be efficacious in nonmood disorders. Anxiety disorders are generally considered nosologically close to mood disorders and several researchers are currently investigating the efficacy of IPT to treat social phobia (also known as social anxiety disorder), posttraumatic stress disorder (PTSD), and panic disorder.

Both individual and group IPT for social phobia are being developed and tested. One particularity of IPT for social phobia (IPT-SP) is that the disorder itself subsumes some aspect of role dysfunction. Because social phobia often has an early onset and a chronic course, the approach of IPT-SP is in many ways similar to that of IPT-D. Lipsitz *et al.* (1999) have added an additional category of 'role insecurity' to the classical four problem areas. This category captures difficulties that are generally milder than those defined by interpersonal deficit. Role insecurity encompasses common symptoms of social phobia such as lack of assertiveness, avoidance of conflict and rejection sensitivity (called 'interpersonal sensitivity' by Stuart and O'Hara). Weissman and Jacobson have adapted IPT in a group format for patients with social phobia, using a 10-session time-limited group. Consistent with the work of Lipsitz, the focus of the treatment is on a therapeutic role

transition to a less impaired state. An open trial by Lipsitz *et al.* (1999) has provided preliminary positive results for IPT-SP and controlled trials are currently under way.

Like social phobia, PTSD is defined by a connection between symptoms and life situation, although in the case of PTSD, by definition, the triggering life events are clearly identified. Krupnick at Georgetown University recently completed a comparison between IPT-PTSD and a waiting-list control group in low-income women attending gynecology clinics (personal communication). IPT was superior to the waiting-list control at the end of the treatment on several measures. A smaller trial, but with a more diverse population in terms of age, ethnicity, and gender distribution, using individual format also showed the superiority of IPT over supportive psychotherapy in measures of PTSD, depression and social functioning (Markowitz, personal communication). Several groups, both in the US and abroad, are currently adapting IPT for panic disorder. However, no manuals or efficacy data have been published to date.

IPT has also been adapted for bulimia nervosa. Although the basic principles of IPT remain unchanged in this adaptation, the four interpersonal problem areas associated with depression may not be as relevant for eating disorders. The maintenance of those areas or the creation of new ones better suited for the treatment of bulimia nervosa requires further exploration. In contrast with IPT for depression, where talk about depression is encouraged, in IPT for bulimia the focus is on the interpersonal relationships and discussion of eating patterns is expressly forbidden in the therapy sessions. Two randomized trials, one using an individual format (Fairburn *et al.*, 1993) and the other a group format (Wilfley *et al.*, 2002) have shown that IPT and CBT have similar efficacy in the treatment of bulimia nervosa. Preliminary results from a multicenter study using an individual format suggests that CBT may be superior to IPT at the end of the acute treatment, but similar at 1-year follow-up.

Currently, other applications of IPT are being studied. These include use of IPT for the treatment of body dysmorphic disorder, somatization disorder, depression following myocardial infarction and in patients with physical disabilities, primary insomnia, and borderline personality disorder. There has also been an increased interest in adapting IPT for administration in other formats. Among these the most popular has been the adaptation to group format for a variety of disorders. Administration of IPT over the phone (Miller and Weissman, 2002) has also become increasingly interesting due to the difficulties of certain patient groups in attending regular therapy sessions (e.g., low income women with young children). IPT is also being adapted to be more consonant with other cultures (Roselló and Bernal, 1999).

Finally, it is important to realize that IPT is not efficacious for all disorders. First, many of the applications described in this section have very limited data on efficacy and still require confirmation by other groups. Second, there have been two negative trials of IPT for the treatment of substance abuse disorders suggesting that certain conditions might require a different treatment approach (Rounsaville *et al.*, 1983; Carroll *et al.*, 1991). Third, it is possible that, similar to the case of clinical trials with medication, some negative studies with IPT may have not been published. If publication bias exists in IPT, this bias may overstate the efficacy of IPT for the treatment of psychiatric disorders. Meta-analytic techniques might be able to assess the existence of such bias, and assess whether IPT has similar efficacy for different disorders or appears to be more efficacious in selected disorders.

Conclusions

Over the last two decades the interest of clinicians and researchers in IPT has grown exponentially and its applications have multiplied. IPT is now a well-established treatment for major depression and it is likely to continue to grow as an alternative to medication and to other psychotherapies. There is growing evidence that IPT can be successfully adapted for other psychiatric disorders and for individuals with very different cultural backgrounds. The International Society for Interpersonal Psychotherapy (ISIPT) has been formed whose mission is to provide information on the application of IPT for a range of mental health disorders and to publicize recent research and clinical findings related to IPT (http://www.interpersonalpsychotherapy.org). Initially the homogeneity of treatment delivery was assured due to the relatively small number of practitioners and applications. A major challenge for IPT will now be to conserve its essence as it is practiced by an increasing number of clinicians, for an increased number of disorders and adapted to an increasing number of cultures.

References

Arieti, S. and Bemporad, J. (1978). *Severe and mild depression*. New York: Basic Books.

Blanco, C., Lipsitz, J., and Caligor, E. (2001). Treatment of chronic depression with a 12-week program of interpersonal psychotherapy. *Americal Journal of Psychiatry*, **158**, 371–5.

Bolton, P., *et al.* (2003). Group Interpersonal Psychotherapy for Depression in Rural Uganda: a randomized controlled trial. *Journal of the American Medical Association*, **289**, 3117–24.

Brown, G. W. and Harris, T. (1978). *Social origins of depression: a study of psychiatric disorder in women*. New York: Free Press.

Brown, G., Harris, T., and Copeland, J. R. (1977). Depression and loss. *British Journal of Psychiatry*, **30**, 1–18.

Browne, E., *et al.* (2002). Sertraline and/or interpersonal psychotherapy for patients with dysthymic disorder in primary care: 6-month comparison with longitudinal 2-year follow-up of effectiveness and costs. *Journal of Affective Disorders*, **68**, 317–30.

Carroll, K. M., Rounsaville, B. J., and Gawin, F. H. (1991). A comparative trial of psycho-therapies for ambulatory cocaine abusers: relapse prevention and interpersonal psychotherapy. *American Journal of Drug and Alcohol Abuse*, **17**, 229–47.

Cohen, M. B., Blake, G., Cohen, R., Fromm-Reichmann, F., and Weigert, E. (1954). An intensive study of twelve cases of manic depressive psychosis. *Psychiatry*, **17**, 103–37.

Coyne, J. C. (1976). Depression and the response of others. *Journal of Abnormal Psychology*, **85**, 186–93.

DiMascio, A., *et al.* (1979). Differential symptom reduction by drugs and psychotherapy in acute depression. *Archives of General Psychiatry*, **36**, 1450–6.

Fairburn, C. G., *et al.* (1993). Psychotherapy and bulimia nervosa: The long-term effects of interpersonal psychotherapy, behavior therapy, and cognitive-behavior therapy. *Archives of General Psychiatry*, **50**, 419–28.

Frank, E., Kupfer, D. J., and Perel, J. M. (1989). Early recurrence in unipolar depression. *Archives of General Psychiatry*, **46**, 397–400.

Frank, E., *et al.* (1990). Three-year outcomes for maintenance therapies in recurrent depression. *Archives of General Psychiatry*, **47**, 1093–9.

Frank, E., Swartz, H. A., and Kupfer, D. J. (2000). Interpersonal and social rhythm therapy: managing the chaos of bipolar disorder. *Biological Psychiatry*, **48**, 593–604.

Frank, J. D. (1973). *Persuasion and healing: a comparative study of psychotherapy*. Baltimore, MD: Johns Hopkins University Press.

Fromm-Reichmann, F. (1960). *Principles of intensive psychotherapy*. Chicago, IL: Phoenix Books.

Henderson, S. (1977). The social network, support and neurosis: the function of attachment in adult life. *British Journal of Psychiatry*, **131**, 185–91.

Kendler, K. S., Karkowski, L. M., and Prescott, C. A. (1999). Causal relationship between stressful life events and the onset of major depression. *American Journal of Psychiatry*, **156**, 837–48.

Klein, D. F. and Ross, D. C. (1993). Reanalysis of the National Institute of Mental Health Treatment of Depression Collaborative Research Program General Effectiveness Report. *Neuropsychopharmacology*, **8**, 241–51.

Klerman, G. L., Weissman, M. M., Rounsaville, B. J., and Chevron, E. S. (1984). *Interpersonal psychotherapy of depression*. New York: Basic Books.

Lipsitz, J. D., Fyer, A. J., Markowitz, J. C., and Cherry, S. (1999). An open trial of interpersonal psychotherapy for social phobia. *American Journal of Psychiatry*, **156**, 1814–16.

Luborsky, L. (1984). *Principles of psychoanalytic psychotherapy: a manual for supportive/expressive treatment*. New York: Basic Books.

Maddison, D. and Walker, W. (1967). Factors affecting the outcome of conjugal bereavement. *British Journal of Psychiatry*, **113**, 1057–67.

Markowitz, J. C., Svartberg, M., and Swartz, H. A. (1998). Is IPT time-limited psycho-dynamic psychotherapy? *Journal of Psychotherapy Practice and Research*, **7**, 185–95.

Merikangas, J., Ranelli, C., and Kupfer, D. (1979). Marital interaction in hospitalized depressed patients. *Journal of Nervous and Mental Disease*, **167**, 689–95.

Meyer, A. (1957). *Psychobiology: a science of man*. Springfield, IL: Charles C. Thomas.

Miller, L. and Weissman, M. (2002). Interpersonal psychotherapy delivered over the telephone to recurrent depressives: a pilot study. *Depression and Anxiety*, **16**, 114–17.

Mufson, L., Weissman, M. M., Moreau, D., and Garfinkel, R. (1999). Efficacy of interpersonal psychotherapy for depressed adolescents. *Archives of General Psychiatry*, **56**, 573–9.

O'Hara, M. W., Stuart, S., Gorman, L. L., and Wenzel, A. (2000). Efficacy of interpersonal psychotherapy for postpartum depression. *Archives of General Psychiatry*, **57**, 1039–45.

Overholser, J. C. and Adams, D. M. (1997). Stressful life events and social support in depressed psychiatric inpatients. In: T. W. Miller *et al.*, ed. *Clinical disorders and stressful life events*. Madison, CT: International Universities Press.

Parker, G. (1979). Parental characteristics in relation to depressive disorders. *British Journal of Psychiatry*, **134**, 138–47.

Paykel, E. S., *et al.* (1969). Life events and depression: a controlled study. *Archives of General Psychiatry*, **21**, 1753–60.

Pearlin, L. I. and Lieberman, M. A. (1977). Social sources of emotional distress. In: R. Simmons, ed. *Research in community and mental health*. Greenwich, CT: JAI Press.

Prigerson, H. G., Frank, E., Reynolds, C. F., and George C. J. (1993). Protective psychosocial factors in depression among spousally bereaved elders. *American Journal of Geriatric Psychiatry*, **1**, 296–309.

Reynolds, C. F. III, *et al.* (1999). Nortriptyline and interpersonal psychotherapy as maintenance therapies for recurrent major depression: a randomized controlled trial in patients older than 59 years. *Journal of the American Medical Association*, **281**, 39–45.

Rosselló, J. and Bernal, G. (1999). The efficacy of cognitive-behavioral and interpersonal treatments for depression in Puerto Rican adolescents. *Journal of Consulting and Clinical Psychology*, **67**, 734–45.

Rothblum, E., *et al.* (1982). Issues in clinical trials with the depressed elderly: case reports and discussion. *American Journal of Psychotherapy*, **37**, 552–66.

Rounsaville, B. J., Glazer, W., Wilber, C. H., Weissman, M. M., and Kleber, H. D. (1983). Short-term interpersonal psychotherapy in methadone maintained opiate addicts. *Archives of General Psychiatry*, **40**, 629–36.

Sullivan, H. S. (1953). *The interpersonal theory of psychiatry*. New York: Norton.

Sloane, R. B., Stapes, F. R., and Schneider, L. S. (1985). Interpersonal therapy versus nortriptyline for depression in the elderly. In: Burrows, G. D., Norman, T. R., and Dennerstein, L., ed. *Clinical and pharmacological studies in psychiatric disorders*, pp. 344–6. London: John Libbey.

Spinelli, M. G. and Endicott, J. (2003). Controlled clinical trial of interpersonal psychotherapy versus parenting education program for depressed pregnant women. *American Journal of Psychiatry*, **160**, 555–62.

Walker, K., MacBride, A., and Vachon, M. (1977). Social support networks and the crisis of bereavement. *Social Science and Medicine*, **11**, 35–41.

Weissman, M. M., Klerman, G. L., Paykel, E. S., Prusoff, B. A., and Hanson, B. (1974). Treatment effects on the social adjustment of depressed patients. *Archives of General Psychiatry*, **30**, 771–8.

Weissman, M. M., *et al.* (1979). The efficacy of drugs and psychotherapy in the treatment of acute depressive episodes. *American Journal of Psychiatry*, **136**, 555–8.

Weissman, M. M., Markowitz, J. C., and Klerman, G. L. (2000). *Comprehensive guide to interpersonal psychotherapy*. New York: Basic Books.

Wilfley, D. E., *et al.* (2002). A randomized comparison of group cognitive-behavioral therapy and group interpersonal psychotherapy for the treatment of overweight individuals with binge-eating disorder. *Archives of General Psychiatry*, **59**, 713–21.

4 Group psychotherapy

Werner Knauss

Introduction

Historical roots and developments

One social setting—different approaches

Group psychotherapy uses a 'natural' social setting—the small, the median, and the large group—to conduct its psychotherapeutic processes. We grow up in *small groups* (among family, peers, friends), we learn and work in *median groups* (in classrooms, committees, teams), and we engage in science, economic activity, and politics in *large groups* (through assemblies, networks, companies, political parties, parliaments, etc.). This chapter will discuss the conditions that are necessary for these natural groupings to become psychotherapeutic. The variety of different approaches to the psychotherapeutic use of groups, ranging from psychoeducation, psychoanalysis, psychodrama, group analysis, and humanistic psychology to cognitive-behaviorism, reflects the different historic roots of group psychotherapy.

So, let us first look at the different theoretical backgrounds, treatment principles, and conceptualization of processes, as well as at the different role played by the group therapist. The effectiveness and efficacy of group psychotherapy, and the indications and contraindications derived from empirical research findings, will be outlined below. As a group analyst, my main focus will be the group-analytic approach to group psychotherapy.

The whole is more than the sum of its parts

A group is more than the sum of its members, just like the meaning of a sentence is more than the line-up of various words. Therefore, we can use three different perspectives in order to understand whole group configurations:

1. The personality of the different members. The intrapsychic world of an individual is made up of internalized networks of relationships (Laing, 1974, p. 16). This internalized network of relationships gets reactivated in a group.

2. The interaction or the interrelatedness between different members. The process of interaction between different, unconscious networks of relationships, reactivated in a group setting, is a focus of attention in all analytically oriented group approaches. This interaction occurs even in other approaches, even when they refrain from using this process of interaction: for instance, cognitive-behavioral approaches tend to avoid it altogether. The sequence, the structure, and the emotional quality of this interaction is used to engender therapeutic processes in all analytically oriented approaches.

3. The system of the group as a whole in its contexts. Each unique group develops through a clash of centripetal and centrifugal forces, which are balanced by its constantly changing structure. Centripetal forces consist of a shared goal and the cohesion or coherence of the group as a whole. While cohesion describes the attractiveness of a group to its members (Levin, 1951), coherence focuses on 'an underlying sense of containment based upon differentiation and understanding' (Pines and Schlapobersky 2000, p. 1452). Centripetal forces ensure the existence of the group and its stability over time. On the other hand, different

norms, different roles and the individual's deviation from group norms are centrifugal forces that initiate change and development. Only if there is a balance between the two forces can the group develop a fluid structure. It is this structure that makes the group a safe enough place for its members to risk making changes.

In order to understand the group process, all three perspectives have to be taken into consideration. Each approach uses these perspectives differently. The political, cultural, and social context of each unique group creates the framework for an unfolding and ever expanding group process.

Brief history

The first psychotherapeutic use of groups was made in the US by medical doctors with the aim of psychoeducation. Pratt (1908, 1922), Lazell (1921), and Marsh (1933) addressed lectures to different groups of patients. The aim was to increase self-control by providing them with more information given about their disease. These lectures were provided in small, median, or large groups. Pratt referred to them as 'thought control classes', Lazell as 'etiology spiel', and Marsh as 'milieu therapy' by social-educational groups (Ettin, 1999, p. 72–8). Similar developments in Vienna were described as 'guidance groups' by Adler. His follower Dreikurs (1932), working in the US, used the same term.

The psychoeducational approach is nowadays used in the application of behavior or cognitive-behavior therapy in groups (cf. Fiedler, 1996; Free, 1999).

In psychoeducational groups, the curative factors are defined as reeducation, socialization, the imbuing of an individual with hope, the raising of morale, and the emotional developments occurring during the teaching process in a group.

Psychoanalysis is the basic theory underpinning group psychotherapy approaches that focus not on teaching and education, but on insight. This insight-through-group experience is pursued through a number of variations on the psychoanalytic theme: group analysis, psychodrama, psychodynamic groups, and various forms of humanistic psychology such as Gestalt therapy (Perls) and transactional analysis (Berne), or encounter groups (Rogers).

The first psychoanalyst to bring together patients suffering from neurotic symptoms in a group using psychoanalytic techniques was T. Burrow (1928), again in the US. His starting point was the perception of humans as a social being and of the group as the natural focus of treatment. His aim was to make conscious both latent and repressed meanings through the here-and-now interaction within a group. Burrow named his method group analysis. He relied on Freud's study, *Group psychology and the analysis of the ego* (Freud, 1921).

Jacob Moreno used the theatre stage to create a scenic understanding of intrapsychic conflictual life. From 1928 onwards, he offered psychodrama demonstrations at Carnegie Hall. Moreno used psychodrama in a small group setting for psychotherapy at the Mount Sinai Hospital in New York City. He developed the method of sociometry (1938) and in 1942 founded the American Society for Group Psychotherapy and Psychodrama. The Society in 1951 became the International Association for Group Psychotherapy, an umbrella organization for all approaches.

In the 1940s, several psychoanalysts used their psychoanalytical understanding to work with patients in a group setting: Lauretta Bender (1937), Louis Wender (1940), Paul Schilder (1940), and Alexander Wolf (1949) worked with resistances and transference processes. They defined the therapist as a symbolic parent and the other patients as representing siblings with the aim of providing social insights through interpersonal exchange: the group 'removes' the problem from the sphere of the individual's symptom formation and suffering. Through group interaction the isolation of the individual, which is seen as an important part of psychoneurosis, is opened up (Schilder, 1936, pp. 612–14).

All these psychoanalytically based group therapy approaches had one thing in common: the method they used was the application of individual psychoanalysis to a group setting with the aim of social integration. The therapeutic emphasis was kept on the individual patient in a small group setting. Samuel Salvson founded the American Group Psychotherapy Association in 1942 and created the International Journal of Group Psychotherapy in 1951.

Moreno, Schilder, and Wolf worked mainly with adults suffering from neurotic illnesses and recommended the exclusion of psychopaths, alcoholics, hypomanic patients, and hallucinating psychotics from groups. Bender and Slavson worked with disturbed children and used puppet play (Bender, 1937, p. 1161) and activity groups primarily to treat overaggressive and excessively withdrawn children. Salvson invented the term group dynamics in 1933.

Group psychotherapy today

Specific psychoanalytic approaches

Three different perspectives can help us to differentiate among the various psychoanalytically based approaches:

◆ psychoanalysis *in* the group
◆ psychoanalysis *of* the group
◆ psychoanalysis *by* the group.

Each of these has a different focus when it comes to the process, the task of the therapist and the curative factors in group psychotherapy.

Psychoanalysis in the group

As already mentioned, the pioneering figures Salvson, Wolf, Schilder, and Bender, as well as Moreno, focused on the process of individual analysis in the context of a group, working through resistances and transference processes to develop the curative factors: insight, sublimation, and catharsis. Their aim was to bring about more conscious personal action and social integration. In this approach, the therapist works like an individual psychoanalyst by using his interpretation of unconscious transference and defense mechanisms, supported by a catalytic group context.

Psychoanalysis of the group

The aftermath of World War II saw the development of new approaches in group psychotherapy, which sought to combine theory and practice in the group as a whole. Again this was based on Freud's ideas on group psychology in which he emphasized the regressive aspects of group life. Here the group is seen as a collective—an organism in which the boundaries between individual consciousnesses is broken down with common fantasies that grip each and every member to a lesser or greater extent.

1. W. Bion (1960) described three basic, unconscious group assumptions as a result of his experiences with groups. These assumptions unify the group as a whole:

   (a) first, *dependency*—the expectation that solutions will be provided by a god-like leader;
   (b) secondly, *fight and flight*—group members seek to flee from battles about differences among them and project them to an outside group;
   (c) thirdly, *pairing*—group members hope for salvation through forming an idealized couple.

   These basic assumptions are shared by the entire group and unconsciously determine its fantasies, communications, and transactions.

They therefore undermine the completion of its tasks as a working group. The transference relationship with the therapist is seen as two-dimensional, as being between the therapist and the group. Technique concentrates on transference interpretations of the whole group, and its relationship with the therapist. Intragroup dynamics are taken in consideration only in what they contribute to the group as a whole. Bion's *Experiences in groups* later resulted in the development of the 'Tavistock Model', which is today also used in the context of organizational consultancy, applying his ideas to corporations and other social institutions.

2. H. Ezriel (1973) perceived group development as directed by a shared, common *group tension* resulting from unconscious, infantile conflicts. Each patient contributes to the shared tension on a latent level. Interpretations concentrate on these ever-changing group tensions, which are seen as a defense against *catastrophic fears*—thus pairing might be seen as a defense against abandonment—clinging together to avert falling into a void, at both an individual and group level.

3. D. S. Whitaker and M. A. Liebermann (1964) perceive the group's interaction as a compromise: unconscious conflicts that emerge during the shared focal conflicts allow only *restricted solutions*. Interpretations are expected to reveal those restricted solutions and their underlying unconscious conflicts with the aim of permitting more productive solutions. Here, for example, the inhibition of rivalry in the group averts potentially dangerous aggression, but also stifles the development of individual strengths.

Psychoanalysis by the group

S. H. Foulkes (1948) developed the *group-analytic approach*, which he described as 'psychoanalysis by the group, of the group, including its conductor' (Foulkes, 1975, p. 3). He was greatly influenced by the social philosophy of the Frankfurt School (Fromm, Adorno, Marcuse, Elias, Fromm-Reichmann et al.,) who tried to integrate the findings of psychoanalysis and sociology (cf. Elliott, 1999, pp. 46–76). Drawing an analogy with the new understanding of the relationship between a neuron and the nervous system, which had been developed by the German neurologist Kurt Goldstein (1934), Foulkes conceptualized the group-analytic process as a dynamic web of communications, the so-called *dynamic matrix*, in which the individual forms a nodal point. 'The whole can adjust to and then compensate for the functional disturbance caused by local damage' (Goldstein, 1934). Here the idea of an 'individual' is—like that of an isolated neuron or electron—a myth, as every individual is part of a web of relationships that define his or her individuality.

In this approach, the therapist follows the group process, encouraging the ever-increasing complexity of communications at various levels mainly by his/her *group-analytic attitude*—i.e., attuning to a multidimensional network of conscious and unconscious, verbal and nonverbal communications. These receive their meaning through a group matrix, which 'determines the meaning and significance of all events . . .' (Foulkes, 1964, p. 292). Here, the group therapist no longer functions as a group leader but as a *group conductor*, frustrating regressive needs and thus replacing the leader's authority by that of the group: all members interpret, analyze, and support each other, including the conductor.

Eclectic or integrative approaches

Interpersonal group psychotherapy

Starting from Yalom (1970/1985), more eclectic or integrative approaches see transference as no more (or less) than one among a number of important aspects of group psychotherapy, conceptualizing it as an interpersonal, perceptional distortion. Insight is sought at four different levels.

1. How others see the patient.
2. What the patient is doing in relationship to others.
3. Why the patient might be doing what he/she is doing.
4. Biographical insight.

Yalom singles out *11 curative factors* in group psychotherapy: the giving of hope, the universality of suffering, altruism, corrective emotional experience, the recapitulation of primary family group (i.e., transference), socialization, imitation, interpersonal learning through feedback, group cohesiveness, catharsis, and existential factors. The therapist offers encouragement to experiment with more satisfying interactions and is supported by feedback from all group members.

Psychodynamic group psychotherapy

Rutan and Stone (2001) developed the concept of psychodynamic group psychotherapy in the US, which offered an integrative approach. Their psychodynamic groups tried to integrate all so-called modern theories of group psychotherapy (Foulkes, 1948; Bion, 1960; Whitaker and Liebermann, 1964; Yalom, 1970/1985; Ezriel, 1973; Agazarian, 1997) with the aim of an 'integrative conceptualization' (Rutan and Stone, 2001, p. 27): this meant the integration of the intrapsychic (character formation, typical defenses, internal object relations), the interpersonal (relational styles and roles, externalization of the internal role through projection and projective identification) the social psychological components (group norms, values, assumptions, and restrictions) of group psychotherapy.

Disturbance-specific application of psychoanalysis

The application of psychoanalysis in groups on three levels (Göttinger model)

Heigl-Evers and Heigl (1973) differentiate among three models of applying psychoanalysis in groups, depending on the ego strength of a group of patients: an *interactional* model is used in the treatment of patients who are severely disturbed. The therapist tries to keep regression to a manageable level by avoiding transference interpretations and by disclosing his or her own feelings and thoughts in response to certain interactions by the patients.

For patients suffering from actual conflicts in relationships, an *analytically oriented* model is provided, which is very similar to the interpersonal theories. This model aims to promote social, interpersonal learning, mainly by providing feedback with minimal interpretation of unconscious fantasies and transference processes. The third model, *psychoanalytic group psychotherapy*, is only used for the working through of unconscious, oedipal conflicts fuelling neurotic symptom formation. A deep level of regression is required for the interpretation and analysis of unconscious defense and transference processes in the group. This is fostered by the therapist's neutrality and abstinence, and by him restricting himself to transference interpretations.

Systems-centered group psychotherapy

Agazarian (1997) implemented general system theory in group psychotherapy by focusing the therapist's and the group's attention on boundary issues and subgrouping factors. The main task, she argued, was to increase communication across boundaries: 'How the group communicates is always more important than what it is communicating about' (Agazarian, 1989, p. 176). In her technique the group leader clarifies subgroup boundaries and encourages very actively interactions that cross boundaries in a respectful way.

Different clinical settings

Outpatient and inpatient treatment

Group psychotherapy can be applied in long-term psychotherapy (of more than 50 sessions) or in short-term psychotherapy (of 20 or fewer sessions). It can be used in an inpatient or an outpatient context, in closed groups (where all group members start and finish the group together), in semi-open groups (with a slow change of membership) or an open group setting (of mainly inpatient groups with an often rapidly changing membership).

Inpatient psychotherapy is widely offered to severely disturbed patients in psychotherapeutic units in general, or in psychiatric hospitals. These psychotherapy units use a variety of group psychotherapeutic approaches.

Practitioners may draw on the therapeutic community (see Chapter 22 'Antisocial personality disorder'), a concept first introduced in England by T. Main (1977, cf. Whiteley, 1994), but structure the understanding of the group dynamics within the whole ward differently:

- The bipolar model (Enke, 1965) differentiates 'a therapeutic room', which is designed for analyzing unconscious conflicts, from 'a reality room', which is designed to allow experimenting and reality testing. The weakness of this model lies in the danger that splitting processes acted out on a ward cannot be integrated by the therapeutic team and so remain apart.

- The integrative model (Janssen, 1985) tries to bring together the different aspects of primitive object relations or part-object relations of the patient by regular and continuing communication of a therapeutic team. These are then reenacted with different individuals or subgroups of the team. The whole network of distorted communications and interactions in different groups or subgroups on a ward can thus be understood as a form of defense and can become conscious through the integrative capacity of the therapeutic team.

- The group-analytic model (Knauss, 2001) uses large group sessions to develop an understanding of the interaction between the two groups on the ward, the patient group and the team group, and between the ward and the social, political, and cultural context of the hospital. Both subgroups need a conductor: the patient group needs one in various group settings (in the therapy group, the art group, the occupational group, the music group, etc.) and the therapeutic team needs an external supervisor in order to understand its own internal dynamics and to preserve its integrating, group-analytic capacity. Therapy mainly takes place as an interaction within and between these two subgroups: the patients' therapy groups and the team group.

Theoretical basis and treatment principles

The dynamic administration

Selection and composition

In all approaches, the selection and composition of the group is crucial in terms of therapeutic efficiency. Most approaches, except for the psychoeducational or cognitive-behavioral ones, follow the general rule that the selection of patients and the composition of the group determine the quality of interaction among group members. These factors, in turn, then provide the foundations for effective treatment.

In all analytical approaches, it is assumed that the composition of the group should be heterogeneous as regards the patients' psychopathology and personality structures. It should also vary in terms of social class, age, and gender, i.e., patients' culturally specific ways of interacting. However, the group should be homogeneous when it comes to the level of frustration its members can cope with or the conflicts they can work through productively (measures of ego strengths). Only for some groups of patients does homogeneity have advantages: these are patients with drug or alcohol addiction, severe psychosomatic illnesses or personality disorders with destructive acting out, as well as psychotic patients or forensic psychiatric patients (Knauss, 1985; Dies, 1993).

In contrast, cognitive-behavioral and psychoeducational approaches prefer groups to be homogeneous groups in terms of symptoms in order to teach patients with similar symptoms about the psychological background of their deviant behavior.

The 'Noah's Ark Principle' ('the animals came in two by two') applies to all approaches:

> Members isolated from the rest of the group by problems, personalities, or histories that no-one else shares are likely to find the experience threatening. We do not put a patient into a position of being isolated by virtue of age, intelligence, ethnicity,

gender, or extreme symptomatology. An impulsive sociopath or sexual deviance would not be well placed except in a group of other such people, at least for the first phase of the therapy.

Pines and Schlapobersky (2000, p. 1454).

The group size recommended by analytic approaches is between five and nine, a size that encourages the development of trust and intimacy. Cognitive-behavioral approaches recommend a group size of between four and six for the training of new skills. However, there may be up to 20 group members present for the teaching part.

The central question remains: Which patient can benefit from which group? 'A central issue is whether or not a particular treatment group is suitable for a specific patient at a given point in the manifestation of symptomatology and the group's current level of development' (Dies, 1993, p. 487).

Preparation and motivation

To prepare patients for the often anxiously awaited experience of group psychotherapy is as important for a positive outcome as the selection and composition of the group (Salvendy, 1993). The point of preparing patients is to reduce anxiety and to motivate them by cognitively and positively pre-structuring the group experience that they want to undergo in order to get better. Anxiety to disclose one's so far private fantasies, needs, weaknesses, and traumatic experiences, often connected with guilt and shame (Seidler, 1997, 2000a,b) can make a patient dread the encounter with that public body, the group. But so can the social isolation caused by the patient's symptom formation. Therefore, it is crucial that the therapist devotes several individual sessions or a waiting group to the patient's preparation and motivation. This strategy is an empirically proven predictor of a successful outcome (Tschuschke and Dies, 1994).

Group rules

One aspect of patient preparation involves familiarizing the patient with the group rules. All analytically oriented approaches operate with the following rules: confidentiality, free-floating association with no conscious exclusion of any fantasy, memory or thought arising in the group process, tolerance towards every verbal communication, the exclusion of body action, and no meetings outside the group session. If such meetings do occur, they have to be discussed in the following group session. The group boundaries have to be clear to all patients: they must know who belongs to the group, the time, place, and duration of group sessions, and the honorarium for each session. It is helpful to mention the possibility of symptom aggravation at the beginning of therapy, which is a sign of resistance to change, because this may prevent patients from dropping out early on. Meetings outside the group and subgroupings are interpreted as resistance to open communication and therefore have to be discussed inside the group.

In order to allow the group to work through a separation, members must announce the termination of their therapy to the group well in advance.

The conceptualization of the group process

Taking the group seriously (Dalal, 1998)?

'The group, the community, is an ultimate primary unit of consideration, and the so-called inner processes in the individual are internalisations of the forces operating in the group to which he belongs' (Foulkes, 1971, p. 212). This means that conscious and unconscious processes in groups are deeply structured by the social unconscious: the group is the primary psychological unit, the individual the primary biological one.

In order to understand all analytic approaches the above theoretical statement by Foulkes, based on the social philosophy of Norbert Elias (1987) and the dynamic psychoneurology of Kurt Goldstein, should to be taken into account.

In those approaches that focus on *psychoanalysis in groups*, the analysis of the individual in a group context, which contributes to individual analysis, is placed at the center.

In approaches that focus on the *psychoanalysis of the group,* as in the Tavistock tradition, the main objectives of analysis are the shared assumptions, tensions, or conflicts of the group as a whole.

In *group-analytic psychotherapy* the shared experience of developing communications within the group is analyzed by the group, including its conductor, at four levels.

1. The current level, which is the working alliance.

2. The transference level.

3. The projective level.

4. The primordial or archaic level.

The aim is not only analysis, but also the translation of unconscious symptom formation into conscious conflicts within and between group members. Group-analytic psychotherapy seeks to create an ever expanding, increasingly complex process of communication. The individual is perceived as a nodal point in the network of group relations, and transference as well as countertransference processes form his or her link to the outside world. The here-and-now conflictual interaction resembles a figure hovering in the background of the dynamic matrix of the group as a whole. 'In learning to communicate, the group can be compared to a child learning to speak' (Foulkes and Anthony, 1968, p. 263).

The basic law of group dynamics

The healing effect of group communication is defined by Foulkes as one of the basic laws of group dynamics: 'The deepest reason why patients . . . can reinforce each others' normal reactions and wear down and correct each others' neurotic reactions is that collectively they constitute the very norm from which, individually, they deviate' (Foulkes, 1948, p. 29). It is the deviation of different individual members from the norm, with each of them going off in a different direction, rather than their submission to the norm, which brings about the development: we seek 'to replace submission by co-operation on equal terms between equals' (Foulkes, 1964, p. 65).

Groups are held together by the need to belong, which is basic when it comes to the development of cohesion. At first, all differences within the group tend to be denied. The regressive process can take two directions: either the group turns into a fused mass, which identifies with an idealized, omnipotent leader, and his or her ideology, or it becomes the sum of isolated individuals who cannot find any meaning in relating. Therefore, submission, idealization, and dependency, which all initially contribute to the cohesion of the group, are simultaneously interpreted as possible defenses against development.

The conductor's analytic attitude frustrates the group members' dependency needs by then setting into motion a process of conscious differentiation. 'The group analyst has to accept the unconscious fantasy of the group which puts the therapist in the position of a primordial leader image and one who is omnipotent, and the group expects magical help from him. But instead of fulfilling this regressive need, the conductor uses it in the best interest of the group, which means that he has to change from a leader of the group to a leader in the group, replacing thereby . . . the leader's authority by that of the group' (Foulkes, 1964, p. 61).

By working through these dependency needs, the deviations from the unifying norms of the group are brought to the fore, and so can be experienced and discussed. This differentiation process runs parallel with the very painful and slow process of accepting the otherness of the other, of being separated. It is advanced by destructive fantasies, which, according to Winnicott (1980), create a differentiation between the self and the other. The major defense against listening to the otherness of the other is a fear of the stranger, of a different world view. 'A functioning group could be seen as a communication process in which competing discourses come into conflict with the aim to free each group member from being stuck in ones own, private discourse, ones own experience of the self and the world and initiates a process of opening up to communicate with other discourses, other ways of being and experiencing which one did not have previous access to' (Dalal, 1998, p. 177).

To achieve this process of differentiation, the group makes use of mirroring (Pines, 1982). Mirroring combines empathy and the notion of being different from the other into a single emotional reaction to one's perception of the otherness of the other. Through mirroring, similarities and differences between group members are explored. If the projective part of the process in mirroring is not fully understood, it can deteriorate into malignant mirroring (Zinkin, 1983). This happens when one group member attempts to change the other, while trying to deny his or her otherness. In case of malignant mirroring, the conductor needs to act with the aim of containing the unbearable pain of separateness.

As the following example illustrates, destructive fantasies play an important part in this differentiation process (cf. Knauss, 1999):

> A patient, a truck driver, disclosed after 20 sessions that he would beat up his wife whenever she said something unpleasant or different from his own view. At this point it was clear that he expected to be thrown out of the group. The communication process stopped, a tense silence emerged, and the whole group was waiting for my reaction. After I had mentioned this process, he was echoed by another patient, a priest, who disclosed that he was sometimes full of destructive, murderous fantasies in which women were slaughtered by a swimming pool. A third patient, a policeman, reported as a resonance to the other two and like in a chain, that he was about to kill his wife, when he discovered that she had a lover. Especially female group members could mirror these destructive fantasies and their acting out as an attempt to bring the otherness of the other under omnipotent control, and as a resistance to the difficult process of respecting the otherness of the other. In a long process of working through and remembering this could be understood as a very painful process of separating from fused, early childhood relationships. Through resonance and the mirror reaction, the group members were able to understand that destructive fantasies and impulses express one's need for unification and support on the one hand, while initiating one's need for differentiation and separation on the other.

A process was set in motion that went from a lack of communication, through resonance and mirroring, to open communication, i.e., from monologue to dialogue. The analytic attitude, the setting and the careful selection and composition of the group all serve to protect the group from actual destruction. They also encourage the creation of a safe place for the communication of destructive fantasies. This means ego development and not only 'ego training in action' (Foulkes, 1964, pp. 82, 129).

Morris Nitsun (1996) has described destructive group forces, naming them the 'antigroup'. He showed that actual destruction is only acted out if the destructive fantasy cannot be verbalized and if the object of the destructive fantasy seeks retaliation. In that case, developmental processes of differentiation between me and not me cannot be set in motion. The creative potential of verbalized, destructive fantasies encourages a differentiation process (Knauss, 1999). It fosters the group members' perception of one another as different subjects with their own rights and needs. The social unconscious of the group, understood as a harbor of all the denied heterogeneity within the group, becomes conscious and brings power relations within and between groups into a shared process of communication. This can also be seen as a process of democratization.

Cohesion, coherence, regression, mirroring, imitation, identification, internalization, resonance, condensation, exchange, sharing, socialization, and polarization, as well as projective identification are group-specific therapeutic factors. The dynamic links between the group structure, the contents of the discussion and the form it takes can become conscious by an ongoing process of mutual interpretations among group members. Only when the communication process gets stuck does the group conductor need to step in with an interpretation or clarification. The conductor therefore follows the group process with curiosity, empathy, and tact, and should not interrupt communication as long as it flows freely. He intervenes solely if the communication process stagnates as a result of overwhelming defense mechanisms.

The group therapist—conductor

In each approach, the therapeutic attitude of the group conductor or group leader is an essential factor. A culture of basic trust can develop only if he takes a largely positive, sincere, and curious attitude towards each patient and the group. This attitude is a precondition for the success of all therapeutic alliances. In analytic approaches, the abstinence and neutrality of the conductor (Knauss, 1994), combined with a sincere effort to understand what is going on, but not to act, is an additional requirement. As mentioned, in a group-analytic approach, the term 'leader' is replaced by the term 'conductor', so as to make clear that the conductor must be 'free from the temptation to play this god-like role, to exploit it for his own needs' (Foulkes, 1964, p. 60). Instead, he must seek to 'wean the group from this need for authoritative guidance . . . ' (Foulkes, 1964, p. 61) and leadership.

This group-analytic attitude contributes fundamentally to the development of a group culture and a climate of tolerance and differentiation within a process of free-floating communication. The transference processes are not only involving the conductor, but also all other group members in a process of multiple, mutual transferences. The same applies to the process of interpretation. The various countertransference processes focus on the dynamic of the unconscious network of relationships existing within the group, creating in the conductor a countertransference to the dynamic matrix of the group as a whole, which he is a part.

The conductor may abandon his role as a 'participant observer' when, and only when, the communication process breaks down due to unconscious conflicts. If the group process does get stuck, however, the conductor must intervene by addressing the process rather than the contents of the communication. When the group stopped communicating after the report of the first patient about his violence towards his wife and was waiting for my reaction to it, I said: 'Do you keep silent and just wait to see how I would react?' This remark on the process opened a space for resonance, chain and mirror reactions in other group members and the communication process, which was blocked by separation anxiety, could continue.

In this commenting-on-process intervention the conductor needs to take into consideration (1) the past outside the group—the 'social history'; (2) the past inside the group—the group's history; (3) the present outside the group—the actual context; and (4) the present inside the group—the actually developing dynamic matrix. The conductor might localize mirror reactions, which can be helpful when it comes to recognizing aspects of oneself and others and to accept the viewpoints of others on oneself. He can also make the group aware of group role configurations, especially if a scapegoating process is taking place, and should always keep in mind the aim of fostering the process of individualization and relating. 'The therapist's task is to follow the interaction, to use interventions sparingly and strategically, to cultivate a reflective curiosity' (Pines and Schlapobersky, 2000, p. 1455). This will include gesture, behavior, body language, and other nonverbal communications that convey feelings when emotions cannot be put into words.

Appropriate *training* is of course required in order to carry out these tasks. Group-analytic training will include theory and a long-term personal therapy by the therapist in a group, as well as long-term and intensive clinical supervision of group-analytic processes.

Scientific exchange and training organizations

In 1952, S. H. Foulkes founded the Group-Analytic Society (London) for the development, exchange and discussion of group-analytic theory, practice, and research. The Group-Analytic Society (London) now provides a network for scientific dialogue between qualified group analysts and researchers from all over the world.

To carry out the specific task of training, senior colleagues of the Group-Analytic Society (London) founded the Institute of Group Analysis, London, in 1972. The scientific journal *Group Analysis* has been published by the Group-Analytic Society (London) since 1967. Numerous other training institutions for group analysis have subsequently been created all over Europe, as well as in Israel and Australia. They are also slowly developing in the US. The European Group Analytic Training Institutions Network has established an International Federation of Training Institutions in Group-analytic psychotherapy.

Brief summary of research findings

What works in groups?

Tschuschke (1999b) analyzed the most important journals for group psychotherapy (i.e., *Group, Group Analysis, International Journal of Group*

Psychotherapy, Journal of Consulting and Clinical Psychology, Small Group Behavior, Small Group Research, The Journal of Psychotherapy: Theory, Practice and Research) during the last 20 years by looking at 117 empirical studies examining mainly the outcome of behavioral or cognitive-behavioral group psychotherapy. He also analyzed 62 empirical studies examining mainly the process of psychodynamic or analytic group psychotherapy. Tschuschke concludes that studies of behavioral or cognitive-behavioral group psychotherapy concentrate on a specific disorder and the outcome for the individual patient, while studies of analytic group psychotherapy concentrate on the development of structural changes during the group-analytic process in patients suffering from various disorders and treated in heterogeneously composed groups. Only in the last 10 years have some studies sought to examine the outcome-process interrelatedness.

We might wish to differentiate between the following:

1. Outcome studies with mainly prepost designs

    (a) either with or without control groups

    (b) comparing different approaches

    (c) comparing different techniques of conducting

    (d) comparing different patient groups.

2. Process-outcome studies examining different process variables by comparing the groups of successful and unsuccessful patients in heterogeneously composed groups.

Randomized controlled trials (RCTs) are difficult to mount and evaluate in the context of group analysis for various reasons:

1. RCTs tend to focus on single rather than multiple disorders (Hall and Mullee, 2000, p. 320). As group-analytic psychotherapy usually works for dynamic reasons with mixed diagnoses in a group, the study of a specific disorder seems to be impossible. Therefore, these studies concentrate on the effects of different group processes on various patients. Only homogeneously composed groups, such as behavioral or cognitive-behavioral groups or group-analytic treatment of addicts or eating disorders, allow the examination of a specific disorder.

2. RCTs tend to be used to evaluate short-term group psychotherapy. Group-analytic psychotherapy is a long-term approach with the aim of bringing about structural changes.

3. 'RCTs necessitate strict protocol and multiple-outcome measures. These are upsetting or irritating to patients and are so unlike work in "natural" clinical settings that lessons from the research are not easily applicable to future clinical practice; efficacy does not equal clinical effectiveness.' (Hall and Mullee, 2000, p. 321).

Consequently, randomized trials comparing two treatments or open trials with a large number of patients treated in a 'natural' setting appear to be more suitable methods than RCTs for evidence-based group psychotherapy. This is despite the fact that 'RCTs provide the only valid—albeit limited—source of evidence for the efficacy of various forms of psychological treatment' (Roth and Fonagy, 1996, p. 19).

Individual versus group psychotherapy

The effect size (ES) in 23 studies using RCTs to compare directly individual and group psychotherapy showed no difference, while both treatment modalities show a big difference in effect size, compared with the control group: for individual psychotherapy it is 0.76 ES and for group psychotherapy 0.90ES (McRoberts *et al.*, 1998).

Group-analytic treatment in eating disorders

A review of the literature on the efficacy of group psychotherapy in the treatment of bulimia nervosa by McKisack and Waller (1997) shows that improvement was associated with long-term groups.

Valbak (2003) undertook an empirical study of long-term group-analytic psychotherapy homogeneously composed with severely disturbed bulimic patients. Its positive results demonstrate that the technique of the treatment has to include the following elements:

1. A careful assessment interview.

2. Consistent monitoring of eating habits and of the connection between self-esteem and outlook.

3. An active response to any ruptures of the therapeutic alliance to prevent dropping-out.

4. An emphasis on continuity, attunement and timing of supportive and confronting interventions.

5. The sustaining of the group matrix as a carrier of hope.

Comparing group analytic and cognitive-behavioral groups

Externalizing patients tend to do better in cognitive-behavioral group psychotherapy, while internalizing patients do better in supportive group psychotherapy (Beutler *et al.*, 1991, 1993).

Severely alcohol abusing patients show more improvement in cognitive-behavioral group psychotherapy, while less severe abusers do better in psychodynamic group psychotherapy (Kadden *et al.*, 1989, 2001; Sandahl *et al.*, 1998). In the case of personality disorders, no difference has been shown between the two treatment modalities (Kadden *et al.*, 2001). Steuer *et al.* (1984) showed that when it comes to depression in the elderly, psychodynamic and cognitive-behavioral group psychotherapy are equally effective in reducing levels of depression. It appears that it is the group that works for these patients, rather than any specific approach.

Sandahl *et al.* (2000) found that there was a significant difference in the way cognitive-behavioral group conductors communicate in comparison with the group analysts' way of communicating in a group: 'cognitive-behaviorally oriented therapists talked more than twice as much as the group-analytically oriented therapists' while 'group members talked 85 percent of the time in the group-analytically oriented groups and 60 percent in the cognitive-behavior therapy' (p. 343). The contents of the communication differs significantly in two categories: while group analysts and patients in group-analytic psychotherapy communicate more on the contents.

Piper *et al.* (1984) showed that long-term group therapy (average 76 sessions) is more effective than short-term group psychotherapy (average 22 sessions). Lorentzen (2000) documented significant progress in the scale of symptoms, interpersonal problems, target complaints, and psychosocial functioning after 100 sessions of outpatient group-analytic psychotherapy. Similar preliminary results are reported by Tschuschke and Anbeh, (2000) who studied a large number of patients (more than 600) in a natural setting with a prepost design, comparing long-term, outpatient analytic group psychotherapy with psychodrama groups. He found for patients in group-analytic psychotherapy an ES of 0.97 for the Global Assessment Functioning Scale and an ES of 2.35 for Target Complaints. The Inventory of Interpersonal Problems showed an ES of 0.62 and the Global Severity Index-SCL90-R showed an ES of 0.67.

Process-outcome studies

The Vancouver/Edmonton Study by Piper *et al.* (1992; 1996a,b; 2001)

This study compared psychodynamic and supportive group psychotherapy in a RCT design on various levels:

♦ The group as a whole

♦ The individual patient

♦ The different styles of conducting

♦ The interpersonal dynamic between patients in the group.

The authors found no significant difference between the two approaches on the level of the group as a whole. The styles of conducting were clearly different.

Patients with more stable object relations (QOR = Quality of Object Relations) benefit more from a psychodynamic approach. Patients with a lower capacity to understand psychodynamic processes (low psychological mindedness) benefit more from other patients. Psychological-mindedness and a high esteem of the group as a whole are the best predictors for a good individual outcome in group psychotherapy.

The Stuttgart Study by Tschuschke and Dies, R. R. (1994)

In this study, five process variables were used to predict who would be the successful and the unsuccessful inpatients in group-analytic psychotherapy. These factors were:

- cohesion
- self-disclosure
- feedback
- interpersonal learning
- reenactment of early family conflicts in the group.

The authors found that:

- cohesion and the feeling to belong to the group are good predictors for success;
- early self-disclosure produces a better outcome;
- more critical feedback was received and given by successful patients;
- insight into the reenactment of infantile conflicts in groups changes the internalized relational network for the better and is linked to an improvement in the quality of object relations.

An intense and positive way of emotionally relating to co-members, which can be fostered by preparing patients for the group process, promotes the capacity to disclose and leads to more frequent and intense feedback from fellow patients. On the other hand, the patient who has a negative emotional relationship to other group members will disclose little and will receive relatively little meaningful feedback. Tschuschke and Dies (1994) conclude that there is 'a complex interdependency among the three therapeutic factors of cohesiveness, self-disclosure and feedback, which promotes a working-through process that is also apparent in the improvement of interpersonal patterns (interpersonal learning-output) within the group and produces enduring intrapsychic changes in objects and self-representations (family re-enactment)'.

Early cohesion and the development of coherency, early disclosure to and confrontation with others, a largely positive alliance with others, and an increasingly noninterventionist group therapist are all linked to a positive outcome for the individual patient (Soldz et al., 1992; Strauß, 1992; Marziali et al., 1997).

Seidler (2000a,b) has found a significant correlation between increased self-relatedness and the reduction of psychosomatic symptoms among inpatients undergoing analytically oriented group psychotherapy. In the beginning of therapy he could observe a shift from somatic symptoms to neurotic symptom formation.

Liebermann (1971) has empirically shown that a well functioning group is able to establish a group culture in which the group members identify with the therapist's therapeutic attitude and thus become more and more therapeutically active.

Kordy and Senf (1992) have shown that being isolated with a specific symptom in a group leads to premature drop-out (as per the Noah's Ark Principle, see above).

A review of the literature dealing with the empirical research of group psychotherapy by Dies (1993) and by Burlingame et al. (2001, 2002) argued that group psychotherapy is effective in cases of alcoholism, anxiety disorders, bereavement, eating disorders, depression, schizophrenia, and sexual abuse.

Cost-effectiveness

The Henderson therapeutic community approach demonstrated its cost-effectiveness for the treatment of severe personality disorders according to an empirical study conducted by Dolan et al. (1996). This outcome paved the way for central funding for similar units in other parts of the UK (cf. Carter, 2002, p. 131).

A retrospective study by Heintzel et al. (2000) produced a key argument in favor of better funding for group psychotherapy by insurance companies. By analyzing 'hard data' such as the use of hospital care, sick leave, medical appointments, and medication, the authors showed that 27 months after the end of therapy, patients who had successfully completed a long-term analytic group psychotherapy had saved more than three times their therapy costs by using far less medical care compared with what they had used in the 27 months prior to it.

Indications and contraindications

The results of empirical research cannot yet provide us with a detailed answer to the question: What works for whom?

Tschuschke (1999) provides an overview of RCT studies that compare the efficiency of individual and group therapy. They are both similarly effective concerning the reduction of suffering from neurotic, psychosomatic, or borderline pathology. Group psychotherapy is more economic and fosters the capacity to develop more satisfying relationships.

Therefore, all patients who can profit from psychotherapy are potentially suitable for group psychotherapy, but assessment must also consider additional factors as follows.

Group psychotherapy should be indicated only after a process in which a patient's motivation and ability for self-disclosure and feedback, as well as their history of previous group interactions, have been carefully assessed. According to Dies (1993), general indications for group psychotherapy include: the motivation to participate and to get emotionally involved, some positive experiences in relating to others in groups in childhood, or at present, some interest in exploring oneself and others and some ability to sympathize or emphasize with others' needs and problems.

Contraindications, therefore, are not confined to symptoms such as acute destructive or self-destructive acting out or acute psychosis. Major problems of self-disclosure, difficulties with intimacy, general personal distrust, and the excessive use of denial are contraindications to group psychotherapy and need a preliminary phase of individual psychotherapy (Knauss, 1985).

Conclusions

Group psychotherapy is an efficient and economic treatment for a great variety of mental disorders. Group psychotherapy uses a natural setting under specific conditions to achieve therapeutic goals. Group psychotherapy is economical not just in economic terms, but also the wealth of potential outcomes: for a large proportion of patients, group psychotherapy does not merely result in a relief of suffering from neurotic, psychosomatic, or borderline symptoms. It also fosters:

- democratization and communication between equals;
- confrontation with the otherness of the other;
- tolerance and an acceptance of the value of diversity;
- differentiation and individuation of each group member within his/her 'own' groups and in relation to other groups.

Thus through sharing, reciprocity, tolerance, and solidarity with the suffering of the other, groups develop a wealth of resources for human development and growth.

References

Agazarian, Y. M. (1989). Group-as-a-whole system theory and practice. *Group*, **13**, 131–54.

Agazarian, Y. M. (1997). *Systems-centered therapy for groups.* New York: Guilford Press.

Bateman, A. W. and Fonagy, P. (2000). Effectiveness of psychotherapeutic treatment of personality disorder. *British Journal of Psychiatry*, **177**, 138–43.

Bender, L. (1937). Group activities in a children's ward as methods of psychotherapy. *American Journal of Psychiatry*, **93**, 1151–73.

Beutler, L. E., *et al.* (1991). Predictors of differential response to cognitive, experiential, and self-directed psychotherapeutic procedures. *Journal of Consulting and Clinical Psychology*, **59**(2), 333–40.

Beutler, L. E., *et al.* (1993). Differential patient treatment maintenance among cognitive, experiential, and self directed psychotherapies. *Journal of Psychotherapy Integration*, **3**, 15–31.

Bion, W. R. (1960). *Experiences in groups*. New York: Basic Books.

Burlingame, G. M., MacKenzie, K. R., and Strauß, B. (2001). Zum aktuellen Stand der Gruppenpsychotherapieforschung I: Allgemeine Effekte von Gruppenpsychotherapien und Effekte störungsspezifischer Gruppenbehandlungen. *Zeitschrift für Gruppenpsychotherapie und Gruppendynamik*, **37**, 299–318.

Burlingame, G. M., MacKenzie, K. R., and Strauß, B. (2002). Zum aktuellen Stand der Gruppenpsychotherapieforschung: II Effekte von Gruppenpsychotherapie als Bestandteil komplexer Behandlungsansätze. *Zeitschrift für Gruppenpsychotherapie und Gruppendynamik*, **38**, 5–32.

Burrow, T. (1928). The basis of group analysis or the analysis of the reactions of normal and neurotic individuals. *British Journal of Medical Psychology*, **8**, 198–206.

Carter, D. (2002). Research and survive? A critical question for group analysis. *Group Analysis*, **35**, 119–34.

Dalal, F. (1998). *Taking the group seriously*. London: Jessica Kingsley.

Dies, R. R. (1993). Research on group psychotherapy: overview and clinical applications. In: A. Alonso and H. J. Swiller, ed. *Group therapy in clinical practice*, pp. 489–90. Washington, DC: American Psychiatric Press.

Dolan, B. M., *et al.* (1996). Cost-offset following specialist treatment of severe personality disorders. *Psychiatric Bulletin*, **20**, 413–17.

Dreikurs, R. (1932). Early experiments with group psychotherapy. *American Journal of Psychotherapy*, **13**, 882–91.

Elias, N. (1987). *Die Gesellschaft der Individuen*. Frankfurt: Suhrkamp.

Elliot, A. (1999). *Social theory and psychoanalysis in transition*, pp. 46–76. London: Free Association Books.

Enke, H. (1965). Bipolare Gruppentherapie als Möglichkeit psychoanalytischer Arbeit in der stationären Psychotherapie. *Zeitschrift für Psychotherapie, Psychosomatik und Medizinische Psychologie*, **15**, 116.

Ettin, M. (1999). *Foundations and applications of group psychotherapy. A sphere of influence*, pp. 72–8. London: Jessica Kingsley.

Ezriel, H. (1973). Psychoanalytic group therapy. In: L. Wolberg and E. Schwartz, ed. *Group therapy 1973: an overview*. New York: Stratton Intercontinental Medical Books.

Fiedler, P. (1996). *Verhaltenstherapie mit Gruppen*. Weinheim: Psychologie-Verlagsunion.

Foulkes, S. H. (1948). *Introduction to group-analytic psychotherapy*. London: Heineman.

Foulkes, S. H. (1964). *Therapeutic group analysis*. London: Allen & Unwin.

Foulkes, S. H. (1971). Access to unconscious processes in the group-analytic group. In: *Selected Papers*, pp. 209–21. London: Karnac Books (first published in *Group Analysis* (1971), **4**, 4–14).

Foulkes, S. H. (1975). *Group analytic psychotherapy: methods and principals*. London: Gordon & Breach.

Foulkes, S. H. and Anthony, E. J. (1965). *Group psychotherapy: the psychoanalytic approach*, 2nd edn. Baltimore, MD: Penguin Books.

Free, L. M. (1999). *Cognitive therapy in groups. Guidelines and resources for practice*. Chichester: John Wiley & Sons.

Freud, S. (1921/1955). *Group psychology and the analysis of the ego*. In: J Strachey, ed. and trans *Standard edition of the complete psychological works of Sigmund Freud*, Vol. 18, pp. 65–143. London: Hogarth Press.

Goldstein, K. (1934; reprinted 1995). *The organism*. London: Zone Books.

Hall, Z. M. and Mullee, M. (2000). Undertaking psychotherapy research. *Group Analysis*, **33**(3), 319–32.

Heigl-Evers, A. and Heigl, F. S. (1973). Gruppentherapie: interaktionell, tiefenpsychologisch–fundiert (analytisch orientiert), psychoanalytisch. *Zeitschrift für Gruppenpsychotherapie und Gruppendynamik*, **7**, 132–57.

Heintzel, R., Beyer, F., and Klein, T. (2000). Out-patient psychoanalytic individual and group psychotherapy in a nationwide catamnestic study in Germany. *Group Analysis*, **33**, 353–72.

Janssen, P. L. (1985). Integrative analytische psychotherapeutische Krankenhausbehandlung. *Forum der Psychoanalyse*, p. 298 ff.

Kadden, R. M., *et al.* (1989). Matching alcoholics to coping skills or interactional therapies: posttreatment results. *Journal of Consulting and Clinical Psychology*, **57**, 680–704.

Kadden, R. M., *et al.* (2001). Prospective matching of alcoholic clients to cognitive-behavioral or interactional group therapy. *Journal of Studies on Alcohol*, **62**, 359–69.

Knauss, W. (1985). The treatment of psychosomatic illnesses in group-analytic psychotherapy—indications and contra-indications. *Group Analysis*, **XVIII/3**, 177–90.

Knauss, W. (1994). Abstinenz: Grenze oder Schranke in der gruppenanalytischen Ausbildung. In: W. Knauss and U. Keller, ed. *9th European symposium in group analysis 'boundaries and barriers'*. Heidelberg: Mattes-Verlag.

Knauss, W. (1999). The creativity of destructive fantasies. *Group Analysis*, **32**(3), 397–411.

Knauss, W. (2001). Gruppenanalyse in der stationären Psychotherapie. *Gruppenanalyse*, **11**, 77–86.

Kordy, H. and Senf, W. (1992). Therapieabbrecher in geschlossenen Gruppen. *Zeitschrift für Psychotherapie, Psychosomatik und Medizinische Psychologie*, **42**, 127–35.

Laing, R. D. (1974). *Die Politik der Familie*. Cologne: Kiepenheuer und Witsch.

Lazell, E. W. (1921). The group treatment of dementia praecox. *Psychoanalytic Review*, **8**, 168–79.

Levin, K. (1951). *Field theory in social science*. New York: Harper & Row.

Liebermann, R. (1971). Reinforcement of cohesiveness in group therapy: behavioural and personality changes. *Archives of General Psychiatry*, **25**, 168–77.

Lorentzen, S. (2000). Assessment of change after long-term psychoanalytic group treatment. *Group Analysis*, **33**, 373–96.

Main, T. (1981). Das Konzept der Therapeutischen Gemeinschaft. In: H. Hilpert *et al.*, ed. *Psychotherapie in der Klinik*, pp. 46–66. Heidelberg-Berlin: Springer.

Marsh, L. C. (1933). Group treatment of the psychosis by the psychological equivalent of revival. *Mental Hygiene*, **15**, 328–49.

Marziali, E., Muroe-Blum, H., and McCleary, L. (1997). The contribution of group cohesion and group alliance to the outcome of group psychotherapy. *International Journal of Group Psychotherapy*, **47**(4), 475–9.

McKisack, C. and Waller, G. (1997). Factors influencing the outcome of group psychotherapy for bulimia nervosa. *International Journal of Eating Disorder*, **22**, 1–13.

McRoberts, C., Burlingame, G. M., and Hoag, M. J. (1998). Comparative efficacy of individual and group psychotherapy: a meta-analytic perspective. *Group Dynamics*, **2**, 101–17.

Nitsun, M. (1996). *The anti-group*. London: Routledge.

Pines, M. (1982). Reflections on mirroring. Reprint in: M. Pines (1998). *Circular reflections*. London: Jessica Kingsley.

Pines, M. and Schlapobersky, J. (2000). Group methods in adult psychiatry. In: M. Gelder, L. Lopez-Ibor Junior, and N. Andreasen, ed. *New Oxford textbook of psychiatry*, Vol. 2, pp. 1442–62. Oxford: Oxford University Press.

Piper, W. F., Debbane, E. G., Bienvenue, J. P., and Garant, J. (1984). A comparative study of four forms of psychotherapy. *Journal of Consultant and Clinical Psychology*, **52**, 268–79.

Piper, W. E., McCallum, M., Joyce, A. S., and Rosie, J. S. (1992). *Adaptation to loss through short-term group psychotherapy*. New York: Guilford Press.

Piper, W. E., Joyce, J. S., and Azim, H. F. A. (1996a). *Time-limited day treatment for personality disorders: interpretation of research design and practice in a group program*. Washington, DC: American Psychological Association.

Piper, W. E., *et al.* (1996b). *Time-limited day treatment for personality disorders: integration of research design and practice in a group program*. Washington, DC: American Psychological Association.

Piper, W. E., MacCallum, M., Joyce, A. S., and Rosie, J. S. (2001). Patient personality and time-limited group psychotherapy for complicated grief. *International Journal of Group Psychotherapy*, **51**, 211–39.

Pratt, J. H. (1908). Results obtained in the treatment of pulmonary tuberculosis. *British Medical Journal*, **2**, 1070–71.

Pratt, J. H. (1922/1963). The tuberculosis class. An experiment in home treatment. Reprint in M. Rosenbaum and M. Berger, ed. *Group psychotherapy and group function*, pp. 111–12. New York: Basic Books.

Roth, A. and Fonagy, P. (1996). *What works for whom? A critical review of the psychotherapy research*. New York: Guilford Press.

Rutan, J. S. and Stone, W. N. (2001). *Psychodynamic group psychotherapy*, 3rd edn. New York: Guilford Press.

Sandahl, C., et al. (1998). Time-limited group psychotherapy for moderately alcohol dependent patients: a randomized controlled clinical trial. *Journal for Psychotherapy Research*, **8**, 361–78.

Sandahl, C., et al. (2000). Does the group conductor make a difference? communication patterns in group-analytically and cognitive behaviourally oriented therapy groups. *Group Analysis*, **33**(3), 333–52.

Salvendy, J. T. (1993). Selection and preparation of patients in organisation of the group. In: H. J. Kaplan and B. J. Sadock, ed. *Comprehensive group psychotherapy*, 3rd edn, pp. 72–84. Baltimore, MD: Williams & Wilkins.

Schilder, P. (1936). The analysis of ideologies as a psychotherapeutic method, especially in group treatment. *American Journal of Psychiatry*, **93**, 601–15.

Schilder, P. (1940). Introductory remarks on groups. *Journal of Social Psychology*, **12**, 83–100.

Seidler, G. H. (1997). From object-relations theory to the theory of alterity: shame as an intermediary between the interpersonal world and the world of psychic structure. *American Journal of Psychotherapy*, **51**, 343–56.

Seidler, G. H. (2000a). *In others' eyes. An analysis of shame*. Madison, WI: International Universities Press.

Seidler, G. H. (2000b). The self-relatedness construct: empirical verification via observation in the context of inpatient group therapy. *Group Analysis*, **33**, 413–32.

Soldz, S., Budman, S., and Demby, A. (1992). The relationship between main actor behaviors and treatment outcome in group psychotherapy. *Psychotherapy Research*, **2**, 52–62.

Steuer, J., et al. (1984). Cognitive-behavioral and psychodynamic group psychotherapy in treatment of geriatric depression. *Journal of Consulting and Clinical Psychology*, **52**, 180–92.

Strauß, B. (1992). Empirische Untersuchungen zur stationären Gruppentherapie. *Zeitschrift für Gruppenpsyhotherapie und Gruppendynamik*, **28**, 125–49.

Tschuschke, V. (1993). *Wirkfaktoren stationärer Gruppenpsychotherapie. Prozess—Ergebnis—Relationen*. Göttingen: Vandenhoeck und Ruprecht.

Tschuschke, V. (1999a). Gruppentherapie versus Einzeltherapie—gleich wirksam?(Individual versus Group Psychotherapy—Equally Effective?). *Zeitschrift für Gruppenpsychotherapie und Gruppendynamik*, **35**(4), 257–76.

Tschuschke, V. (1999b). Empirische Studien mit verhaltenstherapeutischen und psychoanalytischen Gruppenpsychotherapie-Behandlungen. Ein Literatur-Überblick. *Praxis Klinisch Verhaltensmedizin und Rehabilitation*, **48**, 11–17.

Tschuschke, V. and Anbet, T. (2000). Early treatment effects of long-term out-patient group therapies—preliminary results. *Group Analysis*, **33**, 397–412.

Tschuschke, V. and Dies, R. R. (1994). Intensive analysis of therapeutic factors and outcome in long-term inpatient groups. *International Journal of Group Psychotherapy*, **44**, 183–214.

Valbak, K. (2003). Specialised psychotherapeutic group analysis: how do we make group analysis suitable for 'non-suitable' patients. *Group Analysis*, **36**, 73–86.

Wender, L. (1940). Group psychotherapy: The study of its applications. *Psychological Quarterly*, **14**, 708–18.

Whitaker, D. S. and Liebermann, M. A. (1964). *Psychotherapy through the group process*. New York: Atherton Press.

Whiteley, S. (1994). Attachment, loss and the space between: personality disorder in the therapeutic community. *Group Analysis*, **27**(4), 359–82.

Winnicott, D. W. (1980). *Playing and reality*. London: Penguin Press.

Wolf, A. (1949). The psychoanalysis of groups I. *American Journal of Psychotherapy*, **3**, 525–58.

Yalom, I. D. (1970/1985). *The theory and practice of group psychotherapy*, 1st edn. New York: Basic Books (1985, 3rd edn, New York: Basic Books).

Zinkin, L. (1983). Malignant mirroring. *Group Analysis*, **16**, 113–26.

5 Cognitive-behavioral group interventions

David W. Coon, Gia Robinson Shurgot, Zoë Gillispie,
Veronica Cardenas, and Dolores Gallagher-Thompson

This research was supported through the Resources for Enhancing Alzheimer's Caregiver Health (REACH) project, which is funded by the National Institute on Aging (grant no. AG 13289) to DGT, Principal Investigator at this site. Writing of this manuscript was also partly supported by the Office of Academic Affiliations, VA Special MIRECC Fellowship Program in Advanced Psychiatry and Psychology, Department of Veterans Affairs.

Introduction and background

Over the past three decades, cognitive-behavioral therapy (CBT) building on many empirical studies has evolved into one of the predominant forces in psychotherapeutic practice (e.g., Mahoney, 1974; Norcross, 1986; Sanderson and Woody, 1995; Chambless *et al.*, 1996; DeRubeis and Crits-Cristoph, 1998; Nathan and Gorman, 1998; Chambless and Hollon, 1998; Young *et al.*, 2001). More important with regard to the current chapter is the mounting evidence demonstrating the efficacy and utility of cognitive, behavioral, and combined CBT approaches in the group treatment of a variety of mental health problems for a range of age groups (White and Freeman, 2000). For example, this evidence is growing for the treatment of anxiety disorders in children (Silverman *et al.*, 1999; Muris *et al.*, 2002), including posttraumatic stress disorder in Latino immigrant children (Kataoka *et al.*, 2003), and social phobia in adolescents (Hayward *et al.*, 2000; Garcia *et al.*, 2002). Recent research also supports the use of CBT group protocols with adults to treat generalized anxiety disorder (Dugas *et al.*, 2003), obsessive-compulsive disorder (Cordieli *et al.*, 2003), insomnia (Backhaus *et al.*, 2001), and social anxiety in schizophrenics (Halperin *et al.*, 2000), as well as psychological distress in both Chinese HIV patients (Molassiotis *et al.*, 2002) and patients with irritable bowel syndrome (Tkachuk *et al.*, 2003).

Although several recent literature reviews and meta-analyses (e.g., Gatz *et al.*, 1998; Teri and McCurry, 2000; Pinquart and Sörensen, 2001; Sörensen *et al.*, 2003) have helped synthesize many of the successful outcome studies that use CBT with older adult clients, the majority of CBT-based outcome studies and clinical case examples in the treatment literature on older clients are based on individual treatment models. These successful treatment protocols range from later life depression (e.g., Fry, 1984; Steuer *et al.*, 1984; Scogin *et al.*, 1987; Thompson *et al.*, 1987, 2001; Gallagher-Thompson and Steffen, 1994) and generalized anxiety disorder (e.g., Stanley *et al.*, 2003; Wetherell *et al.*, 2003), to sleep disorders (e.g., Morin *et al.*, 1993, 1994; McCurry *et al.*, 1998; Gatz *et al.*, 1998), and family caregiver distress (e.g., Gallagher-Thompson *et al.*, 2000a, 2003; Coon *et al.*, 2003a,b). Despite a limited number of studies focused on group CBT with older adults, there is a growing interest in the development and use of group CBT interventions with older populations to take advantage of some of the inherent benefits of this treatment approach (White and Freeman, 2000; DeVries and Coon, 2002).

In this chapter, we provide an introduction to the use of CBT-based group interventions. We begin by discussing key advantages supporting the rationale of CBT group work with clients and highlight basic CBT techniques that are easily adapted for groups. We then build on these concepts by presenting the essential components of an empirically supported CBT protocol that was developed through our clinical experience and intervention research at the Older Adult and Family Center (OAFC) of the Veterans Affairs Palo Alto Health Care System and Stanford University School of Medicine. This individually based protocol has been easily be adapted for group work with older clients and some of its key components have also been modified and used successfully in psychoeducational skill-building classes for depressed older adults and family caregivers of frail or cognitively impaired elders. To illustrate further these protocols, we include a case example from our clinical intervention research experience conducting CBT-based psychoeducational classes with dementia family caregivers. The chapter closes with a review of several issues that warrant future consideration in both clinical intervention research and clinical practice involving CBT-based group work.

Rationale for cognitive-behavioral therapy group interventions

Toseland, in his book *Group Work with the Elderly and Family Caregivers* (1995), identifies several benefits of group interventions. While his book focuses on older adults and their families, most of the benefits he outlines are easily applicable to other populations: (1) groups have the potential for providing a sense of belonging and affiliation that can help counter social isolation and loneliness and bolster social support; (2) group treatment provides a more objective and emotionally detached perspective that can help clients put problematic experiences in perspective; and (3) group participation offers an opportunity for participants to have their experiences validated and affirmed.

In addition to these aspects, we find that CBT group interventions in particular can provide several advantages for both clients and therapists in comparison not only with individual CBT interventions, but also to groups grounded in other theoretical orientations. CBT groups, which emphasize the development and practice of new coping skills, are less likely to feel stigmatizing to clients with a variety of backgrounds. Sharing perceptions and reactions to their situations allows group members to see that they are not suffering alone and that other people face similar problems, including similar challenges in the development and practice of skills necessary in overcoming their negative mood states (DeVries and Coon, 2002). Moreover, a CBT group format typically helps to empower its members to adopt the belief that self-control of thoughts, behaviors, and feelings is not only desirable, but possible. In many cases, CBT group therapy may provide the first opportunity for many clients to obtain constructive feedback on their behavior from their peers (Freeman *et al.*, 1993), and these interventions allow their members to engage in multiple roles in which they can both give and receive support in the development and implementation of new skills designed to alleviate their distress. This can encourage participants to develop addition interpersonal skills useful in the treatment of most disorders by helping them to learn to give and receive appropriate feedback, and to consider a range of alternative perspectives, creative ideas, and insights (Toseland, 1995; DeVries and Coon, 2002).

CBT group settings also promote collaboration through a number of procedures, including goal setting, agenda setting, role-playing, and creation of homework exercises (Freeman et al., 1993; White, 2000). The collaborative process that occurs in groups also works to combat the resistance that sometimes surfaces in individual therapy. An example of this form of resistance is demonstrated through complaints such as: 'You [the therapist] don't understand what I am going through.' Groups often help overcome this type of resistance as it is much more difficult for older clients to ignore the evidence of their peer participants who have had similar experiences (Freeman et al., 1993). CBT groups can also effectively balance individual and group needs by allowing clients to collaborate actively with leaders and other group members to individualize strategies to better meet the nuances of their situations and experiences (Thompson et al., 2000).

Groups also aid the therapist in other ways such as providing a more accurate assessment of participants' behavioral patterns and coping skills, including their repertoire of interpersonal responses such as the ability to be assertive and give and receive feedback. In groups, therapists do not have to depend solely on client self-reports of how others react to them (Freeman et al., 1993; White, 2000). Finally, group CBT, from a practical perspective, may be a more economical and time effective way to deliver treatment by helping organizations and their clinicians to provide services more quickly to more clients at any one time (Coon et al., 1999; Thompson et al., 2000).

Cognitive-behavioral therapy group interventions: general issues, procedures, and strategies

Most studies investigating the effectiveness of group CBT interventions for the treatment of distress have focused on two types of group approaches: traditional and psychoeducational groups (e.g., Yost et al., 1986; Beutler et al., 1987; Teri and McCurry, 2000; Thompson et al., 2000; DeVries and Coon, 2002). Both approaches use similar techniques, but there are important distinctions between them that are worth highlighting. In psychoeducational groups, sessions are highly structured, with specific topics predetermined for each meeting. The length of time for the treatment is planned to correspond to the amount of material to be covered, and specific, individual issues of the participants are addressed only to the degree that they are relevant to the material presented. In more traditional CBT groups, however, there is more emphasis on the individual problems of each client, with more flexibility in the issues being addressed in the group, which allows for more tailoring of topics, examples, particular intervention techniques, group examples, and homework strategies designed to meet the needs of individual participants (Thompson et al., 2000).

Despite these differences, both psychoeducational and traditional therapy groups are grounded in cognitive and behavioral theories that emphasize the acquisition of various cognitive and behavioral skills for the management of negative emotions. Although the exact strategies and techniques introduced during a group will depend in part on the intended focus of the intervention, there are a few strategies and related tools that are typically viewed as cornerstones to the effective implementation of CBT. In the Introduction to Cognitive-behavioral group therapy for specific problems and populations (White and Freeman, 2000), White (2000) provides an excellent review of key methods and strategies commonly used in group CBT. In sum, participants are often taught to maintain records of their automatic thoughts, to recognize unhelpful and dysfunctional beliefs, and to challenge or replace these ideas with more helpful and functional thoughts. Behavioral change strategies are usually highlighted as well, by helping participants learn to monitor their mood, set behavioral goals, track the frequency of targeted behaviors (such as daily pleasant events or other activity monitoring), and to identify and modify antecedents and/or consequences of the targeted behavior to help reinforce behavioral change (Thompson et al., 2000;

White, 2000; DeVries and Coon, 2002). Problem-solving and relaxation strategies (e.g., meditation, imagery, progressive muscle relaxation, breathing exercises, physical exercise, and biofeedback) are also methods commonly incorporated into CBT-based groups. Arousal hierarchies, including descriptions of anxious triggers and the use of graded exposure exercises, are often central to the treatment of anxiety in CBT groups. Regardless of the group's focus, homework assignments are always introduced with each of these methods and strategies to reinforce skill acquisition and provide important examples for group discussion each week. These homework examples can help to not only foster discussion about barriers to skill development, but also provide models of successful paths to goal attainment. The amount of time spent introducing and explaining these CBT strategies to a group tends to decrease gradually after the first few sessions, and more time begins to be spent on addressing the particular problems each individual group member is experiencing.

Many of today's clients in need of mental health treatment represent a diverse population that encompass individuals with various sociocultural histories and cohort experiences; and, therefore, they may differ in their suitability for different types of CBT group interventions. As a result, clinicians need to conduct thorough assessments to be sure a given treatment is appropriate for each individual (see DeVries and Coon, 2002 and Thompson et al., 2000 for assessment suggestions). For instance, many of today's older adults are not acquainted with the process of psychotherapy, and can hold outmoded beliefs about how group content and process can be used to alleviate their emotional distress. Consequently, it is important to socialize these clients into groups by clarifying goals and expectations, explaining the assumptions of the CBT model that will be used in therapy (which often helps demystify the process), and setting ground rules for participation. Considering the wide range of cohorts of older adults (i.e., World War I, Depression Era, World War II, etc.), it is also essential to be sensitive to the language of different client cohorts. Few older adults today have been heavily influenced by pop psychology and the self-help psychology movements. They are less likely to use 'depression' or 'depressed' as self-descriptors, and more likely to use terms such as 'blue' or 'sad' and to reveal somatic complaints such as sleep interruptions and general fatigue often indicative of negative mood states (Gallagher-Thompson and Coon, 1996). There are also sensory changes in hearing and vision associated with normal aging that can affect the learning and retention of material presented, so adaptations of CBT groups with older adults might include using various forms of auditory and visual presentation, slowing the pace of presentation, and frequently repeating and summarizing the material discussed. Many of these issues may also be applicable to other underserved groups (e.g., ethnic minority clients or disabled persons) that face barriers to treatment, including economic, linguistic, or environmental barriers that negatively impact access, and organizational or provider insensitivity to cultural differences that restricts service availability or acceptability.

Finally, the variety and sequencing of specific procedures, strategies, and techniques used in group CBT interventions can vary considerably depending on the clients' problems, ability levels, personality differences, whether a group has a fixed number of sessions or is ongoing, whether it is closed or open to new clients, and whether the group has a specific or general focus. We frequently suggest a closed group run for a fixed time period of approximately 10–12 weekly sessions, during which the focus of the therapy is on the development of several basic skills. Often, these weekly sessions are subsequently followed up by several monthly boosters to reinforce skill development, enhance maintenance of therapeutic gains, and help with relapse prevention. At the end of the group, the clients are evaluated clinically to determine what worked as well as what was not effective for them. Clients then can choose to discontinue therapy, enter a new group with a different problem focus, or repeat the group to continue to strengthen their development of basic skills (Thompson et al., 2000).

The CBT group interventions presented in the remainder of this chapter build on the empirically supported clinical protocols develop by Thompson and Gallagher-Thompson and their colleagues for brief individual CBT with depressed older adults (e.g., Gallagher-Thompson and Steffen, 1994; Thompson et al., 2001; Laidlaw et al., 2003) and distressed family caregivers of cognitively impaired or physically frail older adults (e.g., Coon *et al.*, 2003a; Gallagher-Thompson *et al.*, 2000a, 2001, 2003). These protocols have been implemented over the past two decades with hundreds of older adults and family caregivers at the OAFC of the VA Palo Alto Health Care System and Stanford University School of Medicine. The next two sections of this chapter provide a succinct overview of two types of CBT groups conducted through the OAFC: a CBT group for depressed older adults and a psycho-educational classes conducted with dementia family caregivers. Treatment manuals relevant to these protocols are currently available from Dolores Gallagher-Thompson (Older Adult and Family Center, VA Medical Center, and Stanford University School of Medicine, 795 Willow Road, Mail Code: 182C/MP, Menlo Park, CA 94025, USA. E-mail: dolorest@stanford.edu).

Group cognitive-behavioral therapy for depressed older adults

The manualized, individual OAFC protocol (Dick *et al.*, 1996; Thompson *et al.*, 1996) and our CBT groups for depressed older adults modify and extend the work of Beck (Beck *et al.*, 1979), Lewinsohn (Lewinsohn, 1974; Lewinsohn *et al.*, 1986) and other CBT theorists (Burns, 1980; Young, 1999) to meet the needs of older adult clients. Our work builds on Beck's theory (Beck *et al.*, 1979) that negative thoughts and beliefs lead to the creation of a negative 'lens' through which appraisal of the world is distorted, resulting in automatic erroneous thinking and negative schemas. In this cognitive model of depression, it is proposed that negative schemas interact with negative life events to produce depressive symptomatology. Treatment focuses on modifying unhelpful thoughts to change affect and behavior by teaching clients to identify their negative thinking patterns, and subsequently, to systematically challenge these negative cognitions to foster more adaptive ways of perceiving situations and themselves.

In contrast to Beck, Lewinsohn's theory (Lewinsohn, 1974; Lewinsohn *et al.*, 1986) states that depression is the result of the repeated absence of pleasant events or activities in the person's life. As the number of pleasant or adaptive behaviors decreases in an individual's daily life, the individual experiences fewer positive social interactions and less pleasure, resulting in behavioral withdrawal, which then becomes a vicious downward cycle into depression, where the individual does less, then feels more depressed, and subsequently, does less again. Consequently, CBT teaches clients to recognize the relationship between engagement in pleasant activities and the maintenance of positive mood by encouraging clients to increase everyday pleasant activities so that negative patterns of withdrawal can be eliminated.

As mentioned earlier, an important initial step in group treatment is to begin to socialize clients into the CBT model by describing the general content and format of the group during the initial contact and in the group's first session. For example, our CBT groups for later life depression have a closed format and run for fixed time periods of 16–20 sessions, with each group session lasting 90–120 minutes. Another key first step is to use various examples relevant to older adults to help introduce the CBT model and demonstrate the relationship between thoughts, behavior, and mood. Chapter 1 of our CBT treatment manual (Dick *et al.*, 1996) provides an example of dysfunctional thinking relevant to older clients that we also use to present the CBT model in our depression groups:

> John is a 66-year-old retired, married man who has weekend plan to finish painting his wife's book cases (*behavior*). Unfortunately, he wakes up with his arthritis really bothering him on Saturday morning (*health*) and is unable to complete the project (*behavior*). As a result, he feels angry and frustrated and a little anxious (*emotions*) about not getting to his work, believing that he is disappointing his wife (*thoughts*). He thinks, 'My wife will think that I do not care about helping her decorate the study (*thoughts*)'. This belief raises his anxiety and frustration about not feeling up to par (*emotion*). This makes it harder for John to figure out how to face the day, and consequently he stays in bed (*behavior*), which in turn only serves to raise his anxiety and strengthen his negative thoughts about his wife's reaction. He ends up feeling 'worn out' and 'blue' (*emotions*).

We use this and similar examples to engage clients in discussing what they might have said, how they might have felt in, and how they would have responded in a similar situation. One of CBT's major tenets makes CBT particularly useful for older individuals who are experiencing numerous and substantive losses, as the experience of loss *per se* does not necessarily lead to depression, but rather it is how loses are perceived and what its meaning is to the individual that determines whether or not depressive symptoms will arise (Thompson *et al.*, 2000).

Once clients seem to understand the CBT model through the use of examples such as the case of John, we discuss the primary goal of the group, which is to decrease and eventually eradicate feelings of depression among its group members. We then emphasize the importance of clients' active participation and collaboration in the group by sharing their difficulties with others in the group, engaging in problem solving with others in the group, and completing homework assignments. We also work with clients to identify up to three target complaints to address over the course of treatment. Common issues that older adults choose to address in groups include loneliness, interpersonal difficulties, problems with functioning related to chronic illnesses, inadequate resources, and severe emotional disturbances.

After the initial group meeting, the rest of the group contacts consist of initial instruction or continued elaboration of specific CBT techniques for the therapist to address that week followed by a group discussion of group members' specific issues. At the beginning of each session, clients are asked to discuss their homework assignments and any problems that emerged since the last group meeting. The therapist then works with the clients to determine whether any specific problems should be added to the agenda. Generally, over the course of therapy, each group member will be given the time to discuss each new technique with the group and to obtain feedback from the group to facilitate mastering of a new technique. Whenever a new technique is introduced in a session, demonstration and practice time is set aside before the end of each session to maximize implementation and homework compliance. Homework assignments typically focus on asking group members to practice part or all of the technique just reviewed in session, and to tailor specific group assignments through group discussions to match each group member's individual goals. Clients take an active role in the design of their homework assignments, based on the collaborative nature of our CBT group interventions. Across sessions, successive approximation is used as a tool to remind clients that reaching goals in treatment is not immediate, but rather that requires continued practice and refinement of skills using the homework assignment to try out these skills in their daily lives. Each group session ends with a summary of what was discussed in the group asking for input from members, as well as the solicitation of questions or comments from group members about previous and current strategies, techniques and homework assignments introduced in the group. Our experience has taught us to protect some group time to actively solicit feedback and questions from the group members given that many older adults, compared with younger group members, are often less likely to ask questions even when they need clarification.

Key techniques

There are three techniques we have found to be essential in the effective implementation of group CBT for depressed older adults: (1) mood monitoring; (2) pleasurable activities; and (3) learning to monitor and refute dysfunctional or unhelpful thoughts. The order and presentation of these different techniques should be adjusted to the needs and characteristics of each group, but we typically encourage the use of mood monitoring and increasing pleasant events, as described by Lewinsohn *et al.* (1986), as the first lessons to be covered in group CBT with depressed older adults. Mood monitoring helps clients gain insight into their situations and to recognize when they are not doing well, when they have improved, and what events are associated with their mood changes (Thompson *et al.*, 2000). Without successful mood monitoring, group members may have a difficult time discovering what tools work for them, as well as what situations are most challenging. Moreover, behavioral interventions are often prescribed during the early stages of treatment because cognitive exercises may be more difficult for clients to understand at first (Persons, 1989). In addition, Beck *et al.* (1979) also recommend increasing the activity level of the clients at the beginning of treatment before tackling cognitive change, as the latter can be more successful when an individual is less depressed or when a stronger therapeutic alliance has been established. Finally, the introduction of cognitive interventions are very useful to explore after clients have faced substantive challenges enacting behavioral homework assignments, as cognitive distortions are often a contributing factor toward diminished homework compliance.

Mood monitoring

Through mood monitoring, group members learn that events can affect their mood positively or negatively, which they can increase pleasant events in their lives, and thus, they can control their mood. The Daily Mood Rating Form is a commonly used self-monitoring mood assessment form. This form asks the client to rate his or her mood daily by filling out three columns that ask for the date, a mood score on a scale from 1 (very depressed) to 9 (very happy), and reasons why the client feels a certain way. This completed form is used to facilitate discussion in group therapy sessions, and as a building block to teach the role of pleasurable activities in improving daily mood. Although this may seem like common knowledge, it is often easy to lose sight of this simple relationship, especially if an individual is experiencing a great deal of depression or anxiety. The concrete realization of this association by monitoring mood on a daily basis can often provide the rationale and incentive for attempting to increase pleasurable events or activities (Thompson *et al.*, 2000).

Pleasant events or activities

Increasing pleasurable activities is a technique that serves to quickly improve mood in a group member who has successfully increased the number of pleasant events occurring each day, and to demonstrate to other group members who have been less accepting of this technique that negative emotions can be positively impacted by increasing one's pleasant activities. The success of this technique is contingent upon selecting activities that are pleasurable, that are not being done on a regular basis, and that can be conducted with minimal difficulty. The Older Person's Pleasant Events Schedule (OPPES; Gallagher and Thompson, 1981) is a useful self-report measure to help develop a list of these activities for older adults. The OPPES (Table 5.1; available in both short and long forms) assesses seven domains that may bring pleasure to older clients including experiencing nature, being in social

situations that are pleasant, spending time alone reflecting and meditating, being praised by others for some activity, giving to others, being involved in activities in which competence is demonstrated, and traditional leisure activities. The OPPES helps tap into the frequency with which activities are conducted over the past month and the degree of pleasure derived from the activity, irrespective of whether the older person engaged in that particular activity. Frequency and Pleasantness scores are then each plotted for the seven domains on a simple graph that offers a quick and easy visual display of how frequently activities were engaged in, in comparison with their degree of pleasantness. This graph serves to identify activities that could be increased or decreased, based upon the degree of pleasure each activity provides for the group member. So, if the frequency of highly pleasurable activities falls far below the degree of pleasure derived from these activities, highly pleasurable activities should be increased. In contrast, if highly unpleasant activities are done more frequently, these unpleasant activities can be decreased in favor of more pleasurable ones.

Daily Thought Records

Dysfunctional thoughts seem accurate and realistic to the individual who produces them, but are essentially counterproductive, dysfunctional, and unhelpful, and when examined carefully, represent an individual's underlying irrational beliefs (Persons, 1989). Beck (1972) labeled these dysfunctional or maladaptive thoughts as automatic because they seem to arise spontaneously and automatically without much effort on the part of the individual. Such dysfunctional thoughts support the core beliefs that lead to problems such as depression and anxiety.

Learning to monitor and refute dysfunctional thoughts is a cognitive technique used to teach the relationship between negative thoughts and feelings, based on the premise that negative emotions are derived from the negative thoughts about a particular situation, and that depressed individuals have distorted negative thoughts about specific situations, themselves, and the future. Common cognitive distortions about situations noted in our older adult clients and many of our family caregivers include the following:

◆ *Name calling* attaches a negative label to self or to others. For example, 'I'm a loser,' 'My husband is a bad parent.'

◆ *Tyranny of the shoulds* are rules clients hold about the way things '*should*' be'. For example, 'I should or have to have a clean house before I go out with my women's group from church.'

◆ *Tune in the negative/ tune out the positive* registers and acknowledges only the negative aspects of a situation and ignores or discounts positive accomplishments.

◆ *This or that (no in-betweens)* views situations in terms of very extreme outcomes. For example, 'I'm either a success or a total failure,' or 'I never get things right, I always mess up.'

◆ *Overinterpreting* is the habit of blowing events out of proportion without all the information and takes a small amount of information provided as the 'whole truth' without confirming its validity. This typically occurs in three different ways: (1) generalization draws conclusions with only a few facts; (2) personalization assumes that others have negative intentions toward or views of the client; and (3) emotional thinking uses feelings as the basis for the facts of the situations (i.e., 'I feel this, then it must be true'.)

◆ *What's the use?* Clients believe that their thoughts or behaviors are not ever effective in changing their situations. For example, 'Whenever I plan a pleasant outing, it never goes as planned, so why try at all?'

◆ *If only* means clients are spending time dwelling on past events and wishing they had said or done something differently. A variant of this is the idea: 'If only things were the way they used to be, I could be happy again.' We find this to be one of the most common patterns observed in depressed older adults who cannot imagine their life being meaningful and enjoyable at all given that certain circumstances are unlikely to change dramatically (e.g., getting one's career or spouse or health back

Table 5.1 Sample items from the Older Persons Pleasant Events Schedule

Please circle one number in each column for each item	How often in the past month?*			How pleasant was it or would it have been?†		
Looking at the stars or the moon	0	1	2	0	1	2
Exploring new areas	0	1	2	0	1	2
Meditating	0	1	2	0	1	2
Planning trips or vacations	0	1	2	0	1	2
Gardening	0	1	2	0	1	2
Going to church or religious services	0	1	2	0	1	2
Seeing beautiful scenery	0	1	2	0	1	2
Listening to music	0	1	2	0	1	2

*0 = not at all; 1 = 1–6 times; 2 = 7 or more times. †0 = not pleasant; 1 = somewhat pleasant; 2 = very pleasant.

after an age-associated loss). We have come to see this as a particularly 'dirty trick' older clients can play on themselves (Dick *et al.*, 1996; Coon *et al.*, 1999).

A useful tool to help learn to monitor and refute dysfunctional thoughts is the Daily Thought Record derived from the work of Beck *et al.* (1979). This form allows group members to learn to identify automatic distortions and to develop rational constructions to replace them. We use the three-column version of the Thought Record to provide our clients with practice in monitoring their unhelpful thoughts about situations and to elicit their emotional reactions associated with those thoughts. After clients have learned to use this tool, we teach them a variety of the following techniques to help challenge these unhelpful thoughts:

- *Action* asks clients to engage in specific behaviors to obtain additional information to help challenge unhelpful assumptions about situations or people.

- *Language* asks older client's to change the actual language they use from negative to positive or harsh to compassionate to help replace negative labels and comments with clear, realistic ones.

- *As if* also changes the tone and language of self-talk, and asks clients to speak to themselves as if someone whose opinion they greatly respect is talking to them.

- *Consider alternatives, in-betweens* instructs clients to think of a ruler that has 0 inches at one end and 12 inches at another. Given there are many inches in between as well as even smaller and smaller measurements, group leaders ask clients to consider the range of alternatives.

- *Scale technique* weighs the advantages and the disadvantages of maintaining a particular thought, emotion, or behavior that is linked to the client's distress.

- *Examine consequences* examines the specific consequences for a particular belief, and helps clients to see that they may have less interest in holding on to certain beliefs.

- *Credit positives* tells clients to spend a few moments thinking of the more pleasant outcomes of events, and positive thoughts, and the positive emotional consequences that result, rather than just dwelling on the negative.

- *Positive affirmations* encourages clients to develop some positive, personal statements to say when feeling overwhelmed with negative thoughts and emotions.

We then present a five-column version of the Thought Record to teach clients how to challenge their cognitive distortions and to evaluate the impact of this technique on the intensity of their emotions. Working on Daily Thought Records in the group setting is extremely productive, both for the individual who is presenting the material as well as for the group members who are participating in the development of appropriate challenges for these unproductive automatic thoughts (Thompson *et al.*, 2000).

In addition to teaching these CBT techniques to improve mood, we instruct our clients on how to use a variety of other CBT strategies based on the particulars of the group as well as the individual needs of its members. These include many of the strategies discussed by White (2000) such as various relaxation exercises, problem-solving skills, and other cognitive techniques such as becoming an inquisitive scientist and examining the evidence, to facilitate behavioral changes (see Dick *et al.*, 1996 and Coon *et al.*, 1999). After all the CBT techniques are taught in the group sessions, termination of the group is openly discussed across the final series of group sessions. As part of the termination process, clients review the CBT skills learned in the group, anticipate and delineate potential danger signals, and work in collaboration with the group leader and other group members to create a maintenance guide that includes all the CBT strategies that worked for them while in therapy, as well as step-by-step procedures to follow in case of a depression relapse. These steps include the initial steps to take to improve mood, and then who to contact and where to go if they do not improve after consistently using their skills on their own.

Psychoeducational skill building classes for family caregivers

Taking care of a relative with health problems, especially older care recipients with dementia, can have detrimental mental and physical health effects for caregivers, including depression, anxiety, anger, and increased risk for health problems (Schulz *et al.*, 1995; Bookwala *et al.*, 2000; Vitaliano *et al.*, 2003). Over the last 15 years, Gallagher-Thompson and her colleagues at the OAFC have developed and refined several empirically supported, CBT-based psychoeducational skill building classes for family caregivers to older adults. Several of these protocols have been shown to significantly reduce various forms of caregiver distress such as depressive symptoms, anger/frustration, and negative coping strategies, as well as to enhance caregiver self-efficacy and positive coping strategies in comparison with either wait-list control conditions (e.g., Gallagher-Thompson and DeVries, 1994; Gallagher-Thompson *et al.*, 2000a, 2001; Coon *et al.*, 2003a) or traditional community support groups (Gallagher-Thompson *et al.*, 2003). Moreover, results from recent outcome studies indicate that these psychoeducational skill building classes can be tailored effectively to meet the cultural needs of Latinas caring for family members with dementia (Gallagher-Thompson *et al.*, 2001, 2003).

In this section, we provide a brief overview of these various CBT-based, manualized psychoeducational classes for family caregivers. These classes, in contrast to our CBT groups for depression, focus on teaching caregivers to cope with the stresses of prolonged caregiving by tailoring cognitive and behavioral change strategies to address the personal situations and needs of distressed caregivers, and by bolstering the caregivers' self-management skills through the use of strategies such as relaxation training, problem solving, or increasing pleasant activities in their lives. Generally, these interventions are conducted in small groups (eight to 10 participants), for structured periods of time (2 hours with a 20-minute break for refreshments and socializing), and duration and frequency (8–10 weekly sessions followed by 2–8 monthly booster sessions). A detailed agenda is set at the beginning of each group meeting, specifying the goals of the class. Homework is reviewed at the beginning of each session, then, a brief presentation about a topic or a new skill is conducted. A brief break then follows, which allows for class leaders to help any members who have difficulty understanding the material. After the break, role-plays and discussions of material just presented occurs in small breakout groups or dyads to facilitate learning, to practice the techniques to be used in the following week, and to troubleshoot any potential difficulties in completing homework assignments. Questions are addressed throughout the group meeting. A brief review at the end of the class highlights any problems that arose in the practice and discussions, reiterates the topics or techniques discussed in that week's class, and reminds caregivers of their homework assignments for the upcoming week.

At the OAFC, we have developed several distinct psychoeducational classes specifically designed for family caregivers: (1) a 'Coping with the Blues' class for increasing life satisfaction (Thompson *et al.*, 1992); (2) a 'Coping with Frustration' class to learn to manage anger and frustration (Gallagher-Thompson *et al.*, 1992); and (3) an 'Increasing Problem-Solving Skills Class' based on the theoretical work of D'Zurilla (1986) that teaches a six-step model for problem solving we adapted for caregivers. Although these psychoeducational classes begin in the same manner, they emphasize distinct CBT techniques to help address different feelings and issues. For instance, the 'Coping with Frustration' class targets caregivers' feelings of anger, frustration, and/or hostility by teaching cognitive techniques, self-talk, and active listening and assertive communication techniques to deal with daily stressors. The emphasis of this class is on learning to identify and modify thoughts that foster feelings of frustration, as well as learning to express feelings appropriately by being assertive in order to reduce the counterproductive use of aggressive or passive communication styles in frustrating situations. In contrast, the 'Coping with the Blues' class contains several components similar to those found in our CBT groups for depressed older adults. This class focuses on addressing feelings of depression by introducing behavioral techniques such as mood monitoring, and helping caregivers

Table 5.2 Coping with Caregiving Psychoeducational Skill Building Class and related homework assignments

	Goals	Homework
Phase 1		
Class 1	Overview of dementia, understanding frustration and caregiver stress, practicing relaxation.	Daily relaxation practice and relaxation diary.
Class 2–4	Identifying antecedents, beliefs, and consequences of frustrating caregiving situations. Identifying unhelpful thoughts about caregiving, changing unhelpful thoughts into adaptive thoughts and linking to new adaptive behaviors.	Relaxation practice and relaxation diary, daily thought records and behavior logs.
Phase 2		
Class 5–6	Understanding different types of communication styles and practicing how to be more assertive in caregiving situations, with professionals and with family members.	Practice assertive communication and Assertiveness Practice Sheet. Daily relaxation practice and daily thought records.
Phase 3		
Class 6–9	Understanding depressive symptoms, and monitoring mood. Identifying and tracking pleasant events and activities, and understanding and overcoming personal barriers to increasing pleasant events to help improve mood. Identify pleasant events to do with care recipient.	Daily mood rating, pleasant events tracking form including obstacles to events. Relaxation diary.
Class 10	Review of major skills taught, listing of problem areas in which skills can be used in the future. Identification of most relevant skills for participants' particular caregiving situations. Discussion of termination and review booster agendas.	Encourage use of all homework, especially that identified as most relevant for caregivers' particular situations.
Phase 4		
8 monthly boosters	Maintain skills learned and fine tune skills.	Apply skills and use homework material and strategies in everyday situations and as new stressors develop.

develop a plan to increase pleasant events in their lives by creating a potential list of pleasant activities, and discussing barriers to adding these pleasant activities into their busy schedules.

More recently our 'Coping with Caregiving' (CWC) class (Gallagher-Thompson *et al.*, 1996) adopted the most useful aspects of these preceding classes and was culturally tailored to help reduce psychological distress among both Latinas and Caucasian female caregivers. Results of a study of 122 Caucasian women and 91 Latinas randomly assigned to either CWC or a traditionally based community support group demonstrated the superiority of the CBT-based CWC class for both groups of women (Gallagher-Thompson *et al.*, 2003). The CWC teaches a limited number of CBT mood management skills through two key approaches that are drawn primarily from the work of Beck (Beck *et al.*, 1979) and Lewinsohn *et al.* (1986). First, an emphasis is placed on reducing the negative affect by teaching caregivers how to relax in stressful situations, appraise the care recipient's behavior more realistically, identify and challenge unhelpful thinking, and communicate more assertively. Second, an emphasis is placed on increasing positive mood through the acquisition of such skills as seeing the contingency between mood and activities, developing strategies to do smaller, everyday pleasant activities, and learning to set self-change goals and reward oneself for accomplishments along the way. Table 5.2 outlines the CWC's key phases and classes and presents their related goals and homework assignments. Although these various psychoeducational classes for caregivers emphasize different cognitive and behavioral techniques during the intensive phase of the treatment, they all end by reviewing and reinforcing the skills taught in class and identifying and discussing problem areas that caregivers think they might face and how they can apply their skills effectively in those future situations.

Homework assignments in group interventions

Homework remains an essential part of group CBT, just as it does in individual treatment. A growing amount of empirical research demonstrates that homework can facilitate therapeutic improvement (e.g., Neimeyer and Feixas, 1990; Burns and Spangler, 2000; Kazantzis *et al.*, 2000), and some of our own empirical work suggests that homework compliance is a significant predictor of treatment outcomes with older adult clients (e.g., Thompson and Gallagher, 1984; Coon and Thompson, 2003). Therefore, we remind therapists to consider that no matter how many insights and changes occur during the session, group members will not solve their problems or improve their depression unless significant cognitive and behavioral changes are made outside of treatment as well. Alleviation of later life distress comes through practicing skills learned in therapy out in the real world by using homework assignments to try out new ways of thinking and more adaptive behaviors (Persons, 1989; White, 2000; Coon and Gallagher-Thompson, 2002; Coon *et al.*, in press).

However, the design of effective homework assignments requires substantial patience, persistence, problem solving, and advance planning on the part of both the group's leader and the group participants to successfully dismantle attitudinal and logistical barriers to its completion. We find that the most effective homework assignments are those that are closely tied to client target complaints and treatment goals, that build on in-session themes, and that are perceived by the older clients as both realistic and important to complete. It is also crucial to allow the group to maintain an active role in making homework decisions, demonstrating CBT's collaborative approach in which the group works together to help one another reach their treatment goals (Thompson *et al.*, 2000). If a high level of teamwork and cooperation are not achieved, group members may lose interest and motivation, or become resentful. Therapists must also quickly establish homework as a priority and foster ongoing adherence from the very beginning of the group. The consistent presence of homework on each session's agenda, both in terms of the review of previously assigned homework as well as the development and reinforcement of next week's assignment sends the right message to clients about its importance and potential utility. Difficulties with homework are likely to increase if the group members are not held accountable for any lack of participation in homework assignments (Thompson *et al.*, 2000; Coon and Gallagher-Thompson, 2002).

Numerous factors can arise and impact homework compliance from practical barriers such as illness and overextension of responsibilities, to memory problems or concerns from the older adult about taking up time in the group to ask for further clarification on an assignment (Coon *et al.*, in press). Some other beliefs that can interfere with homework compliance are the fear that others will require the client to do things that are not actually in the client's best interest or that homework is not a necessary part of the psychotherapeutic process (Persons, 1989). These types of beliefs provide insight into the distortions a client may bring to a group. Another reason for homework noncompliance may be that some group participants are embarrassed to ask questions when they do not understand an assignment, especially in the initial stages of the therapy (Thompson *et al.*, 2000). Often depressed individuals may feel so hopeless that they do not want to try homework assignments because they believe they will not work, or because failure is considered 'certain' (Thompson *et al.*, 2000). It also can be important to use alternative terms for homework assignments as necessary to foster compliance. For some clients, particularly those with little formal education or who performed poorly in school, homework can hold unpleasant connotations or be construed as demeaning. And, homework may increase worry on the part of disabled persons or older adults with sensory limitations that impact reading and writing assignments if modifications have not been introduced and discussed. Therefore, we always encourage therapists and group leaders to collaborate with clients to find more acceptable terms for homework using the group's own language and experience as a backdrop for the discussion. Finding terms such as 'experiments', 'practice sheets', 'journal writing', or 'mind exercise' can help reduce concerns about criticism and support homework completion (Coon *et al.*, in press).

Any difficulty with homework should be addressed immediately in order for the group to be as helpful as possible for its members. We find it is essential to problem-solve with the clients from the very beginning rather than labeling these difficulties as resistance. If clients avoid homework, we engage them in dialogues around the homework tasks and problem-solve to find strategies to foster completion and support skill development. Discussions also should transmit the idea that improvement requires substantive efforts by the client, rather than just the therapist alone (Persons, 1989). One of the most useful and successful ways to combat homework noncompliance is to engage the entire group in helping to figure out how homework assignments can help them (Thompson *et al.*, 2000). Finally, more detailed discussions regarding the use of homework with older adults, including ways to facilitate homework completion and address issues of noncompliance, are available in the literature (Coon and Gallagher-Thompson, 2002; Coon *et al.*, in press).

A case illustration

Latinas Unidas Cuidando y Hablando Abiertamente (Latinas United Caring and Speaking Openly; Gallagher-Thompson *et al.*, 2002), a psychoeducational skill-building class for Latinas caring for loved ones with memory loss met at a local adult day healthcare center, and consisted of six Latina family dementia caregivers and two female co-facilitators. Each participant agreed to attend a total of 13 weekly 2-hour sessions. English was the primary language spoken but occasionally the participants spoke in Spanish to better describe certain thoughts and emotions. Only one caregiver will be described in detail for the purposes of this case illustration, although each participant was asked to attend all of the classes and complete and discuss each of the homework activities described. Please note that the names and details of the class participants have been modified sufficiently to protect their privacy and maintain confidentiality.

One of the participants, Valeria, is a 57-year-old Latina caring for her 64-year-old husband, Ernesto. Ernesto was diagnosed with Alzheimer's disease a little over a year ago, and in this short period of time, he had his driver's license revoked and had lost contact with many of his friends. Valeria came to the group stating that even after 25 years of marriage, she was having a difficult time understanding Ernesto's behavior. The couple's 18-year-old grandson also lives with them, however, he provides very minimal assistance with Ernesto's care.

The first class session explained the goals and guidelines of the group and provided an overview of memory loss and dementia. The caregivers were taught how to rate their current level of stress/tension and were asked to participate in the first of a series of relaxation exercises designed to reduce their stress. Valeria responded well to the class information and willingly completed the homework assignments or *home practice* activities given at the end of each class.

During the second session, the class facilitators with Valeria's permission the Behavior Log (see Table 5.3) see completed as part of her home practice activities on to the whiteboard for the other caregivers to see and use as a way to reinforce their own skill development. Valeria shared with the group how bothered she is when her husband wakes up each morning, and asks her repeatedly 'Where is my grandson?' Although Valeria explains to him that their grandson has left for work, 15 minutes later he looks out of the window at the driveway, notices their grandson's car is missing, and asks Valeria again about their grandson's whereabouts. By the end of the day, Ernesto has asked the same question at least 10 times.

The facilitators asked the class members to brainstorm triggers that might cause or encourage Ernesto's behavior and to provide suggestions to Valeria about what she might change in the environment to eliminate or at least decrease her husband's repetitive questions:

Alicia: I know what you mean when you say it bothers you to hear the same question over and over. That always drives me crazy when my mom does this.

Table 5.3 Behavior log

Please use this log to write down the things your relative does that you would like to change. Or, record each time you do something (associated with caregiving) that increases your stress.

Date/day of Week	Time	Behavior (what your relative does)	How did you feel when this happened?
Monday thru Friday when our grandson goes to work.	When he first wakes up at 10 a.m., then again at about 10.15 a.m., 12.00 p.m.	My husband will ask me over and over where our grandson is. I have to constantly tell him that he is at work.	The first time I have to answer him does not bother me as much. But by the second and third time, I feel angry with him for not remembering what I have said.

Josefina: My husband sometimes does this to me but it does not bother me as much because I try to remind myself that this is part of the disease. They easily can just forget what they heard 5 minutes ago.

Adriana: I have found that something that has helped me is when I leave my husband a note with the information he wants. Just take a yellow post it note and stick it on the window stating: 'Our grandson is at work.'

Josefina: Maybe what he needs is for your grandson to come and say goodbye to him before he leaves to work. If he is asleep, maybe he can leave him a note at his bedside.

Valeria: That is a good idea. I also like the idea of the post it note on the window. I think I might try that.

Facilitator: Yes, these are all good suggestions. Valeria, please continue to complete the behavior log at home and let us know if anything changes.

During a subsequent session when caregivers were asked to complete a more a detailed behavior log for home practice, Valeria volunteered to share her responses (see Table 5.4). She was feeling frustrated and angry because Ernesto continued to insist on wearing the same clothes day after day. The facilitator reminded Valeria and the other caregivers that changing behavior often involves a lot of trial and error, and asked the class once again to brainstorm possible alternative strategies for Valeria to try in the weeks ahead. The group came up with the following four strategies for her to add to her toolbox:

1. Set out fresh clothes for him and reward him when he wears it. Maybe give him a compliment on how nice he looks or make him his favorite breakfast.

2. Hide the outfit he really likes in a place where he cannot find it.

3. Buy him several pairs of the same pants and shirt so that he thinks he is wearing his favorite outfit.

4. When he goes to bed, take his clothes and put them in the laundry machine. Set the machine on the soak cycle so that if he looks for them and notices that they are wet, he will be forced to find something else to wear.

Valeria liked the ideas given by the facilitator and caregivers and agrees to try some of them out. She returns the next week with the completed homework assignment that appears in Table 5.5. Although her husband got irritated after she tried the strategy of putting his clothes in the washer to soak, he did seem to get over it fairly quickly, and then decided it was OK to wear a different outfit.

For the next few weeks, Valeria continued to attend the sessions and participate in the discussions, role-plays, and relaxation exercises. She got along well with all of the women and began to take more risks and open up about her thoughts and feelings. Perhaps the most emotional class meeting for Valerie occurred in Class 7 when she shared that she was 'feeling lousy because Ernesto had lost all of their money.' She was feeling a mixture of anger and guilt, but was having difficulty challenging her unhelpful thoughts about the situation. The facilitator asked Valeria if she would complete a Thought Record with the help of the group regarding this specific situation. Valeria agreed and allowed the facilitator to write the responses on the whiteboard for all the class participants to see and use as a way not only to help Valeria, but also to reinforce their own skill development. She began to see that by taking control of the finances she would be taking better care of both of them. Valeria

Table 5.4 Behavior log

Please use this log to write down the things your relative does (or that you do) that upset you.

Date/day of week	Time	Person present	Trigger	Behavior	Reaction
Everyday	In the a.m.	Myself and husband	He wakes up in the morning and knows that it is time to get dressed.	When he dresses himself in the morning, he insists on wearing the same outfit he has worn for the past five days.	I feel angry because he does not want to look and smell clean.

Table 5.5 Behavior log

Please use this log to write down something your relative does (or that you do) that upsets you and the strategy you used to change it.

Date/day of week	Time	Person present	Trigger	Behavior	Reaction	The strategy I used to change the behavior was:_____
Monday Wednesday	a.m.	Myself and husband	He wakes up in the morning to get dressed. Looks around the bedroom for the shirt and pair of pants.	Asks me where his clothes are. I tell him that they are in the laundry machine being soaked. I hand him a fresh shirt and pair of pants.	He gets mad and tells me that he will be cold if he does not wear his favorite clothes. I tell him he can wear a coat if he feels cold. He says OK, but still is not too happy.	Put the clothes in the laundry machine as soon as he goes to sleep. **What happened after you used this strategy?** He got a little mad but then said it was OK to wear different clothes.

was also reminded that this was not Ernesto's or her fault. Her husband had dementia. The completion of this Thought Record (see Table 5.6) by Valeria and the group also initiated the following discussion about loss:

Facilitator: Valeria, it must be difficult to watch your husband's condition deteriorate. It sounds like he is losing not just his memory, but other things as well.

Valeria: Yes, it is really hard. I felt really bad when his driver's license was revoked. I noticed this was not easy for him to accept because he lost some of his freedom to move around as he wishes. Managing our money was one of the last things he had that made him feel like a man.

Adriana: I know what you mean. I know that for my husband, being in charge of certain things in our household made him feel important during our many years of marriage. I really did not mind that he was controlling about these things because it made me feel safe. Now I am the one having to take control of things that I have no idea how to handle.

Facilitator: I can imagine that it can be scary to have to take on responsibilities that you are not accustomed to. Valeria, I am glad to see that after completing the thought record, you are feeling less guilty. I wonder whether the group can help you think of ways to still allow Ernesto to have some control over some of his money.

Josefina: How about if you give him an allowance? I handle the fiancés for my husband too but he rarely needs money. I just tell him to ask me when he wants some and I will give it to him.

Valeria: I don't know if this will work because it might make him feel like a child who has to ask his mother for an allowance.

Facilitator: Valeria, I can see how this may affect Ernesto's sense of dignity. I am glad that you are thinking of this. Any other ideas?

Adriana: How about if you open up a special bank account for him in which you make small deposits so that he can see that he still has in own money. Let him have an ATM card so that he can have access to his account.

Valeria: You know, I never thought of that. I think that might just work.

Facilitator: Yes, that is a great idea. How are you feeling now Valeria?

Valeria: Much better. I suppose I can arrange it so that he does not feel such a huge sense of loss. He may even feel some relief that he does not have to worry about paying the bills!

The group laughs together.

Exploring future challenges and potential solutions

Both our clinical and intervention research experiences at the OAFC have taught us that group CBT is effective in reducing depression in older adults and alleviating emotional distress in family caregivers to older adults with dementia or physical challenges. CBT group approaches are also emerging as promising treatment options for depression and other disorders such as sleep problems, chronic pain associated with medical conditions, and anxiety disorders that affect both older adults and their younger counterparts (White and Freeman, 2000; DeVries and Coon, 2002). However, there remains a dearth of clinical intervention research on the efficacy and effectiveness of CBT groups with racial and ethnic minority clients (Gallagher-Thompson *et al.*, 2000b; Organista, 2000; Thompson *et al.*, 2000), disabled persons, and rural populations, as well as lesbian, gay, bisexual, and transgendered individuals (Coon and Zeiss, 2003). Organista (2000) and Gallagher-Thompson *et al.* (2000) have decried the neglect of cultural influences in the application of CBT, and have championed the need to culturally tailor group interventions by incorporating culturally appropriate engagement strategies, problem areas, intervention strategies, and homework assignments. There also exists a lack of research regarding the maintenance of therapeutic gains in many of the outcome studies mentioned in this chapter, pointing to the need for clinical outcomes research that follows clients for longer periods of time and helps to identify predictors of long-term gains. Such intervention research should incorporate trials that investigate various options to enhance longer-term outcomes such as the appropriate spacing of in-person booster sessions, telephone follow-ups or internet coaching to reinforce the use of skills acquired during the regular course of therapy. Future research also needs to help us better understand other individual differences that may influence treatment outcomes in different populations (Coon *et al.*, 1999). For example, several variables have emerged in the literature that may influence treatment outcomes with older clients, such as major shifts in depressive mood (M. Thompson *et al.*, 1995), length of time in stressful situations such as family caregiving (Gallagher-Thompson and Steffen, 1994), the quality of the therapeutic alliance (Gaston *et al.*, 1988), and whether significant endogenous symptoms are present (Gallagher and Thompson, 1983). Finally, recent work points to the need to examine the effective integration of technology, including the use of

Table 5.6 Daily Thought Record

Situation *Describe the events that led to your unpleasant feelings*	Current thoughts *Identify your thoughts in the situation*	Emotions *What are you feeling? (sad, angry, anxious, etc.)*	Challenge and replace with more helpful thoughts *What is a more helpful way of thinking about the situation?*	New feelings *What are you feeling now? (sad, angry, anxious etc.)*
My husband cashed his pension check (over $1000) and cannot remember where he put the money. I have looked everywhere and I am just accepting that it is lost. I am trying to decide whether I should arrange to get power of attorney so that I can manage all of the finances.	I cannot allow this to happen again. It is up to me to change this. Taking this one last thing away is really going to hurt him. He has already lost so much and now he is about to lose one more thing that made him happy.	I am angry at him for forgetting where something so important was left. I feel guilty that I am going to be the cause of his sadness and anger.	By taking control of his finances, I will be taking better care of him and myself because we will actually have money. It is not his fault or my fault that he cannot remember where he leaves things. It is the dementia's fault.	I feel a little better. Not as angry with him and myself. I still feel sad that his life has come to this. I feel a little less guilty. I feel understood by the group because they have been through the same thing. That's comforting.

telemedicine strategies into a variety of CBT group treatments (e.g., Hopps *et al.*, 2003; Vincelli *et al.*, 2003). Clinical research into each of these areas combined with the sharing of new developments in the clinical literature by practitioners will help us to continue to better adapt both group and individual CBT interventions for the future.

References

Backhaus, J., Hohagen, F., Voderholzer, U., and Riemann, D. (2001). Long-term effectiveness of a short-term cognitive-behavioral group treatment for primary insomnia. *European Archives of Psychiatry and Clinical Neuroscience,* **251,** 35–41.

Beck, A. (1972). *Depression: causes and treatment.* Philadelphia, PA: University of Pennsylvania Press.

Beck, A. T., Rush, A. J., Shaw, B. F., and Emery, G. (1979). *Cognitive therapy of depression.* New York: Guilford Press.

Beutler, L., *et al.* (1987). Group cognitive therapy and alpraxolam in the treatment of depression in older adults. *Journal of Consulting and Clinical Psychology,* **55,** 550–6.

Bookwala, J., Yee, J. L., and Schulz, R. (2000). Caregiving and detrimental mental and physical health outcomes. In: G. M. Williamson, P. A. Parmelee, and D. R. Shaffer, ed. *Physical illness and depression in older adults: a handbook of theory, research, and practice,* pp. 93–131. New York: Plenum.

Burns, D. D. (1980). *Feeling good: the new mood therapy.* New York: Signet.

Burns, D. D. and Spangler, D. L. (2000). Does psychotherapy homework lead to improvements in depression in cognitive-behavioral therapy or does improvement lead to increased homework compliance? *Journal of Consulting and Clinical Psychology,* **68,** 46–56.

Chambless, D. and Hollon, S. (1998). Defining empirically supported therapies. *Journal of Consulting and Clinical Psychology,* **66,** 7–18.

Chambless, D., *et al.* (1996). Update on empirically validated therapies. *Clinical Psychologist,* **49**(2), 5–15.

Coon, D. W. and Gallagher-Thompson, D. (2002). Encouraging homework completion among older adults in therapy. *Journal of Clinical Psychology/In Session: Psychotherapy in Practice,* **58,** 549–63.

Coon, D. W. and Thompson, L. W. (2003). Association between homework compliance and treatment outcome among older adult outpatients with depression. *American Journal of Geriatric Psychiatry,* **11,** 53–61.

Coon, D. W. and Zeiss, L. M. (2003). The families we choose: Intervention issues with LGBT caregivers. In D. W. Coon, D. Gallagher-Thompson, and L. Thompson, ed. *Innovative interventions to reduce dementia caregiver distress: a clinical guide,* pp. 267–95. New York: Springer.

Coon, D., Rider, K., Gallagher-Thompson, D., and Thompson, L. (1999). Cognitive-behavioral therapy for the treatment of late-life distress. In: Duffy, M., ed. *Handbook of counseling and psychotherapy with older adults,* pp. 487–510. New York: John Wiley and Sons, Inc.

Coon, D. W., Thompson, L., Steffen, A., Sorocco, K., and Gallagher-Thompson, D. (2003a). Anger and depression management: psychoeducational skill training interventions for women caregivers of a relative with dementia. *The Gerontologist,* **43,** 678–89.

Coon, D. W., Gallagher-Thompson, D., and Thompson, L., ed. (2003b). *Innovative interventions to reduce dementia caregiver distress: a clinical guide.* New York: Springer.

Coon, D. W., Thompson, L. W., Rabinowitz, Y. G., and Gallagher-Thompson, D. (in press). Older adults. In: N. Kazantizis, F. P. Deane, K. R. Ronan, and L. L'Abate, L., ed. *Using homework assignments in cognitive-behavior therapy.* London: Brunner-Routledge.

Cordieli, A., *et al.* (2003). Cognitive-behavioral group therapy in obsessive-compulsive disorder: A randomized clinical trial. *Psychotherapy and Psychosomatics,* **72,** 211–16.

Dugas, M. J., *et al.* (2003). Group cognitive-behavioral therapy for generalized anxiety disorder: Treatment outcome and long-term follow-up. *Journal of Consulting and Clinical Psychology,* **71,** 821–5.

D'Zurilla, T. (1986). *Problem solving therapy: a social competence approach to clinical intervention.* New York: Springer.

DeVries, H. M. and Coon, D. W. (2002). Cognitive/behavioral group therapy with older adults. In: F. Kaslow and T. Patterson, ed. *Comprehensive handbook of psychotherapy,* Vol. 2: *Cognitive-behavioral approaches,* pp. 547–67. New York: John Wiley and Sons.

DeRubeis, R. and Crits-Cristoph, P. (1998). Empirically supported individual and group psychological treatments for adult mental disorders. *Journal of Consulting and Clinical Psychology,* **66,** 37–52.

Dick, L. P., Gallagher-Thompson, D., Coon, D. W., Powers, D. V., and Thompson, L. (1996). *Cognitive-behavioral therapy for late-life depression: a client manual.* Palo Alto, CA: Veterans Affairs Palo Alto Health Care System.

Freeman, A., Schrodt, G., Gilson, M., and Ludgate, J. (1993). Group cognitive therapy with inpatients. In: J. Wright, M. Thase, A. Beck, and J. Ludgate, ed. *Cognitive therapy with inpatients,* pp. 121–53. New York: Guilford Press.

Fry, P. (1984). Cognitive training and cognitive behavioral variables in the treatment of depression in the elderly. *Clinical Gerontologist,* **3,** 25–45.

Gallagher, D. and Thompson, L. (1981). *Depression in the elderly: a behavioral treatment manual.* Los Angeles: University of Southern California.

Gallagher, D. E. and Thompson, L. W. (1983). Effectiveness of psychotherapy for both endogenous and non-endogenous depression in older adult outpatients. *Journal of Gerontology,* **38,** 707–12.

Gallagher-Thompson, D. and Coon, D. W. (1996). Depression. In: J. Sheikh, ed. *Treating the elderly,* pp. 1–44. San Francisco: Jossey-Bass.

Gallagher-Thompson, D. and DeVries, H. M. (1994). Coping with frustration classes: development and preliminary outcomes with women who care for relatives with dementia. *Gerontologist,* **34,** 548–52.

Gallagher-Thompson, D. and Steffen, A. M. (1994). Comparative effects of cognitive/behavioral and brief psychodynamic psychotherapies for the treatment of depression in family caregivers. *Journal of Consulting and Clinical Psychology,* **62,** 543–9.

Gallagher-Thompson, D., *et al.* (1992). *Controlling your frustration: a class for caregivers.* Palo Alto, CA: VA Palo Alto Health Care System. (Note: This refers to two English language manuals: a class leader and a class participant version.)

Gallagher-Thompson, D., Ossinalde, C., and Thompson, L. W. (1996). *Coping with caregiving: a class for family caregivers.* Palo Alto, CA: VA Palo Alto Health Care System.

Gallagher-Thompson, D., *et al.* (2000a). Impact of psychoeducational interventions on distressed family caregivers. *Journal of Clinical Geropsychology,* **6,** 91–110.

Gallagher-Thompson, D., *et al.* (2000b). Development and implementation of intervention strategies for culturally diverse caregiving populations. In: R. Schulz, ed. *Handbook on dementia caregiving,* pp. 151–85. New York: Springer.

Gallagher-Thompson, D., Arean, P., Rivera, P., and Thompson, L. W. (2001). Reducing distress in Hispanic family caregivers using a psychoeducational intervention. *Clinical Gerontologist,* **23,** 17–32.

Gallagher-Thompson, D., *et al.* (2002). *Coping with caregiving: reducing stress and improving quality of life.* Stanford, CA: VA Palo Alto Health Care System and Stanford University.

Gallagher-Thompson, D., *et al.* (2003). Change in indices of distress among Latina and Anglo female caregivers of elderly relatives with dementia: site specific results from the REACH National Collaborative Study. *The Gerontologist,* **43,** 580–91.

Garcia Lopez, L. J., *et al.* (2002). Results at long-term among three psychological treatments for adolescents with generalized social phobia (II): Clinical significance and effect size. *Psicologia Conductual,* **10,** 371–85.

Gaston, L., Marmar, C., Thompson, L., and Gallagher, D. (1988). Relationship of patient's pretreatment characteristics to therapeutic alliance in diverse psychotherapies. *Journal of Consulting and Clinical Psychology,* **56,** 483–9.

Gatz, M., Fiske, A., *et al.* (1998). Empirically validated psychological treatments for older adults. *Journal of Mental Health and Aging,* **4,** 9–46.

Halperin, S., Nathan, P., Drummond, P., and Castle, D. (2000). A cognitive-behavioural, group-based intervention for social anxiety in schizophrenia. *Australian and New Zealand Journal of Psychiatry,* **34,** 809–13.

Hayward, C., *et al.* (2000). Cognitive-behavioral group therapy for social phobia in female adolescents: results of a pilot study. *Journal of the American Academy of Child and Adolescent Psychiatry,* **39,** 721–6.

Hopps, S. L., Pepin, M., and Boisvert, J. M. (2003). The effectiveness of cognitive-behavioral group therapy for loneliness via inter-relay-chat among people with physical disabilities. *Psychotherapy: Theory, Research, Practice, Training,* **40**, 136–47.

Kataoka, S. H., *et al.* (2003). A school-based mental health program for traumatized Latino immigrant children. *Journal of the American Academy of Child and Adolescent Psychiatry,* **42**, 311–18.

Kazantzis, N., Deane, F. P., and Ronan, K. R. (2000). Homework assignments in cognitive and behavioral therapy: A meta-analysis. *Clinical Psychology: Science and Practice,* **7**, 189–202.

Laidlaw, K., Thompson, L. W., Dick-Siskin, L., and Gallagher-Thompson, D. (2003). *Cognitive behaviour therapy with older people.* Chichester: John Wiley and Sons Ltd.

Lewinsohn, P. M. (1974). A behavioral approach to depression. In: R. Friedman and M. Katz, ed. *The psychology of depression,* pp. 157–76. New York: Wiley.

Lewinsohn, P., Muñoz, R., Youngren, M., and Zeiss, A. (1986). *Control your depression,* 2nd edn. New York: Prentice Hall.

Mahoney, M. (1974). *Cognition and behavior modification.* Cambridge, MA: Ballinger.

McCurry, S. M., Logsdon, R. G., Vitiello, M. V., and Teri, L. (1998). Successful behavioral treatment for reported sleep problems in elderly caregivers of dementia patients: A controlled study. *Journal of Gerontology,* **53B**, P122–9.

Molassiotis, A., *et al.* (2002). A pilot study of the effects of cognitive-behavioral group therapy and peer support/counseling in decreasing psychologic distress and improving quality of life in Chinese patients with symptomatic HIV disease. *AIDS Patient Care and STDS,* **16**, 83–96.

Morin, C. M., Kowatch, R. A., Barry, T., and Walton, E. (1993). Cognitive-behavior therapy for late-life insomnia. *Journal of Consulting and Clinical Psychology,* **61**, 137–46.

Morin, C. M., Culbert, J. P., and Schwartz, S. M. (1994). Nonpharmacological interventions for insomnia: a meta-analysis of treatment efficacy. *American Journal of Psychiatry,* **151**, 1172–80.

Muris, P., Meesters, C., and van Melick, M. (2002). Treatment of childhood anxiety disorders: a preliminary comparison between cognitive-behavioral group therapy and a psychological placebo intervention. *Journal of Behavior Therapy and Experimental Psychiatry,* **33**, 143–58.

Nathan, P. and Gorman, J., ed. (1998). *A guide to treatments that work.* New York: Oxford University Press.

Neimeyer, R. A. and Feixas, G. (1990). The role of homework and skill acquisition in the outcome of group cognitive therapy for depression. *Behavior Therapy,* **21**, 281–92.

Norcross, J., ed. (1986). *Handbook of eclectic psychotherapy.* New York: Brunner/Mazel.

Organista, K. C. (2000). Latinos. In: J. R. White and A. S. Freeman, ed. *Cognitive-behavioral group therapy for specific problems and populations,* pp. 218–303. Washington, DC: American Psychological Association.

Persons, J. (1989). *Cognitive therapy in practice: a case formulation approach.* New York: W. W. Norton and Company.

Pinquart, M. and Sörensen, S. (2001). How effective are psychotherapeutic and other psychosocial interventions with older adults? A meta-analysis. *Journal of Mental Health and Aging,* **7**, 207–43.

Sanderson, W. and Woody, S. (1995). Manuals for empirically validated treatments. *Clinical Psychologist,* **48**, 7–11.

Schulz, R., O'Brien, A., Bookwala, J., and Fleissner, K. (1995). Psychiatric and physical morbidity effects of Alzheimer's disease caregiving: prevalence, correlates, and causes. *The Gerontologist,* **35**, 771–91.

Scogin, F., Hamblin, D., and Beutler, L. (1987). Bibliotherapy for depressed older adults: a self-help alternative. *The Gerontologist,* **27**, 383–7.

Silverman, W. K., *et al.* (1999). Treating anxiety disorders in children with group cognitive-behavioral therapy: a randomized clinical trial. *Journal of Consulting and Clinical Psychology,* **67**, 995–1003.

Sörensen, S., Pinquart, M., and Duberstein, P. (2003). How effective are interventions with caregivers? An updated meta-analysis. *The Gerontologist,* **42**(3), 356–72.

Stanley, M. A., *et al.* (2003). Cognitive-behavioral treatment of late-life generalized anxiety disorder. *Journal of Consulting and Clinical Psychology,* **71**, 309–19.

Steuer, J., *et al.* (1984). Cognitive-behavioral and psychodynamic group psychotherapy in treatment of geriatric depression. *Journal of Consulting and Clinical Psychology,* **52**, 180–9.

Teri, L. and McCurry, S. (2000). Psychosocial therapies with older adults. In: C. Coffey and J. Cummings, ed. *Textbook of geriatric neuropsychiatry,* 2nd edn. Washington, DC: American Psychiatric Press.

Thompson, L. W. and Gallagher, D. (1984). Efficacy of psychotherapy in the treatment of late-life depression. *Advances in Behaviour Research and Therapy,* **6**, 127–39.

Thompson, L., Gallagher, D., and Breckenridge, J. (1987). Comparative effectiveness of psychotherapies for depressed elders. *Journal of Consulting and Clinical Psychology,* **55**, 385–90.

Thompson, L. W., Gallagher-Thompson, D., and Lovett, S. (1992). *Increasing life satisfaction class leaders' and participant manuals* (revised version). Palo Alto, CA: Department of Veterans Affairs Medical Center and Stanford University.

Thompson, L. W., Gallagher-Thompson, D., and Dick, L. (1996). *Cognitive-behavioral therapy for late-life depression: a therapist manual.* Palo Alto, CA: Veterans Affairs Palo Alto Health Care System.

Thompson, L., Powers, D., Coon, D., Takagi, K., McKibbin, C., and Gallagher-Thompson, D. (2000). Older adults. In: White, R. and Freeman, A., ed. *Cognitive-behavioral group therapy for special problems and populations,* pp. 235–61. Washington, DC: American Psychological Association.

Thompson, L., Coon, D., Gallagher-Thompson, D., Sommer, B., and Koin, D. (2001). Comparison of desipramine and cognitive behavioral therapy in the treatment of late-life depression. *American Journal of Geriatric Psychiatry,* **9**(3), 225–40.

Thompson, M., Gallagher-Thompson, D., and Thompson, L. W. (1995). Linear and nonlinear changes in mood between psychotherapy sessions: implications for treatment and outcomes and relapse risk. *Psychotherapy Research,* **5**, 327–36.

Tkachuk, G. A., Graff, L. A., Martin, G. L., and Bernstein, C. N. (2003). Randomized controlled trial of cognitive-behavioral group therapy for irritable bowel syndrome in a medical setting. *Journal of Clinical Psychology in Medical Settings,* **10**, 57–69.

Toseland, R. (1995). *Group work with the elderly and family caregivers.* New York: Springer.

Vincelli, F., Anolli, L., Bouchard, S., Wiederhold, B. K., Zurloni, V., and Riva, G. (2003). Experiential cognitive therapy in the treatment of panic disorders with agoraphobia: A controlled study. *Cyberpsychology and Behavior: The Impact of the Internet, Multimedia, and Virtual Reality on Behavior and Society,* **6**, 321–8.

Vitaliano, P., Zhang, J., and Scanlan, J. M. (2003). Is caregiving hazardous to one's physical health? A meta-analysis. *Psychological Bulletin,* **129**, 1–27.

Wetherell, J. L., Gatz, M., and Craske, M. G. (2003). Treatment of generalized anxiety disorder in older adults. *Journal of Consulting and Clinical Psychology,* **71**, 31–40.

White, J. R. (2000). Introduction. In: J. R. White and A. S. Freeman, ed. *Cognitive-behavioral group therapy for specific problems and populations,* pp. 3–25. Washington, DC: American Psychological Association.

White, J. R. and Freeman, A. S., ed. (2000). *Cognitive-behavioral group therapy for specific problems and populations.* Washington, DC: American Psychological Association.

Yost, E. B., Beutler, L. E., Corbishley, M. A., and Allender, J. R. (1986). *Group cognitive therapy: a treatment approach for depressed older adults.* New York: Pergamon Press.

Young, J. E. (1999). *Cognitive therapy for personality disorders: a schema-focused approach,* 3rd edn. Sarasota, FL: Professional Resource Press.

Young, J., Weinberger, A., and Beck, A. (2001). Cognitive therapy for depression. *Clinical handbook of psychological disorder,* 3rd edn. New York: Guilford Press.

6 Family therapy

Sidney Bloch and Edwin Harari

The term 'family therapy' covers a variety of approaches. At one extreme it is a method drawn from one or more of a range of theoretically based schools that seeks to help an individual patient who presents with a clinical syndrome. At the other extreme family therapy is a way of thinking about psychotherapy in general; the intervention may involve the individual alone, the nuclear family, or an extended network, but the focus is the relationships between people. According to this view psychopathology reflects recurring, problematic interactional patterns among family members and between the family, and possibly, other social institutions, and may include doctors and helping agencies. Midway between these two positions is one that views the family as acting potentially as a resource or as a liability for an identified patient; different interventions are thus needed to enhance the positive effects of family relationships as compared with those that seek to minimize or negate their noxious effects. As we will elaborate in this chapter such a range of interventions makes it tricky to define and research family therapy.

Historical and theoretical developments

The family has long been recognized as a fundamental unit of social organization in the lives of human beings. Regardless of the specific pattern of family life, the foundational narratives, myths, legends, and folklore of all cultures emphasize the power of family relations to mould the character of the individual and serve as an exemplar of the moral and political order of society.

In the past 150 years new academic disciplines, among them anthropology, sociology, and social history, have devoted much attention to the diverse forms of family structure and function found in different cultures at various historical periods. Constrained perhaps by Western medicine's focus on the individual patient, psychiatry has been tardy in formulating a view of the family other than as a source of genetically transmitted diseases, hence the emphasis on inquiring about the prevalence of mental illness among relatives.

Scattered through Freud's writings are interesting comments about marital and family relationships and their possible roles in both individual normal development and psychopathology (Sander, 1978). Freud's description of unconscious processes such as introjection, projection, and identification explained how an individual's experiences could be transmitted across the generations in a family. Freud's successors elaborated on his formulations, e.g., in 1921 J. C. Flugel published the first detailed psychoanalytic account of family relationships (Flugel, 1921).

Strongly influenced by the work in the UK of Anna Freud, Melanie Klein, and Donald Winnicott, the child guidance movement devised a model of one therapist working with the disturbed child and another with the parents, most often the mother on her own. The two clinicians collaborated in order to recognize how the mother's anxieties distorted her perception and handling of her child, which compounded the child's own developmental anxieties. This work, however, was conducted by psychiatric social workers and only a minority of psychiatrists.

Proliferation of 'schools'

Transgenerational

Things took a different turn in the US. There, Ackerman (1958), who coined the term 'family therapy' in the 1950s, had introduced the idea of working with the nuclear family of a disturbed child using psychodynamic methods. An interest in working with the family, including two or more generations, arose concurrently in several psychiatric centers. Most of the pioneers of so-called 'transgenerational family therapy' were analysts who used many of the concepts of object relations theory that they recast into their own conceptual language.

Thus, Murray Bowen (1971) in his work with psychotic children found that their capacity to differentiate themselves emotionally from their families (especially from mother) while still retaining a sense of age-appropriate emotional belonging was impaired by the legacy of unresolved losses, trauma, and other upheavals in the lives of parental and grandparental generations. Bowen also devised the genogram, a schematic depiction of family structure, with a particular notation for significant family events; this forms a standard part of contemporary family assessment in clinical practice (see pp. 60–2 section on assessment).

Boszormenyi-Nagy and Spark (1984) in their contextual therapy also addressed this transgenerational theme by describing how family relationships between generations and between adults in a marriage were organized around a ledger of entitlements and obligations; this conferred on each person a sense of justice about their position. This, in turn, reflected the experience in childhood of neglect or sacrifices made on a person's behalf for which redress was sought in adult life.

Systems oriented

Bowen had also introduced the principles of systems theory into his work with families. A system may be defined as a set of inter-related elements that function as a unity in a particular environment. General systems theory (GST) was propounded in the 1940s by the German biologist, Ludwig von Bertalanffy (1968); he outlined the principles by which any system (inanimate, animate, or ideational) can be described. Key concepts of GST are hierarchy, the emergence of new properties in the transition from one level of organization to another, and formulations derived from thermodynamics, which describe the exchange of energy between the system and its environment. A family may be considered a partially open system that interacts with its biological and sociocultural environments.

Working with delinquent youth in New York, Salvador Minuchin and his colleagues recognized the relevance of systems thinking to their interventions. The youngsters often came from economically impoverished, emotionally deprived families, headed by a demoralized single parent (most often mother) who alternated between excessive discipline and helpless delegation of family responsibilities to a child or to her own disapproving parent. Such families were understandably mistrustful of words and beyond the reach of conventional 'talking' therapies. Minuchin's emergent structural family therapy came to deploy a series of action-oriented techniques and powerful verbal metaphors that enable the therapist to 'join' the family, and to reestablish an appropriate hierarchy and generational boundaries between the various subsystems (marital, parent/child, siblings).

Later, treating so-called 'psychosomatic families' where the presenting problem was a child suffering from anorexia nervosa, unstable diabetes, or asthma, Minuchin's team noted that unlike the chaotic, leaderless disengaged 'delinquent families' these, while middle-class, intact, and articulate, often were enmeshed. Their members avoided overt expressions of dissent or challenge to ostensible family unity. Typically, marital conflict was detoured through the symptomatic child, resulting in maladaptive coalitions between parent and child, or between grandparent and child, the inclusion of third parties (e.g., a helping agency) into family life. All this led to a loss of appropriate boundaries. Because words were used to avoid change in these well-educated families, Minuchin and Fishman (1981) again looked to actional strategies to challenge their unspoken fears of conflict and change.

Jay Haley's (1976) Strategic Therapy combined aspects of Minuchin's model with ideas of the psychotherapist, Milton Erickson; his hypnotherapy techniques had skillfully exploited the notion that a covert message lurks behind overt communication that defines the power relationship between people. This applies to a patient's ties with his family and their professional helpers.

Another important series of theoretical developments took place in Palo Alto, California, where a group of clinicians gathered around the anthropologist Gregory Bateson (1972) in the 1950s. In his field work, Bateson had noted two relational patterns:

1. Symmetrical, in which each participant's behavior induces the other to do more of what they were already doing as equals. Power struggles in a marriage or between parents and an adolescent, arguments over compliance with medication or family conflict preceding psychotic relapse or an alcoholic binge exemplify such symmetrical escalation; and

2. Complementary, in which participants arrange themselves such that, for example, one is dominant and the other subordinate. The doctor–patient relationship or the parent–child relationship often is of this type, while a pattern of rigid complementarity characterizes the marriages of many patients suffering from chronic anxiety states, agoraphobia, and chronic dysthymia.

The ability to switch from complementary to symmetrical patterns and vice versa, and to alternate between dominant/subordinate and co-equal positions at different times and on various matters are skills that the Bateson approach teaches. It views psychopathology as the product of people getting stuck in once relevant but now dysfunctional modes of relating and problem solving.

Bateson's group also noted that implicit in communication were tacit, nonverbal 'metacommunications' that defined the relationship between the participants. Contradiction or incongruence between these two levels when each message carried great persuasive, moral, or coercive force to the recipient formed part of what they labeled a 'double-bind'. When combined with a tertiary level injunction that forbade escape from the field of communication, this double-bind was proposed as a possible basis for schizophrenic thinking (Bateson et al., 1956, 1962).

Systems oriented: further developments

All these aforementioned system-oriented approaches assume that the family is a system observed by the therapist. However, therapists are not value neutral. As described, in some models they take an active role in advocating and orchestrating specific changes in accordance with a preconceived model of family functioning. Yet these models ignore therapists' biases as well as the relevance of their relationships with families. This probably reflected the determination of certain American family therapists to distance themselves from psychoanalytic theory, and also led them to neglect the family's history, how it altered during the life cycle, and the relevance of past notable events.

In response to these criticisms there was a move away from the here-and-now, problem-focused approach that had characterized most behavioral and communicational views of psychopathology. The Milan

school (Selvini-Palazzoli et al., 1980; see pp. 62–4 in section on course of therapy), whose founders were all psychoanalysts, developed circular questioning, a radically new method of interviewing families. Furthermore, observers behind a one-way screen formulated hypotheses about the family-plus-therapist system and its relevance to the clinical process.

A Norwegian group (Andersen, 1991) developed the 'reflecting team dialogue' in which, following a therapy session, the family could observe the therapists discussing their problem, possible causes, and unresolved factors, which might have led them to seek certain solutions they had persevered with despite obvious lack of success, while neglecting alternative solutions.

Postmodern developments

Family therapists also began to consider that families might be constrained from experimenting with new solutions to difficulties because of the way they had interpreted their past experiences or internalized the explanatory narratives of their family, the expert's, or society at large.

This led to a shift from regarding the family as a social system defined by its organization (i.e., roles and structures) to a linguistic system. According to this view the narrative a family relates about their lives is a linguistic construction that organizes past experience and relationships, and their significance, in particular ways. Other narratives are excluded from consideration. When a family with an ill member talks to health professionals, conversations are inevitably about pathology (a problem-saturated description). The participants ignore times when the problem was absent or minimal, or when they successfully confined it to manageable proportions. A different story might be told if they were to examine the context and relationships that might have led, or could still lead, to better outcomes.

A number of narrative, social constructionist, or solution-focused approaches (the terms are essentially interchangeable) make use of these concepts (De Shazer, 1985; Anderson and Goolishian, 1988; White and Epston, 1990). Philosophically, they align themselves with postmodernism, a movement that challenges the idea that there is a basic truth or grand explanatory theory known only by experts.

Criticism of systems approaches

Many criticisms of the above systems approaches to family therapy have been leveled. These include:

◆ disregard of the subjective and intersubjective experiences of family members;

◆ neglect of the family's history;

◆ denial of unconscious motives that influence individuals in a relationship;

◆ although people are reciprocally connected in a family system the power they exert on one another is not equal (this is highlighted particularly in the problem of violence against women and in various types of child abuse);

◆ inequality and other forms of injustice based on societal attitudes towards differences in gender, ethnicity, class, and the like, are uncritically accepted as 'givens';

◆ minimizing the role of therapeutic relationship, including attitudes family members develop toward the therapist and her feelings towards each of them and to the family as a whole.

This critique has led to an interest in integrating systems-oriented and psychoanalytic concepts, particularly those derived from object relations theory. Attempts at a general level are those of Flaskas and Perlesz (1996), Braverman (1995), and Cooklin (1979), and the feminist perspective (Luepnitz, 2002); specific disorders such as schizophrenia (Ciompi, 1988), and anorexia nervosa (Dare, 1997) have also been targeted. One variant of integration is John Byng-Hall's (1995) masterful synthesis of attachment theory, systems thinking, and a narrative approach.

A further criticism of systems-oriented therapies is their minimizing the impact of material reality such as physical handicap or biological forces in the cause of mental illness, and sociopolitical phenomena such as unemployment, racism, and poverty. These are obviously not merely the result of social constructions or linguistic games. The distress they inflict are real in the extreme.

The 'psychoeducational' approach, 'family crisis intervention', and 'family-sensitive practice' have evolved in the context of the burden that schizophrenia places on the family and the potential for responses of members to influence the course of the illness. This has paved the way for a series of interventions:

- educating the family about what is known regarding the nature, causes, course, and treatment of schizophrenia;
- providing the family with opportunities to discuss their difficulties in caring for the patient and to devise appropriate strategies;
- clarifying conflict in the family not only about the illness but also about other issues;
- regularly evaluating the impact of the illness on the family as individual members and collectively;
- helping to resolve other conflicts not specifically related to the illness, but which may be aggravated by the demands of caring for a chronically ill person.

This type of work may be carried out with several families meeting together. Whatever the case, promising results have been achieved in reducing relapses and frequency of hospital admission (McFarlane *et al.*, 1995).

The limitations of psychoeducational programs for psychiatric disorders and vulnerability to relapse after a psychotic episode have been shown to reflect the emotional climate of the family. It is noteworthy that these potentially disruptive patterns of interaction often are not detectable by the clinician who interviews the patient alone rather than observing him in the context of a family interview (Thompson *et al.*, 2000). Furthermore, the difficulties therapists encounter working with such families vary at different phases of treatment.

While the conventional view claims critical comments are significantly correlated with relapse, it also appears that, at least in some patients with bipolar disorder, a comparative excess of genuinely positive and supportive comments by family members may also be associated with relapse.

Family crisis intervention, initially devised for families with a schizophrenic relative, but since applied to other clinical states, operates on the premise that deterioration in mental state or a request by the family to hospitalize a member may well reflect a change in a previously stable pattern of family interaction. Convening an urgent meeting with patient, spouse, and other key family members, even in a hospital emergency center, is associated with a reduced rate of admission.

Cognitive-behavioral approaches

While integrating some concepts from systems, postmodern, and psychoeducational approaches, cognitive-behavioral therapy emphasizes the importance of identifying and directly modifying dysfunctional ideas and behavioral patterns of family members. When families are in distress they frequently perceive each other's reactions (behavioral and emotional) in a distorted way, which may in turn elicit counterproductive reactions. Persistent deleterious cycles are set up in which family members continually misperceive and/or misinterpret one another and react accordingly. Therapy aims to help family members correct their selective negative biases, negative attributions of one another, negative predictions, dysfunctional assumptions, and unrealistic standards. Cognitive-behavioral therapists work to help family members increase positive behavioral changes, engage in pleasurable activities, and improve communication and problem-solving skills (Epstein and Schlesinger, 2003).

Indications for family therapy

Notwithstanding the application of these various approaches in adult psychiatry for at least three decades, indications remain ill defined compared with other forms of psychotherapy. Moreover, controversy has dogged the subject. This is not altogether surprising. Pioneering family therapists acted perhaps with a touch of hubris when claiming that their innovative approaches were suited to most clinical conditions. Ambitiousness rode high. With the passage of time, a more balanced view evolved that encompasses the notion that a systemic context is advantageous in assessing and treating any psychiatric problem, although it is not axiomatic that family therapy will be the treatment of choice (or even indicated).

We should bear in mind that family therapy is a *mode* of psychological treatment, not a unitary approach with one central purpose. One only has to note the diversity of theoretical models we discussed earlier, with their corresponding variegated techniques. Attempts to link indications to specific models have proved ill advised and contributed little to the field overall.

It has also become clear that conventional diagnoses as listed in DSM-IV or ICD-10 do not serve well as a source to map out indications for family work. DSM-IV has a minimal section, the so-called V diagnoses, covering 'relational problems', which are not elaborated upon at all (American Psychiatric Association, 1994). All we are told is that the problem in relating can involve a couple, a parent–child dyad, siblings, or 'not otherwise specified'. ICD-10 ignores the relational area entirely.

In mapping out indications, we need to avoid the complicating factor of blurring assessment and therapy. A patient's family may be recruited in order to gain more knowledge about his diagnosis and subsequent treatment. This does not necessarily lead to family therapy. Indeed, it may point to marital or to long-term supportive therapy. Thus, we need to distinguish between an assessment family interview and family therapy *per se*.

Finally, a typology of family psychopathology that might allow the diagnostician to differentiate one pattern of dysfunction from another and identify appropriate interventions accordingly is elusive. Here, empirical evidence is inconclusive and clinical consensus lacking. An inherent hurdle is determining which dimensions of family functioning are central to creating a family typology (Bloch *et al.*, 1994). Communication, adaptability, boundaries between members and subgroups, and conflict are a few of the contenders proffered (we offer our own classification below).

It does not help that there are no clear associations between conventional psychiatric diagnoses and family type. Efforts to establish links, such as an anorexia nervosa family (Minuchin *et al.*, 1978) or a psychosomatic family (Clarkin *et al.*, 1979) have not been fruitful. Similarly, work in the area of the family and schizophrenia (e.g., Bateson *et al.*, 1956 and Bowen, 1978) have not yielded durable results. Instead, research supports the view that no particular type of family dysfunction differentiates between specific types of mental illness (as designated on Axis 1 of DSM IV). Rather, having a mentally-ill family member acts as a general stressor on the family that may lead to impaired functioning across a range of family-related activities (Epstein and Schlesinger, 2003). Consistent with the systemic view, such illness-induced family dysfunction may aggravate the course of the illness or complicate its management.

What follows is our attempt to distill past clinical and theoretical contributions, particularly the work of Walrond-Skinner (1978) and Clarkin *et al.* (1979). There are many ways to cut the pie; resultant categories are not mutually exclusive entirely given the considerable overlap in clinical practice; and a particular family may require family therapy based on more than one indication. We also must stress that family dysfunction is obvious in certain clinical situations but more covert in others, and often concealed by a specific member's clinical presentation. Six categories emerge:

1. The clinical problem manifests in explicitly family terms; the therapist readily notes family dysfunction. For example, a marital conflict dominates, with repercussions for the rest of the family or tension between parents and an adolescent child dislocates family life with everyone ensnared in the conflict. In these sorts of situations, the family is the target of intervention by dint of its obvious dysfunctional pattern and family therapy the treatment of choice.

2. The family, nuclear or extended, has experienced a life event, stressful or disruptive in type, which has led to dysfunction or is on the verge of doing so. These events are either predictable or accidental and include, for instance, accidental or suicidal death, financial embarrassment,

serious physical illness, the unexpected departure of a child from the home, and so forth. In all these circumstances, any family equilibrium that previously prevailed has been disturbed; the ensuing state becomes associated with family dysfunction and/or the development of symptoms in one or more members. In some instances, family efforts to rectify the situation inadvertently aggravate it.

3. Continuing, demanding circumstances in a family are of such a magnitude as to lead to maladaptive adjustment. The family's resources may be stretched to the hilt, external sources of support may be scanty. Enduring physical illness, persistent or recurrent psychiatric illness, and the presence in the family of a frail elderly member are typical examples.

4. An identified patient may become symptomatic in the context of a poorly functioning family. Symptoms are an expression of that dysfunction. Depression in a mother or an eating problem in a daughter or alcohol misuse in a father, on family assessment, is adjudged to reflect underlying family difficulties.

5. A family member is diagnosed with a specific condition such as schizophrenia, agoraphobia, obsessive-compulsive disorder, or depression; the complicating factors are the adverse reverberations in the family stemming from that diagnosis. For example, the schizophrenic son taxes his parental caregivers in ways that exceed their 'problem-solving' capacity; an agoraphobic woman insists on the constant company of her husband in activities of daily living; a recurrently depressed mother comes to rely on the support of her eldest daughter. In these circumstances, family members begin to respond maladaptively in relation to the diagnosed relative and this paves the way for a deterioration of his condition, manifest as chronicity or a relapsing course.

6. Thoroughly disorganized families, buffeted by a myriad of problems, are viewed as the principal target of help, even though one member, for instance, abuses drugs, another is prone to violence, and a third exhibits antisocial behavior. Regarding the family as the core dysfunctional unit is the relevant rationale rather than foci on each member's problems individually.

We reiterate that family therapy may be a treatment of choice in all these categories, but not necessarily the only one. Thus, in helping a disturbed family struggling to deal with a schizophrenic son, supportive therapy and medication for the patient is likely to be as important as any family treatment. Similarly, an indication for family therapy does not negate the possibility of another psychological approach being used for one or more members. For instance, an 18-year-old adolescent striving to separate and individuate may benefit from individual therapy following family treatment (or in parallel with it) while the parents may require a separate program to focus on their marital relationship.

Contraindications for family therapy

These are more straightforward than indications; they are self-evident and therefore mentioned briefly.

1. The family is unavailable because of geographical dispersion or death.

2. There is no shared motivation for change. One or more members wish to participate but their chance of benefiting from a family approach are likely to be less than if committing themselves to individual therapy. (We need to distinguish here between poor motivation and ambivalence; in the latter, the assessor teases out factors that underlie it and may encourage the family's engagement.)

3. The level of family disturbance is so severe or long-standing or both that a family approach seems futile. For example, a family that has fought bitterly for years is unlikely to engage in the constructive purpose of exploring their patterns of functioning.

4. Family equilibrium is so precarious that the inevitable turbulence (Goldenberg and Goldenberg, 1996) arising from family therapy is likely to lead to decompensation of one or more members, e.g., a sexually

abused adult may do better in individual therapy than by confronting the abusing relative.

5. A member with a psychiatric condition is too incapacitated to withstand the demands of family therapy. The person in the midst of a psychotic episode or someone overwhelmed by severe melancholia is too affected by the illness to engage in family work.

6. An identified patient acknowledges family factors in the evolution of his problem but seeks the privacy of individual therapy to explore it, at least initially. For example, a university student struggling to achieve a coherent sense of identity may benefit more from her own pursuit of self-understanding. Such an approach does not negate an attempt to understand the contribution of family factors to the problem.

Assessment

Family assessment, an extension of conventional individual psychiatric assessment, adds a broader context to the final formulation. Built up over a series of interviews, the range and pace of the inquiry depends on the features of the case. Its four phases are: history from the patient, a provisional formulation concerning the relevance of family issues, an interview with one or more members, and a revised formulation.

In some cases, it is clear from the outset that the problem resides in the family as a group (see indications); in this context, the phases below are obviously superfluous.

History from the patient

The most effective way to obtain a family history is by constructing a family tree. This provides not only representation of structure but additional information is obtained about important events and a range of family features. Scrutiny of the tree also becomes a source of noteworthy issues warranting exploration and, eventually, of clinical hypotheses.

Personal details are recorded for each member such as age, dates of birth and death, occupation, education, and illness, as are critical events (e.g., migration, crucial relational changes, major losses, and achievements), and the quality of relationships.

An erudite discussion of the family tree—its construction, interpretation, and clinical uses—is presented by McGoldrick and Gerson (1985).

Useful guidelines are to work from the presenting problem to the broader context, from the current situation to its historical origins and evolution, from 'facts' to inferences, and from nonthreatening to more sensitive themes.

Commonly, questions are preceded by a statement such as: 'In order to better understand your problems I need to know something of your background and your current situation'. This is enriched by questions that refer to interactional patterns: 'Who knows about the problem? How does each of them see it? Has anyone else in the family had similar problems? Who have you found most helpful, and least helpful thus far? What do they think needs to be done'. Attitudes of members can thus be explored and light shed on the clinical picture.

The presenting problem and changes in the family

Questions aimed at understanding the current context include: 'What has been happening recently in the family? Have there been any changes (for example, births, deaths, illness, losses). Has your relationship with other members changed? Have relationships within the family altered?'

The wider family context

At this point a broader inquiry flows logically—in terms of members to be considered, and in the time span of the family's history. Information about parents' siblings and their families, grandparents, and a spouse's family may be pertinent. Other significant figures, which may include caregivers and professionals, should not be forgotten.

Apart from information about the extended family's structure, questions about the family's response to major events can be posed: for example, 'How did the family react when grandmother died? Who took it the hardest? How did migration affect your parents?'

Relationships should be explored at all levels covering those between patient and other members and between those members themselves. Conflicted ties are illuminating. Understanding the 'roles' adopted by members is also useful, for example, 'Who tends to take care of others? Who needs most care? Who tends to be the most sensitive to what is going on in the family?'

Asking direct questions about members is informative but a superior strategy is to seek the patient's views about their beliefs and feelings and to look for differences between members; for example: 'What worries your mother most about your problem? What worries your father most?' Several lines of inquiry may reveal differences:

♦ Pursuing sequential interactions: 'What does your father do when you say your depressions are dreadful? How does your mother respond when your father advises you to pull up your socks? How do you react when she contradicts your father?'

♦ 'Ranking' responses: 'Everyone is worried that you may harm yourself. Who worries most? Who is most likely to do something when you talk about suicide?'

♦ Looking for changes in relating since the problem: 'Does your husband spend more or less time with you since your difficulties began? Has he become closer or more distant from your daughter?'

♦ Hypothetical questions dealing with imagined situations: 'How do you think your relationship with your wife will change if you don't improve? Who would be most likely to notice that you were getting better?'

Triadic questions help to gain information about relationships that go beyond pairs; for example: 'How do you see your relationship with your mother? How does your father see that relationship? How would your mother react to what you have told me if she were here today?'

Making a provisional formulation

Two questions about the family arise following the above interview: (1) How does the family typically function, and (2) Do any family features pertain to the patient's problems?

How does the family function?

A schema to organize ideas about family functioning builds from simple to complex observations: structure, changes, relationships, interaction, and the way in which the family works as a whole.

♦ The family tree will reveal the many family *structures* possible—single parented, divorced, blended, remarried, sibships with large age discrepancies, adoptees; unusual configurations invite conjecture about inherent difficulties.

♦ Data will be obtained about significant family *changes* and events. Timing of predictable transitions such as births, departures from home, marriages, and deaths is pertinent. Have external events coincided with these transitions? (times at which the family may be more vulnerable). How have demands placed on the family by such changes been met?

♦ *Relationships* refer to how members interact with one another. This is typically in terms of degree of closeness and emotional quality (e.g., warm, tense, rivalrous, hostile). Major conflicts may be noted as may overly intense relationships.

♦ Particular *interactional patterns* may become apparent. These go beyond pairs. Triadic relationships are more revealing about how a family functions. A third person is often integral to defining the relationship between another pair. A conflict for instance may be rerouted through the third person, preventing any direct resolution. A child may act in coalition with one parent against the other or with a grandparent against a parent.

♦ At a higher level of abstraction, the clinician notes *how the family works as a whole*. Particular patterns, possibly a series of triads, may emerge, which may have recurred across generations. For example, mothers and eldest sons have fused relationships, with fathers excluded, while daughters and mothers-in-law are in conflict.

Idiosyncratic shared beliefs may be discerned that explain much of the way the family does things. 'Rules' governing members' behavior towards one another or to the outside world may flow from these beliefs. For example, a family may hold that 'you can only trust your own family; the outside world is always hostile,' they may therefore avoid conflict at any cost, and prohibit seeking external support.

Evidence of family difficulties may be found at each of these five levels. If they are, the question arises whether these relate or not to the identified patient's problems.

Are family factors involved in the patient's problems?

Links between family functioning and the patient's problems take various forms, but the following categories cover most clinical situations. More than one will often apply: the family as reactive, the family as a resource, and the family in problem maintenance.

The family as reactive

The patient's illness, or its exacerbation, may have occurred at a time of family upheaval. The precipitant for the upheaval may have been the illness itself. An escalating combination of the two may pertain. The illness may have occurred in the face of family stress; it pressurizes the family all the more, and this in turn exacerbates the illness.

The family as a resource

The family may be well placed to assist in treatment. This may be as straightforward as supervising medication, ensuring clinic attendance, and detecting early signs of relapse or providing a home environment that promotes recovery and its maintenance. The family may also call on friends and agencies, professional or voluntary, to offer support.

The family in problem maintenance

Interactions revolving around the patient's illness may act to maintain it in one of three chief ways. First, the illness itself becomes a way of 'solving' a family problem, the best that can be achieved. For example, anorexia nervosa in a teenager due to attend a distant university may lead to her abandoning this plan as she feels unable to care for herself. Were she to leave, parental conflict would become more exposed and her mother, with whom the patient is in coalition against her father, would find herself unsupported. The illness therefore keeps the patient at home and enmeshed in the parental relationship, and also provides a focus for shared concerns and an ostensible sense of unity.

Secondly, maintenance of the illness does not solve a family problem but may have done so in the past. An interactional pattern persists even though it lacks utility. In the previous example, the father's mother died 9 months later. His wife subsequently expressed feelings of closeness, feelings not experienced by him for years; their relationship gradually improved. Both parents, however, continued to treat their daughter as incapable of achieving autonomy, reinforcing her own uncertainty about coping independently if she were to recover.

Thirdly, persistence of illness reflects a perception by the family of themselves and their problems, to which they are bound by the persuasive power of the narrative that they have shaped for themselves; the narrative may have stemmed from the helping professionals' explanatory schemas.

Interview with key informants

The clinician will by now have made an initial assessment of the patient's problems and of the family context. An interview with one or more informants, usually family members, is the next step. Several purposes are served: to corroborate the story, to fill in gaps, to determine influences impinging on the patient, and to recruit others to help. A family meeting is most effective in order to accomplish these goals.

Problems may arise in trying to implement the session. The patient may resist family members being interviewed for all sorts of reasons, e.g., symptoms have been kept secret, the patient regards it as unfair to burden others, he is ashamed of seeing a psychiatrist, he is fearful the family will be blamed or he is suspicious of them. These concerns need ventilating, particularly if the family is pivotal and treatment will be enhanced by their involvement. The patient will agree in most cases. Where the health or safety of a patient or others is threatened, refusal may be overridden on ethical grounds. Otherwise, refusal must be respected. The question of a family session can be raised later after a more trusting relationship has been cemented.

Who should be seen depends on the purpose of the interview; generally, all those living in the household and likely to be affected by the identified patient's illness should participate. Of course, some family members may be living elsewhere but are very much involved. The more family factors pertain, the more desirable the attendance by all members. The patient's views should be sought as he will provide insight into who he considers are key people.

The family interview

The clinician will have garnered substantial information by the time the family is seen. He should reflect on any biases that may have crept into his thinking about the family, and how the situation might influence them to draw him into alliances. This may well happen when conflict prevails. The clinician strives to act neutrally, his sole interest that of 'helping in the situation.' A nonjudgmental stance is paramount.

Introductions are made, names and preferred modes of address clarified. The clinician then explains the meeting's purpose. The details may well influence future participation. Everyone is then invited to share their views about the nature and effects of problems they have encountered.

The clinician may have an idea about how the identified patient's problems relate to family function and can test it out by probing questions and observing of interactions. This idea is typically kept to himself as it is unhelpful to present a hypothesis prematurely. Instead, he seeks details about everyday events and infers patterns thereafter. For example, rather than focusing on 'closeness', he enquires about time spent together by the family, whether intimate experiences are shared, who helps with family tasks, and so on.

Triadic relationships can be scrutinized both through questioning (What does A do when B says this to C?) and observation (What does A do when B and C reveal tensions?). The scope for circular questioning is enhanced if several members participate. A third person may be asked to comment on what two others convey to each other when a particular event occurs. This approach of not asking predictable questions to which the family may by now have stereotypical responses often challenges them to think about their relationships in a fresh way.

Information is elicited that elaborates the family tree. Observations are made concerning family structure and functioning, e.g., who makes decisions, who controls others and in what areas, the quality of specific relationships, conflict, alliances, how clearly people communicate and how they approach problems. The discussion then extends to all spheres of family life: beliefs, traditions, rules, and values.

Throughout the interview the clinician affirms the experiences of all members by not only attending to concerns, but also acknowledging strengths and their efforts to tackle their difficulties.

The interview ends with a summary of what has emerged. The clinician may ask to continue the assessment on a second occasion or may recommend family therapy at this point. If the latter, he then explains its aim and rationale. Arrangements are set for a follow-up session, purportedly the launch of the family therapy *per se*, but in essence a continuation of the 'work' in progress.

Revised formulation

As more information becomes available at each of the aforementioned levels, the initial formulation can be revised as necessary. The five observational levels of structure, transitions, relationships, patterns of interaction, and global family functioning are reexamined in terms of the family as reactive, resourceful, or problem maintaining. Appropriate interventions can be planned, at least for a follow-up session. We are now ready to turn to the course of typical family therapy.

The course of therapy

With the phase of assessment concluded and a family approach agreed upon, therapy begins. We should recall, however, that a family may be referred as a group from the outset on the premise that the problem is inherently a family-based one. In this case, the initial stage incorporates assessment and this is made explicit.

Given the plethora of 'schools' of family therapy, as described earlier, it would be laborious to map out the course of treatment associated with each of them. Instead, we will focus on the approach pioneered by the Milan group (Selvini-Palazzoli *et al.*, 1980) but we should stress that it has undergone much elaboration and refinement over 25 years. Our account tends to highlight the original features. First, we need to comment briefly on the roles the therapist may assume.

Role of the family therapist

Beels and Ferber (1969) who were among the first observers to consider various roles for family therapists, divided them into 'conductors' and 'reactors'; the differentiation remains useful as it transcends schools. The therapist as *conductor* is represented in the work of practitioners such as Satir, Bowen, and Minuchin. Virginia Satir (1967) is a good illustration. With her emphasis on communication, she espoused the notion that the family therapist is a teacher who shares her expertise in optimal communication by setting goals and the direction of treatment. In her case, she guided the family to adopt a new form of language in order to resolve problems in communication that she saw as the root of their troubles. Additionally, the therapist instills confidence, promotes hope for change and makes them feel comfortable in the process.

In Satir and fellow conductors, the therapist is an explicit authority, who intervenes actively in implementing change.

The therapist as *reactor* plays a different role by resonating with, and responding to, what the family manifests. Therapists in the psychoanalytic tradition belong to this group as do what Beels and Ferber label system purists. Typically, the therapist shares observations about patterns of relating that emerge during the sessions. We will illustrate this aspect when describing the Milan approach (Selvini-Palazzoli *et al.*, 1980). We have selected it arbitrarily as we cannot possibly give accounts of every school.

The Milan approach—as illustrative of a course of family therapy applying systems theory

With assessment complete, the therapist (sometimes a pair) meets with the family. With her preparatory knowledge, she shapes a hypothesis about the nature of the family's dysfunction. As a reactor, he has the opportunity, on observing patterns *in vivo*, to confirm her ideas. Such patterns usually emerge from the start making the therapist's job correspondingly easier. Apart from hypothesis testing, another task in this session is to engage the family fully so that they will be motivated to reattend. We could interpolate a dictum here: a primary aim of the first session is to facilitate a second session. A key element in encouraging engagement is for the therapist to promote a sense of curiosity in members so that they raise questions about themselves and the family as a group (Cecchin, 1987).

The chief strategy used is circular questioning, which we touched on in the assessment section (Tomm, 1987). Although it is easy to imagine doing, it is tricky to do well. The main purpose is to address the family's issues indirectly; this avoids pressurizing particular members and perhaps provoking their resistance. For example, the therapist asks questions of an adolescent about how his parents get on with each other; or a mother about how her husband relates to the eldest son; or a grandmother about which grandchild is closest to the parents; and so forth. This mode of inquiry generates illuminating data about individual members and about the family as a group. In this phase, it helps to clarify the hypothesis, to engage participants and affords the therapist greater facility to remain neutral and thus avoid forging alliances with an individual or subgroup. Because the system and not the identified patient is the target of change, the therapist is wary of showing bias. (This does not preclude transient alliances adopted for strategic purposes; these, however, need to be limited in time and distributed throughout the system.)

The therapist and family 'work' together for an hour or so on the basis of promoting curiosity, circular questioning, and neutrality. A number of options then follow. If the therapist is part of a team, her colleagues will have been observing the proceedings through a one-way screen. The family's consent, of course, will have been obtained previously. During a break the team—observers and therapist(s)—systematically pool impressions (Selvini, 1991). This is invariably a rich exchange as team members often note something others may have missed. As a result of these deliberations, a consensus about family functioning evolves. Conclusions are drawn and converted into 'messages'. The therapist returns to the family briefly to convey them. This is akin to the Delphic Oracle. The actual messages and their oracular quality comprise a potent intervention but not necessarily more cogent than interventions in the form of circular questions made earlier. Indeed, the advent of the narrative school has brought with it a de-emphasis on the 'therapist's message' on the premise that 'truth' is a shared construction.

The messages, usually between one and three, are given crisply and with maximal clarity. 'Homework' may be assigned and another session planned (unless termination was set for this point). Messages have several purposes including the promotion of intersessional 'work'. Three or 4 weeks is commonly set aside between meetings, and for good reason. During this time, the family, armed with new ideas, will tackle them in their day to day lives. It is not critical *how* they do so but important *that* they do so. To get back to the point about curiosity, and as Cecchin (1987) has argued, the family's interest in their own functioning should have been so aroused that they will be motivated to continue looking at themselves between sessions.

One of the authors (see Allman *et al.*, 1992) has conducted research on the nature of the message that led to devising a classification. Messages are divisible into three broad groups: supportive, hypothesis related, and prescriptive. In the first, the message has a reassuring, encouraging, or otherwise supportive quality but it is not related to the hypothesis. A complimentary message might be that 'The team were impressed by how open you all were in the session' and a reassuring one that 'This is like a new start for the family; there are bound to be uncertainties'.

Hypothesis-related messages refer to the hypothesis worked out by the therapeutic team, and may assume diverse forms. It may be stated directly, e.g., 'Susan has assumed the role of therapist for her parents and sister in order to prevent the family's disintegration.' There may be reference to change such as 'The team can see John taking responsibility to look after himself; John and his father's improved relationship has allowed this to occur'. The family may be offered options, an outline of possible choices related to the hypothesis, e.g., 'The family could risk being more open or you could continue to keep things to yourselves'. Paradoxical messages are a means to communicate a hypothesis that invites the family to revisit a feature of their functioning so that the family's difficulties are positively promoted and explicitly encouraged, e.g., 'The team sense that your problem is working for the good of your marriage; sticking with your illness can save the marriage'. The paradox may also be split in that the family are told about a divergence of opinion in the team (Papp, 1980). For instance, the family may be informed that some team members believe it too risky for them to communicate openly, whereas others suggest this can be done safely.

Through a prescriptive message the family is given a task directly. This may or may not be related to the hypothesis. For example, the family is urged to meet on their own before the next session in order to explore what inhibits a member from relating closely to the others.

Whatever the form of message, the therapist attempts to de-emphasize the pathological status of the identified patient and to apply what the Milan group refers to as positive connotation. The latter, a brilliant innovation, rests on the premise that all behavior is purposeful, and that the purpose can be construed positively. An adolescent's 'symptom of open grieving' is reframed as serving the family by sparing *them* the anguish of grief. This quality of message calls for creative thinking and flies in the face of the customary view of symptoms as evidence of psychopathology. Again, curiosity enters the picture as the family hears this positive communication concerning an issue that they have hitherto regarded as negative and abnormal.

The above process continues during succeeding meetings and attention is paid to what occurs in the family between sessions. Duration of therapy depends on how entrenched the family dysfunction is rather than on the status of an identified patient's problems. Thus, systemic change is aimed for and the family encouraged to consider a substitute mode of functioning that is feasible and safe. In practice, sessions range in numbers from one to a dozen. If progress has not been achieved by about session 8, it is likely that alternate ways of helping the family and/or the identified patient are called for.

Termination is less problematic than in individual or group therapy. The reason is obvious. The family has come as a living group and will continue to be one after the therapist bows out. In most approaches, even when the therapist is a prominent conductor, the family's own intrinsic resources are highlighted so that these can be drawn on and exploited further upon the therapist's exit. Determining the endpoint is usually straightforward in that there is a shared sense that the work has been accomplished. A hypothesis (or set of) has been introduced, tested, and confirmed. The family system has been carefully examined in order that impediments are recognized and understood and better modes of functioning devised and implemented. The family does not have to leave functioning optimally. Instead, termination occurs when there is agreement that the family is equipped with new options and feels confident to try them out over the long term.

As alluded to earlier, this may be determined alongside a judgment that an identified patient (or other member occasionally) requires another therapy in his or her own right. A clear example is an adolescent who has felt unable to separate and individuate. While family work has explored the system that blocked 'graduation' to adult psychological status, the sense prevails that he could benefit from individual or group therapy by building on changes already achieved. In another example, the parents may conclude, with the therapist's support, that they have an agenda that is not pertinent to their children and therefore best handled in couple therapy.

Problems encountered in therapy

Where assessment has been carried out diligently and motivation for change sustained, treatment proceeds smoothly. This is not to negate a possible crisis buffeting the group. But rather than being derailed, the family is encouraged to regard the crisis as a challenge with which to grapple.

Family treatment does not always succeed. Indeed, deterioration may take place, albeit in a small proportion of cases (Gurman and Kniskern, 1978). What are common difficulties encountered? The nonengaging family is problematic in that while evidence points to the need for family intervention, members cannot participate, usually because they resist letting go 'the devil they know'. In another variation, engagement of particular members may fail. This is particularly so in the case of fathers who tend to see the target of therapy as the identified patient rather than the family as a whole.

Missed appointments may punctuate therapy, often linked to turbulent experiences between sessions or apprehension about what a forthcoming session may reveal. Like any psychotherapy, dropout is possible. On occasion, this is reasonable inasmuch as the indication for family therapy was misconstrued. In other circumstances, dropout is tantamount to failure and may derive from such factors as therapist ineptitude, unearthing of family conflict that they cannot tolerate, and inappropriate selection of a family approach based on faulty assessment.

We have referred to the possible occurrence of a family crisis. Given that the family continues as a living group during treatment, they are exposed to all manner of vicissitudes, and these may disrupt the therapeutic work. For example, an overdose by the identified patient, abrupt marital separation, or a psychiatric admission may take its toll and serve to jeopardize treatment.

In discussing the ending of the treatment, we commented on outcome. Obviously, not all families benefit. The family's dysfunction may be so intractable as to be impervious to change, hypotheses may be 'off the mark', the family may lack adequate psychological sophistication, members may retreat in the face of change because of insecurity, and so forth.

Occasionally, dependency becomes a problem as the family senses a greater security when relying on the therapist. The latter may inadvertently foster dependency by assuming a role of authoritativeness that impedes a growing partnership. The family's own resources are then not given expression.

Finally, a family subgroup may harbor a secret that threatens the principle of open communication between members. The therapist may be inveigled into this group, although he stressed at the onset that keeping secrets is not conducive to the therapeutic process. For example, a call to the therapist from a spouse that she is having an affair that she will not disclose to her husband or children imposes a burden on both therapist and the family work.

Astute judgment is required in these situations. No ready-made prescriptions are available but instead a keen awareness in the therapist that difficulties are possible even in a highly motivated and well selected family. The general principle, however, is to prevent their evolution if at all possible or to recognize them early and 'nip them in the bud'.

Research in family therapy

In appraising the contemporary state of adult family therapy research, the choice is to see the glass as either half full or half empty. We opt for the more optimistic scenario. We need to remind ourselves that adult psychiatry family therapy is a toddler, dating only from the 1970s. During this time, immense strides have been made, particularly in the development of theoretical concepts. Pioneers in the field were chiefly therapists, working with families and tantalized by the nature of the process rather than its effectiveness. In hindsight, this makes sense. Models were completely lacking, the *how* to conduct treatment crying out for creative ideas. As can be seen in the theoretical part of the chapter, these have emerged bounteously, and continue to do so. The result is a rich array of therapeutic approaches, including several comprehensive theoretical contributions (Gurman and Kniskern, 1991). The growth has occurred at a dizzy pace with the inevitable consequence of overload. How can we make sense of the competing offerings? Is integration needed in order to forestall fragmentation of the field? Have we reached the point to reflect on what the terrain looks like? Are we now better placed to carry out outcome studies and to evaluate relative effectiveness? Tough questions and the research pathway is obstructed by many hurdles.

Observers of family therapy research, among them Gurman *et al.* (1986) and Bednar *et al.* (1988) have sought to clarify evolutionary themes and options for further work. Notwithstanding this collective endeavor, we have still not reached the enviable position say of an integrated model such as cognitive-behavioral therapy that, by dint of its relatively integrated status, has been systemically investigated, both its process and outcome, so that we are building up knowledge about how cognitive-behavioral therapy works and for what types of patients.

A complicating aspect of family therapy research is to define components of the approach, namely the therapist assembling a natural group, of varying composition, in which a dominant goal is to alter its functioning. This is altogether a more daunting matter compared with the relatively straightforward task of examining the effectiveness of say a well described treatment given to a single patient presenting with a well defined depressive syndrome.

Even if we were able to design solid outcome studies, we would be left with the conundrum of what constitutes the desired outcome and how to measure it. We can illustrate this by citing the conclusions of Asen and his colleagues (1991) in their investigation of 18 London families. Fundamental differences among the researchers emerged when handling the data. The team had decided to apply a multidimensional set of measures to assess change and at individual, dyadic, and family levels. At follow-up they noticed changes at the first two levels but not in the family as a group. The latter involved ratings of, *inter alia*, communication, boundaries, alliances, adaptability, and competence. The researchers were refreshingly candid in sharing their doubts about how to deal with the findings. Several contradictory interpretations were offered, e.g.: an absence of change in family functioning; the measure of that functioning nonreactive to treatment as it was a trait measure; and an inappropriate model of family therapy applied in the first place. Asen *et al.* concluded that the 'assumptive worlds' of therapists and researchers were being approved rather than the families themselves, a conclusion that makes good sense and an issue continuing to ensnare researchers. (These ethically related dimensions are discussed by Bloch *et al.*, 1994, in *The family in clinical psychiatry*.)

A research team in Oxford (Bloch *et al.*, 1991) encountered similar difficulties in their evaluation of 50 consecutive families treated in an adult family therapy clinic. Whereas two-thirds of the patients were judged to be improved at termination, only half the families were rated as functioning better or much better. Again, like the Asen team, the investigators were left with questions as how to determine what had actually been achieved.

A methodologically simpler way to wrestle with the issue is to focus solely on the identified patient's progress. Hafner *et al.*'s (1990) work exemplifies this choice—a case-controlled evaluation of family therapy in an inpatient setting with subsequent hospital admission data applied as the chief change criterion. Satisfactory as this study is in terms of design, the omission of a family system outcome measure leaves us hankering for more information about the group's functioning following the intervention.

With these tricky matters in mind, let us consider what research in the adult family therapy field needs to sort out. The diffuse question of whether family therapy works or not in this setting is of limited utility, and is reminiscent of the sterile debate that typified psychotherapy outcome research in the wake of Hans Eysenck's throwing down the gauntlet in 1952 (Alexander *et al.*, 1994). While subsequent meta-analyses demonstrated that psychological interventions overall exerted useful effects across a range of conditions, the field was still open to the criticism that efficacy of a specific therapeutic approach for a particular clinical state remained unanswered. The NIMH collaborative study on the treatment of depression was an advance. Family therapy should not repeat the same error and so squander opportunities and time. Instead of posing the futile question of whether family therapy works in adult psychiatry, we should instead ascertain whether a specific approach, whose character is well identified and adherence by therapists to it confirmed, is useful for both the identified patient, with a specific presentation, and the family's functioning, again well defined.

Research has begun to fulfill these desiderata. Many studies exploring interventions in families containing a schizophrenic member have described principles of treatment, the rationale upon which it is based, aspects of the process, and outcome measures in the patient and (in some cases) the family (see, for example, Falloon *et al.*, 1986). Helpful reviews can be found in Dixon and Lehman (1995) and Mueser and Bellack (1995). Although not as advanced as developments in schizophrenia, research conducted in the area of affective disorders has been innovative, and should pave the way for formal outcome studies (see Weber *et al.*, 1988; Keitner, 1990).

The Maudsley study on anorexia and bulimia nervosa aptly illustrates how outcome research can contribute to the clinician (Russell *et al.*, 1987). In a well controlled study, 80 patients were randomized to either family therapy or 'routine individual supportive therapy', following their discharge from an inpatient weight/restoration program. Treatment of the family involved an average 10 sessions, and individual treatment 15 sessions, spaced out over a 1-year period.

Family therapy focused on engaging the family and providing them with information about the eating disorder and the effects of starvation. Parental anxiety was acknowledged and efforts made to help parents take control of their daughter's diet. In parallel with improved physical status, therapy turned progressively to typical adolescent issues of separation and individuation and how these might be accomplished. A structural approach was applied, with systemic and strategic measures incorporated when progress slowed down.

Family therapy of a specific type can be applied to the family as a group in the light of system dysfunction. Thus, while the above research concerning particular psychiatric states, and involving an identified patient, is necessary for progress, this does not preclude outcome studies where the family is the principal target of change. We illustrate this with a particular form of family grief therapy developed in the Center of Palliative Care in the University of Melbourne (Kissane *et al.*, 1998). The model was derived from empirical research on the outcome of family grieving in an oncology setting. A 13-month follow-up yielded five family clusters of which two were distinctly dysfunctional, two functional, and an intermediate group at risk of maladaptive grieving. Three dimensions of family functioning were critical: cohesion, managing conflict, and expressiveness. The investigators then devised a model highlighting the goals of promoting cohesiveness, expressiveness, and optimal management of conflict. A corresponding screening instrument was applied to identify dysfunctional families.

Fifteen therapists were trained to use the emergent treatment guidelines and to work under close supervision in order to ensure that they adhered to the model. The randomized controlled trial (RCT) showed clearly the model's suitability and feasibility. Treatment began prior to the death of a terminally ill parent and extended into the bereavement period. Outcome measures included individual psychosocial morbidity and adaptation and the family's functioning. The model and its practical application are described in detail in *Family focused grief therapy* (Kissane and Bloch, 2002). The findings of the RCT are at the time of writing being subjected to statistical analyses.

This necessarily schematic account of research developments on family therapy in adult psychiatry suggests likely future trends. We can best summarize what research should strive for as: 'Specificity is of the essence'.

While postmodernist foundations of narrative therapies might suggest that they are less amenable to traditional research of the sort we have described, this has not proven to be entirely so. A group of researchers in London studied the accounts by family members of their experiences caring for an acutely psychotic relative, and discerned two patterns of narrative. In one that was described as having meaning, members' stories depicted themes of reparation and restitution and integrated the illness into ongoing family life. In the other, described as frozen or chaotic narratives, members viewed the illness as a series of random events (affinity with Byng-Hall's model—Byng-Hall, 1995; Stern *et al.*, 1999). The clinical implications of these two patterns and their relation to empirical studies of relapse prevention await elucidation.

Psychoeducational interventions for children whose parents suffer from a major affective disorder have been modified to pay attention to the children's narratives of their experiences. Initial findings indicate the possibility of improving the children's resilience and coping with their parents' illness (Focht and Beardslee, 1996). This research approach is promising in terms of its preventative potential and could be extrapolated to the adult sphere.

Training

From a few charismatic figures practicing idiosyncratic, innovative methods of family therapy, the field has developed into an immense, skillfully marketed enterprise in many countries, particularly the US, with hundreds of books, scores of training courses, several dozen journals, and a year-round program of local, national, and international conferences and workshops (Liddle, 1991).

Formal training may occur in one of three contexts (Goldenberg, I. and Goldenberg, H., 1996).

1. University-based, degree-granting programs view family therapy as a distinct profession, with its own corpus of knowledge, and offer diploma, masters, PhD, and postdoctoral training.

2. Free-standing institutes also tend to see family therapy as a distinct discipline and provide part-time training, usually of shorter duration than most university-based programs. A prerequisite for entry in most of these is that the candidate has completed basic training in one of the health professions.

3. Within university-affiliated hospitals and clinics that provide professional training in psychiatry, psychology, social work, and occupational therapy, many provide a brief course in the theory and practice of family therapy as part of general professional training.

Although there is a vast spectrum of training experiences to which students are exposed, most programs include:

1. Live supervision of clinical work with the supervisor (and often other students) observing the trainee and family from behind a one-way screen. Some clinicians consider the one-way screen to be dehumanizing and too objectifying of the family as well as adding to the trainee's performance anxiety. They advocate instead a model of co-therapy (trainee and supervisor), often with other students sitting in the interview room in full view of the family.

2. Video recording of the trainee's work, which is then reviewed by her in the presence of supervisor and fellow students is widely used. Tapes of particular models conducted by eminent therapists are also popular.

Whether training requires familiarity with concepts and techniques of a variety of schools or whether it is preferable to develop expertise in only one school remains debatable. Free-standing institutes tend to be run by therapists of a particular school, so that after a generally cursory overview of the field training is restricted to a specific model. This is even more likely when the program is part of general education in psychiatry, psychiatric nursing, psychology, and social work.

Diversity of schools and training reflects an uncertainty as to whether family therapy is a distinct profession, a method of conceptualizing psychopathology, or a set of therapeutic methods to add to the armamentarium of the mental health professional. This issue is further compounded by the aforementioned trend toward integrating psychodynamic, attachment, systems, feminist, and narrative approaches.

References

Ackerman, N. W. (1958). *The psychodynamics of family life*. New York: Basic Books.

Alexander, J., Holtzworth-Munroe, A., and Jameson, P. (1994). The process and outcome of marital and family therapy: research review and evaluation. In: A. Bergin and S. Garfield, ed. *Handbook of psychotherapy and behaviour change*, 4th edn, pp. 595–630. New York: Wiley.

Allman, P., Bloch, S., and Sharpe, M. (1992). The end-of-session message in systemic family therapy: a descriptive study. *Journal of Family Therapy*, **14**, 69–85.

American Psychiatric Association (1994). *Diagnostic and statistical manual of mental disorders*, 4th edn (DSM-IV). Washington DC: American Psychiatric Association.

Andersen, T. (1991). *The reflecting team: dialogues and dialogues about dialogues*. New York: W. W. Norton.

Anderson, H. and Goolishian, H. A. (1988). Human systems as linguistic systems: preliminary and evolving ideas about the implications for clinical theory. *Family Process*, **27**, 371–393.

Asen, K., *et al.* (1991). Family therapy outcome research: a trial for families, therapists, and researchers. *Family Process*, **30**, 3–20.

Bateson, G. (1972). *Steps to an ecology of mind*. New York: Ballantine Books.

Bateson, G., Jackson, D. D., Haley, J., and Weakland, J. H. (1956). Toward a theory of schizophrenia. *Behavioural Science*, **1**, 251–64.

Bateson G., Jackson, D. D., Haley, J., and Weakland, J. H. (1962). A note on the double-bind. *Family Process*, **2**, 154–61.

Bednar, R., Burlingame, G., and Masters, K. (1988). Systems of family treatment: substance or semantics? *Annual Review of Psychology*, **39**, 401–34.

Beels, C. and Ferber, A. (1969). Family therapy: a view. *Family Process*, **8**, 280–332.

von Bertalanffy, L. (1968). *General systems theory: foundation, development, applications*. New York: Braziller.

Bloch, S., Sharpe, M., and Allman, P. (1991). Systemic family therapy in adult psychiatry: a review of 50 families. *British Journal of Psychiatry*, **159**, 357–64.

Bloch, S., Hafner, J., Harari, E., and Szmukler, G. (1994). *The family in clinical psychiatry*. Oxford: Oxford University Press.

Boszormenyi-Nagy, I. and Spark, G. M. (1984). *Invisible loyalties: reciprocity in intergenerational family therapy*. New York: Brunner-Mazel.

Bowen, M. (1978). *Family therapy in clinical practice*. New York: Jason Aronson.

Braverman, S. (1995). The integration of individual and family therapy. *Contemporary Family Therapy*, **17**, 291–305.

Byng-Hall, J. (1995). *Rewriting family scripts. Improvisation and systems change*. London: Guilford Press.

Cecchin, G. (1987). Hypothesizing, circularity, and neutrality revisited: an invitation to curiosity. *Family Process*, **26**, 405–13.

Ciompi, L. (1988). *The psyche and schizophrenia. The bond between affect and logic*. Cambridge, MA: Harvard University Press.

Clarkin, J., Frances, A., and Moodie, J. (1979). Selection criteria for family therapy. *Family Process*, **18**, 391–403.

Cooklin, A. (1979). A psychoanalytic framework for a systemic approach to family therapy. *Journal of Family Therapy*, **1**, 153–65.

Dare, C. (1997). Chronic eating disorders in therapy: clinical stories using family systems and psychoanalytic approaches. *Journal of Family Therapy*, **19**, 319–51.

De Shazer, S. (1985). *Keys to solution in brief therapy*. New York: W. W. Norton.

Dixon, L. and Lehman, A. (1995). Family interventions for schizophrenia. *Schizophrenia Bulletin*, **21**, 631–43.

Epstein, N. B. and Schlesinger, S. E. (2003). In: M. Reineeke, F. Datrilio, and A. Freeman, ed. *Treatment of family problems in cognitive therapy for children and adolescents*, 2nd edn, pp. 304–37. Guilford Press: New York.

Falloon, I., Boyd, J. L., and McGill, C. (1986). *Family care of schizophrenia: a problem-solving approach to the treatment of mental illness*. New York: Guilford Press.

Flaskas, C. and Perlesz, A. (ed.) (1996). *The therapeutic relationship in systemic therapy*. London: Karnac.

Flugel, J. C. (1921). *The psychoanalytic study of the family*. London: Hogarth Press.

Focht, L. and Beardslee, W. R. (1996). "Speech after long silence": the use of narrative therapy in a preventive intervention for children of parents with affective disorders. *Family Process*, **35**, 407–22.

Friedmann, M. S., McDermutt, W. H., Solomon, D. A., Ryan, C. E., Keitner, G. I., and Miller, I. W. (1997). Family functioning and mental illness: a comparison of psychiatric and nonclinical families. *Family Process*, **36**, 357–67.

Goldenberg, I. and Goldenberg, H. (1996). *Family therapy. An overview*. Pacific Grove, CA: Brooks-Cole.

Gurman, A. and Kniskern, D. (1978). Deterioration in marital and family therapy: empirical, clinical, and conceptual issues. *Family Process*, **17**, 3–20.

Gurman, A. and Kniskern, D. (ed.) (1991). *Handbook of family therapy*, Vol. II. New York: Brunner-Mazel.

Gurman, A., Kiniskern, D., and Pinsof, W. (1986). Research on marital and family therapy. In: S. Garfield and A. Bergin, ed. *Handbook of psychotherapy and behaviour change*, 3rd edn, pp. 565–624. New York: Wiley.

Hafner, J., MacKenzie, L., and Costain, W. (1990). Family therapy in a psychiatric hospital: a case-controlled evaluation. *Australian and New Zealand Journal of Family Therapy*, **11**, 21–5.

Haley, J. (1976). *Problem-solving therapy*. San Francisco, CA: Jossey-Bass.

Jenkins, H. (1989). Precipitating crises in families: patterns which connect. *Journal of Family Therapy*, **11**, 99–109.

Keitner, G. (ed.) (1990). *Depression and families: impact and treatment*. Washington DC: American Psychiatric Press.

Kissane, D. and Bloch, S. (2002). *Family focused grief therapy*. Milton Keynes, UK: Open University Press.

Kissane, D., Bloch, S., McKenzie, M., McDowall, A., and Nitzan, R. (1998). Family grief therapy: a preliminary account of a new model to promote healthy family functioning during palliative care and bereavement. *Psycho-Oncology*, **7**, 14–25.

Langsley, D. G., Pitman, F. S., Machotka, P., and Flomenhaft, K. (1969). Family crisis therapy: results and implications. *Family Process*, **7**, 145–58.

Liddle, H. (1991). Training and supervision in family therapy: a comprehensive and critical analysis. In: A Gurman and D. Kniskern, ed. *Handbook of family therapy*, Vol. II, 2nd edn, pp. 638–97. New York: Brunner-Mazel.

Luepnitz, D. A. (2002). *The family interpreted: psychoanalysis, feminism and family therapy*. New York: Basic Books.

McFarlane, W. R., Link, B., Dushay, R., Marchal, J., and Crilly, J. (1995). Psychoeducational multiple family groups: four-year relapse outcome in schizophrenia. *Family Process*, **34**, 127–44.

McGoldrick, M. and Gerson, R. (1985). *Genograms in family assessment*. New York: Norton.

Minuchin, S. and Fishman, H. C. (1981). *Family therapy techniques*. Cambridge, MA: Harvard University Press.

Minuchin, S., Rosman, A., and Baker, L. (1978). *Psychosomatic families: anorexia nervosa in context*. Cambridge, MA: Harvard University Press.

Mueser, K. and Bellack, A. (1995). Psychotherapy and schizophrenia. In: S. Hirsch and D. Weinberger, ed. *Schizophrenia*, pp. 626–48. Oxford: Blackwell Science.

Papp, P. (1980). The Greek chorus and other techniques of paradoxical therapy. *Family Process*, **19**, 45–58.

Rosenfarb, I. S., Miklowitz, D. J., Goldstein, M. J., and Harmon, L. *et al*. (2001). Family transactions and relapse in bipolar disorder. *Family Process*, **40**, 5–14.

Russell, G. F., Szmukler, G., Dare, C., and Eisler, I. (1987). An evaluation of family therapy in anorexia nervosa and bulimia nervosa. *Archives of General Psychiatry*, **44**, 1047–56.

Sander, F. (1978). Marriage and family in Freud's writings. *Journal of the American Academy of Psychoanalysis*, **6**, 157–74.

Satir, V. (1967). *Conjoint family therapy*. Palo Alto, CA: Science and Behaviour Books.

Selvini, M. and Selvini Palazzoli, M. (1991). Team consultation: an indispensable tool for the progress of knowledge. Ways of fostering and promoting its creative potential. *Journal of Family Therapy*, **13**, 31–52.

Selvini-Palazzoli, M., Boscolo, L., Cecchin, G., and Prata, G. (1980). Hypothesising-circularity-neutrality: three guidelines for the conductor of the session. *Family Process*, **19**, 3–12.

Stern, S., Doolan, M., Staples, E., Szmukler, G. L., and Eisler, I. (1999). Disruption and reconstruction: narrative insights into the experience of family members caring for a relative diagnosed with serious mental illness. *Family Process*, **38**, 353–69.

Stierlin, H. (1989). The psychosomatic dimension: relational aspects. *Family Systems Medicine*, **7**, 254–63.

Thompson, M. C., Rea, M. M., Goldstein, M. J., Miklowitz, D. J., and Weisman, A. G. (2000). Difficulty in implementing a family intervention for bipolar disorder: the predictive role of patient and family attributes. *Family Process*, **39**, 105–20.

Tomm, K. (1987). Interventive questioning: Part II. Reflexive questioning as a means to enable self-healing. *Family Process*, **26**, 167–83.

Walrond-Skinner, S. (1978). Indications and contra-indications for the use of family therapy. *Journal of Child Psychology and Psychiatry*, **19**, 57–62.

Weber, G., Simon, F., Stierlin, H., and Schmidt, G. (1988). Therapy for families manifesting manic-depressive behaviour. *Family Process*, **27**, 33–49.

White, M. and Epston, D. (1990). *Narrative means to therapeutic ends*. New York: W. W. Norton.

7 Psychodynamic couple therapy

David E. Scharff and Jill Savege Scharff

Introduction

Psychodynamic couple therapy is an application of psychoanalytic theory. It draws on the psychotherapist's experience of dealing with relationships in individual, group, and family therapy. Psychodynamic couple therapists relate in depth and get firsthand exposure to couples' defenses and anxieties, which they interpret to foster change. The most complete version of psychodynamic therapy is object relations couple therapy based on the use of transference and countertransference as central guidance mechanisms. Then the couple therapist is interpreting on the basis of emotional connection and not from a purely intellectual stance. Object relations couple therapy enables psychodynamic therapists to join with couples at the level of resonating unconscious processes to provide emotional holding and containment, with which the couple identifies. In this way they enhance the therapeutic potential of the couple. From inside shared experience, the object relations couple therapist interprets anxiety that has previously overwhelmed the couple, and so unblocks partners' capacity for generative coupling.

The development of couple therapy

Couple therapy developed predominantly from psychoanalysis in Great Britain and from family systems theory in the US. At first the limitations of classical psychoanalytic theory and technique inhibited psychoanalysts from thinking about a couple as a treatment unit. In reaction to that inadequacy for dealing with more than one person at a time, family systems research developed. However, many of the early systems theorists were also analytically trained or had been analyzed, and so psychoanalysis had an influence on systems theory contributions to family therapy, and its extension to couple therapy in the US (J. Scharff, 1992). But it was not until object relations theory enriched the field of psychoanalysis in Great Britain that a form of psychoanalysis readily applicable to couples emerged.

Until then, psychoanalytic theory had stressed the innate drives of sexuality and aggression (Freud, 1905). Freud made little reference to the effect of the actual behaviors of parents on children's development, unless abuse had occurred (Breuer and Freud, 1893–95). True, Freud's later structural theory dealt with the role of identification with selected aspects of each parent in psychic structure formation, but these identifications were seen as resulting from the child's fantasy of family romance and aggression towards the rival, not from the parents' characters and parenting styles (Freud, 1923). It was as though children normally grow up uninfluenced by those they depend on until the Oedipus complex develops. Even then, the psychoanalytic focus was squarely on the inner life of the individual.

In the US, family systems theorists understood that spouses became part of an interpersonal system, and then devised ways of changing the system. However, without an understanding of unconscious influence on behavior, they could not address the irrational forces driving that system. In addition, they remained more interested in family systems than in couple systems for many years.

In Great Britain

Object relations theory emerging in Great Britain was also an individual psychology, but as it was being developed to address the vicissitudes of the analyst–analysand relationship, it lent itself well to thinking about couples, as shown by Enid Balint and her colleagues and students at the Family Discussion Bureau of the Tavistock Centre. As object relations theory continued to develop in Great Britain, it provided the theoretical foundation needed for the psychodynamic exploration of marital dynamics being explored at the Tavistock Institute of Marital Studies in the 1950s and 1960s (Pincus, 1955; Bannister and Pincus, 1971). Then in 1957, it was the publication of Henry Dicks (1967) landmark text, *Marital tensions*, integrating Fairbairn's theory of endopsychic structure and Klein's concept of projective identification that gave the crucial boost to the development of a clinically useful couple therapy. At that time, two therapists treated husband and wife separately, and reported on their sessions at a shared meeting with a consultant. The team could then see how the individual psychic structures of marital partners affect one another. This observation led Dicks to realize that the psychic structures interact at conscious and unconscious levels through the central mechanism of projective identification to form a 'joint marital personality,' different from, and greater than, the personality of either spouse. In this way, partners rediscover lost aspects of themselves through the relationship with the other. Later, Dicks and his colleagues realized that it was more efficient for a single therapist to experience the couple's interaction firsthand, and couple therapy as we know it today had arrived (Dicks, personal communication).

In the Americas

The next boost to couple therapy came from psychoanalysis in South America where modern concepts of transference and countertransference were being analyzed in detail. Racker (1968) thought that countertransference was the analysts' unconscious reception of a transference communication from the patient through projective identification. He said that this countertransference might be of two types, concordant or complementary. The concordant identification is one in which the analyst resonates with a part of the patient's ego or self. The complementary identification is one in which the analyst resonates with a part of the patient's object. Let's say that the patient who was abused by his father feels easily humiliated by aggressive men in authority positions. He feels like a worm in front of the analyst whom he glorifies, and he defends against this feeling of weakness and insignificance by boasting about his income. If the analyst feels envious and impoverished in comparison, he is identifying with the patient's ego (concordant identification). If the analyst responds by puncturing the boastful claims, he is identifying with the patient's object derived from his experience with his father (complementary identification). After Racker, analysts could understand their shifting countertransference responses as a reflection not just of the transference, but of the specific ego or object pole of the internal object relationship.

This insight from psychoanalysis deepened appreciation for the way that a relationship is constructed, each partner to the relationship resonating with aspects of projective identifications to a greater or lesser degree. Applying this insight to the couple relationship between intimate partners, couple therapists could better understand how partners treated one another. They also had a way of using their unique responses to each couple to understand how the partners connected with their therapist.

In North America in the 1960s, Zinner and Shapiro (1972) went against the systems theory mainstream to study the family systems of troubled adolescents in relation to their individual psychic structures, using Dicks's ideas as the explanatory linking concept. Focusing on the parents as a couple Zinner (1976) extended Dicks's ideas on marital interaction to explore marital issues as a source of disruption to adolescent development. Their research findings provided further support for the value of couple therapy. Another boost came in the 1970s from developments in the understanding and treatment of sexuality (Masters and Johnson, 1970; Kaplan, 1974; D. Scharff, 1982). Object relations theory of couple therapy now included an object relations approach to sexual intimacy (J. Scharff and D. Scharff, 1991). And in the 1990s, research on attachment processes stemming from the pioneering work of Bowlby, revealed that early infant attachment bonds influence the attachment patterns of adults, which have a profound effect on the life of couples and on the attachment styles of their children. Several clinicians and researchers have applied infant and adult attachment concepts to study the complex attachment of couples (Clulow, 2000; Bartholomew *et al.*, 2000; Fisher and Crandall, 2000).

Theoretical basis of psychodynamic couple therapy

Fairbairn's model of psychic structure

Fairbairn held that the individual is organized by the fundamental need for relationship throughout life. The infant seeks relationship with the mother (or primary caretakers) but inevitably meets with some disappointment, as when the mother cannot be available at all times or when the infant's distress is too great to be managed. The mother who is beckoning without being overly seductive, and who can set limits without being persecuting or overly rejecting, infuses the infant's self with feelings of safety, plenty, love, and satisfaction. The mother who is tantalizing, overfeeding, anxiously hovering, excessively care taking, or sexually seductive is exciting but overwhelming to the infant, who then feels anxious, needy, and longing for relief. The mother who is too depressed, exhausted, and angry to respond to her infant's needs has an infant who feels rejected, angry, and abandoned. The mother who gets it more or less right, has an infant who feels relaxed, satisfied, and loved.

When a frustrating experience occurs, the infant takes into the mind, or introjects, the image of the mother as a somewhat unsatisfying internal object, whether of an exciting or rejecting sort. The infant's next response is to split off the unbearably unsatisfying aspects from the core of this *rejecting internal object* and repress them because they are too painful to be kept in consciousness. However, whenever a part of an object is split and repressed, a part of the ego or self that relates to it is also split off from the main core of the ego along with the object. This now repressed relationship between part of the ego and an internal object is characterized by an affect. *The rejecting (or antilibidinal) object is connected to affects of sadness and anger. The exciting object is connected to affects of longing and craving.* Remaining more in consciousness connected to the central ego is *the ideal object characterized by affects of satisfaction.*

This produces three tiers of three-part structures in the self: central, rejecting, and exciting internal object relationships in the ego, and within each internal object relationship, a part of the ego, the object, and the affect that binds them.

In health, these elements of object relations organization are in internal dynamic flux, but in pathologically limited states, one or another element takes over at the expense of others in a relatively fixed way. So one person can be frozen into an angry rejecting stance towards others if dominated by

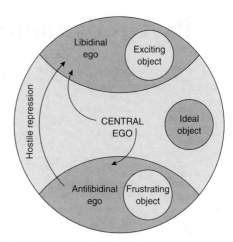

Fig. 7.1 Fairbairn's model of psychic organization. The central ego in relation to the ideal object is in conscious interaction with the caretaker. The central ego represses the split-off libidinal and antilibidinal aspects of its experience along with corresponding parts of the ego and relevant affects that remain unconscious. The libidinal system is further repressed by the antilibidinal system when anger predominates over longing as shown here, but the situation can reverse so that the libidinal system can act to further repress the antilibidinal system when an excess of clinging serves to cover anger and rejection. Copyright David Scharff. Reproduced courtesy of Jason Aronson.

rejecting object qualities; another can be fixed in an excited, seductive and sexualized way of relating. In some trigger situations, one of these ordinarily buried ways of relating can take over in an automatic and repetitive way (Figure 7.1).

Klein and Bion's theory of projective and introjective identification

Klein proposed that people relate unconsciously and wordlessly by putting parts of themselves that feel dangerous or endangered into another person by projection. This unconscious mechanism characterizes all intimate relationships beginning with the infant–parent relationship and continuing throughout life. Through facial gesture, vocal inflection, expressions of the eyes, and minute changes in body posture each of us continuously communicates subtle unconscious affective messages even while communicating a different message consciously, rationally, and verbally. These affective messages are communicated from the right frontal lobe of the brain of one person to the right brain of another below the level of consciousness, but they fundamentally color the reception of all communications (Schore, 2001). They transmit parts of oneself to the interior of the other person where they resonate with the recipient's unconscious organization (a *projective identification*) and may evoke identification with the qualities of the projector. The recipient of a projective identification takes in aspects of the other person through introjective identification (Figure 7.2).

For instance, a child who fears his own anger will place it in his mother, identify her with his own anger, and then feel as afraid of her as he felt of his own temper. Or a weak wife who longs for strength but also fears it, chooses a tyrannical husband whose power she regards with a mixture of fear and awe. A husband who is afraid that being sympathetic implies weakness locates tenderness in his wife or children, where he both demeans it and treasures it.

Bion (1967) described the continuous cycle of projective and introjective identification that occurs mutually between mother and infant. He studied the maternal process of *containment*, in which the parent's mind receives the unstructured anxieties of the child where they unconsciously resonate with the parent's mental structure, and the parent then feeds back more structured, detoxified understanding that in turn structures the child's mind. In this way, the child's growing mind is a product of affective

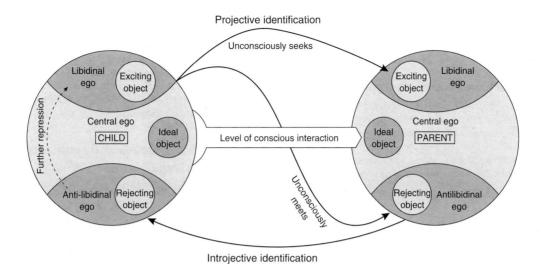

Fig. 7.2 Projective and introjective identification in a marriage. Let's read this diagram of a couple relationship from the husband's point of view. A husband craves affection from an attractive but busy wife. He hopes she will long for him as he longs for her, but she is preoccupied and pushes him away. He responds by rejecting her before she can reject him and he squashes his feelings of love for her. To put this in technical terms, his exciting object relationship seeks to return from repression by projective identification with his wife's exciting object relationship. Instead, it is further repressed by her rejecting object relationship with which he identifies in self-defense. His rejecting object relationship is reinforced as a result and so increases the unconscious secondary repression of his exciting object relationship. His rejecting object is enhanced and his exciting object is crushed. In the marriage with healthy unconscious fit, his rejecting and exciting objects would have been modified and reintegrated into the central ego. Copyright David Scharff. Reproduced courtesy of Jason Aronson.

and cognitive interaction with the parents. The same thing happens in couples: continuous feedback through cycles of projective and introjective identification is the mechanism for normal unconscious communication that is the basis for deep primary relationships. Bion (1961) also described *valency*, the spontaneous emotional clicking of strangers in a group setting, governed by fit between their unconscious needs. A couple is a special small group of two who click as strangers and choose to become intimate, based on their unconscious needs.

Dicks

Dicks (1967) built his theory of marriage by integrating these elements from Fairbairn and Klein (to which we later added the contributions from Bion on valency and containment). Marriage is a state of continuous *mutual projective identification*. Interactions of couples can be understood both in terms of the conscious needs of each partner and in terms of shared unconscious assumptions and working agreements. Cultural elements are the most obvious determinants of marital choice—the sharing of backgrounds or values that are part of conscious mate selection—but Dicks's research showed that the long-term quality of a marriage is primarily determined by *unconscious fit* between the internal object relations sets of each partner.

Winnicott's theory of the parent–infant relationship

To the foundation found in Dicks's integration of theories of Fairbairn and Klein, we have added other aspects. First, we have drawn from Winnicott's (1960) study of the infant–mother relationship (see Figure 7.3). He described three basic elements, the environmental mother, the object mother, and the psychosomatic partnership. The *environmental mother* offers an 'arms around' holding within which she positions the baby, providing a context for safety, security, a sense of well being, and growth. Within this 'arms around' envelope, the *object mother* offers herself as a direct object for use by the baby in a 'focused' relationship in which each incorporates the other as an internal object. There is a transitional zone between the contextual and the focused aspects of the infant–mother relationship. The *psychosomatic partnership* between parent and infant begins in pregnancy as a primary somatic connection with psychological aspects

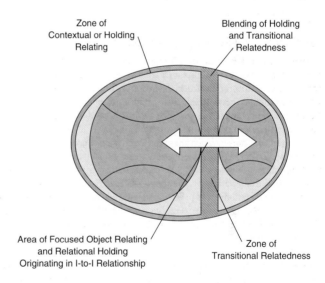

Fig. 7.3 Winnicott's conception of the mother–infant relationship showing contextual holding, transitional space, and focused relating. Focused (or centered or I-to-I) relating occurs in and across the transitional space. Transitional space is in contact with both contextual (or arms-around) relating and focused relating, and is also the zone that blends the two. Transitional space is also the space between inside and outside world for the mother and for the infant, and the space of exchange between their individual inner worlds. Copyright David and Jill Scharff. Reproduced courtesy of Jason Aronson.

based on the parents' fantasies of their unborn child and their imagined roles as parents. As the infant develops and becomes known as a person, the somatic element is subsumed in a psychological connection, which however, always retains vestiges of the original somatic one, and therefore can lead to the somatizing of psychological conflict. In later life the original psychosomatic partnership is the foundation of adolescent and adult sexual relationships (D. Scharff, 1982; J. Scharff and D. Scharff, 1991). In safety and intimacy enjoyed in the context of a committed sexual relationship, the partners experience a focused interpenetration of mind and body. They become each other's internal objects, drawing from internal object relationships that preceded their finding each other, and then modifying them in the light of new experience so as to build new internal organizations.

Attachment theory and couple therapy

Bowlby (1969, 1973, 1980) took an ethological approach to explore Fairbairn's proposition that relationships are the driving force in human motivation. Reviewing studies of mother-infant behavior across many animal species, he found that all primate infants show instinctual behaviors—rooting, sucking, clinging, crying, and smiling—and that these behaviors had nothing to do with aggression release or sexual pleasure. In Bowlby's theory, these instinctual patterns had to do with ensuring protection, proximity, and emotional connectedness, and that when these *needs for proximity* were not met, pathology resulted. Bowlby's theory came to be called attachment theory.

Ainsworth and her colleagues developed a research model for use with humans to explore and refine this early attachment theory. They designed a test called the 'Strange Situation' in which mother and baby are subjected to brief separations with and without a stranger present. They then study, score, and categorize the baby's reactions *on reunion* with the mother (Ainsworth *et al.*, 1978). Infants attachment style at a year can be classified into four groups: secure, anxious-insecure, avoidant-insecure, and disorganized/disoriented. If the baby treats the returning mother directly and confidently—even if the baby expresses angry protest at her absence—the attachment bond is coded as *secure*. If the baby clings, protests, and resists separating again, the coding is *anxious-insecure*; if the baby turns away and more or less shuns the mother, the coding is *anxious-avoidant*. If the infant moves away and then towards the mother, darts glances at her while avoiding her, and shows a chaotically rapid alternation of fear and need, the coding is *disorganized/disoriented*. This *disorganized/disoriented* group is associated with trauma and aggression perpetrated on the infant by the parent, or communicated to the infant unconsciously. It is of particular interest that an infant develops an attachment bond that is specific to each parent or caretaker. For instance, an infant can be securely attached with the mother and disorganized with the father.

Fonagy *et al.* (2003) argued that attachment is not an end in itself but a context in which the self develops out of its relationships to others, a point of view similar to Sutherland (1990). They held that, within those relationships, an important variable is the mother's capacity to mirror her child's feelings and yet mark them as belonging to the child and not to herself. Her capacity to reflect upon and *mentalize* her infants' experience helps the child to read the feelings and intentions of others, discover and regulate affect experienced in interaction, and develop a sense of personal agency and selfhood.

Recently, Main has developed a way of coding attachment styles in adults through analysis of their verbal narrative coherence as they describe their own histories (Main and Solomon, 1987; Main, 1995). Whether the content of these histories is secure or insecure is not the point. It is the style of the telling that determines the coding. An adult's attachment classification predicts the infant's attachment bond to that adult with a high degree of accuracy, even before the birth of the child.

Following these developments, researchers have begun to apply attachment theory to the study of couple dynamics. Clulow and colleagues at the Tavistock Marital Studies Institute have described *complex attachments* between couples (Clulow, 2000; Fisher and Crandall, 2000). Each partner provides an attachment object *for* the other while needing to be attached *to* the other. These patterns change with time and circumstance for a couple. Bartholomew and her colleagues have described various attachment patterns that correlate with healthy relationships and with those that are at risk for abuse or violence. For instance, a couple in which both parties code for secure attachment is at least risk, while a couple in which both partners show insecure, preoccupied, and anxious attachments is at greater risk, and the risk level is magnified when there are disorganized and fearful patterns (Bartholomew *et al.*, 2000).

Couples often experience distance or argument as a rejection that is analogous to the emotional separation that an infant feels. Similarly, they experience the interval between therapy sessions as a separation and reunion. This experience of the episodic nature of treatment mirrors the couple's own history of loss and reunion, and drives issues into the transference. This concurrence is then employed to advantage in couple therapy, as therapists interpret reactions to the frame of treatment in the light of the couple's previous experience.

Theory of transference and countertransference in couple therapy

Transference and countertransference are as central to psychodynamic couple therapy as they are to individual analytic therapy. To understand them, we refer to Winnicott's description of the environmental mother responsible for securing the context for safety and growth, and the object mother available to be used as the material for the child's world of inner objects. In the *contextual transference* a patient treats the therapist as a good understanding parent if the transference is positive, and as a misunderstanding, mismanaging parent if negative. In the *contextual countertransference*, the therapist feels taken for granted as a trusted benign parental object when things are going well, and treated with dismissal, suspicion, or seduction if negative. In the *focused transference* a patient may treat her therapist as a critical mother, a cherished sibling, or a seductive father—projections of discrete inner objects to which the patient's self relates. Or she may deal with her therapist as an ignorant child, greedy baby, or irresponsible adolescent—hateful or craving parts of her self that she puts into the therapist. In the *focused countertransference*, the therapist feels treated in a certain specific way—hated, desired, attacked, or shunned—depending on the discrete ego or object pole of the inner object relationship being lived out through projective identification (J. Scharff and D. Scharff, 1991).

In individual therapy, in the early phase as the patient negotiates entry into the therapeutic space and establishes whether it is safe and secure, the contextual transference is central. As therapy evolves, and with increasing trust in the contextual transference, discrete focused transferences emerge. The therapist receives these discrete object transferences and resonates with them, the resulting countertransference providing access to the internal organization of the patient and becoming the vehicle for their resolution (J. Scharff, 1992).

Similarly, in couple therapy, the contextual transference is important from the beginning, but it emanates not only from each partner individually, but more importantly from their holding of each other—that is from their shared environmental holding. Because the partners have a problem that leads to seeking help, by their own definition their shared holding has been insufficient. This deficit is further communicated to the therapist through their contextual transference. Figure 7.4 shows the transference situation and its origins in the contextual holding (which we sense in their joint marital personality) and through their centered holding (which is the sum of their patterned mutual projective identifications and use of each other as internal objects). Together they project aspects of their separate and shared unconscious life into the therapist, who receives them as countertransference. While individual transferences certainly occur in couple therapy, we understand these principally as compensations for what each partner misses in the couple relationship. In treating couples, we use countertransference to understand deficits in the couple's shared holding that make it difficult for them to provide safety, meet each other's needs, and contain anxiety (see below, example of evaluating a couple).

The *internal couple* is an unconscious psychic structure consisting of two internal objects in the relationship. It represents each person's accumulated experience and fantasies about couples—loving couples, hateful couples, couples with the impossibility of linking, couples who cannot differentiate, sexual and asexual couples. Each therapist carries an internal couple, a constellation comprising the sum of his or her experiences growing up with couples, and an essential determinant of the therapist's countertransference to a couple. Any couple in therapy resonates unconsciously with a facet

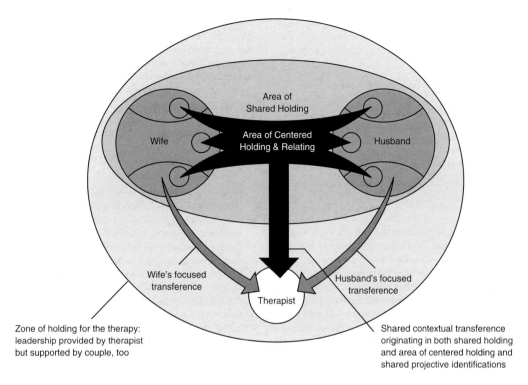

Fig. 7.4 Transference and countertransference in couple therapy. While focused transferences emanate from the individual partners, the most important source of couple transference is the shared contextual transference that conveys strengths and deficits in their shared holding capacity. Couple therapists' countertransference is most usefully interpreted as resonating with this area of transference. Copyright Jill and David Scharff. Reproduced courtesy of Jason Aronson.

of the therapist's internal couple, and this is unique to that couple and that therapist.

Technique in couple assessment and therapy

The frame

In assessment and in subsequent therapy, couple therapists begin by setting a firm, but flexible frame bounded by frequency and length of sessions for an agreed-upon fee, and maintained by a professional attitude that guarantees the couple confidentiality, respects ethical boundaries between therapist and couple, shows concern, interest, tact, and good timing. Couples' attempts to alter the frame are understood as communications about the holding provided by their couple relationship and their individual psychic structures in the present, and in their family of origin in the past.

Holding and containment

Couple therapists maintain a position of involved impartiality while creating a psychological space for work in which to offer safety and security (therapeutic holding) and begin the process of containment (mental receptivity, digestion, and unconscious resonance).

Following affect, gathering history, and working with the unconscious

They look for aspects of object relations history, not by getting a preprogrammed history or a genogram, but by asking for history at moments of heightened affect so as to understand the here-and-now expression of early experience. In this way, history provides the context and language for understanding inner object relations and their effect on current interactions, both in therapy and in the couple's life. Couple therapists track affect in the session because it reveals split-off object relations that are problematic for the couple.

Working with countertransference

Couple therapists use countertransference to detect transference that drives these core-affective moments. They analyze the feelings that are stirred in them by the couple they are treating and look for a match between their own responses and reactions the partners have now or in their families of origin. Responding to one member of the couple, the therapist arrived from inside his own experience at an idea of how that person's partner might be feeling. Resonating variously with a projected part of the ego or the object of one or another internal object relationship in wife or husband, over time therapists figure out the object relations set of each of member of the couple by receiving mirror images in their own object relations set.

Working with dreams and fantasies

Work with dreams and fantasy is another avenue through which therapists reach the unconscious levels of the couple relationship. If a partner reports a fantasy, the therapist asks more about it and helps the partner share reactions and other fantasies. When a partner tells a dream in couple therapy, it is regarded as a communication from both partners, both of whose associations to the dream are valued. All elements are combined in arriving at understanding conveyed through tactful interpretation of defense, anxiety, and inner object relations.

In assessment

In assessment, interpretations are tried out at several levels—from making links between memory and current experience, which the couple has kept apart, to making deeper interpretations about the defensive aspects of mutual unconscious projective identifications or the persistence of childhood patterns of interaction. This tests the couple's defenses and their capacity for therapy. A formulation is then given to support the therapy recommendations. Enough must be said so that the couple can get a taste of therapy and decide if it will be helpful, but it is too soon to know much, and too soon to say all that is apparent in case it might be overwhelming.

Table 7.1 Techniques of couple therapy

Maintain the frame
Hold attitude of involved impartiality
Track the affect
Take object relations history at core affective moments
Assess attachment style
Assess projective identificatory system
Use countertransference to detect transference
Integrate sex therapy
Work with dreams and fantasies
Interpret defensive patterns and subgroupings
Understand basic anxieties.

In therapy

In ongoing therapy, couple therapists continue their efforts to understand and interpret at moments of readiness. They offer continuing psychological holding and containment in a shared collaborative effort to promote growth and healing through understanding. Interpretation of conflict, defense, and understanding of basic anxieties take center stage. Working through the issues over and over in different guises takes the couple into the late phase of therapy. By the time the couple is able to support each other, identify issues, share feelings, dreams, and fantasies, detect the unconscious factors that are interfering, and maintain an intimate bond, they are ready to terminate, equipped with skills for dealing with the developmental challenges that may come their way.

Example of assessment with a couple

The following vignette illustrates the assessment process with a couple, in this case meeting with us as a co-therapy assessment team. A therapist working alone is equally likely to be effective, but for teaching purposes we have chosen a co-therapy example because it readily shows the effects of transference.

Assessing the couple's attachment style

Michelle and Lenny sought consultation because he wanted to get married and she wanted to break up. Their demeanor in the session was teasing, perverse, flippant, seductive, and yet highly entertaining. Michelle was taunting of Lenny, who appeared to delight in her no matter how she demeaned him. They explained that she was cruel only to him, and their friends did not enjoy their act, but as she said, 'He does bring it out in me.' When David Scharff asked why they were still together, Lenny answered, 'I'm the rock in the river, and I stay there while she runs up and down the river.' He thought of himself as being steadfast like a rock, but she accused him of being immovable as a rock. Michelle claimed to have all the vitality for the couple, and while Lenny agreed that he got liveliness from her, he also saw her as flighty.

Michelle had an avoidant attachment style, while Lenny had an anxiously clinging one. Their projective identificatory system was stuck in a pattern in which he idealized her vitality and his steadfastness, while she held him in contempt for being stubbornly passive and for idealizing her. Despite her contempt for his adoration, she desperately needed him to idealize her (as she did not love herself) and he needed her to bring him life.

Noting the projective identificatory system of the couple

Michelle's flamboyantly bright blue shirt with red, green and yellow leaves met an echo in Lenny's blue polo shirt with faint yellow and green stripes and a touch of red. David Scharff, struck by the similarity and difference in their dress, asked about the shirts.

Michelle burst out laughing at the ridiculousness of his comment. She said, 'It's a total coincidence! I bought that shirt for him. He would never buy it. It's not his personality; it's mine.'

However Lenny said, 'I like it, even 'tho I would probably buy the solids.'

The shirts gave a vivid image of their system of mutual projective identification. Lenny had the more solid version of the colorful personality

that he took in from the relationship with Michelle. She got stability from him even though she denigrated it as immovability. He got vitality from her, and tolerated her scorn as the price. Michelle said he came from an indulgent family that did not challenge him, while she came from a disorganized, intellectual family that felt special. Lenny added that in his family, he learned from his mother and sisters that men weren't good to women. He had grown up dedicated to setting that right.

Using transference and countertransference

As the session evolved, the therapists used the transference–countertransference exchange to understand and speak more effectively to the perverse quality of the couple's relationship.

Jill Scharff noted aloud that David Scharff had grown uncharacteristically quiet and seemed sleepy in comparison with her, much as Lenny seemed quiet compared with Michelle. She presumed that this difference between her and him was a countertransference response to the interior of the couple's relationship. She said aloud that she noticed that while she was quick to pick up on what was being said, he seemed uncharacteristically sleepy, perhaps responding to what was not being said. She said that she expected that his state of mind could be understood in a way that would allow more understanding of Michelle and Lenny's situation. That allowed David Scharff to shake himself back to a state of awareness and say what he had felt. He said that together Michelle's contradictions of his observations and Lenny's tolerance of her verbal abuse had defeated him—put him psychologically out of commission. Now, with Jill Scharff's supportive prompting, he was able to make this unconscious defeat conscious, and to say that Michelle's upbeat tone seemed to be the wrong music for the words she spoke about the death of the relationship. Michelle was quick to laugh off his comment that her words 'sounded like a dirge', but Lenny responded seriously. He said, 'It's like the jazz bands at a New Orleans funeral.'

Lenny's capacity to respond with another rich metaphor like this showed the emotional attunement and strength that must have been part of his appeal for Michelle, and encouraged us to predict a good capacity for work in ongoing therapy.

Asking about the couple's sexual intimacy
We asked directly about the couple's sexual life.

Michelle, nonplussed for the first time, said, 'You talk about it, honey!'

It quickly emerged that Michelle hated sex because she hated her body, but Lenny's steadfast caring and careful handling had enabled her to tolerate intercourse for the first time in her life, while enjoying other aspects of sex. Her tone changed instantly as she described the situation: she still had vaginismus—tightness of the pelvic musculature that produced pain on penetration—and she was not orgasmic in intercourse, but she had learned to have orgasms in the shared situation. Gratefully and straightforwardly, she gave Lenny credit in this area.

This discussion filled in another piece of the puzzle. Sex secured their attachment. In this area, Lenny was a good enough object (like a rock) who could modify Michelle's rejection of sexual experience (like water running past it) so that sex could be a pleasure for both of them. We recommended an extended evaluation for understanding the dynamic of their pursuit and avoidance at the surface and their unconscious connectedness at emotional depth, with a view to helping them decide whether to pursue couple therapy.

Integration of sex therapy techniques in couple therapy

Frank discussion of sexual functioning should be part of every couple evaluation. Matter-of-fact queries about sex from the beginning open a space for the frank discussion of sexual material as the therapeutic relationship deepens. Couples may accept superficially reassuring information about their sexual life at first, but later convey disappointment. They need their couple therapist to have a working knowledge of sexuality. Couple therapists must be fully informed on sexual development and dysfunction, sex research advances, and contemporary clinical approaches to extend those formulated by Masters and Johnson (1970), such as Kaplan's (1974) integration of behavioral sex therapy and psychodynamic couple therapy, and D. Scharff's (1982) developmental object relations approach to sexuality, sexual dysfunction, and sexual dysjunction on a couple's intimacy.

Couples' sexual difficulties derive from several areas: deficits in learning about sexual function—often because of cultural or family strictures concerning sex; problems in individual emotional development of one or both partners that produce difficulty in the sexual arena; and marital strain that takes its toll on a couple's sexual function. Life events and transitions— the moment of commitment or marriage, the birth of a first child or a child of one particular gender, adolescents leaving home, job loss, or the onset of menopause—may trigger anxieties that impinge on sexual function. Finally, physiologic factors interfere with sexual function: age, disease, or medication—especially psychotropic medications. Any of these factors that introduce difficulty in sex usually produce repercussions on the couple's overall relationship.

When sexual difficulty is the most significant feature of a couple's problem, or when it runs in parallel with overall difficulty and has not yielded to couple therapy, the couple therapist needs to use behavioral sex therapy techniques, integrated into the overall psychodynamic approach (Kaplan, 1974; J. Scharff and D. Scharff, 1991). The couple agrees to limit their sexual interaction to a graded series of exercises conducted in private. Exercises begin with nude massages, excluding breasts and genitals. Each session is reviewed with the therapist who looks for patterns of difficulty that provide an opportunity to work psychodynamically. Linking small failures in the exercises to the couple's overall difficulties and histories, the therapist interprets the underlying unconscious individual and couple issues, and integrates them in the subsequent assignments. Couples gradually move along the gradations of sexual exchange until they are ready for intercourse. Complete sexual function now has embedded in it both the therapist's contextual support and the therapist's collaborative effort to interpret themes that have precluded or inhibited sexual passion.

Working with dreams in couple therapy

Dreams offer partners a unique opportunity for working on unconscious communication inside the self and the couple's system. Dreams inform couples about the partners' internal self-and-object relations at the same time that they give important clues about the way each spouse uses the other as an external object. A dream from only one spouse obviously reflects the inner object relations of that one person, but told in couple therapy, that dream is regarded as a communication on behalf of the couple, and so it often leads to exploration of issues in both partners. When both partners report dreams, a richly interlocking texture of conscious and unconscious understanding is possible.

A clinical example of dream analysis in sex therapy

The following example illustrates both the course of sex therapy and the crucial role of dreams in helping a couple to move beyond therapeutic impasse. When working with dreams, couple therapists elicit the associations of both the dreamer and the partner and connect the elements of the dream to affect, personal history, sexual desire, and the intimate relationship.

Dr and Mrs T, both 35, were referred to me (DES) after adopting an infant girl. Trying unsuccessfully to conceive during the preceding infertility evaluation, Dr T had experienced impotence occasionally. The couple's shared low sexual desire had become apparent to the social worker during the subsequent adoption evaluation. Dr T mentioned two events that he had found traumatic: he had been involved in boarding school homosexual encounters; and his father had suddenly left his mother 7 years previously. Mrs T, who had older brothers, was pushed to be as athletic as the boys, which left her feeling shaky as a woman. In an individual session,

I encouraged Dr T to tell his wife about his performance anxiety and erectile difficulty. Seeing them in a couple session, I said that they shared an avoidance of sexuality because of uneasiness about themselves as sexual people. I described how shared low sexual desire derived from their internal couples—his of a warring couple, and hers of a family repressing feminine sexuality. They agreed to my recommendation for psychodynamic sex therapy to treat the sexual difficulty itself and to explore and resolve their emotional distance.

Insecure and avoidant aspects of the couple's attachment had been projected into their sexual bond. Both of them were open and trusting. I felt good about them and I was hopeful for their progress. It was not long before I recognized that my hope for them was my countertransference to an excited object transference, and it would soon meet the usual fate of disappointment.

My bubble burst when Dr T found obstacles to scheduling our work. Frustrated, I confronted Dr T more insistently than Mrs T had done. He finally changed his schedule, and reported with a sense of relief that he had passed a crisis of commitment. He felt for the first time different from his father.

The early exercises went well as the couple relaxed into them. They felt a new investment in each other. But when genital stimulation was prescribed, Dr T continually reported feeling no arousal, and drew a blank. To help the couple move past the impasse, I looked to their unconscious. I asked Dr T if he had had any dreams. He promptly obliged:

'I dreamt that a teacher I hardly knew at medical school came over and sat next to me. He was too arrogant to do that in real life. Last week I read that he had killed himself. We used to worry about suicide when my wife's brother was depressed but he didn't die. We also worried that her brother had organic causes for depression, just as I worry my impotence is organic.'

I said that as Dr T could masturbate normally, his erectile function was not organically impaired. So we should look to the dream for understanding the source of his impotence.

Mrs T said, 'I worry he doesn't find me attractive. I never feel sexy like a real woman. I was a runner who developed late and didn't menstruate until I was 23. I think I got stuck at age 16.'

I said that they both felt deficiencies about their bodies like most adolescents do, and that the dream showed that it felt like a life-or-death matter to them. The dream also suggested that they felt I was like an arrogant, unavailable medical school teacher, and could therefore not be trusted to be on their side.

The following exercise sessions were no different. Dr T felt no arousal even with genital stimulation, and actually lost arousal in masturbation exercises. I was losing hope for them. I thought, 'Perhaps they were not treatable after all!' To put this in technical terms, I absorbed their doubts in my countertransference through my introjective identification, and so began to feel my hope for them 'killed off.' I now experienced them as a failed exciting internal couple. It crossed my mind that if they left treatment without improvement, I would be relieved. To use language identified with their metaphors, I felt 'sick of treating them' and 'had lost my desire' to help. Here, in resonance with my internal couple was a replay in my countertransference of their unconscious problem. I felt seduced by them as exciting objects, and then let down by the failure they also feared.

Then Dr T brought a second dream, assuring me it was unrelated to therapy:

I was standing with some people in a large room with our backs to the wall. We were going to be executed one by one. At first, I felt defeatist. I took off my jacket just as I did a moment ago here. I thought, 'I hope they'll hurry.' Then I thought, 'I don't want to die. So, fight!' They were demonstrating killing us with carbon monoxide on a bed—which is how my old teacher killed himself. I asked to use the telephone and called my mother. There was no answer, but I just walked out the door of the room. I took off my shirt because it was a giveaway. It was 2 a.m. I began to run through a strip mall. A motorcycle cop caught up with me, but just then a bad guy came out and shot at him. The cop chased him and I got away.

Dr T's associations to the dream showed that the execution or asphyxiation that he feared was connected to the smothering anxiety of the sexual exercises that I assigned, for which he stripped, and which he carried out on a bed. When I said that the cop and the teacher he feared were standing for me, he said, 'No doubt about that! I am beginning to realize I am afraid of being controlled by you and by my wife if she controls my penis.' He said that the building in which he faced execution was like the boarding school he attended, leading us to talk about his pain on leaving home in adolescence. He explained that he had wanted away from his mother, but once he got to school he missed her and felt unprotected from the sexual teasing of older boys. He remembered that, as he left home, he suddenly realized that his parents had a sexual life.

In the dream, Dr T called his mother as he had done then when threatened by loneliness and homosexual seduction at boarding school. I realized that his resistance to therapy was a fearful reaction to me as a potentially seductive older boy and as a mother he might need too much.

> Responding to Dr T's realization that his parents had a sex life, Mrs T now said, 'Well, they did have another child after you left, your sister, and we named our daughter after her. When I realized that my husband was afraid of me suffocating him in bed if I became sexual, I kept sex under wraps, which suited me anyway because I was so frightened of it. He would treat me as though I were a cop like his mother. We are both afraid of being sexual, and so we've been afraid of you, or rather of what we asked you to do for us. But I think I can stand my fright if my husband will try to stand his.'

Mrs T's reluctance to engage sexually stemmed from her fear that being sexual would make her become a rejecting mother. Like her husband she was afraid of a controlling woman who emasculates her incompetent husband. Therapy addressed this shared internal couple and the unconscious fear it evoked.

In the exercises following this session, Dr T was easily aroused for the first time, and the treatment followed a rapidly successful course, to sexual satisfaction, and eventually to a much-desired pregnancy.

What broke the logjam? Dr and Mrs T recognized the dovetailing of their projective identifications. They revisited their adolescent anxieties about becoming sexual beings. They each found a critical parent in the transference and worked on it. They discovered that they were in the grip of a paralyzed internal couple. Dr T allowed the image of his parents as a sexual couple to resurface, which gave him permission to be a sexual person and reassure his wife that she was desirable. The recovery of an unconscious sexual internal couple facilitated the actual couple's re-entry into the intimate life of the marriage. Given enough time, commitment, and a willingness to work with dreams and fantasies, many couples respond as well.

Challenges to the couple therapist

Working with trauma in couple therapy

Childhood physical abuse, sexual abuse, and traumatic medical intervention at a young age, significantly affect individual development by creating traumatic nuclei and gaps in the psyche. Adult survivors of trauma may visit trauma on their partners or avoid anything that might cause it recurrence. Sexual abuse will often—but not always—show up as sexual symptomatology in the couple, even if they have been able to have a relatively normal sexual life before marriage or early in the marriage (Scharff and Scharff, 1994). Adult trauma, too, will handicap couples, especially if it reawakens memories of childhood injury. Adults who were traumatized in childhood are at increased risk for adult trauma.

> Tony and Theresa came to therapy after Tony lost his right arm and shoulder to amputation to abort a life-threatening infection in the upper arm following an injection there for asthma. Although his employer offered to support physical therapy and the fitting of a prosthetic arm, Tony resisted rehabilitation and became immobilized with depression. Theresa and he grew increasingly angry at each other over the next year. Exploring their anger, the therapist learned that in growing up, they had suffered physical violence. Each had taken the role of defending their siblings from physical attacks from their parents, and been hit frequently in the process. When they married, they had vowed never to fight, and now would go so

far as to punch the wall and break their fists rather than strike each other. They would break a bone, or break up as a couple, rather than risk expressing anger directly, lest they lose all control and hurt each other.

The trauma experienced in adulthood brought this couple's shared history of childhood physical abuse to the forefront. Early in their marriage, their adult attachment seemed secure, but now trauma threatened to overwhelm their current recovery and brought out the old insecurity. Trauma to one partner can overwhelm the couple's holding and containment for one another. A therapist must spend time as witness to the trauma before it is possible to help the couple work in a symbolic, reparative way (Scharff and Scharff, 1994; D. Scharff, 2002).

Working with the difficult couple

The difficult couple is the one that the therapist dreads seeing. A therapist may be unable to tolerate silence, another cannot stand relentless fighting, yet another may be allergic to sweetness that masks hostility. Another type of difficult couple is the one in which one of the partners is sure that the other is being sided with by the therapist. The therapist who is committed to involved impartiality may feel extremely upset by accusations of unfairness and fail to interpret the sibling rivalries being fought out, probably because of painful feelings towards her parents over sibling issues of her own. Whatever specific form it takes, the difficult couple gets to the therapist's internal parental couple and stirs unease and sometimes despair (J. Scharff, 1992). The therapist's capacity for holding and containment is stretched to the limit. Only when the therapist is open to experiencing fully in the countertransference the hopelessness that underlies the couple's defense of being difficult is there some hope of recovery (D. Scharff and J. Scharff, 1991). On the other hand, sometimes the best course is to acknowledge a lack of fit and refer the couple. What may present a problem for one therapist may be easier for another. On the other hand the difficult couple may dump all their negativity with one therapist and appear to do well with the next one but in fact the partners have not developed the capacity to integrate good and bad objects.

Managing resistance to couple therapy

Sometimes one member of a couple does not want therapy, but it is usually possible to get the couple in for a single consultation session in which to work on the reasons for refusing treatment. The psychodynamic couple therapist does not use persuasion or paradoxical prescription to get the couple into treatment, but accepts that these must be a good reason for the resistance and tries to make it conscious and understandable so as to free the couple to make a choice based on a good experience of the value of reflection. Once a couple therapy contract is made, couple therapists work with the couple, not with the individual partners. They establish that way of working and hold to it as a standard from which to negotiate frequency, experiment with requests for individual sessions, and learn.

Working with the couple when there is an affair

The couple dealing with infidelity is filled with disappointment, envy, rage, and sadness. The first task of the couple therapist is to hold all the feelings that the marriage could not. Then she wants to know details of the affair because the attraction of the lover and the keeping of a secret contain important information about repressed object relations that cannot be expressed and contained within the marriage. Splitting good and bad objects between spouse and someone else is a major defense, and it does not stop with the end of the affair. Some couple therapists insist that the affair be stopped, on the grounds that they do not want to sanction a duplicitous life, but most therapists accept the marriage and its infidelity as the patient. They work to see whether the marriage is to continue, at which point the lover must indeed be renounced. Intimate partners cannot work on their relationship while one of them has another intimate partner. Even though the affair is a betrayal and a threat to the marriage, it is often also an attempt to maintain the marriage by getting needs met elsewhere. Sometimes a partner reveals the secret to the therapist on the phone or in an individual session to which both partners have agreed. In this case it is best to acknowledge that a problem has arisen, and ask for more individual sessions to work it through. The therapist does not want to force a confession, but if the marriage is to continue in couple therapy, she learns about the meaning of the affair and the need for secrecy in individual terms, and works towards a planned revelation in the couple setting. Individual work like this may result in ending the couple therapy, or it may become a prelude to it.

Handling acute couple distress

Acute distress arises for instance when there is a sudden revelation of an affair, death of a newborn, suicide threat, acute psychotic reaction, and acute intoxication from substance abuse. Acute distress calls upon the couple therapist for an emergency appointment of sufficient length to assess the situation, give the couple time to express their distress, and let the therapist develop the necessary holding capacity and make the necessary arrangements—or refer to a colleague who can do so. Medication, removal of a violent member from the home, emergency care, and couple consultation may work together to avoid a hospitalization. Speed is essential for taking advantage of the healing potential of the crisis in the system. Enough time is essential for demonstrating the possibility of understanding their overwhelming emotion. And a second appointment within the week should be confirmed before the couple leaves the session.

Termination

The couple in therapy has had some rehearsal for termination when ending each time-limited session and facing breaks in treatment due to illness, business commitments, or vacations. Couple therapists work with the couple's habitual way of dealing with separations in preparation for the final parting, for which they will be ready when the above goals have been met. The couple relives issues from earlier phases of the treatment, now with a greater capacity for expressing feelings, allowing difference, recovering from difficult moments, dealing with loss, respectfully confronting and understanding defensive positions, and mastering anxiety (Table 7.2).

Table 7.2 Criteria for termination

The therapeutic space has been internalized as a reasonably secure holding capacity
Unconscious projective identifications have been recognized, owned, and taken back
The capacity to work together as life partners is restored
Intimacy and sex are mutually gratifying
The holding environment extends to the family
The needs of each partner are separate and distinct
Or, the loss of the marriage is accepted, understood, and mourned

---

References

Ainsworth, M. D. S., Blehar, M., Waters, E., and Wall, S. (1978). *Patterns of attachment: a psychological study of the strange situation*. Hillsdale, NJ: Erlbaum.

Bannister, K. and Pincus, L. (1971). *Shared fantasy in marital problems: therapy in a four-person relationship*. London: Tavistock Institute of Human Relations.

Bartholomew, K., Henderson, A., and Dutton, D. (2000). Insecure attachment and abusive relationships. In C. Clulow, ed. *Adult attachment and couple psychotherapy*, pp. 43–61. London: Brunner/Routledge.

Bion, W. R. (1961). *Experiences in groups and other papers*. London: Tavistock.

Bion, W. R. (1967). *Second thoughts*. London: Heinemann.

Bowlby, J. (1969). *Attachment and loss*, Vol. 1: *Attachment*. London: Hogarth Press. New York: Basic Books.

Bowlby, J. (1973). *Attachment and loss*. Vol. 2: *Separation: anxiety and anger*. London: Hogarth Press. New York: Basic Books.

Bowlby, J. (1980). *Attachment and loss*. Vol. 3: *Loss: sadness and depression*. London: Hogarth Press. New York: Basic Books.

Breuer, J. and Freud, S. (1893–1895). *Studies on hysteria*. In: J. Strachey, trans. and ed. *The standard edition of the complete psychological works of Sigmund Freud*, Vol. 2, pp. 1–305. London: Hogarth Press, 1955.

Clulow, C., ed. (2000). *Adult attachment and couple psychotherapy*. London: Brunner/Routledge.

Dicks, H. V. (1967). *Marital tensions: clinical studies towards a psychoanalytic theory of interaction*. London: Routledge and Kegan Paul.

Fisher, J. and Crandell, L. (2000). Patterns of relating in the couple. In: C. Clulow, ed. *Adult attachment and couple psychotherapy*, pp. 15–27. London: Brunner/Routledge.

Fonagy, P., Gergely, G., Jurist, E. L., and Target, M. (2003). *Affect regulation, mentalization, and the development of the self*. New York: Other Press.

Freud, S. (1905). *Three essays on the theory of sexuality*. In: J. Strachey, trans. and ed. *The standard edition of the complete psychological works of Sigmund Freud*, Vol. 7, pp. 135–243. London: Hogarth Press, 1953.

Freud, S. (1923). *The ego and the id*. In: J. Strachey, trans. and ed. *The standard edition of the complete psychological works of Sigmund Freud*, Vol. 19, pp. 3–66. London: Hogarth Press, 1961.

Kaplan, H. S. (1974). *The new sex therapy*. New York: Brunner/Mazel.

Main, M. (1995). Recent studies in attachment: overview, with selected implications for clinical work. In: S. Goldberg, R. Muir, and J. Kerr, ed. *Attachment theory: social, developmental, and clinical perspectives*. Hillsdale, NJ: Analytic Press.

Main, M. and Solomon, J. (1987). Discovery of an insecure disorganized/disoriented attachment pattern: procedures, findings and implications for the classifications of behaviour. In: M. Yogman and T. Brazelton, ed. *Affective development in infancy*. Norwood, NJ: Ablex.

Masters, W. H. and Johnson, V. E. (1970). *Human sexual inadequacy*. Boston: Little, Brown.

Pincus, L., ed. (1955). *Marriage: studies in emotional conflict and growth*. London: Methuen.

Racker, H. (1968). *Transference and countertransference*. New York: International Universities Press.

Scharff, D. E. (1982). *The sexual relationship: an object relations view of sex and the family*. London: Routledge. (Reprinted 1998: Northvale, NJ: Jason Aronson.)

Scharff, D. E. (2002). The interpersonal sexual tie to the traumatic object. In: J. S. Scharff and S. Tsigouaris, ed. *Self hatred in psychoanalysis*, pp. 47–68. London: Routledge.

Scharff, J. S. (1992). *Projective and introjective identification and the use of the therapist's self*. Northvale, NJ: Jason Aronson.

Scharff, J. S. and Scharff, D. E. (1991). *Object relations couple therapy*. Northvale, NJ: Jason Aronson.

Scharff, J. S. and Scharff, D. E. (1994). *Object relations therapy of physical and sexual trauma*. Northvale, NJ: Jason Aronson.

Schore, A. N. (2001). The right brain as the neurobiological substratum of Freud's dynamic unconscious. In: D. E. Scharff, ed. *The psychoanalytic century: Freud's legacy for the future*. New York: Other Press.

Sutherland, J. D. (1990). Reminiscences. In: J. S. Scharff, ed. *The autonomous self: the work of John D. Sutherland*, pp. 392–423. Northvale, NJ: Jason Aronson.

Winnicott, D. W. (1960). The theory of the parent–infant relationship. *International Journal of Psycho-Analysis*, **41**, 585–95.

Zinner, J. (1976). The implications of projective identification for marital interaction. In: H. Grunebaum and J. Christ, ed. *Contemporary marriage: structure, dynamics, and therapy*, pp. 293–308. Boston: Little, Brown.

Zinner, J. and Shapiro, R. (1972). Projective identification as a mode of perception and behavior in families of adolescents. *International Journal of Psycho-Analysis*, **53**, 523–30.

8 Cognitive-behavior therapy with couples

Frank M. Dattilio

Introduction

Cognitive-behavioral therapy with couples (CBTC) clearly emerged in the past decade as a powerful and effective approach, whether as a mode of integration with other forms of therapy (Dattilio, 1998; Dattilio and Epstein, 2003) or as an independent modality.

It was Albert Ellis who first considered the viability of the application of CBTC (Ellis and Harper, 1961). Ellis and his colleagues acknowledged the important role that cognition plays in marital dysfunction. Ellis offered the premise that relationship dysfunction occurs when partners maintain unrealistic beliefs about their relationship and render extreme negative evaluations of the sources of their dissatisfaction (Ellis, 1977; Ellis *et al.*, 1989). In the 1960s and 1970s, behavior therapists had experimented with applying the principles of learning theory to address problematic behaviors of both adults and children. Many of the behavioral principles and techniques that were used in the treatment of individuals were subsequently applied to distressed couples, and then later to families. For example, Stuart (1969), Liberman (1970), and Weiss *et al.* (1973) presented the use of social exchange theory and principles from operant learning to facilitate more satisfying interactions among couples who complained of distress. This set the stage for the subsequent research that led marital therapists to recognize the importance of intervening with cognitive factors and behavioral interactional patterns. Prior to the major theories of family therapy, it was noted that cognitions could be used as auxiliary components of treatment within a behavioral paradigm (Margolin and Weiss, 1978); however, it was the 1980s that cognitive factors became a real focus of the couples research and therapy literature. Cognitions began to be addressed in treatment in more direct and systematic fashion than what was being proposed in other theoretical approaches to couples therapy (Epstein and Eidelson, 1981; Epstein, 1982; Weiss, 1984; Baucom, 1987; Fincham *et al.*, 1987; A. T. Beck, 1988; Baucom *et al.*, 1989; Dattilio, 1989). As modified distortion and inappropriate perceptions became the focus with couples, therapists began to direct more of their attention toward the inferences and beliefs that partners held about each other and toward their possible use in finding solutions to relationship impasses (Epstein and Baucom, 1989; Baucom and Epstein, 1990; Epstein, 1992; Dattilio and Padesky, 1995). Cognitive assessment and intervention methods were borrowed from individual therapy and adapted for use with couples. As in individual therapy, cognitive-behavioral marital interventions were designed to enhance the partners' abilities to evaluate and modify their own problematic cognitions, as well as to develop skills for communicating and solving problems constructively (Baucom and Epstein, 1990; Epstein and Baucom, 2002).

Although substantial empirical evidence has been accumulated from treatment outcome studies to indicate the effectiveness of CBTC, most studies have focused primarily on behavioral interventions and only a handful have examined the impact of cognitive restructuring procedures (refer to Baucom *et al.*, 1998, for a complete review).

The growing use of cognitive-behavioral methods by couple therapists may be attributed to several factors: research that has supported their efficacy; clients, who generally value a proactive approach to solving problems and building skills, respond positively to them; emphasizes the methods a collaborative relationship has between therapist and client; and finally, the ideas are highly compatible with other modalities of therapy. Recent enhancements of CBTC (Epstein and Baucom, 2002) have broadened the contextual factors that are taken into account, such as aspects of the couple's physical and interpersonal environment (e.g., extended family, the workplace, neighborhood violence, national economic conditions). The approach continues to evolve through the creative efforts of its practitioners and the ongoing research that keeps expanding its applicability to the field.

A cognitive-behavioral model of case conceptualization

Case conceptualization is paramount in CBTC, especially when attempting to understand the dynamics between two people. Much of the conceptualization used follows the basic theory of dysfunctional schemata, which is outlined in detail below.

Automatic thoughts, underlying schemata, and cognitive distortions

Baucom *et al.* (1989) developed a typology of cognitions that have been applied to distressed relationships. Although each type is a normal form of human cognition, all are susceptible to being distorted (Baucom and Epstein, 1990; Epstein and Baucom, 2002). These types include: (1) *selective attention*, an individual's tendency to notice particular aspects of the events occurring in his or her relationship and to overlook others; (2) *attributions*, inferences about the factors that have influenced one's own and one's partner's actions (e.g., concluding that a partner failed to respond to a question because he or she wants to control the relationship); (3) *expectancies*, predictions about the likelihood that particular events will occur in the relationship (e.g., that expressing feelings will result in the partner's being verbally abusive); (4) *assumptions*, beliefs about the natural characteristics of people and relationships (e.g., a wife's generalized assumption that men do not need emotional attachment); and (5) *standards*, beliefs about the characteristics that people and relationships 'should' have (e.g., that partners should have no boundaries between them, sharing all of their thoughts and emotions with each other). Because there is typically so much information available in any interpersonal situation, some degree of selective attention is inevitable. Nonetheless, the potential to form biased perceptions of each other must be addressed. Errors in these inferences can often have negative effects on couple relationships, especially when an individual attributes another's actions to negative motives (e.g., malicious intent) or misjudges how the other will react to one's own actions. Assumptions are commonly adaptive when they are realistic representations of people and relationships, and many standards that individuals hold, such as moral standards concerning the avoidance of abuse of others, contribute to the quality of relationships. Nevertheless, inaccurate or extreme assumptions and standards can lead individuals to inappropriate interaction.

Beck and associates (e.g., A. T. Beck *et al.*, 1979; J. Beck, 1995) refer to moment-to-moment stream-of-consciousness ideas, beliefs, or images as *automatic thoughts*; for example, 'My wife shares our personal business with others. She doesn't care about my feelings regarding privacy.' Cognitive-behavior therapists have noted that individuals commonly accept automatic thoughts at face value rather than examining their validity. Although all five of the types of cognition identified by Baucom *et al.* (1989) can be reflected in an individual's automatic thoughts, cognitive-behavioral therapists have emphasized the moment-to-moment selective perceptions and the inferences involved in attributions and expectancies as being the most apparent within an individual's awareness. Assumptions and standards are thought to involve broader underlying aspects of an individual's world view and are considered to be schemata in Beck's cognitive model (A. T. Beck *et al.*, 1979; J. S. Beck, 1995; Leahy, 1996).

The cognitive model proposes that the content of an individual's perceptions and inferences is shaped by relatively stable underlying *schemata*, or cognitive structures, such as the personal constructs first described by Kelly (1955). Schemata include basic beliefs about the nature of human beings and their relationships, which are assumed to be relatively stable and may become inflexible. Many schemata about relationships and the nature of couples' interactions are learned early in life from primary sources, such as family-of-origin, cultural traditions and mores, the mass media, and early dating or other relationship experiences. The 'models' of self in relation to others that have been described by attachment theorists appear to be forms of schemata that affect individuals' automatic thoughts and emotional responses to significant others (Johnson and Denton, 2002). In addition to the schemata that partners bring to a relationship, each member develops schemata specific to the current relationship.

Schemata about relationships are often not articulated clearly in an individual's mind, but nonetheless exist as vague concepts of what is or should be (A. T. Beck, 1988; Epstein and Baucom, 2002). Previously developed ideas affect how an individual currently processes information in new situations, perhaps, for example, influencing what the person selectively perceives, the inferences he or she makes about causes of others' behavior, and whether the person is pleased or displeased with the relationship. Existing schemata may be difficult to modify, but repeated new experiences with significant others have the potential to change them (Epstein and Baucom, 2002; Johnson and Denton, 2002).

In addition to automatic thoughts and schemata, A. T. Beck *et al.* (1979) identified *cognitive distortions* or information-processing errors that contribute to cognitions' becoming sources of distress and conflict in individuals' lives. In terms of Baucom *et al.*'s (1989) typology, such errors result in distorted or inappropriate perceptions, attributions, expectancies, assumptions, and standards.

There has been much more research on attributions and standards than on the other forms of cognition in Baucom *et al.*'s (1989) typology (see Epstein and Baucom, 2002, for a review of findings). A sizable amount of research on couples' attributions has indicated that spouses in distressed relationships are more likely than those in nondistressed couples to attribute the partner's negative behavior to global, stable traits; negative intent; selfish motivation; and a lack of affection (see Bradbury and Fincham, 1990 and Epstein and Baucom, 2002, for reviews). In addition, spouses in distressed relationships are less likely to attribute positive partner behaviors to global, stable causes. These biased inferences can contribute to pessimism about improvement in the relationships and to negative communication and faulty problem solving. One area of research on schemata has focused on potentially unrealistic beliefs that individuals may hold about marriage (Epstein and Eidelson, 1981). Baucom *et al.* (1996a) assessed the relationship standards that individuals hold about boundaries between partners, distribution of control/power, and the degree of investment one should have in the relationship. They found that those who were less satisfied with the manner in which their standards were met within the relationship were more distressed and communicated more negatively with the partner.

Deficits in communication and problem-solving skills

A considerable amount of empirical evidence shows that distressed couples exhibit a variety of negative and ineffective patterns of communication involving their expression of thoughts and emotions, listening skills, and problem-solving skills (Walsh, 1998; Epstein and Baucom, 2002). Expression of thoughts and emotions involves self-awareness, appropriate vocabulary to describe one's experiences, freedom from inhibiting factors, such as fear of rejection, and a degree of self-control (e.g., not succumbing to an urge to retaliate against the person who upset you). Effective problem-solving pivots on the abilities to define the characteristics of a problem clearly, generate alternative potential solutions, collaborate with one's spouse in evaluating the advantages and disadvantages of each solution, reach consensus about the best solution, and devise a specific plan to implement the solution.

Weaknesses in communication and problem solving may develop as a result of various processes, such as maladaptive patterns of learning during socialization in the family-of-origin, deficits in cognitive functioning, forms of psychopathology, such as depression, and past traumatic experiences in relationships that have rendered an individual vulnerable to disruptive cognitive, emotional, and behavior responses (e.g., rage, panic) during interactions with significant others. Research has indicated that spouses who communicate negatively in their relationships may exhibit constructive communication skills in external relationships with others, suggesting that chronic issues in the intimate relationship are directly impeding positive communication (Baucom and Epstein, 1990).

Excesses of negative behavior and deficits in positive behavior between spouses

Negative and ineffective communication and problem-solving skills are not the only forms of problematic behavioral interaction with distressed couples. Members of close relationships commonly direct a variety of types of nonverbal behavior toward each other (Baucom and Epstein, 1990; Epstein and Baucom, 2002); that is, positive and negative acts that are instrumental (perform a task to achieve a goal, such as completing household chores) or actions intended to affect the other person's feelings (for example, giving a gift). Although there are typically implicit messages conveyed by taciturn behavior, it does not involve the explicit expression of thoughts and emotions. According to the research, partners in distressed relationships direct more negative acts and fewer positive ones toward each other than do members in nondistressed relationships (Epstein and Baucom, 2002). Furthermore, members of distressed couples are more likely to reciprocate negative behaviors, resulting in an escalation of conflict and distress. Consequently, a basic premise of CBTC is that the frequency of negative behavior must be reduced and the frequency of positive behaviors increased. This is particularly important because negative behaviors tend to have a greater impact on the experience of relationship satisfaction than do positive behaviors (Gottman, 1994; Weiss and Heyman, 1997). Negative behaviors have also received more attention from therapists; however, although clients may be distressed in the absence of such behaviors, they still long for more rewarding relationships (Epstein and Baucom, 2002).

Couple theorists and researchers have to this point focused on microlevel positive and negative acts, but Epstein and Baucom (2002) propose that in many instances, an individual's relationship satisfaction is based on more macrolevel behavioral patterns. Some core macrolevel patterns involve *boundaries between and around a couple* (e.g., less or more sharing of communication, activities, and time), *distribution of power/control* (e.g., how the partners attempt to influence each other and how decisions are made), and the *level of investment* of time and energy each spouse commits to the relationship. As noted earlier, individuals' relationship standards concerning these dimensions are associated with relationship satisfaction and communication. The literature suggests that these behavior patterns are core aspects of salubrious interaction (Walsh, 1998; Epstein and Baucom, 2002).

Epstein and Baucom (2002) have also described negative interaction patterns that commonly interfere with the partners' fulfillment of their needs within the relationship. These patterns include mutual (reciprocal) attack, demand/withdrawal (one person pursues and the other withdraws), and mutual avoidance and withdrawal. Epstein and Baucom suggest that often therapists must help clients to reduce these patterns before they will be able to work collaboratively as a couple to resolve issues in their relationship.

Deficits and excesses in experiencing and expressing emotions

Although the title 'cognitive-behavior' does not refer to a couple's emotions, assessment and modification of problematic affective responses are core components of this therapeutic approach. Epstein and Baucom (2002) provide a detailed description of problems that involve either deficits or excesses in the experiencing of emotions within the context of an intimate relationship, as well as in the expression of those feelings to a significant other. The following is a brief summary of those emotional factors in couple's problems.

Some individuals do not pay much attention to their emotional states, and this can result in their feelings being overlooked in close relationships; or alternatively, emotions that are not monitored may suddenly demand expressed attention and be in a destructive fashion, such as in verbally abusive or physically assaultive ways. The reasons for an individual's lack of emotional awareness vary, but they likely include having learned in their family-of-origin that expressing feelings is inappropriate or dangerous, harboring a current fear that expressing even mild emotion will lead to losing control of one's equilibrium (perhaps associated with posttraumatic stress disorder or some other type of anxiety disorder), or maintains the expectation that one's spouse simply does not care how he or she feels (Epstein and Baucom, 2002).

In contrast, some individuals have difficulty with regulating their emotions, and they experience strong emotions in response to even relatively minor life events. Unregulated experience of emotions such as anxiety, anger, and sadness, can result in decreased relationship satisfaction. The person who cannot regulate emotions may also interact in ways that heighten conflict. Factors contributing to unregulated emotional experience may include past personal trauma (e.g., abuse, abandonment), growing up in a family in which others failed to regulate emotional expression, and forms of psychopathology, such as borderline personality disorder (Linehan, 1993).

In addition to the degree to which an individual *experiences* emotions, the degree and manner in which he or she expresses emotions to significant others can affect the quality of the couple's relationship. Whereas some individuals inhibit their expression, others express feelings in an uncensored manner. Possible factors in the expression of unregulated emotions include past experiences in which strong emotional displays were the only means of effectively gaining attention, temporary relief from intense emotional tension, and limited skills for self-soothing.

An inhibited spouse may find it convenient to not have to deal with the other person's feelings, but others will be frustrated by the lack of communication, and may pursue the partner, with the result that a demand/withdraw pattern develops. Spouses who receive unregulated emotional expressions commonly find it distressing and either respond aggressively or withdraw from the partner. Although unbridled emotional expression may be intended to engage others to meet needs, the pattern often backfires (Epstein and Baucom, 2002; Johnson and Denton, 2002).

Practice principles

Methods of clinical assessment

Individual and conjoint interviews with couples, self-report questionnaires, and the therapist's behavioral observation of the couple's interactions are the three primary modes of clinical assessment (Dattilio and Padesky, 1990;

Snyder *et al.*, 1995; Epstein and Baucom, 2002). Consistent with the concepts that are described above, the goals of assessment are to: (1) identify strengths and problematic characteristics of the individuals, the couple, and the environment; (2) place current individual functioning in the context of their developmental stages and changes; and (3) identify cognitive, affective aspects of couple interaction that could be targeted for intervention. For a more detailed discussion of these ideas, the reader is referred to the extensive coverage of procedures in such sources as Baucom and Epstein (1990), Dattilio and Padesky (1990), and Epstein and Baucom (2002).

Initial conjoint interview(s)

One or more conjoint interviews with the couple are an important source of information about past and current functioning. Not only do such interviews provide information about the couple's memories and opinions concerning characteristics and events in their family-of-origin; they also furnish the therapist an opportunity to observe the couple's interactions. While it is time that people may modify their usual behavior in front of a stranger, even during the first interview the couple is likely to exhibit some aspects of typical patterns, especially when the therapist engages them in describing the issues that have brought them to therapy. CBT's approach during the assessment phase uses initial impressions to form hypotheses that must later be tested by gathering additional information in subsequent sessions.

The therapist generally begins the assessment phase by meeting with both partners in order to observe their relationship process and to form hypotheses about patterns that may be contributing to the relationship's dysfunction. The systems theorists refer to this as 'learning their dance' (Dattilio, 1998).

During the initial conjoint interview, the therapist asks the couple about their reasons for seeking treatment. Each spouse's perspective is important, both with respect to the concerns and the changes that are deemed necessary. The therapist also inquires into the couple's history (e.g., how and when the couple met, what initially attracted them to each other, when they married, when children were born, and any events that they believe have influenced their relationship over time). By applying a stress and coping model to the assessment, the therapist systematically explores demands that the couple has experienced based on individual characteristics (e.g., a spouse's residual effects from childhood abuse), relationship dynamics (e.g., unresolved differences in the partners' desires for intimacy and autonomy), and their environment (e.g., heavy job commitments). The therapist poses questions about resources that the couple has available to cope with outlined demands, and any factors that have influenced their use of resources; for example, a belief in self-sufficiency that blocks some people from seeking or accepting help from outsiders (Epstein and Baucom, 2002). Throughout the interview, the therapist gathers information about the spouses' cognitions, emotional responses, and behaviors toward each other. For example, if a husband becomes withdrawn after his wife criticizes his parenting, the therapist may draw this to his attention and ask what thoughts and emotions he just experienced after hearing his wife's comments. The husband might reveal automatic thoughts such as, 'She doesn't respect my opinion. This is hopeless,' and feelings of perhaps anger and despair.

Questionnaires/inventories

Cognitive-behavior therapists commonly use standardized questionnaires to collect information regarding the spouses' views of themselves and their relationships. Often therapists ask spouses to complete several questionnaires before the conjoint and individual interviews, so the therapist can build the interview on the questionnaire responses. Obviously, individual's reports on questionnaires are subject to biases, such as externalizing blame for relationship problems and presenting oneself in a socially desirable light (Snyder *et al.*, 1995); nevertheless, the judicious use of questionnaires can be an efficient means of quickly surveying a couple's perceptions of a wide range of issues that might otherwise be overlooked during interviews.

In addition, some couples are more apt to be able to express themselves in writing than verbally. Issues that come to the fore on a questionnaire can be explored in greater depth in subsequent interviews and behavioral observation. Following are some references that contain representative questionnaires that may be useful for assessment within a cognitive-behavioral model, even though many were not developed specifically from that perspective. Resources for reviews of a variety of other relevant measures include Fredman and Sherman (1987), Jacob and Tennenbaum (1988), Grotevant and Carlson (1989), and Touliatos *et al.* (1990).

A variety of measures have been developed to provide an overview of key areas of couple relationships, such as overall satisfaction, cohesion, communication quality, decision-making, values, and level of conflict. Examples include the Dyadic Adjustment Scale (Spanier, 1976) and the Marital Satisfaction Inventory—Revised (Snyder and Aikman, 1999). Because the items on such scales do not provide specific information about each spouse's cognitions, emotions, and behavioral responses regarding a relationship problem, the therapist must inquire about these during interviews. For example, if scores on a questionnaire indicate limited cohesion between spouses, a CBTC may ask the couple about: (1) their personal standards for types and degrees of cohesive behavior; (2) instances of behavior that did or did not feel cohesive; and (3) positive or negative emotional responses to those actions. Thus, questionnaires can be helpful to a therapist in identifying areas of strength and concern, but a more in-depth analysis is needed to understand specific types of positive and negative interaction and the factors affecting them.

Individual interviews

A separate interview with each spouse is often conducted subsequent to gathering information about past and current functioning, including life stresses, psychopathology, overall health, and coping strengths. Often, partners are more open about describing personal difficulties, such as depression, abandonment in a past relationship, and the like, without the spouse present. Such interviews provide the clinician with an opportunity to assess possible psychopathology that may be influenced by problems in the couple's relationships (and in turn may be affecting spousal interactions adversely). Given the high co-occurrence of individual psychopathology and relationship problems (L'Abate, 1998), it is crucial that couple therapists either be skilled in assessing individual functioning or be ready to make referrals to colleagues who can assist in this task. The therapist can then determine whether conjoint therapy should supplement individual therapy. As noted earlier, therapists must set clear guidelines for confidentiality during individual interviews. Keeping secrets, such as a spouse's ongoing infidelity, places the therapist in an ethical bind and undermines the work in conjoint sessions; consequently, couples are informed that the therapist will not keep secrets that affect the well-being of the spouse. This is particularly important as, once the therapist is privy to a secret, it automatically constitutes collusion and affects therapeutic objectives. On the other hand, when the therapist learns that a spouse is being physically abused and appears to be in danger, the focus shifts toward working with that person to develop plans to maintain safety and to exit the home and seek shelter elsewhere if the risk of abuse increases.

Behavioral observation

In a cognitive-behavioral approach, assessment is ongoing throughout the course of treatment, and the therapist observes the relationship during each session. These relatively unstructured behavioral observations are often supplemented by a structured communication task during the initial conjoint interview (Baucom and Epstein, 1990; Epstein and Baucom, 2002). Based on information the couple provides, the therapist may select a topic that the couple considers to be unresolved and ask them to spend several minutes discussing it while the therapist observes. The couple might be asked merely to express their feelings about an issue and respond to each other's expression in any way they deem appropriate, or they may be asked to try to resolve the issue in the allotted time frame. Typically, the therapist

leaves the room to minimize the potential of influencing their interactions. In this case; video or audiotaping may be used. Such taped problem-solving discussions are used routinely in couple-interaction research (Weiss and Heyman, 1997), and even though spouses often behave somewhat differently under these conditions than at home, they commonly become engaged enough in the discussion that pertinent aspects will emerge.

Assessment feedback to the couple

CBT is a collaborative approach in which the therapist continually shares his or her thinking with the clients and develops interventions designed to address their concerns. After collecting information via interviews, questionnaires, and behavioral observations, the therapist meets with the couple and provides a concise summary of the patterns that have emerged, including: (1) their strengths; (2) their major presenting concerns; (3) life demands or stressors that have produced adjustment problems for the family; and (4) constructive and problematic macrolevel patterns in their interactions that seem to be influencing their presenting problems. The therapist and couple then identify their priorities for change, as well as some interventions that may alleviate the problems. This is a vital time for the therapist to explore potential challenges to couple therapy, such as fear of changes that partners anticipate, will be stressful and difficult for them, and to work with them on steps that can be taken to reduce both. The therapist also needs to consider the shift that will occur within the relationship and how it will affect the overall homeostasis. (See section on Challenges.)

Clinical change mechanisms and specific therapeutic interventions

Educating couples about the cognitive-behavioral model

It is extremely important to educate couples about the cognitive-behavioral model of treatment (Dattilio and Padesky, 1990) if one is employing it. The structure and collaborative nature of the approach necessitates that the couple clearly understand the principles and methods involved. The therapist initially provides a brief didactic overview of the model and periodically refers to specified concepts during therapy. In addition to presenting such 'mini-lectures' (Baucom and Epstein, 1990), the therapist often asks spouses to engage in bibliotherapy, reading portions of relevant popular books, such as A. T. Beck's (1988) *Love is never enough* and Markman *et al.*'s (1994) *Fighting for your marriage*. The couples also should be aware that homework assignments will be an essential part of treatment and that bibliotherapy is one type that will help orient them to the treatment model. In this way, all parties stay attuned to the process of treatment and the notion of taking responsibility for their own thoughts and behaviors is reinforced.

The therapist informs the spouses that he or she will structure the sessions in order to keep the therapy focused on achieving the goals that they agreed to pursue during the assessment process (Dattilio, 1994, 1997; Epstein and Baucom, 2002). Part of the structuring process involves the therapist's and the couple's setting an explicit agenda at the beginning of each session. Another aspect is the establishing of ground rules for client behavior inside and outside sessions; some examples include that individuals should not tell the therapist secrets that cannot be shared with other family members, that all family members should attend each session unless the therapist and spouses decide otherwise, and that abusive verbal and physical behavior is unacceptable.

Interventions to modify distorted and extreme cognitions, emotions, and behaviors

A prerequisite to modifying spouses' distorted or extreme cognitions about themselves and each other is increasing their ability to identify their automatic thoughts. After introducing the concept of automatic thoughts—those that spontaneously dart through one's mind—the therapist coaches the couple in observing the thought patterns during sessions that are associated with their negative emotional and behavioral responses to each other. In the cognitive-behavioral model, monitoring one's subjective experiences is a skill that can be developed further if necessary. In order to improve the skill of identifying one's automatic thoughts, clients are typically asked to keep a small notebook handy between sessions and to record a brief description of the circumstances in which they felt distressed about the relationship or become engaged in conflict. This log also should include a description of any automatic thoughts, as well as the resulting emotional and behavioral responses to other family members. A modified version of the Daily Records of Dysfunctional Thoughts (A. T. Beck *et al.*, 1979) was initially developed for the identification and modification of automatic thoughts in individual cognitive therapy. Through this type of record keeping, the therapist is able to demonstrate to couples how their automatic thoughts are linked to emotional and behavioral responses and to help them understand the specific macrolevel themes (e.g., boundary issues) that upset them in their relationship. This procedure also increases the spouses' understanding that their negative emotional and behavioral responses to each other are potentially controllable through systematic examination of the cognitions associated with them. Thus, the therapist is coaching each spouse in taking greater responsibility for his or her own responses. An exercise that often proves quite useful is to have couples review their written logs and *identify* the *specific* links among thoughts, emotions, and behavior. The therapist then asks each person to explore alternative cognitions that might produce different emotional and behavioral responses to a situation.

Identifying cognitive distortions and labeling them

It is helpful for spouses to become adept at identifying the types of cognitive distortions involved in their automatic thoughts. It can be effective to have each partner refer to the list of distortions outlined in the next section and to label any distortions in the automatic thoughts that he or she logged during the previous week. This can be done by using the Daily Dysfunctional Thought Sheet (Figure 11.5, p. 118). The therapist and client can discuss the aspects of the thoughts that were inappropriate or extreme, and how the distortion contributed to any negative emotions and behavior at the time. Such in-session reviews of written logs over the course of several sessions can increase family members' skills in identifying and evaluating their ongoing thoughts about their relationships.

If the therapist believes that a spouse's cognitive distortions are associated with a form of individual psychopathology, such as clinical depression, he or she must determine whether or not the psychopathology can be treated within the context of the couple relationship, or if the individual needs a referral for individual therapy. As noted earlier, procedures for assessing the psychological functioning of individual spouses are beyond the scope of this chapter, but it is important that couple therapists become familiar with the evaluation of psychopathology and make referrals to other professionals as necessary.

Common cognitive distortions

Arbitrary inference

Conclusions that are made in the absence of supporting substantiating evidence; often involved in invalid attributions and expectancies. For example, a man whose wife arrives home from work a half-hour late concludes, 'She must be doing something behind my back.' Distressed spouses often make negative attributions about the causes of each other's positive actions.

Mind reading

This is a type of arbitrary inference in which an individual believes he or she knows what another person is thinking or feeling without communicating directly with the person. For example, a husband noticed that his wife had been especially quiet and concluded, 'She's unhappy with our marriage and must be thinking about leaving me.'

Selective abstraction

Information is taken out of context and certain details are highlighted while other important information is ignored. For example, a woman whose husband fails to answer her greeting in the morning concludes, 'He is ignoring me,' even though the husband had cleared a place for her at the breakfast table when she entered the room.

Overgeneralization

An isolated incident is considered to be a representation of similar situations in other contexts, related or unrelated; often contributes to selective attention. For example, after having an argument with her husband, a wife concludes, 'All men are alike!'

Magnification and minimization

A case or circumstance is judged as having greater or lesser importance than is appropriate; often leading to distress when the evaluation violates the person's standards for the ways family members 'should' be. For example, an angry husband becomes anxious and enraged when he discovers that his wife used their emergency credit card for miscellaneous purchases so he complains, 'She has no regard for our finances.'

Personalization

External events are attributed to oneself when insufficient evidence exists to render a conclusion; a special case of arbitrary inference commonly involves misattributions. For example, a wife states, 'My husband has little respect for me, therefore, I must be a loser.'

Dichotomous thinking

Also labeled '*polarized thinking*,' experiences are classified into mutually exclusive, extreme categories, such as complete success or total failure; commonly contributing to selective attention, as well as to violation of personal standards. For example, a husband has spent several hours working on cleaning the couple's cluttered basement and removed a considerable number of items for inclusion in a yard sale. However, when the wife enters the basement, she looks around and exclaims, 'What a mess! When are you going to make some progress?'

Labeling

The tendency to portray oneself or another person in terms of stable, global traits, on the basis of past actions; negative labels are an integral part of attributions that couples often make about the causes of each other's actions. For example, after a husband has made several errors in the household budgeting and in balancing their checkbook, the wife concludes, 'He is a careless person,' and she does not consider situational conditions that may have led to those errors.

Testing and reinterpreting automatic thoughts

The process of restructuring automatic thoughts involves the spouse considering alternative explanations. Such consideration will require that, the spouse examine evidence concerning the validity of various thoughts and/or their appropriateness in a given situation. Identifying a distortion in one's thinking or finding an alternative way to view relationship events may have an impact on emotional and behavioral responses to one's relationship. The following types of questions can be helpful in guiding each spouse in examining his or her thoughts:

♦ From your past experiences or the events occurring recently in your relationship, what evidence exists that supports this thought? How could you get some additional information to help you judge whether or not your thoughts are appropriate?

♦ What might be some alternative explanations for your partner's behaviors? What else might have led him/her to behave that way?

♦ Several types of cognitive distortions have been offered that can influence a person's views of other family members and can contribute to becoming upset with them. Which cognitive distortions, if any, do you see in the automatic thoughts you had about . . . ? For example, a woman who believed that her husband was being unrealistic in his demands reported the automatic thoughts, 'He enjoys punishing me. I have no autonomy.' In turn, this interpretation contributed to her anger and resentment toward him. The therapist helped the woman to see that she was, in essence, mind reading, and that it would be important to inquire more about her husband's feelings to reach an accurate conclusion. The therapist encouraged her to ask her husband to describe his feelings, and he said that although he felt guilty about his demandingness, he believed that he would never receive any attention from her unless he behaved in this way. The wife was able to hear that her inference might not have been accurate, and the therapist related that the couple probably would benefit from problem-solving discussions to address the issue of what types of demands are appropriate. Similarly, the therapist coached the wife in examining her automatic thought, 'He enjoys pushing me,' leading her to recount several instances in which her husband was less demanding and more caring. Thus, the wife acknowledged that she had engaged in dichotomous thinking. The therapist discussed with the couple the danger of thinking and speaking in extreme terms, which are unrealistic, because very few events occur 'always' or 'never.' Even so, this is a common distortion found among couples in conflict.

Thus, gathering and weighing the evidence for one's thoughts are an integral part of CBTC. Couples are able to provide valuable feedback that will help each other evaluate the validity or appropriateness of their cognitions, as long as they use good communication skills (described later). After individuals challenge their thoughts, they should rate their belief in the alternative explanations and in their original inference, perhaps on a scale from 0 to 100. The 'new' revised thoughts may not be assimilated unless they are considered credible on a deeper level.

Testing predictions with behavioral experiments

Although an individual may use logical analysis successfully to reduce his or her negative expectancies concerning events that will occur in couple or family interactions, often first-hand corroboration is needed. CBT often guides couples in devising 'behavioral experiments' in which they test their predictions about particular actions leading to certain responses from other members. For example, a man who expects that his wife and children will resist including him in their leisure activities when he gets home from work can make plans to try to engage with the family when he arrives home during the next few days and see what happens. When these plans are hatched during the conjoint therapy sessions, the therapist can ask the wife, in this case, what she predicts their responses will be during the experiment. The wife may anticipate potential obstacles to success and appropriate adjustments can be made. In addition, when a spouse commits to participating in good faith and the commitment is voiced and witnessed, the likelihood of the experiment's success is increased.

The use of imagery, recollections of past interactions, and role-playing techniques

When spouses attempt to identify during their therapy sessions thoughts, emotions, and behavior that emerged in incidents outside sessions, they may have difficulty recalling pertinent information regarding the circumstances and each person's responses. This is particularly true when the couples' interaction was emotionally charged. Imagery and/or role-playing techniques may be extremely helpful in recalling memories regarding such situations. In addition, these techniques often rekindle spouses' reactions, and what begins as a role-play may quickly become an *in vivo* interaction.

For example, the use of deep breathing and relaxation exercises have been used to help spouses recall a particular argument and/or a scenario that upset them. Having them imagine the room that they were in along with the clothes that they were wearing may be helpful in recalling their automatic thoughts at the time. Although recounting past events can provide

important information, the therapist's ability to assess and intervene with spouses' problematic cognitive, affective, and behavioral responses to each other as they occur during sessions affords the best opportunity to changing relationship patterns (Epstein and Baucom, 2002). Imagery sometimes helps to accomplish this goal.

Couples can also be coached in switching roles during role-playing exercises in order to increase empathy (Epstein and Baucom, 2002). For example, spouses can be asked to exchange roles as they recreate a recent argument concerning finances. Focusing on the other person's frame of reference and subjective feelings provides new information that can modify one spouse's view of the other. Thus, in this example, when the husband played the role of his wife he was able to understand better her anxiety about money and her conservative behavior about spending it, which had its roots in her experience of poverty growing up.

Many distressed couples have developed a narrow focus on problems in their relationship by the time they seek therapy, so the therapist may ask them to report their recollections of the thoughts, emotions, and behaviors that occurred between them when they met, dated, and developed amorous feelings toward each other. The therapist can focus on the contrast between past and present experiences as evidence that the couple was able, at one time, to relate in a more satisfying way and may be able to regenerate positive interactions with some appropriate effort.

Imagery techniques should be used with caution and skill, and probably should be avoided if there is a history of abuse in the relationship. Similarly, role-play techniques should not be used until the therapist feels confident that the couple will be able to contain strong emotional responses and refrain from abusive behavior toward each other.

Downward arrow

The 'downward arrow' is a technique used by cognitive therapists (e.g., A. T. Beck *et al.*, 1979; J. S. Beck, 1995) to track the associations among an individual's automatic thoughts, in which an apparently benign initial thought may be upsetting owing to its being linked to other more significant thoughts. For example, a husband may report experiencing anxiety associated with the automatic thought: 'My wife will leave me if I do not bring home enough money.' The intensity of the emotional response becomes clarified when the therapist asks a series of questions such as, 'And if that happened, what would it mean to you?' or 'What might that lead to?' The husband responds with, 'It will mean I'm a failure.' Couples can evaluate how likely it is that the expected catastrophe will occur. In some cases, this will lead to modification of the individual's underlying catastrophic expectancy; in other cases, it may uncover a real problem in the relationship, such as a need for the wife to consider the emphasis that she places on money.

The downward arrow technique also is used to identify the assumptions and standards underlying one's automatic thoughts. This is accomplished by identifying the initial thought, having the individual ask himself or herself, 'If so, then what?' and moving downward until the individual locates the relevant core belief. Thus, the husband in the above example might also have developed a general insecurity and an issue regarding his sense of self-worth.

Interventions to modify behavior patterns

The major forms of intervention used to reduce negative behavior and to increase positive behavior are: (1) communication training regarding expressive and listening skills; (2) problem-solving training; and (3) behavior change agreements. These are briefly described below, and readers can consult texts such as Guerney (1977), Robin and Foster (1989), Dattilio and Padesky (1990), Jacobson and Christensen (1996), and Epstein and Baucom (2002) for detailed procedures.

Communication training

Improving couples' skills for expressing thoughts and emotions, as well as for listening effectively to each other, is one of the most common forms of intervention therapy. In CBTC, it is viewed as a cornerstone of treatment because it can have a positive impact on problematic behavioral interactions, reduce partners' distorted cognitions about each other, and contribute to the regulated experience and expression of emotion. Therapists begin by presenting instructions to couples about the specific behaviors involved in each type of expressive and listening skill. Speaker guidelines include acknowledging the subjectivity of one's own views; describing one's emotions, as well as one's thoughts; pointing out positives, as well as problems; speaking in specific rather than global terms; being concise so that the listener can absorb and remember one's message; and using tact and diplomacy (e.g., not discussing important topics when one's partner is preparing to retire for the evening). The guidelines for empathic listening include exhibiting attentiveness through nonverbal acts (e.g., eye contact, nods), demonstrating acceptance of the speaker's message (the person's right to have his or her personal feelings) whether or not the listener agrees, attempting to understand or empathize with the other's perspective, and reflecting back one's understanding by paraphrasing what the speaker says. Each spouse receives handouts describing the communication guidelines so that he or she can refer to them during sessions and at home. Over time, it is hoped that these guidelines will become part of the couple's repertoire.

Therapists often model good expressive and listening skills for clients. They may use videotape examples, such as those that accompany Markman *et al.*'s (1994) book *Fighting for your marriage*. During sessions, the therapist coaches the couple or family in following the communication guidelines, beginning with discussions of relatively benign topics so negative emotions will not interfere with constructive skills. As the clients demonstrate these skills, they are asked to practice them as homework, with increasingly conflictual topics. As couples practice communication skills, they gain more information about each other's motives and desires, which will then aid them in diffusing distorted cognitions about each other. Following the guidelines may also bolster each individual's perception that the other is respectful and motivated by goodwill.

Problem-solving training

Cognitive-behavioral therapists also use verbal and written instructions, modeling, and behavioral rehearsal and coaching to facilitate effective problem solving with couples. The major steps involve achieving a clear and specific definition of the problem in terms of behaviors that are or are not occurring, generating specific behavioral solutions to the problem without evaluating one's own or one's spouse's ideas, weighing the advantages and disadvantages of each alternative solution and selecting a solution that appears to be feasible and attractive to all members involved, and agreeing on a trial period for implementing the selected solution and assessing its effectiveness. Homework is integral to learning and integrating skills (Dattilio, 2002; Epstein and Baucom, 2002).

Behavior change agreements

Contracts that are used to exchange desired behavior still have an important role in CBTC. Therapists try to avoid making one spouse's behavior change contingent on another's, so the goal is for each person to identify and enact specific behavior that would likely be pleasurable to the other, regardless of what actions the other spouse takes. The major challenge facing the therapist is to encourage the spouses to avoid 'standing on ceremony' by waiting for others to take the initiative to be positive. Brief didactic presentations on negative reciprocity in distressed relationships on the fact that one can only have control over one's own actions, and on the importance of making a personal commitment to improve the relationship atmosphere may help to reduce individuals' reluctance to make the first positive contribution. An example of using a behavior change agreement may involve the therapist negotiating for equal effort on the part of both spouses to take the initial step forward conjointly. This is with the attempt to have each partner focus on the change they need to make with themselves rather than what they want their spouse to change. A verbal or sometimes even a written agreement that both spouses sign may help to solidify their commitment to taking the first step forward conjointly.

Interventions for deficits and excesses in emotional responses

Although CBT is sometimes characterized as neglecting emotions, this is not the case, and a variety of interventions are used, either to enhance the emotional experiences of inhibited individuals or to moderate extreme responses (see Dattilio, 2002; Epstein and Baucom, 2002, for detailed procedures). For couples who report experiencing little emotion, the therapist can establish clear guidelines for behavior inside and outside of sessions in which expressing oneself will not lead to recriminations as well as use downward-arrow questioning to inquire about underlying emotions and cognitions, coach the person in noticing internal cues to his or her emotional states, repeat phrases that have emotional impact on the person, refocus attention on emotionally relevant topics when the individual attempts to change the subject, and engage the individual in role-plays concerning important relationship issues in order to elicit emotional responses. Individuals who experience intense emotions that affect him or her and significant others adversely, can be helped by the therapist compartmentalizing emotional responses by scheduling specific times to discuss distressing topics. The therapist may also coach the individual in self-soothing activities such as relaxation techniques, attempt to improve the person's ability to monitor and challenge upsetting automatic thoughts, encourage him or her to seek social support from others, develop the ability to tolerate disturbing feelings, and enhance skills for expressing emotions constructively so others will pay attention.

Homework

Homework assignments are a central feature of CBTC. Because the actual therapy sessions are limited to only 1 or 2 hours per week, outside activities that support the treatment process are essential if the new behavior is to become permanent. Self-help assignments can serve as a strategy to reinforce what is learned in the treatment process. Homework is also an integral part of the collaborative process between the therapist and spouses. Assignments typically include the techniques and strategies listed throughout this chapter. Such assignments may also be tailored to specific problems and to accommodate results from the collaborative processing during the therapy session that week. For a detailed overview of homework assignments in couple and family therapy, the reader is referred to Dattilio (2002).

Challenges

In a recent text by R. E. Leahy (2003), the issue of roadblocks in cognitive therapy is addressed across various populations. The discussion of couples highlights the factors that may interfere with the levels of engagement and progress in therapy. Epstein and Baucom (2003) outline several factors, including partners' negativity and hopelessness about change in the relationship, discomfort about participating in conjoint therapy, distress about changing the homeostasis in the relationship, failure to take personal responsibility for change, and individual psychopathology.

Dattilio (2003) further outlines a number of roadblocks that therapists may encounter when working with couples, one of which he labels 'Therapists Roadblocks,' which are obstacles that may include the therapist's own resistance or defense mechanisms that emerge during the course of treatment. Sometimes, the therapist varies the work through his or her own issues from his or her family-of-origin or his or her own marriage. It is one of the less recognized roadblocks that occur during the course of treatment. Nonetheless, these are issues that may impede progress in therapy and every therapist should be aware of it. Another is unrealistic expectations that the couple may develop during the course of treatment, particularly early on. Setting realistic expectations is essential in couples therapy so that spouses don't become overzealous about what they anticipate being able to accomplish in treatment. One way of overcoming such obstacles is to be as realistic and flexible as possible as to what can be accomplished in treatment and when to discuss this collaboratively with the couple. Other areas of roadblocks may involve cultural obstacles. Therapists must and should familiarize themselves with various cultural aspects in the literature as well as with environments from which individuals hail in order to avoid stumbling blocks due to cultural issues. Racial issues go hand-in-hand with this topic, although this is reported to be less an issue in the literature than with cultural matters.

Environmental forces may also expose couples to issues that inhibit or impede change during the course of treatment. This may involve family members or other aspects of their environment that work against the process of treatment. Psychopathology is clearly one of the major hurdles in treatment with couples, particularly significant psychopathology that exists with one or both partners. Personality disorders particularly raise a challenge for a therapist and need to be addressed in more specific detail, perhaps on a one-to-one basis. If not, it is strongly recommended that spouses are referred out for individual psychotherapy.

Factors such as low intellectual and cognitive functioning that can affect the previous treatment are also areas that draw concern. These also may yield individuals who are not particularly amenable to treatment. In addition, it is stated by Dattilio (2003) that the inadequate use of homework assignments may also be a roadblock, particularly with not allowing couples enough out-of-session assignments to support and reinforce that which is obtained during the course of treatment. Homework, which is discussed in the aforementioned section is a hallmark of CBT and is something that very much should be used strategically on a regular basis.

Therapists need to be aware of such challenges in order for headway to be made in treatment. Many of the aforementioned techniques and interventions may be used to address these challenges during the course of therapy with couples.

Research

Effectiveness of cognitive-behavioral therapy with couples

CBT has received more extensive evaluations in controlled outcome studies than any other form of couple or family therapy, and a review of outcome studies that employed stringent criteria for efficacy indicated that cognitive-behavioral treatment is efficacious for reducing relationship distress (Baucom et al., 1998). Most studies on couples therapy have been restricted to evaluations of the behavioral components of communication training, problem-solving training, and behavioral contracts, and they have found that these interventions are more effective in reducing distress than wait-list control and placebo conditions. A small number of studies with other approaches such as emotionally focused and insight-oriented couple therapies (e.g., Snyder et al., 1991; Johnson and Talitman, 1997) suggest that they have comparable or, in some cases, better outcomes than behaviorally/oriented approaches, but there is a need for additional research. Only a few studies have examined the impact of adding cognitive restructuring interventions to behavioral protocols (e.g., Baucom et al., 1990). Typically, some cognitive interventions have been substituted for behaviorally/oriented sessions in order to keep the total number of sessions equal across the treatments that are compared. In Case studies in couples and family therapy (Dattilio, 1998), cognitive-behavioral strategies are integrated with more than 16 modalities of couple and family therapy. A review of those studies indicate that combined CBT was as effective as the behavioral conditions, although cognitively/focused interventions tend to produce more cognitive change whereas behavioral interventions are more apt to foster modified behavioral interactions (Baucom et al., 1998). Dattilio and Epstein (2005) has noted that there is a need for research on a truly integrated CBT that targets each couple's particular cognitive, behavioral, and affective problems in proportion to their intensity, rather than providing a fixed number of sessions of each type of intervention to all couples. Also, Whisman and Snyder (1997) argue that tests of cognitive interventions have been limited by a failure to assess the range of problematic cognitions (selective attention, expectancies,

attributions, assumptions, and standards) identified by Baucom et al. (1989). Studies also have been limited to samples of predominantly white, middle-class couples, so the effectiveness with other racial and socio-economic groups is unknown. Thus, research on the effectiveness of CBT for couples has been encouraging; however, there are still areas that need to be investigated.

Overall, CBT has proven its effectiveness with difficult couples and is also destined to be a modality that is frequently used by mental health practitioners in the future. It is already regarded by many in the field as integrating nicely with other modalities of couples treatment.

References

Baucom, D. H. (1987). Attributions in distressed relations: how can we explain them? In: S. Duck and D. Perlman, ed. Heterosexual relations, marriage and divorce, pp. 177–206. London: Sage.

Baucom, D. H. and Epstein, N. (1990). Cognitive-behavioral marital therapy. New York: Brunner/Mazel.

Baucom, D. H., Epstein, N., Sayers, S., and Sher, T. G. (1989). The role of cognitions in marital relationships: definitional, methodological, and conceptual issues. Journal of Consulting and Clinical Psychology, 57, 31–8.

Baucom, D. H., Sayers, S. L., and Sher, T. G. (1990). Supplementing behavioral marital therapy with cognitive restructuring and emotional expressiveness training: an outcome investigation. Journal of Consulting and Clinical Psychology, 58, 636–45.

Baucom, D. H., et al. (1996a). Cognitions in marriage: the relationship between standards and attributions. Journal of Family Psychology, 10, 209–22.

Baucom, D. H., Epstein, N., Rankin, L. A., and Burnett, C. K. (1996b). Assessing relationship standards: the Inventory of Specific Relationship Standards. Journal of Family Psychology, 10, 72–88.

Baucom, D. H., Shoham, V., Mueser, K. T., Daiuto, A. D., and Stickle, T. R. (1998). Empirically supported couples and family therapies for adult problems. Journal of Consulting and Clinical Psychology, 66, 53–88.

Beck, A. T. (1988). Love is never enough. New York: Harper and Row.

Beck, A. T., Rush, A. J., Shaw, B. F., and Emery, G. (1979). Cognitive therapy of depression. New York: Guilford Press.

Beck, J. S. (1995). Cognitive therapy: basics and beyond. New York: Guilford Press.

Bradbury, T. N. and Fincham, F. D. (1990). Attributions in marriage: Review and critique. Psychological Bulletin, 107, 3–33.

Dattilio, F. M. (1989). A guide to cognitive marital therapy. In: P. A. Keller and S. R. Heyman, ed. Innovations in clinical practice: a source book, Vol. 8, pp. 27–42. Sarasota, FL: Professional Resource Exchange.

Dattilio, F. M. (1994). Families in crisis. In: F. M. Dattilio and A. Freeman, ed. Cognitive-behavioral strategies in crisis intervention, pp. 278–301. New York: Guilford Press.

Dattilio, F. M. (1997). Family therapy. In: R. L. Leahy, ed. Practicing cognitive therapy: a guide to interventions, pp. 409–50. Northvale, NJ: Jason Aronson.

Dattilio, F. M. (1998). Case studies in couples and family therapy: systemic and cognitive perspectives. New York: Guilford Press.

Dattilio, F. M. (2002). Homework assignments in couple and family therapy. Journal of Clinical Psychology, 58(5), 570–83.

Dattilio, F. M. (2003). Techniques in family therapy. In: R. E. Leahy, ed. Overcoming roadblocks in cognitive therapy. New York: Guilford Press.

Dattilio, F. M. and Epstein, N. B. (2003). Cognitive-behavioral couple and family therapy. In: G. Weeks, G. Sexton, and M. Robbins, ed. Handbook of family therapy: theory, research and practice, pp. 147–75. New York: Brunner Routledge.

Dattilio, F. M. and Epstein, N. B. (2005). The role of cognitive-behavioral intervention in couple and family therapy. Journal of Marital and Family Therapy, 31(1), 2–12.

Dattilio, F. M. and Padesky, C. A. (1990). Cognitive therapy with couples. Sarasota, FL: Professional Resource Exchange.

Ellis, A. (1977). The nature of disturbed marital interactions. In: A. Ellis and R. Grieger, ed. Handbook of rational-emotive therapy, pp. 170–6. New York: Springer.

Ellis, A. and Harper, R. A. (1961). *A guide to rational living*. Englewood Clips, NJ: Prentice-Hall.

Ellis, A., Sichel, J. L., Yeager, R. J., DiMattia, D. J., and DiGiuseppe, R. (1989). *Rational-emotive couples therapy*. New York: Pergamon Press.

Epstein, N. (1982). Cognitive therapy with couples. *American Journal of Family Therapy*, 10, 5–16.

Epstein, N. (1992). Marital therapy. In: A. Freeman and F. M. Dattilio, ed. *Comprehensive casebook of cognitive therapy*, pp. 267–75. New York: Plenum Press.

Epstein, N. and Baucom, D. H. (1989). Cognitive-behavioral marital therapy. In: A. Freeman, K. M. Simon, L. E. Beutler, and H. Arkowitz, ed. *Comprehensive handbook of cognitive therapy*, pp. 491–513. New York: Plenum Press.

Epstein, N. and Baucom, D. H. (2002). *Enhanced cognitive-behavioral therapy for couples: a contextual approach*. Washington, DC: American Psychological Association.

Epstein, N. B. and Baucom, D. H. (2003). Overcoming roadblocks in cognitive-behavior therapy with couples. In: R. Leahy, ed. *Roadblocks in cognitive therapy*. New York: Guilford Press.

Epstein, N., and Eidelson, R. J. (1981). Unrealistic beliefs of clinical couples: their relationship to expectations, goals and satisfaction. *American Journal of Family Therapy*, 9(4), 13–22.

Fincham, F. D., Beach, S. R. H., and Nelson, G. (1987). Attribution processes in distressed and nondistressed couples: 3. Causal and responsibility attributions for spouse behavior. *Cognitive Therapy and Research*, 11, 71–86.

Fredman, N. and Sherman, R. (1987). *Handbook of measurements for marriage and family therapy*. New York: Brunner/Mazel.

Gottman, J. M. (1994). *What predicts divorce?* Hillsdale, NJ: Lawrence Erlbaum.

Grotevant, H. D. and Carlson, C. I. (1989). *Family assessment: a guide to methods and measures*. New York: Guilford Press.

Guerney, B. G., Jr. (1977). *Relationship enhancement*. San Francisco: Jossey-Bass.

Jacob, T. and Tennenbaum, D. L. (1998). *Family assessment: rationale, methods, and future directions*. New York: Plenum.

Jacobson, N. S. and Christensen, A. (1996). *Integrative couple therapy: promoting acceptance and change*. New York: Norton.

Johnson, S. M. and Denton, W. (2002). Emotionally focused couple therapy: creating secure connections. In: A. S. Gurman and N. S. Jacobson, ed. *Clinical handbook of couple therapy*, 3rd edn, pp. 221–50. New York: Guilford Press.

Johnson, S. M. and Talitman, E. (1997). Predictors of success in emotionally focused marital therapy. *Journal of Marital and Family Therapy*, 23, 135–52.

Kelly, G. A. (1955). *The psychology of personal constructs*. New York: Norton.

L'Abate, L. (1998). *Family psychopathology: the relational roots of dysfunctional behavior*. New York: Guilford Press.

Leahy, R. (1996). *Cognitive therapy: basic principles and applications*. Northvale, NJ: Jason Aronson.

Leahy, R. (2003). *Roadblocks in cognitive therapy*. New York: Guilford Press.

Liberman, R. P. (1970). Behavioral approaches to couple and family therapy. *American Journal of Orthopsychiatry*, 40, 106–18.

Linehan, M. M. (1993). *Cognitive-behavioral treatment of borderline personality disorder*. New York: Guilford Press.

Margolin, G. and Weiss, R. L. (1978). Comparative evaluation of therapeutic components associated with behavioral marital treatments. *Journal of Consulting and Clinical Psychology*, 46, 1476–86.

Markman, H. J., Stanley, S., and Blumberg, S. L. (1994). *Fighting for your marriage*. San Francisco: Jossey-Bass.

Robin, A. L. and Foster, S. L. (1989). *Negotiating parent-adolescent conflict: a behavioral-family systems approach*. New York: Guilford Press.

Snyder, D. K. and Aikman, G. G. (1999). The Marital Satisfaction Inventory—Revised. In: M. E. Maruish, ed., *Use of psychological testing for treatment planning and outcomes assessment*, pp. 1173–210. Mahwah, NJ: Erlbaum.

Snyder, D. K., Wills, R. M., and Grady-Fletcher, A. (1991). Long-term effectiveness of behavioral versus insight-oriented marital therapy: A 4-year follow-up study. *Journal of Consulting and Clinical Psychology*, 59, 138–41.

Snyder, D. K., Cavell, T. A., Heffer, R. W., and Mangrum, L. F. (1995). Marital and family assessment: a multifaceted, multilevel approach. In: R. H. Mikesell, D. D. Lusterman, and S. H. McDaniel, ed. *Integrating family therapy: handbook of family psychology and systems theory*, pp. 163–82. Washington, DC: American Psychological Association.

Spanier, G. B. (1976). Measuring dyadic adjustment: new scales for assessing the quality of marriage and similar dyads. *Journal of Marriage and the Family*, 38, 15–30.

Stuart, R. B. (1969). Operant-interpersonal treatment for marital discord. *Journal of Consulting and Clinical Psychology*, 33, 675–82.

Touliatos, J., Perlmutter, B. F., and Straus, M. A., ed. (1990). *Handbook of family measurement techniques*. Newbury Park, CA: Sage.

Walsh, F. (1998). *Strengthening family resilience*. New York: Guilford Press.

Weiss, R. L. (1984). Cognitive and strategic interventions in behavioral marital therapy. In: K. Hahlweg and N. S. Jacobson, ed. *Marital interaction: analysis and modification*, pp. 309–24. New York: Guilford Press.

Weiss, R. L. and Heyman, R. E. (1997). A clinical-research overview of couples interactions. In: W. K. Halford and H. J. Markman, ed. *Clinical handbook of marriage and couples interventions*, pp. 13–41. Chichester: Wiley.

Weiss, R. L., Hops, H., and Patterson, G. R. (1973). A framework for conceptualizing marital conflict, a technology for altering it, some data for evaluating it. In: L. A. Hamerlynck, L. C. Handy, and E. J. Mash, ed. *Behavior change: methodology, concepts, and practice*, pp. 309–42. Champaign, IL: Research Press.

Whisman, M. A. and Snyder, D. K. (1997). Evaluating and improving the efficacy of conjoint couple therapy. In: W. K. Halford and H. J. Markman, ed. *Clinical handbook of marriage and couples interventions*, pp. 679–93. Chichester: Wiley.

9 The arts therapies

Joy Schaverien and Helen Odell-Miller

Introduction: the arts therapies

In the arts therapies—art therapy, music therapy, drama therapy, and dance movement therapy, as well as psychodrama—an art form is applied as a form of psychotherapy in clinical treatment. Collectively these professions, excluding psychodrama, are known as the arts therapies. They are based on the dual premise that the arts have a healing potential and that they offer a means of access to unconscious material. Within the framework of a therapeutic relationship they offer different experiences from other forms of psychotherapy, which rely on the spoken word—'the talking cure', as the main channel for mediation.

Each of these art forms has been introduced into clinical practice through a different route. Moreover the training and history of each is different in countries within Europe and in the USA. The authors are a British art and music therapists and therefore it is inevitable that this will influence our accounts. However, the bibliography is intended to redress this and it includes selected references for the other modalities and other countries: for drama see Jones (1996), Jenkyns (1996), and Doktor (1995); dance see Chodorow (1991), Payne (1993); and psychodrama see Moreno (1977), Holmes and Karp (1992), and Holmes (1992). The development of art therapy in Britain is recorded by Waller (1991); in Europe, Waller (1998); in the USA, Junge and Asawa (1994) and Rubin (2001).

Music therapy, art therapy, and drama therapy are now established professions in the UK, and State Registered under the Health Professions Council (HPC). In July 2002 there were 1886 Registered arts therapists in the UK and 18 postgraduate training courses, all validated by universities. Many of these universities also now offer Masters and PhD level degrees in the arts therapies. Of the 1886, 1065 were art therapists, 422 music therapists, and 397 drama therapists. In addition to this there are also a smaller unspecified number of dance movement therapy practitioners registered with the Association for Dance Movement Therapy who were not eligible to register with the HPC at the time of writing.

A brief summary of the three State Registered Professions in the Department of Health (2002) briefing document reveals their common purpose and states simply that:

> *Art therapists* provide a psychotherapeutic intervention which enables clients to effect change and growth by the use of art materials to gain insight and promote the resolution of difficulties. *Drama therapists* encourage clients to experience their physicality, to develop an ability to express the whole range of their emotions and to increase their insight and knowledge of themselves and others. *Music therapists* facilitate interaction and development of insight into clients' behavior and emotional difficulties through music.

As a result of state registration arts therapists in the UK are increasingly included in government policy and planning mechanisms, for example in *Meeting the Challenge, a Strategy for the Allied Health Professions*, published in November 2000, which aimed to increase understanding of the roles Allied Health Professions.

Art therapy and art psychotherapy

Joy Schaverien

Theoretical basis

Art therapy is also sometimes known as art psychotherapy and this dual title reflects some of the perceived differences, and at times lively debates, within this profession.

Art therapists, as other psychotherapists, owe a debt to Freud and Jung and their successors. However, their initial inspiration was the art form and therefore the route to clinical practice has been rather different than the traditional psychoanalytic path. This influences the theoretical base of the practice.

In Britain the first art therapists were artists who became interested in working in psychiatric hospitals, at first as volunteers. In the 1950s art therapists worked in studios in the large psychiatric hospitals that provided inpatient treatment for a variety of psychiatric disorders. These artists knew that art was a significant factor in healing for some of their patients. They were untrained in psychiatry and psychotherapy and there was little theory to confirm their intuition and so they deferred to the knowledge and experience of the medical practitioners. Much creative collaboration took place in this way, for example, between the artist and art therapist Adamson (1984) and the psychiatrist Cunningham-Dax (1953). The art therapist created an attentive presence and a studio environment for patients to make art but they did not interpret the pictures (Lyddiatt, 1971; Thomson, 1989). If the medical director or the resident psychiatrist took an interest, the patients would take their pictures to him for interpretation.

It was similar with Champernowne (1969, 1971), a Jungian analyst, who founded a therapeutic community for the arts called *Withymead* (see Stevens, 1986) in the west of England. Here many British art therapists, including Nowell Hall (1987) and Edwards (1989), began their lifelong professional interest in art therapy. Champernowne too considered that the art therapist would elicit material but, she as the psychotherapist, attended to its significance within the treatment. This hierarchical division of roles fostered a split between the facilitation of the art process and an analysis of its meaning.

In the USA the history was a little different in that the more significant influence in the early days of the profession was Freud. Naumberg (1953) was a pioneer, working and writing in the 1950s to bring together art and psychotherapy. She discussed the transference and the therapeutic relationship, which in Britain at that time received little attention. Kramer (1958, 1971) also in the USA was more inclined to the former position and has probably stayed closer to the art process for the many years that she has continued her dual practice as an artist and art therapist. Rubin discusses the importance of these and other early figures in the USA (Rubin, 2001).

Since those early days a great deal has changed in the training, professionalism, and therefore the international recognition of art therapy as a mode of treatment. However, the legacy of this history is to be found in the creative theoretical debates that continue within the profession today. The question of where the healing in art therapy lies is often a factor. An artificially polarized characterization of the debates might represent three different categories of art therapy, in which the artwork and the therapeutic relationship take different positions. Elsewhere (Schaverien, 1994, 2000) I have differentiated these by according them the titles of art therapy, art psychotherapy, and analytical art psychotherapy. This artificial division is intended to draw out some of the differences in the practice. The same art therapist might offer all of these forms of art therapy at some time. I propose imagining each of the three categories to be a picture made up of a figure–ground relationship.

1. *Art therapy.* In art therapy the picture and its creation is the foreground of the therapeutic process. The therapeutic relationship would be the background from which the art process emerges. The art therapist is a facilitator and witness but does not usually interpret the artwork.

2. *Art psychotherapy.* In art psychotherapy the therapeutic relationship is the foreground and the picture the background. The pictures illustrate the therapeutic relationship or recount some aspect of the history in visual form. They may even record the transference but are essentially the backdrop for the person-to-person transference and countertransference relationship. Here the picture may sometimes be used as an illustration of the state of the artist but attention to the therapeutic relationship may reduce its power.

3. *Analytical art psychotherapy.* In analytical art psychotherapy the two are interchangeable. The pictures interrelate with the person-to-person transference and countertransference dynamic but neither figure nor ground has priority; they are of equal status, creating an alternating focus, which integrates the picture fully within the transference.

The hypothetical practitioner of art therapy might consider the art to be healing in itself and therefore the art therapist is the 'midwife', providing the right conditions for this to take place. This practitioner might provide a combination of art materials, space, and quiet attention so that a natural healing process will be facilitated. Little interpretation or intervention is needed from the art therapist. Such an approach has been written about in an original way by Simon (1992, 1997). There is little doubt that this process has worked admirably for many of the more disturbed inpatient populations of large psychiatric hospitals over many years (see Skailes, 1997; Wood, 1997; Maclagan, 1997). Criticisms might be:

- that respect for autonomy of the image, which this approach fosters, may result in the artworks being overidealized, or

- that when the content of the artwork is overwhelming to the artist it needs to be discussed (its implications need to be mediated verbally in order for its archetypal power to be depotentiated).

To continue this artificial separation of the theoretical positions I turn to the practitioner of art psychotherapy. This person might consider mediation of the dual facets of the therapeutic relationship—the transference and the artwork—through the spoken word to be essential. The criticism of this approach might be that too much emphasis on the therapeutic relationship reduces the image to a mere description of psychological states. Consequently, the artwork is reduced rather than given its full power of expression.

There is agreement between art therapists, from whatever theoretical position, that the process of making art is healing. It is the means of its mediation that is sometimes questioned. In the first case the archetypal power of the image may be overwhelming and in the second it may be reduced. The analytical art psychotherapist might aim to take account of both through attention to the transference–countertransference dynamic. This is because the integration of the material that is evoked within the artwork needs to take place. Interpretation of the pictures as well as analysis of the artist's relation to them is vital if experience is to be mediated to the point at which the unconscious becomes conscious. This approach is not without its critics and timing is crucial; if the image is interpreted too

soon—before it has had time and space to work its nonverbal healing—the patient may experience this is an intrusion. Therefore the process needs to be addressed according to the needs and ability of each patient.

The questions that exercise art therapists could be summarized as those regarding whether the healing lies in the art alone or whether it occurs when art is mediated within a therapeutic relationship. Similar creative debates are to be found in the literature of the other arts therapies.

Treatment principles: practice settings, diagnostic categories, and assessment

The cultural context is considered to be important and, in therapeutic practice, attention is given to the inner world, the intrapersonal experience, and outer world, the sociocultural context in which the therapy takes place. In the state sector in Britain art therapists work in all kinds of settings in the National Health Service (NHS), in community mental health teams, psychiatric and general hospitals, social services, psychotherapy departments, prisons, palliative care, and child and family departments. They also work in private clinics and in private practice but this is less common than the state sector.

In the USA and in Europe the client groups and treatment principles are similar but the training and licensing requirements are different. For example, in some countries it is more common for the art therapist to work in private practice. In order to be licensed to practice there is a requirement of a recognized qualification as a psychologist or psychotherapist as well as an art therapy qualification. What is common is that art therapists throughout the world work with similar patient populations and client groups. They employ a range of behavioral and psychodynamic approaches depending on the interest of the individual practitioner and the needs of the client group (see Rubin, 1987 for the diversity of approaches to art therapy). Art therapists work with individuals, adults and children, and with patient groups, institutional groups, and families.

The integration of art materials within a consulting room involves thought about the layout of the room and the messages conveyed by their presence. Most art therapists work in a room that can accommodate a certain amount of mess. There is usually a wide selection of art materials available as well as a table and chairs. A sink is a useful asset in the art room so is a large selection of different sizes of paper, clay, and sometimes a potter's wheel and kiln. Storage is an important consideration as it is usual for the art therapist to keep the artwork for the patient or art therapy group in a folder, or folders, between sessions. Therefore a plans chest or set of storage shelves gives an important nonverbal message about the ways in which the artworks are valued. It is clear that, as a form of psychotherapy, art therapy makes a different impression on the prospective client from the moment they enter the room.

The assessment for art therapy will include an interview and then possibly several sessions of art therapy to see if making art becomes meaningful for the person. Thus the response to the expectation of engaging with art materials will be significant.

Art therapy may be particularly relevant for those whose condition is not immediately amenable to verbal expression, for those who cannot speak their pain. Art offers a medium for symbolic expression in states that cannot be symbolized in any other way. However, it is significant that not all art is symbolic. Therefore in assessment attention will be given to the way the person relates to the art as well as to the therapist. Understanding of the difference between sign and symbol is important in order to observe this. Art therapists often work successfully with patients suffering from psychotic illnesses and eating disorders. In each of these disorders the problem centers on a concrete form of relating and the lack of ability to symbolize. Through the unconscious use of the art materials and images produced in art therapy a relationship is built where the ability to symbolize may develop (Killick and Schaverien, 1997).

Case example

In order to give a sense of the processes involved, here is a brief case vignette from private practice. Ms A, a single woman in her early forties, was referred for art therapy by her general medical practitioner. She had no previous history of psychiatric problems and had a successful professional life. However, since her mother died a few months earlier she had been suffering from anxiety and depression. Ms A explained that, as the eldest of three girls and the only unmarried daughter, she and her mother had always had a close relationship. She was therefore shocked after her mother's death when something in her snapped. A family friend had remarked that Ms A was lucky because she had had a happy childhood and she was shocked to find herself denying it. Subsequently she became overwhelmed as memories of her mother's physically abusive behavior flooded her conscious mind. She tried to tell her sisters but they did not appear to remember the incidents in question or to believe her. Thus Ms A began to doubt the validity of her own memories and yet the impact was such that she knew them to be true.

For the first sessions she seemed almost unaware of my presence and ignored the art materials as she recounted a number of painful memories. She kept repeating them; as if trying to establish the validity of these recollections. In the fourth session, indicating the art materials, I suggested that she might find it helpful to put the incidents down on paper so that she could show me what had happened. At first she tentatively drew the scene she wanted to describe using diagrammatic figures to demonstrate. She explained the layout of the room and the relative positions of her mother and herself. As she spoke my role was that of facilitator and witness of her account.

The content of the pictures, in this case, is less important than their long-term effects. At last there was someone to whom she could report the incidents of injustice that she was remembering. On one occasion there were three figures in the picture. The third was not discussed and it was drawn in a rather tentative manner. As this figure was not mentioned in Ms A's account of what the picture revealed I pointed it out to her and asked her what that figure was doing. It was as if it was the first time Ms A had noticed that figure, although she had drawn it. She stopped and then after a shocked silence she told me that she now remembered that her father had witnessed the abuse without intervening. Therefore, although it was the mother who was beating the child the father was complicit. This was the first awareness of his involvement and it was the picture that brought it to the fore.

Gradually over the weeks these incidents multiplied and so the pictures. Each week I would keep the picture for her in a folder in the art room. Over the 2 years of this therapy she would return to her pictures often and compare them. She would notice things about them that had previously been unnoticed. Very gradually they did not have the same power for her as before. She could look at them without the overwhelming affect that had accompanied the remembering of the incidents.

Ms A could have told me of the memories of these incidents. In fact to begin with she did; however, it was important for her to be able to externalize them. Once they were on paper they were outside of her. In this way she could stand back from her own experience and witness it herself. She was able to see and come to terms with them. I propose that it was in the making and the viewing of these rather rudimentary pictures that a process of transformation in her psychological state came about.

Art therapy process of Ms A and the development of art therapy theory

In *The revealing image* (Schaverien, 1991) a series of processes was identified that take place with the making and processing of an artwork within a therapeutic relationship. The first of these is the scapegoat transference. This is a transference of attributes and states that is made to the artwork in the process of its creation. Like the original scapegoat, in the Bible, the artwork comes to embody affect that could find no other concrete form. It holds the affect 'out there' separate from the person who created it. Thus the person can view it as separate from her. This was the case with Ms A, her pictures became a scapegoat that embodied the emotion associated with the events that could find no other satisfactory form of articulation. She was able to put the terrible traumatic events outside on paper and view them herself. At first she was identified with the image but gradually a separation differentiation took place through a series of five stages that have previously been

identified (Schaverien, 1991, p. 106). These are outlined below as they are processes common in art therapy.

1. *Identification.* This is the state immediately after the picture is made. There is a strong connection between the artist and the work, and words at this time cannot add to the experience of looking at the image and taking in what it reveals.

2. *Familiarization.* As the picture is viewed the artist begins to become familiar with its content, to understand and become conscious of the impact of all that it reveals. This is the beginning of a differentiation of the elements that the picture reveals. This is still a very private process between the artist and her work.

3. *Acknowledgment.* The artist now begins to acknowledge consciously the implications of the picture. Speculation takes place about other possible previously unconscious aspects of the picture. Now discussion with the therapist is possible and interpretations may be received.

4. *Assimilation.* This is the stage of reintegration of the material that is held in the picture. It is now owned and the implications assimilated. This is an additional contemplative stage that takes place between the artist and the picture.

5. *Disposal.* This stage is a result of the previous stages. The picture that holds powerful affect cannot merely be left unattended and thought needs to be given to the ways in which such a picture is dealt with after the previous processes. Thus during the therapy the therapist might keep the picture safely for the patient. Before the therapy ends it is necessary to make decisions about what will happen to the pictures. There are a number of options: the patient might take the pictures with her, leave them behind in the art room, or destroy them. The point is that a conscious decision needs to be made about their disposal and its implications, rather than just leaving it unspoken. (Schaverien, 1991, p. 106).

It is both possible, and even at times of benefit, to the patient, to dispose finally of artwork by leaving it with the therapist or by destroying it—providing—and this is an important point—its contents are previously integrated within the personality. Ms A experienced all these stages over the time that we worked together. In keeping the pictures in my room in a plans chest, within a folder, they were safely held there until the time when she had acknowledged and psychologically assimilated their content. Finally, the pictures no longer carried so much power; the incidents that they bore no longer troubled her as she had become familiar with the feelings associated with them. This permitted a separation from their impact to develop. Thus it is that the concrete nature of the artwork, its physical form, offers a means of mediating for which no other means of articulation can be substituted.

Brief summary of research findings

There is an increasing research-based literature on art therapy emerging in both the UK and the USA. In the USA diagnostic assessments and psychological profiling through pictures generated for the purpose are more common than in Britain. This indicates a difference in the present developments and research bases in the two countries. The interested reader is referred to *Art Therapy: the Journal of the American Art Therapy Association, The Arts in Psychotherapy*, and *Inscape* for up to date research.

During the last 15 years, a consistent body of art therapy literature in Britain has developed, starting with *Art as therapy* (Dalley, 1984) and *Images of art therapy* (Dalley *et al.*, 1987). In 1997 the profession of art therapy achieved State Registration in the UK. This was the result of long and persistent negotiations within the NHS by members of the council of the British Association of Art Therapists. Waller (1991) has documented the history of this up to 1982, when art therapy first became a recognized profession within the NHS. Wood (1997) has traced the history with specific reference to patients with a history of psychosis and this has been developed in her, as yet unpublished, research (Wood, 2000), which documents the process of art therapy with patients with a history of psychosis.

A critical approach to the processes involved has developed and it is no longer enough to claim, for example, merely that art is healing in itself.

Such statements need to be backed up by critical argument and clinical research. The existing research means that such claims are beginning to be substantiated with clinical data and theoretical discourse (Gilroy, 1992; Gilroy and Lee, 1995; Gilroy and McNeilly, 2000). Case and Dalley (1990, 1992) describe art therapy with children, informed by psychoanalytic theories. Maclagan's interest 'outsider art' as well as art therapy is developed in a number of papers including Maclagan (1989, 1997). I have explored the particular effects of the concrete nature of the pictures in the transference and countertransference relationship. My research is informed by Jungian theory and in particular *The psychology of the transference* (Jung, 1946), psychoanalytic theories and the philosopher Cassirer (1955a,b, 1957; Schaverien, 1991). Further, in *Desire and the female therapist* (Schaverien, 1995) the 'aesthetic countertransference' is explored in relation to the gaze of the artist and the return gaze of the picture.

In the USA the founders, Naumberg whose approach was psychoanalytic, Kramer whose approach is very centered on the art in art therapy, and Rhyne whose Gestalt art experience influenced many. The next generation includes Rubin (1987) whose book *Approaches to art therapy* was influential and McNiff (1994). Then there is a flurry of activity in the present including Malchiodi and Hyland Moon. However, most art therapists draw on the particular theories that seem to apply to their own client group or experience of art in therapy.

Indications and contraindications

It might be assumed that those who are 'good at art' or who have attended a fine art program would be the most suitable candidates for art therapy. However, this is not always the case as such a person might be too skilled at concealing to benefit from the process. It is partly the unexpected nature of what is produced that makes art therapy so effective and lack of skill or previous ability contribute to this. When there is a need for the unconscious material to press to the fore through visual expression previously unskilled people may find themselves surprisingly visually articulate. It is as if, when the unconscious needs to express itself, the ability is there.

It has sometimes been thought that art therapy should be restricted and not applied with patients in psychotic states. However, this has been widely challenged by research in art therapy where it has become clear that this client group, if appropriately understood and monitored, benefits from the experience of nonverbal expression in a contained setting. A number of art therapists have written in detail about this (see Killick, 1991; Killick and Greenwood, 1995; Killick and Schaverien, 1997; Wood, 2000).

Summary and future developments

Art therapy has come a long way since its beginnings in hospitals and it now operates from an increasingly strong theoretical research base. We look forward to publications such as that planned by Andrea Gilroy (2004 forthcoming) whose book with regard to art therapy that is evidence based will be a welcome addition to the field.

Music therapy
Helen Odell-Miller

Introduction and context of music therapy services

Music therapists are most commonly employed in special needs education services, or in health service settings, as part of psychological treatment services or therapy services in which increasingly arts therapies departments are established particularly in Mental Health and Learning Disability NHS Trusts. Increasingly in line with NHS modernization, music therapists work in community-based teams, as part of community mental health or learning disability teams or within Primary Care Trust. Referral is usually by doctors, nurses, psychologists, occupational therapists, and psychotherapists. As arts therapists are allied health professionals, there should usually be an Resident Medical Officer for any case. Some music therapists work privately or are funded by the Charity sector such as the National Autistic Society, Alzheimer's Disease Society, Music Space, and Nordoff-Robbins. International patterns of employment and the levels of established music therapy vary from country to country, and few countries have State Registered Music Therapists. In the UK all professional training is at postgraduate level. In some countries in Europe there is no agreement about what constitutes basic training for a music therapist. In the USA most music therapy training is at undergraduate level with some at postgraduate level. A variety of theoretical approaches, is found and some from behavioral schools particularly in the USA. In some European countries such as Belgium and Denmark training is established within a strong psychoanalytic framework. This variety means that it is difficult to give a true international view. However, where possible this is given and as music therapy is more established in the UK than in most countries, the perspective here focuses upon UK practice.

What is music therapy?

In music therapy, patients are offered the opportunity make live music, either improvised or precomposed, on instruments and with voice, with the music therapist who is a trained musician and music therapist. Music therapy can also involve listening to taped or pre-composed music with therapeutic intent.

No musical ability is required by the patients, although cases showing the benefits of treatment range from those who are accomplished musicians to those who have no previously acquired musical skills. The patient's expression through music and the therapist's attunement, through their training as a musician and therapist, facilitates the development of other therapeutic processes.

Musical improvisation is often the focus of the therapy, particularly in the UK, where the underlying rationale is that active music making reflects the patient's current state. This in turn can lead to an understanding of internal and external, interpersonal and intrapersonal changes, which may be desirable. A variety of instruments is used including tuned and untuned percussion, piano, and single line instruments. In other countries, particularly the USA there is a predominance of receptive techniques where listening to music, such as in Guided Imagery in Music (GIM) is the focus of the therapeutic process (Bonny, 1978). However, the method of live musical improvisation or community-based performance (Pavlicevic and Ansdell, 2004) with therapeutic intent, is most predominant in Europe.

In this method, owing to the time element and rhythmic dimensions of music, an immediate intense experience of the 'here-and-now' is provided by music therapy. Interactions can be 'played out' within improvisations, and it is fundamental to this way of working that the therapist responds to this. It is also important to recognize when music-making might be encouraging defenses, such as when a patient becomes fixed upon musical structures, for example steady repetitive duple-time phrases, instead of expressing feelings of distress and chaos in a more irregular rhythmic pattern.

The role of the music therapist is crucial in facilitating the patient's expression, particularly when the latter seems stuck or tentative. This is sometimes understood in symbolic terms as a parental role. For example, in some cases, harmonic input from the piano can inhibit patients from being able to work through their own problems. However, there are times when the opposite is true and the basis for someone exploring a problem is that a musical dialog with a supportive role taken by the therapist is necessary. Here, considerations of transference and countertransference are essential.

Theoretical considerations

During the last 20 years, music therapists have become more concerned with finding a theoretical framework in order to understand therapeutic processes in more depth, but also in order to relate to other disciplines such as neurology, psychiatry, medicine, psychology, psychoanalysis, and musicology.

Music therapists have particularly contributed to an understanding of early interaction, and ideas from music therapy might be particularly useful to the psychoanalyst or psychotherapist working with regressed or less verbal patients. The music therapist, similarly to a mother in early mother–baby interactions can respond to the tiniest nuances to show listening, understanding, and meaning, without words.

As Davies and Richards (2002) write in their book about analytically informed group music therapy:

> If that gaze is withheld or unavailable, the infant is at a loss and left with the terrifying sense that there may be no recognition or containment of her intense feelings. The same can be said of sounds. An existence in which a carer relates to her child in silence, or what the child perceives as silence, is equally traumatic. When the carer cannot listen to or be moved by the baby's voice, she and her baby together cannot develop the idiosyncratic shared vocabulary of sounds that needs to be at the heart of their interactions. At the early stage the overwhelming need is for communication, recognition, response and sharing of feeling, long before there are words available to make statements or explain ideas.
>
> Davies and Richards (2002, pp. 17–18)

Stern (1985) uses musical metaphor to describe processes that have always been in the music therapists' vocabulary such as 'affect attunement' and therefore already we see that much can be gained by paying attention to the forms of interaction music offers.

In the same book Davies and Richards (2000) also draw attention to inventiveness, another prelinguistic phenomenon often lost in adulthood, and of the directness that music encompasses along with its capacity for embracing of emotional complexity and contrast. They draw attention to a discussion about music by Langer (1942) where she celebrates the ambivalence of music, and as a result, its capacity to be true to life because music cannot be directly translated into words.

The uniqueness of music therapy is often marked by its emphasis and focus on live improvised music. In order to enhance the understanding of the relationship between therapist and patient within this complex dynamic, music therapists have drawn upon psychoanalytic theory, particularly concepts of transference, countertransference, object relations, and attachment theory during the last two decades. In Odell-Miller (2001), this influence is addressed, and literature referring to the debate between music therapists regarding this subject is summarized. More recently (Odell-Miller, 2003), music therapists have also begun to address what it is about music therapy process that could influence psychoanalysis. This topic is discussed here in the light of music therapy, but the arguments might well apply to other arts therapies, as highlighted in the book *Where analysis meets the arts* (Searle and Streng, 2001).

It is useful here to describe the universal element that links music therapy with psychoanalytic thinking. Each discipline is concerned with encouraging the spontaneous expression of the person: in music therapy this takes the form of musical improvisation while in psychoanalysis this takes the form of free association.

In considering the history of music therapy it will be seen that while the origin of musical improvisation as a focus for the music therapy relationship owes much to this particular art form, the actual function of music therapy has developed in two directions. The first has gradually incorporated the psychoanalytic concepts of transference, countertransference, and projective identification into the music therapist's therapeutic vocabulary as a means to try and understand the musical relationship between the patient and the therapist. The second has tried to maintain an entirely musical understanding of the relationship between therapist and patient (Ansdell, 1995). Without describing in detail where the specific differences between these approaches lie it might be suggested that in the first

approach music therapy could be in danger of becoming a mere adjunct to psychoanalysis, while in the second approach the value of the therapy might be too dependent on musical analysis, without looking at a wider clinical picture.

Priestley (1994), a British music therapist was the first to articulate some of the connections between psychoanalysis and music therapy in the early 1970s, and interestingly at that time her ideas were taken up in Germany rather in Britain. I suggest that this is because music therapy in Britain was founded by musicians, and upon musical and developmental theories as mentioned above, and that therapists were not ready for this viewpoint. One example of Priestley's use of music as an extension to psychoanalytic theory is found in her ideas about musical structure, and its function as taking the place of a superego function when working with repressed emotion. This has been taken up by others such as Nygaard-Pederson (2002) in Eschen (2002).

Relating through music is a different experience than that of words, and the structure of music including rhythm, pitch, duration, and timbre, and its emotional and interactive nature offers something unique particularly for those who find words difficult. However, despite this unique quality, music therapy has sometimes been thought of as a form of modified psychotherapy, which uses a mode of nonverbal communication to facilitate the relationship and rapport between patient and therapist, but in this way of thinking there is a danger that the music is seen as an adjunct, thus missing the very essence of its therapeutic value. Existing literature also reflects more of a 'middle ground' using the term *psychoanalytically informed* approach where the detail of how music therapists *integrate* psychoanalytic theory into the practice of music therapy in varying ways is explored. Examples are numerous, but there has been debate about the balance of music and psychoanalytic thinking, and the danger of the loss of music if psychoanalytic theory 'takes over'. There is also debate about the richness and clinical rigor that psychoanalytic thinking can bring to the music therapy relationship, and whether it is possible to define musical transference and countertransference. Some examples of texts that together summarize the development of how music therapy draws upon psychoanalytic theory are given here (Woodcock, 1987; Towse, 1991; John, 1992; Priestley, 1994; Brown, 1999; Streeter, 2000; Odell-Miller, 2001; Davies and Richards, 2002).

To conclude this section, we might wonder what music therapy might have to offer psychoanalysis, as we know Freud, while rather puzzled by music as discussed in Odell-Miller (2001), derived his early theories from practicing hypnosis. Here the patient loses him or herself in terms of becoming out of touch with conscious processes through hypnosis. Musicians might play a whole piece of music as if in a trance, where there is little conscious recollection of the experience of having played a piece of music. This points towards the fact that musical interaction might have something to offer in the realm of dreams and repressed emotion and memory as a way of speeding up or 'unsticking' the verbal and thinking processes.

A recent text (Wigram *et al.*, 2002) comprehensively summarizes research in the field from an international perspective, and current models and frameworks of practice. It is clear from this that there is a growing trend for music therapists to take a more psychotherapeutic approach in all clinical fields, although in the USA developmental and behavioral approaches are still more prominent. The clinical fields where music therapy is seen to be most beneficial are learning disabilities (particularly adults and children on the autistic spectrum), psychiatry (particularly schizophrenia and dementia), and new areas are those of palliative care, including bereavement and personality disorders. In the field of autism music therapists have worked with the theoretical and clinical ideas of Ann Alvarez. Music therapy, and other arts therapies could therefore be seen to challenge psychoanalytic orthodoxy, while also developing through its influence. Rather than viewing music therapy and other arts therapies, with their emphasis on action through art forms, as a form of acting out or intrusion within the psychoanalytic arena, these therapies can have a positive influence in this arena. Particularly where there are nonverbal or regressed states encountered, a musical or nonverbal relationship might enhance and perhaps challenge some established aspects of psychoanalysis as suggested by Alvarez (2002).

Clinical considerations

Music therapy is an effective treatment for people with communication disorders or difficulties. This might relate to their diagnosis but also to their current state, perhaps of not having easy access to words and therefore a less verbal approach is indicated.

In all fields careful consideration is given as to the appropriateness of different methods and approaches, and with those who are psychotic or who have dementia a more directive, structured, and less 'psychoanalytic' approach may be necessary. A useful textbook with clear guidance from around the world is found in *Improvisational models of music therapy* (Bruscia, 1987). Similarly, in a more recent book *The dynamics of music psychotherapy* (Bruscia, 1999) an international perspective is given illustrated by case studies about the particular approaches used in a psychodynamic framework by music therapists around the world, with examples showing a range of techniques ranging from song-writing, song and instrumental improvisation, and receptive techniques. From this it is clear that cultural and historical considerations vary enormously and there are no absolute models or protocols that are always practiced with a certain patient group, although researchers are constantly trying to articulate approaches and outcomes more clearly.

A brief summary of research and evidence-based practice in music therapy and other arts therapies

Emerging clinical evidence and research findings suggest that music therapy might be as effective as other treatments, particularly in some fields such as dementia and autism (Wigram *et al.*, 2002), so there is much to be gained from multidisciplinary exchange.

Many patients seeking therapy have been deprived of relationships, and musical interaction can often give the direct experience of recognizing and showing that this deprivation has been heard, processed, and given meaning. This can happen in a way that words might not be able to address owing to their inherent lack of 'affect' in some cases, or total absence, in others.

The growing body of research and evidence base in the arts therapies is in the form of both qualitative and quantitative research projects. The ongoing evidence base is reflected in the professional journals and books published and also in conference proceedings worldwide. In the UK, for example The Royal College of Psychiatrists has included arts therapies research presentations in recent conferences and there are also arts therapies research centers beginning on a small scale, but growing at universities such as Goldsmiths College, University of London, Hertfordshire University, Sheffield University, and Anglia Polytechnic University, Cambridge.

The Department of Health publication in the UK *Treatment choice in psychological therapies and counselling* (2001) mentions arts therapies as additional treatments for people needing psychological treatments, alongside therapies such as psychotherapy, cognitive-behavior therapy, and cognitive analytic therapy. Although the evidence base is too large to summarize here, important key documents are listed and a few projects can be mentioned. For example in a recent HEFCE report *Promoting research in nursing and allied health professions*, arts therapies evidence in the field of autism and dementia is mentioned (Odell-Miller, 1995; Wigram, 2000). Specific outcomes are that music therapy increases levels of engagement significantly in a long stay ward for older people with mainly diagnoses of dementia. Furthermore in a controlled study, music therapy shows higher mean levels of engagement in the same population than in reminiscence therapy treatment, although the results were not statistically significant. The study also showed that music therapy treatment applied weekly shows general increased levels of engagement in this population than when music therapy is applied randomly (Odell-Miller, 1995).

There is a wealth of literature in a variety of fields forming an evidence base now including palliative care, learning difficulties and the autistic spectrum, trauma, forensic psychiatry, eating disorders, adult mental health, dementia, and other areas.

Wilkinson *et al.* (1998) show that regular drama and dance therapy sessions in a controlled study can reduce levels of depression in a small sample size group study. Wigram (2000) sites several studies that show how music therapy increases levels of communication for people with autism, and Odell-Miller (2002a), while finding that a randomized controlled trial did not show significant results (for many practical and methodological reasons), show in a qualitative analysis, that the specific relationship and rapport with the arts therapist and the arts media are central to the patient's perception of how arts therapies work in the field of adult mental health.

Case example

To illustrate the music therapy clinical process, this case pays particular attention to the psychotherapeutic aspects of the process. The case vignette is of a 35-year-old man with manic depression, who was seen individually for music therapy over a period of 4 years. The case is written up in detail in the book *Where psychoanalysis meets the arts* (Searle and Streng, 2001). Early sessions consisted of music, which seemed symbiotic in nature, where the music therapist seemed drawn into the countertransference as a nurturing maternal figure. One example of change taking place literally musically, but helped by an understanding of the countertransference is as follows. In session 9 the patient reveals a very destructive aspect of himself, expressing loud violent-sounding cymbal playing for 4 minutes. During this, the therapist plays the drum, trying to provide some rhythmic structure and stability, while at the same time supporting him in his need to express himself and release tension. This was a turning point in the therapy—as the therapist provided rhythmic language through improvised drum beats in order to help the client find order within chaos, at the same time as validating his emotional state by showing this in her playing, reflecting the powerful 'affect' in the room. If taped, examples of intense cymbal playing, sounding loud and uncontrolled could be heard. The therapist gradually used more regular drum beating and also some irregular in order to support the patient in this form of expression. There is also a 'rallentando' at the end, precipitated by a gradual subtle slowing down of the therapist's drum beats in order to encourage the music to end, as a boundary was necessary. The qualities of music that enable 'real' time to be experienced through musical interaction are vital here. The patient had been using the cymbal in this way for 4 minutes. It was important for the destructive side of his life to be expressed with the therapist in the session in order to help him in the therapy, and for the therapist to survive this and to return the following week. At this point verbal interpretation was not appropriate, but in the following weeks the experience provided the material for the possibility of helpful interpretation as described in the full case discussion in Odell-Miller (2001). It is difficult to see how this crucial experience of playing the cymbal, or something like it, could have taken place without the musical context, unless some destruction to objects or people had taken place.

The second musical example, of an interaction from the last few months of his therapy, shows a supportive role taken by the therapist from the piano, using predictable harmonic progressions to follow support and interact with the patients playing on a metallophone. There is a sense of integration here, and acknowledgment of an interaction—a consideration by the patient of this relationship both musically and socially. At the start of therapy he had no way of showing consideration for others, was suicidal and depressed, had been violent towards his ex-wife, was estranged from his three sons, and he found it difficult to relate to the therapist. Sessions moved between music and words, re-creating some patterns of relating (which seemed to represent early relationships), which were very significant due to the fact that his mother suffered from schizophrenia and had been unable to look after him. He became able to respond to the therapist's music and there was a sense of two people able to 'give and take': neither merged nor 'cut off'. This musical experience led to further understanding of his feelings and behaviors, and provided the basis for interpretation and understanding.

For example, a lullaby quality of many early sessions was prevalent. While the patient's music was often still somewhat rigid, by the end of the therapy, there were points of fluidity. After 4 years of individual weekly music therapy he managed to stop his destructive violent behavior in relationships, and said he was helped by the improvisations. We see here the importance of the active relationship with the therapist, while maintaining the therapeutic boundaries of the sessions. The understanding of the patient's life events was possible with improvisation being a vehicle for expression and integration of previously unintegrated states. The therapy took place in a day clinic and is described in detail in Odell-Miller (2001).

Improvisation

We see from this case that improvisation is a creative act, difficult to describe in words, and its inclusion is central to music therapy technique. When people are ill, physically or mentally, they often atrophy—they feel unconnected within themselves and with their surroundings. This is supported by research findings, which found that people with learning disabilities, schizophrenia, autism, and other related disabilities lacked synchronicity within themselves, and in relation to interactions with others, in comparison with nonpathological populations. The possibilities for re-creating synchronicity are particularly potent within musical improvisation, and it can also offer something essential to the relationship between patient and therapist, where there is less radical impairment, but where words and thinking are temporarily unavailable. Many psychotherapists are increasingly interested in this interactive area as being essential to the therapeutic process, for example as shown in the Interpersonal Theories of the Conversational Model.

Improvisation allows for the patient to become spontaneously involved in an interaction that can take on its own shape and form with the therapist's input guiding this. It can take on a dream-like quality. Patients are often surprised at the manner or mood of their expressions, pointing towards a similar process to the unconscious, at work. Articulating this in words has always been a problem for music therapists and while psychoanalytic theory has supplied some mechanisms for doing this, the very nature of what the following definition of musical countertransference is describing, indicates in itself what music therapy might offer to psychoanalysis. It lies at the heart of what musical interactions can articulate in terms of atmosphere, and implication: those things that cannot be easily spoken.

> Musical counter-transference takes place in a shared clinical improvisation. As the therapist you realise that you are playing in a certain way in response to the patient, which previously you had been unaware or unconscious of. You are then subsequently able to make use of this musical experience. This would be by consciously altering your musical style; which could be called a musical interpretation; and/or after the music has finished, making a verbal interpretation during discussion arising from the musical interaction. This interpretation helps the patient understand how they may have influenced your response
>
> Odell-Miller (2001).

It seems clear that people for whom music therapy rather than another treatment is helpful, are likely to be those who find independent listening and thinking difficult and need a transitional space (the therapy session), and some assistance in which to do this (the music therapist). For example, a live musical interaction through improvisation is like an active communication that requires some effort, but at the same time taps into the spontaneous flexibility of the brain to adapt and even manipulate its surroundings. It is well known that mood can change following a musical experience. Many can make these connections alone, and understand meaning within those moments, but for some, a live interactive experience through music therapy might be the only way of thinking and feeling and developing an identity. The value of improvisational music therapy rather than passive listening therapy is in the fact that it encourages thinking and feeling, and helps relate to others, for people who may need some assistance with this.

The emphasis upon nonverbal interaction and active participation mirrors some of the recent developments in psychological therapies such as the cognitive therapies. Not much has been said here of Jungian psychology. This is because there is more widely known about its tribute to art as a central element of unconscious processing as written about by many including and art therapist and Jungian analyst Schaverien (2001). Casement makes a case for psychoanalysis to become less focused upon the content of words and linguistic analysis and more upon the expressing dimension of how communication is happening and upon what the patient is trying to bring to our attention. Good psychoanalytic practice naturally strives for this, but where fragile interaction, and an intense awareness of rhythms, timbres, and tempo are necessary, music therapy provides a framework that includes listening, attending, attuning, responding, and interpreting, within an attitude that can be reflective, vital, and thoughtful all at once.

References

Adamson, E. (1984). *Art as healing.* London: Coventure.

Alvarez, A. (2002). *Levels of Meaning in Psychoanalytic Work: Areas of Overlap with Music Therapy.* The Shirley Foundation Lecture. 10th World Conference of Music Therapy. Oxford University.

Alvin, J. (1975). *Music therapy.* London: Hutchinson.

Ansdell, G. (1995). *Music for life.* London: Jessica Kingsley.

Bonny, H. (1978). GIM Monograph No 2. The Role of Taped Music Programs in the GIM Process. Baltimore: ICM Press.

Brown, S. (1999). Some thoughts on music, therapy and music therapy. *British Journal of Music Therapy*, **13**(2).

Bruscia, K. (1987). *Improvisational models of music therapy.* Philadelphia: Barcelona Pub.

Bruscia, K. (1999). *The dynamics of music psychotherapy.* London: Jessica Kingsley.

Case, C. and Dalley, T., ed. (1990). *Working with children in art therapy.* London: Routledge.

Case, C. and Dalley, T. (1992). *The handbook of art therapy.* London: Tavistock/Routledge.

Cassirer, E. (1955a). *Language*, Vol. 1. *The philosophy of symbolic forms.* New Haven, CT: Yale University Press.

Cassirer, E. (1955b). *Mythical thought*, Vol. 2. *The philosophy of symbolic forms.* New Haven, CT: Yale University Press.

Cassirer, E. (1957). *The phenomonology of knowledge*, Vol. 3. *The philosophy of symbolic forms.* New Haven, CT: Yale University Press.

Champernowne, I. (1969). *Art therapy as an adjunct to psychotherapy.* London: Inscape 1. *Journal of the British Association of Art Therapists.*

Champernowne, I. (1971). *Art and therapy: an uneasy partnership.* London: Inscape 3. *Journal of the British Association of Art Therapists.*

Chodorow, J. (1991). *Dance therapy and depth psychology.* London: Routledge.

Condon, W. S. and Ogston, W. D. (1966). Sound film analysis of normal and pathological behaviour patterns. *Journal of Nervous and Mental Disease*, **143**(4), 338–47.

Cunningham Dax, E. (1953). *Experimental studies in psychiatric art.* London: Faber and Faber.

Dalley, T. (1984). *Art as therapy.* London: Tavistock.

Dalley, T., *et al.* (1987). *Images of art therapy.* London: Routledge.

Darnley-Smith, R. and Patey, H. (2002). *Music therapy.* London: Sage.

Davies, A. and Richards, E. (2002). *Music therapy and group work: sound company.* London: Jessica Kingsley.

Department of Health. (2000). *Meeting the Challenge: A Strategy for the Allied Health Professions.* Ref No. 22586.

Department of Health. (2001). *Treatment Choice in Psychological Therapies and Counselling.* Ref No. 23454.

Edwards, M. (1989). Art, therapy and romanticism. In: A. Gilroy and T. Dalley, ed. *Pictures at an exhibition: selected essays on art and art therapy.* London: Tavistock/Routledge.

Eschen, J. (2002). *Analytical music therapy.* London: Jessica Kingsley.

Gilroy, A. (1992). Research in art therapy. In: D. Waller and A. Gilroy, ed. *Art therapy: a handbook.* Buckingham: Open University Press.

Gilroy, A. (2005). *Art therapy research and evidence based practice*. London: Sage.

Gilroy, A. and Lee, C. ed. (1995). *Art and music: therapy and research*. London: Routledge.

Gilroy, A. and McNeilly, G. (2000). *The changing shape of art therapy*. London: Jessica Kingsley Publishers.

Hobson, R. (1985). *Forms of feeling: the heart pyschotherapy*. London: Routledge.

Holmes, P. (1992). *The inner world outside: object relations theory and psychodrama*. London: Tavistock/Routledge.

Holmes, P. and Karp, M. (1991). *Psychodrama: inspiration and technique*. London: Tavistock/Routledge.

Jenkyns, M. (1996). *The play's the thing: exploring text in drama and therapy*. London: Routledge.

John, D. (1992). Towards music psychotherapy. *Journal of British Music Therapy*, **6**(1), 10–13.

Jones, P. (1996). *Drama as therapy: theatre as living*. London: Routledge.

Jung, C. G. (1946). The psychology of the transference. In: *Collected Works, 16*. London: Routledge.

Junge, M. P. and Asawa, P. P. (1994). *A history of art therapy in the United States*. American Art Therapy Association.

Killick, K. (1991). The practice of art therapy with patients in acute psychotic states. London: Inscape. *Journal of the British Association of Art Therapists*. (Winter).

Killick, K. and Greenwood, H. (1995). Research in art therapy with people who have psychotic illnesses. In: Gilroy, A. and Lee, C. (eds) *Art and music: therapy and research*. London: Routledge.

Killick, K. and Schaverien, J., ed. (1997). *Art, psychotherapy and psychosis*. London: Routledge.

Kramer, E. (1958). *Art therapy in a children's community*. Illinois: Thomas.

Kramer, E. (1971) *Art as therapy with children*. London: Elek.

Langer, S. (1942). *Philosophy in a new key*. Cambridge, Mass: Harvard.

Lyddiatt, E. M. (1971). *Spontaneous modelling and painting: a practical approach in therapy*. New York: St Martin's Press.

Maclagan, D. (1989). Fantasy and the figurative. In: A. Gilroy and T. Dalley, ed. *Pictures at an exhibition*. London: Tavistock/Routledge.

Maclagan, D. (1997). Has 'psychotic' art become extinct? In: K. Killick and J. Schaverien, ed. *Art, psychotherapy and psychosis*. London: Routledge.

McNiff, S. (1994). *Art as medicine*. London: Piatkus.

Moreno, J. L. (1977). *Psychodrama*. Beacon, NY: Beacon House (first published 1946).

Naumberg, M. (1953). *Psychoneurotic art: its function in psychotherapy*. New York: Grune & Stratton.

Nowell Hall, P. (1987). Art therapy: a way of healing the split. In: T. Dalley *et al.*, ed. *Images of art therapy*. London: Tavistock.

Nygaard-Pederson, I. (2002). Analytical music therapy with adults in mental health and in counselling work. In: J. Eschens, ed. *Analytical music therapy*. London: Jessica Kingsley.

Odell-Miller, H. (1995). Approaches to music therapy in psychiatry with specific emphasis upon the evaluation of work within a completed research project with elderly mentally ill people. In: Wigram, Saperston and West, (eds). *The art and science of music therapy: a handbook*, pp. 83–110. Harwood Academic Publications.

Odell-Miller, H. (2001). Music therapy and its relationship to psychoanalysis. In: Y. Searle and I. Streng (eds). *Where analysis meets the arts*. London: Karnac Books.

Odell-Miller, H. (2003). Are words enough? Music therapy as an influence in psychoanalytic psychotherapy. In: L. King & R. Randall ed. pp. 153–66. *The Future of Psychoanalytic Psychotherapy*. London: Whurr.

Odell-Miller, H. (2002a). *Background to arts therapies*. Unpublished Briefing Paper prepared on behalf of Arts Therapies Professions.

Odell-Miller, H., Hughes, P., Mortlock, D., and Binks, C. (2002b). *An investigation into the effectiveness of the arts therapies (art therapy, dramatherapy, music therapy, dance movement therapy) by measuring symptomatic and significant life change for people between the ages of 16–65 with continuing mental health problems*. Addenbrookes NHS Trust & Anglia Polytechnic University.

Pavlicevic, M. (1997). *Music therapy in context: music meaning and relationship*. London: Jessica Kingsley.

Pavlicevic, M. and Ansdell, G. (2004). *Community music therapy*. London: Jessica Kingsley.

Pavlicevic, M. and Trevarthon, C. (1989). A musical assessment of psychiatric states in adults. *Psychopathology*, **22**, 325–34.

Payne, H. (1993). *Handbook of inquiry in the arts therapies*. London: Jessica Kingsley.

Priestley, M. (1994) *Essays on analytical music therapy*. USA: Barcelona Pub.

Rhyne, J. (1973). *The Gestalt art experience*. Chicago, IL: Magnolia Street Publishers.

Rubin, J. (2001). *Approaches to art therapy*. London: Brunner/Routledge (first edition published in 1987).

Schaverien, J. (1991). *The revealing image: analytical art psychotherapy in theory and practice*. London: Tavistock/Routledge.

Schaverien, J. (1994). Analytical Art Psychotherapy: Further reflections on theory and practice. *Inscape, Journal of the British Association of Art Therapists*, **2**, 41–9.

Schaverien, J. (1995). *Desire and the female therapist: engendered gazes in psychotherapy and art therapy*. London: Routledge.

Schaverien, J. (2000). The triangular relationship and the aesthetic countertransference in Analytical Art Psychotherapy. In: A. Gilroy and G. McNeilly, ed. *The changing shape of art therapy*.

Schaverien, J. (2001). Art and analytical psychology. In: Y. Searle and I. Streng (eds). *Where analysis meets the arts*. London: Karnac Books.

Searle, Y. and Streng, I. (2001). *Where analysis meets the arts*. London: Karnac Books.

Simon, R. (1992). *The symbolism of style*. London: Tavistock/Routledge.

Simon, R. (1997). *Symbolic images in art as therapy*. London: Routledge.

Skailes, C. (1997). The forgotten people. In: Killick, K. and Schaverien, J., ed. *Art, psychotherapy and psychosis*. London: Routledge.

Stern, D. (1985). *The interpersonal world of the infant*. USA: Basic Books.

Stevens, A. (1986). *Withymead*. London: Coventure.

Streeter, E. (2000). Finding a balance between psychological thinking and musical awareness in music therapy—a psychoanalytic perspective. *Journal of British Music Therapy*, **13**(1).

Thomson, M. (1989). *On art and therapy*. London: Virago.

Towse, E. (1991). Relationships in music therapy: do music therapy techniques discourage the emergence of transference? *British Journal of Psychotherapy*, **7**(4), 323–30.

Waller, D. (1991). *Becoming a profession: the history of art therapy in Britain 1940–82*. London: Tavistock/Routledge.

Waller, D. (1998). *Towards a European art therapy: creating a profession*. Buckingham: Open Universities Press.

Wigram, T. (2002). *Meeting Health Care Needs of Children and Adults with Learning Disability, Motor Disorders and Pervasive Developmental Disorders including Autism, Asperger Syndrome and Rett Syndrome by treatment with Music Therapy: Efficacy within the Criteria of Evidence-based Practice*. Paper prepared in response to the Department of Public Health, Consultant Paediatricians, Purchasers and Providers of Healthcare Services in a Hertfordshire NHS Trust.

Wigram, T. (2002). Indications in music therapy: evidence from assessment that can identify the expectations of music therapy as a treatment for Autistic Spectrum Disorder (ASD): meeting the challenge of evidence based practice. *British Journal of Music Therapy*, **16**(1), 11–28.

Wigram, T., Nygaard Pederson, I., and Bonde, L. O. (2002). *A comprehensive guide to music therapy: theory, clinical practice, research and training*. London: Jessica Kingsley.

Wilkinson, N., Srikumar, S., Shaw, K., and Orell, M. (1998). Drama and movement therapy in dementia: A Pilot Study. *The Arts in Psychotherapy* **25**(3), 195–201.

Wood, C. (1997). The history of art therapy and psychosis 1938–95. In: K. Killick and J. Schaverien, ed. *Art, psychotherapy and psychosis*. London: Routledge.

Wood, C. (2000). Art, psychotherapy and psychosis: the nature and politics of art therapy. Unpublished PhD Dissertation University of Sheffield.

Woodcock, J. (1987). Towards group analytic music therapy. *Journal of British Music Therapy*, **1**(1), 16–22.

10 Psychotherapy integration

Rutger Willem Trijsburg, Sjoerd Colijn, and Jeremy Holmes

In this chapter we shall consider psychotherapy integration not just as a specific therapeutic modality, but also as a theoretical and research viewpoint that encompasses several of the distinct psychotherapeutic approaches reviewed in this section. Psychotherapy integration will thus be considered as a general 'tendency' within contemporary psychotherapy, and a modality in its own right.

We start by describing the historical background of psychotherapy integration. After defining the several theoretical approaches in psychotherapy integration, integrative treatment modalities and 'common factors' will be discussed. Some examples of clinical applications and empirical evidence on the effectiveness of treatment modalities will also be given.

Historical overview and theoretical background

In the opening address of the Second Psychoanalytic Congress in 1910, Freud stated that the psychoanalytic technique has to be altered in phobic patients, because 'these patients cannot bring out the material necessary for resolving their phobia so long as they feel protected by obeying the condition which it lays down'. Only after they can do without the protection of their phobia, does 'the material become accessible, which, when it has been mastered, leads to a solution of the phobia' (Freud, 1910/1975, p. 145).

The integrative implication of Freud's comment is the possibility that the 'protection of the phobia' may not be removed by interpretation alone, and that a preliminary, concurrent, or even alternative approach involving exposure, may also be necessary.

Polarization of different psychotherapeutic camps, rivalry, misunderstanding, 'straw-man-ism', and dogmatic pseudocertainties have characterized battles between different psychotherapeutic modalities, especially between behaviorism and psychoanalysis. The fundamental theoretical antitheses lie between therapeutic monism and therapeutic eclecticism, and between specificity and universality (Karasu, 1986).

Monism versus eclecticism

Therapeutic monism (called sectarianism by Karasu, 1986) is based on the premise that psychotherapeutic modalities have unique qualities differentiating them from other modalities. Each treatment modality, it is held, uses specific and unique therapeutic approaches, producing greater effectiveness compared with other methods, sometimes related to specific diagnostic categories or problems [e.g., cognitive-behavioral therapy (CBT) in obsessive-compulsive disorder, q.v.], or to effects not dealt with by other methods (e.g., psychoanalysis's view that it alone can bring about 'structural' as opposed to 'symptomatic' change).

At worst, therapeutic monism leads to: (1) downplaying the significance of interventions and processes that are relevant to all psychotherapeutic treatments; (2) Procrusteanism—i.e., offering potential patients only one type of treatment, irrespective of the presenting problem and personality of the sufferer, and withholding more appropriate treatments; and

(3) splitting of the professional world, power struggles, and denigration other treatments.

Eclecticism, by contrast, is based on an empiricist view of treatment, and is concerned with developing ways of predicting change under specific circumstances irrespective of the model. Seeking the best treatment for the person and the problem, it is essentially pragmatic (Norcross and Newman, 1992). Dissatisfaction with 'grand theories' and technical procedures derived from these theories ('a plague on all your houses'), as the motive force behind eclecticism (or technical eclecticism), is sometimes construed as atheoretical and even antitheoretical, leading to syncretism (the uncritical and unsystematic application of procedures; Norcross and Newman, 1992). Eclecticism distances itself from 'schoolism', and disavows any claims for itself as a separate school, but, rather, uses treatment interventions shown to be effective, irrespective of the particular theory from which they derive.

This chapter is not anti-'monism'—indeed there is good evidence that therapists who stick to one model, albeit flexibly, get better results than either model-hopping eclecticists or rigid monists (Beutler and Consoli, 1992). Effective eclectic psychotherapy needs to be based on a thorough problem analysis and a well-founded treatment plan, leading to optimal use of various interventions. In short, neither monism nor eclecticism is contrary to good clinical practice, nor can either lay exclusive claim on effectiveness.

Specificity versus universality

The specificity model is based on a natural science paradigm, and implies that under optimal circumstances, particular interventions will result in the intended effects. The universality model draws on anthropology and sociology and assumes that any socially sanctioned method of healing believed to be effective, and applied within a healing relationship by a healer to a sufferer seeking relief, may produce changes in feelings, attitudes, and behavior (Frank and Frank, 1991, pp. 2–3).

The model of psychotherapeutic specificity—or 'drug metaphor' (Shapiro, 1995)—in psychotherapy has provided the main paradigm for outcome studies in psychotherapy. Given that professionals are required to deliver psychotherapeutic treatments that are scientifically supported, to uphold professional standards, and to offer financially and ethically acceptable services, it is necessary to offer treatments of proven effectiveness. Governments, insurance companies, and patients increasingly insist on this.

Cognitive-behavioral therapists have led the way in using the specificity paradigm in psychotherapy. Methodologically sound studies, especially randomized controlled trials (RCT), of cognitive-behavioral treatments have shown that psychological therapies stand up well in comparison with drug treatments in psychiatry. This led the American Psychological Association's Society of Clinical Psychology's (Division 12) Task Forces (now the 'Standing Committee of Science and Practice') to develop lists of so-called 'validated' therapies (Task Force on Promotion and Dissemination of Psychological Procedures, 1995; Chambless *et al.*, 1996, 1998; Chambless and Hollon, 1998).

Although the ideal of a list of *validated treatments* was changed into the less definitive and dogmatic concept of *empirically supported therapies*, the work of the Standing Committee remains problematic (e.g., Lambert and Barley, 2002; Norcross, 2002a; Elliott *et al.*, 2004; Lambert *et al.*, 2004). It has inspired another APA Division Task Force (APA Division of Psychotherapy Task Force) to come up with a list of 'empirically supported therapy *relationships*' (Norcross, 2002a). This contrast between 'therapy' (i.e., a drug-like 'pure' treatment) and 'relationship' (i.e., a possible component of any effective therapy) vividly illustrates the antithesis between specificity and universality.

One of the more problematic aspects of the RCT model is that the evidence does not consistently or clearly show the superiority of one school over another (Lambert, 1992; Lambert and Bergin, 1994; Lambert and Ogles, 2004). Others, however, conclude that the way in which these critics used meta-analysis led them to a premature, or even false, determination that treatments are equally effective. For example, research techniques may not have been sophisticated enough to show differences in effectiveness, or similar outcomes may have been reached via different pathways.

Frank and others (Karasu, 1986; Frank and Frank, 1991) have argued that the crucial factor in any helping situation is the quality of the *relationship* between helper and recipient. The relationship is influenced by many factors. For patients these comprise, among others motivation, trust, hope, and idealization. In therapists, powers of suggestion, persuasion, warmth, empathy, involvement, directivity, and expert status. Interactional factors include contact, bond, agreement, rapport, and contract. Such interactional and relationship factors are important in every psychotherapeutic treatment.

In line with the 'drug metaphor' model these universal factors are viewed as 'nonspecific', because, in comparison with the specific factors, they are considered to be therapeutically neutral. However, here the drug metaphor breaks down, because both specific *and* nonspecific factors are based on psychological mechanisms (Lambert and Bergin, 1994; Lambert and Ogles, 2004). For instance, Lambert and Bergin (1994) showed that 'placebo therapy' (e.g., minimal attention) produces better outcomes than no-treatment or waiting-list controls. Nonspecific factors are often inadequately operationalized in placebo treatments, thus it is not clear to what extent 'minimal attention' compares with more intensive 'specific' attention. This leaves the question open how great the differences in effectiveness between active and 'placebo' treatments would be if nonspecific factors would be adequately defined, operationalized, trained, applied, and checked for adherence and competence (Arkowitz, 1992). Indeed, it would then be difficult still to view these factors as nonspecific instead of specific (Lambert and Bergin, 1994). In conclusion, it is inherently impossible for psychotherapeutic treatments to employ specific factors to the exclusion of nonspecific factors, and vice versa.

Another aspect has arisen from variance studies in treatment delivery in RCT. Initially these studies treated such differences as 'error' variance (Lambert, 1989; Lambert and Barley, 2002). Determined attempts were made to minimize individual differences between therapists within a treatment condition, e.g., by training therapists to offer the prescribed treatment using manuals, by supervision, and by monitoring adherence and competence. However, therapist variability appears to be the rule rather than the exception (Luborsky *et al.*, 1985; Shapiro *et al.*, 1989). For instance, Luborsky *et al.* (1985) found that interactional variables, especially the quality of the working alliance, were responsible for differences between therapies, more so than the quality of the individual therapies. The conclusion is that, irrespective of model, the role of the individual therapist and the working alliance with the patient cannot be neglected in psychotherapy (Lambert, 1989; Lambert and Barley, 2002).

These and other considerations have led to the redefining of nonspecific aspects of psychotherapy as 'common factors', i.e., those that were held in common by most or every psychotherapeutic treatment (Lambert and Ogles, 2004).

A model

To summarize the argument so far, neither monism and specificity, nor eclecticism and universality can grasp clinical reality in its totality. A historical/ structural model can explain their various roles (see Figure 10.1).

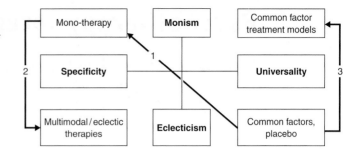

Fig. 10.1 Psychotherapeutic models (after Karasu, 1986).

Figure 10.1 shows that first, at the time of the founding of modern, scientific, 'Western' psychotherapy (to begin with Freud), common factors, originating in the prescientific era (Frank and Frank, 1991), were replaced by monistic (scientific) treatments of psychiatric disorders. Examples of this are psychoanalysis and CBT. Secondly, the plethora of these approaches gave rise to eclectic therapies. One example of this is multimodal therapy (Lazarus, 1976, 1989, 1992, 1997). Lastly, with the growing 'postmodern' scientific awareness of the importance of common factors and the realization that most so-called 'monistic' therapies in reality consist of a mixture of change-producing strategies, theoretical models were developed and new types of treatment were designed, including the Common Factor Model of Arkowitz (1992), interpersonal therapy (see Chapter 3 this volume), cognitive analytic therapy (CAT; Ryle, 1999), psychodynamic interpersonal therapy (Margison, 2002), the Cyclical Psychodynamic Model (Wachtel, 1997; Wachtel and Seckinger, 2001) among others.

The impact of different groups of interventions can be analyzed in this model. It is reasonable to assume that interventions from the monistic and the universal models are complementary. Thus specific interventions add value to the common factors and reinforce their effects (Strupp and Hadley, 1979). Equally, common factors reinforce the effects of specific interventions. Also, adding specific interventions derived from other models to a monomethodical approach may enhance the effects of the latter. In their turn, monomethodical approaches are necessary for the development of new interventions which then find their way into eclectic psychotherapies. There is currently an overall trend towards psychotherapy integration, or at least cross-fertilization, which advocates dialogue between theoreticians, researchers, and practitioners from different therapeutic orientations.

Integrative trends in clinical practice

Surveys of therapists' orientations show that integrative approaches are the most commonly practiced. Thus one-half to two-thirds of providers prefer to offer their clients a variety of interventions from major theoretical schools rather than a single modality (Lambert *et al.*, 2004). A recent survey of Dutch psychotherapists (Trijsburg *et al.*, in press) showed that therapists with various primary orientations used the full range of interventions to varying degrees. Figure 10.2 shows that subjects with a primary cognitive or behavioral orientation use more directive interventions than those with a primary client-centered, experiential, psychoanalytic, or psychodynamic orientation, whereas the latter use more nondirective interventions. Psychotherapists with a primary integrative and eclectic orientation are positioned in between and show a mixture of both nondirective and directive interventions. Importantly for our argument here, self-attributed monotherapists of all orientations appeared to use interventions derived from other theoretical schools.

Power emphasizes the 'accidental' nature of model-specific theories and interventions, and argues that free association and transference might just as well have been be applicable to CBT as to psychoanalysis had the history of psychotherapy been different. Similarly, Alford and Beck (1997) argue that CBT is

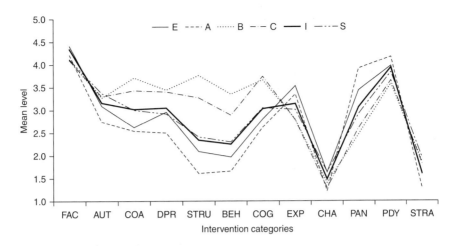

Fig. 10.2 Mean scoring level of the intervention categories for six psychotherapeutic orientations. Reprinted from Trijsburg, R. W., Lietaer, G., Colijn, S., Abrahamse, R. M., Joosten, S., and Duivenvoorden, H. J. (2004). Construct validity of the Comprehensive Psychotherapeutic Interventions Rating Scale. *Psychotherapy Research*, **14**, 346–66. A = Psychoanalytic–psychodynamic; B = Behavioral; C = Cognitive; E = Client-centered—experiential; I = Eclectic—integrative; S = Systemic; AUT, Authoritative support; BEH, Behavioral; CHA, Chair work (experiential procedures); COA, Coaching; COG, Cognitive; DB, Directive-Behavioral; DPR, Directive Process; EXP, Experiential; FAC, Facilitating; PAN, Psychoanalytic; PDY, Psychodynamic; STRA, Strategic; STRU, Structuring.

as much an integrative as a monotherapy. Eclecticism is surveyed from a psychoanalytic perspective by Gabbard and Westen (2003) who describe a range of different interventions considered likely to produce change, including working not just with the unconscious and defense mechanisms, as in classical theory, but also with conscious conflicts and using such 'facilitative' strategies as support and humor which would be more likely to emerge from a cognitive therapy or humanistic background.

The trend toward eclectic and integrative psychotherapies is evidenced by the formation of societies that support the idea of psychotherapy integration (the Society for the Exploration of Psychotherapy Integration, SEPI and the Society of Psychotherapy Research, SPR), journals, and handbooks (Norcross and Goldfried, 1992; Stricker and Gold, 1993; Snyder and Ingram, 2000). Lambert *et al.* (2004) stated that the encyclopedic *Handbook of psychotherapy and behavior change* 'has been eclectic from its inception in 1967 and its first publication by Bergin and Garfield in 1971' (p. 7).

Approaches in psychotherapy integration

Norcross and Newman (1992) differentiated three forms of integration: technical eclecticism, theoretical integration, and the common factors approach. All three combine aspects of psychotherapeutic treatment originating from different sources.

Holmes and Bateman (2002) similarly differentiate organizational integration (making available a range of therapies so that the patient can be assigned to whatever fits his or her needs best), theoretical integration (showing how similar phenomena may be described in different languages, e.g., psychoanalysis's 'internal objects' and CBT's 'schemata'), and practical integration (a pragmatic use of whatever therapeutic approach seems useful for a particular patient and problem). The latter, they argue, often characterizes the work of 'mature clinicians' of whatever basic persuasion, who feel free to borrow elements from other orientations when clinical need dictates.

Messer (1992) describes the latter as 'assimilative integration'. This form of integration advocates a firm grounding in one system of psychotherapy and 'a willingness to incorporate or assimilate, in a considered fashion, perspectives or practices from other schools' (p. 151).

Below, we discuss technical eclecticism, theoretical integration, and the common factors approach. In each case we define the model, and give

examples of treatment models and their applications. It has to be noted that most integrationists, e.g., Norcross and Newman (1992), stress the importance of combining specific interventions, shown to be effective in empirical research, with common factors in treatments. Nor are the three forms of integrationism mutually exclusive. Other aspects of integration, e.g., the combination of psychotherapy with drug therapy (q.v. Chapter 39), are discussed elsewhere in this volume.

Technical eclecticism

Technical eclecticism is empirically oriented. Technical eclecticists combine different empirically supported interventions in any given treatment. Examples are the treatment models developed by (1) Beutler's systematic eclectic psychotherapy (SEP; e.g., Beutler and Consoli, 1992; Beutler and Harwood, 2000; Beutler *et al.*, 2002a), and (2) Lazarus' multimodal therapy (e.g., Lazarus, 1976, 1989, 1992, 1997). Essentially, different practical approaches are used and combined without adopting wholesale the theoretical model behind these interventions.

Example of an eclectic treatment model: systematic eclectic psychotherapy

Beutler's SEP starts from the need for pragmatic forms of eclectic treatments and is based on the belief that different interventions are effective for different types of patients in different phases of treatment. It seeks its inspiration in clinical practice, empirical research, and the philosophy 'that psychotherapy is a social-influence or persuasion process in which the therapist's operational theory forms the content of *what* is persuaded, and the therapist's technology functions as the *means* of influence. The quality of the therapeutic relationship is thought to define the limiting influence of the procedures used' (Beutler and Consoli, 1992, p. 266).

Essentially, SEP represents a model of treatment selection that encompasses both established common factors as well as specific procedures. It formulates indications and contraindications for the application of these procedures. SEP contends that operational theories from different origins are applicable in different types of patients, provided that such theories permit the therapist to offer the patient an explanation of change, a perspective on change, and treatment goals that can be reached. One advantage of this approach is that theoretical integration at the explanatory level is not necessary; instead the theoretical (explanatory) considerations will have to be translated into the (descriptive) language of social persuasion theory.

The model emphasizes:

1. *Matching* of patient and therapist. SEP states that some communalities in the backgrounds of therapists and patients are necessary for patients to develop initial trust in the therapist. Equally, differences of viewpoint matter, in that it is through difference that new experience arises. Also, the severity of problems is important in formulating a treatment plan, as the initial patient motivation is directly dependent on the extent to which suffering is acute and immediate or long term and chronic.

2. *Tailoring* procedures to patient characteristics. Special attention is given to the reactance and the coping style of patients, in deciding how directive, or exploratory to be. Thus more extravert practically oriented patients may respond better to a directive style, while the reverse is true for introverted people (Beutler *et al.*, 2002a).

3. *Strategic change.* For therapy to be successful, SEP states that intermediate goals (e.g., fostering the working alliance, identification of patterns in behavior, thoughts, feelings, and interpersonal relationships, change efforts, and termination) need to lead to structural change in the patient's psyche and that these in turn need to be reflected in changes in behavior and relationships.

Case example of an eclectic treatment

Mr A, a 48-year-old married man asked for help ostensibly in order to 'work through some issues from the past'. In fact he had been feeling depressed for at least a year, and was unhappy in his 25-year-old marriage. He stated that he felt angry with, and controlled by, his wife, and seriously was considering leaving her.

He was an only child, brought up by a single mother, who married when he was 10 to a stepfather who had no time for Mr A. At 16 he left home to join the armed services. He felt that he had been dominated by his mother and always had to do her bidding, and the same pattern repeated itself in his marriage. When, several years previously, his wife had an affair he decided he would do anything to keep her, and took responsibility for what happened on the grounds that he had been neglecting her.

The assessment interview focused on his chronically low self-esteem, difficulty in asserting himself, anxious attachment to the insecure base of his mother and then his wife, and unresolved oedipal conflicts around separation from the mother figure in the absence of a 'good enough father' with whom to identify.

The early sessions of therapy included systemic therapy techniques in the form of role-play, in which Mr A rehearsed what he would like to say to his wife. His compliance and dependency were evident in that it was clear that he was asking her permission to leave, even though he was well aware she wanted the marriage to survive. Using a cognitive therapy technique he was asked as homework to list on paper the pros and cons of asking his wife's permission for something basically unpalatable to her.

The therapist also felt that Mr A was unhappy with role-play, but went along with it in a compliant slightly sulky fashion, reminiscent of his attitude to those in authority.

This countertransference response—a psychoanalytic concept—was then used to illustrate Mr A's hostile dependency, a theme that he worked on in subsequent sessions.

Therapy was eclectic in the sense that techniques from three distinct therapeutic techniques were combined in order to produce an appropriate 'tailor-made' therapy for this patient. He needed help in his immediate marital crisis (systemic); he needed to understand the dynamics underlying his long-term relationship difficulties (psychoanalytic); and he needed the structure provided by a homework assignment (CBT). These approaches were synergistic in the sense that dynamic themes manifested themselves in the way in which Mr A responded to the systemic and cognitive-behavioral interventions.

Theoretical integration

Colijn (1995) uses a culinary metaphor to explain the difference between eclecticism and integrationism: eclectic therapists assemble a meal by putting together different dishes on one plate, whereas integrationists will create a new dish, based on several ingredients (p. 436). Thus theoretic integration draws on apparently antithetical existing theories, but synthesizes them to produces a new structure with its own theoretical basis. Examples of this are Ryle's CAT (Ryle, 1990), Wachtel's integration of psychoanalytical and behavioral treatment in the 'Cyclical Psychodynamic' model (Wachtel, 1997), and the transtheoretical model of Prochaska (e.g., Prochaska and DiClemente, 1992; Prochaska and Norcross, 2002).

Example of an integrative treatment model: cognitive analytic therapy

Ryle (1990) decided to bring together the best of cognitive-behavior and psychoanalytic practice into a well-structured time-limited therapy applicable for work in third-party funded settings. Key features of CAT include:

1. The use of the 'psychotherapy file', a pen and paper form filled in by the patient, which aims to identify 'snags, traps, and dilemmas' that have led to the need for help. For example, a dilemma relevant to Mr A above might encapsulate dysfunctional dichotomous thinking such as 'either I am submissive, stay close to those that matter to me, but must bend to their will, or I assert myself but run the risk of antagonizing those I love and ending up alone'.

2. An initial four-session assessment phase at the end of which a written and diagrammatic formulation is arrived at collaboratively between patient and therapist. This 'sequential diagrammatic formulation', unique to CAT, is based on the idea that neurotic procedures are often self-sustaining. For example, someone whose core belief is that they are unlovable will shy away from close involvement with others and thus reinforce his view that no one cares about him. The importance of the CAT diagram is that it shows the patient in 'black and white' what they are up to, and also how their own attitudes contribute to the problem that hitherto has been attributed either to a hostile world or to malevolent fate.

3. Homework assignments between sessions, with analogue scales agreed between therapist and patient to monitor progress.

4. A nondirective atmosphere in the sessions in which the therapist responds to whatever material the patient brings.

5. The use of transference and countertransference to identify 'reciprocal role relationships'—i.e., an attachment/object-relations model in which the patient occupies one of a limited range of relational strategies such as victim/abuser, placator/bully, isolate/clinger. Mr A might well describe have described himself as assuming a placatory/secretly resentful role. Therapy then tries to help extend the range of possibilities, in CAT terminology called 'exits', in Mr A's case to find ways to be assertive but not enraged.

6. A strong emphasis on working through termination, after 16 or 24 sessions, culminating in a collaborative 'good-bye' letter summarizing the course of therapy, its achievements and work for the future.

Thus CAT brings together elements from CBT (1, 2, 3 above) and psychoanalysis (4, 5), but also adds its own theoretical and practical stamp. The shared formulation and goodbye letters are unique to CAT, as are the notion of reciprocal role procedures, and a psycholinguistic emphasis on the 'interpersonal gesture' and finding a language to name it.

The discussion of CAT raises the question of at what point a therapy ceases to be 'integrative' and becomes a 'monotherapy' in its own right. A comparable case might be that of dialectical behavior therapy (DBT, q.v.), designed originally to reduce self-harming borderline personality disorder. DBT uses ideas derived from behavior therapy, CBT, and Zen Buddhism, but is in fact a highly prescribed set of therapeutic procedures specific to itself.

Case example of an integrative treatment based on the cyclical psychodynamic model (Wachtel and Seckinger, 2001)

The model of cyclical psychodynamics (Wachtel, 1997) was originally conceptualized as a way to bring together cognitive-behaviorist and psychoanalytical points of view, but was later extended to incorporate systemic, and even social and cultural dimensions. The model focuses on the vicious circles originating in early childhood experiences, and investigates the ways in which these patterns are reinforced in actual daily life.

Mr J came into therapy with a presenting problem of a pigeon phobia. Because pigeons are ubiquitous in New York, almost every dimension of Mr J's social and professional life was affected by his phobia. Avoiding pigeons was almost a full-time occupation. As a consequence of his phobia, Mr J was severely limited in both his social and occupational activities. He was not completely socially isolated, but he had a ready-made excuse whenever he felt the slightest bit anxious about socializing. The limitations and restrictions in his life could thereby be experienced by him not as a product of deeper anxieties, which he was initially quite hesitant to approach, but as an unfortunate side-effect of his pigeon phobia.

In exploring the origins of Mr J's pigeon phobia, Mr J's earliest relevant memory was not directly about pigeons but about a parakeet, a friend's pet that had bitten him when he was about 9 years of age. The event was not experienced as significant at the time (it was just a minor nip), but about 6 months later Mr J began to show signs of anxiety around birds in general, which before long became a terror specifically of pigeons. The momentous occurrence that intervened during those 6 months was Mr J's mother's becoming seriously ill with a progressive degenerative disease. Her illness, which led to her being in and out of hospitals for the next 20 years, was devastating for the family, but although its impact was vividly palpable, Mr J's parents decided it would be best not to tell him about it. When she was home and bedridden, and very obviously severely weakened, they would say things such as that she had a very bad cold or a flu. When she was hospitalized, they would give some minimizing explanation, and convey that she would be home in just a few days, which rarely came to pass.

The therapist's understanding of Mr J's phobia, which was communicated to Mr J, was that in large measure it was a way, in the course of his growing up, of his being able to convey to his parents how frightened he was. The atmosphere in the home was such that there was no space for him to convey *what* he was anxious about (that was a taboo topic) but via the phobia he could at least convey that he *was* anxious. The nip by the parakeet thus provided a language for his fear; as the memory of it resonated, it became the foundation for a psychological structure that served to provide some way of addressing his terror in the face of the family prohibition on discussing the mother's illness.

In approaching Mr J's phobia, the therapist assumed that helping to understand its meaning would be useful to him. The explorations that led to the understanding were of value in a number of ways. They provided a model of open and mutual engagement with a problem that was in sharp contrast with Mr J's experience growing up; they helped him to *make sense* of his experience and, simply by virtue of that, to feel somewhat more in control of his life; they also provided an opening and a rationale for addressing the larger set of issues that had become entwined with Mr J's phobia. Mr J manifested a pervasively avoidant way of living that was aided and justified *by* the phobia. The fantasy of 'I would if only I could' of the phobia as *the* explanation for his social and occupational avoidance, was an important target for therapeutic work, which needed to be addressed first before moving on to Mr J's social and occupational anxieties.

Nonetheless, and consistent with much evidence, the best way to help him get over the phobia *per se* was straightforward systematic desensitization. Hierarchies were created along dimensions such as the number of pigeons Mr J encountered and how far from the pigeon or pigeons Mr J was, and a desensitization procedure based on the hierarchy was applied. Mr J made significant progress with a combination of imaginal and *in vivo* desensitization, but the nature of his resistance was quite interesting. For more insight-oriented therapists, the use of methods such as systematic desensitization is often seen as compromising or impeding the process of exploration. In Mr J's case, however, much of the resistance was in the opposite direction, Mr J using wanting to talk and explore as a means of avoiding the systematic desensitization. Thus, the systematic desensitization, as a path to overcoming the phobia, threatened the rest of the defensive psychological structures that had evolved *around* the phobia.

As the work proceeded, systematic desensitization and work on Mr J's social skills were intertwined with more insight-oriented work that examined the anxieties, inhibitions, and conflicted anger and identifications in relation to his parents.

The systematic desensitization, far from being mechanical and manualized, was often a source of new associations and directions for exploration. The psychodynamic exploration, far from being neutral or focused exclusively on the 'inner world' or 'psychic reality', was engaged throughout with the choices Mr J was making in his life and the realities he confronted as a result of still earlier choices and their consequences. The cyclical psychodynamic vantage point aimed to free Mr J from the specific symptoms that constituted his presenting complaint and, to the degree that he embraced such an aim, to help him expand the possibilities that life offered him by fostering the kind of insight psychodynamic working through can provide.

Common factors

The third approach is the *common factors approach*, which aims at utilizing and combining aspects that are common to all psychotherapies. Therapeutic warmth would be one such example (described by Gabbard and Westen, 2003, as a 'facilitative factor'). This approach is advocated by, among others, Beitman (1987, 1992), Frank and Frank (1991), Arkowitz (1992), and Garfield (1995). Colijn's (1995) culinary metaphor would imply here that meals have to be served hot.

Example of a common factors treatment model: Arkowitz' common factors therapy for depression

The common factors therapy for depression developed by Arkowitz (1992) is based on the view that efficacy studies fail to show differential effectiveness of different therapies. Moreover, it is often shown that attention-placebo controls are effective in their own right. Because depression is associated with low social support, the therapeutic relationship with all its supportive elements can be very important for patients. Arkowitz's idea was to develop a systematic—as opposed to the unsystematic attention-placebo treatments—psychotherapeutic treatment based on common factors. He based this treatment on Frank's ideas about helping relationships. The most important elements for a common factor treatment are:

1. A warm and positive relationship.
2. The application of procedures believed to be effective (e.g., support, encouragement, acceptance, opportunity for emotional expression).
3. A plausible explanation of symptoms, and a treatment rationale connecting the therapeutic procedures alleviating these symptoms.
4. Inducing positive expectations of the treatment.

Arkowitz articulated guidelines based on existing treatment manuals, and on Rogers' work (the necessary and sufficient conditions of change, i.e., empathy, genuineness, and unconditional positive regard, cf. 'Empathy, positive regard, and congruence' section). Other therapist behaviors include encouraging affective expression, providing empathic reflections of thoughts and feelings, and providing realistic support and encouragement.

Arkowitz' guidelines can be viewed as a common factors treatment because the therapist is explicitly advised *not* to engage in specific interventions derived from specific theories, e.g., interpretations, active attempts to correct negative and distorted thinking, a persistent focus on interpersonal conflict, or specific behavioral instructions or assignments.

The common factors approach delineated by Arkowitz is reminiscent of the general model of supportive therapy (cf. 'Common factors in practice: supportive psychotherapy' section, see below) but differs in that it is specifically designed for milder depression and explicitly eschews designating itself as a modality—even as a 'nonmodal modality'!

Common factors in practice: supportive psychotherapy

Supportive psychotherapy (ST) is nevertheless perhaps best seen as the day-to-day clinical manifestation of the common factors approach described above. ST is paradoxical in that it is widely practiced by mental health professionals, and yet is the least theorized, recognized, regulated, or researched. It is provided to clients by psychiatric nurses, psychiatrists, counselors, social workers, general practitioners (family physicians), and clinical psychologists, often in combination with pharmacotherapy and social interventions.

Rockland (1989) and Van Marle and Holmes (2002) provide accounts of the theoretical, research, and clinical aspects of ST—minimal though they are compared with other modalities. The aims of ST are to enhance coping; to maximize strengths; and to maintain the positive aspects of the status quo, including preventing deterioration, especially in the case of clients with major mental illnesses. Regression in the service of personality restructuring is discouraged. Dependency on the therapist is assumed, but kept within manageable bounds by titrating a 'minimal necessary intervention' (i.e., contact frequency) against clinical need.

Therapists accept that they may need to act as an 'auxiliary ego' for the patient, and to facilitate major life decisions in the areas of housing, employment, marriage, and the use of medication. There is always an attempt to bolster and buttress the patient's ego strengths, and to counter-act tendencies to self-destructiveness.

The development of transference, especially negative and regressive transference, is discouraged by the relative nonopacity of therapists who, within limits, will allow themselves to be more 'real' than in traditional psychoanalytic approaches. This might entail making 'joining' remarks, offering limited self-revelation, and occupying a more definite professional role as a doctor or psychologist, rather than cultivating psychoanalytic neutrality. Equally, a CBT therapist working in ST would put much less pressure on the client to complete homework tasks, or carry out challenging psychological 'experiments' to test their assumptions as compared with their formal CBT practice.

The indications for ST include any psychiatric illness where the ego is felt to be too fragile for exploratory or regressive therapy. Thus patients with psychotic illnesses, severe personality disorders or somatization disorders may all be candidates for ST, often after a period of more formal therapy has been tried and failed. Equally, as the patient matures, ST can be a precursor to more intensive monotherapy.

Case example of a supportive psychotherapy after 'failed' psychoanalytic therapy

Mrs B, a married high school teacher in her 30s, suffered from major depressive disorder and borderline personality disorder and was referred for psychoanalytic psychotherapy. She had had a very disturbed period in her 20s, spending 2 years in an inpatient psychiatric unit. Her arms were a mass of self-inflicted scars. Her capacity to cope with her daily life of work and looking after her small son were severely compromised and she spent most of her weekends in bed, recovering from the week and being waited on hand and foot by her dutiful and desperate husband.

Initially she embarked willingly on therapy but soon became increasingly suspicious and paranoid in the traditional psychoanalytic context. She did not like lying down on the couch, and felt that her therapist was laughing at her. She wondered if the smoke alarms were in fact secret microphones spying on her. She found the therapist's silence at the start of sessions unbearable, and his attempts to link current difficulties with her bleak and highly 'unsupportive' childhood (her mother ill with depression and her father sexually abusive of her) far-fetched and absurd.

Therapy increasingly approached an 'impasse' and things came to a head when Mrs B had to be readmitted to hospital as her depressive features worsened and she became suicidal.

At this point the therapist decided to switch to ST. Mrs B's sessions were reduced from thrice to once weekly, she sat up face-to-face, he initiated the sessions by asking her each time 'how are things going', and was generally smiley and supportive, using warmth and humor as much as was possible. He helped her identify her strengths and construed as 'heroic' (without irony) her capacity to negotiate her job, motherhood, and a marriage given her major mental illness. The first few minutes of the session were often spent discussing neutral topics such as the book she happened to be reading,

holiday plans, or films she had seen. The therapist made practical suggestions when she brought problems concerning the upbringing of her son.

Therapy continued for the next 10 years during which time she left her unsatisfactory marriage, made a much better match, looked after her son effectively, found a less demanding part-time job, and had no further hospital admissions. The frequency of sessions gradually reduced from weekly, to fortnightly to monthly to bi-monthly.

Conceptualizations of common factors

Several conceptualizations of common factors are in existence (e.g., Karasu, 1986; Grencavage and Norcross, 1990; Lambert and Bergin, 1994; Lambert and Ogles, 2004; Trijsburg *et al.*, in press). These are based on theoretical considerations (Karasu, 1986), study of the literature (Grencavage and Norcross, 1990), empirical findings (Lambert and Bergin, 1994; Lambert and Barley, 2002; Lambert and Ogles, 2004), and on surveys (Trijsburg *et al.*, in press).

Karasu

Karasu's (1986) system is based on three concepts: affect induction, cognitive control, and behavioral regulation.

Affect induction

This is viewed by Karasu as the primary instrument of primitive healing procedures. To this end, séances are held, often in groups led by healers, and with the aid of rhythmic music, chanting, dance, the use of intoxicating or hallucinatory drugs and exhaustion (e.g., lack of sleep). This results in trancelike states, accompanied by diminished resistance and heightened sensitivity to suggestions. By using suggestion, evil forces, demons, and spirit possession, held to lie at the root of the individual's sufferings, will be mastered or exorcized. The sufferer will be reconciled with life and his or her own situation.

Affect induction, Karasu claims, has found its way into official psychotherapy, e.g., in flooding and implosion (behavioral techniques) or as a catharsis (in the early days of psychoanalysis) and in so-called 'chairwork' (Gestalt, experiential therapy). However, most applications of affect induction can be found in the periphery of official psychotherapy, e.g., in bioenergetics, primal scream, and Morita therapy. Karasu argues that without working through, affect induction in itself does not lead to permanent psychological change. Nevertheless many treatment modalities use more subtle forms of affect induction, based on the assumption that affective experiences during treatment are superior in their effects than purely intellectual or cognitive experiences (Elliott *et al.*, 2004).

Cognitive control

This is used by more sophisticated therapies to render more permanent the transient changes conjured up by affect induction in primitive healing. Cognitive explanations and beliefs in primitive healing are based on irrational convictions. Moreover, the context is one of a highly charged and unexamined dependent relationship (Ehrenwald, 1966). According to Karasu, cognitive control is integral to any psychotherapeutic modality, implying the acquisition of new perceptions and patterns of thinking, leading to growing self-consciousness and understanding.

Behavioral regulation

This is self-evidently the trademark of behavior therapy. But learning to act differently is also implicit in nonbehavioral treatment modalities, e.g., psychoanalysis and client-centered psychotherapy. 'Insight' without behavioral change is considered by psychoanalysts to be a sign of intellectual rather than emotional understanding. Behavior therapists induce behavioral change by direction, suggestion, and advice. In contrast, psychoanalysts and client-centered therapists refrain from engaging in such direct methods, but would challenge patients where there appear to be difficulty in generalizing from insights gained in therapy into everyday life.

Grencavage and Norcross

Grencavage and Norcross (1990) collected publications concerned with common factors and counted the number of times each factor was named. Through this procedure they delineated five categories of common factors: patient characteristics, therapist characteristics, change processes, structure of the treatment, and the therapeutic relationship (see Table 10.1).

There is general agreement in the literature about the relevance of these five overarching topics, although most schools, competing in the psychotherapeutic market-place, stress their supposedly unique techniques for achieving change. According to Grencavage and Norcross, the relationship forms the bedrock of therapeutic change. They subdivide the elements contributing to the relationship into several components: client characteristics (e.g., positive expectation and hope or faith), therapist qualities (e.g., warmth, empathic understanding, and acceptance), treatment structure (e.g., a healing setting and communication), and relationship elements (e.g., development of working alliance and engagement). The research literature (q.v. Chapter 38 Psychotherapy Research, this volume) consistently shows that the therapeutic relationship is a crucial determinant of good outcomes in therapy. Apart from this, most authors agree on the importance of a degree of abreaction, the acquisition and practicing of new behaviors, and the offering of a treatment rationale.

Lambert and Bergin

Lambert and Bergin divide common factors into support, learning, and action factors. Theirs is a phasic model, in which support precedes changes in belief system and attitudes, which in their turn lead on to behavioral changes. Table 10.2 summarizes what they see as the relevant components of effective psychotherapy.

Lambert and Barley (2002) summarized the findings, based on more than 100 studies, underpinning the explanatory model of improvement in psychotherapy as a function of therapeutic factors (Lambert and Bergin, 1994). Extratherapeutic factors (e.g., diagnostic variables and the availability of social support) explain 40% of improvement, specific therapeutic techniques 15%, expectancy (placebo) 15%, and common factors, 30%. The latter group (also called 'relationship factors'), consists of therapist variables (e.g., interpersonal style, personal attributes), facilitating conditions (e.g., empathy, warmth, and positive regard), and the therapeutic relationship (e.g., working alliance). These relationship (or common) factors largely resemble the support factors summarized in Table 10.2, and appear to predict a larger proportion of outcome variance than specific factors (summarized in Table 10.2 as learning and action factors).

Trijsburg et al.

Another approach to common factor research derives from a field survey of Dutch psychotherapists (Trijsburg et al., in press). In this study, 1142 psychotherapists of different psychotherapy orientations rated 72 interventions from the Comprehensive Psychotherapeutic Interventions Rating Scale. Factor analysis revealed specific and common factors. The specific factors were: behavioral, cognitive, experiential, psychoanalytic, psychodynamic, strategic interventions, and 'chair work' (i.e., 'gestalt-humanistic'). The common factors were: facilitating, authoritative support, coaching, directive process, and structuring interventions (see Table 10.3).

Besides the facilitating factor, already established in the literature, authoritative support, coaching, directive process, and structuring interventions were more unexpected findings of this study. They are transmodal and in part confirm the lists produced by Karasu, Grencavage and Norcross, and Lambert and Bergin. This study shows that specific interventions themselves, traditionally associated with specific therapeutic approaches, are in fact common to several schools, thereby underlining the view that the combination between specific and common factors are both essential for therapeutic change.

Table 10.1 Common factors, mentioned in 50 publications (1936–89)

Client characteristics—6%	*Therapist qualities—21%*
Positive expectation/hope or faith	General positive descriptors
Distressed or incongruent client	Cultivates hope/enhances expectancies
Patient actively seeks help	Warmth/positive regard
Change processes—41%	Empathic understanding
Opportunity for catharsis/ventilation	Socially sanctioned healer
Acquisition and practice of new	Aceptance
behaviors	
Provision of rationale	*Treatment structure—17%*
Foster insight/awareness	Use of techniques/rituals
Emotional and interpersonal learning	Focus on 'inner world'/exploration of
Feedback/reality testing	emotional issues
Suggestion	Adherence to theory
Success and mastery experiences	A healing setting
Persuasion	There are participants/an interaction
Placebo effect	Communication (verbal and nonverbal)
Identification with the therapist	Explanation of therapy and
Contingency management	participants' roles
Tension reduction	*Relationship elements—15%*
Therapist modeling	Development of alliance/relationship
Desensitization	(general)
Education/information provision	Engagement
	Transference

From Grencavage, L. M. and Norcross, J. C. (1990).

Table 10.2 Sequential listing of factors common across therapies that are associated with positive outcomes

Support factors	Learning factors	Action factors
Catharsis	Advice	Behavioral regulation
Identification with therapist	Affective experiencing	Cognitive mastery
Mitigation of isolation	Assimilation of problematic experiences	Encouragement of facing fears
Positive relationship	Changing expectations for personal effectiveness	Taking risks
Reassurance	Cognitive learning	Mastery efforts
Release of tension	Corrective emotional experience	Modeling
Structure	Exploration of internal frame of reference	Practice
Therapeutic alliance	Feedback	Reality testing
Therapist/client active participation	Insight	Success experience
Therapist expertness	Rationale	Working through
Therapist warmth, respect, empathy, acceptance, genuineness		
Trust		

From Lambert, M. J. and Bergin, A. E. (1994, p. 163).

Some common factors and their effectiveness

Therapist attitudes and behaviors

Empathy, positive regard, and congruence

Empathy, positive regard, and congruence were formulated by Rogers (1951) as the necessary and sufficient conditions of therapeutic change.

Table 10.3 Common factors according to the Confirmatory Factor Analysis of items of the Comprehensive Psychotherapeutic Interventions Rating Scale

Facilitating	Authoritative support	Coaching	Directive process	Structuring
Empathy	Collaboration	Supportive encouragement	Self-disclosure	Setting and following the agenda
Acceptance	Direct reassurance	Therapist as expert	Exploration of activities	Assign homework
Involvement	Responsibility outside patient	Therapy rationale	Explain direction in session	Review homework
Warmth	Reformulation of problem	Explicit guidance	Summarizing	Scheduling and structuring activities
Rapport		Active control Advice and guidance Didactic approach	Challenging	Self-monitoring

From Trijsburg et al., in press.

Although referring to a basic attitude toward patients, these three conditions can be translated into concrete therapist behaviors, which then can be measured and correlated with outcome.

Empathy may be defined as 'understanding the client's frame of reference and way of experiencing the world' (Bohart *et al.*, 2002, p. 89). The construct is multifaceted and complex. It comprises attitudinal and behavioral, as well as cognitive and affective elements. Empathy operates in the dialogue between the therapist and the patient, and influences both of them. Empathy can be expressed in many ways, e.g., restating what the patient has said in different words, thus adding meaning or depth, or asking questions. The nonverbal aspects of communicating empathy, it's timing and wording, are highly important. In order to be effective, empathic understanding needs to be accurate and sensitive in confirming the experiences and feelings of the patient. Perhaps due to the multifaceted character of the construct, many different measures of empathy have been developed, e.g., observer-, client- and therapist-rated instruments, global measures as well measures that tap empathy on a moment-to-moment basis.

A meta-analysis of the effects of empathy on the outcome of treatment (Bohart *et al.*, 2002) based on 47 studies and 190 separate tests of the empathy-outcome association in 3026 clients, yielded a weighted effect size of $r = 0.32$. This is a medium effect but which surpasses the effect sizes from studies of working alliance. Interestingly, empathy was at least as, and maybe somewhat more, effective in cognitive-behavioral therapies than in experiential, psychodynamic and other therapies. The authors suggest, somewhat paradoxically, that empathy may be more important in directive treatments, thus providing 'an effective ground for intervention' (p. 96).

Rogers's concept of *positive regard* is also complex and multifaceted. Its meaning is conveyed through many similar terms, e.g., affirmation, respect, acceptance (nonpossessive) warmth, support, caring, and prizing (Farber and Lane, 2002). In their 2004 research summary, Orlinsky *et al.* (2004) grouped positive regard under the heading of 'therapist affirmation versus negation', defined as 'personal rapport in a relationship . . . manifested in the feelings that persons have towards one another (e.g., liking, warmth, trust vs. wariness, aloofness, resentment)' (p. 353). In their 1994 review Orlinsky *et al.* concluded that therapist affirmation is positively correlated with outcome in 56% of process-outcome correlations (41% not significant, 3% negative). In the 2004 review Orlinsky *et al.* (2004) concluded that therapist affirmation is positively correlated with outcome in 56% of process-outcome correlations (41% nonsignificant, 3% negative). In the 2004 review they reported on 12 addition al studies and concluded that 'a clear majority of findings showed affirmative therapist behaviour related to positive outcome'.

Congruence involves 'both a self-awareness on the part of the therapist, and a willingness to share this awareness' (Klein *et al.*, 2002). Related concepts are openness, self-congruence, genuineness, and transparency. Again, this is a complex concept, involving, maybe more so than with empathy and positive regard, the quality of the relationship between therapist and patient. The empirical evidence on the association between congruence and

outcome can be evaluated as mixed (Orlinsky *et al.*, 1994, 2004; Klein *et al.*, 2002). Klein *et al.* (2002) reported 34%, and Orlinsky *et al.* (1994) 38% positive results. As Orlinsky *et al.* (1994) found five studies published in the 1980s, and three in the period 1993–2001, there seems clearly to be a diminished interest in research on congruence in relation to outcome. Nevertheless, Klein *et al.* (2002) concluded that congruence, perhaps in interaction with empathy and positive regard, is likely to exert a positive influence on outcome.

Self-disclosure

Historically, self-disclosure has been viewed as an aspect of genuineness or transparency in client-centered therapy, defined as the functional use of personal information (Carkhuff, 1969). This definition implies that self-disclosures relate to verbal expressions and not to nonverbal behavior or personal characteristics of therapists (Hill and Knox, 2002). Clearly there is an important distinction between gratuitous personal revelations on the part of the therapist ('I found myself getting depressed too, after my mother died last year'), and self-disclosure that aims to illustrate that the therapist has a 'thinking mind' and a specific point of view ('what you said just now made me feel quite sad, and made me think how easily we tend to underestimate the impact of bereavement in our lives').

Although self-disclosure is usually associated with client-centered therapy, current developments in psychoanalytic psychotherapy and CBT, suggest that the judicious and thoughtful use of self-disclosures may help in furthering the responsiveness of patients and in strengthening the therapeutic alliance, thereby leading to more effective treatments. For instance, some contemporary psychoanalysts acknowledge the current trend towards more therapist disclosure (Ehrenberg, 1995; Renik, 1995; Bernstein, 1999). Although Wolpe (1984) stated that therapist disclosure is not a behavior therapy technique, the possibility of a 'dyadic effect', meaning that therapist disclosure has the potential to encourage client disclosure, is acknowledged in behavior therapy (Pope, 1979). The dyadic effect can be explained by modeling (Bandura, 1970) and by social exchange theory. Other indications for self-disclosure in behavior therapy include applying modeling and behavioral rehearsal (Lazarus, 1985), or when the patient shows behavior toward the therapist resembling maladaptive behaviors toward other people (O'Leary and Wilson, 1975).

Hill and Knox (2002) offer several practice guidelines, related to intrapersonal self-disclosures, summarized below:

- therapists should generally disclose infrequently;

- the most appropriate topic involves professional background, and the least appropriate include sexual practices and beliefs;

- disclosures should be used to validate reality, normalize, model, strengthen the alliance, or offer alternative ways to think and act;

- therapists should avoid using disclosures that are for their own needs, remove the focus from the patient, or otherwise interfere with the therapeutic process or the therapeutic relationship.

Working with resistance

Resistance, originally a psychoanalytic concept is defined in at least three ways in the literature: as a patient characteristic, as a response to accurate but unpalatable interventions applied by the therapist, or as a characteristic of the therapeutic relationship.

Resistance is a core element in psychoanalytic theory, and is inherent to the 'basic rule' of free association, which is designed to overcome it. Traditionally, the psychoanalytic model views resistance as being located at the level of the patient. However, newer models hold that resistance may be viewed as relationally determined (Trijsburg, 2003).

Treatment modalities that view resistance as being avoidable, rather than intrinsic to the therapeutic process, tend to apply specific strategies to improve compliance. Examples include structuring the treatment, stressing the gradualness of change (including setbacks), and structuring homework (Goldfried, 1982). However, noncompliance may also be thought as manifesting the problem behavior that brought the patient to therapy in the first place. Behavior therapy and CBT have developed specific techniques for conceptualizing and overcoming resistance. The following aspects of resistance can be distinguished (Goldfried, 1982): (1) resistance as a manifestation of patient's problems; (2) resistance resulting from other problems than the one treated; (3) resistance due to pessimism in the patient; (4) resistance arising from fear of changing; (5) resistance due to overburdening the patient; (6) resistance resulting from the patient not being motivated to change (defined by Jacobson and Margolin, 1979, in terms of costs–benefits: as long as benefits lag behind costs in terms of work to be done, there will be obstacles in the way of change, i.e., resistance); (7) reactance, i.e., an emotional response to demands.

The concept of (interpersonal) reactance, colloquially 'contrariness', deserves special mention. This concept derives from empirical research on persuasion theory and models of interpersonal influence (Brehm and Brehm, 1981) and refers to the tendency to respond in an oppositional manner if someone feels thwarted in his or her autonomy. Directive interventions in reactant patients increases the risk of treatment failure. When confronted by such situations, interventions low in directiveness and paradoxical interventions may result in better effects.

Treatment techniques developed for the situations described above are *switching the focus* of treatment from the therapeutic work outside of therapy to therapy itself; *changing the treatment goals*; *reformulation of the problem*, often in more positive terms, enabling the patient to get a different view of the problem (e.g., when resistance results from anticipatory anxiety, the therapist may normalize anxiety, may stress the importance of anxiety as a signal of change, or as a challenge to experiment with the feeling), *ambiguous assignment*; and *paradoxical interventions*.

Ambiguous assignments are those that are given ultratentatively, suggesting that the assignment may or may not prove to be effective, relevant, or sensible, or may be too difficult for the patient (e.g., formulated as a rhetorical question 'I'm thinking of this assignment, which may be quite helpful to address this problem. However, I'm wondering if this assignment is not too difficult for you? If you're interested, I can tell you how it goes. You want to hear about it?'). Also, the therapist confesses that the assignment may well be ill timed, the patient may not have enough time to follow the assignment up, etc. In this way, the patient has a chance to escape, without having failed the assignment. The hope is that he may become interested and still perform the task, thereby gaining positive feedback from accomplishment.

Paradoxical interventions often take the form of apparently unfitting interventions related to symptomatic behavior (e.g., 'prescribing the symptom', e.g., to an agoraphobic 'I think it is important that you go continue not to venture outside, not even for a second'), cognitions (e.g., the instruction make an anticipated catastrophe worse by exaggerating it in one's mind), or to relational behaviors (e.g., the task of having an argument with one's spouse at a predetermined point in time). In the Trijsburg *et al.* (in press) study, paradoxical interventions and the ambiguous task assignment clustered in the 'strategic interventions' factor.

Other interventions, found in the Trijsburg *et al.* (in press) study to belong to a factor of 'authoritative support', may also be useful when therapy reaches an 'impasse' (a psychoanalytic concept, q.v.), e.g., *direct reassurance*, *placing the responsibility for a problem outside the patient*, and *collaboration*.

Relationship variables

Working alliance

Two currently important models of the working alliance concept, i.e., Luborsky's two-factor model (Luborsky, 1976) and Bordin's pantheoretical model (Bordin, 1976). Luborsky distinguishes 'Type I' and 'Type II' working alliance. Type I working alliance defines the therapist as warm, helping, and supporting. Type II relates to the cooperation between therapist and patient. Research suggests that Type I working alliance is more important in the opening phase of therapy, whereas the Type II will be dominant in the later phases of treatment (Horvath *et al.*, 1993).

In Bordin's (1976) view the central part of the working alliance is the active collaboration between patient and therapist. The working alliance involves three aspects, i.e., agreement on the therapeutic goals, agreement on the tasks to be done as the therapeutic work, and an emotional bond between the patient and the therapist.

Earlier studies showed the working alliance to be an important predictor of outcome, which is similar across various treatment modalities (Horvath and Symonds, 1991; Horvath and Greenberg, 1994; Martin *et al.*, 2000). Estimations of the effect size (ES), based on correlational analyses, vary between ES = 0.22 (Martin *et al.*, 2000), and ES = 0.26 (Horvath and Symonds, 1991). The study reported in Norcross (2002b), using partly overlapping data with earlier studies, resulted in an effect size of ES = 0.21 (weighted by sample size; Horvath and Bedi, 2002).

Horvath and Bedi (2002) suggest that the therapist's ability to maintain open and clear communication is related to the quality of the alliance. On the negative side, poor or deteriorating alliances are reported in therapists that take charge in the early phase of therapy, who are perceived by their clients as 'cold', or who offered insight or interpretation prematurely.

Repairing alliance ruptures

In all psychotherapeutic modalities, the working alliance is important, not as a goal in itself, but a means to an end, e.g., working through the transference neurosis, bringing about self-exploration, behavior change, or changes in a system. Where this goes wrong, therapy is in jeopardy. Alliance rupture and repair are therefore crucial to successful therapeutic work.

From a psychodynamic perspective, failure to repair minute-to-minute, or gross alliance ruptures, characterizes the unattuned care-giving characteristic of pre-borderline states. Via projective identification (q.v.) the therapist will characteristically be induced into such mis-attunements. Working with alliance ruptures in therapy help the patient to trust himself and his relationships with others, possibly for the first time in his or her life.

Over the past 10 years, Safran and Muran developed several techniques that may be helpful in overcoming ruptures in the therapeutic alliance. Their views were summarized in a 'relational treatment guide' (Safran and Muran, 2000). The authors distinguish between ruptures in the therapeutic process at the level of tasks and goals, and at the level of the therapeutic bond. They describe interventions that may help repairing these ruptures. The interventions are described in Table 10.4, and will be discussed in the following paragraphs.

Disagreements on tasks and goals

Disagreements on tasks and goals can be approached in direct and in indirect ways.

Direct approaches are: (1) explaining the therapeutic rationale; (2) microprocessing; and (3) exploring core relational themes. *Indirect* approaches to disagreements on tasks and goals are (4) reframing the meaning of tasks and goals, and (5) changing tasks and goals.

1. Explaining the therapeutic rationale. Disagreement on tasks and goals may result from (simple) misunderstandings or a lack of understanding in the patient. In case of a misunderstanding, the therapist may

Table 10.4 Therapeutic alliance rupture intervention strategies

	Direct	Indirect
Disagreements on tasks and goals	Therapeutic rationale and microprocessing tasks Exploring core relational themes	Reframing the meaning of tasks and goals Changing tasks and goals
Problems associated with the relational bond	Clarifying misunderstandings Exploring core relational themes	Allying with the resistance New relational experience

From Safran and Muran (2000, p. 17).

(once again) explain procedures or tasks, or clarify the reasons why a particular procedure is applied. One example would be to discuss the importance of monitoring behavior between sessions, or why particular exercises may be helpful to the patient. In psychodynamic treatments the therapist may explain the nature of free association, or the reasons why the therapist refrains from giving advice. Explanations are focused on the content and procedural aspects of treatments.

2. Microprocessing. Some patients may not have understood a question or explanation. This could be a simple misunderstanding, or due to unconscious resistance. At first, many patients react to the question 'could you tell me what's on your mind?' with something like, 'Nothing. What do you expect me to say?' Microprocessing techniques that may be helpful here could be exercises that may help patients understand the type of inner experiences that are important in therapeutic change (e.g., focusing, Gendlin, 1996, or the reconstruction of automatic thoughts). For example, when a patient was challenged about her apparent reluctance to talk about painful experiences as a child, she explained that she felt that she did not want to 'keep whining about things in the past', and was afraid her therapist would dislike her for this. She admitted that she always feared people thinking about her as being a whining and sulking person.

3. Exploring core relational themes. The tone of voice, nonverbal behavior, and the attitude of a patient may point to aversion, distrust, or skepticism and the collaboration in early phases of the treatment.

4. Reframing (an indirect approach to disagreements on tasks and goals) derives from the strategic (systemic) approach, and was described above as 'reformulation, often in more positive terms' (cf. 'Working with resistance' section). An example of this would be exposure to social situations in a social phobic patient. As exposure may induce feelings of anxiety and shame, the patient may react to an assignment of this kind with fear or aversion. Reformulation in terms of finding an opportunity to observe one's reactions (self-monitoring) in the situation, instead of just running the risk of being humiliated, may help the patient to accept the assignment.

5. Changing tasks and goals, another indirect approach, implies the empathic consideration of the therapist with respect to the problems patients may have with seemingly unfitting or too difficult tasks or goals (cf. 'Working with resistance' section). This could lead the patient to formulate more relevant goals and tasks. Also, the patient will then have the experience of being in charge, which in turn may also lead to increasing motivation to take on more difficult assignments later in the treatment.

Problems associated with the relational bond

Problems associated with the relational bond can be approached in direct and in indirect ways. *Direct* approaches are (1) clarifying misunderstandings, and (2) exploring core relationship themes. *Indirect* approaches are (3) going along with the resistance, and (4) new relationship experience.

1. Misunderstandings can be clarified in a *direct* way, if the therapist is able to be open about what may have caused the misunderstanding. Acknowledgement of one's own role in causing the misunderstanding

and explaining this to the patient are necessary for this clarification to be effective. Clarifications need to be given in the here-and-now, and need not lead to disclosure about personal problems in the therapist, nor need they have to lead to interpretations of possible inner conflicts of the patient. One example would be the patient that falls silent during a session, seems no longer interested or absent. The therapist may ask what happened, and this could lead the patient to hint at being hurt by something the therapist has said. Repairing the rupture would imply that the therapist recognizes what s/he could have contributed to the patient's feelings (e.g., 'I'm sorry if I said something that distressed you. What went through your mind when I said that?', or 'You know, I think I said that wrong. What I should have said is: 'I'm worried that the vacation might not turn out well for you').

2. Every rupture in the relational bond may eventually lead to the exploration of core relational themes. For instance, a therapist treating a stubborn, reticent, and sometimes unpleasant patient, sooner or later may feel tempted to 'forget' an appointment, or to say something out of place, which then of course will have rejecting implications (Horvath and Bedi, 2002). Focusing on these ruptures in the relational bond enables the therapist and patient to discuss the relational theme in terms of earlier experiences, to gain insight in these experiences, and to achieve therapeutic changes.

3. Allying with the resistance, an indirect approach, conceives of the negative attitude in the patient as his or her best answer in the situation. For example, the patient might say: 'I don't like talking about this. You always bring this up, and every time I know you are going to do this, and I don't want it. I want to stop this. I'm leaving'. Saying 'I think you find it difficult to talk about this' might merely exacerbate the rupture. Instead, the therapist could say something like 'You have made your point. It is obvious that you don't want to discuss this, and you have a perfect right to talk or not talk about whatever you like in your session'.

4. A second indirect approach is to attempt to create a new relational experience by the therapist's nonintrusive presence in the therapy, especially when things are very difficult. Here the nonintrusive presence of the therapist may be essential to prevent the working alliance from breaking down. Examples might be affect-storms, panic attacks, acute depersonalization, states of narcissistic injury, or persistent silence. In this type of situation, the therapist may stay in the background, acting as a '*holding environment*' (Winnicott, 1976).

Safran and Muran's (2000) view of rupture–repair clearly goes beyond 'schoolism'. Theirs is a truly integrative approach, in that they show that different theoretical views may each contribute in important ways to the maintenance of a good working alliance. For instance, self-disclosure and focusing derive from the client-centered approach, reframing from a strategic and systemic viewpoint, and exploring core relationship themes from the psychodynamic approach.

The number of studies of the effectiveness of repairing alliance ruptures is still limited. In their review, Safran *et al.* (2002, p. 251) concluded that there is preliminary evidence available that: (1) indicates that ruptures occur fairly frequently in psychotherapy; (2) supports the importance of specific procedures (e.g., nondefensive behavior of the therapist) in resolving ruptures; (3) indicates that for some patients, the development of an alliance characterized by rupture–repair cycles over the course of treatment, is associated with positive outcome; and (4) indicates that poor outcome is associated with disruptive patterns (therapists responding in a hostile way to hostile patients).

Integration in practice

Indications for integrative therapy

If integrative therapy (IT) is seen by its advocates as combining the best from all the traditional monotherapies then indications would be many, contraindications few. Also, given the lack of specificity of IT and the fact that it covers a range of different approaches including supportive therapy, eclectic therapy, aspects of the work of the mature monotherapy clinician, together with explicitly 'integrative' therapies such as interpersonal psychotherapy (combining psychodynamic, systemic, and supportive), DBT (CBT, behavioral therapy, and Zen), and CAT (analytic, DBT, and interpersonal) defining the indications is no easy task. The practice of IT is more likely to arise from adventitious conditions such as the habits and orientation of the therapist, the psychotherapeutic culture of a particular center and its often charismatic leaders, and the demands of those responsible for funding the therapy, rather than the specific needs of the client.

Nevertheless, indications might be considered as follows:

◆ when traditional monotherapies have failed

◆ where the presenting problem and its developmental background are uncertain, and a number of different approaches may be needed before it is clear which direction the client needs to go

◆ where the therapist lacks experience in monotherapies but has basic 'common factors' counseling skills

◆ where the patient is too disturbed for monotherapy and is more suitable the common factors approach embodied in ST

◆ where the client has a number of different problems which need to be tackled sequentially by the same therapist, e.g., agoraphobia (therapist uses CBT), marital difficulties (therapist performs couple therapy) and depression (therapist uses interpersonal psychotherapy) (although monotherapy enthusiasts would try to find the common theme behind all three, low self-esteem, or lack of assertiveness for instance, and address therapy to that).

In a stepped care approach it would be conceivable to start with an 'evidence-based' monotherapy, aimed at the central problem of the patient, and to add other therapeutic approaches only when the complexity (e.g., comorbidity, chronicity) of the patient's problems would demand such extensions. As indicated above, an integrative approach is especially suitable for more complex relationship-based treatments for character problems or personality disorders.

Contraindications and possible pitfalls of integrative therapy

The main contraindication arises from the fact that IT can become a 'defense' on the part of both therapist and client against recognizing the need for monotherapy. Thus a patient may 'offer' the therapist a number of disparate difficulties—e.g., difficulty in sustaining long-term relationships, uncertainty about choice of career, and bulimic symptoms. The integrative therapist might be tempted to take each of these in turn and 'work' on them, with varying degrees of success, rather than seeing all three as manifestations of a developmental disorder associated with disturbed care-giving in childhood, which would respond best to monotherapy, e.g., psychoanalytic, or 'schema-focused' CBT.

Offering IT in this circumstance would be a pitfall. This relates to the problem of 'model-hopping' in IT. Monotherapies have clearly developed theories and procedures for dealing with difficulty, encapsulated in such psychoanalytic concepts as impasse and working through. If the therapist changes tack every time the therapy meets resistance then conflicts will be skirted around and core problems left untouched.

A related problem concerns the ethical dimension of therapy. IT is perhaps inherently less clearly defined in its procedures and processes than monotherapies. Therapy that encourages warmth and empathy, and does not necessarily conceptualize countertransference or enactment, may lend itself to therapeutic abuse more easily than monotherapies (although we know of no specific empirical evidence to support this suggestion). The therapist who offers his female client a 'supportive' hug at the end of a session, or tells her how attractive she is in order to counteract her feelings of low self-esteem, or offers her sex therapy to help with her anorgasmia, in addition to psychoanalytic therapy and 'chair work', may have placed more than one foot on the 'slippery slope' that leads ultimately to the abuse of clients by therapists. Good supervision and reflective practice are an essential part of IT, as they are of all psychotherapeutic work.

Future developments

Psychotherapy integration is a tendency present both within the traditional psychotherapy schools, which incorporate therapeutic ideas and methods from other orientations, and in the dialogue between therapy schools, which ultimately will lead to new forms of therapy. This tendency is likely to continue to grow, as the focus on evidence-based treatments gradually shift from empirically supported diagnosis–treatment combinations, to evidence-based relationship and contextual factors. Also, the growing number of studies into the dose–effect relationship in psychotherapy, closely related to managed care policy making (Lambert and Ogles, 2004) are likely to stimulate psychotherapy integration, as cognitive therapies discover the need for more extended treatments, and psychoanalytic therapies the need for greater brevity. More and more, the 'pure-form' psychotherapy modalities will be stimulated to integrate relevant therapeutic practices from other schools as well as common factors. Whether this will lead to one common general theory of psychotherapy is a question for future theoreticians and researchers to determine, some of whom we hope may be readers of this volume.

References

Alford, B. and Beck, A. (1997). *The integrative power of cognitive therapy*. New York: Guilford Press.

Arkowitz, H. (1992). A common factors therapy for depression. In: J. C. Norcross, and M. R. Goldfried, ed. *Handbook of psychotherapy integration*, pp. 402–32. New York: Basic Books.

Bandura, A. (1970). *Principles of behavior modification*. New York: Holt, Rinehart and Winston.

Beitman, B. D. (1987). *The structure of individual psychotherapy*. New York: Guilford Press.

Beitman, B. D. (1992). Integration through fundamental similarities and useful differences among schools. In: J. C. Norcross and M. R. Goldfried, ed. *Handbook of psychotherapy integration*, pp. 202–31. New York: Basic Books.

Bernstein, J. W. (1999). The politics of self-disclosure. *Psychoanalytic Review*, **86**, 595–605.

Beutler, L. E. and Consoli, A. J. (1992). Systematic eclectic psychotherapy. In: J. C. Norcross and M. R. Goldfried, ed. *Handbook of psychotherapy integration*, pp. 264–99. New York: Basic Books.

Beutler, L. E. and Harwood, T. M. (2000). *Prescriptive psychotherapy: a practical guide to systematic treatment selection*. New York: Oxford University Press.

Beutler, L. E., Harwood, T. M., Alimohamed, S., and Malik, M. (2002a). Functional impairment and coping style. In: J. C. Norcross, ed. *Psychotherapy relationships that work. Therapist contributions and responsiveness to patients*, pp. 145–70. Oxford: Oxford University Press.

Beutler, L. E., Moleiro, C. M., and Talebi, H. (2002b). Resistance. In: J. C. Norcross, ed. *Psychotherapy relationships that work. Therapist contributions and responsiveness to patients*, pp. 129–43. Oxford: Oxford University Press.

Bohart, A. C., Elliott, R., Greenberg, L. S., and Watson, J. C. (2002). Empathy. In: J. C. Norcross, ed. *Psychotherapy relationships that work. Therapist contributions and responsiveness to patients*, pp. 89–108. Oxford: Oxford University Press.

Bordin, E. (1976). The generalizability of the psycho-analytic concept of the working alliance. *Psychotherapy: Theory, Research and Practice*, **16**, 252–60.

Brehm, S. S. and Brehm, J. W. (1981). *Psychological reactance: a theory of freedom and control*. New York: Academic Press.

Carkhuff, R. R. (1969). *Helping and human relations*. New York: Holt, Rinehart and Winston.

Chambless, D. L. and Hollon, S. D. (1998). Defining empirically supported therapies. *Journal of Consulting and Clinical Psychology*, **66**, 7–18.

Chambless, D. L., *et al.* (1996). An update on empirically validated therapies. *The Clinical Psychologist*, **49**, 5–18.

Chambless, D. L., *et al*. (1998). Update on empirically validated therapies, II. *The Clinical Psychologist*, **51**, 3–16.

Colijn, S. (1995). Van inquisitie naar oecumene. De integratief/eclectische trend in Nederland [From inquisition toward oecumene. The integrative/eclectic trend in the Netherlands]. *Tijdschrift voor Psychotherapie*, **21**, 433–8.

Ehrenberg, D. B. (1995). Self-disclosure: therapeutic tool or indulgence? *Contemporary Psychoanalysis*, **31**, 213–28.

Ehrenwald, J. (1966). *Psychotherapy: myth and method. An integrative approach*. New York: Grune and Stratton.

Elliott, R., Greenberg, L. S., and Lietaer, G. (2004). Research on experiential psychotherapies. In: M. J. Lambert, ed. *Bergin and Garfield's handbook of psychotherapy and behavior change*, 5th edn, pp. 493–539. New York: Wiley.

Farber, B. A. and Lane, J. S. (2002). Positive regard. In: J. C. Norcross, ed. *Psychotherapy relationships that work. Therapist contributions and responsiveness to patients*, pp. 175–94. Oxford: Oxford University Press.

Frank, J. D. and Frank, J. B. (1991). *Persuasion and healing; a comparative study of psychotherapy*, 3rd edn. Baltimore: The Johns Hopkins University Press.

Freud, S. (1910/1975). *The future prospects of psycho-analytic therapy*. In: *Standard edition of the complete psychological works of Sigmund Freud*, Vol. 11, pp. 139–51. London: Hogarth Press.

Gabbard, G. and Westen, D. (2003). Rethinking therapeutic action. *International Journal of Psychoanalysis*, **84**, 823–42.

Garfield, S. L. (1995). *Psychotherapy: an eclectic-integrative approach*, 2nd edn. New York: Wiley.

Gendlin, E. T. (1996). *Focusing-oriented psychotherapy: a manual of the experiential method*. New York: Guilford Press.

Goldfried, M. R. (1982). Resistance in clinical behavior therapy. In: P. L. Wachtel, ed. *Resistance. Psychodynamic and behavioral approaches*, pp. 95–113. New York: Plenum Press.

Grencavage, L. M. and Norcross, J. C. (1990). Where are the communalities among therapeutic common factors? *Professional Psychology: Research and Practice*, **21**, 372–8.

Hill, C. E. and Knox, S. (2002). Self-disclosure. In: J. C. Norcross, ed. *Psychotherapy relationships that work. Therapist contributions and responsiveness to patients*, pp. 255–65. Oxford: Oxford University Press.

Holmes, J. and Bateman, A. (2002). *Integration in psychotherapy. Models and methods*. Oxford: Oxford University Press.

Horvath, A. O. and Bedi, R. P. (2002). The alliance. In: J. C. Norcross, ed. *Psychotherapy relationships that work. Therapist contributions and responsiveness to patients*, pp. 37–69. Oxford: Oxford University Press.

Horvath, A. O. and Greenberg, L. S. (1994). *The working alliance: theory, research, and practice*. New York: Wiley.

Horvath, A. O. and Symonds, B. D. (1991). Relation between working alliance and outcome in psychotherapy: a meta-analysis. *Journal of Counseling Psychology*, **38**, 139–49.

Horvath, A. O., Gaston, L., and Luborsky, L. (1993). The therapeutic alliance and its measures. In: N. E. Miller, L. Luborsky, J. P. Barber, and J. P. Docherty, ed. *Psychodynamic treatment research. A handbook for clinical practice*, pp. 247–73. New York: Basic Books.

Jacobson, N. S. and Margolin, G. (1979). *Marital therapy. Strategies based on social learning and behavioral exchange principles*. New York: Brunner/Mazel.

Karasu, T. B. (1986). The specificity versus nonspecificity dilemma: toward identifying therapeutic change agents. *American Journal of Psychiatry*, **143**, 687–95.

Klein, M. H., Kolden, G. G., Michels, J. L., and Chisholm–Stockard, S. (2002). Congruence. In: J. C. Norcross, ed. *Psychotherapy relationships that work. Therapist contributions and responsiveness to patients*, pp. 195–215. Oxford: Oxford University Press.

Lambert, M. J. (1989). The individual therapist's contribution to psychotherapy process and outcome. *Clinical Psychology Review*, **9**, 469–85.

Lambert, M. J. (1992). Psychotherapy outcome research: implications for integrative and eclective psychotherapists. In: J. C. Norcross and M. R. Goldfried, ed. *Handbook of psychotherapy integration*, pp. 94–129. New York: Basic Books.

Lambert, M. J. and Barley, D. E. (2002). Research summary on the therapeutic relationship and psychotherapy outcome. In: J. C. Norcross, ed. *Psychotherapy relationships that work. Therapist contributions and responsiveness to patients*, pp. 17–32. Oxford: Oxford University Press.

Lambert, M. J. and Bergin, A. E. (1994). The effectiveness of psychotherapy. In: A. E. Bergin and S. L. Garfield, ed. *Handbook of psychotherapy and behavior change*, 4th edn, pp. 143–89. New York: Wiley.

Lambert, M. J. and Ogles, B. M. (2004). The efficacy and effectiveness of psychotherapy. In: M. J. Lambert, ed. *Bergin and Garfield's handbook of psychotherapy and behavior change*, 5th edn, pp. 139–93. New York: Wiley.

Lambert, M. J., Bergin, A. E., and Garfield, S. L. (2004). Introduction and historical overview. In: M. J. Lambert, ed. *Bergin and Garfield's handbook of psychotherapy and behavior change*, 5th edn, pp. 3–15. New York: Wiley.

Lazarus, A. A. (1976). *Multimodal behavior therapy*. New York: Springer.

Lazarus, A. A. (1985). Setting the record straight. *American Psychologist*, **40**, 1418–19.

Lazarus, A. A. (1989). *The practice of multimodal therapy. Systematic, comprehensive, and effective psychotherapy*. Baltimore: Johns Hopkins University Press.

Lazarus, A. A. (1992). Multimodal therapy: technical eclecticism with minimal integration. In: J. C. Norcross and M. R. Goldfried, ed. *Handbook of psychotherapy integration*, pp. 231–63. New York: Basic Books.

Lazarus, A. A. (1997). *Brief but comprehensive psychotherapy. The multimodal way*. New York: Springer.

Luborsky, L. (1976). Helping alliances in psychotherapy. In: J. L. Cleghorn, ed. *Successful psychotherapy*. New York: Brunner/Mazel.

Luborsky, L., McLellan, A. T., Woody, G. E., O'Brien, C. P., and Auerbach, A. (1985). Therapist success and its determinants. *Archives of General Psychiatry*, **42**, 602–11.

Margison, F. (2002). Psychodynamic interpersonal therapy. In: J. Holmes and A. Bateman, ed. *Integration in psychotherapy*, pp. 107–24. Oxford: Oxford University Press.

Martin, D. J., Garske, J, P., and Davis, M. K. (2000). Relation of the therapeutic alliance with outcome and other variables: a meta-analytic review. *Journal of Consulting and Clinical Psychology*, **68**, 438–50.

Messer, S. B. (1992). A critical examination of belief structures in integrative and eclectic psychotherapy. In: J. C. Norcross and M. R. Goldfried, ed. *Handbook of psychotherapy integration*, pp. 130–65. New York: Basic Books.

Norcross, J. C. (2002a). Empirically supported therapy relationships. In: J. C. Norcross, ed. *Psychotherapy relationships that work. Therapist contributions and responsiveness to patients*, pp. 3–16. Oxford: Oxford University Press.

Norcross, J. C., ed. (2002b). *Psychotherapy relationships that work. Therapist contributions and responsiveness to patients*. Oxford: Oxford University Press.

Norcross, J. C. and Goldfried, M. R., ed. (1992). *Handbook of psychotherapy integration*. New York: Basic Books.

Norcross, J. C. and Newman, C. F. (1992). Psychotherapy integration: setting the context. In: J. C. Norcross and M. R. Goldfried, ed. *Psychotherapy integration*, pp. 3–45. New York: Basic Books.

O'Leary, K. D. and Wilson, G. T. (1975). *Behavior therapy: application and outcome*. Englewood Cliffs, NJ: Prentice Hall.

Orlinsky, D. E., Grawe, K., and Parks, B. K. (1994). Process and outcome in psychotherapy—Noch einmal. In: A. E. Bergin and S. L. Garfield, ed. *Handbook of psychotherapy and behavior change*, 4th edn, pp. 270–376. New York: Wiley.

Orlinsky, D. E., Rønnestad, M. H., and Willutzki, U. (2004). Fifty years of psychotherapy process-outcome research: continuity and change. In: M. J. Lambert, ed. *Bergin and Garfield's handbook of psychotherapy and behavior change*, 5th edn, pp. 307–89. New York: Wiley.

Pope, B. (1979). *The mental health interview*. New York: Pergamon Press.

Prochaska, J. O. and DiClemente, C. C. (1992). The transtheoretical approach. In: J. C. Norcross and M. R. Goldfried, ed. *Psychotherapy integration*, pp. 300–34. New York: Basic Books.

Prochaska, J. O. and Norcross, J. C. (2002). Stages of change. In: J. C. Norcross, ed. *Psychotherapy relationships that work. Therapist contributions and responsiveness to patients*, pp. 303–13. Oxford: Oxford University Press.

Renik, O. (1995). The ideal of the anonymous analyst and the problem of self-disclosure. *Psychoanalytic Quarterly*, **64**, 466–95.

Rockland, L. H. (1989). *Supportive therapy: a dynamic approach*. New York: Basic Books.

Rogers, C. R. (1951). *Client-centered therapy*. London: Constable.

Ryle, A. (1990). *Cognitive analytic therapy*. Chichester: Wiley.

Safran, J. D. and Muran, J. C. (2000). *Negotiating the therapeutic alliance. A relational treatment guide*. New York: Guilford Press.

Safran, J. D., Muran, J. C., Samstag, L. W., and Stevens, C. (2002). Repairing alliance ruptures. In: J. C. Norcross, ed. *Psychotherapy relationships that work. Therapist contributions and responsiveness to patients*, pp. 235–54. Oxford: Oxford University Press.

Shapiro, D. (1995). Finding out about how psychotherapies help people change. *Psychotherapy Research*, **5**, 1–21.

Shapiro, D. A., Firth-Cozens, J., and Stiles, W. B. (1989). The question of therapists' differential effectiveness: a Sheffield psychotherapy project addendum. *British Journal of Psychiatry*, **154**, 383–5.

Snyder, C. R. and Ingram, R. E., ed. (2000). *Handbook of psychological change: psychotherapy processes and practices for the 21st century*. New York: Wiley.

Stricker, G. and Gold, J. R. (1993). *Comprehensive handbook of psychotherapy integration*. New York: Plenum Press.

Strupp, H. H. and Hadley, S. W. (1979). Specific vs. nonspecific factors in psychotherapy. *Archives of General Psychiatry*, **36**, 1125–36.

Task Force on Promotion and Dissemination of Psychological Procedures (1995). Training in and dissemination of empirically validated psychological treatments: Report and recommendations. *The Clinical Psychologist*, **48**, 3–23.

Trijsburg, R. W. (2003). Weerstand [Resistance]. In: R. W. Trijsburg, S. Colijn, E. Collumbien, and G. Lietaer, ed. *Handboek Integratieve Psychotherapie*, IV 3.6, pp. 1–30. Utrecht: De Tijdstroom.

Trijsburg, R. W. *et al.* (in press). Construct validity of the Comprehensive Psychotherapeutic Interventions Rating Scale (CPIRS). *Psychotherapy Research*.

Van Marle, S. and Holmes, J. (2002). Supportive psychotherapy as an integrative psychotherapy. In:. J. Holmes and A. Bateman, ed. *Integration in psychotherapy*, pp. 175–94. Oxford: Oxford University Press.

Wachtel, P. L. (1997). *Psychoanalysis, behavior therapy, and the relational world*. Washington DC: American Psychological Association (APA).

Wachtel, P. L. and Seckinger, R. A. (2001). De cyclische psychodynamische benadering [Cyclical Psychodynamics]. In: R. W. Trijsburg, S. Colijn, E. Collumbien, and G. Lietaer, ed. *Handboek Integratieve Psychotherapie*, VII.9, pp. 1–24. Utrecht: De Tijdstroom.

Winnicott, D. W. (1976). *The maturational processes and the facilitating environment. Studies in the theory of emotional development*. London: Hogarth Press.

Wolpe, J. (1984). Behavior therapy according to Lazarus. *American Psychologist*, **39**, 1326–7.

II

Psychotherapy in psychiatric disorders

11 Cognitive-behavior therapy for mood disorders

Willem Kuyken, Ed Watkins, and Aaron T. Beck

Cognitive-behavioral therapy (CBT) for mood disorders is based on a cognitive theory of mood disorders with solid empirical foundations for its basic tenets, sets out principles that emerge from practice, theory, and research, and has been subjected to numerous outcome studies that have led it to be a 'treatment of choice.' CBT uses a combination of behavioral and cognitive techniques to help a person cope with symptoms, find better ways to deal with life problems, and to change the patterns of thinking, beliefs, and responses presumed to underlie the maintenance of depression (see A. T. Beck *et al.*, 1979 for the seminal exposition; Moore and Garland, 2003, for more chronic and recurrent depression; Young *et al.*, 2003, for schema-focused approaches). This chapter focuses primarily on a form of cognitive therapy developed by Professor Aaron T. Beck over 30 years ago and which has spawned a number of derivatives that address particular aspects (e.g., McCullough, 2000; Segal *et al.*, 2002; Moore and Garland, 2003). We cannot do justice to the depth of clinical and research innovation and will therefore signpost key publications throughout the chapter and provide an 'Indicated Reading List' at the end of the chapter.

We first describe a case example and refer to this case throughout the chapter to illustrate CBT for mood disorders (see Box). We then describe the cognitive and behavioral theories that underpin CBT approaches for depression using this as the basis for describing the main therapeutic approaches to mood disorders as well as their evidence base. Key practice principles in CBT are applied specifically to mood disorders. Some common themes and issues in working as a CBT practitioner with clients with mood disorders are identified, discussed and illustrated through the case example. Finally, we set out future directions for CBT practitioners and researchers.

Mood disorders comprise affective, cognitive, behavioral, and somatic elements. In the case illustration of Sheryl (see Box) these were persistent low mood, guilt, and anhedonia (affective), negative automatic thoughts and ruminative thinking (cognitive), social withdrawal (behavioral), and sleep disturbance (somatic). Sheryl had suffered from mood disturbance throughout her adult life and had developed a range of negative beliefs about depression: 'suffering depression is shameful,' 'my experience is unique,' 'nobody will understand,' 'this state will last forever,' and 'the future is bleak and hopeless.'

The family of mood disorders is a heterogeneous group of conditions that share in common mood regulation difficulties. The classification of mood disorders are described comprehensively in the *Diagnostic and statistical manual of psychiatric disorders* (DSM), 4th edn (American Psychiatric Association, 1994). We will refer to three broad groups of mood difficulties. The first, unipolar major depression, refers to an episode where mood is seriously compromised (e.g., at least 2 weeks of depressed mood or loss of interest/anhedonia) and evidence of four additional depressive symptoms (e.g., loss of energy, low self-worth, guilt, suicidal ideation, sleep disturbance, appetite disturbance). The second, bipolar depression is characterized by one or more manic or mixed episodes, usually accompanied by depressive episodes. The third, dysthymia refers to at least 2 years of depressed mood more days than not, accompanied by additional depressive symptoms that do not meet the threshold for major depression.

To date, CBT approaches have focused primarily on unipolar depression. However, the last 10 years has seen the development of CBT expertise for bipolar disorder (Basco and Rush, 1996; Newman *et al.*, 2002) and more recently adaptations for atypical depression (Jarrett *et al.*, 1999) and dysthymia (Arnow and Constantino, 2003).

Practitioners working with people with mood disorders draw several further distinctions that are important in understanding the presenting issues and in making treatment choices. The first distinction refers to the severity of disorder, which is usually mapped on to the continuum from mild to moderate to severe (with or without) psychotic features. The severity of the disorder is judged by the number of symptoms, the severity of particular symptoms, and the degree of functional impairment. A person with mild depression may report only five symptoms, each with mild presentations and producing little or no social or occupational disability. A person with severe depression may report most of the symptoms to a significant degree and may be incapacitated at home or in a psychiatric inpatient setting. This may include mood-congruent psychotic features such as delusions (e.g., of being punished) or hallucinations (e.g., berating voices).

A further distinction is whether the depression is the first episode or part of a recurrent pattern of depressive episodes. The diathesis-stress formulation and treatment of depression is probably different for these two presentations. Similarly, the age of first onset is important, as earlier onset is associated with more problems in adulthood, poorer prognosis, and greater likelihood of eventual suicide (Rao *et al.*, 1999; Fombonne *et al.*, 2001). In recurrent depression, the person's experience over time is important. Do episodes of depression arise through a gradual onset or more rapidly? Do the episodes last weeks, months, or even years? Is recovery gradual, sporadic or rapid? Between episodes does the person feel well and function fully or does s/he experience ongoing residual symptoms of depression?

The final categorizations that are sometimes used are of 'chronic' and 'treatment-resistant/refractory' depression. While nosologically contentious, some consensus exists that practitioners and researchers tend to use these to refer to the group of people who have unremitting depression that begins in adolescence/early adulthood and lasts over years (chronic depression) (McCullough, 2000; McCullough *et al.*, 2003) or who do not respond to established evidence-based approaches.

These finer-grained categorizations are important because CBT theory and practice are adapted for different forms of depression. Therefore, through a thorough assessment process, a cognitive therapist would formulate diagnostic opinions that shape intervention choices (see Box for the diagnostic opinions for Sheryl).

Theoretical conceptualizations of mood disorders

CBT theories of mood disorders move beyond description to explain and predict depressive phenomena. We cannot do full justice to CBT theories of depression here and interested readers are referred to recent reviews (see: A. T. Beck, 1996; Ingram *et al.*, 1998; Clark *et al.*, 1999). In brief, CBT theories of mood disorders are based on several assumptions. First, a diathesis-stress biopsychosocial model is implicated in the development and maintenance of emotional disorders. That is to say, biological, psychological, and social factors can all be involved in both diathesis, predisposing someone to mood disorders, as well as acting as stressors that precipitate the onset/relapse of mood disorders. Second, maladaptive beliefs about the self, the external world and the future are shaped through formative developmental experiences. Third, these maladaptive beliefs lie dormant and are activated only when precipitated by resonant situations. Fourth, when precipitating situations occur, the beliefs interact with the situation through processes of selective attention and inference, and generate negative mood reactions. These negative beliefs and emotions lead to behavioral consequences that serve to maintain negative mood (A. T. Beck, 1976b; A. T. Beck *et al.*, 1979). Figure 11.1 shows this original model, and provides an illustration by describing a typical situation–belief–emotion–behavioral cycle for Sheryl.

This basic cognitive model has been significantly elaborated and refined on the basis of over 30 years of empirical work (see: Clark *et al.*, 1999). One significant refinement is the suggestion that maladaptive cognitive processing, including negative beliefs, becomes activated only *after the onset of depressive mood problems* when dysphoric states are present (Miranda and Persons, 1988; Teasdale and Cox, 2001). In the onset and maintenance of mood disorders, depression is *fuelled* by a stream of negative ruminative automatic thoughts (e.g., 'My high functioning façade is breaking down,' 'My family think I am weak,' 'I will be unable to cope with a family Christmas') that are congruent with underlying higher-order modes (e.g., 'self-as-weak') and dysfunctional assumptions (e.g., 'If my high functioning façade breaks down people will think I am weak').

A second significant refinement is the concept of core modes that become activated in depression. Core modes are interlocking information processing systems that draw on the parallel processing from cognitive, affective, and sensory processing modules (Teasdale and Barnard, 1993; A. T. Beck, 1996). Once instated in depression, these core modes have a self-maintaining property as mode-consistent biases of attention, overgeneralized memories, higher-order self-schemas, ruminative thinking, and sensory feedback loops from unpleasant bodily states 'interlock' in self-perpetuating cycles of processing. The more often a person has suffered depression, the more easily these core modes become automatic and easily activated (Segal *et al.*, 1996). The content of depressive core modes tends to be organized around themes of loss, defeat, failure, worthlessness, and unloveability.

Several theoretical reformulations argue that core modes are *directly* linked to depressive affective and motivational symptoms (Teasdale *et al.*, 1993;

Sheryl: a case illustration of a woman with recurrent major depression

Sheryl is a 44-year-old married woman, who presented with major, chronic, recurrent depression. A detailed assessment revealed an early onset of dysthymia at age 12 and a first episode of major depression at age 17. Her primary care physician has prescribed a selective serotonin reuptake inhibitor, which was augmented with lithium when Sheryl did not respond. She is currently unemployed, having been laid off 5 months ago from her job. Sheryl reports a difficult childhood, during which she felt little support or love from her parents. Her father suffered from depression and substance dependence, and died when she was aged 16 through suicide (although this information only became available some way through therapy). Sheryl has four children. Two of the children (male aged 23, female aged 23) were the children of her first husband who was alcohol dependent. He physically and sexually abused Sheryl, escalating to a point where Sheryl took refuge in a women's center. The younger two children (female aged 17 and male aged 12) are children by her second husband, with whom she currently lives. Her husband works as an engineer and she describes him as supportive.

Sheryl presented with the following issues: (1) increasing social withdrawal; (2) suicidal thoughts; (3) loss of her job and lack of success in finding a new job; (4) conflict with her 17-year old daughter; and (5) lack of self-worth. Sheryl's goals for therapy were: (1) to return to work; (2) increase her sense of self-worth; and (3) manage her daughter's problematic behavior more effectively.

The DSM-IV diagnostic impressions were as follows:

- *Axis I*: major depressive episode, recurrent, severe; dysthymia (early onset)

- *Axis II*: avoidant personality traits

- *Axis III*: migraine

- *Axis IV*: occupational problems (unemployed); economic problems (low income); other psychosocial problems (conflict with 17-year-old daughter)

- *Axis V*: GAF (current): 55

  GAF (highest in last year): 55

Use of standardized measures of depression severity, hopelessness and anxiety, Beck Depression Inventory-II, Beck Hopelessness Scale and Beck Anxiety Inventory suggested depression and hopelessness in the severe range and anxiety in the moderate range. Item analysis, with follow-up questioning suggested suicidal ideation but no suicidal intent. The assessment further indicated that that the onset of depression would be quite sudden, with Sheryl moving rapidly from normal functioning to feeling overwhelmed, often triggering a suicide attempt. On several occasions this had required hospitalization. Episodes tended to be of several months duration with a gradual recovery. Between episodes Sheryl was able to function normally, but careful assessment indicated that this was more apparent than real, with significant residual depressive symptoms that she did not disclose to others or indeed acknowledge fully to herself: fatigue, irritability, negative intrusive thoughts, and feelings of guilt.

Sheryl's nonresponsiveness to initial pharmacotherapy suggests combination CBT and pharmacotherapy as the next treatment approach.

Activating Event
A stressful event that is resonant to the person's idiosyncratic beliefs
{Laid off from work}

Beliefs Activated
Depressive beliefs about the self, the external world and the future
{Self: 'I am useless'
External world: 'Others will discover that I am useless and reject me'
Future: 'I will never succeed; the future is hopeless'}

Emotions
Emotions that result from and then reciprocally interact with activated beliefs
{Despondency}

Behavior
Behavioral orientations and actual behaviors resulting from beliefs and emotions
{Withdrawal}

Fig. 11.1 Illustration of basic cognitive model of depression, with case example.

Power and Dalgleish, 1997), while lower order maladaptive beliefs are linked to depression only *indirectly* through the core modes. Maladaptive beliefs are secondary dysfunctional assumptions (e.g., 'I have to put on a strong façade, or people will reject me'), rules for living (e.g., 'don't show weakness'), and attitudes (e.g., 'weak people are pathetic') that are closely linked to core modes (e.g., 'self-as-weak'). Various commentators have noted this distinction between higher-order self-schemas and lower-order maladaptive beliefs as reflecting the difference between emotional and intellectual belief, 'hot' and 'cold' cognition (Teasdale, 1993; J. S. Beck, 1995; Young *et al.*, 2003), or as clients have described it to us 'I know it in my gut rather than in my head.'

Related to core modes are cognitive and behavioral compensatory strategies that enable a person to cope with the negative consequences of core modes. The strategies are usually part of a spectrum of normal coping strategies but have become problematic because they have become inflexible and therefore inadvertently maintain core modes and maladaptive beliefs. In their most primitive form perceived threat triggers compensatory strategies to mobilize for action or inhibit into inaction. Examples of dimensions of compensatory strategies include:

avoid intimacy—appropriate intimacy—overly intimate

passive-aggressive—appropriate assertiveness—aggressiveness

abdicate control to others—appropriate use of control—authoritarianism

A table and schematic diagram summarize the reformulation of depression (Table 11.1 and Figure 11.2).

Activating events (internal or external) activate orienting schemas, which in turn activate the patterns of cognitive processing (dynamic cognitive structures) that are core modes or interlocked 'minds-in-place.' The cognitive features that make up depression (e.g., ruminative thinking, negative appraisals, memory biases) are produced once a negative core mode is instated. The characteristics and relationship between core modes, maladaptive beliefs, and compensatory strategies are shown in Table 11.1 and Figure 11.3.

In parallel with the emphasis on compensatory strategies in cognitive accounts, recent behavioral conceptualizations of depression have highlighted the importance of avoidant behaviors in depression, particularly within the behavioral activation (BA) approach. BA was initially developed as part of a component analysis of the active components of CBT, and only reflected the behavioral components of CBT (Jacobson *et al.*, 2001; Hopko *et al.*, 2003). After BA was found to be as effective as BA plus thought challenging and as effective as full CBT in treating major depression (Jacobson *et al.*, 1996), the treatment was further elaborated (see: Martell *et al.*, 2001), drawing on behavioral approaches to depression (e.g., Ferster, 1973). Central to the BA conceptualization of depression is the concept of secondary avoidant behaviors in response to the symptoms of depression produced by

Precipitating Event
A stressful internal or external event

Orienting Schemas
Attentional processes focus on personal and negative stimuli

Cognitive Structures
Core modes comprising higher-order negative self-referent structures

Cognitive Products
Ruminative thinking
Cognitive errors
Negative appraisals
Overgeneral autobiographical memory functioning

Fig. 11.2 Cognitive model of depression.

Table 11.1 Core modes, dysfunctional assumptions, and compensatory strategies in depression

	Core modes	Maladaptive beliefs	Compensatory strategies
Characteristics	Higher-order schema about the self, others and world Associated sensory feedback loops Directly linked to affect Closed and resistant to change Easily activated Maintained by maladaptive beliefs and compensatory strategies	Propositional level of meaning Secondary to core modes Less direct links to affect or bodily states Maintain and maintained by compensatory strategies	Maintain homeostasis between inputs and internal states Activated by affective thermostat Can be cognitive or behavioral Adaptive in origin Maladaptive in avoiding, maintaining and/or compensating for core modes Maintained by and maintain core modes
Typology	*Loss/defeat*: Sense of loss and/or defeat *Competence/power*: Perceived difficulty being able to function competently, capably or independently *Worth*: Sense of self as having no value *Unloveability/unacceptability*: Sense of self as unacceptable/ unlovable to others	Attitudes Assumptions Rules	Emotional constriction—emotional lability Autonomy—sociotropy Cognitive flexibility Approach-avoidance Perfectionism Avoid intimacy—overly intimate Passive-aggressiveness—authoritarianism
Examples	Self-as-incompetent/powerless/repugnant Others-as-rejecting/domineering World-as-threatening	It is terrible to be weak *Positive assumption*: If I am full of bravado, my family will think I am okay *Negative*: If my family discover the 'real me' they will reject me I should constantly strive to be the ideal mother, strong, capable and self-contained	All or nothing thinking Rigid, monolithic thinking Emotional avoidance Social withdrawal

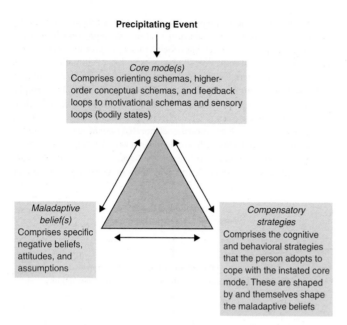

Fig. 11.3 Schematic diagram of cognitive reformulation of depression.

negative events: BA proposes that unhelpful secondary coping responses lead to the maintenance of depression. Typically, unhelpful secondary coping responses involve attempts to escape from an aversive environment (e.g., arguments, confrontations, reminders of loss) or to avoid aversive situations or emotional states (risk of failure or embarrassment), that is, secondary coping responses are compensatory strategies. Avoidance behaviors include being passive, withdrawal, rumination, complaining, or avoiding new activities. Because these behaviors reduce exposure to aversive situations they are negatively reinforced and become more prevalent, reducing the frequency and narrowing the range of other behaviors, which in turn reduces contact with positive reinforcers and increases the risk for depression.

Cognitive model of bipolar disorder

As in the original cognitive model for depression, cognitive approaches to bipolar disorder emphasize a diathesis-stress biopsychosocial model and focus on the importance of maladaptive beliefs and automatic thoughts. Although a comprehensive cognitive model of bipolar disorder is yet to be delineated, recent attempts to develop cognitive behavioral approaches for bipolar disorder have all focused on evidence suggesting that psychosocial stressors and adverse cognitive styles interact with an inherent biological vulnerability to produce manic and depressed episodes (Newman *et al.*, 2002). The biological vulnerability appears in part to be hereditary, with bipolar disorder running in families, and genetic factors demonstrated in twin and adoption studies. Recent theories have suggested that biological vulnerability to bipolar disorder may result from dysregulation in the BA system, which is a putative neurobiological motivational system that regulates goal-directed approach to potential reward and is proposed to influence positive affect, energy, and attention.

Other evidence suggests that bipolar episodes occur in response to stressful life events, whether disruptions in daily routines (Malkoff-Schwartz *et al.*, 1998), negative life events, or even goal attainment. Typically, it appears that negative life events predict bipolar depression, while goal attainment predicts mania; however, the relationship is not always straightforward, with negative events producing mania in the context of increased BA.

Cognitive-behavioral approaches to bipolar disorder emphasize that an individual's cognitive style and behavioral coping strategies in response to stressful life events mediates the extent to which the biological vulnerability is expressed in a full-blown bipolar episode. Consistent with this, Reilly-Harrington *et al.* (1999) report that negative attributional styles increase vulnerability to both manic and depressive symptoms following stressful life events.

Similarly, the response to prodromes of mania and depression is considered an important factor in the cognitive-behavioral model. Prodromes are the early signs and symptoms that can precede a full-blown episode, which the cognitive model assumes to be activated by the interaction between stressful life events and biological vulnerability. For example, disruptions in daily routine coupled with biological vulnerability may lead to reduced sleep. The cognitive-behavioral approach to bipolar disorder predicts that the particular thinking patterns and coping strategies instated in response to prodromal symptoms will determine whether a full bipolar episode will occur. As in models of unipolar depression, particular patterns of affect, cognition, and sensory input (e.g., depressed mood or hypomania) are hypothesized to activate associated schemas or core modes, which, in turn, will bias information processing towards information consistent with the schema, further fuelling the mood states. Thus, a patient in a hypomanic state will have positively valenced schemas activated, which will be characterized by processing that emphasizes goal attainment and potential rewards, while downplaying potential risks and problems. The particular schemas and modes that are activated in response to stress are hypothesized to determine which life events an individual will be more vulnerable to and to determine what form their response to stress will take. The activation of more adaptive, less extreme schemas and modes will lead to more stable mood, while less adaptive, more extreme schemas will produce further emotional dysregulation. For example, extreme beliefs about need for achievement and autonomy would be hypothesized to increase risk for depression and/or mania in patients with a biological vulnerability when exposed to potentially triggering events. In the case of perceived failure, such beliefs may lead to low self-worth and depressed mood, while in the context of perceived success such beliefs may lead to more grandiose thoughts about the self, feeding into hypomania.

Schemas and modes will also determine the strategies chosen to respond to stressful events and prodromes, e.g., achievement-related schemas would lead to overdriven behavior to compensate for lost time. Helpful coping strategies act against the prevailing prodrome, e.g., reduced arousal in hypomania, whereas unhelpful coping strategies further reinforce the initial stages of the bipolar episode, fuelling more extreme mood swings, e.g., rushing around doing many things at once (Lam *et al.*, 2001). The specific schemas and modes available to be activated in any individual by stressful events or prodromes will depend upon his or her early learning history, as well as upon experiences in adolescence and adulthood, often linked to the onset and consequences of the bipolar disorder (e.g., beliefs such as 'I am a difficult person' and 'I am defective' following from the emotional fallout of mood swings).

Cognitive models of bipolar disorder also highlight the self-fulfilling nature of the disorder, with the consequences of a bipolar episode further contributing to the maintenance of the episode. For example, impulsive spending may lead to financial problems, irritability coupled with poor concentration may lead to problems at work or the loss of employment and promiscuous behavior may lead to problems in intimate relationships. All of these episode-related difficulties could then act as further stressors to interact with the underlying biological vulnerability to further generate bipolar symptoms. Furthermore, bipolar disorder is associated with a great deal of loss (e.g., lost potential, lost employment prospects, lost relationships), self-blame for impulsive acts committed during mania, and stigma, which can act as further stressors and/or further reinforce dysfunctional beliefs.

Thus, in summary, cognitive models of bipolar disorder emphasize: (1) underlying biological vulnerability (emotional dysregulation) and underlying cognitive vulnerability (dysfunctional schemas); (2) that these vulnerabilities interact with stressful life events to determine prodromes and patient's responses to prodromes; (3) less adaptive schemas will lead to less adaptive coping strategies and the exacerbation of prodromes into full-blown episodes; and (4) The consequences of episodes further exacerbate stressful life events and underlying cognitive vulnerabilities.

The advantages of these theoretical formulations to the CBT practitioner are that they introduce a more integrative model of mood disorders that provides clear rationales for why and how a broad range of CBT interventions might impact on cognition, behavior, and affect.

Does cognitive-behavioral therapy for mood disorders work? Efficacy and process-outcome research

CBT has been demonstrated to be a generally effective treatment for depression in the large number of studies that have accumulated since the original study by Rush et al. (1977). CBT produces a greater improvement in symptoms than no treatment or waiting-list controls (Dobson, 1989) and demonstrates equivalent efficacy to pharmacotherapy for depression, although many studies did not employ a drug–placebo control condition or monitor plasma medication to check on the adequacy of pharmacotherapy (e.g., Blackburn et al., 1981; Hollon et al., 1992; Blackburn and Moore, 1997).

What about CBT compared with other psychotherapies? The large multisite National Institute of Mental Health (NIMH) Treatment of Depression Collaborative Research Program (TDCRP) trial (Elkin et al., 1989), which compared CBT, interpersonal psychotherapy, imipramine, and a placebo control, found that although there were few significant differences between treatments, for more people with more severe depression, pharmacotherapy and interpersonal therapy did better than CBT, with CBT only doing as well as placebo control on several outcome measures. This result has been much debated, with questions about differences in the skill in application of CBT across sites. Other studies comparing CBT with interpersonal or psychodynamic therapies for depression found CBT as effective as psychodynamic/interpersonal (PI) therapies (see: Leichsenring, 2001). However, the people in the NIMH-TDCRP study tended to have more severe depression than the other studies. More recent evidence attests to the efficacy of CBT for people diagnosed with depression, across a wide range of depression severity (DeRubeis et al., 1999).

One randomized controlled trial (RCT) compared CBT with BA (Jacobson et al., 1996; Gortner et al., 1998). The BA component of CBT focused on monitoring daily activities, assessment of pleasure and mastery, graded task assignment, cognitive rehearsal, problem solving, and social skills training. There were no significant differences between BA, BA plus modification of automatic thoughts (AT) and a full CBT treatment, at completion of treatment, 6-month follow-up (Jacobson et al., 1996), or 2-year follow-up (Gortner et al., 1998).

How well does CBT work for more chronic and severe depression? A recent trial examined CBT with and without nefazodone for chronic depression, operationalized as major depression lasting at least 2 years or a current major depression superimposed on preexisting dysthymia (Keller et al., 2000). This version of CBT, Cognitive-Behavioral Analysis System of Psychotherapy (CBASP) differs from classical CBT in its explicit focus on the consequences of client's interpersonal behavior through the use of a situational analysis protocol, which helps clients to identify whether their expectations and behaviors help or hinder movement towards their goals (see: McCullough, 2000). This trial found that CBASP and nefazodone in combination produced more remission in chronic depression (48%) than either nefazodone (29%) or CBASP alone (33%) (Keller et al., 2000). One limitation of this study was that treatment-resistant participants, that is, people who had not responded to previous antidepressants or psychotherapy, were excluded, i.e., the study lacked an important subgroup of chronic depression.

Nonetheless, if replicated, this study would suggest that a combination of CBT and pharmacotherapy may be most appropriate for chronic depression.

One potential benefit of CBT for depression is that it reduces relapse/recurrence to a greater extent than antidepressant medication. Given that recurrence is a significant problem for people with major depression (Judd, 1997a,b), treatments that reduce relapse/recurrence are urgently needed. A number of studies report that after 1 or 2 years follow-up, relapse rates following treatment for depression with CBT were lower than for people treated with pharmacotherapy, when both treatments are stopped at termination (Kovacs et al., 1981; Simons et al., 1986; Evans et al., 1992; Shea et al., 1992; Gortner et al., 1998) (see also meta-analysis: Gloaguen et al., 1998). However, interpretation of these findings needs to be cautious because different studies used different criteria for relapse; Beck Depression Inventory scores greater than 16 or 'treatment reentry for depression' (Kovacs et al., 1981; Simons et al., 1986), compared with fulfilling criteria for major depression (Shea et al., 1992). Clearly, diagnosis of major depression is the most stringent criterion, while reentry into treatment is problematic as people in the CBT condition may still be symptomatic but attempting to deal with their symptoms themselves. Furthermore, an important comparison group is antidepressant continuation; people maintained on antidepressant appear to do as well as people who received a brief course of CBT (Evans et al., 1992). Blackburn and Moore (1997) in a randomized acute trial for recurrent major depression compared acute antidepressant treatment followed by maintenance antidepressants, acute CBT treatment followed by maintenance CBT and acute antidepressant treatment followed by maintenance CBT. All three groups showed clinical improvements during the acute and maintenance phases of treatment, with no significant differences between the three groups. CBT is therefore as effective in preventing the recurrence of depression as continued antidepressant medication.

More recently, several trials have specifically investigated the role of CBT treatments as relapse prevention for people whose depression was in remission rather than as an intervention for current depression. Fava et al. (1994, 1996, 1998) have developed a version of CBT to be used after successful treatment of an acute episode by pharmacotherapy. This therapy protocol involves a combination of CBT focused on residual symptoms of depression, life-style modification, and well-being therapy. Residual symptoms of depression are known to predict increased risk of relapse and therefore targeting such symptoms may well help reduce future episodes of depression. RCTs suggest that CBT for residual depression results in significantly less relapse/recurrence over 2 years (25%) than standard clinical management in the absence of antidepressant medication (Fava et al., 1998). Paykel et al. (1999) further demonstrated that compared with clinical management alone, clinical management plus CBT reduced relapse in 158 people with recent major depression that had partially remitted with antidepressant treatment.

An alternative approach to preventing relapse/recurrence has specifically targeted people with a history of recurrent depression who are currently in remission. Based on the hypothesis that these people tend to be caught up in ruminative depressive processing at times of potential relapse/recurrence, Teasdale et al. (1995) proposed that using mindfulness meditation, which fosters a relationship to thoughts and feelings antithetical to such rumination, might prevent future episodes of depression. Therefore, elements of a mindfulness-based stress reduction program (Kabat-Zinn, 1990) were incorporated into CBT to create mindfulness-based cognitive therapy (MBCT). MBCT is delivered in weekly group training sessions, in which participants practice and develop a moment-by-moment nonjudgmental awareness of sensations, thoughts, and feelings, through the use of formal and informal meditation exercises. These awareness exercises are further practiced during homework (see: Segal et al., 2002). For people with a history of three or more episodes of major depression, MBCT significantly reduced risk of relapse/recurrence over 1 year compared with treatment as usual (Teasdale et al., 2000). Without a further component trial, it is not possible to determine whether it was the mindfulness element or the CBT element or the combination thereof that was effective in this treatment.

In recent years, several RCTs have shown that compared with standard clinical management (including the prescription of mood stabilizers), standard clinical management plus CBT can reduce the recurrence of future bipolar episodes in people with bipolar disorder (e.g., Perry et al., 1999; Lam et al., 2000, 2003; Scott et al., 2001). These trials have focused on CBT as an adjunct to mood stabilizers.

What works for whom?

Understanding the process and mechanisms of successful CBT for mood disorders is essential to developing more efficacious, more effective, and more appropriately targeted treatments for depression. The cognitive model (A. T. Beck, 1976a) predicts that CBT should produce specific changes on measures of cognitions, that these changes in cognitions are unique to CBT and that these changes in cognitions should predict symptomatic improvement.

One approach to testing this model is to examine changes on questionnaires designed to assess cognitive-specific changes, such as the Dysfunctional Attitude Scale (DAS: Weissman and Beck, 1978) and the Attributional Style Questionnaire (ASQ: Peterson et al., 1982). Several studies have found that people receiving pharmacotherapy for depression achieved similar changes in mood and cognitive processes as people receiving CBT, suggesting that cognitive changes were secondary to mood change (e.g., Imber et al., 1990). However, Seligman et al. (1988) found that CBT significantly improved explanatory style on the ASQ and that change in explanatory style correlated with change in depressive symptoms. However, without comparing CBT with other therapies, it was not possible to determine whether this change was unique to CBT or just secondary to symptomatic improvement. DeRubeis et al. (1990) found that change from pretreatment to mid-treatment on the ASQ and DAS predicted change in depression from mid-treatment to posttreatment for depressed patients in a CBT group but not in a pharmacotherapy group, suggesting that cognitive change is associated with improvement in CBT but is not alone sufficient to produce symptom relief.

There are general problems with the use of questionnaire measures to investigate cognitive change. Self-report responses are vulnerable to demand effects, response biases and the mood of the reporter may influence which items are endorsed, as many items differ in hedonic tone. Furthermore, it is not clear how well self-report questionnaires measure underlying cognitive structures and processes, such as schema, which are hypothesized to be important in the development of depression. There is also evidence to suggest that the specific cognitive biases associated with depression can only be observed when people are tested in a negative mood (Teasdale and Dent, 1987; Dent and Teasdale, 1988; Miranda et al., 1988).

More supportive of the cognitive change hypothesis, recent research found that a significant minority of people diagnosed with depression undergoing CBT showed 'sudden gains', where there was substantial symptom improvement in one between-session interval (Tang and DeRubeis, 1999). Such sudden gains are associated with better long-term outcomes, with people who experienced sudden gains significantly less depressed than those not experiencing sudden gains at 18-month follow-up. In CBT, sudden gains seemed to be preceded by critical sessions in which substantial cognitive changes occurred. However, as the sudden gains effect has recently been found in supportive-expressive psychotherapy for depression (Tang et al., 2002), the exact mechanism underpinning sudden gains (i.e., different mechanisms for different therapies versus nonspecific treatment effects) remains unresolved.

Recent studies have suggested that changes in the style of processing depression-related information, rather than just changes in thought content, might be important in the mechanism of CBT. Teasdale et al. (2001) found that in people with residual depression, CBT reduces an absolutist all-or-nothing thinking style, which, in turn, was found to mediate the effects of CBT on preventing relapse. Similarly, CBT successfully reduces relapse in people who report increased 'metacognitive awareness' at the end of treatment (defined as the ability to view thoughts as mental events in a wider context of awareness) (Teasdale et al., 2001). Thus, these studies suggest that CBT may prevent relapse by shifting the mode or style of processing. However, these studies have exclusively focused on residual depression with relapse as the outcome measure, leaving the generalizability of these findings to acute depression unresolved.

Interestingly, successful CBT for acute depression produces significantly greater reductions in 'cognitive reactivity' (operationalized as increases in dysfunctional attitudes following a negative mood induction) than successful pharmacotherapy for depression (Segal et al., 1999). Together with Teasdale et al.'s findings, this result is consistent with the notion that CBT helps people to acquire compensatory or metacognitive skills (Barber and DeRubeis, 1989) that regulate their cognitive responses to sad mood and stressful events.

An alternative approach to examining the process of change in CBT is to study the effects of specific techniques on outcome. Several therapy process-outcome studies suggest that homework is perceived as helpful and contributes significantly to change in cognitive therapy (Burns and Nolen-Hoeksema, 1991; Detweiler and Whisman, 1999; Burns and Spangler, 2000). Concrete symptom-focused methods of CT predict subsequent symptom reduction when assessed early in treatment (DeRubeis and Feeley, 1990). These concrete methods involved setting an agenda, asking for specific examples, labeling cognitive errors, examining evidence, and monitoring thoughts. However, less focused, more abstract approaches, such as exploring the meaning of thoughts and discussing the therapy, did not predict improvement.

What predicts whether someone will respond to CBT for depression (a prognostic indicator) and whether someone will respond better to CBT than to another treatment (a prescriptive indicator)? Various client variables predict poor outcome to CBT (see: Hamilton and Dobson, 2002), including increased severity and chronicity of the depression and perfectionistic beliefs (Shahar et al., 2003), although these variables predict poor outcome for all interventions. Married clients do better with CBT than single clients (Jarrett et al., 1991). People with avoidant personality disorder may respond better to CBT than to interpersonal therapies (Barber and Muenz, 1996), although higher levels of endorsement of avoidant beliefs predicts poorer outcome in CBT (Kuyken et al., 2001).

In summary, there is now a large and converging body of evidence to indicate that CBT is an effective acute treatment for unipolar depression and is an effective relapse prevention treatment for unipolar depression, and, potentially, a relapse prevention treatment for bipolar disorder. While early studies failed to show that changes in cognition precede symptom changes in CBT, more recent work suggests that sudden gains are preceded by important shifts in beliefs and that CBT effects changes in the process (rather than the content) of cognition. Process-outcome research suggests that CBT can be made more effective by explicitly and concretely teaching patients metacognitive skills in generating specific plans and evaluating their own thoughts.

Key practice principles in cognitive-behavioral therapy for depression

Cognitive therapy for depression will follow the key practice principles of all CBT treatments (see Chapter 2 by Grant et al.). In the rest of this section, we will elaborate on how the key principles are applied to depression, using the case example of Sheryl as an illustration.

Cognitive therapy focuses on current problems and is goal oriented

When treating depression, identifying, operationalizing, and prioritizing current problems and goals is a core aspect of therapy. Such goals direct the therapy and need to be reviewed regularly. These goals should be clear, mutually agreed, specific, and detailed in ways that are helpful to the therapy (including cognitive, affective, and behavioral elements). Identifying specific problems and goals can help patients to feel that their problems are more manageable and more optimistic about change. The problem and goal list for Sheryl are shown in the box and were reviewed at session 8, 16, and at the final session of therapy.

Cognitive therapy is based on a cognitive formulation of the presenting problems

CBT case formulation has been defined as 'as a coherent set of explanatory inferences about the factors causing and maintaining a person's presenting problems that is derived from cognitive theory of emotional disorders' (Bieling and Kuyken, 2003) or as 'the linchpin that holds theory and practice together' (Butler, 1998). A case formulation should guide treatment and serve as a marker for change and as a structure for enabling practitioners to predict beliefs and behaviors that might interfere with the progress of therapy. The case formulation provides a psychological explanation that can help the therapist and client understand what is maintaining the depression and a clear rationale for intervention. There have been several attempts to provide individualized case formulation systems firmly based in cognitive theory that can be used by cognitive therapist in day-to-day practice and in treatment process and outcome research (Muran and Segal, 1992; Linehan, 1993; Persons, 1993; J. S. Beck, 1995; Needleman, 1999).

A CBT formulation rubric for clients with mood disorders makes use of the main elements of a standard case formulation as well as using cognitive theory in its explanatory elements (Figure 11.4). Standard case formulation rubrics describe: (1) the presenting issue(s); (2) predisposing factors; (3) precipitating factors; (4) perpetuating factors; and (5) protective factors. A general depression formulation rubric and the formulation for Sheryl are shown in Figure 11.4.

The formulation for Sheryl ties together in a coherent way how her presenting problems are explainable in CBT terms. It was essential to be able to explain her social withdrawal, low self-worth and conflict could be understood developmentally in terms of what had acted as predisposing and precipitating factors and crucially what core modes, dysfunctional assumptions, and compensatory strategies were maintaining her presenting problems. This formulation was continually revised and updated as new information became available and formed part of the rationale for intervention choices.

Cognitive therapy is based on active collaboration

From the first meeting the client and therapist engage in a process of 'collaborative empiricism' (J. S. Beck, 1995). The therapist takes an active stance, supporting the client in working towards the therapy goals. The initial building of collaboration with Sheryl involved a preliminary description of her depression in biological, cognitive, behavioral, and affective terms (Greenberger and Padesky, 1995). With Sheryl describing her symptoms and the therapist mapping these out on a whiteboard it was possible to build a descriptive picture in CBT terms.

Cognitive therapy tends to be short to medium term

Cognitive therapy for depression typically involves 16–20 meetings, although brief versions have been developed for particular circumstances (e.g., Bond and Dryden, 2002) and more sessions are indicated for chronic and recurrent depression (e.g., Moore *et al.*, 2003). Initial sessions tend to be frequent (either twice a week or weekly) to initiate the change process, manage suicide risk, and achieve symptom relief, and later sessions tend to be less frequent (monthly and perhaps even 3-monthly) to consolidate gains and prevent relapse.

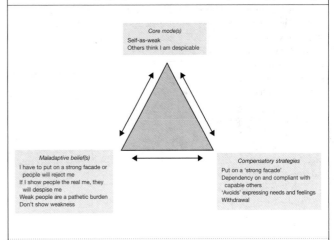

CBT Case Formulation

Name: Sheryl

Presenting issue(s) *[i.e., agreed list of problems and goals.]*

Problem list
1) Increasing social withdrawal
2) Lack of self-worth
3) Loss of her job/lack of success in finding a new job
4) Conflict with her 17-year-old daughter

Goal list
1) Return to work
2) Increased sense of self-worth
3) Improved ability to manage teenage daughter

Predisposing factors *[i.e., factors that have increased the person's vulnerability to experiencing their current problems. These can be biological (e.g., comorbid physical conditions such as migraine), psychological (e.g., recurrent flashbacks of a previous trauma), or social (e.g., chronic financial problems), and can be distal (e.g., loss of parent at age 16) or proximal factors (e.g., escalating conflict with daughter over the last 6 months) increased vulnerability to presenting issues.]*

Mother: perceived as 'capable,' discouraged expression of feelings, would react negatively to children becoming 'demanding.'
Father: alcohol dependent, verbally undemonstrative, committed suicide when Sheryl was aged 16.
Siblings: large number of siblings. Older brother with cerebral palsy.
First husband: abusive, emotionally, physically and sexually.
Coexisting physical health problem: migraine.
Ongoing stress of managing teenage daughter's behavioral problems.

Precipitating factors *[i.e., internal or external events that triggered presenting issues.]*

Being made redundant from her job

Perpetuating Triangle *[i.e., factors that maintain the presenting problems.]*

Core mode(s)
Self-as-weak
Others think I am despicable

Maladaptive belief(s)
I have to put on a strong facade or people will reject me
If I show people the real me, they will despise me
Weak people are a pathetic burden
Don't show weakness

Compensatory strategies
Put on a 'strong facade'
Dependency on and compliant with capable others
'Avoids' expressing needs and feelings
Withdrawal

Protective Factors *[i.e., 'what is right with the person,' elaborating the person's personal and social resources.]*

Good interpersonal skills
Strong relationship with current husband
Capable as a mother and in her work
Committed to addressing her problems

Fig. 11.4 Cognitive-behavioral formulation diagram for depression.

Cognitive therapy draws on a wide range of cognitive and behavioral techniques to change thinking, beliefs, and behaviors

The first class of therapeutic approaches focus on the client's behavior. The rationale is that for some people behavior monitoring, BA, and behavioral change can lead to substantive gains. For example, people with more severe depression often become withdrawn and inactive, which can feed into and exacerbate depression. The person withdraws, and then labels him/herself as 'ineffectual,' thereby fuelling the depression. By focusing on this relationship and gradually increasing the person's sense of daily structure and participation in masterful and pleasurable activities the person can take the first steps in combating depression (A. T. Beck et al., 1979). Other behavioral strategies include scheduling pleasurable activities, breaking down large tasks (e.g., finding employment) into more manageable graded tasks (e.g., buying a newspaper with job advertisements, preparing a resume . . .), teaching relaxation skills, desensitizing a person to feared situations, role-playing, and assertiveness training. To maximize the likelihood of success, plans need to be operationalized at a very concrete, detailed level, including consideration of when, where, how, and with whom the plans will be implemented, as well as potential obstacles and how to overcome them. It is important to note that within CBT, these behavioral techniques are used with the 'collaborative empiricism' approach, such that before plans are implemented, thoughts and beliefs relevant to the activity (e.g., 'It is pointless to try', 'I won't succeed', 'I am too tired', 'I am not interested') can be set out as hypotheses to be tested. Recent adaptations to CBT suggest that the changes in behavioral contingencies may be particularly important in treating severe and recurrent depression (see: McCullough, 2000; Martell et al., 2001).

The second class of therapeutic approaches focus on the client's negative automatic thoughts and maladaptive beliefs. Cognitive techniques are designed to increase clients' awareness of these thoughts, challenge them by evaluating their basis in reality, and providing more adaptive and realistic alternative thoughts. The Dysfunctional Thought Record is used as a primary tool for developing this skill (Figure 11.5). Repeated practice at dealing with negative thinking is required for thought challenging to become a robust skill. Useful approaches to challenging automatic thoughts include listing evidence from past experience that supports and refutes each hypothesis, generating alternative explanations, checking whether a thought may reflect a cognitive error, and reattributing negative events to factors other than the client's personal inadequacy.

In cognitive theory maladaptive beliefs (e.g., 'If I drop my façade, others will despise me') and higher-order core mode beliefs (e.g., 'self-as-weak') underlie automatic thoughts and are the next focus of cognitive interventions. Careful questioning about and exploration of client's unrealistic and maladaptive beliefs is carried out to examine if beliefs are based in reality, and to correct the distortions and maladaptive beliefs that perpetuate emotional distress. The advantages and disadvantages of the assumptions are explored and the possibility of adopting more functional, alternative rules is discussed. Early, often childhood, events that may have led to the adoption of these rules are explored and can be challenged, for example by using imagery to relive the event coupled with questions to introduce new perspectives. For Sheryl growing up in her family of origin a family maxim was 'stiff upper lip' or 'don't show weakness.' Behavioral plans designed to act against assumptions are a powerful way to change beliefs by providing personal experience that counters the assumption. For Sheryl this involved a process of applying the same standard to herself that she applied to other people, i.e., 'a 'capable' person can be both strong and vulnerable and it is OK to show both these sides of the coin.'

Core modes require a further set of therapeutic strategies (J. S. Beck, 1995; Young et al., 2003). For example, when core modes such as 'self-as-weak' are identified, more adaptive beliefs (e.g., 'I am basically capable and likeable') can be established through Socratic questioning, examining advantages and disadvantages of the old and new core beliefs, acting 'as if' the new core beliefs were true, using coping cards, developing metaphors, subjecting the beliefs to tests across the person's life history and reconstructing associated memories and images (J. S. Beck, 1995). For many clients, automatic images, rather than thoughts, are powerfully associated with emotions and behaviors. Images are central to the sequelae of trauma and to psychiatric disorders such as posttraumatic stress disorder (PTSD) and other anxiety disorders that are often comorbid with depression. Images are handled in similar ways, but instead of verbally evaluating and challenging images, more visual techniques are used (J. S. Beck, 1995).

Date	The situation	Emotion	Automatic thoughts	Rational response	What was the outcome?
	What were you doing or thinking about?	*What did you feel? How bad was it (0–100)?*	*What exactly were your thoughts? How far did you believe each of them (0–100%)?*	*What are your rational answers to the automatic thoughts? How far do you believe each of your rational responses right not?*	*How do you feel (0–100)? What can you do now?*

Daily Record of Thoughts and Feelings
Name _____
Week ending _____

Fig. 11.5 Dysfunctional thought record. From Beck, A. T., Rush, A. J., Shaw, B. F., and Emery, G. (1979). *Cognitive therapy for depression*. New York: Wiley. Copyright 1979 by Wiley. Reprinted with permission.

The third range of approaches takes place between therapy sessions as homework assignments. Homework is an essential element of cognitive therapy, aimed at building understanding and coping skills throughout the week, increasing self-reliance and rehearsing adaptive cognitive and behavioral skills. Homework moves the discussions in session from abstract, subjective discussion of issues to real day-to-day experiences. The therapist acts as coach, guiding and debriefing the client from week to week. Homework assignments are tailored to the individual, are set up as no-lose propositions, and may range from the therapist suggesting a relevant book, to the person undertaking a long procrastinated assignment (e.g., telephoning a friend to resolve an area of unspoken conflict), while monitoring the thoughts and images that come to light in preparing for the assignment (e.g., 'the friend will be angry towards me'). As therapy progresses, the client takes on more responsibility for setting and reviewing the homework.

Having outlined the principles that underpin cognitive therapy, we aim to convey a sense of how cognitive therapy works in practice. We will outline a typical therapy session, as well as the progression of therapy as a whole, illustrating this through the case of Sheryl.

A typical cognitive therapy session

This involves checking how the client has been doing, reviewing the previous session, setting an agenda, working through the agenda items, setting homework, reviewing/summarizing the session, and eliciting feedback. The therapist will usually ask the client for a brief synopsis of the time since they last met, and as far as possible will try to enable a linking of both positive and negative experiences to thoughts and behaviors. For example, in one session when Sheryl's depression had moved from the severe to the moderate range, she attributed this change to 'being able to see the depressive thinking as a part of the depression rather than as a part of me.' A session would then review the homework from the previous session, again seeking to link progress or lack of progress to the therapy goals. For example, following session 1 Sheryl was asked to monitor her hour by hour activity, assigning mastery and pleasure scores (–5 to +5) to each activity. At the subsequent session Sheryl appeared demoralized and linked this to her diaries indicating that no event was associated with any mastery or pleasure. Having explored her meaning in more detail, this proved to be an opportunity to introduce the idea of depressive cognitive distortions (see Table 11.2): it became clear that she was discounting any positives (e.g., 'anyone can get their kids to school in the morning').

The session then moves on to the further agenda items. As they work through the items, the therapist and client seek to examine how the issues can be understood in terms of the cognitive formulation and how the issues relate to the therapeutic goals. Once there is a hypothesis about how the issue can be meaningfully understood, an appropriate intervention can be suggested. This is done collaboratively, with the therapist setting out the rationale and proceeding where there is a clear basis for collaboration. Sheryl's tendency to present a high functioning façade to her family was based on the belief 'If I tell them how I feel they will think I am weak.' Through collaborative empiricism and homework, it emerged that when Sheryl spoke to her husband about how she was feeling, he was understanding, amused (you're not as good at pretending as you think you are) and relieved (it emerged that he lived in fear he would return home to find her following a suicide attempt). This sort of collaborative empiricism provides the basis for socializing to the cognitive model and the beginnings of thought challenging. As the therapist and client work through the agenda items, the therapist makes use of frequent capsule summaries. These serve to ensure therapist and client agree about what has been said, provides a chance to review the session as it proceeds and build a strong therapeutic relationship. Because people with mood disorders experience negatively distorted thinking, they may see the therapy and the therapist in negative ways (e.g., Sheryl would often say, 'I don't deserve this help'). Capsule summaries can elicit these distortions and provide an opportunity to challenge this undermining negative thinking.

At the end of the session, the therapist asks the client for a summary of the session (e.g., 'What do you think you can take away from today's session that might be useful to you?'). The therapist and client agree homework that will move the client on towards his or her goals and problem solve any anticipated difficulties with the homework. Finally, the therapist asks for any feedback, both positive and negative, on the session (e.g., 'What did you like and not like about how today went so that we can ensure next time things are working well for you?').

A typical cognitive therapy for depression

This might comprise four phases. The first involves ensuring a sound therapeutic relationship, socializing the client to cognitive therapy and establishing the problem/goal list. The therapist aims for some symptom relief very early (preferably in session 1), to build a sense of hope about the therapeutic process. With Sheryl this early phase was quite straightforward

Table 11.2 Cognitive distortions

Distortion	Example
All-or-nothing thinking: the person sees things in black-and-white categories.	'My performance is not perfect, so I must be a total failure.'
Overgeneralization: the person sees a single negative event as a never ending pattern of defeat.	'I'm always messing up everything.'
Mental filter: the person picks out a single negative detail and dwells on it exclusively.	The person notices that s/he have put on a few pounds and thinks, 'I am overweight, I am horrible,' ignores other parts of their life—that they have a nice smile, people like them, they are holding down a job or raising a family.
Fortune telling: the person makes negative predictions about the future without realizing that the predictions may be inaccurate.	'I'll never get a job or have a relationship.'
Emotional reasoning: the person assumes that negative emotions necessarily reflect the way things are.	'I feel hopeless, therefore everything is hopeless.'
Shoulds, musts, and oughts: the person tries to motivate themself with shoulds and shouldn'ts, as if they had to be whipped and punished before they could be expected to do anything.	'I shouldn't sit here, I should clean the house.'
Personalization: the person sees themself as the cause of some negative external event, for which they in reality are not primarily responsible.	For example, if someone yells at you, you might think 'I did something wrong,' but maybe the other person is having a bad day or has a bad temper.
Discounting the positives: the person dismisses positive information about themselves or a situation.	For example, 'Being a mother who takes care of my kids is not an example of being capable because every mother does this.'

as she had been waiting some time to see a CBT therapist and had used this time to read a self-help book (*Mind over mood*, by Greenberger and Padesky, 1995) and to consider her goals for therapy. The CBT model made sense of her symptoms and this provided early relief from the experience of being overwhelmed by her symptoms. She also read several first person accounts of depression for people who suffer depression, which was helpful in making her feel less isolated and in countering some of her negative beliefs about depression (e.g., Lewis, 2002; McDonnell, 2003).*

The second phase involves behavioral strategies that will activate the client and begin to provide more significant symptom relief. This phase was more problematic because Sheryl tended to discount positive reinforcers and at difficult times passivity acted as a negative reinforcer. Changes in behavior for Sheryl operated in parallel with changes in beliefs. The third phase typically involves identifying and evaluating the client's thoughts and behaviors that are involved in maintaining the presenting problems. As appropriate, client and therapist work together to challenge maladaptive thought patterns (e.g., all-or-nothing thinking) and develop more adaptive ways of thinking. Similarly, maladaptive behaviors (e.g., avoidance) are identified, evaluated, and alternative behaviors are tried out. Sheryl described the main gains during this phase as a greater acceptance of 'the committee meeting in my mind,' regular use of thought records to break down and challenge negative thinking styles and the building up of alternative higher-order beliefs around 'self-as-capable.' An important aspect of this work involved dropping her high functioning façade and being able to ask for help when she needed it, and challenging the associated negative automatic thoughts ('they'll think I'm pathetic'). The third and final phase of therapy focuses on relapse prevention. The goal of cognitive therapy is to enable clients to 'become their own cognitive therapist,' anticipating problematic situations, challenging their maladaptive thinking in these situations and experimenting with new and more adaptive ways of thinking and behaving. The therapist increasingly assumes the role of consultant to the 'client cognitive therapist,' reviewing what *the client learned* in therapy, reinforcing the client's effective problem solving, supporting the client in preparing for setbacks and supporting the client with learning effective problem-solving skills. Sessions tend to become less frequent and discontinue as the client and therapist have confidence that the therapeutic goals have substantively been attained and the client has the cognitive and behavioral skills to manage both everyday and anticipated future problems. The CBT case formulation should enable a good prediction of what future difficulties are most likely to prove problematic. This is used to rehearse how the client might manage these difficulties and thereby prevent future relapse if these difficulties occur.

Behavioral approaches to mood disorders are further elaborated in BA for depression (see: Martell *et al.*, 2001). Practically, BA focuses on the context and functions of thoughts and behaviors rather than their form or content. The formulation for any client will be focused on variability and situatedness rather than stability, examining what differences in environment and behavior influence the client's feelings and their success at achieving goals. Every session the client and therapist will monitor the relationship between situation/action and mood and do a fine-grained analysis of day-to-day activity as it relates to mood.

For example, when making plans, it is useful to ask questions such as 'Under what conditions have you failed and under what conditions have you not failed?', and use the information arising to manipulate situational contingencies to maximize success. Similarly, when dealing with negative thoughts, BA focuses on their context and consequences rather than challenging them directly. Thus, if the thought 'I'm a failure' regularly

occurs when a client is faced with a potentially difficult situation and has the consequence of stopping her from approaching and dealing with the situation, it may be hypothesized that the thought has the conditioned function of avoiding risk. In BA, a core aspect of therapy involves identifying these avoidance patterns, using the mnemonic TRAP (Trigger, Response, Avoidance Pattern) and coaching clients to get back on track by developing alternative coping using the mnemonic TRAC (Trigger, Response, Alternative Coping). In this case, the alternative coping would be to approach the feared situation despite the presence of the thought.

Changes in routine, such as sleeping late in the day, missing meals, and changes in patterns of social contact, can further maintain depressed mood, and, therefore, BA focuses on building clients back into more regular routines. To reduce passive coping and to increase awareness of the effects of behaviors on outcome, clients are encouraged to be proactive. In particular, clients are coached to act in line with their goals rather than their feelings. For example, if the goal was to have better self-esteem, the behaviors associated with better self-esteem would be determined in detail, e.g., more assertive, more eye contact, more erect and dignified posture, and plans made for the client to act out these behaviors as if they had better self-esteem. Clients are given the rationale that it is easier and faster to change their actions, over which they have direct control, which may in turn influence their feelings (to change from the 'outside-in'), than to change their feelings in order to act differently (e.g., acting when it feels right, i.e., from the 'inside-out'). Clients are encouraged to divorce action from their mood state and to learn that they rather than their mood can control their actions by acting even when they don't feel like acting.

Throughout BA, the mnemonic 'ACTION' is used to focus clients on the key principles:

Assess the function and context of a behavior

Choose to activate or avoid

Try out behavior chosen

Integrate behavior into a routine

Observe the outcome of the behavior

Never give up.

In BA the first sessions will be used to socialize into the model, provide a rationale and establish rapport. The main body of the sessions will use whatever behavioral approaches are appropriate to the idiosyncratic functional analysis of each client. The final sessions will work on relapse prevention by reviewing what has been learnt, reviewing patterns of avoidance identified and drawing up a response plan to maintain activation strategies.

Cognitive therapy for bipolar disorder: key practice principles

CBT for bipolar disorder adapts the classic cognitive therapy approach for depression in several ways (see: Basco *et al.*, 1996; Lam *et al.*, 2000). First, there is psychoeducation explaining the diathesis-stress model, outlining the joint role of medication and psychological treatment in reducing acute episodes. Therapists help clients to recognize that bipolar disorder involves a biological vulnerability, perhaps in the form of heritable changes in brain chemistry, which interact with stress to produce episodes of mania or depression. Cognitive therapy is emphasized as a means of reducing stress by learning improved coping skills and through testing personal perceptions that can themselves be stressful (e.g., self-critical thoughts).

Second, clients are taught self-monitoring and self-regulation skills, with an emphasis on identification and early recognition of prodromes and development of good coping strategies in response to prodromes. An idiosyncratic evaluation of early, late, and middle warning signs of an impending episode are drawn up with each client and useful coping plans made for each symptom. Encouraging clients to keep daily activity schedules and mood charts can be very helpful in facilitating effective self-monitoring, and ensuring that potential episodes are caught early enough.

---

* When recommended thoughtfully to clients (and therapists), these books can greatly increase understanding and hope by illustrating the feelings, thoughts, behaviors, and somatic features that make up 'the territory of depression.' Clients find them compelling because they are written by people who have experienced mood disorders first hand. For example, Gwyneth Lewis writes of her depression: 'Under the duvet, an internal ice age had set in. I had permafrost around my heart. This is what dying of cold must be like, once the numbness has started (Lewis, 2002, p. 1).

Typical prodromes for mania include reduced sleep/need for sleep, increased goal-directed activity, reduced anxiety, increased optimism, irritability, increased libido, increased sociability, racing thoughts, and distractibility. Typical prodromes for depression include reduced interest in people or activities, feeling sad or depressed, disturbed sleep, tiredness, low motivation, increased worry, and poor concentration. For mania prodromes, engaging in calming activities, increasing rest, reducing stimulation and decreasing activity would be useful strategies, whereas increasing levels of activity, enjoying the 'high', and 'making up for lost time' would be unhelpful strategies likely to increase the risk of a full-blown manic episode. Similarly, for depression prodromes, keeping busy and maintaining routines are associated with better outcomes, while cutting down on activities, withdrawing from other people and going to bed are associated with worse outcomes. For each client, an individual case formulation is required to determine the idiosyncratic prodromes and the most functional responses, as there is a great degree of individual variability. For example, some clients report changes in sensory experiences, such as colors becoming brighter or noises sharper, or increased pleasure at the sensation of moving at speed, when they are becoming hypomanic. For such clients, behavioral plans would need to modulate their experience of such sensations, e.g., pacing their exposure to stimulating environments such as art galleries, museums, shopping malls, and temporarily reducing travel by car, plane, or train.

Third, behavioral plans are made to promote good sleep and good daily routine, in recognition of the evidence that disruptions in sleep and working routine are implicated in the onset of bipolar episodes (Healy and Williams, 1989; Malkoff-Schwartz et al., 1998). Maintaining regular times to go to bed and get up, as well as meal times, can significantly help to stabilize mood. Clients learn to balance their activity schedules, not to do too much or too little, and to pace their own activities. The role of social activity needs to be carefully monitored and paced—social withdrawal is a warning sign for depression, while increased social contact can be overstimulating and feed into the development of mania. The roles of medication, substance, and alcohol use also need to be explored in detail with clients as potential risk factors for episodes. For a number of clients, discontinuation of their mood stabilizer is associated with the recurrence of a bipolar episode, as is very apparent from reviewing their life history—for these clients, explicit recognition of what their own experience tells them about the effectiveness of medication can be very productive. Given the high rates of alcohol and substance abuse in bipolar disorder, close monitoring of usage and explicit plans to keep use to a level that is not associated with the spiraling of mood is also important. As with all plans with bipolar clients, such plans need to be arrived at collaboratively and from an open exploration of the advantages/disadvantages of the options.

Fourth, as in CBT for unipolar depression, therapists challenge unhelpful automatic thoughts and clients use Daily Thought Records. However, as well as challenging negative thoughts associated with depression, therapists can also challenge excessively positive thoughts that may be involved in the development of mania. When focusing on hypomanic thoughts, it is important to be open, giving clients plenty of autonomy in their responses, as well as to review with clients the consequences of hypomanic thoughts, in order to overcome reluctance to dwell on positive thoughts. For example, clients can be taught to examine grandiose thoughts such as 'I know better than everyone else' and check whether these thoughts accurately reflect their past experience, and whether such thoughts are dependent upon their mood. Similarly, clients can be encouraged to examine the longer-term costs and benefits of their more-impulsive and grandiose thoughts. For example, questions such as 'How many of your ideas still seem a good idea a week later? If this is genuinely a good idea, it should still be a good idea next week. Can you try and leave it for a week?' can help to reduce impulsivity.

It is useful here to explore client's ambivalence about their manic episodes—many bipolar clients experience the initial stages of mania as positive, as they are no longer depressed, feel more confident, have more energy, and are more creative, but also report that more extreme mania is distressing because they feel out of control, act in self-destructive ways, and, in some cases, experience extreme anxiety and/or unpleasant psychotic experiences. As the cognitive model would expect, however, the information processing biases afforded by the hypomania mean that clients tend to focus on the positives of their mood state and forget the negative experience of the mania. Exploring both sides of the mania with clients in a Socratic way can be very helpful for facilitating rapport and for helping clients maintain the perspective necessary to motivate themselves to maintain therapy plans during an incipient hypomania.

Finally, as in standard CBT, therapy works to challenge dysfunctional assumptions that increase risk of relapse. Bipolar clients display the same dysfunctional assumptions as clients with unipolar major depression in the context of a depressed episode. However, bipolar clients also have more idiosyncratic assumptions centering on highly driven and extreme goal-attainment beliefs, e.g., 'I should be happy all the time', 'If I put in enough effort, I should be able to achieve everything I want'. Bipolar clients with these attitudes are more likely to engage in extreme goal-pursuing behavior ('trying to make up for lost time'), which is likely to disrupt their sleep and daily routines precipitating further episodes. Cognitive therapy can identify such beliefs collaboratively with clients and then explore how realistic and useful such beliefs are. Final sessions can also productively explore the losses and stigma that clients have incurred as a result of their illness and help clients to work through these issues, by grieving for these losses and developing more functional views. As the losses and stigma associated with bipolar disorder are genuine, Socratic questions more helpfully focus on people's approach to this reality (e.g., 'What constructive lessons can I learn from my past?' 'How can I go forwards from here in a way that makes my life worthwhile?'), rather than by challenging the evidence for the losses. Clients' own self-stigma can be challenged, particularly the relatively common beliefs that they are defective. Such beliefs often arose during adolescence when clients had difficult relationships with family and peers, as a consequence of mood swings that occur as the first manifestation of the illness. It is particularly helpful to refocus clients on their strengths and to encourage them to consider and pay attention to the multiple roles they occupy (e.g., parent, son, friend, worker) rather than exclusively focus on the label of bipolar disorder.

Difficult situations, challenges, and what to do about them

In this section, we will briefly consider what to do when faced with some of the most common difficulties and challenges that occur during CBT for depression, particularly when it is severe, chronic, and recurrent.

Suicide and hopelessness

Suicidal thoughts, intentions, and suicidal attempts are common in depression and contribute to the significant mortality associated with depression (Brown et al., 2000). Furthermore, suicidal impulses fluctuate greatly and can rapidly and powerfully emerge in clients to even apparently minor setbacks. Thus, therapists need to be constantly alert for suicidal thoughts and plans, and for the concomitant hopelessness and sense of being trapped that often develops into suicidal thinking. Expressions suggestive of suicidal intent such as 'I can't take it any more', 'It is all pointless', changes in affect, such as increased calmness and resignation, and changes in behavior such as increased secretiveness should be explored. The Beck Hopelessness Scale provides an excellent measure of suicide risk and scores of 8 and above are associated with significantly increased risk of suicide attempts as well as eventual suicide (A. T. Beck et al., 1989). Suicidal intent and plans need to be directly and explicitly discussed with the client.

The first step in dealing with suicidal intent is to minimize the immediate risk of a suicide attempt. Reducing the risk will involve understanding the motives for wanting to attempt suicide. Typical motives include wanting to escape a situation that is perceived as intolerable and never going to change and/or attempting to engineer some interpersonal response, whether it be a 'cry for help' or an impulsive attempt to hurt others. Once the therapist and client are able to discuss the possible reasons for wanting to attempt suicide, with the therapist empathizing with the client's position, it is then possible to explore whether the situation is as intolerable and unchangeable as perceived. Socratic questioning can instill hope by helping clients to see that there might be alternative interpretations of their situation and that they have alternative options to deal with the problem. Drawing out both reasons for dying and reasons for living, including the advantages and disadvantages of each option, can help to produce a more objective view of the situation.

The most important practical step at this juncture is to work with clients on reducing their access to the means of killing themselves (e.g., pills, guns, etc.). As many suicidal attempts are impulsive, the simple expedient of removing the means significantly increases survival rates. A close analysis of previous attempts at suicide can reveal the series of events that escalate into a suicide attempt, and help to identify the decision points and key contingencies to target with further behavioral plans. For example, for many clients, the decision to try to reduce negative feelings through drugs or alcohol can be a critical step towards suicidal behavior. The therapeutic relationship is also an important tool, with therapists trying to keep clients involved and curious about the process of therapy and maintaining continuity between sessions, perhaps by explicitly asking the client to agree to not harm themselves in that time.

Once there is some progress at helping clients to consider the possibility of alternative views of their difficult situation, the next step is to facilitate problem solving in order to reduce the crisis or difficulties that contribute to the hopelessness. Problem solving is typically impaired in suicidal and depressed clients, and, thus, explicit attempts to define problems in specific detail and to work on generating alternative responses can be powerful.

Client does not respond to cognitive-behavioral therapy

As an active empirical therapy, it is important for therapists to monitor their client's progress—if after four to eight sessions of CBT, there seems to be no improvement, a comprehensive review is necessary. Several factors could conspire to impair improvement. First, the client may not be convinced by attempts at thought challenging. It is essential to check whether clients experience any changes in belief and emotion following a discussion of their thoughts. If there is no change, the therapist needs to explore what is maintaining the client's negative beliefs and what doubt's or objections he or she has about alternative interpretations or disconfirming evidence. It is also important to check that the challenging of thoughts is both emotive and experiential: that is, clients have their 'hot' cognitions activated, and the exploration of evidence and alternatives draws richly on their own personal experience rather than on dry abstractions. Second, it may be that the therapist is not being flexible enough and not selecting the approaches that best match the idiosyncratic concerns and abilities of the client. The more therapy can reflect and build from the client's own way of speaking, thinking, and acting, the more likely it is to be meaningful and helpful to the client.

Third, therapy may not work if it is not focused on the core problem or appropriate mechanisms identified in the formulation or if the formulation is incorrect. Careful assessment and formulation can help to avoid this difficulty and can remedy such an impasse when it occurs. However, depressed clients can be avoidant and find it difficult to share important information with a therapist because they find it shaming or have little trust of others. Turning to the example of Sheryl, there was little improvement in mood over the first six sessions, which focused on behavioral change with the intention of preparing her to return to work, even though she was making progress on this goal. Only in session 6 following the increased stress occasioned by her daughter's acting out and cutting, did Sheryl disclose her father's suicide when she was herself a teenager and the way that she felt shame and responsibility for his suicide. Her interpretations of this event and its implications for Sheryl's ongoing relationships (e.g., compliant, fearful of tipping others over the edge, perception of herself as weak and a burden) seemed central to her depression. Only when the formulation took

into account this information did therapy begin to focus on core issues underlying her low self-worth.

Beliefs and thoughts of the therapist

The cognitions of the therapist are important in the progress of therapy, and, often, difficulties in therapy will be associated with, and exacerbated by unhelpful therapist thoughts. Unhelpful thoughts include therapists becoming too pessimistic about clients, therapists making negative interpretations of clients such as blaming them for not getting better, the therapist having self-critical thoughts about their own competence, and therapists having underlying assumptions of their own activated in therapy. It is important that therapists monitor their own thoughts and spend time reviewing them before and after therapy sessions, both individually, and, where possible, in supervision.

Past history of trauma or abuse

Depression is often associated with a past history of abuse or experience of trauma (Hill, 2003). Recent evidence suggests that CBT adapted for people with people with chronic depression and a history of early abuse is efficacious and superior to pharmacotherapy alone (Nemeroff et al., 2003). Histories of abuse can often lead to emotions such as shame and humiliation (see later section for more detail). Where clients have comorbid PTSD, adapting CBT for this disorder may make treatment more effective. Sheryl had distressing intrusive images of when her ex-husband raped her, which she found scary and shaming. Teaching her coping skills such as relaxation to deal with the strong feelings that accompanied these memories helped Sheryl to feel more confident about confronting these issues. The use of imaginal exposure coupled with cognitive restructuring was then used to work through and process the upsetting events.

Interpersonal difficulties

Clients with chronic and severe depression often have difficulties with other people, including oversensitivity to other's responses, avoidant social behavior (e.g., reduced eye contact, submissive posture), passivity, anger, defensiveness, reduced assertiveness, and overly aggressive assertiveness. Furthermore, people with depression can elicit interpersonal cycles that maintain and accentuate their problems (Hammen, 2003). Therapists should be keenly tuned into how this might arise in the therapeutic relationship and seek to use this as further 'grist to the mill' for the cognitive-behavioral approach. For example, with Sheryl the therapist needed to monitor the risk of becoming overly controlling when Sheryl's behavior became passive and dependent. Skillfully noting these behavioral patterns, formulating the contingencies, and adopting an approach that leads to desired behavioral outcomes can provide a vehicle for change (McCullough, 2000). Furthermore, skillful use of feedback and capsule summaries will help develop a more accurate collaborative formulation of interpersonal-related cognitions and provide an opportunity to identify possible misinterpretations that therapists and clients are making.

Therapy also provides a forum for clients to practice changes in interpersonal behavior in a relatively safe environment, for example, less social avoidance, increased assertiveness, and disclosure of difficult feelings such as anger and self-hatred. Empathic, nonjudgmental yet ecologically valid responses from the therapist to these changes in behavior can be powerful learning experiences for clients, for example, discovering that one can be angry with someone else without them hating you. With Sheryl, a lot of her interpersonal difficulties came from finding it difficult to express her concerns and feelings to others. In her childhood, her parents had tended to discourage her from expressing her feelings and respond negatively when she did, to the extent that when her father killed himself, it strongly reinforced and exacerbated Sheryl's views that she should not express her feelings. With her teenage daughter, this meant that Sheryl was loath to express concerns and lay down rules, which in turn, led to further unhappiness when her daughter's behavior became unmanageable. Therapy focused on building up more assertive behaviors from Sheryl.

Common difficult themes: low self-esteem, self-hatred, shame, and humiliation

Many depressed clients suffer from an underlying negative view of the self, accompanied by destructive emotions such as shame and humiliation (Gilbert *et al.*, 1996). These negative self-evaluations and the associated intense emotions are distressing to clients and often lead to interpersonal difficulties and dysfunctional behavior, by sapping motivation, increasing sensitivity to criticism, and by increasing passivity, avoidance and concealment. These difficulties will be manifest in therapy, interfering with forward therapeutic momentum. The depressed client who has an exaggerated sense of inferiority such as Sheryl (e.g., 'self-as-weak,' 'Others think I am despicable,' 'I am worse than everyone else') may well be loath to openly discuss their thoughts and feelings with a therapist, as this will be perceived as another shaming situation, confirming her personal inadequacy.

Low self-esteem is an overlapping construct with shame. In CBT, low self-esteem has been usefully conceptualized as a global negative self-judgment, which is further maintained by the adoption of dysfunctional rules of living, typically extreme rules for self-validation (e.g., 'I need to do everything perfectly'), which in turn lead to unhelpful compensatory behaviors, such as avoidance, concealment of feelings and overvigilance for success and failure. With Sheryl, her extreme rules included 'I need to make sure everyone else is happy' 'I should avoid upsetting other people at all costs', leading to a hypervigilance for other people's emotional responses and a lack of assertiveness.

Similar treatment issues arise for shame, humiliation, and low self-esteem. First, the therapist has to be sensitive to the potential effects of their choice of words and their nonverbal body language on clients who are highly sensitive to perceived criticism and likely to respond defensively. The client's concerns and sense of shame/inferiority needs to be gently explored, with an implicit recognition and explicit acknowledgment that she may be keeping upsetting or shaming material back and may find it difficult to talk about certain events. Rather than forcing a client to talk about these difficult themes directly, it may be more useful to look at her predictions about what would happen if she disclosed her 'secrets', and to respond with empathic reflections about how difficult or painful she must be finding this. With Sheryl, she predicted that expressing how she really felt and talking about what had happened to her, would lead to other people rejecting her. Talking about her father's suicide and the rape by her ex-husband tested this belief in the session.

Behaviors maintaining low self-esteem and shame can be identified (e.g., looking out for failure rather than for success; safety behaviors that prevent clients from discovering that they are okay just being themselves) and reduced, and, in contrast, more positive behaviors encouraged. The advantages and disadvantages of holding on to feelings of shame and humiliation can also be discussed, particularly in reference to getting revenge.

For all these themes, particular techniques may be helpful: (1) using a positive data-log so that the client is deliberately focusing and recording their positive qualities, positive interactions, and positive achievements every day, to counterbalance their bias towards negative views of the self, and (2) reviewing evidence for and against the negative view of the self, particularly through behavioral experiments and through a detailed life review in which periods of the client's past are examined to see if there is any evidence against the negative view of themselves or alternative interpretations for negative events that previously supported the sense of worthlessness. With Sheryl, a detailed examination of her childhood and adolescence helped to generate alternative explanations for her parents lack of emotional warmth and support for her: (1) they were overwhelmed with caring for her siblings, including her older brother who suffered from cerebral palsy, and (2) her father and possibly also her mother were suffering from depression themselves. Examples of when she had close emotionally-open relationships with people were used to counter her negative self-beliefs—e.g., her close school friend, her good relationship with her grandmother. In the same way, the various factors contributing to her father's suicide could be more objectively evaluated. Such interventions often require experiential approaches including imagery and role-play and sessions need to be organized that there is sufficient time for intense emotions to settle before the session finished. Other useful approaches might include helping clients to focus on being compassionate and forgiving towards themselves.

Future directions

The last three decades have seen CBT for mood disorders develop as a treatment of choice for unipolar depression and a promising intervention for bipolar disorder. We would predict that the next 25 years will see a range of exciting developments in CBT research and practice. In the area of outcome research, the most obvious area for advancement is where promising initial research suggests that CBT may prove to be an evidence-based approach: depression that is comorbid with personality disorders, PTSD, and substance misuse, dysthymia and bipolar disorder. Similarly, psychotherapy outcome research is needed to examine how cognitive therapy fares when it is adapted to different populations (e.g., older adults) and to different service settings (e.g., primary care). As we increasingly recognize depression as a potentially chronic relapsing condition, efforts to address depression in young people are urgently required. Given the scale of depression as a public health problem (Murray and Lopez, 1997), alternative formats (e.g., Internet-facilitated group therapy) are required.

In a climate of managed health care, evidence-based practice, and practice guidelines, researchers, practitioners, and policy makers are increasingly asking the question 'What works best for whom?'. Beyond the comparative outcome studies, this sets the stage for interesting psychotherapy process and psychotherapy process outcome research. The mechanisms by which cognitive therapy is effective are not well understood, and this research will inform practice and health care policy. The stepped care approach to planning services and interventions is likely to be important here, as we become increasingly knowledgeable about what works for whom and through what mechanism. Cognitive therapy for depression is amenable to contemporary stepped care approaches, whereby clients are assessed and offered increasingly specialized, intensive, and complex interventions based on an algorithm of clinical need and optimal cost-effectiveness. Using the range of established cognitive therapy approaches, steps might graduate from bibliotherapy (Jamison and Scogin, 1995), to computer-based approaches (Wright *et al.*, 2002), to brief psychoeducational approaches in primary care, to brief group approaches in secondary care to more in depth and extended individual or group cognitive therapy in either secondary or tertiary care (DeRubeis and Crits-Christoph, 1998).

The recent focus on primary and secondary prevention of mood disorders is welcome and there is much mileage in building on initial successes (e.g., Jaycox *et al.*, 1994; Segal *et al.*, 2002). The acceptability of cognitive therapy to many children and adolescents with depression and to people with recurrent depression combined with an increasing acknowledgment that primary and secondary prevention are high priority healthcare areas suggests we are likely to see much innovative and important work in this area.

Cognitive therapy is established as a mainstream psychotherapy of choice and training, supervision and accreditation are areas that require further development that extends and builds on existing best practice. There is an increasing body of cognitive therapy practitioners and researchers who are well placed to continue this work.

Suggested further reading

Beck, A. T., Rush, A. J., Shaw, B. F., and Emery, G. (1979). *Cognitive therapy of depression*. New York: Guilford Press.

Beck, J. S. (1995). *Cognitive therapy: basics and beyond*. New York: Guilford Press.

Bieling, P. J. and Kuyken, W. (2003). Is cognitive case formulation science or science fiction? *Clinical Psychology: Science and Practice*, **10**, 52–69.

Clark, D. A., Beck, A. T., and Alford, B. A. (1999). *Scientific foundations of cognitive theory and therapy of depression*. New York: Wiley.

Hamilton, K. E. and Dobson, K. S. (2002). Cognitive therapy of depression: pretreatment patient predictors of outcome. *Clinical Psychology Review*, **22**, 875–93.

Martell, C., Addis, M., and Jacobson, N. (2001). *Depression in context: strategies for guided action*. New York: Norton.

McCullough, J. P. (2000). *Treatment for chronic depression: cognitive behavioral analysis system of psychotherapy*. New York: Guilford Press.

Moore, R. G. and Garland, A. (2003). *Cognitive therapy for chronic and persistent depression*. Chichester: Wiley.

Newman, C. F., Leahy, R. L., Beck, A. T., Reilly-Harrington, N. A., and Gyulai, L. (2002). *Bipolar disorder: a cognitive therapy approach*. Washington, DC: American Psychological Association.

Segal, Z. V., Williams, J. M. G., and Teasdale, J. D. (2002). *Mindfulness-based cognitive therapy for depression: a new approach to preventing relapse*. New York: Guilford Press.

References

American Psychiatric Association (1994). *Diagnostic and statistical manual of mental disorders*, 4th edn (revised edn). Washington, DC: American Psychiatric Association.

Arnow, B. A. and Constantino, M. J. (2003). Effectiveness of psychotherapy and combination treatment for chronic depression. *Journal of Clinical Psychology*, **59**, 893–905.

Barber, J. P. and DeRubeis, R. J. (1989). On second thoughts: where the action is in cognitive therapy. *Cognitive Therapy and Research*, **13**, 441–57.

Barber, J. P. and Muenz, L. R. (1996). The role of avoidance and obsessiveness in matching patients to cognitive and interpersonal psychotherapy. Empirical findings from the treatment for depression collaborative research program. *Journal of Consulting and Clinical Psychology*, **64**, 951–8.

Basco, M. R. and Rush, A. J. (1996). *Cognitive-behavioral therapy for bipolar disorder*. New York: Guilford Press.

Beck, A. T. (1976a). *Cognitive therapy and emotional disorders*. New York: Meridian.

Beck, A. T. (1976b). *Cognitive therapy and emotional disorders*. New York: International Universities Press.

Beck, A. T. (1996). Beyond belief: a theory of modes, personality and psychopathology. In: P. M. Salkovskis, ed. *Frontiers of cognitive therapy*, pp. 1–25. New York: Guilford Press.

Beck, A. T., Rush, A. J., Shaw, B. F., and Emery, G. (1979). *Cognitive therapy of depression*. New York: Guilford Press.

Beck, A. T., Brown, G., and Steer, R. A. (1989). Prediction of eventual suicide in psychiatric-inpatients by clinical ratings of hopelessness. *Journal of Consulting and Clinical Psychology*, **57**, 309–10.

Beck, J. S. (1995). *Cognitive therapy: basics and beyond*. New York: Guilford Press.

Bieling, P. J. and Kuyken, W. (2003). Is cognitive case formulation science or science fiction? *Clinical Psychology: Science and Practice*, **10**, 52–69.

Blackburn, I. M. and Moore, R. G. (1997). Controlled acute and follow-up trial of cognitive therapy and pharmacotherapy in out-patients with recurrent depression. *British Journal of Psychiatry*, **171**, 328–34.

Blackburn, I. M., Bishop, S., Glen, A. I. M., Whalley, L. J., and Christie, J. E. (1981). The efficacy of cognitive therapy in depression—a treatment trial using cognitive therapy and pharmacotherapy, each alone and in combination. *British Journal of Psychiatry*, **139**, 181–9.

Bond, F. W. and Dryden, W. (2002). *Handbook of brief cognitive behaviour therapy*. Chichester: Wiley.

Brown, G. K., Beck, A. T., Steer, R. A., and Grisham, J. R. (2000). Risk factors for suicide in psychiatric outpatients: a 20 year prospective study. *Journal of Consulting and Clinical Psychology*, **68**, 371–7.

Burns, D. D. and Nolen-Hoeksema, S. (1991). Coping styles, homework, compliance and the effectiveness of cognitve-behavioural therapy. *Journal of Consulting and Clinical Psychology*, **59**, 305–11.

Burns, D. D. and Spangler, D. L. (2000). Does psychotherapy homework lead to improvements in depression in cognitive behavioral therapy or does improvement lead to increased homework compliance? *Journal of Consulting and Clinical Psychology*, **68**, 46–56.

Butler, G. (1998). Clinical formulation. In: A. S. Bellack and M. Hersen, ed. *Comprehensive clinical psychology*, pp. 1–24. New York: Pergamon Press.

Clark, D. A., Beck, A. T., and Alford, B. A. (1999). *Scientific foundations of cognitive theory and therapy of depression*. New York: Wiley.

Dent, J. and Teasdale, J. D. (1988). Negative cognition and the persistence of depression. *Journal of Abnormal Psychology*, **97**, 29–34.

DeRubeis, R. J. and Crits-Christoph, P. (1998). Empirically supported individual and group psychological treatments for adult mental disorders. *Journal of Consulting and Clinical Psychology*, **66**, 37–52.

DeRubeis, R. J. and Feeley, M. (1990). Determinants of change in cognitive therapy for depression. *Cognitive Therapy and Research*, **14**, 469–82.

DeRubeis, R. J., *et al.* (1990). How does cognitive therapy work—cognitive change and symptom change in cognitive therapy and pharmacotherapy for depression. *Journal of Consulting and Clinical Psychology*, **58**, 862–9.

DeRubeis, R. J., Gelfand, L. A., Tang, T. Z., and Simons, A. D. (1999). Medications versus cognitive behavior therapy for severely depressed outpatients: mega-analysis of four randomized comparisons. *American Journal of Psychiatry*, **156**, 1007–13.

Detweiler, J. and Whisman, M. A. (1999). The role of homework assignments in cognitive therapy for depression: potential methods for enhancing adherence. *Clinical Psychology: Science and Practice*, **6**, 267.

Dobson, K. S. (1989). A meta-analysis of the efficacy of cognitive therapy for depression. *Journal of Consulting and Clinical Psychology*, **57**, 414–19.

Elkin, I., *et al.* (1989). National Institute Of Mental Health Treatment of Depression Collaborative Research Program—general effectiveness of treatments. *Archives of General Psychiatry*, **46**, 971–82.

Evans, M. D., *et al.* (1992). Differential relapse following cognitive therapy and pharmacotherapy for depression. *Archives of General Psychiatry*, **49**, 802–8.

Fava, G. A., Grandi, S., Zielezny, M., Canestrari, R., and Morphy, M. A. (1994). Cognitive-behavioral treatment of residual symptoms in primary major depressive disorder. *American Journal of Psychiatry*, **151**, 1295–9.

Fava, G. A., Grandi, S., Zielezny, M., Rafanelli, C., and Canestrari, R. (1996). Four-year outcome for cognitive behavioral treatment of residual symptoms in major depression. *American Journal of Psychiatry*, **153**, 945–7.

Fava, G. A., Rafanelli, C., Grandi, S., Canestrari, R., and Morphy, M. A. (1998). Six-year outcome for cognitive behavioral treatment of residual symptoms in major depression. *American Journal of Psychiatry*, **155**, 1443–5.

Ferster, C. B. (1973). A functional analysis of depression. *American Psychologist*, **28**, 857–70.

Fombonne, E., Wostear, G., Cooper, V., Harrington, R., and Rutter, M. (2001). The Maudsley long-term follow-up of child and adolescent depression 1. Psychiatric outcomes in adulthood. *British Journal of Psychiatry*, **179**, 210–17.

Gilbert, P., Allan, S., and Goss, K. (1996). Parental representations, shame interpersonal problems, and vulnerability to psychopathology. *Clinical Psychology and Psychotherapy*, **3**, 23–34.

Gloaguen, V., Cottraux, J., Cucherat, M., and Blackburn, I. M. (1998). A meta-analysis of the effects of cognitive therapy in depressed patients. *Journal of Affective Disorders*, **49**, 59–72.

Gortner, E. T., Gollan, J. K., Dobson, K. S., and Jacobson, N. S. (1998). Cognitive-behavioral treatment for depression: relapse prevention. *Journal of Consulting and Clinical Psychology*, **66**, 377–84.

Greenberger, D. and Padesky, C. A. (1995). *Mind over mood: change how you feel by changing the way you think*. New York: Guilford Press.

Hamilton, K. E. and Dobson, K. S. (2002). Cognitive therapy of depression: pretreatment patient predictors of outcome. *Clinical Psychology Review*, **22**, 875–93.

Hammen, C. (2003). Interpersonal stress and depression in women. *Journal of Affective Disorders*, **74**, 49–57.

Healy, D. and Williams, J. M. G. (1989). Moods, misattributions and mania—an interaction of biological and psychological factors in the pathogenesis of mania. *Psychiatric Developments*, **7**, 49–70.

Hill, J. (2003). Childhood trauma and depression. *Current Opinion in Psychiatry*, **16**, 3–6.

Hollon, S. D., *et al.* (1992). Cognitive therapy and pharmacotherapy for depression—singly and in combination. *Archives of General Psychiatry*, **49**, 774–81.

Hopko, D. R., Lejuez, C. W., Ruggiero, K. J., and Eifert, G. H. (2003). Contemporary behavioral activation treatments for depression: procedures, principles, and progress. *Clinical Psychology Review*, **23**, 699–717.

Imber, S. D., *et al.* (1990). Mode-specific effects among 3 treatments for depression. *Journal of Consulting and Clinical Psychology*, **58**, 352–9.

Ingram, R. E., Miranda, J., and Segal, Z. V. (1998). *Cognitive vulnerability to depression*. New York: Guilford Press.

Jacobson, *et al.* (1996). A component analysis of cognitive-behavioral treatment for depression. *Journal of Consulting and Clinical Psychology*, **64**, 295–304.

Jacobson, N. S., Martell, C. R., and Dimidjian, S. (2001). Behavioral activation treatment for depression: returning to contextual roots. *Clinical Psychology: Science and Practice*, **8**, 255–70.

Jamison, C. and Scogin, F. (1995). The outcome of cognitive bibliotherapy with depressed adults. *Journal of Consulting and Clinical Psychology*, **63**, 644–50.

Jarrett, R. B., Eaves, G. G., Grannemann, B. D., and Rush, A. J. (1991). Clinical, cognitive, and demographic predictors of response to cognitive therapy for depression—a preliminary report. *Psychiatry Research*, **37**, 245–60.

Jarrett, R. B., *et al.* (1999). Treatment of atypical depression with cognitive therapy or phenelzine—A double-blind, placebo-controlled trial. *Archives of General Psychiatry*, **56**, 431–7.

Jaycox, L. H., Reivich, K. J., Gillham, J., and Seligman, M. E. P. (1994). Prevention of depressive symptoms in school children. *Behavioural Research and Therapy*, **32**, 801–16.

Judd, L. L. (1997a). Prevalence, correlates, and course of minor depression and major depression in the national comorbidity survey—Discussion. *Journal of Affective Disorders*, **45**, 28–9.

Judd, L. L. (1997b). The clinical course of unipolar major depressive disorders. *Archives of General Psychiatry*, **54**, 989–91.

Kabat-Zinn, J. (1990). *Full catastrophe living: how to cope with stress, pain and illness using mindfulness meditation*. New York: Delacorte.

Keller, M. B., *et al.* (2000). A comparison of nefazodone, the cognitive behavioral-analysis system of psychotherapy, and their combination for the treatment of chronic depression. *New England Journal of Medicine*, **342**, 1462–70.

Kovacs, M., Rush, A. J., Beck, A. T., and Hollon, S. D. (1981). Depressed outpatients treated with cognitive therapy or pharmacotherapy—a one-year follow-up. *Archives of General Psychiatry*, **38**, 33–9.

Kuyken, W., Kurzer, N., DeRubeis, R. J., Beck, A. T., and Brown, G. K. (2001). Response to cognitive therapy in depression: The role of maladaptive beliefs and personality disorders. *Journal of Consulting and Clinical Psychology*, **69**, 560–6.

Lam, D. H., *et al.* (2000). Cognitive therapy for bipolar illness—a pilot study of relapse prevention. *Cognitive Therapy and Research*, **24**, 503–20.

Lam, D., Wong, G., and Sham, P. (2001). Prodromes, coping strategies and course of illness in bipolar affective disorder—a naturalistic study. *Psychological Medicine*, **31**, 1397–402.

Lam, D. H., *et al.* (2003). A randomized controlled study of cognitive therapy for relapse prevention for bipolar affective disorder—outcome of the first year. *Archives of General Psychiatry*, **60**, 145–52.

Leichsenring, F. (2001). Comparative effects of short-term psychodynamic psychotherapy and cognitve-behavioural therapy in depression: a meta-analytic approach. *Clinical Psychology Review*, **21**, 401–19.

Lewis, G. (2002). *Sunbathing in the rain: a cheerful book about depression*. London: Falmingo, Harper Collins.

Linehan, M. M. (1993). *Cognitive-behavioral treatment of borderline personality disorder*. New York: Guilford Press.

Malkoff-Schwartz, S., *et al.* (1998). Stressful life events and social rhythm disruption in the onset of manic and depressive bipolar episodes—A preliminary investigation. *Archives of General Psychiatry*, **55**, 702–7.

Martell, C. R., Addis, M. E., and Jacobson, N. S. (2001). *Depression in context: strategies for guided action*. New York: Norton.

McCullough, J. P. (2000). *Treatment for chronic depression: cognitive behavioural analysis system of psychotherapy*. New York: Guilford Press.

McCullough, J. P., *et al.* (2003). Group comparisons of DSM-IV subtypes of chronic depression: Validity of the distinctions, Part 2. *Journal of Abnormal Psychology*, **112**, 614–22.

McDonnell, F. (2003). *Threads of hope: learning to live with depression. A collection of writing*. London: Short Books.

Miranda, J. and Persons, J. B. (1988). Dysfunctional attitudes are mood-state dependent. *Journal of Abnormal Psychology*, **97**, 76–9.

Moore, R. G. and Garland, A. (2003). *Cognitive therapy for chronic and persistent depression*. Chichester: Wiley.

Muran, J. C. and Segal, Z. V. (1992). The development of an idiographic measure of self-schemas: an illustration of the construction and the use of self-scenarios. *Psychotherapy*, **29**, 524–35.

Murray, C. J. L. and Lopez, A. D. (1997). Global mortality, disability, and the contribution of risk factors: Global Burden of Disease Study. *Lancet*, **349**, 1436–42.

Needleman, L. D. (1999). *Cognitive case conceptualisation: a guidebook for practitioners*. Mahwah, NJ: Lawrence Erlbaum.

Nemeroff, C. B., *et al.* (2003). Differential responses to psychotherapy versus pharmacotherapy in patients with chronic forms of major depression and childhood trauma. *Proceedings of the National Academy of Sciences USA*, **100(4)**, 14293–6.

Newman, C. F., Leahy, R. L., Beck, A. T., Reilly-Harrington, N. A., and Gyulai, L. (2002). *Bipolar disorder: a cognitive therapy approach*. Washington, DC: American Psychological Association.

Perry, A., Tarrier, N., Morriss, R., McCarthy, E., and Limb, K. (1999). Randomised controlled trial of efficacy of teaching patients with bipolar disorder to identify early symptoms of relapse and obtain treatment. *British Medical Journal*, **318**, 149–53.

Persons, J. B. (1993). Case conceptualization in cognitive-behavior therapy. In: K. T. Kuelehwein and H. Rosen, ed. *Cognitive therapy in action: evolving innovative practice*, pp. 33–53. San Franscisco, CA: Jossey-Bass.

Peterson, C., *et al.* (1982). The Attributional Style Questionnaire. *Cognitive Therapy and Research*, **6**, 287–99.

Power, M. J. and Dalgleish, T. (1997). *Cognition and emotion: from order to disorder*. Hove, UK: Psychology Press.

Rao, U., Hammen, C., and Daley, S. E. (1999). Continuity of depression during the transition to adulthood: a 5-year longitudinal study of young women. *Journal of the American Academy of Child and Adolescent Psychiatry*, **38**, 908–15.

Reilly-Harrington, N. A., *et al.* (1999). Cognitive styles and life events interact to predict bipolar and unipolar symptomatology. *Journal of Abnormal Psychology*, **108**, 567–78.

Rush, A. J., Beck, A. T., Kovacs, M., and Hollon, S. D. (1977). Comparative efficacy of cognitive therapy and imipramine in the treatment of depressed outpatients. *Cognitive Therapy and Research*, **1**, 17–37.

Scott, J., Garland, A., and Moorhead, S. (2001). A pilot study of cognitive therapy in bipolar disorders. *Psychological Medicine*, **31**, 459–67.

Segal, Z. V., Williams, J. M. G., Teasdale, J. D., and Gemar, M. (1996). A cognitive science perspective on kindling and episode sensitization in recurrent affective disorder. *Psychological Medicine*, **26**, 371–80.

Segal, Z. V., Gemar, M., and Williams, S. (1999). Differential cognitive response to a mood challenge following successful cognitive therapy or pharmacotherapy for unipolar depression. *Journal of Abnormal Psychology*, **108**, 3–10.

Segal, Z. V., Williams, J. M. G., and Teasdale, J. D. (2002). *Mindfulness-based cognitive therapy for depression: a new approach to preventing relapse*. New York: Guilford Press.

Seligman, M. E. P., *et al.* (1988). Explanatory style change during cognitive therapy for unipolar depression. *Journal of Abnormal Psychology*, **97**, 13–18.

Shahar, G., Blatt, S. J., Zuroff, D. C., and Pilkonis, P. A. (2003). Role of perfectionism and personality disorder features in response to brief treatment for depression. *Journal of Consulting and Clinical Psychology*, **71**, 629–33.

Shea, M. T., *et al.* (1992). Course of depressive symptoms over follow-up: findings from the National Institute of Mental Health Treatment of Depression Collaborative Research Program. *Archives of General Psychiatry*, **49**, 782–7.

Simons, A. D., Murphy, G. E., Levine, J. L., and Wetzel, R. D. (1986). Cognitive therapy and pharmacotherapy for depression: sustained improvement over one year. *Archives of General Psychiatry*, **3**, 43–8.

Tang, T. Z. and DeRubeis, R. J. (1999). Reconsidering rapid early response in cognitive behavioral therapy for depression. *Clinical Psychology: Science and Practice*, **6**, 283–8.

Tang, T. Z., Luborsky, L., and Andrusyna, T. (2002). Sudden gains in recovering from depression: are they also found in psychotherapies other than cognitive-behavioral therapy? *Journal of Consulting and Clinical Psychology*, **70**, 444–7.

Teasdale, J. D. (1993). Emotion and 2 kinds of meaning—cognitive therapy and applied cognitive science. *Behaviour Research and Therapy*, **31**, 339–54.

Teasdale, J. D. and Barnard, P. J. (1993). *Affect, cognition, and change: re-modelling depressive thought*. Hove, UK: Erlbaum.

Teasdale, J. D. and Cox, S. G. (2001). Dysphoria: self-devaluative and affective components in recovered depressed patients and never depressed controls. *Psychological Medicine*, **31**, 1311–16.

Teasdale, J. D. and Dent, J. (1987). Cognitive vulnerability to depression—an investigation of 2 hypotheses. *British Journal of Clinical Psychology*, **26**, 113–26.

Teasdale, J. D., Segal, Z., and Williams, J. M. G. (1995). How does cognitive therapy prevent depressive relapse and why should attentional control (mindfulness) training help. *Behaviour Research and Therapy*, **33**, 25–39.

Teasdale, J. D., *et al.* (2000). Prevention of relapse/recurrence in major depression by mindfulness-based cognitive therapy. *Journal of Consulting and Clinical Psychology*, **68**, 615–23.

Teasdale, J. D., *et al.* (2001). How does cognitive therapy prevent relapse in residual depression? Evidence from a controlled trial. *Journal of Consulting and Clinical Psychology*, **69**, 347–57.

Weissman, A. N. and Beck, A. T. (1978). Development and validation of the Dysfunctional Attitudes Scale: a preliminary investigation. In Chicago.

Wright, J. H., *et al.* (2002). Development and initial testing of a multimedia program for computer-assisted cognitive therapy. *American Journal of Psychotherapy*, **56**, 76–86.

Young, J. E., Klosko, J., and Weishaar, M. E. (2003). *Schema therapy: a practitioner's guide*. New York: Guilford Press.

12 The psychoanalytic/psychodynamic approach to depressive disorders

David Taylor and Phil Richardson

Introduction and orientation

The psychoanalytic approach to human psychology is based upon two major paradigms. The first is biological (Sulloway, 1979). Men and women are viewed as possessing what have been described as 'stupendous and fundamental' biological drives. The individual must employ and satisfy these motivations and affects—hunger, sex, fear, aggression, love, and hate—in order to manage the tasks of the life cycle. The biological paradigm of psychoanalysis is particularly important when considering depression, because it gives full recognition to the power and substantiality of those drives and affects. Abnormalities in these drives and affects play a large part in the pathogenesis of depressive states.

The second paradigm is based upon a view of the human as a being saturated with meanings, intentions, and purposes. Fulfilling the basic aims of life, including having and rearing offspring, always involves operating through and within kinship and other groups. Success will depend upon capacities for achieving intermediate aims, such as finding and keeping a love object. At least some degree of harmonization of the 'stupendous and fundamental' drives with those organizations connected with the higher faculties is necessary for an individual to be capable of *loving* and *working*. These are capacities that Freud argued had become life aims in their own right. A damaged capacity to develop, sustain, and achieve aims of this central kind is a crucial part of the causal sequence leading to depression. In turn, depression, once established, will lead to further deterioration in these ego functions.

Psychoanalytic/psychodynamic accounts of depression

Modern psychodynamic views of depression see it as a complex disorder of functioning, with its origin in infancy and childhood. The earliest years are an intense formative time when both innate and environmental factors will determine the development, or absence, of crucial psychological and relational capacities. The unique make-up and experiences of individuals over the unfolding life cycle leads to a vulnerability, which in turn, through final common pathways, culminates in depressive syndromes with familiar constellations of symptoms. The difficulties in loving and working, which potentially arise out of an unsatisfactory childhood situation, operate as intermediate and partial factors in a complex interaction with life events.

There is considerable agreement between the various psychoanalytic accounts of depression that have been developed over the century since Freud and Abraham began their investigations. There are also some differences. Different constituents have been focused upon as if they were the whole. Probably each theory has a contribution to make to getting an overall picture. Some theories, for example, emphasize the diminished sense of personal efficacy and potency (e.g., Bibring, 1953). Others focus on problems with the individual's sense of self (e.g., Kohut, 1971), while still others consider as crucial the role of conflicts between impulses of love and hate (e.g., Jacobsen, 1946; Klein, 1935). Depressive disorders, arising out of individual lives and histories, are complex conditions.

While these differences may arise in part from focusing upon different aspects of the same entity, they extend into important questions of etiology. For instance, both Kohut and Winnicott, albeit in rather different terms, proposed that idealization of the self and others is a developmentally normal stage *en route* to normal self-esteem. Klein, on the other hand, thought that many of the problems with diminished self-esteem, failed grandiosity or narcissism that are seen in depression, which undoubtedly go on to cause problems of their own, are secondary to more basic conflicts between loving and hating impulses towards external objects.

Other differences concern the emphasis given to genetic, constitutional, or endogenous versus environmental factors. Also important is how and to what extent early feeding and nurturing experiences influence the content and form of adult thinking, feeling, and relating. There are different positions on methods of reconstructing the subjective world of infants and their relationships. While the implications of some psychoanalytic accounts of depression are limited to the disorder, others are more far-reaching. Some suggest that the mental operations seen in depression have a central role in normal development as well, and what began as a set of ideas and observations about depression has grown into a general theory of emotional development.

What follows is an account of the main themes in the foremost psychoanalytic/psychodynamic accounts of the nature and origin of depression.

Depression and mourning as reactions to loss

Freud, as his title *Mourning and Melancholia* (1917) indicates, was linking together these two processes as being different kinds of reaction to the same kind of event, involving a loss. This can be the loss of a love object, or perhaps more usually in the case of melancholia (a variety of major depressive disorder) some less tangible loss or injury involving an individual's wishes, ideals, beliefs, or hopes, all of which contributes to a sense of self.

There are important points of difference between mourning and melancholia. Although it is quite common to mourn for a lost self, in mourning in general it is the world that is felt to have lost meaning. In melancholia by contrast it is the self that is experienced as reduced and impoverished. In mourning, as well as there being some anger, there are also prominent feelings of sadness and longing, and some characteristic forms of sympathetic identification with the lost object. In melancholia, there exists a higher level of anger and destructiveness, which may be turned upon the self dangerously as in suicide.

Mourning has an adaptive function, whereas melancholia is maladaptive. Freud viewed mourning as an active psychological process rather than simply a passive registering of the loss or bereavement. Recollections of the lost or abandoning love object are 'worked over' repeatedly. This is an involuntary process that involves picturing the bereaved in periods of intense longing and psychological absorption (*hypercathexis* was the term coined by Freud's translators). Although emotionally painful, it is through this means that the reality of the loss is slowly accepted, and the tie to the object relinquished or modified, until eventually the resources of the individual are freed once more, so that a new adaptation becomes possible. In melancholia there is less obvious evidence of relinquishment and less consequent adaptive development.

The inner world and its objects

As well as having made specific contributions to the understanding of grief and depression, *Mourning and Melancholia* marked a period in psychoanalysis when earlier models based upon viewing the psyche as a 'mechanism' were succeeded by object relations theories. All versions of object relations theory are based on the idea that relationships in infancy and childhood with parental and sibling figures are essential in their own right. With regard to our particular subject, disruptions and abnormalities in early nurture and feeding relationships, and in the way they are internalized, give rise to a susceptibility to depressive disorders in the adult.

The distinctive feature of psychoanalytic object relations theories is their concern with the phenomenon of an inner, subjectively imbued world of thought, imagination, and representation. The inner world is constructed through the internalization of the earliest relationships with parents and siblings. What is encountered—and what is perceived—in the world is shaped, and shapes, the inner models of emotional life. According to psychoanalytic accounts, the interplay of these interactions can be seen in our inner world of thoughts, feelings, imagined discourses, and dreams.

Clinical illustration

Mr A's marriage was spoiled by powerful feelings of anger and hostility that he couldn't account for. He feared that they were out of control and were destroying his marriage, leaving him struggling, depressed, abandoned, and bleak. The patient felt that his wife was 'addicted' to her family. In particular, he hated the attention that she lavished on her sister who was still breast feeding her 3-year old son. Mr A felt that his quarrelling was compulsive. 'I just cannot stop having a go about her sister,' he said, after he had quarreled again about his wife's attachment to her. His wife, N, had become angry and called him an Inquisitor. He had smashed a valuable bowl. That night he had a dream.

'There was only a flat and sandy island with water all around. There had been a nuclear explosion. The ground was contaminated by radioactive fall-out. Everything was finished. There was no chance of escape for me and the other people there. N was among them and she had decided to leave me. I was crying, 'Do you really like hurting me? You are doing this because I have put all my hope with you.'

The analyst saw this dream as depicting the condition of Mr A's inner world and the nature of his unconscious fantasy life. Using a model based upon the notion of powerful conflicts between love and hate, the nuclear explosion could be understood as representing the patient's angry explosions at being passed over, as he experienced it, in favor of his wife's family. The radioactivity represented their emotional fall-out.

The atmosphere in the dream is that of a nuclear winter. Nothing good in his inner world is felt to survive the massiveness of his rage. No sense of life remains, no good relationships nor hope for the future seem possible. The prevailing thrust of the internal relationships, as well as the actual argument connected with them, has become the intended infliction of hurt. The patient experiences himself as abandoned to his desolate fate. In this way, the complex affects of depression are considered to arise meaningfully out of this conflict of powerful feelings.

The condition of the internal representation of the primary love objects—in infancy, mother and her breast, and father—is a central issue in some psychoanalytic accounts of depression. Important functional capacities within the individual's psyche are located in the internal object. These are connected with providing support and love, and the ability to manage feelings. The ego's attempt to spare the love object from harm is a central theme in the syndrome of depression. If the love object at the center of the ego is felt to be hurt, damaged, or weakened—for instance by high levels of internal hostility or rivalry—then the individual feels bad or damaged: the stability of the ego is diminished. Being loved or unloved is linked with the moral distinction between good and bad. This intertwining of the most important dimensions in emotional life is central in depression.

The outward form taken by these core inner issues varies greatly. Blatt (1974) has identified two main types of depression characterized by different stances towards the object and the self. In what Blatt terms the *anaclitic* form of depression, the person feels that if they are able to restore a particular relationship with an external love object, by whatever means necessary—pleading, cajoling, threatening, then their happiness, and sense of personal worth and goodness, will be restored. The individual's efforts are devoted to changing the outside world, which is felt to hold the key to restoring well-being. The case described in the illustration above is of this type.

In contrast, the person manifesting the *introjective* form of depression is focused upon their inner world where they are concerned with whether their natures and impulses are good or bad, and with trying to sort out their inner relationship with important figures in their lives. 'Was I good or bad in my relationship with father or mother?' 'Was mother or father good or bad?' 'How, and on what terms, can they be preserved or looked after?' are the sorts of unspoken questions that lie behind these self-examinations. Whereas those with the anaclitic form may be thought of as preoccupied with the possibilities of cure by the power of another's love, the introjective individual believes in a cure by moral effort.

The critical agency and the depressive super-ego

Noting the exaggeration of moral judgement that occurs in depression, Freud was concerned to understand how and why floridly unrealistic beliefs that the self is harmful and bad can become so prominent. He described the setting up of *a critical agency* as a 'grade' within the ego that 'henceforth will judge the ego'. Subsequently, he combined his earlier idea of an ego-ideal (*v.i.*) with the critical agency, to arrive at the notion of the super-ego. The super-ego is therefore one part of the individual's mind acting upon another part of that same mind. It is this attribute of being capable of 'action within' that makes it such an important concept in depression. It covers a much wider range of conscious and unconscious operations than those we customarily recognize as the work of conscience.

We know through introspection that there are two kinds of mental experience: awareness and self-awareness. Self-awareness is consciousness of being aware. Conscience is a subspecies of self-awareness, where the feeling of not having lived up to one's ethical or moral values results in guilt. This is mature conscience in its familiar form. But even in relatively normal and healthy people an inner voice is often too ready to criticize, blame, and accuse the self. In those with a predisposition to depression it is often *as if* someone within the individual's mind was judging and observing in a spoiling, superior, sadistic, or overindulgent way.

Sometimes the familiar forms of super-ego functioning such as the conscience are manifestations of the highest ethical or moral values. However, often super-ego functioning consists of the postulation of morals as a camouflage: it is moralism rather than morals that holds sway. Indeed, Freud went further when he recognized that the super-ego quite regularly functioned as a psychologically primitive set of omnipotent, defensive, narcissistic functions, which are capable of operating in a way that damages an individual's mental functioning.

With the frighteningly destructive power of the melancholic super-ego in mind, Freud pointed out that the greatest danger facing the ego in melancholia was losing the approval or love of the super-ego and, by implication, gaining its hatred. This kind of super-ego functioning is what makes melancholia into such a serious mental illness. It has the power to degrade the ego's capacity for mature thought and judgement into, quite literally, murderous impulses directed at the self or sometimes at others.

At first in psychoanalysis the normal super-ego was approached from the angle of its being a part of *child* development. However, subsequent psychoanalytic work was concerned with working out the *infantile* origins of this severe depressive super-ego. Klein (1933) reported fearful fantasies of hostile figures in the play of children between $2^3/_4$ and 4 years (some of whom were depressed: for example, Erna), which she controversially considered to be manifestations of the super-ego originating in the first months of postuterine life. These had the primitive ferocity found in melancholia, which existed as well in lower-key forms in chronic depressive states. Klein considered that the nature of these fantasies indicated that they derived from the infant's earliest relationship with the mother's breast. This early super-ego is not an exact copy of the real character of the child's parents but is shaped as well by fantasies about them colored by the child's own angry and hateful feelings. These amalgams of reality and fantasy then come home to roost within the child, where they may operate as a source of persecution. To a certain extent, this is viewed as normal: the ordinarily hungry and screaming infant becomes frightened after a while, as it feels its world has become imbued with its angry and destructive feelings.

Later developments in this line of work have included ideas about the existence of an 'ego-destructive super-ego', which, through countless inner attacks—in the form of contemptuous thoughts about others as well as about the self—can produce stupor-like states, and erode connections between thoughts and ideas (Bion, 1962; O'Shaughnessy, 1999).

Jacobson (1954), following the early work of Rado (1927), while agreeing with Klein about the importance of primitive destructive objects in depression, disagreed about their origin. Jacobson argued that severe disillusionment about the parents in the first year of life damages the infantile ego and initiates a premature formation of the super-ego. As a consequence, she reasoned, it is not possible for the maturing individual to give up the tendency to cling to what is essentially an idea of a magical power based upon infantile beliefs. By continuing the struggle with the love object intrapsychically, the self maintains its utter dependence on it. It becomes the victim of the super-ego: in its fantasy life it is tortured as if it were a helpless and powerless child by a cruel condemning mother. The enduring hope is of gaining the approval of this powerful entity so that it will relent, and offer softness and support, as originally the mother's breast had done.

Jacobson underlined the distinction that exists between representations of the deflated and worthless parents, and those who are perceived as inflated and punishing ones—good or bad. The child, and later the adult, still hopes to regain love and security from the 'God-like parents' by pleading, by atonement and abasement. But the parents, who in infancy were felt to be omnipotent, are not only turned into bad hostile punishing beings; once deprived of their power they appear low, bad, defiled, empty, and castrated—parents from whom nothing can be expected. This deflation and destruction of the parental images inevitably leads to self-deflation and self-destruction.

The infantile phases of development and depression

Abraham (1911) was the first to propose that issues connected with the infant's feeding relationship with mother are central in depression. Longing, disappointment, and disillusionment arising from these earliest desires are at the center of much depressive feeling. Deutsch (1932) also thought that the deeper dispositional elements in depression can be traced to the earliest ego frustrations, separations, and disappointments. Depressive reactions can be found in the early postnatal separations from the object, while early manic reactions could be traced to the restoration of the same object.

One of Klein's (1935) additions to the original work on mourning and melancholia was the hypothesis that the reaction to any loss occurring later in the life cycle will be influenced by revived aspects of the reaction to loss at the earliest stages of development. Weaning—losing the breast—was regarded as the prototype of all later losses. However, the repeating sequences of hunger, feeding, satisfaction, and the comings and goings of people (the father or the siblings and the mother's own comings and goings) were also seen as powerful additional stimuli to the baby's rapidly increasing capacity to recognize the breast (and the mother) as separate from, rather than as part of him. Giving up the beliefs and attitudes associated with a split world, experienced in terms of the exclusive possession of wholly good objects and the expulsion of wholly bad ones, precipitates a phase of mourning and grief. The infant experiences the forerunners of the adult emotions of concern and regret at its inability to protect the mother from its demands. Klein termed this constellation of feelings 'the depressive position.'

The early loss of the object during weaning may result in depression in later life, if the infant has not been able to establish a loved object securely within at the early period of development. While it was recognized that good maternal care or, alternatively, a depriving, severe, or cruel upbringing, had a big effect upon the child's capacity to internalize a good object, the focus of these investigations was upon the development of the inner world of the infant and, in this internal world, the role of its aggressive, hostile, and loving feelings. In a subsequent development Bion (1962) examined the function of the mother as an essential environmental factor in the infant's psychological development.

The mother's mental functioning, the nature of the mother-and-baby's rhythms of comings and goings, of the repeated cycles of hunger, feeding, and satisfaction, and of the presence of other people, are key parts of the infant's environment as is the infant's own temperament. Day-to-day features of the maternal environment, as well as major traumatic events such as early maternal death or extended separations, influence whether the deep-seated and passionate wishes of early infancy can be relinquished in favor of the infant's being able to connect with the mother on a basis of reality. When things go well this internal reality is of a mother who is able to console and feed as well as to let the child wait. It is also one where the nature of the mother's relationship with the father is accepted. When the representation of the mother is less benign and reliable the individual may nurse unrealistic hopes based upon compensatory exaggerations of the unsatisfied wishes and needs of infancy and so be vulnerable to a depressive illness when these break down in adulthood.

The role of orality in depression

Even after a normal development, much of the original power of the oral needs, wishes, and longings of infancy persists into adult life. Although their mode and totality of expression is suppressed, they continue to exercise a determining influence upon the psyche. Food is always intimately bound-up with love and vice versa. Relinquishing love objects later in life revives the intense pangs involved in leaving behind the earliest oral satisfactions and fantasies. Surmounting the power of the oral needs, wishes, and longings of unrequited infantile need and love is a major developmental and emotional challenge.

The role of aggression and ambivalence

The intimate relationship that exists between aggression, emotional ambivalence, and depression has been repeatedly emphasized in psychoanalytic studies (Abraham, 1911, 1924; Freud, 1917; Klein, 1935, 1940). Abraham (1911, 1916), based upon observations made in the course of the psychoanalytic treatment of patients with psychotic depression, concluded that the patients' capacity to love was being overwhelmed by feelings of hatred about which they were often acutely anxious. Freud suggested that in states of depression, aggressivity towards others is held back and turned upon the self. Depression, anxiety, and self-reproach then ensue because the self has become identified with the lost object. However, there is no consensus on the precise nature of the role of aggression in the etiology of depression. Bleichmar (1996) described the four main psychoanalytic positions on the role of aggression in the following way:

◆ As a necessary part of the human condition and a fundamental factor in every depression (for example, Klein, 1935, 1940).

◆ As part of a larger configuration that consists of frustration, rage, and failed attempts to gain a desired end. When for external or internal reasons the ego is unable to attain its goals, aggression is turned towards a fused representation of self and object (*v.i.*), with an ensuing loss of self-esteem.

◆ As a by-product of a diminished self-esteem as the outcome of primary fixations to experiences of helplessness especially in childhood (e.g., Bibring, 1953).

◆ As a secondary phenomenon in response to what is primarily a failure in a parental external object, which gives rise to pain and narcissistic rage (*v.i.*) (e.g., Kohut, 1971).

Constitutional and genetic factors

In the history of psychoanalytic thought, several constitutional or temperamental factors—considered to be inherited, at least in part—have been put forward as predisposing to later difficulties. Deutsch (1951), in a discussion of the pre-psychotic personality of manic-depressives, suggested a specific ego-weakness manifesting as a vulnerability and intolerance towards frustration, hurt, and disappointment. Klein (1930) thought that there were innate differences between individuals in terms of their tolerance of anxiety stirred up in the course of development as well as in terms of aggressiveness and envy. When these feelings are pronounced they give rise to difficulties in making secure internalizations of good objects. However, there is always a difficulty in determining the direction of the effect.

Most psychoanalytic accounts of the contribution of nature and nurture to the development of neurosis and mental illness were formulated before the advent of modern genetics. We now know more about environmental and genetic factors, and their complex interactions. The issue now before us is the way in which nature *plus* nurture leads to the phenomena we are examining. However, one of the challenges is identifying the psychological correlates—the psychological manifestations at the level of character—of the genetic factors contributing to depression.

Narcissism and the self

Various phenomena in depression are recognized under the central psychoanalytic concept of narcissism. Some of the descriptive usages of the term refer to states of the ego—the self—and the ego-ideal, which are of central importance in depression. These range from a normal degree of self-regardingness, confidence, and morale (with a realistic view of the self as competent, and at least to a degree lovable), through to an increased preoccupation with the self. In this second state, the self may be experienced as inadequate, weak, and marginal on the one hand or self-admiring and perfect (with omnipotent control over the self or others) on the other. These different states of mind are all positioned on the narcissistic dimension of attitudes to the self.

The terms 'narcissistic injury' or ' narcissistic wound' tend to be associated with the idea of traumatic insults to the natural expectations of the self. However, these terms are also employed when referring to the kind of hurt suffered by the vain or conceited. The term 'narcissistic' also designates a constellation in the personality of traits of selfishness, ruthlessness, contemptuousness, and superiority. Some quite major personality shifts or orientations, such as withdrawal from the outside world to a preoccupation with the self or internal objects, and fusions or identifications of self and objects are also called narcissistic.

Most of these usages, while to some degree descriptive, have developmental or etiological implications that vary according to the theoretical model employed. For example, Jacobson stressed the 'narcissistic breakdown' of the depressed person as the central psychological problem. By this she meant the loss of self-esteem, feelings of impoverishment, helplessness, weakness, and inferiority that is so often felt. However, the meaning she is giving to the term 'narcissistic breakdown' can only be fully understood in the context of her overall view of depression as a condition arising out of early disappointment, and the sort of parental images that she postulates this gives rise to.

In an attempt to reduce the lack of definition arising from the conceptual range and power of the term 'narcissism', Jacobsen introduced the term 'self-representation' meaning the 'concept' of the self—the unconscious and preconscious images that people have of the body, self, and personality.

Bibring (1953) also emphasized the centrality of the sense of helplessness and powerlessness in depression. In Bibring's view the subject's *representation* of his incapacity to attain goals is more important in the etiology of depression than object loss *per se*. Of course, this representation may include the inability to achieve the presence of the love object. The representation of self-incapacity arises out of a fixation to experiences of helplessness and powerlessness. Each time the depressive person feels he cannot fulfill his aspirations, all previous experiences—either real or imaginary—in which the feeling of helplessness dominated will be reactivated.

The view taken of the nature of narcissistic attitudes and positions is one of the major differences between psychoanalytic accounts of depression. Kohut (1971) suggested that the development of the sense of the self was an independent line in development that is damaged in those vulnerable to depression. Parents who can provide phase-appropriate idealizing, grandiose, and narcissistic attitudes towards the child are key to satisfactory development of self-esteem. Also, the parents need to be satisfactory models for these narcissistic wishes. Kohut felt that a parent's failure to meet such needs—either by failing themselves, or being depressed, excessively critical, or denigrating, or by the absence of the sort of overvaluation that parents normally invest in children, interferes with the development of what is often termed 'healthy narcissism'.

In contrast, Klein felt that while there are healthy forms of narcissism—certain kinds of pride and self-respect, for instance—other forms, including superiority and self-idealization, are the outcomes of defenses against primitive impulses of aggression and rivalry towards early providing figures. These result in confusions and acquisitive identifications between the self and object.

Identification

Identification plays a crucial part in depression. In the phrase, the 'shadow of the object falls on the ego' Freud was expressing vividly the idea that the effects of aggression and frustration were being directed at the ego when, in reality and originally, they have been felt about the lost object. The self identifies with the object in the sense that it treats itself as if it were that object. Through this means it sustains the belief that the object lives. This preserves its relationship with an object whose loss cannot be faced. This is sometimes described as a narcissistic form of identification because of the sense of being in the individual's interest rather than those of the object.

Identification is encountered in other phenomena in depression. For example, in Klein's depressive position, the child's sympathetic identification with the mother is based upon the child's love and concern about fantasized damage done to the object. The ego, by sharing and suffering the imagined pain of the object, seeks to spare that with which it is in sympathy. Klein thought that some of the self-hatred found in depression is based upon the ego's dislike of, and despair at, the nature of its own hostile impulses.

Research evidence

Evidence concerning psychoanalytic approaches to depression may be considered from two angles. First, there are many empirical research approaches that bear upon the broad psychoanalytic propositions outlined in the earlier 'Psychoanalytic/psychodynamic accounts of depression' section on the inner structure of depression and etiological factors influencing the development and course of depression. Unfortunately, it is beyond the scope of this chapter to examine these further but it is an essential part of the scientific enterprise to consider how the findings of observational studies may be *corroborated and drawn together by* what is postulated about the inner world in depression.

The second contribution of research is the employment of outcome evaluation tools in the form of efficacy and effectiveness studies to form a view of the value of psychoanalytic approaches as treatments of depression. These will now be reviewed.

The efficacy and effectiveness of treatments for depression

Introduction

The term 'psychodynamic psychotherapy' encompasses all those therapeutic approaches, derived originally from psychoanalysis and depth psychologies, in which the dynamic role of unconscious processes and the significance of the therapeutic relationship are central. While psychodynamic psychotherapies vary a lot the ideas of psychoanalytic and depth psychology are common denominators underlying the approach to treatment.

In any appraisal of research evidence it is important to bear in mind any limits that follow from the test conditions employed. Most efficacy studies of treatments for depression have studied short courses of treatment with short follow-ups and inadequate concealment of treatment allocation, conducted with patient populations who offer good prospects of responsiveness (e.g., minimal comorbidity), thereby optimizing the chance of the treatment concerned being shown in a good light. However, depression is usually a long-term condition marked by relapse. Effectiveness studies of therapy conducted in real clinical practice with clinically representative populations have been less frequently reported. The treatment periods required with such populations are longer than those used by efficacy studies (Morrison *et al.*, 2003).

A recent systematic review of controlled trials for treatment-refractory depression (Stimpson *et al.*, 2002) found few randomized controlled trials (RCTs), and none involving psychological treatments, which met more exacting criteria for methodological adequacy. The paucity of outcome research on psychological and drug treatments whose test conditions are adequate in terms of the nature of the clinical problem is the key fact, especially with respect to long-term refractory depression. This conclusion applies to trials of psychodynamic psychotherapy also.

The RCT evidence that is available suggests that both antidepressant medication and psychological therapies generate an improvement over the short term of approximately 12–13 points on the Beck scale (NICE Depression Guideline, 2004). Among the psychological therapies, this type of evidence is strongest for cognitive-behavioral therapy (CBT) and interpersonal psychotherapy (Department of Health 2001; NICE Depression Guideline 2004). There is also evidence in favor of couple therapy on systemic lines when compared with medication, for a clinically-representative sample of depressed patients (Leff *et al.*, 2000).

The increasing influence of evidence-based approaches in public sector health care has lead to more studies of psychodynamic therapy using RCT methodology in the past 10 years (Fonagy *et al.*, Open Door Review of Outcome Studies in Psychoanalysis and Psychoanalytic Psychotherapy, Second Edition 2002).

Studies of the efficacy of psychodynamic therapy as a treatment of depression

The Sheffield Psychotherapy Project (Shapiro *et al.*, 1994) compared 8 or 16 weeks of an 'exploratory therapy' (a form of psychodynamic-interpersonal therapy) with 'prescriptive psychotherapy' (somewhat resembling CBT) for depressed patients. The two therapies were found to be equally effective, but patients with more severe depression did better with 16 weeks of therapy. The patients were followed-up for a year when 57% of treatment responders had fully, and 32% partially, maintained their gains, and 11% had relapsed. This study has been replicated (Barkham *et al.*, 1994).

The work of Guthrie and her colleagues evaluating the effectiveness of Hobson's brief psychodynamic-interpersonal therapy (Guthrie *et al.*, 1998, 1999) has been extended to the treatment of patients who have made suicide attempts (Guthrie *et al.*, 2001). Relative to a treatment-as-usual control condition, patients who had self-poisoned and presented to emergency services, showed significant reductions in suicidal ideation and reduced Beck Depression Inventory scores at 6 months follow-up following four sessions of home-based psychodynamic-interpersonal therapy. These results indicate the potential benefit of a psychodynamic treatment approach to an important clinical problem associated with depressive symptomatology.

An RCT of home-based brief therapy for depressive symptoms has been reported by Cooper *et al.* (2003). Women suffering from postnatal depression received either routine care or one of three psychotherapies (nondirective, CBT, and psychodynamic) over a 10-week period and were then assessed up to 5 years postpartum. Unlike patients receiving nondirective and CBT, only the psychodynamically treated group showed a significant reduction in depression (Structured Clinical Interview for DSM-IIIR) relative to the controls at post-treatment. By the 9-month follow-up, however, the benefit of treatment was no longer apparent. These results were compatible with therapy speeding a recovery, which would, in the majority of cases, have occurred spontaneously over time.

Gallagher and Thompson (Thompson *et al.*, 1988; Gallagher-Thompson and Steffen 1994), reported studies that establish the empirical validity of psychodynamic psychotherapy for depressed patients over the age of 65 years. These compared the relative benefits of brief psychodynamic therapy and CBT for elderly depressed patients and for their clinically depressed caregivers (Gallagher-Thompson and Steffen, 1994). Psychodynamic psychotherapy had clearer effects for those depressed caregivers who were newer to the caregiving tasks while CBT seemed to offer most for longstanding caregivers, findings that suggest treatment-specific effects.

The combination of psychodynamic psychotherapy with antidepressant medication has been evaluated using RCT methodology. Within the test conditions employed combined treatment appears to offer a benefit over and above drug treatment alone. Burnand *et al.* (2002), for example, showed a significant incremental benefit of psychodynamic psychotherapy over clomipramine alone in 74 patients with major depression. The therapists who were nurses had a 6-month manual-based training. Benefits were evident on clinical and health economic measures (accounting for hospitalization rates and days lost from work). The cost saving was $2311 (US) per patient over the treatment period.

Further evidence for the benefit of a combined psychotherapy–medication approach has been provided by de Jonge *et al.* (2001). Sixteen sessions of 'short psychodynamic supportive therapy' improved the outcomes of patients with major depression on a variety of measures of depression and quality of life over a 6-month period. Promising though the results of both these studies seem, the absence of long-term follow-up assessments should be noted.

Few other trials of psychodynamic therapy as a treatment for depression have been carried out by neutral researchers. Some investigators sympathetic to other therapies have used dynamic therapy as a comparator (e.g., Bellack *et al.*, 1981). Roth and Fonagy (prev. citation) caution that these trials were unlikely to have employed psychodynamic psychotherapy administered by appropriately trained practitioners and their results may not derive from a proper test.

The results of psychotherapy research in general

The generic efficacy of psychotherapy compared with no treatment has been established for a long time. Study after study, meta-analysis after meta-analysis, has validated psychotherapy as an evidence-based treatment. 'The available research has led to one basic conclusion: psychotherapy in general has been shown to be effective. Positive outcomes have been reported for a wide variety of theoretical positions and technical interventions. The reviews cover data from mildly disturbed persons with specific limited symptoms as well as from severely impaired patients . . .' (Lambert, 1992, p. 97). Throughout this literature the size of the effect is remarkably stable, and is comparable with that found in education and with psychoactive medication (see Lambert and Bergen, 1994 for a complete review).

Research more specific to the method

Psychodynamic and psychoanalytic approaches are simultaneously types of therapy and a research methodology. This is not only true from the practitioner's point of view. The patient seeking help may well be motivated as much by a need to 'research' and understand his or her own life as by the need for symptomatic relief. At a certain point in the course of a psychodynamic psychotherapy, customary distinctions between cure and knowledge may cease to operate. A deeper understanding of oneself may in and of itself be a kind of cure, which, as well as helping to modify symptoms, can lead to benefits such as the growth of an active capacity to reflect upon internal states. This may be an important part of what is needed to recover the capacity to act, or to make relationships. Operating together synergistically, developments such as these may lead the individual to become both more engaged and more resilient—to become more capable of the demands involved in having a life, and less vulnerable to breakdown in the future.

Establishing the justification for therapeutic claims of this sort involves moving beyond theory-neutral treatment trials to investigate the question of whether specific treatments possess specific elements capable of leading to types of change not available otherwise. Theory-informed research strategies, perhaps involving clinical case studies, and well-designed longitudinal effectiveness studies may be required to investigate unrealized or unoperationalized functions of the personality. These may provide information about therapeutic possibilities that can complement that obtained from Type I RCTs.

An example of the potential value of retrospective longitudinal effectiveness studies comes from a body of research that has sought to investigate the clinical impression that improvement may continue after psychodynamic psychotherapy ends, in some instances even after a period of possible deterioration. Sandell's (1987) important study demonstrated patients gaining in strength and capacity after treatment had ended. A carefully designed naturalistic long-term follow-up study showed that a clinically representative group of patients with significant depressive symptomatology had, after long-term psychoanalytic psychotherapy, moved into the normal range of scores (Leuzinger-Bohleber *et al.*, 2002). At follow-up, they were doing better in terms of days off work than the normal population. This study included in-depth interviews that made it possible to discern distinct and differing patterns of change in the way that various personality types managed their thoughts and feelings. These patterns included the demonstrable emergence of reflective functioning.

The therapeutic possibilities of a reflective, insightful personality function are one reason, if reasons should be needed, for wanting to study the interior, subjective side of experience. Most depressed patients, as well as experiencing symptoms are preoccupied with what they feel are failures to fulfill their wishes or live up to their standards. On closer acquaintance, these states often appear to be concerned with failed or lost relationships. Most important are the absent or lost love objects, stretching back to childhood relationships with mother or father or other aspects of upbringing. There are often concerns about the goodness of others' motives and dispositions as well as with one's own. Thus many depressed patients have ideas as to why and how they came to be depressed. As the patient's view of what has been affectively significant in his or her life is the raw material out of which potent ego functioning may arise it is important to have considered to what extent they are right in these ideas. A realistic knowledge of inner life and cure can be closely connected.

Key practice points

Values and aims

In the view of psychoanalysis, men and women are subject to a wide variety of internal states and emotions arising out of their lives so far that are often difficult to manage. The treatment is based on the idea that the patient can internalize a vital yet subtle capacity to learn about and use these states of mind in the further conduct of their lives. This involves a therapeutic process based upon the repeated and sustained understanding of the functioning of areas of their personality hitherto unexplored. This process takes place within a specialized relationship with an analyst/therapist (Milton, 2001).

The therapeutic benefit arises as a by-product of personal growth rather than as a result of self-conscious learning techniques or by striving for change directly. An overforceful, overdirected search for 'improvement' can be counterproductive.

The setting and its continuity

Most patients will be helped by an assessment consultation before they start treatment. This gives an opportunity to work out whether they want to embark upon a treatment that requires active engagement in a process that can be emotionally challenging as well as supportive.

Before treatment begins the therapist tells the patient about the basic form of the treatment and agrees a regular time for the sessions. Most often this takes the form of once-weekly sessions of 50 minutes each. In more intensive forms of treatment the sessions may be two to five times weekly. The regularity and consistency of the setting provides parameters within which the patient can relate and the therapist work. The therapist needs to make sure that the sessions will not be interrupted. Alterations of frequency, time, and the room should be kept to a minimum. Well in advance

the therapist tells the patient of holiday breaks. Of course, there may be circumstances when the therapist has to cancel or rearrange sessions; the patient should not be unrealistically protected from all of the irregularities ordinarily encountered in life.

When people become emotionally important it is normal to be sensitive to their absence. Most people, but particularly those with a disposition to depression, are vulnerable to interpersonal situations hinting of emotional deprivation or loss, and react to separations. Those liable to depression are insecure in their relationships. As a result they may find it difficult to manage the combination of separateness and dependence that is part of therapy. However, these difficulties stirred up by the course of therapy provide an opportunity for new learning. A key part of the therapist's work is the recognition and understanding of the patient's feelings about the breaks, gaps, limitations, and frustrations inherent in the therapeutic encounter. Therefore the patient's reactions, which may include distress, anxiety, emotional coolness, withdrawal, anger, or the recurrence of previously remitting depression shouldn't be damped down or avoided.

The therapist's process of understanding may allow the depressed patient to renew contact with a good, containing, and understanding external object when previously the patient felt unable to find good experience. When this happens the therapist takes on some of the resonance of a primary good object—the mother and her breast, or father—for the patient. This ameliorates the patient's internal world, which will have been felt to have become a source of pain containing unresponsive, abandoning, damaged, or dead objects.

Clinical illustration

Ms H returned for her first session after a gap over the Christmas break. After a pause she said in a hoarse voice that she had a 'flu'. Judging by her haggard look it seemed likely that the state of suffering was emotional as well as viral. The patient began to cry. She said she was worried that she was worrying her sister, who was as a consequence losing weight. The therapist interpreted whether the patient was making herself ill because of her guilt about her sister but the patient became still—almost statue-like—not saying anything further for 20–30 minutes.

During this time the therapist essayed a number of comments, which led nowhere. The main burden of these was that the patient was having to face many painful things in her life where she was unable to help or affect matters. Her father was mentally ill, and her mother was dead, and she'd been unable to avert the bad outcome she now had to live with. Perhaps nobody could have done so. Perhaps these losses had been in her mind especially at Christmas, a time of families. He suggested that she felt it important to show him what she'd felt. Speaking didn't seem enough.

She then spoke of a relative who had invited her to his house. Speaking crossly, she said she was unable to go because she got a panic attack at the very thought of being in a room with a child whom she might have to look after. She had then been left with her sister, whom she felt had had such a horrible time and whom she was now exposing to her broken-down state. The therapist, who really felt not able to bear the increasing pain of this account, interrupted and spoke of the patient's crossness with her difficulties—with herself being vulnerable. This crossness, he suggested, made her more needy not less.

The patient fell silent again. Eventually the therapist just said quietly that she must have found Christmas hard. Unlike his earlier more complicated interpretations this simple statement seemed to strike a chord. The patient could talk more easily, apparently now feeling that she'd be listened to, and also seeming to feel that she was being understood. She seemed to take a different, softer attitude to her experiences of the holiday. It was better to cry, she said. Today before she came, she'd been trying to cry but no relief came. It had been a horrible year. All her family were failures. As she left at the end of the session she asked, 'What's the date of the next session?'. It turned out that this had not been fixed, as the therapist thought it had.

This illustration shows how the duration of the Christmas break cannot be interpreted away. Instead the patient has to convey her feelings more directly, and the therapist has to accept this, until eventually the patient gets the sense that the message has made its mark. Then she is able to feel helped by an understanding that is simple. The fact that the time of the next session hadn't been fixed suggests that the therapist might have been finding the painfulness of the feelings encountered in the treatment of very traumatized and depressed patients difficult. The patient's inquiry after her next session, however, reveals her basically positive response to the work of the session even when—or perhaps *because*—she has been conveying, with the utmost power the hopelessness of her situation and the uselessness of the therapy.

The therapist's sensitivity to what it is like to wait when feeling in need is essential, as it forms the basis of understanding that can safeguard the patient and the treatment. Reactions to gaps can threaten the patient's stability and their experience of the therapy as providing something meaningful.

The psychoanalytic focus

Psychoanalytic psychotherapy, especially when treating patients who are depressed, is preferentially concerned with areas of personal functioning involving loving, hating, destroying, repairing, and so on, in relation to others who are, or who have been, of central emotional significance. In depression, feelings of disappointment, love, anger, criticism, neglect, or undermining destructiveness are turned inwards in ways that end up causing suffering, or victimhood. This can be seen in all aspects of a person's ways of communicating, relating, and thinking.

The patient making more meaningful contact with these sorts of feelings and intentions is the key to recovery. As a result of the way the analyst and the patient work together on these sorts of issues, there is a tendency for the patient to find they can perceive and engage with their world with an enlarged repertoire.

Clinical illustration

A depressed patient with a history of severe emotional deprivation in infancy was just coming to be able to realize that she was locked as if without air in a bleak, lifeless, emotionally responseless world. In one session when the atmosphere of claustrophobic desolation was palpable the patient was able, almost for the first time, to refer openly to its impact upon her. She managed to say, 'Just a few moments ago I had this feeling of wanting to flail my arms about, to slap myself.' As if to spare the analyst, she added, 'I feared that it might disturb you'. Actually, although she was speaking quietly and gave no sign of acting upon her impulse, this whole sequence was electric. It had nothing of the 'as if' about it.

It was an achievement for this patient to be able to speak of this bleak state and its self-directed expression. The analyst's thoughts about the first origins of patient's feelings was that her mother had often been stuporose and neglectful. It was easy to imagine the patient as an infant who had been left emotionally to experience an emptiness, or absence, made asphyxiating by the accumulation of her own unmet expectations and needs. The impulse to flail her arms may arise from a situation that is intolerable but at least it draws it to the attention of others. However, the analyst's just referring the patient's impulse back to a reconstructed original infantile situation with her mother would not help by itself. What is more important is the analyst's awareness of the *potential* this expression of impulse has now for the patient's future emotional growth.

Making and monitoring contact

Making emotional contact with the depressed patient is a first task of the therapy. Although particularly important in the early stages, this is something that requires attention in each and every session regardless of the phase of the therapy. Many depressed patients have experienced developmental injuries, or much personal adversity and loss. The therapist's sensitivity to the impact of these on the patient's functioning is important. Environmental adversity commonly can take the form of early losses, a chaotic upbringing with many caregivers, gross maltreatment and neglect, or childhood sexual abuse. However, less obvious, yet no less damaging, injuries can arise from more subtle disappointments and humiliations such as cold care and emotional unavailability. Equally, patients can suffer a great deal from the damaging consequences of their own psychological defenses or internal object relations.

While differences in theory and in training affect the 'what and why' of interpretation it is important that whatever their orientation the therapist employs open-minded formulation rather than imposes theory-driven formulae. The goal is to understand the person rather than the material. However, making emotional contact depends on more than the therapist's knowledge and sensitivity. It is powerfully affected by factors operating in the patient. Nuances in the patient's activity, in a way of relating—for example, by being subtly reproachful and angry, or alternatively appealing, or distressed, or by active biases in a way of understanding the therapist's communications, will all affect the way the therapist can function. For example, the therapist may be nudged into becoming moralistic, judgmental, or sometimes excessively sympathetic.

One of the therapist's most important tasks is to monitor the effect the patient is having on his or her way of thinking and relating in order to understand what this may indicate about the patient's way of operating. Where therapists are inexperienced or in training, supervision is essential. Experienced therapists and analysts should continue the discipline of reflective practice through regular case presentation with colleagues.

Meaningful connection in thought, feeling, and relationships

The focus upon depressive symptoms, which may have been the patient's first, or ostensible, occasion for seeking help, tends to recede once therapy has become established. While sometimes it is important to work out just how the conflicts and difficulties may have led to particular symptoms, this focus may lose meaning for the patient. Instead patients become more concerned with their lives, and the working over of significant feelings, events, and relationships that are tacitly understood as having provided the ground out of which depressive symptoms have developed. The emphasis on symptoms may return, or new symptoms develop, because of external stresses, breaks in therapy, some failure of understanding, in reaction to the opening up of previously unexplored areas, or as the ending of therapy comes into sight.

Mental pain and guilt

Excessive mental pain is characteristic of depression. However, having a normal capacity to suffer mental pain is as important in the personal sphere as being able to feel physical pain is for bodily self-preservation. It is for this reason that when mental pain is present in the depressed patient the therapist tries to bring it and its causes into the open, rather than to smooth it away or deny it. At the same time, however, the therapist will try to moderate excessive pain through giving the pain its proper proportion and by understanding its nature and origin.

As we have seen the pain of object loss is a common element and some melancholia's are based upon the extreme painfulness of relinquishing a lost object. As the object is felt to be dead this means that to maintain the connection with the love object the patient must feel dead too. Significant loss of an object or belief system disrupts the relationship with the internal good object, which as described above, is central to the ego's stability. As already described, the therapist with their comments and interpretations tracks the inner feelings connected with these states and this ameliorates mental pain.

Some of the painful mental suffering characteristic of depression arises from the sado-masochistic nature of those internal object relations associated with a punishing super-ego. They can involve cycles of punishing the self and the object. Some depressed patients by taking up positions of martyrdom or victimhood achieve a hidden gratification by making others seem to inflict pain or reject them. The therapist need to be able to identify and describe these positions so that ultimately the patient will be able to also.

Sometimes causing oneself to suffer pain masochistically may obscure a more deeply feared pain originally felt at the hands of others and this needs to be understood.

In patients with chronic forms of depression, the capacity to suffer painful conflicts may be numbed to defend against these underlying pains. This leads the person to avoid *any* change or growth because of the danger that it is felt to represent. In chronic depressions, states of dulled, partial breakdown are clung to because they offer some functioning and equilibrium, albeit at the cost of restricted capacities and continued disability. No matter how unresponsive, stuck, or chronic the patient's adjustment may appear to be, it is important to recollect that it may be based upon a precarious internal situation.

Internalization and termination

An important step in the consolidation of these changes is based upon the patient's internalization of the therapist's consistent attitude towards life experiences and the mental states associated with them. Some internalizing of this kind of functioning may be seen in the patient while therapy is ongoing but it is only consolidated after the ending of therapy.

The ending of the therapy can provoke a crisis in which the belief in the goodness of the object is once more called into question. The successful working through of the loss represented by the ending of therapy involves a mourning process that, if it is successfully negotiated, will be succeeded by the more stable internalization of the therapist's function as a dynamic element in the patient's own personality.

Difficult situations and their solutions

The necessity for emotional first aid in the depressed

Therapists may find themselves in situations with depressed patients where they urgently need to enable the patient to recover their interest in staying alive. Through interpretive understanding they need to alleviate, first-aid fashion, those mental processes (especially super-ego processes) that are most powerfully causing suffering. Interpretation is also needed to support those capacities that enable the patient to begin to think about what has happened in their life and inner world. Therapists treating seriously depressed patients need not feel that they must rely upon interpretation alone. They should feel authorized to take emergency action and to seek help as clinically appropriate.

As indicated already there is some research evidence supporting the value of combining medication with psychodynamic psychotherapy. This should be used when the depression is life-threatening.

While there may be few situations in psychodynamic psychotherapy where antidepressants are actively contraindicated, many patients feel that medication diminishes their contact with themselves, or in other ways alters their mental functioning in ways that they dislike. The UK Committee on the Safety of Medicines (2003) recently advised that several SSRIs should not be used with young people because of the reports of increased suicidal and aggressive feelings.

Negative therapeutic reactions

Negative reactions to improvement are characteristic in depressive states and working them through is an important part of the therapeutic process. These reactions have many origins. Most frequently, there is a part of the patient's mind, often taking the form of a destructive super-ego formation, which retaliates as if it had been left out or as had found its dominance threatened when things seem to get a bit better. These parts of the mind need recognition and understanding just as much as any other.

However, the therapist will need to be alert to these reactions, to be able to accept them, and understand the dynamics that may be operating. There may be deep-seated masochistic trends in the personality that require illumination before improvement can be regarded as at all stable. At other times, the desire to reverse the child–parent relation, to get power over the parents (the therapist) and to triumph over them gives rise to deep-seated guilt feelings and cripples any of the patient's endeavors. Stupor-like states may express as well as defend against the more violent of these reactions.

As described above for some patients a compromise within a psychic retreat permits a kind of limited life at the price of accepting a level of disability. This is equivalent to paying protection money: 'consenting to be robbed so as not to be murdered'. The sacrificing of resourcefulness it exacts leads to an emotional version of the disability benefits trap.

Suicidal states

In the treatment of the seriously depressed it is not uncommon for dangerous suicidal states to follow periods of improvement. These dangerous reactions, customarily explained in terms of a release of the previous condition of inhibition, may take the form of direct urges to murder or attack others. Other times the patient feels urges towards self-murder. Both of these can be very frightening to the patient, as well as potentially dangerous. Obviously, following improvement the therapist needs to be alert to the possibility of reactions of this sort.

Patients may sense something aggressive or explosive developing within them. The therapist may be able to anticipate the signs of anxiety and concern about these incipient developments and use interpretation to modify the way they emerge.

Clinical illustration

Mr C a depressed borderline man tended to pick rows with petty officials when he would go into loud tirades full of violent imagery. As he became more isolated and desperate, the violence increased; he began to pick arguments with the police and to risk arrest. The therapist understood this as the patient's only way of communicating that his violence was getting out of hand. He suggested that the patient was choosing to do battle with someone who he was sure could protect themselves and perhaps might protect him also. This interpretation, along with realism about the aggressivity of the disputes, served as a point of contact for the patient. Gradually, as he was able to extend the depth of his meaningful communication with the therapist his circumstances improved but his inner poverty became more difficult to hide from. He brought a dream in which he was hanging below the arch of a bridge over some black and icy waters (he lived near a river). This dream alerted the therapist to the risk of a suicidal depression developing in Mr C. He interpreted that the patient had been able to find a bridge between himself and the therapist, a bridge towards a better life. However, he might feel that it wasn't recognized that this meant contact with an inner life which felt like icy waters not an easy feeling of security.

The therapist's ability to judge when the patient feels their impulses are getting out of control is of great value. Sometimes speaking of this will enable a discussion between the therapist and the patient about the correct course of action. In these situations the patient is often very split and the sane part of the patient can be an ally in estimating the severity and in the management of the situation. For example,

It seems to me that you have enough from today's session to get through to next week but it may be this isn't so. What do you think? . . . You can always phone, should things get more difficult . . . . Perhaps, you feel that you need more help in managing this and we need to recognize this?

It can be seen from the above how part of the *therapist's* appraisal of the risk will be an assessment of the patient's contact with him or her, and the reliability of the understanding between them. When the patient is secretively or openly in the grip of a dangerously destructive part of themselves the therapist may need to intervene, or ask colleagues to intervene, to detain the patient compulsorily.

Of course, it is important for those involved in this work to face the fact that the patient's complete safety cannot be guaranteed whatever steps are taken. Regrettably suicides or homicides occur. They create anger, deep-seated guilt, and blame, which have a major psychological impact on those involved. Tactful, supportive, and understanding discussion is—after a while—helpful.

Countertransference issues

As patients with depression often have difficulties with handling aggressive or hostile feelings they behave in ways that evoke these in others. The patient's consistent seeking of the passive role, the martyred saint or the victim can stir up guilt, or rage, in those who want to be helpful. This dynamic may operate powerfully in those with 'treatment-resistant' depression. Other depressed patients subtly invite a somewhat critical or moralizing stance. This may be to confirm the illusion that all that is lacking in the patient is more of an effort.

Depressed patients can stir up wishes to rescue and cure. They can also stir-up powerful feelings of despair, hopelessness, and rejection. In suicidal patients the therapist commonly experiences a wish to keep them alive, however, the therapist may sometimes wish that the patient would end it all. It is important to think about both these feelings. A part of the patient that wishes to live and prosper may be evoked in the therapist or when despair and hatred is evoked the patient may be at risk of suicide.

Much can be learnt from these, to some degree, inevitable reactions. As indicated above therapeutic processes are greatly improved by seeking supervision from a more experienced and knowledgeable colleague or by clinical presentations and discussions in general. If countertransference reactions are beginning to deform the work, then case supervision can make the difference between success and failure.

'Comorbidity'—panic disorder, alcohol, and substance misuse

It has been estimated that between 14% and 37% of patients with major depressive disorder have panic attacks (Pini *et al.*, 1997; Fava *et al.*, 2000), whereas 40–70% of patients with panic disorder at some point will meet the criteria for major depressive disorder. Rudden *et al.* (2003) in a series of psychodynamic treatment studies have examined the co-occurrence of these conditions and were able to make valuable recommendations about what needs to be understood and interpreted. This sort of understanding equips the therapist to work out strategies for responding to phobic patients who, for instance, are unable to attend their sessions when this means venturing out in the dark.

There is a connection between dependence disorders and depression. Alcohol dependence and other substance misuse often overlies significant depression as well as other disturbance. Their treatment presents particular challenges. A small proportion of patients diagnosed with depression are defending against some underlying psychotic or borderline decompensation. This may emerge as the patient becomes more known in therapy. It may take the form of 'nothing happening' in the therapy. These eventualities need to be recognized and responded to accordingly.

Drop-out

In most instances, the threatened drop-out needs to be responded to by understanding what is going on and in a spirit of confident thoughtfulness and persistence, through interpretation. Some kind of 'therapist testing crisis' often seems to need to happen, and to be surmounted, if the treatment of patients with significant depression is to be successful. The testing may employ destructive despair, phobia, noncontact, nonresponse, increase of depression, or suicidality. In these situations the therapist's 'not taking the patient's "no" for an answer' requires great clinical judgement and expertise, to be able to distinguish when it is necessary and when it is neither indicated nor appropriate. The patient's consent is a *sine qua non* for psychotherapeutic treatment. A small number of patients make a decision that this form of therapeutic probing and disturbing is not for them, and the decision needs to be respected.

Conclusions

From the dynamic point of view much remains to be discovered about the etiology, prevention, and treatment of depressive disorders. The findings and ideas of the future cannot be fully anticipated. However, it is possible to guess about future directions by extrapolating on the basis of existing trends. These include:

- *The nature of the disability in depressive disorders.* Discussions of the burden of depressive disorder have concentrated upon the impact of

symptoms, distress, social or occupational malfunctioning, hospitalization, increased mortality, and suicide. These are important, but a more penetrating conceptualization of personal functioning leading up to depression as well as that following from it is needed. Better recognition of key psychological functions such as the ability to form life projects and core relationships might lead to more measures based upon functional capacity rather than symptoms. Such instruments would be valuable in the further study of depression and its treatment.

- *The disease entity approach to depressive syndromes.* The study of depressive disorders is organized around the use of diagnoses based on symptom pictures. Developmental perspectives, and dynamic psychopathological approaches based upon the study of personality functioning and object relations, may be able to contribute more to our understanding of the factors determining prognosis and the degree of treatment responsiveness or resistance.

- *Within the framework of the nosological approach a more adequate dynamic classification of depression is needed.* Blatt (1974) and Bleichmar (1996) have made helpful contributions. The current authors are developing a dynamic dimensional model to be based upon the experience of treating long-term depressed patients with a degree of treatment resistance.

- *Gene–environment expression.* First identifying and then tracking the development of the psychological, temperamental phenotype expressions as outcomes of gene–environment interaction, and their role in the genesis of depression, will be of great potential value in working out ways of preventing depressive disorders.

- *Treatment studies.* The psychoanalytic understanding of those elements contributing to chronicity, and resistance to treatment, are more deeply understood now than they were a century ago. As a result of clinical psychoanalytic research, we may now have sufficient understanding to improve the outlook for those who suffer from the more damaging and intractable forms of depression. This possibility needs to be tested.

References

Abraham, K. (1911). Notes on the psychoanalytic investigation and treatment of manic-depressive insanity and allied conditions. *Selected Papers on Psycho-Analysis*, 1927. London: Hogarth.

Abraham, K. (1916). The influence of oral erotism on character-formation. *Selected Papers on Psycho-Analysis*, 1927. London: Hogarth.

Abraham, K. (1924). A short study of the development of the libido. *Selected Papers on Psycho-Analysis*, 1927. London: Hogarth.

Barkham, M., Rees, A., Shapiro, D. A., Agnew, R. M., Halstead, J., and Culverwell, A. (1994). Effects of treatment method and duration and severity of depression on the effectiveness of psychotherapy: Extending the Second Sheffield Psychotherapy Project to NHS settings. Sheffield University SAPU Memo 1480.

Bellack, A. S. *et al.* (1981). Social skills training compared with pharmacotherapy and psychotherapy in the treatment of unipolar depression. *American Journal of Psychiatry*, **138**, 1562–7.

Bibring, E. (1953). The mechanics of depression. In *Affective Disorders*. New York International Press.

Bion, W. R. (1962). *Learning from experience.* London: Heinemann.

Bion, W. R. (1963). *Elements of psycho-analysis.* London: Heinemann.

Blatt (1974). Levels of object representation in anaclitic and introjective depression. *Psychoanal. Study Child*, **29**, 107–57.

Bleichmar (1996). Some subtypes of depression and their implications for psychoanalytic treatment. *International Journal of Pschyoanalysis*, **77**: 935–62.

Burnand, Andreoli, Kolatte, Venturini, and Rosset (2002). Psychodynamic psychotherapy and clomipramine in the treatment of major depression. *Psychiatric Service*, **53**(5), 25–6.

Cooper, B. and Cooper, P. J. (2003). The impact of post-partum depression on child development. In: I. Goodyear, ed. *Aetiological Mechanism in Developmental Psychopathology*. Oxford: Oxford University Press.

Department of Health (2001). *Treatment choice in Psychological therapies and counselling*. London: HMSO.

Deutsch, H. (1932). *Psychoanalysis of the neurosis*. London: Hogarth.

Deutsch, H. (1951). Abstract of panel discussion of mania and hypomania. *Bulletin of the American Psychoanalytic Association*, 7(3).

Fava, M., Rankin, M., Wright, E. C., Alpert, J. E., Nierenberg, A. A., Pava, J., and Rosenbaum, J. F. (2000). Anxiety disorders in major depression. *Comparative Psychiatry*, 41, 97–102.

Fonagy, P. *et al.* (2002). *Open Door Review of Outcome Studies in Psychoanalysis and Psychoanalytical Psychotherapy*, 2nd edn.

Freud, S. (1917). Mourning and Melancholia. *S. E.*, 14.

Freud, S. (1926). *Inhibitions, Symptoms and Anxiety. S. E.*, 20.

Gallagher-Thompson, D. and Steffen, A. M. (1994). Comparative effects of cognitive-behavioral and brief psychodynamic psychotherapies for depressed family caregivers. *Journal of Consulting and Clinical Psychology*, 62, 543–49.

Guthrie, E., Moorey, J., Margison, F., Barker, H., Palmer, S., McGrath, G., Tomenson, B., and Creed, F. (1999). Cost-effectiveness of brief psychodynamic-interpersonal therapy in high utilizers of psychiatric services. *Archives of General Psychiatry*, 56, 519–26.

Guthrie, E. *et al.* (1998). Brief psychodynamic interpersonal therapy for patients with severe psychiatric illness which is unresponsive to treatment. *British Journal of Psychotherapy*, 15, 155–66.

Guthrie, E. *et al.* (2001). Randomised controlled trial of brief psychological intervention after deliberate self poisoning. *British Medical Journal*, 323, 135–8.

Jacobsen, E. (1943). Despression: the Oedipus complex in the development of depressive mechanism. *Psychoanalytic Quarterly*, 12, 541–60.

Jacobsen, E. (1946). The effect of disappointment on the ego and superego formation in normal and depressive development. *Pyschoanalytical Review*, 33, 129–47.

Jacobsen, E. (1954a). Psychotic identifications. *Journal of the American Psychoanalytical Association*, 2(4).

Jacobsen, E. (1954b). Transference problem in the psychoanalytic treatment of a severely depressed patient. *Journal of the American Psychoanalytical Association*, 2(4).

de Jonge, P. *et al.* (2001). Case complexity in the general hospital. *Psychosomatics*, 42, 204–12.

Klein, M. (1930). The importance of symbol formation in the development of the ego. *International Journal of Psychoanalysis*, 11, 24–39.

Klein, M. (1933). The early development of conscience in the child. *Psychoanalysis Today*. Lorand, ed. New York: Covici-Friede.

Klein, M. (1935). A contribution to the psychogenesis of the manic depressive states. *International Journal of Psychoanalysis*, 16.

Klein, M. (1940). Mourning and its relation to manic depressive states. *International Journal of Psychoanalysis*, 21.

Kohut, H. (1971). Analysis of the Self. New York: IUP.

Lambert, M. J. (1992). Psychotherapy outcome research: implications for integrative and eclectic theories. In J. C. Norcross and M. R. Goldfried, ed. *Handbook of Psychotherapy Integration* New York: Basic Books.

Lambert, M. J. and Bergin, A. E. (1994). The effectiveness of psychotherapy. In: A. E. Bergin and S. L. Garfield, ed. *Handbook of Psychotherapy and Behaviour Change*. New York: Wiley.

Leff, J., Vearnals, S., Brewin, C., Wolff, G., Alexander, B., Asen, E., Drayson, D., Jones, E., Chisholm, D., and Everitt, B. (2000). The london depression intervention trial: an RCT of anti-depressants vs. couple therapy in the treatment and maintenance of depressed people with a partner: clinical outcomes and costs. *British Journal of Psychiatry*, 177, 95–100.

Leuzinger-Bohleber, M. and Target, M. (2002). *Outcomes of Psychoanalytic Treatment*. London: Whurr Publishers.

Lydiard, B., Otto, M., and Milrod, B. (2000). Panic disorder. In G. Gabbard, ed. *Treatment of Psychiatric Disorders*, 3rd edn, p. 45. Washington, DC: American Psychiatric Association Press.

Milton, J. (2001). Psychoanalysis and cognitive-behavioural therapy: rival parameters or common ground. *International Journal of Psychoanalysis*, 82(3), 431–47.

McPherson, S., Richardson, P. H., and Leroux, P. (2003). Clinical effectiveness in psychotherapy and mental health. 23. London: Karnac.

Morrison, C. *et al.* (2003). The external validity of efficacy trials for depression and anxiety. *Psychology and Psychotherapy*, 76, 109–32.

NICE Depression Guideline (2004).

O'Shaugnessy, E. (1999). Relating to the super-ego. *International Journal of Psychoanalysis*, 49, 691–98.

Pini, S., *et al.* (1997). Prevalence of anxiety disorders comorbidity in bipolar depression, unipolar depression and dysthymia. *Journal of Affective Disorder*, 42, 145–53.

Rado, S. (1927). Das Problem der Melancholie. *Int. Zeitschr. F. Psychoanal.*, 13, trans. 1928 in *International Journal of Psychoanalysis*, 9.

Rosenfeld, H. (1959). An investigation into the psycho-analytic theory of depression. *International Journal of Psychoanalysis*, 40, 105–29.

Roff, A. and Fonagy, P. (1996). *What Works for Whom*. New York: The Guilford Press.

Rudden, M., Busch, F. N., Milrod, B., Singer, M., Aronson, A., Roiphe, J., and Shapiro, T. (2003). Panic disorder and depression: a psychodynamic exploration of comorbidity. *International Journal of Psychoanalysis*, 84, 997–1015.

Sandell, R. (1987). Effects of psychoanalysis and long-term psychotherapy. In: M. Leuzinger-Bohleber and M. Target, ed. (2002). *Outcomes of Psychoanalytic Treatment*.

Shapiro, D. A., Barkham, M., Rees, A., Hardy, G. E., Reynolds, S., and Start-up, M. (1994). Effects of treatment duration and severity of depression on the effectiveness of cognitive/behavioural and psychodynamic/interpersonal psychotherapy. *Journal of Consulting and Clinical Psychology*, 62, 522–34.

Stimpson, N., Agrawal, N., and Lewis, G. (2002). Randomised controlled trials investigating pharmacological and psychological interventions for treatment-refractory depression. *British Journal of Psychiatry*, 181, 284–94.

Sulloway, F. J. (1979). *Freud: The Biologist of the Mind: Beyond the Psychoanalytic Legend*. Fontana: Bungay.

Thompson, L. W. *et al.* (1998). Personality disorder and outcome in the treatment of late-life depression. *Journal of Geriatric Psychiatry*, 21, 133–46.

UK Committee on the Safety of Medicines (2003).

Weston, D. and Morrison, K. (2001). A multi-dimenstional meta-analysis of treatments of depression, panic and generalized anxiety disorder: an empirical examination of the status of empirically supported psychotherapies. *Journal of Consulting and Clinical Psychology*, 69, 875–89.

Winnicott, D. W. (1955). The depressive position in normal emotional development. *British Journal of Medical Psychology*, 28, Pt. 2 & 3.

Winnicott, D. W. (1957). *The Child and The Family*. London: Tavistock.

13 Anxiety disorders

Robert L. Leahy, Lata K. McGinn, Fredric N. Busch, and Barbara L. Milrod

Introduction

Anxiety disorders are one of the most common psychological disorders found in national surveys of the prevalence of psychiatric problems. Many anxiety disorders are persistent rather than episodic, with a large percentage of patients with generalized anxiety, social anxiety disorder (SAD), or obsessive-compulsive disorder (OCD) reporting difficulties lasting years. In many cases, the existence of an anxiety disorder will precede the emergence of a later depressive disorder, perhaps because there is a common diathesis or because the demoralization of having a long-lasting anxiety disorder contributes to self-criticism, withdrawal, loss of rewards, and general feelings of helplessness and hopelessness. Indeed, many individuals suffering from these anxiety disorders rely on alcohol or other drugs as anxiety management, thereby complicating their problems.

In this chapter we have brought to the reader two quite different theoretical and clinical orientations to understanding and treating anxiety disorders—specifically, cognitive-behavioral therapy (CBT) and psychodynamic therapy. We attempt to provide theoretical models and clinical strategies drawn independently from these models. Because of the differences in these models, we have chosen to let them stand independently from one another and leave it to the reader to explore the possibility of clinical integration.

Cognitive-behavioral theory and model of anxiety disorders

The behavioral and cognitive models of phobia and anxiety have witnessed a substantial development over the last 35 years. More detailed descriptions of specific models of each anxiety disorder are provided in this chapter. However, earlier models of acquisition of phobia were initially based on the model of classical conditioning, outlined by Pavlov. The supposition was that neutral stimuli were inadvertently 'paired' with noxious outcomes (*such as injury or unpleasant experiences*), and that these associations were learned and the previously neutral stimulus was later avoided. Mowrer (1939, 1960) later viewed this simple associationist model as inadequate to explain the maintenance of fear of situations that were avoided, as the simple associationist model would imply that the strength of the fear should decline with longer avoidance. Mowrer posited a two-factor theory (*explained below*) that accounted for the acquisition of fear through classical associationist conditioning and the maintenance of fear through the anxiety reduction repeatedly experienced through escape of avoidance in the presence of anticipation of the feared stimulus.

Utilization of exposure paradigms—whereby the patient was urged to engage in exposure to the feared stimulus without the opportunity to escape—was expected to lessen the anxiety or fear as the patient experienced no harm during the exposure. Initially Wolpe advocated a form of reciprocal inhibition, pairing 'responses' such as relaxation, assertion, or the sexual response, in the presence of the feared stimulus. The rationale is that relaxation would be incompatible with fear and would replace fear as a response. Subsequent research on exposure to feared stimuli indicated that relaxation was not an important or even useful component of exposure.

The behavioral model emphasized the development of response and stimulus hierarchies that reflected increasingly more anxiety or fear for specific stimuli. Therapists were urged to begin with modeling their own exposure to the feared stimulus, while the patient later imitated this coping behavior. Use of exposure—while preventing escape or neutralization—would provide the patient with an experience of habituation to the feared stimulus and—in cognitive terms—the disconfirmation that the stimulus needed to be avoided because it conferred danger. This model was expanded to the treatment of specific phobia, SAD, and OCD.

Beck and Emery's cognitive model stressed both the biological preparedness of certain fears and the cognitive distortions associated with these fears. Thus, Beck was able to identify the role of the individual's interpretations, e.g., catastrophic interpretations of events or symptoms ('*I won't be able to stand it*', '*I'll get so anxious I will die*'), mislabeling ('*I am crazy*'), and fortune-telling ('*something terrible will happen*'). The initial cognitive approach advocated by Beck stressed the use of exposure in the context of identifying the patients' predictions and testing them out through behavioral exposure.

Subsequent cognitive and behavioral models attempted to specify specific cognitive components for each of the anxiety disorders—indeed, arguing for a specific refined model for each diagnostic category. As a consequence of this greater specificity of the model, we describe how the CBT model is applied for each of the anxiety disorders in this chapter.

The psychodynamic understanding and treatment of anxiety disorders

Having developed several psychological models of anxiety, psychoanalysts have only recently begun to focus on the treatment of specific anxiety disorders. Systematic placebo-controlled studies of specific anxiety disorders with psychodynamic approaches have not yet been accomplished. Nevertheless, psychodynamic theory has significant clinical explanatory potential for anxiety disorders through its focus on intrapsychic conflicts, unconscious fantasies, defense mechanisms, and the compromise function of symptoms, factors that are not central to other psychological or neurobiological theories. In addition, the clinical techniques of focus on the transference, examining the emotional impact of the patient's developmental history, exploring the meaning of symptoms, and the technique of using free association provide a broad array of therapeutic tools for potentially lessening symptoms and vulnerability to recurrence of disorders.

For systematic studies to be performed, psychoanalysts and psychoanalytic researchers must develop specific treatments, described in treatment manuals, for anxiety disorders focusing on dynamics specific to each of these disorders, as well as the particular treatment approaches tailored to these dynamics. As of the writing of this chapter, manuals of this sort for anxiety disorders have only been developed for panic disorder (Wiborg and Dahl, 1996; Milrod *et al.*, 1997) and posttraumatic stress disorder (PTSD) (Lindy *et al.*, 1983; Weiss and Marmar, 1993; Marmar *et al.*, 1995). As will be discussed below, preliminary studies using these manuals suggest that the psychodynamic approach is a promising treatment for panic disorder (Wiborg and Dahl, 1996; Milrod *et al.*, 2000, 2001) and PTSD (Lindy *et al.*, 1983).

In this section, we shall describe basic psychodynamic principles that can be used to develop psychodynamic models and treatment approaches to specific anxiety disorders.

Relevant core dynamic concepts

In order to understand psychodynamic theories and approaches to anxiety disorders, it is useful to review certain core dynamic concepts.

Traumatic anxiety versus signal anxiety

Freud (1926/1959) described two types of anxiety: the traumatic form, in which the ego is overwhelmed by anxiety and stimuli that it cannot contain, and a signal form ('signal anxiety'), which alerts the ego to the presence of wishes, impulses, or feelings that are considered dangerous.

The tripartite model of the mind

According to the 'structural theory', developed by Freud (1923/1961), the mind is divided into three relatively stable 'structures' with discrete functions: the ego, the id, and the superego. The id subsumes the instinctual drives that emerge as the individual's needs and wishes, conscious or unconscious. The ego mediates between the drives and external reality, in part through the operation of defenses (see below). The superego includes the conscience and moral ideals and precepts, with both rewarding and punishing functions.

Defenses

Signal anxiety triggers characteristic defense, means of warding off or disguising dangerous wishes and impulses to render them less threatening. If the ego is ineffective at warding off the danger felt from internal wishes and unconscious fantasies (Shapiro, 1992), traumatic anxiety, in the form of overwhelming anxiety or panic, can result. Another outcome might be that the patient develops symptoms that bind anxiety, such as a phobia or obsessions. By attaching the anxiety to specific symptoms, it will be experienced as more controllable, and the frightening unconscious wishes are more disguised. In phobias, for example, the internal fear converts to a specific external danger that can be avoided (see Specific phobia section below).

The unconscious

In psychoanalytic theory, mental life operates on both conscious and unconscious (out of awareness) levels (Breuer and Freud, 1895/1955). Wishes, fantasies, and impulses that may be considered dangerous to the ego are frequently unconscious, and it is their potential emergence into consciousness that is experienced as threatening. Anxiety disorders arise in part from unconscious factors.

Compromise formation

In order to diminish the risk from threatening fantasies or impulses, the ego synthesizes a compromise between the wish and the defense that is being employed to avert the threat from the wish (Breuer and Freud, 1895/1955). Psychiatric symptoms, as well as fantasies and dreams, are compromise formations that symbolically represent both the wishes and the defenses.

The pleasure principle

According to Freud's formulation, individuals unconsciously avoid unpleasurable feelings and fantasies via the mental operation of repression and other defenses (Freud, 1911/1958). In subsequent writings, Freud (1920/1955) modified the idea of the pleasure principle to include the notion that discharging intense emotions was more fundamental than the pursuit of pleasure. According to the psychoanalytic theory of the pleasure principle, anxiety disorder symptoms are less distressing than the unconscious conflicts underlying the symptoms.

Representations of self and others

Over the course of development, people internalize representations (mental images and concepts) of themselves and others, and themselves in relation to others. Patients with anxiety disorders often have representations of others (object representations) as being demanding, controlling, threatening, and anxiety inducing. These object representations add to the experience of fantasies and feelings as dangerous. Anger is often experienced as a danger to attachments, and attachments feel insecure.

Neurophysiological vulnerability and psychodynamic factors in anxiety disorders

Evidence suggests that neurophysiological vulnerabilities may trigger a psychological state that can increase the potential of an individual to develop an anxiety disorder. A temperamental fearfulness can affect the individual's perceptions of themselves and others, as well as the sense of safety of feelings and fantasies. Kagan and colleagues (Rosenbaum et al., 1988; Biederman et al., 1990; Kagan et al., 1990) identified a group of behaviorally inhibited children who demonstrated fear responses in the setting of environmental novelty. Children felt to be at risk for the development of panic disorder (offspring of parents with panic disorder and agoraphobia) were found to have high rates of behavioral inhibition compared with a control group, and children with behavioral inhibition were likewise found to have an increased rate of anxiety disorders. Thus, this fearfulness may have a genetic origin that in interaction with a particular set of psychological and environmental factors can trigger the development of anxiety disorders.

Psychodynamic treatment of anxiety disorders

Psychodynamic psychotherapy operates through the identification of the unconscious and conscious fantasies and conflicts underlying anxiety disorder symptoms, bringing them into the therapeutic dialogue, where they can be understood and rendered less threatening. These fantasies can be brought to the surface by exploring the meanings of symptoms, the stressors that precede or exacerbate symptom onset, and the fantasies and feelings that emerge in the relationship with the therapist (the transference). As these fantasies and conflicts are rendered less catastrophic, the symptoms often diminish and resolve. An important component of this form of therapy is helping patients to become aware of, more tolerant of, and more effective in expressing their drives and wishes.

Exploration of underlying dynamic meanings of symptoms provides important clues about unconscious fantasies and conflicts that fuel anxiety symptoms. Although patients with anxiety disorders share general sets of symptoms, individual variations in the syndromes are an important source of information about unconscious significance. For instance, one patient's fear of choking during panic attacks when drinking liquids was linked to intense, exciting, and frightening struggles for control with her father when she was a child regarding how much food and drink she should have at the dinner table. The exploration of this symptom led to an understanding of angry and sexualized feelings in her relationship with her father that she experienced as dangerous, yet needed to reexperience over and over in the form of symptoms. Circumstances preceding symptom onset, feelings experienced other than anxiety, and defense mechanisms employed provide additional clues about the psychological origins of symptoms.

Use of the transference is a core component of psychoanalytic treatment. In the phenomenon of transference, components of central relationships are unconsciously experienced as deriving from current relationships (Freud, 1909/1953). This process takes place with the therapist as well. Understanding the patient's fantasies about the therapist and the treatment can be of value in any form of treatment, but from a psychodynamic perspective, the transference situation has far-reaching effects, and necessarily influences therapeutic outcome.

For example, a patient's fear that he will be abandoned by significant people in his life if he expresses his rage or frustration can be examined in the context of a stable, reassuring relationship with the therapist. Therapists also explore with patients how current perceptions or misperceptions of others, including the therapist, are linked with perceptions of significant others in childhood. For instance, patients who experience others and the therapist as shaming them may describe having experienced shaming behavior from their parents. Fantasies and dreams provide crucial information about intrapsychic conflicts, as well as the transference.

There is an emphasis in psychodynamic psychotherapy on monitoring one's own reactions to patients, referred to as the countertransference (Gabbard, 1995). Negative, critical, or distancing behavior, of which the therapist may or may not be aware, can have a disruptive impact on the therapeutic alliance, and can limit the impact of any treatment. Although awareness of one's own reactions to a patient is of value in any treatment, psychodynamic psychotherapists scan their own reactions as additional clues to understanding patients. For instance, the therapist may be aware of his own discomfort and avoidance when a patient with PTSD appears to be on the verge of discussing a particularly painful aspect of the trauma she experienced. Not all reactions to patients, however, are induced by particular patient behavior and attitudes, and psychodynamic psychotherapists attempt to learn about the various feelings different patients, conflicts, and disorders may elicit in them. With patients with anxiety disorders, therapists should be particularly concerned about fantasies and fears of exacerbating a patient's anxiety symptoms.

Specific phobia

Diagnostic features

The defining characteristics of specific phobia are intense fear of anxiety in the presence of a specific stimulus or situation, where this fear results in impairment or discomfort, and the individual realizes that the fear is excessive. Typical specific phobias include fears of animals, blood or injection, heights, water, insects, rats, and other stimuli or experiences. About 11% of the general population has a lifetime prevalence of specific phobia (Wittchen et al., 1994).

Evaluation

Specific phobia is intense fear and arousal in the presence of a specific stimulus or feared object (such as heights, animals, water). This is distinguished from panic disorder (where the fear is that the individual's arousal will go out of control and cause a medical emergency or insanity) and from SAD where the individual fears that the symptoms of anxiety will be observed by others resulting in humiliation or embarrassment. Specific phobia is also distinguished from PTSD in that patients with PTSD fear intrusive memories or images. Specific phobia can be evaluated by use of a variety of instruments, including the Fear Questionnaire (Marks and Mathews, 1979) and the Fear Survey Schedule (Wolpe and Lang, 1964).

Theoretical models

The most widely used theoretical model of specific phobia is based on learning theory. Since Watson's (1919) observations of a conditioned fear of furry objects in a young child (by pairing shock with a rabbit), behavior therapy has viewed specific phobia as resulting from a learned association of a negative consequence paired with a neutral stimulus. This classical, or Pavlovian, model was later modified in the two-factor theory of 'conservation of fear' proposed by Mowrer (1960). According to Mowrer, the initial fear was established through classical conditioning (e.g., the neutral stimulus of the stove was paired with the negative experience of being burned). However, avoidance of the stove in the future was based on operant conditioning—that is, when the individual approached the stove there was an increase of fear. Avoiding or escaping was associated with reduction of fear (thereby negatively reinforcing the operant of escape or avoidance through the consequence of fear reduction). The two-factor model thus accounted for the acquisition of fear through classical conditioning and the avoidance of feared stimuli through the negative reinforcement of reducing fear through the operants of escape of avoidance. Fear was thereby 'conserved'.

The implication of the classical and operant models was that fear could be overcome by direct exposure without escape. In addition, Wolpe (1958) introduced the idea of responses incompatible with fear or anxiety with the concept of 'reciprocal inhibition'. This refers to the fact that certain responses (or experiences) (e.g., relaxation, sexual behavior, and assertiveness) are incompatible with the response of fear. By pairing these incompatible responses (e.g., inducing relaxation in the presence of the feared stimulus) the individual can decondition the learned fear. Related to this model is the use of habituation techniques and extinction—that is, repeated exposure of the stimulus will reduce its potentiating effect (habituation) or repeated exposure without reinforcement (e.g., escape is negatively reinforcing) reduces the acquired associative link of the conditioned stimulus (CS) (e.g., the stove) with the learned (conditioned) response (e.g., fear).

While recognizing the value of conditioning and negative reinforcement for escape and avoidance, there has been a growing recognition of the importance of 'prepared' behaviors (Seligman, 1971), innate fears, or innate predispositions. According to these Darwinian influenced ethological models there are certain stimuli that the human infant is predisposed to fear. These stimuli reflect dangers in the evolutionary expected environment—that is, the primitive environment of danger from predators, natural catastrophes, and abandonment. For example, research on the distribution of fears in various cultures reveals that the same stimuli are largely equally feared and that these stimuli reflect primitive dangers. This nonrandom distribution of fears, with heights, water, animals, thunder/lightening topping the list, suggests that human infants and children are preadapted to fear events that confer danger. The Dunedin study in New Zealand offers further support to the ethological model of fear. In this study a large number of children were followed from early infancy to early adulthood and records of their fears and their experiences with feared events was obtained. Contrary to the 'learned fear' model proposed by associationist and operant theories, children who previously have suffered injuries from falling were *less* afraid of falling in the future. The learning models would have predicted the opposite—but the ethological model suggests that fears may be protective and innately predisposed. Moreover, an overwhelming high percentage of parents of children who feared water were afraid of the water on the very first presentation of a pool of water. Now, despite the argument that fears may be predisposed through evolution, the ethological model argues for some plasticity—that is, fears can be unlearned through exposure.

The cognitive model of specific phobia suggests that, in addition to the two-factor theory and the ethological model, there are specific cognitions and behaviors that may add to fear and avoidance. These include beliefs that the threat/danger of a stimulus is related to the fear that it elicits (see Ost, 1997; Ost and Hugdahl, 1981) and that safety behaviors may protect the individual from the threat. Examples of these cognitive distortions in fear include the following: 'If I am anxious, then it must be dangerous' and 'I must get rid of the anxiety immediately'. Safety behaviors include superstitious behaviors or thoughts that attempt to neutralize the fear or provide some protection from the fear. Examples of safety behaviors that fearful individuals may utilize include repeated self-assurance (praying, self-talk), magical rituals (wearing specific clothing on an airplane), hypervigilant scanning of the environment (e.g., checking for sounds and movements on an airplane), collecting information about danger (e.g., checking the weather forecasts or safety records of airlines), and requiring someone to accompany them when in the presence of a feared stimulus. The cognitive model of specific phobia suggests that these safety behaviors act as a disattribution error—that is, 'The only reason that I am safe is that I engaged in my safety behaviors'. Thus, safety behaviors might reduce the efficacy of the exposure used in behavioral treatment—a supposition now supported by empirical data.

Empirical support for treatments

There is overwhelming support for the efficacy of behavioral exposure treatment for specific phobia—in some cases, over 90% of patients being effectively treated with exposure treatment with some use of anxiety management techniques (Ost, 1997). Most fears can be successfully treated in fewer than five sessions, with massed practice or prolonged exposure yielding more rapid results.

Rationale for treatment and interventions

Given the importance of the role of avoidance and escape in the maintenance of fear, behavioral treatments rely on repeated exposure to feared stimuli. The rationale for treatment is to identify the feared situations or stimuli, introduce the use of relaxation techniques (if needed), and engage the patient in gradual but prolonged exposure to the stimulus. We have found it helpful to educate the patient about the evolutionary significance of phobias—that is, that most of the stimuli that are feared (e.g., heights, water, insects, animals) would confer danger in a primitive environment where these feared stimuli were present and dangerous. This preparedness of phobia leads to the emergence of a fear later, but that the use of behavioral exposure can reverse this process. The two-factor theory of anxiety 'conservation' outlined by Mowrer (1939, 1960) can be helpful in understanding that fears may be acquired through being 'paired' with a noxious experience, but that they are maintained or conserved through the anxiety reduction of escape or avoidance.

Strategies and techniques

Behavioral treatment of specific phobia follows a set pattern of interventions. During the assessment phase the therapist evaluates which stimuli or situations are avoided or experienced with discomfort. The Fear Survey is a useful assessment measure as is the Initial Fear Evaluation for Patients (Leahy and Holland, 2000). The patient's Fear Hierarchy (see Leahy and Holland) provides information for the assessment of a ranking or hierarchy of feared situations as well as the rating of degree of fear and whether the situation is actually avoided. Although anxiety management (such as breathing exercises and relaxation) are helpful, they are not necessary for exposure to the feared stimulus.

Brief plan of treatment

Socialization to treatment begins with providing the patient with the *Information for Patients about Specific Phobia* (Leahy and Holland, 2000) or by informing the patient of the nature of acquired and predisposed fear. Patients often find the Darwinian model provides them with a demystifying and nonstigmatizing explanation of their fear. Initial interventions involve training the patient in relaxation techniques (deep muscle relaxation, breathing, meditative techniques). Patients are trained in identifying Subjective Units of Distress (SUDs), rating their fear or anxiety from 0 to 100% (or 0–10), with higher numbers corresponding to greater fear. Imaginal exposure is used whereby the patient begins with imagining, in session, the least feared situation in the hierarchy and holding this image in mind until SUDs are reduced by 50% or more and then moving up the hierarchy to gradually more feared stimuli. *In vivo* exposure involves actual exposure to the feared stimulus. It is useful to obtain initial SUDs right before, during, and after the exposure and to elicit predictions from the patient about what he or she fears will happen (e.g., 'the elevator will crash' or 'I will drive off the bridge').

Safety behaviors are important impediments to exposure efficacy and these can be identified by asking patients if they do anything to make themselves feel safer. For example, asking the patient, 'When you drive across the bridge, when you are afraid, do you do any of the following to make yourself feel safer—talk to yourself, avoid looking to the side, clench the steering wheel, slow down, or anything else?'

As the patient is able to tolerate situations higher in the hierarchy the therapist can indicate that continued exposure—far beyond normal experiences with the stimulus—should be continued after treatment has been completed. For example, a patient with a fear of elevators should be told to continue taking elevators up and down for weeks—even when it is not necessary—in order to overpractice exposure. Any 'setbacks' or 'relapses' should be followed by re-initiating the program of exposure. Relaxation should be continued on a daily basis in order to reduce physiological arousal.

Case example

The patient was an executive in his fifties who had suffered from fear of heights for 9 years—with this fear increasing in the past 3 years. The patient indicated that he feared crossing bridges, climbing mountains, driving in the mountains, and standing close to the edge of precipices. He indicated very little fear of flying and pointed out that his fear of heights was due to his fear that he might lose control of the vehicle or himself and fall over the side. He utilized a number of safety behaviors that he believed lessened his fear, including having his wife drive or accompany him as a passenger ('She could take over the driving'), planning far ahead so as to anticipate trouble, avoiding looking to the side of the bridge, clenching the steering wheel, driving very slowly, alternating with the break and accelerator, talking to himself, avoiding the rear-view mirror, and avoiding bridges or heights totally.

The therapist explained to the patient both the Darwinian model and the learning theory model and provided him with the information sheet from Leahy and Holland (2000). He was quite skeptical of both models and said he would take a 'wait and see attitude'. The therapist encouraged this and suggested, 'Let's collect some data about what happens with your fear as we proceed'. A fear hierarchy for heights was obtained and the first intervention was imaginal exposure for thinking about specific bridges. The in-session imaginal exposure suggested little initial fear, so the imagined stimulus was changed to thinking about himself standing at the edge of a cliff. This immediately increased fear, which abated with prolonged exposure.

Specific safety behaviors were targeted. The therapist explained how these safety behaviors made him believe that he could not face the situation without these magical behaviors and thoughts and then relinquishing them would be important. The therapist utilized a role-play where the therapist played the role of the safety behavior thoughts (e.g., 'You need to clench the steering wheel or you will go over the side') while the patient argued against these thoughts. Furthermore, the patient was asked to imagine and later actually produce the opposite behaviors of his safety behaviors. For example, rather than clenching the wheel, he was asked to loosen his grip, rather than driving slower, he was to drive normally, rather than avoid the rear view mirror, he was to look at it on and off, and rather than avoiding looking over the side, he was to gaze on and off over the side. These were first practiced with imaginal training and later with *in vivo* training. Finally, he was to write out his predictions of what would happen and the actual outcome for various exposures.

Closer questioning revealed that the patient was inadvertently hyperventilating by taking very deep breaths during these experiences. Apparently he had 'heard' that you should take deep breaths to calm yourself. It was explained that this might add to his sense of light-headedness and that he should breathe normally.

After seven sessions (spaced over a 3-month period) after the initial intake, the patient had engaged in all of the feared behaviors in his hierarchy, including driving across numerous long bridges, driving for hours in the mountains, and standing at the edge of cliffs. These exposures became boring in themselves, but he was encouraged to continue to look for further opportunities after his treatment was completed.

Psychodynamic model for specific phobia

From the psychodynamic viewpoint, specific phobias develop from the ego's response to the threatened emergence of forbidden aggressive or sexual wishes. When these wishes trigger signal anxiety, certain defense mechanisms characteristic of phobias are activated to repress and disguise these wishes: displacement, projection, and avoidance (Gabbard, 2000). For example, in Freud's case of Little Hans (Freud, 1909/1955), a child developed a phobia of horses, which in Freud's view had come to symbolically represent his father. The child's fear of aggressive and competitive wishes toward his father was displaced (to horses) and projected: the horse was going to damage him, rather than that he was going to damage the horse (father). Then the anxiety could be diminished by the avoidance of horses. Thus, the phobic symptom symbolically replaced the anxiety from unconscious wishes.

Psychodynamic treatment of specific phobia

In psychodynamic psychotherapy, the therapist seeks to elucidate the meanings of the specific symptom, and the defenses that contribute to it, and uses them as guides for disentangling the unconscious threatening wishes. Exploring the circumstances surrounding symptom onset and what comes to mind about a specific symptom aids in this process. In this context the frightening unconscious wishes can be brought into consciousness and rendered less threatening. For example, when Freud communicated to Hans his aggressive and competitive wishes toward his father, his phobic symptoms resolved.

Obsessive-compulsive disorder

Diagnostic features

The DSM-IV [American Psychiatric Association (APA), 1994] defines obsessions as

> persistent and recurrent thoughts, ideas, images, or impulses that are experienced as intrusive and inappropriate, that are not simply excessive worries about real-life problems, and that cause marked anxiety or distress (e.g., thoughts of killing a child, becoming contaminated). The person recognizes that they are a product of his own mind and attempts to suppress or ignore the obsessions or to neutralize them with some other thought or action.

Compulsions are defined as

> repetitive behaviors (e.g., checking the stove, handwashing) or mental acts (e.g., counting numbers) that the person feels driven to perform in response to an obsession or according to rigid rules. The compulsion is aimed at preventing or reducing distress or preventing some dreaded situation; however, the compulsions are either unrealistic or clearly excessive.

Insight into illness is no longer necessary for the diagnosis so long as the excessiveness or senselessness of obsessions and compulsions is recognized at some point during the course of the disorder.

Diagnostic and assessment measures

OCD may be diagnosed using semistructured clinical interviews such as the Structured Interview for the DSM (SCID-P; Spitzer *et al.*, 1987) or the Anxiety Disorders Interview Schedule (ADIS-IV; DiNardo and Barlow, 1988; DiNardo *et al.*, 1993). Dimensional measures may also be used to assess for the severity and content of symptoms. The Yale-Brown Obsessive-Compulsive Scale is the most widely used rating scale in assessing severity of OCD symptoms (Y-BOCS; Goodman *et al.*, 1989a,b). Other rating scales include the Mandsley Obsessive–Compulsive Inventory (Hodgson and Rachman, 1977), the Padua Inventory (Sanavio, 1988), the Obsessive-Compulsive Inventory (Foa *et al.*, 1998b), and the Compulsive Activity Checklist (Freund *et al.*, 1987). Finally, two recent questionnaires, the Obsessional Beliefs Questionnaire and the Interpretation of Intrusions Inventory, have been developed by an international consortium of researchers to identify and rate cognitive aspects of intrusive thoughts and obsessions (Obsessive Compulsive Cognitions Working Group, 1997, 2001).

Other measures to assess for general severity of illness include the Beck Anxiety Inventory (BAI; Beck *et al.*, 1988a) and the Beck Depression Inventory (BDI; Beck *et al.*, 1988b). Patients may also be given general measures of disability such as the Sheehan Disability Scale (Leon *et al.*, 1992) to assess the degree to which the symptoms are interfering with the patient's functioning.

Treatment forms utilized over the course of treatment included the automatic and revised thought log, the obsession-compulsion monitoring form, the imaginal and *in vivo* exposure form, and the exposure monitoring form (McGinn and Sanderson, 1999).

Cognitive-behavioral models of obsessive-compulsive disorder

Behavioral models: two-stage theory

Mowrer's two-stage theoretical model of the acquisition and maintenance of fear and avoidance behaviors (Mowrer, 1939, 1960) has been further elaborated to explain the onset and maintenance of symptoms in OCD (Dollard and Miller, 1950). This model proposes that a stimulus that does not automatically elicit anxiety or fear (*a neutral stimulus*) becomes associated with a stimulus (*an unconditioned stimulus or UCS*) that naturally elicits anxiety or fear (*an unconditioned response or UCR*) by being paired with it. Through this pairing, the previously neutral stimulus (*the CS*) now becomes capable of eliciting fear or anxiety on its own (*the conditioned response or CR*). Obsessive fears, which take the form of recurrent and intrusive thoughts, images, ideas, or impulses are proposed to develop via this conditioning process. For example, Jim may become anxious about eating meat if he develops salmonella poisoning. Eating meat (*NS*) becomes associated with salmonella poisoning (*UCS*) and becomes capable of eliciting fear on its own (*CS*).

In explaining how fear or anxiety maintains itself, the model proposes that individuals develop avoidance and escape behaviors (*e.g., avoid eating meat, repetitively wash hands if they come into contact with meat*) to reduce the anxiety elicited by the CS (*e.g., meat*), and by doing so, become negatively reinforced by the cessation of anxiety that follows. In other words, despite the fact that the CS (*e.g., meat*) is no longer paired with the initial traumatic stimulus or UCS (*e.g., salmonella poisoning*), the conditioned fear response continues because the individual is negatively reinforced by the experience of reduced anxiety that follows the escape or avoidance behaviors, including compulsive rituals. As a result, the fear response does not extinguish because the individual does not learn that the CS is no longer paired with the UCS and that it is not dangerous in and of itself. Compulsive rituals are conceptualized as avoidance behaviors that are developed to reduce this elicited anxiety. Because obsessions are intrusive, passive avoidance and escape behaviors are usually insufficient in alleviating the anxiety associated with their arousal. Hence, active avoidance behaviors (*compulsions*) are developed by individuals in order to reduce the anxiety created by the CS (*in this case, meat*), and are maintained by their success in doing so.

Evidence for Mowrer's two-stage theory of the development of fear is insufficient. Not only do a majority of patients with anxiety disorders, including OCD, deny a link between symptom onset and specific traumatic events (Rachman and Wilson, 1980), this model does not take into account other modes of onset reported by patients such as informational learning (*e.g., becoming fearful of germs after hearing about a news report on the breakout of* Escherichia coli *among school children*) or observational learning (*e.g., growing up with a parent who is constantly afraid of catching a disease*) (Foa and Kozak, 1986).

By contrast, there is far more support for Mowrer's two-stage conceptualization of the maintenance of fear. Studies have demonstrated that environmental cues trigger anxiety (Hodgson and Rachman, 1972; Hornsveld *et al.*, 1979) and that obsessions increase distress (Rabavilas and Boulougouris, 1974; Boulougouris *et al.*, 1977). Research has also demonstrated that performing handwashing and checking rituals following an urge to ritualize leads to decreases in anxiety (Hodgson and Rachman, 1972; Roper *et al.*, 1973; Roper and Rachman, 1976; Hornsveld *et al.*, 1979).

Cognitive theories

Cognitive models generally hypothesize that a faulty appraisal style may underlie the dysfunction in obsessional thinking (Beech and Liddell, 1974; Carr, 1974; A. T. Beck, 1976; McFall and Wollersheim, 1979; Guidano and Liotti, 1983; Foa and Kozak, 1985; Reed, 1985; Salkovskis, 1985; Pitman, 1987; Wegner, 1989; Warren and Zgourides, 1991). Having obsessions is not believed to be dysfunctional in and of itself. In fact, research shows that up to 90% of the 'normal' population report having cognitive intrusions (Rachman and de Silva, 1978). Although several cognitive theories have been used to explain OCD symptoms (A. T. Beck, 1976; Beech and Liddell, 1974; Carr, 1974; McFall and Wollersheim, 1979; Guidano and Liotti, 1983; Foa and Kozak, 1985; Reed, 1985; Salkovskis, 1985; Pitman, 1987; Wegner, 1989; Warren and Zgourides, 1991), the two most comprehensive cognitive theories are described here in some detail (Foa and Kozak, 1985; Salkovskis, 1985). For a summary account of other cognitive theories, interested readers are invited to read Riggs and Foa (1993), Steketee (1993b), or Jakes (1996).

Foa and Kozak's information processing model

Based on Lang's model (1979), Foa and Kozak (1985) conceive of fear as an 'information network' that exists in memory. This memory network contains representations about fear cues, fear responses, and their meaning. According to them, all anxiety disorders have the following impairments in these networks: (1) faulty estimate of threat (e.g., perceiving danger or threat when there is objectively none); (2) excessive negative 'valence' for the feared event (e.g., excessive degree of affective response); (3) extreme response to danger or threat (e.g., physiological reactivity); and (4) persistence of fears (e.g., continuing to perceive danger despite evidence to the contrary).

Foa and Kozak suggest that, although all anxiety disorders have specific impairments in their memory network, OCD differs from other anxiety disorders in that their inferential judgments about harm appear to be impaired. Accordingly, an individual suffering from OCD will conclude that an event or situation is dangerous unless it is proven safe without a doubt. Furthermore, even if information suggests that a situation is not dangerous, or even if harm does not occur after exposure to a certain event or situation, individuals with OCD still fail to learn from direct experience and will fail to conclude that the particular event or situation is safe. As a result, rituals designed to reduce the occurrence of harm do not provide ultimate safety and must be performed repeatedly.

Foa and Kozak also indicate that specific types of fears are unique to OCD (Riggs and Foa, 1993). Some individuals with OCD develop excessive connections between anxiety and a particular stimulus (e.g., garbage can), and overestimate the threat harm related to the feared stimulus (e.g., I will catch a disease if I take out the garbage). Other individuals fear the meaning of certain acts (e.g., books should always be lined up in order of height) and not the stimulus itself (e.g., book). In other words, it is the asymmetry that induces the anxiety in this case and not the books themselves.

While there is some support for the notion that individuals with OCD tend to overestimate threat, no clear evidence yet exists to suggest that they exhibit a stronger negative valence for feared situations (Steketee, 1993a) and preliminary research disproves the observation that individuals with OCD have higher physiological reactivity than normals (Foa et al., 1991). Other theoretical propositions espoused by Foa and Kozak (1985) (e.g., persistence of fear) have yet to be tested.

Salkovskis' cognitive model

According to this model (Salkovskis, 1985, 1989) intrusive obsessional thoughts by themselves do not lead to increased anxiety or distress. However, in individuals with OCD whose underlying belief systems are characterized by responsibility and self-blame, such thoughts trigger (secondary) negative automatic thoughts that lead to anxiety or distress. In other words, individuals with OCD experience dysfunctional, anxiety-provoking automatic thoughts (e.g., my baby will die) in the presence of intrusive obsessions (e.g., obsessional image of baby dying), which in turn, are based on certain core assumptions and beliefs they hold (e.g., if I have an obsession, it will come true, I bear responsibility for harm; only immoral people have such thoughts). Hence, the dysfunction lies not in the obsessions themselves but in the way these obsessions are processed or appraised. Owing to this faulty appraisal, these individuals experience greater anxiety in response to the obsessions, find it more difficult to dismiss them or ignore them, and end up ritualizing in order to alleviate the anxiety associated with obsessions. In this model, ritualized or compulsive behaviors are performed in order to reduce this sense of responsibility and self-blame, which in turn, reduces the distress associated with the obsessions.

According to Salkovskis (1985, p. 579), the OCD patient's exaggerated sense of responsibility and self-blame is characterized by the following dysfunctional assumptions: (1) 'having a thought about an action is like performing the action;' (2) 'failing to prevent (or failing to try to prevent) harm to self or others is the same as having caused the harm in the first place;' (3) 'responsibility is not attenuated by other factors (e.g., low probability

of occurrence);' (4) 'not neutralizing when an intrusion has occurred is similar or equivalent to seeking or wanting the harm involved in that intrusion to happen;' (5) 'one should (and can) exercise control over one's thoughts'.

Preliminary research supports Salkovskis' contention that individuals with OCD have an increased sense of responsibility and self-blame regarding harm (Salkovskis, 1989). A recent study found that change in beliefs preceded change in OCD symptoms in cognitive and behavior therapy, which also provides support for the cognitive model (Rheaume and Ladouceur, 2000). However, critics argue that appraisals and neutralizing behaviors do not completely explain why obsessions become abnormal and further contend that the proposed themes of responsibility and self-blame explain some obsessive-compulsive themes (e.g., aggressive, sexual, blasphemous thoughts) better than others (e.g., contamination fears, cleaning rituals) (Jakes, 1996). Finally, critics also note that a successful intervention (e.g., reducing the sense of responsibility and self-blame) does not imply causation (i.e., that an increased sense of responsibility caused the obsessions to occur in the first place) (Jakes, 1996). For instance, although the Rheaume and Ladoucer found that change in beliefs preceded change in treatment, their study found that successful treatment with both cognitive and behavior therapy also led to a subsequent change in beliefs.

Psychodynamic model of obsessive-compulsive disorder

Psychodynamic focus on OCD, while significant in the early development of psychoanalysis, has been limited in recent years (Esman, 1989, 2001). As with panic disorder and social phobia, struggles with angry and competitive feelings and fantasies are considered central to the development of the disorder, with a focus on fears of loss of control. The punitive superego, characteristic of these patients, increases the danger they feel from the potential experience of these feelings. In the psychoanalytic literature, OCD has been described as occurring alongside a regression to an earlier stage of ego development, in which the individual fears that her thoughts and fantasies might damage someone else. Defenses include undoing, in an attempt to symbolically and magically make restitution for angry feelings via compulsive behaviors. Also, patients tend to intellectualize or become preoccupied to avert the experience of frightening feelings.

OCD symptoms have also been described as representing a compromise formation. For instance, Freud (1909/1961) described a patient who became obsessed with whether to remove a stone from the road that he feared might lead to damage of the carriage of the woman he loved, who would subsequently be driving on the road. He removed the stone from the center of the road, where he feared her carriage might hit it, symbolically protecting her, but then decided that this was absurd and replaced the stone, as he struggled with his ambivalence and aggressive feelings. Thus, as noted above, the compulsive act may attempt to undo aggressive fantasies and do penance to avert guilt and anxiety. Salzman (1985, p. 13) summarizes the obsessive compulsive dynamic as a need for control in all aspects of life: 'The obsessive compulsive dynamism is a device for preventing any feeling or thought that might produce shame, loss of pride or status or a feeling of weakness or deficiency whether such feelings are aggressive, sexual or otherwise.'

Some recent authors (Brandchaft, 2001; Meares, 2001) have focused on the impact of disruptions in the infant and child–caregiver relationship as a source of obsessive and compulsive symptoms. In this view, the aggression and guilt described above are secondary to developmental traumas from unresponsive and/or unempathic caretakers. Obsessional preoccupations represent both the experience of the insecure relationships with parents and attempts to control the ongoing threat of loss of the attachment figure; Meares (2001) specifically relates parental overprotectiveness to the failure of the child to test adequately his conceptions of the environment and reality, predisposing the child to magical thinking and OCD.

Empirical support for treatments

Traditionally considered to be refractory to treatment, many treatments now effectively treat OCD. Treatments that have demonstrated efficacy include cognitive and behavioral therapies and serotonergic medications. Psychodynamic psychotherapy and many psychotropic medications have not proven effective in treating OCD (Knight, 1941; Black, 1974; Malan, 1979; Perse, 1988) and hence should not be considered first-line treatments.

Behavior therapy

Over 30 uncontrolled and controlled research trials conducted over many sites throughout the world attests to the effectiveness of behavior therapy (*i.e., exposure and response prevention*) as a treatment for OCD (see McGinn and Sanderson, 1999; Barlow, 2002; Griest and Baer, 2002 for a review). These and other trials, conducted to examine the efficacy of exposure and response prevention, generally show that between 50% and 75% of patients with obsessions and compulsion exhibit a substantial decrease in their symptoms, and a majority appear to maintain gains in treatment even years after they discontinue treatment (for a comprehensive and detailed review of studies demonstrating the efficacy of behavior therapy, please see Foa *et al.*, 1985, 1998a; Steketee, 1993b; Foa and Kozak, 1996; Abramowitz, 1997; Foa and Franklin, 2001; Griest and Baer, 2002). A meta-analysis by Abramowitz (1997) examining only controlled trials confirms the finding that combined exposure and response prevention leads to a substantial improvement in patients with OCD, and finds that the effectiveness of behavioral treatments increase with therapist-guided, direct exposure (Abramowitz, 1997). Another meta-analysis demonstrated the efficacy of behavior therapy over placebo and reported a large average effect size of 1.46 for behavior therapy (van Blakom *et al.*, 1994). In addition, a recent summary of five studies showed that many patients did not meet criteria for OCD following treatment, and demonstrated minimal relapse following treatment discontinuation (Steketee and Frost, 1998). Finally, preliminary findings show that results from controlled trials appear to be generalizable to outpatient, fee-for-service settings (Kirk, 1983; Franklin *et al.*, 2000).

Overall, recent controlled trials demonstrate that behavior therapy may be as or more effective than medication alone, and that behavior therapy is associated with a comparably lower rate of relapse (Rachman *et al.*, 1979; Marks *et al.*, 1980; Mawson *et al.*, 1982). Further confirmation comes from a meta-analysis conducted by Abramowitz (1997) who found an overall advantage of behavior therapy over selective serotonin reuptake inhibitors in the studies reviewed. Studies also suggest that combining medication and behavior therapy may not confer a benefit over behavior therapy alone but may be more beneficial than medication alone, especially in preventing relapse (Marks *et al.*, 1988; Cottraux *et al.*, 1990; van Balkom *et al.*, 1998; Simpson *et al.*, 1999; Kozak *et al.*, 2000).

An examination of the relative efficacy of behavioral techniques for the treatment of obsessive thoughts indicates that obsessive thoughts respond primarily to exposure (Mills *et al.*, 1973; Foa *et al.*, 1980a, 1984) and that combined *in vivo* and imaginal exposure appear to be superior at maintaining long-term gains, particularly for those patients who cognitively avoid their catastrophic fears (Foa *et al.*, 1980b). Exposure appears somewhat less effective in the treatment of pure obsessionals (patients who present with obsessive ruminations but no compulsions) (Emmelkamp and Kwee, 1977; Stern, 1978; Kasvikis and Marks, 1988; Steketee, 1993b; Salkovskis and Kirk, 1997). However, experts believe that many pure obsessionals may present with covert rituals that are not classified as such and hence the untreated rituals may serve to hinder the treatment of obsessions (Steketee, 1993b). Efficacy studies also indicate that ritualized behaviors and thoughts respond primarily to response prevention (Mills *et al.*, 1973; Foa *et al.*, 1980b, 1984; Turner *et al.*, 1980).

Cognitive therapy

A number of case reports initially suggested that cognitive therapy is an effective treatment for OCD (Salkovskis, 1983; Headland and McDonald, 1987; Salkovskis and Westbrook, 1989; Roth and Church, 1994), especially when used adjunctively with behavioral techniques such as exposure and response prevention (Salkovskis and Warwick, 1985, 1986; Kearney and Silverman, 1990; Freeston, 1994). Evidence from early controlled studies confirmed that cognitive strategies used in rational-emotive therapy are

effective in reducing OCD symptoms but found that they did not confer an accrued benefit over exposure and response prevention (Emmelkamp *et al.*, 1988; Emmelkamp and Beens, 1991).

More recently, several controlled trials using Beck's cognitive model not only confirmed that cognitive strategies are effective in treating OCD but found that they may be as effective as behavioral strategies when used alone (Van Oppen *et al.*, 1995; Jones and Menzies, 1998; Cottraux *et al.*, 2001). A meta-analysis combining only controlled trials confirms the finding that cognitive strategies are at least as effective as behavioral treatments (Abramowitz, 1997). Finally, a study by Freeston *et al.* (1997) demonstrated that combined cognitive restructuring, exposure, and response prevention was substantially better than a wait-list control, and produced an 84% success rate that was maintained a year later.

Cognitive therapy has also been used to treat patients who are resistant to behavior therapy alone (Salkovskis and Warwick, 1985, 1986), especially pure obsessionals or patients without overt rituals who tend not to respond well to just exposure and response prevention (Salkovskis and Kirk, 1997). However, more controlled research trials are needed to determine better the effectiveness of cognitive therapy as a treatment for OCD.

Treatment rationale and strategies

Symptoms treated within a cognitive-behavioral framework include the obsessive thoughts, images, impulses, or urges, and the compulsions that may take the form of ritualized thoughts or behaviors. Also targeted in treatment are the secondary automatic thoughts that develop among patients with OCD (*e.g., I am a bad person for having such thoughts*). Essentially, two primary goals of cognitive-behavioral strategies are to (1) alleviate the anxiety associated with obsessions, thereby reducing the frequency and persistence of these thoughts, images, impulses, or urges, and (2) reduce compulsions and alleviate feelings of relief associated with compulsions.

Before treatment is initiated, detailed information is obtained on the nature and exact count of the patient's external (*e.g., knives*) and internal (*e.g., images*) triggers of obsessive anxiety, catastrophic fears (*e.g., my baby will die*), compulsive rituals (*e.g., checks 25 times a day*), and passive avoidance or escape behaviors (*e.g., does not cook*).

Psychoeducation

Following assessment, the first phase of treatment is initiated where patients learn strategies to normalize their obsessions and compulsions and manage their anxiety. In *psychoeducation*, the patient is directly educated about the disorder, including the definition, demographics, etiology, treatment, etc. Educating patients enables them to learn that they suffer from an illness shared by others and reduces their sense of shame about their symptoms. Self-help books are also prescribed to complement strategies learned in therapy and patients are encouraged to join organizations in order to receive ongoing education and support.

Cognitive restructuring

Cognitive restructuring (A. T. Beck, 1976; J. S. Beck, 1995; Salkovskis and Kirk, 1997) attempts to modify the secondary dysfunctional automatic thoughts (*e.g., I am a bad person for having such thoughts*) that individuals with OCD have following their obsessional images, thoughts, urges, or impulses (*e.g., images of mother being stabbed*). Automatic thoughts stemming from maladaptive beliefs about responsibility and self-blame are restructured as well as those arising from other beliefs identified in OCD and anxiety disorders in general, including vulnerability to threat, perfectionism, morality, rigidity, doubt, and uncertainty (see McGinn and Sanderson, 1999 for a review). As these automatic thoughts are rigorously and continually replaced by thoughts based on empirical evidence and rational examination (*e.g., imagining that my baby is stabbed does not make me a bad person, I love my baby and I cannot control all the thoughts that pass through my head*), anxiety declines, and consequently, obsessions and compulsions gradually lessen over time. Successful cognitive restructuring leads to the modification of underlying beliefs to reflect an appropriate degree of responsibility, blame, vulnerability to threat, and so on.

Exposure

During the second phase of treatment, exposure techniques (Riggs and Foa, 1993; Steketee, 1993b) break the association between obsessions and anxiety by directly exposing patients to the anxiety triggers rather than by challenging the dysfunctional automatic thoughts that follow obsessions or precede rituals. Exposure may be conducted in imagination or *in vivo* or both, depending on which is indicated and/or practical to implement (see McGinn and Sanderson, 1999 for a full description and indications of imaginal versus *in vivo* exposure). Typically, individuals are exposed systematically over a prolonged period of time to increasingly anxiety-provoking phobic stimuli (*e.g., garbage*) that trigger obsessive anxiety (*e.g., I will die from salmonella poisoning if I take the garbage out*) until their anxiety reaction is eliminated. The success of systematic exposure is attributed to the fact that as patients tolerate prolonged confrontation with anxiety triggers without trying to escape or neutralize the thought with some other thought or action, they learn that their catastrophic fears do not occur (*in this case, contact with garbage does not lead to salmonella poisoning and eventual death*), and as a result, their anxiety associated with these obsessions ultimately dissipates. As they become habituated to anxiety triggers (*e.g., contact with garbage does not create anxiety*), patients experience a reduction in obsessive thoughts. Because exposure is done in a systematic, hierarchical fashion, patients learn to tolerate manageable levels of anxiety as they confront low-grade phobic situations and then ultimately face more anxiety-provoking stimuli.

Response prevention

Exposure is administered in conjunction with response prevention (Riggs and Foa, 1993; Steketee, 1993b), which attempts to block compulsions (*e.g., not washing hands after touching garbage*). The goal of response prevention is to break the association between ritualized behaviors and thoughts and the subsequent feelings of relief or reduced anxiety. Rituals are identified, patients are given a rationale for response prevention, presented with specific rules, and are generally assisted by family members to comply. Although many graded forms of response prevention may be administered (*e.g., reducing number of rituals*), the ultimate goal is complete cessation of ritual performance. Strategies recently developed to help individuals engage in response prevention (*e.g., response cost for performance of rituals*) may also be used to facilitate response prevention (McGinn and Sanderson, 1999). If possible, response prevention begins in the first treatment session. By the end of treatment, patients are presented with guidelines for 'normal behavior' because many do not know what constitutes normal behavior (*e.g., what amount of handwashing is appropriate*).

Acute treatment is discontinued when obsessions and compulsions become infrequent and do not impair functioning. Strategies to maintain gains and prevent relapse are implemented and treatment is slowly tapered over time.

Case illustration

Michele is a 28-year-old woman who presented with longstanding obsessive fears of becoming contaminated by germs. She washed her hands multiple times a day and used gloves to attend to the simplest of household chores. More recently, she reported developing obsessive fears about her baby coming to harm. Michele began to ritualistically repeat a series of numbers (*e.g., '6, 6, 6, 6, 6, 6'*), phrases (*'I repent'*), and images (*e.g., imagined her baby playing with his toys*) fairly continuously throughout the day. She dropped out of graduate school during her first semester, could not leave the house without her baby, stopped cooking (*'I can't touch knives'*), and cleaning (*'I feel the germs will seep into my pores'*).

During the initial treatment session, Michele was given a simple but detailed description of OCD, including facts and figures on demographics, prevalence, etiology, and so on. The cognitive-behavioral model was explained to Michele along with a description of the strategies she would learn in treatment. The importance of completing in between sessions was emphasized and her husband was identified as a co-therapist to facilitate completion of weekly assignments. Michele was prescribed Foa and Wilson's book (1991) titled *Stop obsessing! How to overcome your obsessions and compulsions* and was encouraged to join the Anxiety Disorders Association of America (www.adaa.org) and the Obsessive Compulsive Foundation (www.ocfoundation.org).

Using a thought log, Michele learned to identify and monitor secondary automatic thoughts during periods of obsessive anxiety. Michele learned that these habitually occurring thoughts and images typically followed obsessional thoughts and stimuli and typically led to anxiety and the urge to ritualize. Illustrative automatic thoughts were identified such as 'if I eat this meat, I (or my baby) will get germs and die,' 'the fact that I imagined my baby getting stabbed means that he will die unless I think of him safely playing with his toys,' or 'I am immoral for thinking that he is dead.' It soon became evident that these thoughts reflected her underlying dysfunctional beliefs that she was fundamentally evil, vulnerable to creating and experiencing harm, was personally responsible for any misfortune that befell her or her family and incapable of coping well during adversity. As her maladaptive automatic thoughts were replaced to reflect an appropriate degree of responsibility and vulnerability to harm, and as her beliefs about her morality and ability to cope were modified through rational self-examination, her anxiety associated with obsessions and compulsions began to decline. Within a few weeks, Michele's obsessions and compulsions became less frequent. As a result of daily practice in her own environment, Michele grew adept at restructuring her cognitions and soon began to feel confident that she could reduce her anxiety on her own.

Her list of anxiety triggers was now organized hierarchically from least to most anxiety provoking on a scale of 1–100 (*e.g., garbage, meat, knives*) and a working hierarchy was created to reflect increasing contact (and anxiety) with each item (*e.g., imagining touching garbage, touching garbage*). Prolonged, systematic exposure was initiated with the least anxiety-provoking item until she habituated to it, after which she was exposed to the next item and so on. For example, Michele first imagined touching garbage, then touched the lid with gloves, then without gloves. When she was successfully able to handle garbage using her bare hands with minimal anxiety, the next item on her overall hierarchy was selected (*e.g., knives*) and was again organized hierarchically to reflect increasing contact (and anxiety) with that item (*e.g., looking at a picture of a knife, imagining holding a knife, looking at a knife*. As Michele also presented with obsessive fears that could not be implemented through *in vivo* exposure (*e.g., obsessions of baby being stabbed*), she was exposed to increasingly anxiety-provoking scenes in her imagination until her anxiety declined (imaginal exposure).

Because Michele could not tolerate the anxiety associated with completely abstaining from rituals at the outset, a graded response prevention was formulated and administered in conjunction with exposure. Michele was prohibited from performing rituals to neutralize the anxiety associated with items currently or previously the subject of exposure but was permitted to ritualize to items to which she had yet to be exposed.

Although Michele was able successfully to tolerate exposure and was able to abstain from performing rituals during exposure sessions, she found it difficult to conduct exposure and refrain from performing rituals at home, even with her husband's assistance. To facilitate response prevention, a weekly contingency plan was instituted wherein Michele rewarded herself for conducting exposure sessions at home (*e.g., bought herself a CD*) and a response cost was instituted when she performed rituals (*e.g., was not able to watch her favorite show, had to send money to a despised politician*). Self critical thoughts were also modified to reduce feelings of excessive guilt on the occasions she inadvertently performed rituals.

Michele's overall mood improved as her anxiety began to decline. As Michele's obsessions and compulsions declined to manageable levels and she was able to go about her daily life with minimal impairment, sessions now focused on helping her maintain gains and prevent relapse. For example, Michele was encouraged to take charge of her continued treatment with less and less guidance from the therapist, understand the difference between symptom recurrence and relapse, learn how to cope with symptom recurrence, and encouraged to pursue new activities to fill in the long gaps of time that she had previously spent performing her rituals. Sessions were tapered down to biweekly, and then monthly sessions and so on as Michele learned to manage her symptoms on her own. Michele was encouraged to identify stressors that led to increased symptoms and contact the therapist if she experienced a resurgence in between sessions.

Psychodynamic treatment of obsessive-compulsive disorder

Although with our present state of knowledge treatment of severe OCD should be primarily psychopharmacological or cognitive-behavioral (Stein, 2002), psychodynamic approaches can provide additional understanding and insights into the illness, particularly in milder or more moderate forms (Gabbard, 2000, 2001). Patients may benefit from exploring the meanings and defensive functions of obsessions and compulsions. Shame or embarrassment about symptoms and the fantasies associated with them can interfere with treatment. The atmosphere of safety with the therapist and the therapist's nonjudgmental exploratory stance can aid the patient in easing his intense self-criticisms and more openly discussing his symptoms. Identifying and reducing these sources of resistance to treatment can also increase compliance with medication and CBT. OCD symptoms are highly disruptive of relationships; problematic interactions with others secondary to the symptoms can be productively examined in the transference–countertransference work of the therapy (Gabbard, 2000, 2001).

Case example

Linda was a 40-year-old single woman who presented with multiple rituals and obsessional thoughts for many years that had become disruptive of her daily routine in the preceding 3 months. These included knocking on wood, checking the stove and locks, and being preoccupied with Zodiac signs to try to gain information as to whether something terrible was about to happen to her, spending about an hour a day on these rituals. In addition, Linda felt threatened by a very close relationship with her boyfriend, fearful of his betraying and rejecting her despite his expressing interest in marrying her. She had lost her job 4 months prior to presentation, apparently unrelated to her OCD symptoms, and was concerned about finding a new one. Although sertraline provided some relief, her symptoms continued at a reduced level and her fears about her boyfriend persisted.

Linda reported a difficult childhood with a father whom she experienced as neglectful or only interested her academic achievement. Although she made many efforts to gain his affection through her schoolwork she felt that he still rejected her. Her mother was an anxious and preoccupied woman, and Linda believed that she had to take care of her mother rather than receive maternal comfort. Furthering her problems, social unrest in her country of origin forced the family to move to the US when she was age 11. Thus she had to cope with the loss of friends and her home, and adapt to a strange new environment, a task that she found at times to be overwhelming.

The therapy explored the many functions of Linda's symptoms. She and her therapist noted that her feelings of helplessness and uncertainty that were triggered by the loss of her job reminded her of the upheaval she experienced when she had to leave her home as a child. The checking behavior was a coping mechanism to control these feelings of helplessness, by displacing them to potential fantasied disasters (*fire, burglary*) that she could avert by her rituals. In addition, Linda felt deeply threatened by her growing ties to her boyfriend and possible marriage. In particular, she felt certain at times that he would reject her once she committed to him, just as her father rejected her despite her efforts. She attempted to ward off this expected disaster with her rituals as well with horoscope checking, which focused on whether others with her sign were having problems with relationships. Helping Linda to understand the origins of her fears and the function of her obsessions and compulsions aided in the further reduction of her symptoms. In particular, helping her to tolerate her feelings of

helplessness, and linking them to the anxiety and frustration of her childhood traumas, led her to feel less threatened by her current life challenges.

Social anxiety disorder

DSM-IV definition

The hallmark feature of SAD (*formerly social phobia*) is excessive and persistent anxiety (*or panic attacks*) in situations in which the person is exposed to unfamiliar people or subjected to scrutiny by others while performing specific tasks (*e.g., public speaking, eating in a restaurant*). Such individuals fear that they will act in a way (or display visible anxiety symptoms) that will be humiliating or embarrassing. DSM-IV (APA, 1994) require that individuals recognize that their fears are excessive or unreasonable. According to the DSM, exposure to the feared social situation almost invariably provokes anxiety and hence these situations are avoided or endured with dread. As a result, these symptoms create significant distress and impairment in functioning. Individuals with SAD suffer from extreme loneliness and isolation and report impairment in social, occupational, marital, and other spheres of their life.

Commonly feared situations include formal speaking or interactions (70%), informal speaking or interactions (46%), problems with assertion (31%), and being observed by others (22%) (Holt *et al.*, 1992). Individuals with SAD may fear one or two specific social situations such as public speaking, but the vast majority present with evaluative fears in multiple social situations. Finally, a small proportion of individuals fear almost any social contact with others and if such broad-based fears are present, the individual is classified as having Generalized Social Anxiety Disorder (APA, 1994).

Diagnostic and assessment measures

SAD may be diagnosed using semistructured clinical interviews such as the Structured Interview for the DSM (SCID-P; Spitzer *et al.*, 1987) or the Anxiety Disorders Interview Schedule (ADIS-IV) (DiNardo and Barlow, 1988; DiNardo *et al.*, 1993). These interviews also help clinicians rule out other disorders that may explain the presenting symptoms and rule in other disorders that may co-occur with SAD. The Fear of Negative Evaluation Scale (FNE) and the Social Avoidance and Distress Scale (*SADS*) may be used in conjunction with diagnostic tools to measure concerns with social-evaluative threat and distress and avoidance in situations (D. Watson and Friend, 1969). The Leibowitz Social Anxiety Scale (*LSAS*) is a newer scale and is widely used to assess the range of performance and social difficulties experienced by individuals with social anxiety (Liebowitz, 1987). Behavioral assessment tests are also frequently used. Such tests typically ask individuals to role-play a social situation (*e.g., give a speech or converse with a stranger*) while the therapist monitors their discomfort level on several indices, including their subjective rating of distress, as well as behavioral (*e.g., speed of performance*), and psychophysiological (*e.g., heart rate is monitored*) measures.

The BAI (A. T. Beck *et al.*, 1988a) may also be used to measure general anxiety levels and given the high rate of depression among individuals with social anxiety, the BDI (A. T. Beck *et al.*, 1988b) is often administered. The Sheehan Disability Scale (Leon *et al.*, 1992) may also be used to assess the degree to which the symptoms are interfering with the patient's functioning.

Treatment forms utilized over the course of treatment included the automatic and revised thought log, the imaginal and *in vivo* exposure form, and the exposure monitoring form (McGinn and Sanderson, 1999; Leahy and Holland, 2000).

Cognitive-behavioral models of social anxiety disorder

Behavioral models

In explaining how social anxiety may be acquired and maintained, Mowrer's two-stage theory proposes that direct experience with a traumatic experience (*e.g., a socially embarrassing interaction*) (*UCS*) that naturally elicits anxiety (*UCR*) may lead to the development of social anxiety via classical conditioning. According to this model, anxiety becomes conditioned to social situations (neutral stimuli) via association with the initial traumatic social situation (*UCS*). Hence, these social situations (*now CS*) become capable of producing fear on their own. Through higher-order conditioning and stimulus generalization, the number of social cues that lead to anxiety increases over time, and thereby creates significant impairment over time.

In explaining the maintenance of social anxiety, this model suggests that avoidance of social situations perpetuates social anxiety in the long run. By avoiding social situations, individuals experience a temporary reduction in anxiety, which serves to reinforce the avoidance behavior. However, this avoidance prevents them from learning that negative social consequences do not always occur, and hence their fears continue unabated. In other words, by avoiding the social situations, individuals with social anxiety fail to realize that the CS (*social situations*) is no longer paired with the UCS (*initial traumatic social situation*) and hence the fears do not get extinguished.

Current behavioral models of social anxiety suggest that social fears may be the result of an evolutionarily determined preparedness to associate fear with anger, criticism, rejection, or other means of social disapproval, which have important implications for the survival of the organism (Seligman, 1971; Barlow, 2002). However, biological and psychological vulnerabilities are cited as necessary predisposing factors in the development of SAD. Contemporary models also recognize that social anxiety may develop via multiple routes (Barlow, 2002). For example, Barlow suggests that for vulnerable people, relatively minor negative social or performance situations may also lead to anxiety. Further, although research suggests that many individuals link their onset to an initial traumatic event, a significant proportion implicate recall vicarious learning experiences in the development of their anxiety (Ost and Hugdahl, 1981).

Cognitive models

Contemporary models emphasize the role of cognitive processes in the development and maintenance of SAD and note that the hallmark symptom of SAD, the fear of negative evaluation, is itself a cognitive feature (Heimberg and Barlow, 1991; Butler and Wells, 1995; Clark and Wells, 1995; Barlow, 2002). Cognitive models propose that social anxiety is maintained by dysfunctional thinking and biased information processing. Specifically, this models suggest that individuals with SAD believe they are in danger of revealing anxiety symptoms or behaving ineptly, and that such behavior will have disastrous consequences in terms of loss of status, loss of worth, and rejection (Clark and Wells, 1995; Rapee and Heimberg, 1997; Turk *et al.*, 2001). Dysfunctional assumptions underlying such cognitions include perfectionistic standards of performance and an excessive need for approval and typical core beliefs include self-schemas of incompetence or undesirability and beliefs that others are inherently critical and evaluative (Leahy and Holland, 2000; Turk *et al.*, 2001). Such dysfunctional beliefs are perpetuated because individuals with SAD disregard or overlook positive feedback, avoid social situations altogether or use safety-seeking behaviors to reduce their anxiety, thereby preventing disconfirmation of negative beliefs. In addition, cognitive models have emphasized the role of self-focused attention in the maintenance of social anxiety. According to this model, individuals with social anxiety are not focused on external events such as the task at hand or an ongoing conversation and instead, are more likely to imagine what others are thinking of them or how they look and sound to others. In a self-fulfilling prophecy, this self-focused attention leads to poorer social performance and increases the likelihood of negative appraisals by observers.

The cognitive model has received empirical support from several experimental studies. Research studies have demonstrated that individuals with SAD report more negative and fewer positive thoughts during social interactions, more thoughts about the impressions they are creating on others, underestimate their own performance, overestimate the degree to which their anxiety is visible, and tend to interpret negatively ambiguous

social situations (Stopa and Clark, 1993, 2000; Clark and Wells, 1995; Heimberg and Juster, 1995; Leary and Kowalski, 1995; Rapee, 1995; Wells *et al.*, 1998; Wells and Papageorgiou, 1999). Research also suggests that such individuals tend to interpret catastrophically mild negative feedback, are more likely to remember negative feedback and will be more likely to respond to treatment if the fear of negative evaluation is modified.

Empirical support for cognitive-behavior therapy

Prior to the introduction of social phobia into the diagnostic nomenclature, few studies examined the efficacy of psychotherapy treatments for this condition. Since its introduction into the DSM-III (APA, 1980), numerous studies have been undertaken to determine the efficacy of psychotherapy treatments for SAD. A growing body of evidence now suggests that cognitive-behavioral treatments are efficacious in treating SAD and have been found to be superior to waiting-list conditions (see Hope *et al.*, 1993; for a complete review, Taylor, 1996; Turk *et al.*, 2002). Studies have also found that the effects of CBT are maintained in the long run, even for periods up to 5 years following therapy discontinuation.

Behavior therapy

Exposure is considered to be the essential ingredient in all anxiety disorders, including SAD. Numerous studies demonstrate that exposure alone is an effective treatment for SAD (Fava *et al.*, 1989) and that its effects are superior to progressive muscle relaxation (PMR) training (Alstroem, 1984; Al-Kubaisy *et al.*, 1992), pill placebo (Turner *et al.*, 1994), wait-list control (Butler *et al.*, 1984; Newman *et al.*, 1994), and a control therapy comprising of psychoeducation, self-exposure instructions, and unspecified anxiolytic mediation (Alstroem, 1984).

Cognitive therapy

Different forms of cognitive therapy including Beck's cognitive therapy, Ellis's rational emotive therapy, and Meichenbaum's self-instructional training have demonstrated efficacy in the treatment of SAD (see Coles *et al.*, 2002 for a review). It is noted, however, that with few exceptions, most cognitive therapies include behavioral techniques such as behavioral experiments and exposure and hence are not a pure test of cognitive restructuring (Juster and Heimberg, 1995). Further, it is unclear if cognitive therapy adds efficacy beyond the effects of exposure alone (Hope *et al.*, 1993; Turk *et al.*, 2002).

However, because the fear of negative evaluation, the hallmark of social phobia, is essentially a cognitive construct, several researchers believe that cognitive interventions may play a more important role in the treatment of SAD than in other anxiety disorders (Butler, 1989). Further, in light of studies that show that exposure alone has no substantial impact on the fear of negative evaluation (Butler *et al.*, 1984) and that fear of negative evaluation has a strong relationship to treatment outcome (Mattick and Peters, 1988; Mattick *et al.*, 1989), it suggests that altering distorted thoughts related to these fears may be significantly related to treatment outcome. Finally, some research suggests that, although exposure plus cognitive restructuring does not increase efficacy of treatment above and beyond exposure alone, the combined treatment is associated with lower relapse rates once treatment is discontinued, suggesting that the addition of cognitive restructuring may be protective in the long run (Heimberg and Juster, 1995).

Psychodynamic model of social phobia

There are clinical and psychodynamic similarities between panic disorder and social phobia. Clinically, social phobia shares the symptoms of anticipatory anxiety, panic-like symptoms, or panic attacks in feared situations, and phobic avoidance of feared situations. In addition, the two disorders may share a similar neurophysiological vulnerability, as behavioral inhibition described by Kagan *et al.* (1990) is associated with social phobia as well as panic disorder. Parents of children with behavioral inhibition have been found to be at greater risk for the development of anxiety disorders, particularly social phobia (Rosenbaum *et al.*, 1991a,b).

Whether through physiological predisposition, developmental stressors, traumatic experiences, or a combination of these factors, these patients typically have internalized representations of parents, caretakers, or siblings who shame, criticize, ridicule, humiliate, abandon, and embarrass them. These perceptions are established early in life and then are repeatedly projected on to persons in the environment who are avoided, for fear of their being critical and rejecting. Avoidance adds to difficulties in developing coping strategies.

As with panic patients, in patients with social phobia, anger is threatening due to fears of rejection by important attachment figures. For social phobics, anger and disdain for others are typically denied and projected on to others in order to avoid acknowledging these feelings (Gabbard, 1992; Zerbe, 1994). However, with this projection, the patient views others as critical and rejecting of him, triggering social anxiety. Additionally, patients experience guilt about their anger at others for being critical or rejecting, and for their own aggressive yet denied wishes for attention. Social anxiety can serve as a punishment for this guilt.

In addition to conflicts with the experience of anger, social phobic patients struggle with intense feelings of inadequacy. Alongside their low self-esteem, they can develop a compensatory grandiosity, with fantasies of others being very responsive or adoring of their specialness (Kaplan, 1972). This is typically associated with a desire to exhibit oneself sexually (Fenichel, 1945), which must be denied. This grandiosity adds to the recurrent disappointments that these patients experience in social situations, and may intensify the pain and anger they experience in response to rejection.

As with other psychological symptoms, from a psychodynamic view, social phobia also represents a compromise formation. Social phobics are conflicted about the wish to exhibit themselves sexually, and social anxiety is both an expression of the conflict, and a punishment for the wish. Avoidance of social situations aids in avoidance of the conscious experience of these wishes. Similarly, anxiety and avoidance punishes the individual for angry feelings and fantasies. Efforts at idealization of self or others attempt to ward off painful feelings of low self-esteem but then add to the potential for disappointment.

Psychodynamic treatment of social phobia

The therapist must be particularly alert to the patient's shameful feelings in treatment of social phobia. The patient may anticipate that the therapist will be as critical and rejecting of him as he expects others will be. This can be used as an opportunity to explore an early transference reaction to the therapist and to examine the patient's fantasies that he experiences as conflicted. In particular, angry fantasies and exhibitionistic wishes may emerge. The therapist explores the patient's fears upon entering a social setting, and why the patient may have difficulty confronting these fears. This inquiry will often aid or encourage the patient to confront his social anxiety directly.

Cognitive-behavior therapy

An extensive body of research supports the efficacy of combining cognitive restructuring and exposure. These studies show that CBT is more effective than waiting-list control groups (Kanter and Goldfried, 1979; Butler et al., 1984; DiGiuseppe et al., 1990; Hope et al., 1995), an educational-supportive control therapy (Heimberg et al., 1990, 1993, 1998; Lucas and Telch, 1993), and pill placebo (Heimberg et al., 1998). To date, Heimberg's Cognitive-behavioral Group Therapy (CBGT) for SAD has received the widest empirical support and is included in a list of empirically supported treatments by the Society of Clinical Psychology's (Division 12 of the American Psychological Association) Task Force on Promotion and Dissemination of Psychological Procedures (Heimberg et al., 1990; Chambless et al., 1998). A number of well-designed studies demonstrate that CBGT is efficacious in the treatment of SAD (Gelernter et al., 1991; Heimberg et al., 1985, 1990, 1998; Heimberg et al., 1993). These studies demonstrate that the CBGT is comparable with medications, such as phenelzine, and superior to other treatments such as an educational-supportive group psychotherapy and pill placebo (Lucas and Telch, 1993; Heimberg et al., 1998). Group and individual version of treatment do not appear to vary with regard to efficacy

(Lucas and Telch, 1993). Social effectiveness therapy, another combined treatment that combines social skills training and exposure, has also received empirical support but has not met required criteria for placement on the list of empirically supported treatments (Turner et al., 1994, 1996).

Some studies show that combining exposure and cognitive restructuring is more effective than either treatment alone (Butler et al., 1984; Mattick and Peters, 1988) while others show that combining treatments does not add to the efficacy of exposure alone (Butler et al., 1984; Hope et al., 1995; Taylor, 1996). Further, a number of review articles and meta-analyses demonstrate that CBT is not more effective than exposure alone (Feske and Chambless, 1995; Taylor, 1996; Turner et al., 1996; Gould et al., 1997). Meta-analytic reviews suggest that exposure is associated with the largest effect sizes and that exposure alone and exposure combined with cognitive restructuring are not significantly different with regard to effect sizes, drop out or relapse rates (Feske and Chambless, 1995; Taylor, 1996; Gould et al., 1997). Further, dismantling studies suggest that exposure alone is at least as effective as exposure plus cognitive restructuring (Hope et al., 1995).

Treatment plan and strategies

The goal of cognitive-behavioral strategies is to alleviate the anxiety and avoidance behaviors associated with the social or performance situations. When possible, group treatment is the format of choice for patients with social anxiety because it is cost-effective, gives participants the opportunity to learn vicariously, see others with similar problems, and make a public commitment to change (Sank and Shaffer, 1984; Heimberg, 1991). Group treatment also provides the opportunity for multiple role-play partners and a range of people to provide evidence to challenge distorted thoughts (Sank and Shaffer, 1984; Heimberg, 1991).

Treatment is initiated once the therapist has established the diagnosis of social anxiety and assessed the extent to which symptoms create distress and impair functioning. The therapist identifies key cognitive, behavioral, and physical symptoms of anxiety, lists all the social situations that patients endure with dread or avoid altogether along with the safety-seeking behaviors they employ to cope with their anxiety in social situations.

Psychoeducation

During the psychoeducation phase, which typically takes one session to complete, the goal is to provide information about SAD, correct myths, and foster optimism. Toward this end, the therapist discusses the nature and evolutionary function of social anxiety, educates the patient on symptoms, demographics, and etiology of SAD and outlines the various treatments that have demonstrated efficacy in remediating symptoms. Finally, the therapist presents the cognitive-behavioral model of treatment and provides a brief overview of the different components of treatment.

Relaxation training

Relaxation training is employed when hyperarousal is a prominent feature in the patient's symptomatology. The goal of relaxation training is to decrease hyperarousal and regulate breathing in individuals with social anxiety to help them stay calm and focused during social encounters. PMR is used to reduce the physiological components of anxiety and is based on the Jacobsonian technique of alternating muscle contraction and relaxation (Bernstein and Borkovec, 1973; Brown et al., 2001). Patients are trained to discriminate between muscle tension and relaxation and the goal of discrimination training is to facilitate rapid relaxation to individual muscle groups by enabling patients to detect sources and early signs of muscle tension and substitute the learned relaxation response. Once the patient has mastered PMR using all muscle groups (typically over a span of 2 weeks), relaxation exercises are shortened to key muscle groups and strategies such as relaxation-by-recall and cue-controlled relaxation are used to generalize effects to problematic social situations (see McGinn and Sanderson, 1999, for a review).

Like PMR, breathing retraining is used to reduce the somatic component of anxiety. Specifically, patients learn diaphragmatic breathing to counteract the shallow, irregular, and rapid breathing patterns often exhibited by individuals under anxiety or stress. The latter is characterized by the use of chest muscles (thoracic breathing) and is associated with an increase in respiration rate (hyperventilation). By contrast, in abdominal or diaphragmatic breathing, the process of breathing is even and nonconstricting, as the inhaled air (oxygen) is drawn deep into the lungs and exhaled (carbon dioxide) as the diaphragm constricts and expands. This type of breathing involves movement in and out of the abdominal rather than the chest muscles, and allows for the most efficient exchange of oxygen and carbon dioxide with the least effort (see Schwartz, 1987, for a complete description). Breathing retraining is believed to reduce respiration rate and cause changes in autonomic functioning, thereby leading to overall relaxation (Clark *et al.*, 1985).

Cognitive restructuring

Typically, cognitive restructuring is used in conjunction with exposure exercises in the treatment of SAD. Goals include modifying negative cognitions about the self (*e.g., defectiveness, undesirability*), modifying unrealistic standards of performance (*e.g., perfectionism*), and modifying view of others as extremely evaluative and critical. Automatic thoughts regarding feared and avoided situations are elicited, cognitive distortions are identified, and rational responses are developed before individuals engage in simulated or actual *in vivo* exercises. Then, individuals are instructed to use cognitive restructuring techniques before, during, and after each exposure exercises in order to facilitate exposure tasks.

Cognitive restructuring may be particularly useful for patients who do not exhibit behavioral avoidance of feared situations. Such individuals may use cognitive maneuvers to avoid anxiety (*e.g., distract themselves, withdraw into themselves*) thus preventing the experience of full-blown anxiety during social or performance tasks. Others may distort social or performance encounters (*e.g., see them as unsuccessful*) despite objective evidence to the contrary.

Attention refocus

As attention is often disrupted in individuals with social anxiety, attention strengthening and refocusing exercises are also utilized to help patients refocus their attention on the task at hand instead of on the mental representation of how they appear to others, and away from the expected negative feedback they expect from others. The goal of these exercises is to help patients refocus attention on the task at hand (*e.g., a conversation with a stranger*), which is believed to lead to better performance and an increased likelihood of positive feedback from others. Patients are taught to sustain their attention by practicing tasks requiring concentration such as reading increasingly complex materials over increasing lengths of time. Next, patients learn to practice the task with an increasing list of distractions. Finally, patients apply attention strengthening exercises to social or performance situations and are encouraged to focus attention on the other person or the social task at hand. With increasing awareness, patients learn how to refocus attention on the task even if attention habitually comes back to the self.

Social skills training

Social skills training is employed only if individuals demonstrate social skills deficits. Goals during this phase include creating an awareness of the social environment, and enhancing interpersonal and/or presentation skills as needed. The process of skills training includes initial instruction on the skill and subsequent demonstration of the skill by the therapist. After the therapist teaches and models the required behaviors, the client is typically asked to rehearse the behavior during the session following which corrective feedback and positive reinforcement are offered until the individual has mastered the required skill. Flexibility exercises are also used to address the rigid behavioral style common to individuals with social anxiety.

Systematic exposure

The goal of systematic exposure includes breaking the association between social situations and fear and breaking the association between escape and avoidance of social situations and subsequent feelings of relief. Exposure may be conducted in imagination (imaginal exposure), directly during social situations (*in vivo*) or in 5–10-minute role-plays of anxiety-provoking situations during treatment sessions (simulated exposure). In a group format, other group members serve as role-play partners in addition to the therapist. Outside 'actors' may also be brought in to serve as role-play partners in both individual and group formats. Props may be used to make the simulated exposures as realistic as possible. For example, a patient may be required to stand at a podium while giving a talk or food may be brought in if a patient has a fear of eating in public.

Anxiety-provoking situations using exposure exercises are based on fear and avoidance hierarchies that contain rank-ordered situations rated for fear, avoidance, and fear of negative evaluation by others. These can range from initiating a conversation with a stranger to giving a presentation at a staff meeting. Nonperfectionistic, behavioral goals should be set for exposure tasks which may require some negotiation as patients with social anxiety tend to have unrealistic or unmeasurable goals (*e.g., I should feel no anxiety, or I should be responsible for filling in all the pauses in a conversation*) (Heimberg, 1991). During exposure, anxiety levels and automatic thoughts are monitored periodically and the exposure task is continued until the anxiety decreases or plateaus and the goal(s) have been met. The patient's performance and anxiety level, as well as the automatic thoughts and rational responses used during exposure are then discussed, with the goal of identifying self-statements that increase their anxiety and those that decrease it to facilitate future performance. Individuals are not permitted to use escape or avoid behaviors during exposure in order to prevent the anxiety from reducing prematurely. Subtle avoidance behaviors such as distraction or safety-seeking behaviors are also eliminated.

Although *in vivo* exposure is described as the treatment of choice for anxiety disorders in general (Barlow and Beck, 1984), simulated exposure techniques form an important part of treatment for social anxiety for multiple reasons (Heimberg, 1991). One reason is because *in vivo* exposure exercises are harder to design and implement in the treatment of social anxiety. Unlike simple exposure exercises such as driving over a bridge for a panic disorder patient, patients with social anxiety must perform a complex sequence of interpersonal behaviors during the phobic situation, and expose themselves to a variety of feared interpersonal consequences. *In vivo* exposure are not only more complicated but are also less easily available to socially anxious patients who may have cut themselves off from most social contacts. Because social situations are intrinsically unpredictable, it is also harder to design *in vivo* exercises in advance, and harder to ensure that patients repeat the same social situation or expose themselves to easier situations before difficult ones. Finally, the success of *in vivo* exposure usually comes from prolonged exposure to the feared situation, which leads to habituation of anxiety. Because several social or performance situations involve a brief exchange, patients with anxiety cannot remain in the situation until the anxiety peaks and then reduces. However, in order to facilitate transfer-of-training to real-life social or performance situations, *in vivo* exposure exercises are generally assigned to patients during each session. Specific homework assignments are negotiated with patients and are coordinated with simulated exposure tasks conducted during sessions.

Typical exposure situations include initiating or maintaining a conversation with members of the same or opposite sex, asking for a date, writing, eating, drinking, working or playing while being observed, assertion and interaction with authority figures, job interviews, participating in small or large groups, parties, meetings, and public speaking. Other exposure situations include joining ongoing conversations, giving and receiving compliments, making mistakes in front of others, revealing personal information, expressing opinions, and drawing attention in front of a crowd.

Acute treatment is discontinued when social anxiety is significantly reduced and does not impair functioning. Strategies to maintain gains and prevent relapse are implemented and treatment is slowly tapered over time.

Case illustration

James is a 32-year-old computer analyst who described his social anxiety as a curse passed down from generations. He recalled that he was shy as a child and never spoke up in class. He remembers rejecting a variety of career options including his dream to become a musician. He feels that he was trapped behind what he called an 'invisible barrier' and feels that he never allowed people to see his 'true' personality. Although he is attractive, James was afraid of dating and had never had a meaningful relationship until he was actively pursued by a woman whom he ultimately married. He decided to begin treatment after he was promoted to the position of a manager. He initially turned down the position but after he read an article on SAD in *Time* magazine, James decided to accept the new position and pursue treatment.

Although James had begun the process of reading on SAD, the psycho-education phase reinforced his growing understanding of his condition. Realizing that he had a disorder that could be treated effectively quickly reduced the symptoms of depression he had been experiencing for the past 2 years. He began to feel optimistic that he could be helped and expressed an eagerness to continue with treatment. James was assigned self-help books such as Ronald Rapee's *Overcoming shyness and social phobia* (1998) and was encouraged to join the Anxiety Disorders Association of American (www.adaa.org).

James reported that he had been experiencing increased physical tension as he had accepted the new position. To combat these symptoms, he was taught deep muscle relaxation and breathing retraining and was instructed to practice exercises daily. As he mastered the exercises over the next few weeks, James was encouraged to use them as and when he needed before he faced anxiety-provoking situations.

Although James had many social or performance-based situations that triggered anxiety, his decision to accept the promotion at work necessitated a focus on interpersonal situations at work related to his new position. Using a thought log, James learned to identify and monitor automatic thoughts during periods of social anxiety at work or in anticipation of social encounters in his new position. Representative automatic thoughts were identified such as 'he will think I am stupid,' 'I am going to mess up,' 'they will be able to see that I am nervous,' 'they will be waiting for me to fall on my face,' 'they won't listen to me,' and 'I will not be able to cope with the stress of this new job.' Once James was able to identify his own auto-matic thoughts, he was encouraged through guided discovery and Socratic questioning to consider the fact that he did not know for sure what others were thinking, and to help broaden his perceptions away from the most cata-strophic predictions (*e.g., he may not notice that I am nervous, she may be thinking that I am better than the previous manager*). His perfectionistic standards of performance (*e.g., I cannot expect that I will be able to be an effective manager immediately*) and his belief that others were critical and evaluative (*e.g., she will think I am a loser*) were also modified. Within a few weeks, James grew skilled at identifying and challenging his automatic thoughts using Socratic questioning. As a result of daily practice, he began to notice a reduction in anxiety, particularly during moments when he anticipated social encounters at work.

Using a fear and avoidance hierarchy, the therapist and James identified key interpersonal situations that he would face in his new position. Key situations such as interfacing with clients and his team at work in his new position were transformed into specific, behavioral tasks such as meeting clients face to face, calling clients on the telephone, holding a meeting with his staff, asking his staff to conduct tasks, and so on. Once these tasks were rated it became clear that even the smallest task (*e.g., calling clients on the telephone*) was creating more than a moderate level of anxiety (*e.g., over 50 on a scale of 1–100*). Consequently, imaginal exposure and anxiety provok-ing tasks unrelated to his place of employment were first used in initial exposure sessions. For example, James practiced exposure with tasks such as asking strangers for the time (30) for directions (35), asking acquaint-ances for simple favors (40), imagining talking to clients on the telephone (45) before he confronted more anxiety-provoking tasks at work. In addi-tion, other exposure tasks such as mispronouncing a word in front of others (60) and slipping and falling in front of strangers (75) were used later on in the hierarchy to help James learn that he was capable of coping even if he did place himself in a position where negative evaluation might occur.

By integrating cognitive restructuring into exposure, James was able to acknowledge that he could not expect to become a skilled manager right-away and consequently, was able to set nonperfectionistic goals during exposure. Simulated exposure exercises were also used with the therapist and James role-playing key situations. For example, other individuals were bought in to the session to simulate work meetings during an exposure session.

As James did not possess leadership skills, exposure sessions were often preceded by sessions where requisite skills were practiced during sessions through instruction, modeling, behavior rehearsal, corrective feedback, and positive reinforcement. James was also assigned to read books on leader-ship and effective communication strategies in the workplace. Finally, to refocus his attention on conversations with clients and staff instead of on how he appeared to them, James was taught attention refocusing exercises. He was required to read increasing long and complex articles on computer programming, first under optimal conditions such as in his home after his wife went to bed, and then under increasingly distracting situations such as with music on, in the subway and so on. Finally, James learned to become aware of situations in which his attention wandered away from the task at hand (*e.g., a conversation with a client*) and learned to apply the new skills to refocus his attention away from the mental representation of himself and towards the task at hand.

James was encouraged to use cognitive restructuring before and after exposure situations to ensure that his fear of negative evaluation changed as a result of successful exposure. He was also encouraged to use exposure situations as behavioral experiments in which to test out irrational predic-tions. James was also encouraged to continue using daily relaxation exer-cises but was not permitted to use them during exposure sessions, in order to prevent his anxiety from reducing artificially. He practiced social and attention skills prior to exposure and soon began to feel less anxious, more confident about his ability to handle his new job and his ability to cope with his symptoms.

As his symptoms reduced and he was able to perform effectively at work, other social and performance situations were targeted in treatment. Acute treatment was discontinued once his overall symptoms reduced to man-ageable levels, his social functioning was no longer impaired, and he was able to guide his own treatment. Strategies to maintain gain and prevent relapse now became the focus of treatment and session were tapered to monthly sessions until James was able to manage on his own.

Panic disorder and agoraphobia

Diagnostic features

Panic disorder is defined by the occurrence of panic attacks, which are marked by intense physical sensations (heart palpitations, shakiness, sweat-ing, shortness of breath, sensation of choking, chest pain, nausea, dizziness, feelings of detachment or unreality (depersonalization or derealization), fear of losing control or going insane, fear of a medical crisis (e.g., heart attack), numbness or tingling, and hot or cold flashes (APA, DSM IV)). Agoraphobia is characterized by fear of open spaces, places where exit is blocked or other stimuli (such as heights, bright sunlight), where the fear is that the situation may elicit a panic attack. The lifetime prevalence of panic disorder is 1.5–3.8%, with females twice as likely to manifest this disorder. Age of onset for panic disorder with agoraphobia is in the early twenties.

Evaluation

Panic disorder is distinguished from SAD in that in SAD the main fear is that others will see the individual's anxiety and that this will be a humiliat-ing experience. Panic disorder is distinguished from OCD in that in OCD the main fear is of making mistakes or being contaminated or leaving some-thing undone—rather than the fear of the consequences of one's own anxi-ety, as is characteristic of panic disorder. Although in the general population there are many individuals who manifest agoraphobia without prior history of panic disorder, it is individuals with both panic disorder and agoraphobia who are more likely seek treatment.

People with panic disorder and agoraphobia are 18 times more likely to try to commit suicide than people without any psychiatric disorder (Weissman *et al.*, 1989) and are more likely to have an increased risk of cardiovascular disease, including aneurysm, congestive heart failure, and pulmonary embolism (Coryell *et al.*, 1982, 1986). These people eventually have a risk of stroke that is twice the rate for other psychiatric disorders (Weissman *et al.*, 1990; McNally, 1994).

Theoretical models

Many of the situations that are feared by the agoraphobic are situations that might confer greater danger in an evolutionary adaptive environment (Leahy and Holland, 2000). For example, situations that might elicit panic attacks are open spaces (greater vulnerability to predators), closed spaces (vulnerability to suffocation or being trapped), bright sunlight (more visible to predators), and heights (danger of falling). Although the fear in panic disorder is of the consequences of one's own anxiety symptoms (that is, the fear of going insane, losing control, or a medical crisis) it may be that this 'fear of fear'—elicited in these specific situations was adaptive to primitive ancestors. There is a reasonably high heritability component for panic disorder, suggesting a genetic link of some importance.

The cognitive-behavioral theoretical model is derived from the work of A. T. Beck *et al.* (1985), Clark (1986), and Barlow (1988). The initial physiological arousal—rapid breathing, dizziness, or sweating—may, in some cases, be due to greater exertion, fatigue, undiagnosed illness, life stressors—that are often underestimated by the panicker. This initial 'panic attack' is accompanied by a catastrophic interpretation—'I am going crazy'—leading to hypervigilance for other signs of anxious arousal. This increased self-focus on one's own arousal increases the likelihood of arousal being detected or escalated—leading to false confirmations that another panic attack is imminent. Many panickers rely on 'safety behaviors'—such as being accompanied by another person, stiffening one's posture, 'taking deep breaths' (that augment the hyperventilation syndrome). Situations that 'trigger' increased arousal—such as open spaces, heights, closed spaces, or behaviors that trigger arousal (exercise) are anticipated with dread or tolerated with increased discomfort.

Empirical support for treatment

Gould *et al.* (1995) have provided a meta-analysis of 48 controlled studies of cognitive-behavioral treatment of panic disorder with agoraphobia. The authors concluded from this analysis that CBT was highly effective in yielding panic-free outcomes, with an effect size of 0.88 (compared with an effect size of 0.47 for pharmacological treatment). The range of percent of patients who received CBT who were panic free after treatment was between 32% and 100%. In most of the studies reviewed, the percentage of panic free exceeded 80%. When CBT was compared with an emotion-focused approach, the former was significantly more effective than the latter (Shear *et al.*, 2001).

Rationale for treatment and interventions

Strategies and techniques

The plan of treatment involves a variety of interventions including socialization to treatment (explaining the CBT model of panic and agoraphobia and the use of bibliotherapy), anxiety management techniques (rebreathing, PMR, time-management), construction of a fear hierarchy (including external stimuli—for example, open areas, heights, closed spaces, and interoceptive stimuli—feelings of dizziness or hyperventilation sensations), and gradual exposure to stimuli in the hierarchy. In addition, identifying catastrophic predictions, eliminating safety behaviors, and setting up behavioral experiments to disconfirm negative predictions about anxious arousal are important cognitive components of treatment.

We utilize the patient information forms from the Leahy and Holland (2000) manual on treatment of depression and anxiety disorders. Many patients find the schematic presented above to be especially useful in demystifying the nature of panic disorder. Behavioral anxiety management techniques (such as relaxation training, activity scheduling, and rebreathing) are helpful in reducing overall level of arousal, but are not sufficient in themselves to eliminate panic disorder or anticipatory anxiety about having panic attacks. It is important to convey to the patient that reducing anxious arousal is not the same thing as decatastrophizing anxiety—as some anxious arousal will be inevitable, it is important to develop a different interpretation and response to the anxiety. Indeed, in explaining the cognitive-behavioral treatment plan, the therapist should be careful to inform the patient that increasing anxious arousal—through exposure—and even inducing panic attacks in session—will be essential components of therapy.

The process of exposure, and the role of safety behaviors, is explained to the patient as an opportunity to learn (with new tools that are available) that panic attacks can be induced, experienced, and naturally come to a swift conclusion. This will help disconfirm the belief that panic attacks will lead to something more adverse—such as insanity or medical emergencies. Furthermore, safety behaviors will need to be eliminated as they do not allow disconfirmation of the panic beliefs. Thus, as illustrated in the schematic, the patient utilizing the superstitious safety behaviors (such as holding on to a chair in order to avoid falling) will not experience the liberating experience of learning that his dizziness does not lead to a collapse response even when he is not holding on to the chair.

We utilize imaginal exposure early in treatment to afford the patient with the opportunity of experiencing the feared stimuli within a more comfortable presentation. During imaginal exposure to the situations and sensations of panic, the therapist engages in role-plays with the patient to either elicit the catastrophic predictions (*e.g., I am losing control and I will die*) or to challenge these catastrophic predictions (e.g., *I have had numerous panic attacks and nothing terrible has happened*). Many patients are assisted by using 'flash cards' (e.g., index cards) on which catastrophic predictions are written on one side while rational or calming responses are listed on the other side. Subsequent to imaginal exposure the therapist and patient will move on to more threatening stimuli and will engage in exposure to these situations *in vivo*.

Inducing panic attacks in session, with the explanation of this technique and its rationale, can allow the patient to engage in experiencing the interoceptive stimuli (shortness of breath, dizziness, sweating, or heart racing)—and learn that these sensations are self-limiting. Induction of panic symptoms can be accomplished by practicing rapid breathing or spinning in a chair with the therapist noting the patient's report of subjective units of distress (anxiety level) at short periodic intervals. Some clinicians find it useful to provide the patient with panic-reversal behaviors—such as breathing into a bag slowly, practicing diaphragmatic breathing, or running in place (all of which will establish a balance of carbon dioxide and reduce hyperventilation or dizziness). However, it is also effective to allow the patient the opportunity that riding out a panic attack without utilizing these anxiety management techniques can also be effective.

Case example

The patient was a single woman in her mid-twenties who complained of fearing panic attacks in shopping malls. She indicated that her first panic attack occurred 2 months after her breakup in a relationship when she became intensely anxious while at an indoor shopping mall where she had previously had a discussion about a breakup with her boyfriend. During the initial panic attack she experienced shortness of breath, dizziness, sweating, and a sense that she was about to collapse and feared that she would not be able to get out of the mall without being accompanied by someone. Subsequent to the initial panic attack she began to experience intense anxiety while walking along wide avenues in New York City. As a result of her panic disorder she avoided malls and tried to walk close to buildings to which she could escape from the open space in the event of a panic attack.

The first phase of treatment focused on socialization to the CBT model of panic. This involved providing her with an evolutionary rationale for innately predisposed fears of open spaces. In addition, further evaluation indicated that her safety behaviors included scanning the street or building for quick exits or escape routes, tightening her body while walking, narrowing her focus on specific signs of 'danger', sitting in a chair, exiting the street into a taxi, and trying to 'take deep breaths' (which was based on the incorrect advice of another therapist). She was instructed in diaphragmatic breathing—which she practiced as an initial homework assignment. A fear hierarchy was constructed that consisted of being at the center of a mall (most feared), walking into a mall, walking into a crowded hotel lobby, walking along a wide avenue, fluorescent lights, and bright sunlight. The therapist indicated that these feared stimuli might be related to situations that conferred danger in a primitive environment (being trapped—no exit available—and bright light making her more visible and vulnerable to predators). Initially, she was quite skeptical of this interpretation—but she noted over the week following the first meeting that she felt considerably less anxious.

Noting her safety behaviors was also valuable for her, as it helped explain why she still maintained her fears even after she had experienced some exposure. Specifically, the therapist indicated that she might be inclined to attribute a successful exposure experience to her safety behaviors—rather than to the safety of the situation. She was instructed to keep track of her use of safety behaviors, identify her predictions of what would happen if she relinquished these behaviors (e.g., 'I will collapse' or 'If I do not tighten my body when I am walking, I will lose control and run out'). These predictions were subsequently tested out by either deliberately relinquishing the safety behaviors or actually doing the opposite of her safety behaviors (e.g., purposefully trying to make her body as loose as possible or avoiding looking at any exits and scanning the sidewalk rather than the buildings for safety places).

Gradual exposure to avenues and crowded streets was followed by exposure to hotel lobbies. She was instructed to repeat these exposures for 30 minutes each day—and to view her experience of anxiety as a successful component of her exposure. This was considered important as she had perfectionistic expectations about her anxiety—'I shouldn't feel any anxiety'. This idealized view was challenged by 'You need to have some anxiety or fear during exposure for you to learn that your anxiety will diminish'.

At termination of treatment after 3 months the patient was able to enter and walk through malls with mild anxiety and to cross wide avenues without anxiety. Her mood and confidence had improved substantially and she reported greater confidence in being able to handle any threat of panic in the future.

Psychodynamic model of panic disorder

The model for panic disorder described by Busch et al. (1991) and Shear et al. (1993) weaves neurophysiological factors with psychodynamic concepts and data to develop a psychodynamic formulation for panic disorder. This model was employed for the development of treatment interventions and manualization (Milrod et al., 1997). The authors describe that an inherent tendency toward fearfulness in unfamiliar situations results in a state of fearful dependency on significant others in the child's environment to provide a sense of safety. This anxious attachment causes a narcissistic humiliation for the child, as he cannot feel safe without the help of others, and a propensity toward anger at others for being unable to provide sufficient comfort to relieve his anxious state. Children may also develop a state of fearful dependency in environments in which parents behave in a critical, threatening, or rejecting manner.

Thus these children develop representations of others as abandoning, rejecting, and controlling. Anger at others is fueled by these perceptions, but the child is fearful of experiencing or expressing anger for fear of driving away or damaging the needed parent. Fearful dependency can be triggered again in adulthood by life events that represent danger or separation from a significant other. Angry feelings, which are often unconscious, are experienced as a danger to centrally important relationships, and signal anxiety is triggered. Defenses such as reaction formation, in which anger is converted into positive or helping feelings, or undoing, in which any negative feelings that do emerge into consciousness are taken back, attempt to quell the danger experienced from frightening angry feelings. However, these defenses fail, and patients experience the onset of traumatic anxiety in the form of a panic attack. The panic attack represents a compromise formation, in which the patient can express anger via demands for help from others, can desperately seek help in the setting of feared loss or separation, and can shut out angry feelings considered to be dangerous with a focus on intense, overwhelming anxiety. From the standpoint of the pleasure principle, patients experience a panic attack as less painful than the potential risk of loss of an important attachment figure, or of a conscious awareness of other symbolic meanings that the panic attack carries.

Empirical support for psychodynamic treatment of panic disorder

Case reports and psychological assessments of patients with panic disorder formed the basis for the development of a systematic approach to the psychodynamic treatment for panic disorder (Busch et al., 1991; Milrod et al., 1997). Milrod and Shear (1991) found 35 case reports of successful treatment of panic with psychodynamic psychotherapy or psychoanalysis in the psychoanalytic literature. A 15-session manualized psychodynamic psychotherapy for panic disorder, when combined with clomipramine treatment, was found to reduce the risk of relapse over an 18-month period following treatment termination compared with a group treated with clomipramine alone (Wiborg and Dahl, 1996). This study did not match treatment groups for frequency of therapist contact.

Milrod et al. (2000, 2001) conducted an open trial of panic-focused psychodynamic psychotherapy (PFPP) (Milrod et al., 1997), a manualized psychodynamic treatment that focuses on exploring the underlying unconscious meanings of panic symptoms and associated psychodynamic conflicts. This therapeutic approach was employed as a 24-session, twice weekly treatment intervention for 21 patients with DSM-IV panic disorder, using standardized panic disorder assessment measures recommended by the National Institute of Mental Health Collaborative Report (Shear and Maser, 1994). At study entry, patients had significant panic disorder and agoraphobia, along with functional impairment. Of 17 treatment completers (four patients were dropouts), 16 experienced remission of panic disorder and agoraphobia, and also experienced statistically significant, clinically meaningful improvements in phobic symptoms and psychosocial function, both at treatment termination and at 6-month follow-up following a 6-month no-treatment interval. The results of the open trial suggested that PFPP is a promising treatment for panic disorder. A randomized controlled trial of PFPP in comparison with applied relaxation training (ART) is in progress.

Psychodynamic treatment of panic disorder

In treatment of panic disorder, therapists focus on the conflicts surrounding separation and anger as they emerge in precipitating events, interpersonal relationships, and in the transference. Examining the use of defenses is of value in bringing frightening feelings and fantasies to consciousness (Busch et al., 1995; Milrod et al., 1997). For example, the therapist treating a panic patient can identify the use of reaction formation when a patient is avoiding the experience of anger by being overly helpful to those with whom they are actually angry. For instance, a patient may refer to 'loving to death' a boyfriend whom she actually experiences as depriving and hurtful. Undoing, in which angry feelings are expressed and then taken back, provides an important opportunity to identify and explore the threat the patient experiences from angry feelings. By examining these defenses the therapist can help the patient with the core conflicts in panic, and with the fear of disrupting attachment to others who are considered essential to safety.

Case example

Sarah was a 29-year-old single administrative assistant who presented with the onset of panic disorder 4 months prior to evaluation. In addition to typical symptoms of panic disorder she described clenching her teeth and stomach pain. The symptoms recurred after she returned from a trip abroad with her boyfriend, Dan, that had lasted several months. When they returned they moved to their usual homes in separate towns, which were about a 3-hour drive apart. Although Sarah hoped to marry Dan she became aware of the limitations in his availability to her. They planned to get together every weekend, but he often missed coming to visit her because his job kept him very busy. She became frustrated because she did not feel he was making the effort to set the necessary limits at his job to make sure he could see her. She became increasingly anxious during her discussions with Dan about these issues, leading ultimately to panic attacks. When they were together she described him as very nice to her, and said that they got along quite well. Thus she struggled with whether she was right to see him as putting her secondary to his work, and whether he could be trusted.

Sarah was also struggling with other stresses. She had been laid off prior to the trip and began to feel financial pressure. She also felt lonely, as most of her friends were in the city she had left 2 years previously. Even more so than with her boyfriend, she complained that friends in her new location did not follow up with plans and were not responsive when she needed them.

Sarah described a difficult and tumultuous upbringing. The youngest of four siblings, her father was an alcoholic who withdrew from the family when drunk. Her mother was temperamental, and easily overwhelmed by her children's demands. When she was 7 years old, conflicts between her parents intensified, with her father ultimately leaving the house for a year. Her father's drinking increased when Sarah was an adolescent, and she struggled with rage and her hurt feelings about his behavior. She feared that her father would injure himself in a fall or car accident. At times during her adolescence, she was recruited to bring him home from the bar or take him to a rehabilitation program. She was extremely embarrassed by her father's behavior and worried about what her friends thought of both of them. In her view, he was a caring and interested father during his sober periods who 'disappeared' emotionally and sometimes physically when he was drinking. In part related to her father's alcoholism, the family was in constant financial turmoil. Sarah recalled feeling frightened about whether the family would be able to meet monthly payments.

Sarah entered into a 24-session psychodynamic psychotherapeutic treatment that was part of a research protocol. In the first few sessions it became evident that her panic attacks were precipitated by her separations from Dan. The panic attacks began after their return from their trip and would intensify when he left after they spent the weekend together. In addition, the panic became more severe when he would cancel a visit with her.

Exploration of her relationship with her father provided clues about the difficulty she had with separations. When the therapist was questioning her about her father's 'disappearances' when drinking, she became tearful when expressing anger at her father. Then she suddenly became disparaging of the psychotherapy: 'I dealt with my anger a long time ago. There's no point in dredging it all up again. It's just going to make me feel worse.' The therapist replied that trying to sweep her anger under the rug would not be helpful to her, and her ongoing struggles with her anger likely emerged in her panic. Sarah then revealed that she was fearful that her anger at Dan, when she was disappointed with him, would cause him to reject her. Similarly, she felt that any expression of her own and her mother's and siblings' frustration with her father set off his drinking bouts, and triggered his extended disappearances.

Sarah viewed her needs as potentially driving away her boyfriend and father. After separations from Dan she struggled with her wishes to call him, presuming she would come across as 'too needy'. She feared that Dan would see her as 'high maintenance' and abandon her. She felt that expressions of need were another factor that triggered her father's drinking. Panic occurring at these times included a feeling of desperate aloneness and wishes to contact her mother and others for comfort. However, she attempted to avoid being needy by acting more self-sufficient, leaving her feeling even more isolated. Examining the patient's catastrophic fears of her anger and dependency when separated helped to detoxify these feelings, rendering them less likely to trigger panic.

Discussion about termination, which began in session 16, indicated that she viewed the therapist as another source of support who would suddenly disappear. She reacted to the approaching termination initially with feelings of anger, hurt, rejection, and anxiety. She eventually was able to see the similarities between her feelings about the treatment ending and those she experienced toward her father and boyfriend. She was particularly worried that she would have a recurrence of her panic with no one to help her. Her ability to safely work through these feelings with her therapist added to a reduction in her fears, the resolution of her panic, and an increased ability to manage separations.

Generalized anxiety disorder

Diagnostic features

Generalized anxiety disorder (GAD) is characterized by physiological arousal (restlessness, fatigue, difficulty concentrating, irritability, muscle tension, insomnia) and apprehensive worry. Unlike other anxiety disorders where the fear or anxiety is about a specific event or stimulus, GAD is characterized by worry about several events (e.g., relationships, illness, finances, work). Lifetime prevalence of GAD is about 5% and 1-year prevalence is 4% reflecting the fact that GAD is widespread and chronic (Blazer et al., 1991; Wittchen et al., 1994; Kessler et al., 1999; Newman et al., 2003).

Evaluation

GAD is characterized by worry about a number of different things, the sense that worry is dangerous or out of control and physical arousal and tension. Measures assess the degree of worry in GAD (Penn State Worry Questionnaire), examination of beliefs about worry (Metacognitions Questionnaire), areas or topics of worry (Worry Domains Questionnaire), and the Intolerance of Uncertainty Scale (IUS). GAD status may also be evaluated using the Anxiety Disorders Interview Schedule (Brown et al., 1994) and the Generalized Anxiety Disorder Questionnaire (GAD-Q; Newman et al., 2002).

Theoretical models

The behavioral model of GAD stresses both individual differences in arousal and experiences that are coupled with negative consequences. According to this model, specific events or stimuli become associated through conditioning with anxiety or fear. Treatment implications of the strict behavioral model include emphasis on decreasing anxious arousal through relaxation, coupling this relaxation with the feared stimuli (reciprocal inhibition; Wolpe, 1958), increasing exposure without escape, and enhancing assertion.

The cognitive-behavioral model, developed over the past 15 years, emphasizes the central role of worry in GAD (Borkovec, 1994; Wells, 1997). Worry primarily involves thoughts (rather than images) that are experienced as ego-syntonic, but which are associated with predictions of negative outcomes. In particular, worriers with GAD are more likely to perceive threats that are either not there or are ambiguous (MacLeod et al., 1986; Borkovec, 1994; Matthews and Wells, 1999, 2000), they underestimate their ability to cope with negative outcomes, and their negative predictions are often extreme. Borkovec noted that worriers with GAD often believe that the worry itself will cause negative consequences for them (such as sickness or insanity) and that their worry is 'out of control'. However, worriers also believe that their worry protects and prepares them and, therefore, cannot be easily abandoned.

A recent model of worry as intolerance of uncertainty has gained significant empirical support. Dugas, Ladouceur, Freeston and colleagues have indicated that worriers are often so intolerant of uncertainty that they continue to worry (or seek solutions to hypothetical problems) until the uncertainty can be reduced (Freeston, 1994; Dugas and Ladacoeur, 1998; Dugas et al., 2004). Ironically, though, given the intolerance of uncertainty, this search for a perfect solution above the threshold of certainty will lead to failure, thereby leading to further worry and further search for perfect solutions.

Borkovec and others have proposed that worry is an attempt to avoid negative emotions by relying on abstract, linguistic processing rather than direct emotional processing (Borkovec and Hu, 1990; Borkovec, 1994; Heimberg *et al.*, 2003). When GAD patients engage in worry, they are actually less anxious or aroused, resulting in the inhibition of emotion during the worry phase. This inhibition of emotion regarding unpleasant content prevents 'exposure' or 'emotional processing', resulting in a later rebound of anxiety after the worry abates. Wells and his colleagues have described this as the 'incubation' of anxiety that results from relying on worry.

Developmental histories of GAD patients reveal an interesting pattern of experiences that may give rise to later vulnerabilities related to uncertainty, negative outcome, and concern over the feelings of others. For example, GAD adults report that during childhood that they had more disruptions in attachment relationships, experienced 'reversed parenting' (such that they attended to the emotional needs of a parent who often neglected the patient's needs), unpredictability of outcomes (or noncontingency), and had parents who combined both overcontrol and coldness. Presumably, these socialization experiences would sensitize worriers to the needs of others—for example, GAD patients rank high on empathy and their most common worries relate to interpersonal issues. Moreover, the child growing up in this kind of family would learn to inhibit emotional experience and expression and rely on anticipatory problem solving—either to soothe the emotional needs of the parent or to solve problems that others could not solve or that the child could not rely on to solve.

Most intriguing, in support of the emotional avoidance model, is that worriers as children were the most likely of all anxiety disorder patients to have experienced a physical trauma or threat of physical trauma. Yet, they are the least likely of adult anxiety patients to worry or fear such trauma. This may reflect that worriers engage in focusing on relatively irrelevant concerns as a way of avoiding the more troublesome physical vulnerability.

Empirical support for treatments

There is considerable support that cognitive-behavioral treatments are effective in the treatment of GAD (Gould *et al.*, 2003), with some evidence that treatment gains are maintained 6 months after CBT is completed. Moreover, combining cognitive and behavioral treatment is more effective than behavior therapy alone (Butler *et al.*, 1991).

Rationale for treatment and interventions

Strategies and techniques

Cognitive-behavioral treatments for worry have incorporated a variety of interventions aimed, alternately, at autonomic arousal, stimulus control of worry, uncertainty training, distinguishing between productive and unproductive worry, time management, activity scheduling, problem solving, identifying and challenging automatic thoughts, evaluating estimates of probabilities, mindfulness training, and interpersonal interventions.

Brief plan of treatment

Treatment will include a variety of techniques and evaluations, not necessarily used in a particular sequence. A brief plan might include the following: initial assessment (see above), identifying meta-cognitive beliefs and distinguishing between Type 1 and Type 2 worry (i.e., Type 1 worry that involves negative predictions about the future and Type 2 worry that involves concern that worry may go out of control or cause harm to the self). Worry time is assigned, that requires that the patient delay all worry to a specific time and place, thereby conferring a sense of control and finiteness to the worry. Worries that occur outside of worry time are written on cards and then become the focus of attention during the latter worry time. Predictions of negative outcomes are gathered and tested against actual outcomes.

Cognitive therapy techniques are helpful in addressing specific worries. The therapist can ask the patient to identify the specific worry, identify the emotions associated with the worry, examine the costs and benefits of the worry, consider the outcomes of past worries, weigh the evidence for and against the worry, ask what advice the patient would give to a friend with the worry, and collect evidence about specific predictions.

The patient can be trained in uncertainty tolerance: first, a distinction is made between present and future possible problems. Second, the present problems are reframed as problems to be solved, activating problem-solving strategies and behaviors. Third, 'possible problems' become the focus of uncertainty training, with the patient practicing flooding himself with the thought or image that the bad thing 'could' happen, with instructions to eliminate reassurance. The patient is encouraged to practice living in the present—including mindfulness training, focusing on the present circumstance, and using activities to immerse himself in present experience.

Relaxation and other meditative training may be utilized as anxiety management techniques that may assist in reducing generally higher autonomic arousal. These anxiety management techniques not only reduce the arousal that may exacerbate the worry, but they may also provide the patient with evidence that he or she does have some control over the worry.

Case example

The patient was a 53-year-old manager who complained of worrying all his life. Always someone concerned with being conscientious, he noted that his worry had become more pronounced in the past 15 years, as he had taken on more responsibilities at work that involved deadlines and uncertainty of outcome. He relied on sedatives for sleep, had found antidepressant medication to be unhelpful and had several short experiences in traditional psychotherapy that were not productive.

The general GAD model was explained to him, distinguishing between productive and unproductive worry, and emphasizing the importance of uncertainty tolerance. A distinction was made between worries that can rapidly (almost immediately) be turned into a 'to do' list of specific action versus worries about 'possible' events over which he had almost no control. Specific 'to do' lists were utilized daily, along with tracking actual accomplishments and behaviors on a daily basis. Worry time was set aside for flooding himself with worries and listing these worries. This resulted in a recognition that his worries primarily focused on a few areas—work to be done, meetings he would have, and the concern about being on time.

The worry time was immensely helpful to him and ran against his initial prediction that he would not be able to set aside worries until later. This gave him more of a sense of control. Specific predictions were elicited that characterized these worries—'I won't get the report in' and 'People will be hostile toward me'—and these were tested weekly. Uncertainty training was implemented—with the therapist telling him that much of worry is the intolerance of uncertainty. He was urged to practice both in session and as self-help homework repeating, 'It's possible that I can make mistakes and people will be angry with me'. In addition, he practiced visualizing (as exposure) images of negative outcomes until these outcomes became boring.

On a daily basis the patient was instructed to practice PMR, forming visual images of relaxing settings. In addition, he was encouraged to increase the frequency of aerobic exercise, which he did to a moderate degree.

In regard to his insomnia, he was instructed to avoid naps and to use the bed only for sleep and sex. Thus, he refrained from reading in bed, given this guideline. Like many insomniacs, his sleeplessness was due to mental activity. He was instructed to write out his worries and his action to do list at least 3 hours before bedtime. If he had difficulty falling asleep, he was instructed to practice repeating 'I will never fall asleep'. The rationale for this instruction is that his insomnia was based on a worry—'I might never get to sleep'—that he tried to neutralize by 'trying to sleep'. This generally failed.

Over the course of nine biweekly sessions his worry diminished substantially and his sleep improved. He was urged to continue with the worry time, to do lists, uncertainty training, and practicing feared thoughts at the termination of treatment.

Psychodynamic model of generalized anxiety disorder

From a dynamic perspective, anxiety is linked to the potential emergence of threatening unconscious wishes into consciousness, and to early interpersonal relationships that form an internal psychological template in which attachments are experienced as easily disrupted. In GAD, defenses have been ineffective at neutralizing or disguising unconscious wishes, leading to persistent anxiety, or somatization may be operating as a primary defense. Crits-Christoph et al. (1995, 1996) suggest that early relationships in GAD patients trigger feelings of rejection, potential loss, anger, and a sense of needing to protect the caregiver to maintain the relationship. Ongoing anxiety derives from these conflicted feelings and the sense of unstable relationships. In addition, they hypothesize that past traumas can set off a pattern of generalized worry.

Psychodynamic treatment of generalized anxiety disorder

As in other psychodynamic approaches with anxiety disorders, the therapist explores the content of the patient's specific worries with the goal of determining the particular threatening unconscious wishes that the patient is attempting to manage or displace, in an effort to make the patient's emotional reactions more understandable to him. In addition, early life relationships and traumatic experiences are investigated to determine why the patient views attachments as easily disrupted and the world as unsafe. Further clues can be obtained from experiences of anxiety in the transference. The therapy provides a safe atmosphere in which frightening unconscious wishes and conflicts can emerge and be rendered less threatening, which functions to diminish conscious worrying about the self, relationships, and the world.

Posttraumatic stress disorder

Diagnostic features

PTSD is defined by exposure to a life-threatening or injury-threatening experience in which the individual experienced intense fear, helplessness or horror and after which the individual experienced one of the following: intrusive recollections of images of the event, recurrent distressing dreams, experiencing the event as if it is recurring, psychological distress with exposure to the event, or physiological reactivity to stimuli similar to the event. In addition, there are attempts to avoid the stimulus and increased and recurrent arousal (insomnia, irritability, hypervigilance, etc.) (APA, DSM IV). The lifetime prevalence of PTSD in the National Comorbidity Study was 7.8% (males 10.4% and females 5.0%, with 60% of males and 51% of females exposed lifetime to traumatic events). Younger individuals are at greater risk for PTSD than older individuals.

Evaluation

PTSD differs from panic disorder in that the individual with PTSD has had these symptoms for longer than 1 month following the trauma (versus acute stress disorder) and re-experiences the traumatic event through intrusions, dreams, and a sense of the recurrence of the event (versus panic disorder). Evaluation instruments for PTSD include the Clinician-Administered PTSD Scale (CAPS), the PTSD Symptom Scale, and the Impact of Events Scale-Revised (Weiss and Marmar, 1997).

Theoretical models

The behavioral model of PTSD entails both classical and operant conditioning, following Mowrer's two-factor theory. Specifically, it has been proposed that the original traumatic event results in a learned association of the emotional trauma that has occurred with the stimuli (visual images, sensations, sounds, etc.) of this event. Future encounters or memories of the event activate the traumatic experience, resulting in increased anxiety. Avoidance or even numbing following the event results in decreased anxiety, thereby reinforcing avoidance or escape and consequently maintaining the traumatic association. Foa and her colleagues have expanded on the behavioral model by proposing that PTSD is characterized by a combination of the associations described above and by the meanings given to the experience. This model stresses the importance of the 'fear structure', which includes the problematic interpretations given to the event, such as 'I am never safe', 'I can be killed at any time', 'The

world is not fair', or 'I am all alone'. Foa's model stresses the importance of both information and emotional processing and places the cognitive-affective 'fear structure' at the heart of PTSD. According to this model, attempts to assimilate the feared experience—in order to process it and give it meaning—occur during the intrusive 're-experiencing', but are so overwhelming that complete processing is not obtained. This results in further attempts to avoid and, consequently, emerging interpretations that one is helpless and always vulnerable. Similar to 'shattered assumptions', the traumatic event may have more generalized implications for the individual about the nature of physical and interpersonal security and meaning.

Specific cognitive processes involved in PTSD include dissociative experiences (derealization and depersonalization), increased recall of vivid imagery associated with the trauma, but also a tendency in some cases to have vague or overgeneral recall (Loftus and Burns, 1982; Brewin and Holmes, 2003). McNally provides an extensive review of the literature related to memory processes, 'repressed' memory, and so-called 'traumatic amnesia'. His review casts considerable doubt on sensational claims of 'recovered memory' related to abuse and trauma. Rather, it appears that traumatic events generally are more memorable and account for the intrusive nature of subsequent PTSD. There is mixed evidence for attentional biases—but some evidence suggests that individuals with PTSD manifest the Stroop effect of interference with subliminal stimuli (Harvey et al., 1996). Shame and anger are also often associated with the traumatic experience, mental defeat (a combination of helplessness and dissolution of personal identity, Elhers et al., 2000), negative beliefs associated with depression and PTSD (Foa et al., 1999). Brewin and colleagues have proposed a dual representation model of trauma, suggesting that information is encoded and experienced as verbally accessible memory (VAM) or situationally accessible memory (SAM), with sights, sounds, and sensations experienced at the more 'primitive' level of SAM (Brewin, 1996; Brewin and Holmes, 2003). Thus, effective treatment of PTSD would entail both the verbal or narrative meanings associated with trauma (VAM) and the more concrete stimuli and sensations entailed in SAM. Interpersonal factors are also associated with PTSD, with lack of social support predicting continuation of symptoms (see Brewin et al., 2000). Finally, eye movement desensitization and reprocessing (EMDR) was developed by Shapiro and has been utilized for treatment of PTSD by associating the elicited images of trauma with rapid eye movements produced by the patient following the therapist's hand. Although some studies have found this to be as effective as exposure and anxiety management interventions, the findings are mixed.

Empirical support for treatments

There is considerable support for cognitive-behavioral treatments of PTSD, with some protocols utilizing a combination of various interventions and other utilizing other CBT interventions. It is not unusual for CBT outcome studies to utilize extended or double sessions (60–120 minutes) so as to allow for sufficient exposure and habituation to the feared stimulus. Empirical support for the efficacy of these treatments can be found in numerous reports (Foa et al., 1991, 1995; Tarrier et al., 1999).

Rationale for treatment and interventions

The cognitive-behavioral approach to treatment proposes that the patient must re-experience the traumatic images and stimuli, activate the fear structure associated with the traumatic experience, and learn that the images and stimuli are no longer dangerous. This is based on the model of exposure with response prevention, where exposure entails re-experiencing the images long enough that the patient habituates a fear response and by preventing escape or avoidance during this exposure by prolonging the experience. Thus, the two-factor model of conditioning—stressing both classical conditioning through exposure and operant conditioning (by preventing escape) is the basic rationale. In addition, cognitive restructuring assists the patient in modifying the dysfunctional beliefs that have arisen during this experience.

Strategies and techniques

The approach to treatment involves several components, including psychoeducation of the nature of PTSD (see Leahy and Holland, 2000 for handouts for patients on PTSD), anxiety management techniques (relaxation, rebreathing, stress management), developing a detailed description of the initial traumatic event, identifying specific 'hot spots' associated with increased anxiety (or numbing), repeated exposure to the narrative of the trauma, construction of a fear hierarchy, imaginal or *in vivo* exposure to the elements in the fear hierarchy, identifying the automatic thoughts and 'shattered assumptions' that are associated with the trauma, and cognitive restructuring. Other interventions that are utilized are reducing or eliminating use of alcohol or drugs, reducing avoidant behavior in general, and the use of activity scheduling and longer-term goal setting. In cases of trauma associated with rape or abuse, 'rescripting' of the traumatic experience through imagery and active role-plays can be utilized (see Smucker and Dancu, 1999).

Case example

The patient was a 31-year-old married female who had been exposed to the destruction of the World Trade Center and who pursued treatment 5 months after the event. During the traumatic event, she had been near the buildings and had been caught by the falling debris. She witnessed bodies falling and feared during the experience that she would be killed. She returned to her apartment—not far from the trauma site—and was unable to get in touch with her husband. When she presented for treatment she was depressed, anxious, had recurring images of the explosion, feared watching airplanes in the sky, and was avoiding going near Ground Zero. She had increased drinking since the event, suffered from insomnia, and felt hopeless about the future.

The therapist provided her with information about PTSD (see Leahy and Holland, 2000) and explained to her that she was suffering from PTSD and that the treatment would consist of learning how to understand why she still had the fears and intrusive experiences that she had and to utilize exposure techniques and cognitive therapy techniques to modify her feelings and beliefs. Her automatic thoughts about the event and life at present was that she was 'really' all alone, she could be killed at any moment, life is not safe, and you always have to keep your guard up. The therapist explained to her that the reason that she was re-experiencing these intrusive images was that her mind was trying to assimilate this information but was being overwhelmed with the intensity of the content. Gradual and repeated exposure—first utilizing imaginal and then *in vivo* techniques—would be expected to have an effect on the emotional evocativeness of these images.

Her drinking behavior was an initial focus of treatment, as increased substance abuse has a negative impact on treatment efficacy. She examined the costs and benefits of drinking, how drinking impeded her processing of this experience, and how drinking added to her sense of inability to handle the trauma. Initially, she kept a log of the drinking, including noticing her emotions and situational triggers. After 2 weeks her drinking had been reduced by 80%. Until the drinking had subsided, the exposure and cognitive restructuring was delayed. In addition, like many individuals who are traumatized and who hope to use avoidance as a coping mechanism, her resistance to treatment was also addressed. This included examination of her beliefs that therapy would open up these memories and make things worse. The therapist acknowledged that exposure and examination of her thoughts and feelings would increase anxiety temporarily, but that her current situation of anxiety, depression, nightmares, avoidance, and intrusive imagery was to be weighed against the initial 'costs' of treatment.

The patient was asked to describe in great detail the events of 9–11 and to review with the therapist the particular 'hot spots' that were most difficult. As the patient recalled the events, the therapist noticed a bland and distant style that the patient used in describing events. On further inquiry the patient indicated that these events (falling bodies, debris collapsing around her) were especially troublesome and that the bland style was simply a manner of avoiding the emotional content. The patient was asked to write out a detailed description of the event and read it over and over each day until it became less anxiety provoking. During the therapy session, the particular 'hot spots' were explored, indicating that the patient interpreted these images as indicating that her life was always in danger and that anything can happen to anyone—and that it probably would happen. These feelings of helplessness and danger were then explored using standard cognitive therapy techniques.

For example, the belief that she was helpless was examined by defining helplessness ('unable to do anything'), examining the costs and benefits of this belief, reviewing the evidence and keeping an activity schedule in which pleasure and mastery were recorded. Furthermore, she examined the singularity of this event and considered how her increased awareness of her own mortality might result in greater insight, maturity and wisdom. Exposure to the images of planes flying and endangering her was conducted by having her practice modifying the image by thinking of a plane flying very slowly out to sea, turning back, and then flying again out to sea. This gave her more of a sense of control over the image and reduced her anxiety substantially. Finally, she was encouraged to visit the site of the World Trade Center and to go there every day for 1 week. Initially, this provoked intense anxiety that gave way to sadness and finally to acceptance.

Psychodynamic model of posttraumatic stress disorder

In Freud's conceptualization (1920), trauma pierces the ego's 'stimulus barrier', overwhelming the ego. In an attempt to cope with resulting traumatic anxiety, the ego employs dissociation, minimizing painful feelings through denial, or separating the feelings from thoughts and memories surrounding the trauma. Any intense affect state can create fears of a recurrence of the trauma (Krystal, 1988). In addition, the individual is driven to repeat the trauma in an attempt to assuage feelings of overwhelming helplessness and lack of control.

As with other anxiety disorders, the vicissitudes of anger play an important role in the psychodynamic underpinning of PTSD symptoms. Patients with PTSD experience intense rage at those they view to be responsible for their trauma (Brom *et al.*, 1989). This rage is projected on to others not connected to the event, who are consequently viewed as dangerous, intensifying anxiety. Patients may employ the defense of identification with the aggressor, in which they ally themselves with the individual or group responsible for the trauma (Lindy *et al.*, 1983). This mental operation can help to allay feelings of helplessness and may provide a sense of empowerment. However, identification with the aggressor often triggers guilt, and fears of becoming like the abuser.

Survivor guilt, a core feature of one type of posttraumatic reaction, can occur when an individual survives a traumatic experience in which others have died or have been severely injured. The individual who survives unconsciously identifies with the victims of trauma, but may also develop an unconscious identification with the perpetrators of the trauma, as described above, triggering guilt.

Developmental experiences can affect the risk of developing PTSD in response to a trauma. Traumatic developmental experiences can disrupt the early sense of autonomy and cause a regression from the developmental level that has been attained. Traumatic experiences in adulthood also cause regression, and often reawaken past experiences of disillusionment and anger at parents for failures to protect children from earlier traumas.

Empirical support for psychodynamic treatment of posttraumatic stress disorder

Lindy *et al.* (1983) studied 30 survivors of a fire using a brief (six to 12 sessions) manualized psychodynamic therapy. Nineteen of the survivors met DSM III criteria for PTSD. The patients demonstrated significant improvement and were less symptomatic than a control group of untreated survivors at follow-up. Brom *et al.* (1989) found improvement in patients with PTSD in three treatment groups (psychodynamic psychotherapy, hypnotherapy, and systematic desensitization) compared with a control group. The psychodynamic treatment was more effective with avoidance symptoms compared with the other treatments, which were more effective with intrusive symptoms. A manualized psychodynamically oriented group psychotherapy for Vietnam veterans with PTSD has also been developed (Weiss and Marmar, 1993), but has not been systematically tested.

Psychodynamic treatment of posttraumatic stress disorder

In the psychodynamic treatment of PTSD, efforts are made to explore the precipitating traumatic event to give the patient an opportunity to discharge feelings of rage and terror and to investigate the unconscious significance of the event. Unlike other exposure-based treatments of PTSD (Resick and Schnike, 1993; Foa *et al.*, 1999; Jaycox *et al.*, 2002), therapeutic focus is not on reexperiencing the trauma. Exploration and reexperiencing of a traumatic experience may be harmful or disruptive to some patients, and therapists need to be careful to modulate their exploration to what the patient can tolerate (Krystal, 1988; Gabbard, 2000). It is important to investigate what made this event traumatic to this particular patient, and what factors in the patient's background, including prior traumas, rendered them susceptible to PTSD. The therapist should identify unconscious fantasies of identification with the aggressor related to the trauma. In therapy of all anxiety disorders, but particularly in PTSD, exploration of the patient's need to be punished by the symptoms themselves as a result of intense guilt is essential.

Conclusions

In this chapter we have attempted to outline both cognitive-behavioral and psychodynamic models of treatment. The cognitive-behavioral model has been more extensively validated empirically, although there is now an attempt to provide more empirical validation of the psychodynamic model. The rapid expansion of specific cognitive-behavioral models for specific anxiety disorders suggests that this model will likely undergo further expansion and sophistication in coming years.

Although the focus here has been on the Axis I nature of these disorders, most individuals with anxiety disorders, especially those with long-standing problems, will also present with personality disorders that may complicate the clinical picture. Perhaps for this reason most practicing clinicians utilize an eclectic or integrative orientation—one that may gain from the various models presented in this chapter.

Finally, as most therapists adhere to an eclectic approach, the different issues addressed by the cognitive and psychodynamic approaches may allow the therapists to provide a more comprehensive approach to treatment. Indeed, it has been our experience that few patients in the real world of clinical practice actually present with only a single Axis II anxiety disorder. This comorbidity may challenge the clinician to incorporate not only more than one empirically validated treatment module, but also more than one theoretical approach.

References

Abramowitz, J. S. (1997). Effectiveness of psychological and pharmacological treatments for obsessive-compulsive disorder: a quantitative review. *Journal of Consulting and Clinical Psychology*, **65**, 44–52.

Al-Kubaisy, T., Marks, I. M., Logsdail, S., and Marks, M. P. (1992). Role of exposure homework in phobia reduction: a controlled study. *Behavior Therapy*, **23**(4), 599–621.

Alstroem, J. E. (1984). Effects of four treatment methods on social phobic patients not suitable for insight-oriented psychotherapy. *Acta Psychiatrica Scandinavica*, **70**(2), 97–110.

American Psychiatric Association. (1980). *Diagnostic and statistical manual of mental disorders*, 3rd edn. Washington, DC: American Psychiatric Association.

American Psychiatric Association. (1994). *Diagnostic and statistical manual of mental disorders*, 4th edn. Washington, DC: American Psychiatric Association.

van Blakom, A. J., *et al.* (1994). A meta-analysis on the treatment of obsessive compulsive disorder: a comparison of antidepressants, behavior, and cognitive therapy. *Clinical Psychology Review*, **14**(5), 359–81.

van Balkom, A. J. L. M., *et al.* (1998). Fluvoxamine versus cognitive-behavior therapy in obsessive compulsive disorder. *Journal of Nervous and Mental Disease*, **186**, 492–9.

Barlow, D. A. and Beck, A. T. (1984). *The psychosocial treatment of anxiety disorders*. In: J. B. W. Williams and R. L. Spitzer, ed. Psychotherapy research: Where are we and where should we go? pp. 29–66. New York: The Guilford Press.

Barlow, D. H. (1988). *Anxiety and its disorders: the nature and treatment of anxiety and panic*. New York: Guilford Press.

Barlow, D. H. (2002). *Anxiety and its disorders: the nature and treatment of anxiety and panic*, 2nd edn. New York: Guilford Press.

Beck, A. T. (1976). *Cognitive therapy and the emotional disorders*. New York: International Universities Press.

Beck, A. T., Emery, G., and Greenberg, R. L. (1985). *Anxiety disorders and phobias: a cognitive perspective*. New York: Basic Books.

Beck, A. T., Epstein, N., Brown, G., and Steer, R. A. (1988a). An inventory for measuring anxiety: psychometric properties. *Journal of Consulting and Clinical Psychology*, **56**, 893–7.

Beck, A. T., Steer, R. A., and Garbin, M. G. (1988b). Psychometric properties of the Beck Depression Inventory: twenty-five years of evaluation. *Clinical Psychology Review*, **8**, 77–100.

Beck, J. S. (1995). *Cognitive therapy: basics and beyond*. New York: Guilford Press.

Beech, H. and Liddell, A. (1974). Decision-making, mood states and ritualistic behavior among obsessional patients. In: H. R. Beech, ed. *Obsessional states*. London: Methuen.

Bernstein, D. A. and Borkovec, T. D. (1973). *Progressive relaxation training*. Champaign, IL: Research Press.

Biederman, J., *et al.* (1990). Psychiatric correlates of behavioral inhibition in young children of parents with and without psychiatric disorders. *Archives of General Psychiatry*, **47**, 21–6.

Black, A. (1974). The natural history of obsessional neurosis. In: H. R. Beech, ed. *Obsessional states*, pp. 19–54. London: Methuen.

Blazer, D., George, L., and Winfield, I. (1991). Epidemiologic data and planning mental health services. A tale of two surveys. *Social Psychiatry and Psychiatric Epidemiology*, **26**, 21–7.

Borkovec, T. D. (1994). The nature, functions, and origins of worry. In: G. C. L. Davey and F. Tallis, ed. *Worrying: perspectives on theory, assessment and treatment*, pp. 5–33. Chichester: Wiley.

Borkovec, T. D. and Hu, S. (1990). The effect of worry on cardiovascular response to phobic imagery. *Behaviour Research and Therapy*, **28**, 69–73.

Boulougouris, J., Rabavilas, A., and Stefanis, C. (1977). Psychophysiological responses in obsessive-compulsive patients. *Behaviour Research and Therapy*, **15**(3), 221–30.

Brandchaft, B. (2001). Obsessional disorders: a developmental systems perspective. *Psychoanalytic Inquiry*, **21**(2), 253–88.

Breuer, J. and Freud, S. (1895/1955). *Studies on hysteria*. In: J. Strachey, ed. and trans. *Standard edition of the complete psychological works of Sigmund Freud*, Vol. 2, pp. 1–181. London: Hogarth Press.

Brewin, C. R. and Holmes, E. A. (2003). Psychological theories of posttraumatic stress disorder. *Clinical Psychology Review*, **23**(3), 339–76.

Brewin, C. R. (1996). Cognitive processing of adverse experiences. *International Review of Psychiatry*, **8**(4), 333–9.

Brewin, C. R., Andrews, B., and Valentine, J. D. (2000). Meta-analysis of risk factors for posttraumatic stress disorder in trauma-exposed adults. *Journal of Consulting and Clinical Psychology*, **68**(5), 748–66.

Brom, C., Kleber, R. J., and Defares, P. B. (1989). Brief psychotherapy for post-traumatic stress disorders. *Journal of Consulting and Clinical Psychology*, **57**(5), 607–12.

Brown, T. A., DiNardo, P., and Barlow, D. H. (1994). *Anxiety Disorders Interview Schedule for DSM IV*. Boulder, CO: Graywind Publications.

Brown, T. A., O'Leary, T. A., and Barlow, D. H. (2001). Generalized anxiety disorder. In: D. H. Barlow, ed. *Clinical handbook of psychological disorders*, 3rd edn, pp. 154–208. New York: Guilford Press.

Busch, F. N., Cooper, A. M., Klerman, G. L., Shapiro, T., and Shear, M. K. (1991). Neurophysiological, cognitive-behavioral, and psychoanalytic approaches to panic disorder: toward an integration. *Psychoanalytic Inquiry*, **11**(3), 316–32.

Busch, F. N., Shear, M., Cooper, A. M., Shapiro, T., and Leon, A. C. (1995). An empirical study of defense mechanisms in panic disorder. *Journal of Nervous and Mental Disease*, **183**(5), 299–303.

Butler, G. (1989). Issues in the application of cognitive and behavioral strategies to the treatment of social phobia. *Clinical Psychology Review*, **9**, 91–106.

Butler, G. and Wells, A. (1995). Cognitive behavioral treatments: Clinical applications. In: R. G. Heimberg, M. R. Liebowitz, D. A. Hope, and F. R. Schneier, ed. *Social phobia: diagnosis, assessment, and treatment*, pp. 310–33. New York: Guilford Press.

Butler, G., Cullington, A., Munby, M., Amies, P., and Gelder, M. (1984). Exposure and anxiety management in the treatment of social phobia. *Journal of Consulting and Clinical Psychology*, **52**(4), 642–50.

Butler, G., Fennell, M., Robson, P., and Gelder, M. (1991). Comparison of behavior therapy and cognitive behavior therapy in the treatment of generalized anxiety disorder. *Journal of Consulting and Clinical Psychology*, **59**, 167–75.

Carr, A. T. (1974). Compulsive neurosis: a review of the literature. *Psychological Bulletin*, **81**(5), 311–18.

Chambless, D. L., *et al.* (1998). Update on empirically validated therapies: II. *Clinical Psychologist*, **51**, 3–16.

Clark, D. M. (1986). A cognitive approach to panic. *Behaviour Research and Therapy*, **24**(4), 461–70.

Clark, D. M. and Wells, A. (1995). A cognitive model of social phobia. In: R. G. Heimberg, M. R. Liebowitz, D. A. Hope, and F. R. Schneier, ed. *Social phobia: diagnosis, assessment, and treatment*, pp. 69–93. New York: Guilford Press.

Clark, D. M., Salkovskis, P. M., and Chalkley, A. (1985). Respiratory control as a treatment for panic attacks. *Journal of Behavior Therapy and Experimental Psychiatry*, **16**, 23–30.

Coles, M. E., Turk, C. L., and Heimberg, R. G. (2002). The role of memory perspective in social phobia: immediate and delayed memories for role played situations. *Behavioural and Cognitive Psychotherapy*, **30**(4), 415–25.

Coryell, W. H., Noyes, R., and Clancy, J. (1982). Excess mortality in panic disorder: a comparison with primary unipolar depression. *Archives of General Psychiatry*, **39**(6), 701–3.

Coryell, W. H., Noyes, R., and House, J. (1986). Mortality among outpatients with anxiety disorders. *American Journal of Psychiatry*, **143**(4), 508–10.

Cottraux, J., *et al.* (1990). A controlled study of fluvoxamine and exposure in obsessive-compulsive disorder. *International Clinical Psychopharmacology*, **5**, 17–30.

Cottraux, J., *et al.* (2001). A randomized controlled trial of cognitive therapy versus intensive behavior therapy in obsessive compulsive disorder. *Psychotherapy and Psychosomatics*, **70**, 288–97.

Crits-Christoph, P., Connolly, M. B., Azarian, K., Crits-Christoph, K., and Shappell, S. (1996). Psychodynamic-interpersonal treatment of generalized anxiety disorder. *Psychotherapy*, **33**, 418–30.

Crits-Christoph, P., Crits-Christoph, K., Wolf-Palacio, D., Fichter, M., and Rudick, D. (1995). Brief supportive-expressive psychodynamic therapy for generalized anxiety disorder. In: J. P. Barber and P. Crits-Christoph, ed. *Dynamic therapies for psychiatric disorders (Axis I)*, pp. 43–83. New York: Basic Books.

DiGiuseppe, R., McGowan, L., Simon, K. S., and Gardner, F. (1990). A comparative outcome study of four cognitive therapies in the treatment of social anxiety. *Journal of Rational-Emotive and Cognitive Behavior Therapy*, **8**(3), 129–46.

DiNardo, P. and Barlow, D. H. (1988). *Anxiety Disorders Interview Schedule for DSM IV*. Boulder, CO: Graywind Publications.

DiNardo, P., Moras, K., Barlow, D. H., Rapee, R. M., and Brown, T. (1993). Reliability of the DSM-III-R disorder categories using the Anxiety Disorders Interview Schedule—revised (ADIS-R). *Archives of General Psychiatry*, **50**, 251–6.

Dollard, J. and Miller, N. E. (1950). *Personality and psychotherapy: an analysis in terms of learning, thinking, and culture*. New York: McGraw-Hill.

Dugas, M. J., and Ladouceur, R. (1998). Analysis and treatment of generalized anxiety disorder. In: V. E. Caballo, ed. *International handbook of cognitive-behavioural treatments of psychological disorders*, pp. 197–225. Oxford: Pergamon Press.

Dugas, M., Buhr, K., and Ladouceur, R. (2004). The role of intolerance of uncertainty in the etiology and maintenance of generalized anxiety disorder. In: C. L. Heimbert, Turk and D. S. Mennin, ed. *Generalized anxiety disorder: Advances in research and practice*. New York: Guilford.

Elhers, A. and Clark, D. M. (2000). A cognitive model of posttraumatic stress disorder. *Behaviour Research and Therapy*, **38**, 319–45.

Emmelkamp, P. M. and Beens, H. (1991). Cognitive therapy with obsessive-compulsive disorder: a comparative evaluation. *Behaviour Research and Therapy*, **29**(3), 293–300.

Emmelkamp, P. M. and Kwee, K. (1977). Obsessional ruminations: a comparison between thought-stopping and prolonged exposure in imagination. *Behaviour Research and Therapy*, **15**(5), 441–4.

Emmelkamp, P. M., Visser, S., and Hoekstra, R. (1988). Cognitive therapy vs exposure in vivo in the treatment of obsessive-compulsives. *Cognitive Therapy and Research*, **12**, 103–14.

Esman, A. H. (1989). Psychoanalysis and general psychiatry: obsessive-compulsive disorder as paradigm. *Journal of the American Psychoanalytic Association*, **37**(2), 319–36.

Esman, A. H. (2001). Obsessive-compulsive disorder: current views. *Psychoanalytic Inquiry*, **21**(2), 145–56.

Fava, G. A., Grandi, S., and Canestrari, R. (1989). Treatment of social phobia by homework exposure. *Psychotherapy and Psychosomatics*, **52**(4), 209–13.

Fenichel, O. (1945). *The psychoanalytic theory of neurosis*. New York: W. W. Norton.

Feske, U. and Chambless, D. L. (1995). Cognitive behavior versus exposure treatment for social phobia: a meta analysis. *Behavior Therapy*, **26**, 695–720.

Foa, E. B., Dancu, C. V., Hembree, E. A., Jaycox, L. H., Meadows, E. A., and Street, G. P. (1999). A comparison of exposure therapy, stress inoculation training, and their combination for reducing posttraumatic stress disorder in female assault victims. *Journal of Consulting & Clinical Psychology*, **67**(2), 194–200.

Foa, E. B., Rothbaum, B. O., Riggs, D. S., and Murdock, T. B. (1991). Treatment of posttraumatic stress disorder in rape victims: a comparison between cognitive-behavioral procedures and counseling. *Journal of Consulting & Clinical Psychology*, **59**(5), 715–23.

Foa, E. B., Rothbaum, B. O., and Molnar, C. (1995). Cognitive-behavioral therapy of posttraumatic stress disorder. In: M. J. Friedman, D. S. Charney, and A. Y. Deutch, ed. *Neurobiological and clinical consequences of stress: from normal adaptation to posttraumatic stress disorder*, pp. 483–94. Philadelphia, PA: Raven Press.

Foa, E. B. and Franklin, M. E. (2001). Obsessive compulsive disorder. In: D. H. Barlow, ed. *Clinical handbook of psychological disorders: a step by step treatment manual*, 3rd edn, pp. 209–63. New York: Guilford Press.

Foa, E. B. and Kozak, M. J. (1985). Treatment of anxiety disorders: implications for psychopathology. In: A. H. Tuma and J. D. Maser, ed. *Anxiety and the anxiety disorders*, pp. 421–52. Hillsdale, NJ: Lawrence Erlbaum.

Foa, E. B. and Kozak, M. J. (1986). Emotional processing of fear: exposure to corrective information. *Psychological Bulletin*, **99**, 20–35.

Foa, E. B. and Kozak, M. J. (1996). Psychological treatments for obsessive-compulsive disorder. In: M. R. M. R. F. Prien, ed. *Long-term treatments for anxiety disorders*, pp. 285–309. Washington, DC: American Psychiatric Press.

Foa, E. B. and Wilson, R. (1991). *Stop obsessing!: how to overcome your obsessions and compulsions*. New York: Bantam.

Foa, E. B., Steketee, G., and Milby, J. B. (1980a). Differential effects of exposure and response prevention in obsessive-compulsive washers. *Journal of Consulting and Clinical Psychology*, **48**, 71–9.

Foa, E. B., Steketee, G., Turner, R. M., and Fischer, S. C. (1980b). Effects of imaginal exposure to feared disasters in obsessive-compulsive checkers. *Behaviour Research and Therapy*, **18**(5), 449–55.

Foa, E. B., Steketee, G. S., Grayson, J. B., Turner, R. M., and Latimer, P. (1984). Deliberate exposure and blocking of obsessive-compulsive rituals: immediate and long-term effects. *Behavior Therapy*, **15**(5), 450–72.

Foa, E. B., Steketee, G. S., and Ozarow, B. (1985). Behavior therapy with obsessive-compulsives: from theory to treatment. In: M. Mavissakalian, ed. *Obsessive-compulsive disorder: psychological and pharmacological treatment*. New York: Plenum Press.

Foa, E. B., McNally, R. J., Steketee, G. S., and McCarthy, P. R. (1991). A test of preparedness theory in anxiety-disordered patients using an avoidance paradigm. *Journal of Psychophysiology*, 5(2), 159–63.

Foa, E. B., Franklin, E. B., and Kozak, M. J. (1998a). Psychosocial treatments for obsessive-compulsive disorder: Literature review. In: R. P. Swinson, M. Antony, S. J. Rachman, and M. A. Richter, ed. *Obsessive-compulsive disorder: theory, research and treatment*, pp. 258–76. New York: Guilford Press.

Foa, E. B., Kozak, M. J., Salkovskis, P. M., Coles, M. E., and Amir, N. (1998b). The validation of a new obsessive-compulsive disorder scale: the obsessive-compulsive inventory. *Psychological Assessment*, 10(3), 206–14.

Franklin, M. E., Abramowitz, J. S., Kozak, M. J., Levitt, J. T., and Foa, E. B. (2000). Effectiveness of exposure and ritual prevention for obsessive compulsive disorder: randomized versus non randomized samples. *Journal of Consulting and Clinical Psychology*, 68, 594–602.

Freeston, M. H. (1994). *Characteristiques et traitement de l'obsession sans compulsion manifeste*. Unpublished thesis, Universite Laval, Quebec.

Freeston, M. H., Rhéaume, J., Letarte, H., Dugas, M. J., and Ladouceur, R. (1994). Why do people worry? *Personality and Individual Differences*, 17(6). 761–802.

Freeston, M. H., *et al.* (1997). Cognitive-behavioral treatment of obsessive thoughts: a controlled study. *Journal of Consulting and Clinical Psychology*, 65, 405–13.

Freud, S. (1909/1953). *Fragment of an analysis of a case of hysteria*. In: J. Strachey, ed. and trans. *Standard edition of the complete psychological works of Sigmund Freud*, Vol. 7, pp. 3–122. London: Hogarth Press.

Freud, S. (1909/1961). *Notes upon a case of obsessional neurosis*. In: J. Strachey, ed. and trans. *Standard edition of the complete psychological works of Sigmund Freud*, Vol. 1, pp. 155–318. London: Hogarth Press.

Freud, S. (1911/1958). *Formulations on the two principles of mental functioning*. In: J. Strachey, ed. and trans. *Standard edition of the complete psychological works of Sigmund Freud*, Vol. 12, pp. 213–26. London: Hogarth Press.

Freud, S. (1920/1955). *Beyond the pleasure principle*. In: J. Strachey, ed. and trans. *Standard edition of the complete psychological works of Sigmund Freud*, Vol. 18, pp. 3–64. London: Hogarth Press.

Freud, S. (1923/1961). *The ego and the id*. In: J. Strachey, ed. and trans. *Standard edition of the complete psychological works of Sigmund Freud*, Vol. 19, pp. 1–66. London: Hogarth Press.

Freud, S. (1926/1959). *Inhibitions, symptoms and anxiety*. In: J. Strachey, ed. and trans. *Standard edition of the complete psychological works of Sigmund Freud*, Vol. 20, pp. 77–174. London: Hogarth Press.

Freund, B., Steketee, G. S., and Foa, E. B. (1987). Compulsive Activity Checklist (CAC): Psychometric analysis with obsessive-compulsive disorder. *Behavioral Assessment*, 9, 67–79.

Gabbard, G. O. (1992). Psychodynamics of panic disorder and social phobia. *Bulletin of the Menninger Clinic*, 56(2, Suppl. A), A3–13.

Gabbard, G. O. (1995). Countertransference: the emerging common ground. *International Journal of Psychoanalysis*, 76, 475–85.

Gabbard, G. O. (2000). *Psychodynamic psychiatry in clinical practice*, 3rd edn. Washington, DC: American Psychiatric Press.

Gabbard, G. O. (2001). Psychoanalytically informed approaches to the treatment of obsessive-compulsive disorder. *Psychoanalytic Inquiry*, 21, 208–21.

Gelernter, C. S., *et al.* (1991). Cognitive-behavioral and pharmacological treatments of social phobia: a controlled study. *Archives of General Psychiatry*, 48(10), 938–45.

Goodman, W. K., *et al.* (1989a). The Yale-Brown Obsessive-compulsive Scale. II. Validity. *Archives of General Psychiatry*, 46, 1012–16.

Goodman, W. K., *et al.* (1989b). The Yale-Brown Obsessive-compulsive Scale. I. Development, use and reliability. *Archives of General Psychiatry*, 46, 1006–11.

Gould, R. A., Otto, M. W., and Pollack, M. H. (1995). A meta-analysis of treatment outcome for panic disorder. *Clinical Psychology Review*, 15(8), 819–44.

Gould, R. A., Buckminster, S., Pollack, M. H., Otto, M. W., and Yap, L. (1997). Cognitive-behavioral and pharmacological treatment for social phobia: a meta-analysis. *Clinical Psychology-Science and Practice*, 4(4), 291–306.

Gould, R. A., Safren, S. A., Washington, D. O. N., and Ott, M. W. (2003). Cognitive-behavioral treatments for generalized anxiety disorder: a meta-analytic review. In: D. S. Mennin, ed. *Generalized anxiety disorder: advances in research and practice*. New York: Guilford Press.

Griest, J. H. and Baer, L. (2002). Psychotherapy for obsessive-compulsive disorder. In: D. S. Stein and E. Hollander, ed. *Textbook of anxiety disorders*, pp. 221–33. Washington, DC: American Psychiatric Publishing.

Guidano, V. F. and Liotti, G. (1983). *Cognitive processes and the emotional disorders*. New York: Guilford Press.

Harvey, A. G., Bryant R. A., and Rapee, R. M. (1996). Preconscious processing of threat in posttraumatic stress disorder. *Cognitive Therapy and Research*, 20(6), 613–23.

Headland, K. and McDonald, B. (1987). Rapid audio-tape treatment of obsessional ruminations: a case report. *Behavioural Psychotherapy*, 15(2), 188–92.

Heimberg, R. G. (1991). *A manual for conducting cognitive-behavioral group therapy for social phobia*, 2nd edn. Unpublished manuscript, State University of New York at Albany, Center for Stress and Anxiety Disorders, Albany, NY.

Heimberg, R. G. and Barlow, D. H. (1991). New developments in cognitive-behavioral therapy for social phobia. *Journal of Clinical Psychiatry*, 52(Suppl.), 21–30.

Heimberg, R. G. and Juster, H. R. (1995). Cognitive behavioral treatments: literature review. In: R. G. Heimberg, M. R. Liebowitz, D. A. Hope, and F. R. Schneier, ed. *Social phobia: diagnosis, assessment, and treatment*, pp. 262–309. New York: Guilford Press.

Heimberg, R. G., Becker, R. E., Goldfinger, K., and Vermilyea, J. A. (1985). Treatment of social phobia by exposure, cognitive restructuring and home-work assignments. *Journal of Nervous and Mental Disease*, 173(4), 236–45.

Heimberg, R. G., *et al.* (1990). Cognitive behavioral group treatment for social phobia: comparison with a credible placebo control. *Cognitive Therapy and Research*, 14, 1–23.

Heimberg, R. G., Salzman, D. G., Holt, C. S., and Blendell, K. A. (1993). Cognitive-behavioral group treatment for social phobia: effectiveness at five-year follow-up. Erratum. *Cognitive Therapy and Research*, 17(6), 597–8.

Heimberg, R. G., *et al.* (1998). Cognitive behavioral group therapy vs phenelzine therapy for social phobia. *Archives of General Psychiatry*, 55, 1133–41.

Heimberg, R. G., Turk, C. L., and Mennin, D. S., ed. (2003). *Generalized anxiety disorder: advances in research and practice*. New York: Guilford Press.

Hodgson, R. J. and Rachman, S. J. (1972). The effects of contamination and washing in obsessional patients. *Behaviour Research and Therapy*, 10, 111–17.

Hodgson, R. J. and Rachman, S. J. (1977). Obsessional-compulsive compliants. *Behaviour Research and Therapy*, 15, 389–95.

Holt, C. S., Heimberg, R. G., Hope, D. A., and Liebowitz, M. R. (1992). Situational domains of social phobia. *Journal of Anxiety Disorders*, 6, 63–77.

Hope, D. A., Holt, C. S., and Heimberg, R. G. (1993). Social phobia. In: T. R. Giles, ed. *Handbook of effective psychotherapy*, pp. 227–51. Colorado: Plenum.

Hope, D. A., Heimberg, R. G., and Bruch, M. A. (1995). Dismantling cognitive-behavioral group therapy for social phobia. *Behaviour Research and Therapy*, 33(6), 637–50.

Hornsveld, R. H. J., Kraaimaat, F. W., and van Dam-Baggen, R. M. J. (1979). Anxiety/discomfort and handwashing in obsessive-compulsive and psychiatric control patients. *Behaviour Research and Therapy*, 17, 223–8.

Jakes, I. (1996). *Theoretical approaches to obsessive-compulsive disorder*. Cambridge: Cambridge University Press.

Jaycox, L. H., Zoellner, L., and Foa, E. B. (2002). Cognitive-behavior therapy for PTSD in rape survivors. *Journal of Clinical Psychology*, 58, 891–906.

Jones, M. K. and Menzies, R. G. (1998). The relevance of associative learning pathways in the development of obsessive-compulsive washing. *Behaviour Research and Therapy*, 36(3), 273–83.

Juster, H. R. and Heimberg, R. G. (1995). Social phobia: longitudinal course and long-term outcome of cognitive-behavioral treatment. *Psychiatric Clinics of North America*, 18(4), 821–42.

Kagan, J., *et al.* (1990). Origins of panic disorder. In: J. Ballenger, ed. *Neurobiology of panic disorder*, pp. 71–87. New York: Wiley.

Kanter, N. J. and Goldfried, M. R. (1979). Relative effectiveness of rational restructuring and self-control desensitization in the reduction of interpersonal anxiety. *Behavior Therapy*, **10**(4), 472–90.

Kaplan, D. M. (1972). On shyness. *International Journal of Psychoanalysis*, **53**, 439–54.

Kasvikis, Y. and Marks, I. M. (1988). Clomipramine, self-exposure, and therapist-accompanied exposure in obsessive-compulsive ritualizers: two-year follow-up. *Journal of Anxiety Disorders*, **2**(4), 291–8.

Kearney, C. A. and Silverman, W. K. (1990). Treatment of an adolescent with obsessive-compulsive disorder by alternating response prevention and cognitive therapy: an empirical analysis. *Journal of Behavior Therapy and Experimental Psychiatry*, **21**, 39–47.

Kessler, R. C., DuPont, R. L., Berglund, P., and Wittchen, H.-U. (1999). Impairment in pure and comorbid generalized anxiety disorder and major depression at 12 months in two national surveys. *American Journal of Psychiatry*, **156**(12), 1915–23.

Kirk, J. W. (1983). Behavioural treatment of obsessive-compulsive patients in routine clinical practice. *Behaviour Research and Therapy*, **21**, 57–62.

Knight, R. (1941). Evaluation of the results of psychoanalytic therapy. *American Journal of Psychiatry*, **98**, 434–46.

Kozak, M. J., Liebowitz, M. R., and Foa, E. B. (2000). Cognitive behavior therapy and pharmacotherapy for obsessive compulsive disorder: the NIMH sponsored collaborative study. In: W. K. Goodman and M. V. Rudorfer, ed. *Obsessive compulsive disorder: contemporary issues in treatment*, pp. 501–30. Mahwah, NJ: Lawrence Erlbaum Associates.

Lang, P. J. (1979). A bio-informational theory of emotional imagery. *Psychophysiology*, **16**(6), 495–512.

Leahy, R. L. and Holland, S. J. (2000). *Treatment plans and interventions for depression and anxiety disorders*. New York: Guilford Press.

Leary, M. R. and Kowalski, R. M. (1995). The self presentation model of social phobia. In: R. G. Heimberg, M. R. Liebowitz, D. A. Hope, and F. R. Schneier, ed. *Social phobia: diagnosis, assessment, and treatment*, pp. 94–112. New York: Guilford Press.

Leon, A. C., Shear, M. K., Portera, L., and Klerman, G. L. (1992). Assessing impairment in patients with panic disorder: the Sheehan Disability Scale. *Social Psychiatry and Psychiatric Epidemiology*, **27**, 78–82.

Liebowitz, M. R. (1987). Social phobia. *Modern Problems in Pharmacopsychiatry*, **22**, 141–73.

Lindy, J. D., Green, B. L., Grace, M. C., and Titchener, J. (1983). Psychotherapy with survivors of the Beverly Hills Supper Club fire. *American Journal of Psychotherapy*, **37**, 593–610.

Loftus, E. F. and Burns, T. E. (1982) Mental shock can produce retrograde amnesia. *Memory Cognition*, **10**, 318–23.

Lucas, R. A. and Telch, M. J. (1993, November). *Group versus individual treatment of social phobia*. Paper presented at the 27th Annual Convention of the Association for Advancement of Behavior Therapy, Atlanta, GA.

MacLeod, C., Mathews, A., and Tata, P. (1986). Attentional bias in emotional disorders. *Journal of Abnormal Psychology*, **95**, 15–20.

Malan, D. (1979). *Individual psychotherapy and the science of psychodynamics*. London: Butterworths.

Marks, I. M. and Mathews, A. M. (1979). Brief standard self-rating for phobic patients. *Behaviour Research and Therapy*, **17**(3), 263–7.

Marks, I. M., Stern, R. S., Mawson, D., Cobb, J., and McDonald, R. (1980). Clomipramine and exposure for obsessive-compulsive rituals: I. *British Journal of Psychiatry*, **136**, 1–25.

Marks, I. M., et al. (1988). Clomipramine, self-exposure and therapist-aided exposure for obsessive-compulsive rituals. *British Journal of Psychiatry*, **152**, 522–34.

Marmar, C. R., Weiss, D. S., and Pynoos, R. S. (1995). Dynamic psychotherapy of post-traumatic stress disorder. In: M. J. Friedman, D. S. Charney, and A. Y. Deutch, ed. *Neurobiological and clinical consequences of stress: from normal adaptation to post-traumatic stress disorder*, pp. 495–506. Philadelphia, PA: Lippincott-Raven.

Matthews, G. and Wells, A. (1999). The cognitive science of attention and emotion. In: T. Dalgleish and M. J. Power, ed. *Handbook of cognition and emotion*, pp. 171–92. Brisbane: Wiley.

Matthews, G. and Wells, A. (2000). Attention, automaticity, and affective disorder. *Behavior Modification*, **24**, 69–93.

Mattick, R. P. and Peters, L. (1988). Treatment of severe social phobia: effects of guided exposure with and without cognitive restructuring. *Journal of Consulting and Clinical Psychology*, **56**(2), 251–60.

Mattick, R. P., Peters, L., and Clarke, J. C. (1989). Exposure and cognitive restructuring for severe social phobia: a controlled stud. *Behavior Therapy*, **20**, 3–23.

Mawson, D., Marks, I. M., and Ramm, L. (1982). Clomipramine for chronic obsessive compulsive rituals: two year follow-up and further finding. *British Journal of Psychiatry*, **140**, 11–18.

McFall, M. E. and Wollersheim, J. P. (1979). Obsessive-compulsive neurosis: a cognitive-behavioral formulation and approach to treatment. *Cognitive Therapy and Research*, **3**(4), 333–48.

McGinn, L. K. and Sanderson, W. C. (1999). *Treatment of obsessive compulsive disorder*. Northvale, NJ: Jason Aronson.

McNally, R. J. (1994). *Panic disorder: a critical analysis*. New York: Guilford Press.

Meares, R. (2001). A specific developmental deficit in obsessive-compulsive disorder: the example of the wolf man. *Psychoanalytic Inquiry*, **21**(2), 289–319.

Mills, H. L., Agras, W. S., Barlow, D. H., and Mills, J. R. (1973). Compulsive rituals treated by response prevention. *Archives of General Psychiatry*, **28**, 524–7.

Milrod, B. and Shear, M. K. (1991): Dynamic treatment of panic disorder: a review. *Journal of Nervous and Mental Disease*, **179**, 741–3.

Milrod, B., Busch, F., Cooper, A. M., and Shapiro, T. (1997). *Manual of panic-focused psychodynamic psychotherapy*. Washington, DC: American Psychiatric Press.

Milrod, B., et al. (2000). Open trial of psychodynamic psychotherapy for panic disorder: a pilot study. *American Journal of Psychiatry*, **157**(11), 1878–80.

Milrod, B., et al. (2001). A pilot open trial of brief psychodynamic psychotherapy for panic disorder. *Journal of Psychotherapy Practice and Research*, **10**(4), 239–45.

Mowrer, O. H. (1939). A stimulus-response analysis of anxiety and its role as a reinforcing agent. *Psychological Review*, **46**, 553–65.

Mowrer, O. H. (1960). *Learning theory and behavior*. Wiley: New York.

Newman, M. G., Hofmann, S. G., and Trabert, W. (1994). Does behavioral treatment of social phobia lead to cognitive changes? *Behavior Therapy*, **25**(3), 503–17.

Newman, M. G., et al. (2002). Preliminary reliability and validity of the Generalized Anxiety Disorder Questionnaire-IV: a revised self-report diagnostic measure of generalized anxiety disorder. *Behavior Therapy*, **33**(2), 215–33.

Newman, M. G., Zuellig, A. R., Kachin, K. E., Constantino, M. J., and Cashman, L. (2003). The reliability and validity of the GAD-Q-IV: a revised self-report diagnostic measure of generalized anxiety disorder. *Psychological Medicine*, **33**(4), 623–35.

Obsessive Compulsive Cognitions Working Group. (1997). Cognitive assessment of obsessive compulsive disorder. *Behaviour Research and Therapy*, **35**, 667–81.

Obsessive Compulsive Cognitions Working Group. (2001). Development and initial evaluation of the Obsessive Beliefs Questionnaire and the Interpretation of Intrusions Inventory. *Behaviour Research and Therapy*, **39**, 987–1006.

Ost, L.-G. (1997). Rapid treatment of specific phobia. In: G. C. L. Davey, ed. *Phobias: a handbook of theory, research and treatment*, pp. 227–46. Hoboken, NJ: Wiley.

Ost, L.-G. and Hugdahl, K. (1981). Acquisition of phobias and anxiety response patterns in clinical patients. *Behaviour Research and Therapy*, **19**(5), 439–47.

Perse, T. L. (1988). Obsessive-compulsive disorder. A treatment review. *Journal of Clinical Psychiatry*, **49**, 48–55.

Pitman, R. K. (1987). A cybernetic model of obsessive-compulsive psychopathology. *Comprehensive Psychiatry*, **28**, 334–43.

Rabavilas, A. D. and Boulougouris, J. (1974). Physiological accompaniments of ruminations, flooding and thought stopping in obsessive patients. *Behaviour Research and Therapy*, **12**, 239–43.

Rachman, S. J. and de Silva, P. (1978). Abnormal and normal obsessions. *Behaviour Research and Therapy*, **16**(4), 233–48.

Rachman, S. J. and Wilson, G. T. (1980). *The effects of psychological therapy*. Oxford: Pergamon Press.

Rachman, S. J., et al. (1979). The behavioral treatment of obsessional-compulsive disorders, with and without clomipramine. *Behaviour Research and Therapy*, **17**, 467–78.

Rapee, R. M. (1995). Cognitive behavioral treatments: literature review. In: R. G. Heimberg, M. R. Liebowitz, D. A. Hope, and F. R. Schneier, ed. *Social phobia: diagnosis, assessment, and treatment*, pp. 41–66. New York: Guilford Press.

Rapee, R. M. (1998). *Overcoming shyness and social phobia: a step-by-step guide*. Northvale, NJ: Jason Aronson.

Rapee, R. M. and Heimberg, R. G. (1997). A cognitive-behavioral model of anxiety in social phobia. *Behaviour Research and Therapy*, **35**(8), 741–56.

Reed, G. E. (1985). *Obsessional experience and compulsive behavior: a cognitive structural approach*. Orlando, FL: Academic Press.

Resick, P. A. and Schnike, M. K. (1993). *Cognitive processing therapy for rape victims: a treatment manual*. Newbury Park, California: Sage Publications.

Rheaume, J. and Ladouceur, R. (2000). Cognitive and behavioral treatments of checking behaviours: an examination of individual cognitive change. *Clinical Psychology and Psychotherapy*, **7**, 118–27.

Riggs, D. S. and Foa, E. B. (1993). Obsessive compulsive disorder. In: D. H. Barlow, ed. *Clinical handbook of psychological disorders*, pp. 189–239. New York: Guilford Press.

Roper, G. and Rachman, S. (1976). Obsessional-compulsive checking: experimental replication and development. *Behaviour Research and Therapy*, **14**, 25–32.

Roper, G., Rachman, S., and Hodgson, R. (1973). An experiment on obsessional checking. *Behaviour Research and Therapy*, **11**(3), 271–7.

Rosenbaum, J. F., *et al.* (1988). Behavioral inhibition in children of parents with panic disorder and agoraphobia: a controlled study. *Archives of General Psychiatry*, **45**(5), 463–70.

Rosenbaum, J. F., Biederman, J., Hirshfeld, D. R., Bolduc, E. A., and Chaloff, J. (1991a). Behavioral inhibition in children: a possible precursor to panic disorder or social phobia. *Journal of Clinical Psychiatry*, **52**(Suppl.), 5–9.

Rosenbaum, J. F., Biederman, J., Hirshfeld, D. R., Bolduc, E. A., and Chaloff, J. (1991b). Further evidence of an association between behavioral inhibition and anxiety disorders: results from a family study of children from a non–clinical sample. *Journal of Psychiatric Research*, 25, 49–65.

Roth, A. D. and Church, J. A. (1994). The use of revised habituation in the treatment of obsessive-compulsive disorders. *British Journal of Clinical Psychology*, **33**, 201–4.

Salkovskis, P. M. (1983). Treatment of an obsessional patient using habituation to audiotaped ruminations. *British Journal of Clinical Psychology*, **22**(4), 311–13.

Salkovskis, P. M. (1985). Obsessional-compulsive problems: a cognitive-behavioural analysis. *Behaviour Research and Therapy*, **23**(5), 571–83.

Salkovskis, P. M. (1989). Cognitive-behavioural factors and the persistence of intrusive thoughts in obsessional problems. *Behaviour Research and Therapy*, **27**(6), 677–82.

Salkovskis, P. M. and Kirk, J. (1997). Obsessive-compulsive disorder. In: D. M. Clark and C. G. Fairburn, ed. *Science and practice of cognitive behaviour therapy*, pp. 179–208. New York: Oxford University Press.

Salkovskis, P. M. and Warwick, H. M. (1985). Cognitive therapy of obsessive-compulsive disorder: treating treatment failures. *Behavioural Psychotherapy*, **13**(3), 243–55.

Salkovskis, P. M. and Warwick, H. M. (1986). Morbid preoccupations, health anxiety and reassurance: a cognitive-behavioural approach to hypochondriasis. *Behaviour Research and Therapy*, **24**(5), 597–602.

Salkovskis, P. M. and Westbrook, D. (1989). Behaviour therapy and obsessional ruminations: can failure be turned into success? *Behaviour Research and Therapy*, **27**(2), 149–60.

Salzman, L. (1985). Psychotherapeutic management of obsessive-compulsive patients. *American Journal of Psychotherapy*, **39**(3), 323–30.

Sanavio, E. (1988). Obsessions and compulsions: the Padua Inventory. *Behaviour Research and Therapy*, **26**(2), 169–77.

Sank, L. I. and Shaffer, C. C. (1984). *A therapist's manual for cognitive behavior therapy in groups*. New York: Plenum Press.

Schwartz, M. S. (1987). *Biofeedback: a practitioner's guide*. New York: The Guilford Press.

Seligman, M. E. (1971). Phobias and preparedness. *Behavior Therapy*, **2**(3), 307–20.

Shapiro, T. (1992). The concept of unconscious fantasy. *Journal of Clinical Psychoanalysis*, **1**, 517–24.

Shear, M., Cooper, A. M., Klerman, G. L., Busch, F. N., and Shapiro, T. (1993). A psychodynamic model of panic disorder. *American Journal of Psychiatry*, **150**(6), 859–66.

Shear, M., Houck, P., Greeno, C., and Masters, S. (2001). Emotion-focused psychotherapy for patients with panic disorder. *American Journal of Psychiatry*, **158**(12), 1993–8.

Simpson, H., Gorfinkle, K., and Liebowitz, M. R. (1999). Cognitive-behavioral therapy as an adjunct to serotonin reuptake inhibitors in obsessive-compulsive disorder: an open trial. *Journal of Clinical Psychiatry*, **60**(9), 584–90.

Smucker, M. R. and Dancu, C. V. (1999). *Cognitive-behavioral treatment for adult survivors of childhood trauma: Imagery rescripting and reprocessing*. Northvale, NJ: Jason Aronson.

Spitzer, R. L., Williams, J. B. W., and Gibbon, M. (1987). *Structured clinical interview for DSM–III-R—patient version*. New York: New York State Psychiatric Institute.

Stein, D. J. (2002). Obsessive-compulsive disorder. *Lancet*, **360**, 397–405.

Steketee, G. S. (1993a). Social support and treatment outcome of obsessive compulsive disorder at 9-month follow-up. *Behavioural Psychotherapy*, **21**(2), 81–95.

Steketee, G. S. (1993b). *Treatment of obsessive compulsive disorder*. New York: Guilford Press.

Steketee, G. S. and Frost, R. O. (1998). Cost-effective behavior therapy for obsessive-compulsive disorder. In: E. Sanavio, ed. *Behavior and cognitive therapy today: essays in honor of Hans J Eysenck*, pp. 289–304. Boston, MA: Boston University.

Stern, R. (1978). Obsessive thoughts: the problem of therapy. *British Journal of Psychiatry*, **133**, 200–5.

Stopa, L. and Clark, D. M. (1993). Cognitive processes in social phobia. *Behaviour Research and Therapy*, **31**(3), 255–67.

Stopa, L. and Clark, D. M. (2000). Social phobia and interpretation of social events. *Behaviour Research and Therapy*, **38**, 273–83.

Tarrier, N., Pilgrim, H., Sommerfield, C., Faragher, B., Reynolds, M., Graham, E., *et al.* (1999). A randomized trial of cognitive therapy and imaginal exposure in the treatment of chronic posttraumatic stress disorder. *Journal of Consulting and Clinical Psychology*, **67**(1), 13–18.

Taylor, S. (1996). Meta analysis of cognitive behavioral treatments for social phobia. *Behavior Therapy and Experimental Psychiatry*, **27**, 1–9.

Turk, C. L., Heimberg, R. G., and Hope, D. A. (2001). Social anxiety disorder. In: D. H. Barlow, ed. *Clinical handbook of psychological disorders: a step-by-step treatment manual*, 3rd edn, pp. 114–53. New York: Guilford Press.

Turk, C. L., Lerner, J., Heimberg, R. G., and Rapee, R. M. (2002). An integrated cognitive-behavioral model of social anxiety. In: S. G. Hofmann and P. M. DiBartolo, ed. *From social anxiety to social phobia: multiple perspectives*, pp. 281–303. Needham Heights: Allyn and Bacon.

Turner, S. M., Hersen, M., Bellack, A. S., Andrasik, F., and Capparell, H. V. (1980). Behavioral and pharmacological treatment of obsessive-compulsive disorders. *Journal of Nervous and Mental Disease*, **168**, 651–7.

Turner, S. M., Beidel, D. C., and Jacob, R. G. (1994). Social phobia: a comparison of behavior therapy and atenolol. *Journal of Consulting and Clinical Psychology*, **62**(2), 350–8.

Turner, S. M., Cooley Quille, M. R., and Beidel, D. C. (1996). Behavioral and pharmacological treatment for social phobia. In: M. R. Mavissakalian and R. F. Prien, ed. *Long term treatments of anxiety disorders*, pp. 343–71. Washington, DC: American Psychiatric Press.

Van Oppen, P., *et al.* (1995). Cognitive therapy and exposure in vivo in the treatment of obsessive compulsive disorder. *Behaviour Research and Therapy*, **33**(4), 379–90.

Warren, R. and Zgourides, G. D. (1991). *Anxiety disorders: a rational-emotive perspective*. Elmsford, NY: Pergamon Press.

Watson, D. and Friend, R. (1969). Measurement of social-evaluative anxiety. *Journal of Consulting and Clinical Psychology*, **33**(4), 448–57.

Watson, J. B. (1919). *Psychology from the standpoint of a behaviorist*. Philadelphia: Lippincott.

Wegner, D. M. (1989). *White bears and other unwanted thoughts: suppression, obsession, and the psychology of mental control*. New York: Penguin.

Weiss, D. S. and Marmar, C. R. (1993). Teaching time-limited dynamic psychotherapy for post–traumatic stress disorder and pathological grief. *Psychotherapy Research*, **30**, 587–91.

Weissman, M. M., Klerman, G. L., Markowitz, J. S., and Ouellette, R. (1989). Suicidal ideation and suicide attempts in panic disorder and attacks. *New England Journal of Medicine*, **321**(18), 1209–14.

Weissman, M. M., Markowitz, J. S., Ouellette, R., Greenwald, S., and Kahn, J. P. (1990). Panic disorder and cardiovascular/cerebrovascular problems: results from a community survey. *American Journal of Psychiatry*, **147**(11), 1504–8.

Wells, A. (1997). *Cognitive therapy of anxiety disorders: a practice manual and conceptual guide*. New York: John Wiley and Sons.

Wells, A. and Papageorgiou, C. (1999). The observer perspective: biased imagery in social phobia, agoraphobia, and blood/injury phobia. *Behaviour Research and Therapy*, **37**, 653–58.

Wells, A., Clark, D. M., and Ahmad, S. (1998). How do I look with my minds eye: perspective taking in social phobic imagery. *Behaviour Research and Therapy*, **36**(6), 631–4.

Wiborg, I. M. and Dahl, A. A. (1996). Does brief psychodynamic psychotherapy reduce the relapse rate of panic disorder? *Archives of General Psychiatry*, **53**, 689–94.

Wittchen, H. U., Zhao, S., Kessler, R. C., and Eaton, W. W. (1994). DSM-III-R generalized anxiety disorder in the National Comorbidity Survey. *Archives of General Psychiatry*, **51**(5), 355–64.

Wolpe, J. (1958). *Psychotherapy by reciprocal inhibition*. Stanford, CA: Stanford University Press.

Wolpe, J. and Lang, P. J. (1964). A Fear Survey Schedule for use in behaviour therapy. *Behaviour Research and Therapy*, **2**, 27–30.

Zerbe, K. J. (1994). Uncharted waters: psychodynamic considerations in the diagnosis and treatment of social phobia. *Bulletin of the Menninger Clinic*, **58**(2, Suppl. A), A3–20.

14 Schizophrenia

D. Turkington, B. Martindale, and G. R. Bloch-Thorsen

Introduction

Schizophrenia is a major cause of disability worldwide with a roughly stable prevalence of approximately 1%. The outcome in Western society has generally been viewed as being poor with a tendency to regular relapse or chronicity in the majority. There would appear to be no convincing evidence as yet of any explanatory underlying disease process. It would seem most likely that schizophrenia represents the syndromal manifestation of a variety of diverse accumulated insults to psychological functioning. These would include combinations of the following stressors: genetic, biological, environmental, and psychological. The different combinations of these elements in each individual formulation will contribute to the form and content of the actual psychotic symptoms displayed. This chapter will attempt to outline how the different main psychological treatment modalities (psychodynamic, cognitive-behavioral, and family) conceptualize and work with these diverse presentations of positive, negative, and linked affective symptoms. Process of therapy along with models of therapy effect will be described. Possible pitfalls will be outlined with strategies to overcome these. The evidence base supportive of each intervention will be stated. The chapter will end with a discussion of future research and training directions in relation to implementation.

Historical overview (from exorcism to Freud, Leff, and Kingdon)

Psychological interventions for schizophrenia probably began with exorcisms in primitive societies where possession by an evil spirit was deemed to be the cause of the problems. This concept has not gone away and even today some patients and carers seeing a frightening and inexplicable change in their psychotic relative, will request exorcism. This can lead to problems in the therapeutic alliance and in such cases therapists of all modalities would need to explore the patient's models of illness and treatment before deciding on how to proceed. Following the years of magical treatments and simple incarceration (which would again appear to be on the increase) moral management of schizophrenia began with the founding of the Retreat at York in the UK by William Tuke in 1792. Moral treatment included respect for the patient, pleasant grounds for recreation, and adequate facilities for sheltered occupation (Tuke, 1889). Psychological models of psychosis really began with Freud. In his early investigations into paranoia, he theorized that paranoia was a 'neurosis of defense' and that the chief defense mechanism was projection (Freud, 1895). Later he analyzed the persecutory delusions of Schreber from the latter's memoirs (Freud, 1911). In this analysis, as well as extending the theory of paranoia, Freud investigates the inter-relationships of narcissism and the vicissitudes of the sexual drives and gender identity in psychosis especially in the face of frustrations and disappointments. Harry Stack Sullivan, influenced by object relations theory, extended this model and ended up by concluding that schizophrenia was a functional psychological disorder in which symptomatic improvement could be expected with psychotherapy (Sullivan, 1962). Fromm-Reichman (1950) stressed that patients

with schizophrenia exhibited a degree of motivation for engagement in therapy despite a pervasive distrust of others due to adverse early life events. Meyer (1950) echoed this therapeutic optimism in his biopsychosocial model of mental illness and his acceptance of a need for an autobiographical anamnesis or history to clarify symptom onset and dysfunctional adaptive styles. Until the development of psychoeducational family work, which evolved less than 30 years ago, very little research had been published on the use of family interventions within the field of schizophrenia. The view of the role of the family in inducing, developing, and sustaining schizophrenia changed over the years. This was related to changes in illness models from biological to personal weakness to posttraumatic. Researchers such as Bateson *et al.* (1956), Fromm-Reichmann (1950), and Lidz *et al.* (1957) stated that the parents of patients with schizophrenia were cold, dominant, conflict inducing, weak, or giving double communications. Statements such as this were not inclined to develop a good carer perspective on the possible benefits of family therapy. This situation was worsened by the dearth of any valid research evidence. In the late 1960s the English psychiatrists George Brown and John Birley (Brown and Birley, 1968) asked the crucial question 'Why is it that some persons with schizophrenia manage to cope well after the initial episode of psychosis while others do not?' They believed that extraneous factors influenced the subsequent course and therefore wanted to investigate environmental factors. They discovered that a family milieu with excessive criticism, hostility, overinvolvement, and lack of warmth toward the patient contributed to an increased risk of relapse (high expressed emotion family, high EE). Variables found to reduce relapse were warmth, acceptance and positive comments towards the patient (low expressed emotion family, low EE). Falloon *et al.* (1985) and Leff and Vaughan (1985) stressed in their ground breaking work just how crucial the family environment was in relation to the issue of relapse in schizophrenia.

Although a cognitive approach was being used in the nineteenth century by such renowned psychiatrists as Esquirol (1938), it did not achieve prominence again until Beck in 1952 described a seminal case. In this paper he described the use of a psychodynamic formulation with cognitive and behavioral techniques to achieve symptomatic improvement and eventual remission in a patient with a systematized persecutory delusion. Treatment manuals later followed (Kingdon and Turkington, 1994; Fowler *et al.*, 1995). Integrative cognitive models of symptom emergence and maintenance were only developed much more recently (Garety *et al.*, 2001). The new millenium has seen the further development of interpersonal therapy, cognitive remediation, and cognitive analytical therapy in the treatment of schizophrenia. As psychodynamic therapy was the first approach to be developed followed by family therapy and then, more recently, cognitive-behavioral therapy (CBT) this order will be followed in describing techniques throughout this chapter.

Conceptualization

The psychodynamic model

Descriptively, all psychodynamic models of psychosis would concur with most other models of psychosis that various aspects of 'normal' synthetic mental functioning have become disturbed. In keeping with the usual meaning of psychosis, it is various aspects of 'reality' that the mind cannot synthesize or integrate.

Where psychodynamic models diverge significantly from many other models is the centrality of the theory that psychotic phenomena are the result of a balance of dynamic mental forces that have purposes and functions for the individual. These may include unconscious motivation, meaningfulness, and meaningfulness avoided for defensive reasons. Psychodynamic models are often compatible with aspects of other models, providing no model intends to be reductionistic (Robbins, 1993). For example, there is no need in the psychodynamic model to rule out the likelihood that variations in the genetic or other biological substrates of the brain or early environmental and neurodevelopment factors can contribute to differences between individuals in their capacity to handle cognitive or emotional loads (Grotstein, 1995).

Information reaches the mind from many sources, for example, the eyes, ears, and skin. Thoughts and memories are themselves sources of data for the mind to process. If the mind is in a state where it is 'threatened' by that information or has already been overwhelmed, 'psychotic' dynamic mechanisms may be utilized in an attempt (unconscious motivation) to rid one of that information with its unacceptable meaning or further overwhelming affect. The consequences of these processes result in the symptoms and signs of psychosis.

In psychosis it is common for the sensory and mental apparatus (that are usually sources of information) to be used by the psychotic aspects of mind as routes by which information about reality, including the 'reality' of unacceptable internal thoughts and feelings can seem to be eliminated from awareness. Hence the vast range of areas of potential disturbance, e.g., auditory hallucinations, tactile phenomena, and disorders of thought and ideation often attributed to other minds (resulting in persecutory psychotic phenomena).

Psychotic psychodynamic mechanisms

Many psychodynamic and other practitioners now recognize that persons with psychosis have both intact aspects of their minds or personalities and other aspects that have been taken over by the psychotic process. Bion (1957) described these very well in his paper 'Differentiation of the psychotic from the non-psychotic personalities'. The nonpsychotic aspects of the personality are able to take in and integrate reality, such as information provided by the sensory and thinking apparatus. By contrast psychotic aspects of the person, unwilling or unable to tolerate mental pain or frustration, 'attack' those aspects of either the mind itself or the perceptual sources of these unwelcome realities (Bion, 1959). Both may coexist in complex relation with one another as in the following vignette:

A 66-year-old widow Y, with diminishing resources of all kinds, was increasingly overwhelmed by the belief that she was being subjected to attempts to steal all her possessions by persons who tried to enter her flat through gas pipes and cracks in the floorboards. This lady went to the mental hospital to complain rather than the police station. [This case also illustrates the attempt to project (*externalize*) the source of her diminishing resources, as she found it too painful to be aware of her own increasing frailty including her aging body.]

So in psychodynamic models, the psychotic manifestations are part of an active process that is in a dynamic relationship with the nonpsychotic aspects of the person often competing for supremacy.

A core mechanism in the psychodynamics of psychosis is the active breaking of the links between elements of information or thoughts and (in fantasy) and expelling the resulting fragments in a desperate attempt at safety (fragmentation or splitting and projection). This results in 'bizarre experiences'. A simplified example of hallucinatory voices may assist:

A woman went on holiday without her partner and had sexual relations with others. Although she made no connection herself to the aforementioned facts, on her return she broke down into a psychosis with prominent persecutory and denigratory auditory hallucinations calling her a 'slut'.

This could be understood as a relatively unsuccessful dynamic attempt by psychotic processes to eliminate the unbearable 'reality' of her own harsh

internal thoughts (voice) about her behavior (her conscience). Psychoanalysts use the term 'psychotic mechanisms' when they are referring to psychological defenses that attempt to bypass—or even eliminate reality. They are akin to certain dream processes such as those in which the reality of time and space can be disregarded (for example, in a dream one can be in opposite sides of the world at the same time, or be several persons all in one). These contrast with 'neurotic' mechanisms when painful reality is retained. In this example the woman was unconsciously ridding herself of her thoughts that she might have been uncaring and self-centered in her behavior. Here the elimination/projection uses a fantasy of eliminating of internal issues via the auditory sensory apparatus so they appear to come from the external world. By a process of unconscious identification, the thoughts 'projected' into the minds of others are unbearable to those of others too. So the others (the voice persons) are in turn maliciously trying to force the ideas back into her. In psychosis these are experienced as concrete factual experiences and not thoughts or ideas. In neurosis, the person might present with perhaps anxiety or depression, obsessional behaviors or compulsive thoughts or punitive guilt—the common feature is that knowledge (thought) of the behavior is not being eliminated from the mind but being reacted to with other mechanisms of dealing with a painful awareness.

The example may also assist in understanding the psychodynamic model for the impoverishment/blunting of affect (negative symptoms) that is often seen in more chronic psychoses. The person mentioned above was unconsciously desperately trying not to experience affects such as loss of self-esteem or the damage to the relationship with her partner, let alone guilt, concern, and remorse. The person is therefore very restricted in the sort of life that can be led because of this much reduced (fluctuating) capacity to manage affects and reflection. This is often referred to as ego depletion or ego impoverishment. As a result of evacuation/ejection of substantial aspects of one's mind and the perceptual apparatus, the personality is depleted (impoverished).The ejected fragments continue as alienated or 'bizarre' objects experienced as having a personality—such as a television set, or camera usually trapping the person in a persecutory world, occasionally comforting (Hinshelwood, 1989).

The psychodynamic model of psychosis also has a major contribution to play in the understanding of interpersonal processes in psychosis. For example, it has been established from much replicated research that living in a household where there is 'high EE' in relatives is associated with a much greater risk of psychotic relapse (Leff and Vaughan, 1985). When therapy leads to the successful containment of such emotions by relatives the relapse rate is very considerably reduced. Migone (1995) has made useful attempts to bridge the empirical atheoretical concept of expressed emotion in terms of the three phases of projective identification espoused for example by Ogden (1979). In the first phase, unwanted or threatening mental contents, e.g., feelings of inadequacy or guilt or fears of criticism in relatives are projected (as a result they may criticize the patient or become excessively involved in order to compensate for these unwelcome feelings). In the second phase, the projecting relative(s) places 'interpersonal pressure' (through expressed emotion) so that the other (e.g., the psychotically vulnerable person) fits the projection, e.g., he or she is worthy of criticism (e.g., he is lazy). The latter cannot contain the projections and over time decompensates and/or projects back into the relatives (e.g., accuses the family or family member) arousing further feelings in a negative circular fashion that cannot again be contained in the relatives. The main emphasis of this psychoanalytic explanation of expressed emotion, is that of unbearable feelings in the family member(s) who try to eject outside of him or herself and locate in the person vulnerable to psychosis. It is vital to emphasize that psychoanalysts are referring to unconscious processes, otherwise these concepts will be misused and families will be blamed.

Unfortunately, these ideas, which are based on careful observations, are themselves vulnerable to the possibility of blaming family members by inexperienced professionals rather than understanding. It is important to be clear that it is unconscious mechanisms and unacceptable feelings or thoughts that are being inferred in the psychodynamic model. These cannot necessarily be immediately accepted into consciousness even through empathic interpretation.

A developmental perspective

Psychodynamic theorists continue to consider that vulnerability to psychosis is strongly correlated to prior mental development (Holmes, 2001). There is now compelling research evidence for the importance of a combination of both genetic and formative family environmental factors and their interaction in altering vulnerability to psychosis favorably and unfavorably. The evidence stems especially from the work of Tienari *et al.* (1994) in a long-term project that evaluated both genetic and adoptive family mental health functioning. A large number of adopted away children from mothers with schizophrenia and a control group of adopted children with biological mothers without psychosis were studied. Alanen (1997) gives a thorough review and synthesis of the psychodynamic theories on the 'origin' of schizophrenia. The developmental view does not exclude the clinical observations that occasionally psychotic breakdowns can occur in persons with previously well functioning personalities in the face of massive stresses (see CBT conceptualization).

Family therapy conceptualization

The theoretical model that underpins the use of psychoeducational family therapy in schizophrenia is the vulnerability/stress model. This model explains the onset of the disease, its course, and social manifestations as being due to complex interactions between biological, environmental, and behavioral factors. The psychoeducational therapist or family group leader does not stress or address this model in treatment. The model is acknowledged as being a theoretical model and is handled with openness and a pragmatic attitude in therapy. According to the vulnerability/stress model the symptoms of schizophrenia are the consequence of psychobiological vulnerability combined with environmental stress. This psychobiological vulnerability makes the patient less able to handle the type of stress of normal adolescence. This helps families not to feel at fault for the development of the psychosis. It also takes care of the fact that for many patients developing schizophrenia it is not possible to find stressors or traumas that can explicitly explain why this person became psychotic. This also explains why some but not all children in the same family climate developed the illness, i.e., the children had different degrees of vulnerability to develop psychosis. The model also takes care of the fact that in certain families schizophrenia is very common due to genetic factors. The development of schizophrenia can take years from the first early signs to the emergence of clearly recognizable psychotic symptoms. It is considered that the onset of the illness occurs when the patient's stress tolerance has been exceeded. It may therefore be theoretically possible to prevent or at least delay the emergence of psychotic symptoms through education and stress management for patients who are recognized to be vulnerable or who are in the early stages of a psychotic prodrome. Research in this area would suggest that the delayed emergence of psychotic symptoms can be achieved in this way (Birchwood *et al.*, 1997; Johannessen *et al.*, 2001; McGorry *et al.*, 2002). Psychoeducational family therapy is proven to reduce relapse following a first episode of schizophrenia when the patient lives with a high EE family. It is not yet known whether these high EE families have been so before the development of the psychosis or whether having a psychotic family member creates stress in the family that produces the typical interactional styles of the high EE family. Some current research is pointing more towards the latter explanation (Johannessen *et al.*, 2001).

Cognitive-behavioral therapy conceptualization of schizophrenia

The process of CBT with the schizophrenic patient is linked to a conceptualization of the illness that is influenced by Bleuler (1911), Freud (1911), and Zubin and Spring (1977). Bleuler stressed that the schizophrenias were a group of psychotic disorders with a variety of presentations and differential outcomes. Freud stressed that psychotic symptoms had meaning and the vulnerability stress hypothesis of Zubin and Spring indicated how genetic, obstetric, infectious, personality, and other vulnerabilities interacted with stressors to initiate the emergence of the psychotic prodrome. More recently cognitive therapists (Kingdon and Turkington, 1998) have viewed the schizophrenias as consisting of five overlapping subgroups on the basis of a comprehensive review of their clinical casework.

Sensitivity disorder

Sensitivity disorder (which approximates to Carpenter *et al.*, 1988, deficit syndrome) or Crow's (1980) Type II schizophrenia. This subgroup of the schizophrenias is usually described as being genetically weighted and with a gradual slide into a psychotic prodrome in adolescence. There usually appears to be minimal amounts of stress that trigger this and the presenting clinical appearance is of core negative symptoms such as alogia and affective blunting. The delusions and hallucinations linked to affective blunting are regarded as being held with less emotional investment and conviction than when affective blunting is not present (Kirkpatrick *et al.*, 1996). These hallucinations and delusions are often highly responsive to basic CBT interventions such as reality testing and the use of coping strategies once the patient has engaged. These Type I delusions are present in the order of 50% of cases of schizophrenia.

Anxiety psychosis

In comparison with the above presentation the Type II delusion is less frequent. The Type II delusion is protective of underlying painful affect, such as depression, shame, or guilt. The Type II delusion usually arises after a period of intense and incremental anxiety often in middle life and is typical of a different subgroup of the schizophrenias, the *anxiety psychosis*. In this type of schizophrenia the Type II delusion usually presents as a systematized persecutory or grandiose delusion in the absence of negative symptoms. Sensitivity disorder and anxiety psychosis both tend to be responsive to CBT. The anxiety psychosis, however, often requires a longer intervention and peripheral questioning and reality testing alone are rarely effective. Clarification of the meaning of the delusion in the case formulation linked to work on the related underlying 'hot' schema seems to be necessary. Such patients will often show a degree of depression, guilt, or shame as the delusion begins to recede and the underlying hot schema is exposed (Turkington and Siddle, 1998). Whereas a good symptomatic improvement can be achieved with sensitivity disorder by a trained Community Psychiatric Nurse within a relatively brief intervention the anxiety psychosis will require 20–40 sessions with an experienced cognitive therapist if a substantial and durable benefit is to be achieved.

Traumatic psychosis

The third subgroup of the schizophrenias would appear to be *traumatic psychosis*. This is a group in which trauma is involved in the etiology of the psychotic disorder and flavors the psychotic symptoms. Often these patients have suffered from sexual assault early in life and borderline traits can be present in the personality. It would appear that any form of trauma can, however, precipitate a traumatic psychosis under certain circumstances and in relation to certain vulnerabilities. It has been reported that two-thirds of female chronic hallucinators with schizophrenia have suffered from childhood sexual assault (Heins *et al.*, 1990). The hallmark of the traumatic subgroup is the presence of derogatory and command hallucinations. Linked schemas are often those of 'badness', 'worthlessness', or 'being evil'. Patients holding such core maladaptive beliefs about their own value often tend to believe these derogatory hallucinations, which are trauma synchronic and they develop varying levels of depression. The cognitive therapy conceptualizations of these cases rely on cognitive models of trauma (Ehlers and Clarke, 2000) and of hallucinations (Morrison, 1998). Progress and therapy depends on the development of a clear formulation followed by the reliving of the trauma while using coping strategies to deal with stressful psychotic symptoms. Work with linked schemas allows improvement in self-esteem and self-efficacy leading to improved engagement with therapy. Such patients are often revolving door patients who seem to derive less benefit from antipsychotic medication than do sensitivity disorder and anxiety psychosis. Owing to the coexisting variable levels of depression, self harm and eventual suicide is not uncommonly the outcome unless psychotherapy is made available.

Drug-induced psychosis

Perhaps the most difficult subgroup to work with is that with coexisting ongoing hallucinogen dependence. This group, which we have labeled *drug-induced psychosis* often, tend to have linked dysfunctional personality traits if not personality disorder. Those who are antisocial and rebelling against family and society in general often use hallucinogens such as strong cannabis, amphetamine, and LSD to perpetuate psychotic symptoms. This often leads to high EE in family members and poor adherence to all forms of treatment. These factors tend to act as maintaining factors for maintenance of psychotic symptoms. There is some evidence that CBT can be of benefit to this subgroup but it would appear to need to be linked to motivational interviewing in the early stages (Barrowclough *et al.*, 2001). Coexisting family therapy to work with the maintaining factor of high EE would seem to be indicated.

Catatonia

The last subgroup within this conceptualization is now relatively rare in the UK. *Catatonia* of schizophrenic origin is now only rarely seen outside institutional settings, usually in liaison settings as a result of infectious or inflammatory origin. These patients are now usually seen on neurology wards, the bulk of the remainder of catatonic presentations, which are linked to functional psychosis, are now usually affective. Schizophrenic catatonia would appear to be the most organically weighted (Wilcox and Nasrallah, 1987) of these subgroups and, although research is sparse in this area, would seem to have least to gain from CBT and other psychological interventions.

Summary

Schizophrenia is therefore best conceptualized in relation to its psychological treatment by CBT on the basis of the above five subgroups. All of these have there own unique and overlapping mechanisms of symptom production and maintenance. Individual CBT would appear to be strongly effective in sensitivity disorder, anxiety psychosis and traumatic psychosis. It is a more difficult task but still likely to be a crucial intervention within drug related psychosis.

Research

Research into psychodynamic approaches

The first study comparing psychoanalytic psychotherapy with medication in psychosis was in Pennsylvania (Bookhammer *et al.*, 1966) and was with young, first admission patients with psychotic illness. Tentative conclusions were that the particular form of intensive psychotherapy was about equal in effectiveness with medication. However, the research therapy was carried out in the presence of an audience, which may well have had intimidating elements (Karon, 1989).

The Wisconsin study (Rogers *et al.*, 1967) was mainly a client-centered approach with patients seen twice a week for up to 2.5 years compared with two control groups treated with medication. Although many findings were not impressive, after termination the psychotherapy patients had nearly a 100% reduction in bed usage in the following year from 117 versus 219 days (but significant only to $P = 0.1$). The study was probably underpowered to test the hypothesis that length of stay was altered by the treatment. Findings related increasing warmth, empathy, and genuineness in the therapeutic relationship with other positive outcomes.

The California project, is most often quoted as showing definitively that medication is the indispensable treatment of choice and that psychoanalytic psychotherapy is ineffective (May, 1968). The same inexperienced psychiatrists treated a total of 228 different patients by five different methods (psychotherapy without medication, psychotherapy with medication, medication alone, ECT, and milieu therapy). Although some aspects of research design were impressive, a major limitation was the absence of any quality control measures of the therapy and therapists. In addition, the ending of therapy and the final evaluations both took place on the very day of discharge from hospital! This is hardly a neutral time for a patient with schizophrenia patient in psychotherapy. It could be said that this study showed that psychotherapy of schizophrenic patients by *inexperienced* therapists in a *hospital* setting is not beneficial, but few other conclusions could safely be drawn.

In the Massachusetts study (Grinspoon, 1972) Karon (1989) highlights again the poor quality control of the therapists who were not experienced with either chronic schizophrenic patients nor with the economic and ethnic culture of the patients they were treating. More than half the patients had received ECT or insulin comas and all had been in a state hospital for more than 3 years. Behavioral measures did not improve for the psychotherapy patients but 68% were able to live outside hospital compared with 37% of the (nonrandomized) control group.

The trial of treatment of schizophrenia in which quality control of the psychotherapy itself was most carefully protected is that by Karon and Vandenbos (1981) in Michigan. Although numbers were small (36), the patients tended to be severe cases from seriously socially disadvantaged backgrounds. The main problem with this study is that the control group patients were moved from the admitting hospital, if they did not improve sufficiently for discharge, to a state hospital albeit with better auxiliary facilities than the admitting hospital. This was in contrast to the two groups involved in psychotherapy that remained in the admitting hospital in order to be able to receive the psychotherapy. With this important proviso, blind evaluations at 6 months showed that the results of the inexperienced therapists could be accounted for solely by medication effects as in the California study above (May, 1968). However, at this stage the quality controlled experienced psychotherapists had significantly better results in terms of reduction in hospitalized days and measures of thought disorder, whether or not medication was administered. By 12 months the patients of the inexperienced but supervised therapists were functioning better than the control group on medication. At the end of 20 months, psychotherapy (average 70 sessions) was more effective than medication, with the patients of the experienced therapists showing a balanced improvement across all measures.

Two years after termination, psychotherapy patients had half the number of hospitalization days compared with the medication control group and patients of experienced therapists did better than those of the inexperienced. Changes in thought disorder seem to be a better predictor of longer-term ability to function outside hospital than short-term behavioral criteria, supporting other researchers' findings.

There is a consistency in all the studies quoted above that psychotherapy patients spend less time in hospital than those in medication alone group controls. The Michigan study had a number of cost evaluations that were positive in the long term for the psychotherapy group. In addition, only 33% of the latter needed welfare payments compared with 75% of those of the medication-only controls. Karon (1989) stresses that the cost benefit–findings would have been completely opposite if the evaluations were only done at 6 months of treatment.

Therapeutic alliance

One important point is the question of therapeutic alliance. In a psychotherapy research project that is often quoted as unfavorable to psychotherapy (Gunderson *et al.*, 1984), the drop-out rate was very large (69%). A good measure is needed to evaluate whether the patient is generally and genuinely co-operating in the therapy (in the same way that a trial of medication would need to have some accurate means of knowing that the patient was taking it).

Overall the results of the early research into brief periods of psychoanalytic psychotherapy for persons with psychosis was not very encouraging. Further, more detailed reviews have been conducted by the following authors (Karon, 1989; Mueser and Berenbaum, 1990; Martindale *et al.*, 2000).

It is disappointing that there has not been much recent research into treatments that offer a predominantly psychoanalytic treatment that takes account of the deficiencies in the pioneering trials just mentioned. What is clearly needed is research that aims to discover more effective ways of achieving a therapeutic alliance in the psychoanalytic psychotherapy of psychosis, that has much better quality controls of the therapists, that is of sufficient duration to study the longer-term goals associated with the goals of psychoanalytic psychotherapy. In addition there have been substantial developments in psychoanalytic theory and technique in recent decades that are likely to have given many therapists more effective clinical methods of working with the psychotic persons. For a detailed case example that also discusses a considerable amount of contemporary theory see Pestalozzi (2003).

The psychoanalytic method with patients in psychotic states has to be very different from the psychoanalytic method with patients who are in more integrated states. Certainly, techniques that may provoke further regression are not indicated and the therapy needs a good deal of structure and the active establishment of sufficient interpersonal 'relatedness' with sufficient trust and mutual respect. This approach represents a considerable change from the practice during the time when much of the older research in psychoanalytic psychotherapy with psychosis was conducted. This older research had a number of limitations that have been extensively commented on from different perspectives.

In contemporary times, psychoanalytic understanding and psychoanalytic psychotherapy is most widely incorporated into the need-adapted approach that is practiced widely in Scandinavia (Alanen *et al.*, 1991). Here a range of interventions are used according to a comprehensive ongoing evaluation, including a psychodynamic understanding of each patient's specific situation. The full range of approaches are based on the establishment of a secure therapeutic relationship, which may move into more formal psychoanalytic therapy.

Two persons with similar forms of hallucinations and delusions will vary enormously in their motivation and in the life situation in which they have developed a psychosis. Need-adapted treatment decisions will center on these individual differences and contexts. Randomized controlled trial research would tend towards focusing on a particular treatment and evaluating outcome of the symptoms that were *common to* a group of patients. The randomized controlled trial design, by its nature, draws inferences from groups the membership of which is determined by randomization between two (or more) alternatives that can be described as in 'equipoise' (i.e., there is a plausible case for either option being superior). By contrast, the 'need-adapted approach' is based on a competing principle that informed choice is based on the idea that an idiographic assessment of need for *each individual* and the type of treatment is paramount. This could well mean that in two patients with similar psychotic symptoms, assessment might lead to a decision to recommend on *other* clinical grounds, a focus on medication in one, a family intervention in another and individual psychoanalytic therapy in other control trials of need-adapted approaches are therefore difficult to design. An additional problem is that need-adapted approaches are integrated ones with the overall therapy being dependent on several interventions over time rather than a single one. For example, therapy would not only hope to reduce psychotic symptomatology but aim to reengage and accompany the patient on a number of developmental trajectories that he or she has fallen away from sometimes over a period of years preceding the psychosis or as a consequence. Evaluative research therefore needs to be conducted over a period of some years rather than months.

Research into family interventions

Recent meta-analysis confirms the efficacy of family therapy in the prevention of relapse with an NNT in terms of relapse prevention in the first year of 6.5 (Jones *et al.*, 2000). (NNT stands for the average Number Needed to Treat in this case to prevent a single relapse.) Psychoeducational family therapy has a track record of 30 years of research. Many different programs have

been offered but those proven useful have all had some common elements as described by Dixon and Lehman (1995). These are as follows:

1. Schizophrenia is regarded as an illness.

2. The family environment is not implicated in the etiology of the illness.

3. Support is provided and families are enlisted as therapeutic agents.

4. The interventions are part of a treatment package used in conjunction with routine drug treatment and outpatient clinical management.

The programs usually consist of educating about the illness itself, including course, treatment, and outcome. There are regular meetings where different problem-solving methods and communication skills are learned. Other benefits of the program include support, understanding, and containment.

All research on family intervention has taken into consideration the fact that the direct goal in the treatment program is to reduce the negative expressed emotions in the families and thereby reduce the stress for the patient. This will create a healthier milieu and prevent relapse. Brown *et al.* (1972) created a research instrument, the Camberwell Family Interview (CFI), a semistructured interview lasting 90 minutes, to score the intensity of the critical comments, hostility, and overinvolvement in the families. During the last 10 years several review articles have been published, including Barbato and D'Avanzo (2000) and Pitschel-Walz *et al.* (2001) who summarized more than 30 published studies, including almost 2000 families. Although the programs differ in length from 2 to 24 months and some of them address single families and some multifamilies, a highly significant majority show a significant effect on relapse rates.

Defining relapse can be difficult. One approach is to use symptom thresholds but this can be highly subjective and depending on interpretation. Hospitalization depends on access to hospital beds and the availability of crisis teams, work on unemployment figures, and so on. All this taken into consideration, the conclusion of the meta-analysis of these studies confirms an effect on relapse equal to that of medication. Pitchel-Walz *et al.* (2001) conclude in their article: 'this meta analysis clearly indicates that including relatives in treatment programs is an effective way of reducing relapse rates and rehospitalization rates in patients with schizophrenia.' 'Psychoeducation for patients and their families should become a basic part of a comprehensive psychosocial treatment package that is offered to all patients with schizophrenia.' The conclusion of Barbato and D'Avanzo (2000) concurs with the above.

However, there are reasons to believe that the benefits of psychoeducational therapy are effective mainly in high EE families where a substantial number of sessions are given. Also, there are only sufficient numbers to confirm the benefits in male chronic patients.

Family therapy does not claim to reduce general levels of symptomatology or achieve a reduced burden of care, but it has been shown to be cost-effective due to the large proportion of schizophrenia costs, which are consumed by repeated hospitalization (Davies and Drummond, 1994). Implementation of family therapy in the UK has been a problem in that nurses who have trained in this modality on return to their Community Mental Health Teams have often found themselves unable to delivery family therapy to schizophrenic patients. The reason for this has been due to high case loads, lack of appropriate supervision, and the need for crisis work (Leff, 2000). Reducing expressed emotion (excessive criticism or overinvolvement) using behavioral family therapy does seem to reduce relapse when high EE is present in carers who spend more than 35 hours per week of face to face contact with the schizophrenic relative (Leff and Wing, 1971). McCreadie and Robinson (1987), however, stressed that a low EE family could be an active therapeutic factor in relation to the patient's schizophrenic illness and that reduction of the carer's high EE may not be the effective therapeutic ingredient. He also noted that many families who are assessed to be of high EE at the time of acute admission, subsequently revert to low EE status, once the stress of the acute relapse of the admission was over. Irrespective of these criticisms, family therapy has been recommended in the UK National Institute for Clinical Excellence Guidelines (National Institute for Clinical Excellence, 2002) and now must be provided by Mental Health Trusts where indicated. In comparison, individual psychoeducation has an NNT for prevention of relapse in the first year of 9.5 but there is some evidence of a risk of increase in suicidal ideation (Carroll *et al.*, 1998). It would appear that the great weight of evidence is that family therapy can reduce relapse in certain patients with schizophrenia, it therefore seems necessary to supply an individual intervention to the patient with schizophrenia to improve symptomatology to complement the effect of family therapy in relapse.

The benefits of CBT as shown by NNTs (a binary outcome measure) are confirmed by studies of effect size (a continuous measure). CBT has been shown to have a large effect size on residual psychotic symptoms in schizophrenia by the end of therapy (effect size 0.65) with more gains at short-term follow-up (effect size 0.9) (Gould *et al.*, 2001). It would appear, however, that the literature shows a moderate effect size for other psychological modalities (supportive counseling and befriending) in overall symptoms of schizophrenia at the end of therapy. The befriending group, however, were more significantly worse off at short-term follow-up. The benefits of CBT are apparent in terms of hallucinations and delusions (Tarrier, 1998), negative symptoms, and depression (Sensky *et al.*, 2000) as well as overall symptoms (Kuipers *et al.*, 1997). Brief CBT has also been delivered within a randomized trial and shown to improve adherence leading to improved symptomatology at the end of therapy and at short-term follow-up (Kemp *et al.*, 1996, 1998). As well as this significant and durable effect on all the residual symptoms of schizophrenia, brief CBT has been shown to translate into community settings (Turkington *et al.*, 2002). In this pragmatic trial community psychiatric nurses were trained over a 10-day period in CBT of schizophrenia and delivered this both to patients (six sessions) and carers (three sessions). Overall symptoms, insight, and depression were all significantly improved by the end of this brief CBT intervention. When CBT is delivered in the community by psychiatric nurses, by the end of therapy there is a moderate effect on depression within schizophrenia (NNT = 9) and a moderate effect on insight (NNT = 10). There is a weak effect on overall symptoms (NNT = 13), but no detectable effect on positive or negative psychotic symptoms. It would seem that the strong effects achieved with 20 session expert cognitive therapy does translate into the community but with differential effects of moderate size. Cognitive remediation is a form of retraining in relation to the cognitive deficits of schizophrenia and has also been shown to be effective (Wykes *et al.*, 2002). It would appear potentially to be an ideal supplement in relation to the benefits of CBT in patients with sensitivity disorder. If CBT can deliver symptomatic improvement and improve adherence with antipsychotic medication and if family therapy can reduce relapse, what then is the role for psychodynamic psychotherapy?

Key practice principles

Psychodynamic

Psychodynamic approaches (see Conceptualization) are based on the psychoanalytic model of mental functioning with its principal tenets of (1) unconscious processes dominating mental life, and (2) the centrality of the outcome of earlier life experience in determining capacities to integrate affects and also determining attitudes to key persons in contemporary relationships (transference).

Projections, containment, and countertransference

In recent decades, substantial shifts have occurred in technique in individual psychodynamic therapeutic work with those vulnerable to psychosis. These shifts stem from an increase in understanding of the particular unconscious processes occurring in psychosis—especially the powerful consequences of 'psychotic' projections into the minds of therapists (leading to countertransference). This has resulted in a shift from a relatively exclusive focus on insight in the patient as being the factor that leads to therapeutic change, to (1) a greater focus on better containment in the mind of the professional of the experience of the patient, and (2) a much more serious awareness of the fragility of the patient's integrative capacities in the face of the strength of the need to project. This has been reinforced by the older research that

demonstrated the high dropout rate and low therapeutic alliance in traditional (insight orientated) psychoanalytic therapy with persons with psychosis (Gunderson *et al.*, 1984). Other important research has highlighted that contrary to what was expected, supportive interventions can lead to important psychic change (Wallerstein, 1995). Further developments have occurred as a result of a) deeper understandings of what is meant by containment in the countertransference.

> In a psychoanalytic sense, the word 'containment' refers to the process whereby the therapist detects that the patient is unconsciously attempting to recruit him into acting a role in his inner drama. Containment refers to the psychotherapeutic skill of being able to accept and emotionally and cognitively digest or 'metabolize' the patient's projections, in the service of understanding him. It involves withstanding and tolerating the impact of the process (in the countertransference). He may eventually understand sufficiently to help the patient work through and find better ways of managing what are usually unconscious impulses and desires that he is dealing with by projection. These wishes, emotions and impulses have never before been properly acknowledged or integrated into the patient's self.
>
> Jackson (2001)

The emphasis on containment of projections in the countertransference in psychosis work has meant that psychoanalytic ideas have far more value in all kinds of mental health settings, as the following vignette will convey.

> Patient A was admitted in a seriously suicidal and very psychotic state. She did not respond to medication over many weeks. When consultation was sought, the nurses mentioned how contemptuous she was of them. This was difficult for them to bear. Exploration revealed that the patient had for many years felt contemptuous of the seeming inability of her parents to even acknowledge her difficulties and had given up on them. In the consultation it transpired that, somewhat in contrast to other patients, the staff knew little about A's difficulties and background, and that A was unconsciously assuming the staff to be useless like her view of her parents. The focus of work had up till now been almost exclusively pharmaceutical, with the danger of the staff traumatizing the patient through accusing the patient of being uncooperative rather than trying to make sense of her contempt, which would be likely to be a major feature of formal individual or family therapy offered.

Although this vignette stems from work on an inpatient ward, the understanding of these sorts of experiences could apply to any mental health setting, or therapeutic format (individual, group, family, or therapeutic milieu). Psychoanalytic observers have been much impressed by the extent to which cognitive therapists recognize the power of unconscious schema in determining relationships (Padesky, 1994) and symptoms.

Personal meaning in psychotic symptoms

Psychoanalytic practitioners will be less concerned with tackling individual symptoms, than with trying to understand the meaning of the symptoms and their relevance to the overall longer-term treatment goals as will be clear from the following patient with a *delusional belief*:

> A 25-year-old man, B, was admitted with the dominating symptom (which did not trouble HIM!) of being in love with a famous female model from another country. He believed that she was in love with him too and demonstrated how he could always call her up when he wanted and they would TALK and make love etc. A psychodynamically informed picture emerged. The sudden onset of this psychotic delusion had relieved the man of the lonely broken hearted state he had been in for weeks.

The medical approach in this case had been to find the right medication that would remove the delusion without consideration that the delusion had a psychological function (meaning and meaning to be avoided) and therefore that their recommendations of medication would be opposed. If successful in countering the delusion, B would be likely to return to the status ante in which he was very seriously distressed. A psychoanalytic approach would be to focus on establishing long-term relationship(s) in which the patient might in time feel sufficiently secure to get some attention for his developmental insecurities (which might possibly result in the patient wanting to take some medication, which he had been resisting for psychodynamically obvious reasons). The setting for the treatment for this young man would result from an evaluation of the best combination of social/therapeutic milieu, group, family, or individual therapy if resources were available. Whichever setting or psychotherapeutic modality, analytic, cognitive, or systemic, a psychodynamic assessment of change would not be satisfied very much only with the absence of delusions, but would be assessing whether B had been able to manage the affects involved in social and more intimate relations with women without psychotic deterioration.

Applied psychoanalytic approaches with patient B would involve:

1. Supporting B to reengage with activities that he could manage that were less problematic in order to minimize 'collateral' damage from the breakdown and thus reengaging on some areas where continuing development could occur.

2. Working at a pace that B could manage on making conscious the difficulties that antedated the breakdown as the issues that he needed help with. This was not easy work as B had long internalized in his character what one might call prepsychotic denial of problems. This was in keeping with his long experience in his formative years of his parents' difficulties in keeping their minds open to the fact of his vulnerability and his underlying lack of confidence and to the trauma that stemmed from their divorce with its multiple implications for him. In the countertransference it was difficult for community staff to cope with B's indifference and dismissiveness of therapeutic needs and they felt pressured into going along with a leave him alone or give up attitude when he would miss appointments and seem unconcerned. In time it was possible to engage with him gradually as to how vulnerable he indeed felt with the staff to being abandoned or forgotten when he did begin to mention worries and problems. This case illustrates well the continuity between his flagrant delusion that 'successfully' rescued him from his too painful state and earlier ways of denying difficulties.

Systematized delusion within a normal personality

A psychodynamic approach would not accept without very careful evidence that a systematized delusion could arrive out of an entirely normal personality. It is most likely that most parts of the personality *appear* intact to others, but on careful evaluation there are areas of the mind that cannot bear certain realities and copes with them in a psychotic way. These might well be quite hidden until an event highlights the problem.

A 45-year-old man, D, sought analytic help as part of a decision in mid-life to train as a nurse. On the surface he had maintained a reasonably stable marriage and had four children and had not had previous mental health assistance. The analysis seemed to be proceeding well but after some time the analyst gave 6 months notice that for health reasons, he was not going to continue to be available. The patient was unable to function at the end of this period and sunk into a black unremitting serious depression in which suicide seemed an option. Starting with a new therapist revealed a long-standing delusional belief that had not been consciously communicated. This was that the patient had really become an integral part and equal member of the first therapist's family. A key event in the patient's history was that when he was 7 his mother had left him for some months with his father while she went with his siblings but not him to another part of the country. This had had a radical effect on his self-esteem and left him with powerful envious feelings towards those that stayed with his mother. The delusional belief about his relationship with his therapist had protected him from these unmanageable and violent feelings of being different from the therapist's family members. His decision to work in the nursing field was partly based on a projection of fears of his own needs for care as he grew older and feared he could not rely on his family.

A further example of a delusion operating unconsciously in an otherwise fairly normal personality was a 40-year-old woman, who suffered from anxiety and panic attacks only in relation to a narrow aspect of her work with a voluntary organization for persons with mental health problems. It transpired that these symptoms were related to an omnipotent delusion that she should be able to attend to all the suffering persons that came to her attention and no one should be turned away. In other ways this person was highly effective and creative.

Psychodynamic therapy in both these cases involved a long process.

1. Of helping the nonpsychotic part of the persons to hold on to awareness that the psychotic part of the personality with its delusion beliefs

did not in fact want to come to attention. This was because of the painful feelings of loss, frustration, and destructive envy (in the first case), and that through the delusional belief these feelings would never need to be experienced.

2. Whereby the psychotic parts of the patients tried to recreate their delusional beliefs with the therapists (this is called the psychotic transference).

3. A great deal of careful monitoring was required by the therapists that they did not unwittingly go along with unrealistic expectations. They needed to be sure that they did not also overlook or unduly prevent frustration, disappointment, and envious attacks becoming conscious within the treatment relationship so that integration of these feelings into the personality of the patients was possible with expansion of nonpsychotic capacities.

The following is an example of a psychotic transference that one would normally expect to develop in such a patient:

A 40-year-old female veterinary surgeon C was in a forensic psychiatric hospital for a number of years after she had experienced several psychotic episodes. Her index offense for this admission had been to attempt to pierce a young child in the eye with a needle. Many aspects of her personality were intact, she was sociable and involved in ward life, was competent at intellectual games and kept well informed of events in the world outside. She maintained, however, that she was only in the hospital because the doctors had been poisoning her with their injections for many years and that she was in great pain as a result of these injections.

Over the years the focus had indeed been on a pharmaceutical approach, which had clearly not been successful.

She was offered a weekly session with a psychotherapist and soon developed a psychotic transference in which she had the expectation that the function of her therapist would be to take her side to tell the medical staff of the mistake that doctors had made over many years. The therapist was also to inform the doctor in charge that C was really a brilliant person who prior to admission had invented and written a thesis on new rules for tennis that would make her famous. (It was hypothesized that the attack on the child was related to unbearable envy of the future of the child, in the face of the unbearable truth of her mental illness recurring.)

It cannot be predicted what would have happened if this woman had been given a psychologically informed approach many years ago. However, what was striking in her records is the complete absence of any sign of a member of staff having engaged with her on a long-term basis to try and process anything of her breakdown and the painful consequences of this, which was all so forcefully attributed to the staff.

Tactile hallucinations in a traumatic case

Mr E was a 19-year-old who had found his first girlfriend in bed with another male friend. He quickly decompensated into a very distressing psychotic state. After receiving psychodynamic psychotherapy much of his mind and his previous functioning recovered but he kept his distance from girls. He was left with tactile somatic hallucinations in his 'thighs', which were especially prominent before going to sleep. The sensations felt like something alien getting inside trying to control him and were sometimes accompanied by 'a knocking at the windows and ornaments on the mantel piece rattling'—'just as if someone was trying to get in!'

He had been unconsciously trying to be rid of sexual thoughts and traumatic memories. The somatic hallucinations in his thighs were an expression of the failure of this evacuation. They were 'trying to get back in'.

E mainly complained about this and hoped that the problem would be 'taken away' and he spent much time seeking expert advice on adjusting antipsychotic medication.

Painstaking work over many months led Mr E to be clear that he was trying to cope with his trauma by happily believing that he could get on with his life 'without girls or any wish for an intimate sexual relationship' (getting rid of the problem). Without apparent conscious connection, he would also tell his therapist frequently how unfulfilled and meaningless he felt his life to be and how distressed he was at seeing others progress in a blissful fashion in their personal lives.

Through slow psychodynamic work, E and his therapist were able to bring these two previously disconnected aspects of his mind in relation to one another. Against much opposition, he could see that any thoughts of a sexual relationship were painfully connected with memories of being interfered with, 'messed about', and let down. He was terrified of a further major psychosis (i.e., he had a double trauma). The ornaments rattling on the edge of the shelf were an unconscious desymbolized expression of repeating the breakdown—the fall—if he let back in the thoughts a sexual girlfriend that he had 'thrown out of the window'.

Key practice principles of family therapy in schizophrenia

Psychoeducative family therapy differs from individual therapy and from therapies based on psychodynamic understandings and methods. The theories in family work do not oppose psychodynamic or psychoanalytic views and a patient can fruitfully receive individual therapy based on a psychodynamic understanding at the same time as he joins family groups. The group leader can be analytical, systemically, or cognitive-behaviorally trained. Often it is easier for a nonanalytic therapist to conduct the sessions, but it is also possible for a psychodynamically oriented therapist to lead family groups as long as the models are not mixed.

The atmosphere in family work is of cooperation, education and practical, pragmatic problem solving. The therapist also reveals more of himself and his private life than one does in psychodynamic psychotherapy.

In the session one not only deals with practical matters, but when one deals with psychological matters one does so in a pragmatic way. If the patient talks about hallucinations, one tries to find out what situation triggers them, and what can be helpful in dealing with them. The suggestions can vary from changing medication to talk more about it with the individual therapist, and often a combination of suggestions is pursued.

The same attitude is held towards delusions, anxiety, depression, or any other psychiatric symptoms that come into the open.

People with psychosis, and especially schizophrenia can for a phase of their lives suffer from cognitive impairment, and are specially vulnerable to unclear, communication. Psychoeducative family work stresses clear communication, that one is talking for himself and not practicing mind reading. The problem-solving methods used, also are easy to follow when your mind is not optimally functioning. The therapist uses the blackboard and written messages.

This is not only respectful towards the patient and the family, but is a service appreciated on many levels.

Case: parents

Mr and Mrs Field came to the therapist's office for the first time. Their only son had been admitted to the acute ward 3 days before, after he had spent 3 weeks in bed unable to rise and to go to the university where he studied biology.

What Mr Field expressed as his main concern was whether their son Eric would be able to get well enough to pass his exam in 6 weeks. He had always been an excellent student and, although he had been a bit mixed up and withdrawn for the latest month, he had to his father's knowledge attended lectures and been studying diligently for the last 3 weeks.

The mother sat looking down during the father's speech, using the handkerchief often at the corner of her eyes. She looked at the therapist and asked what he thought. Was it serious? How would it be for him being at the hospital? Had they done the right thing admitting him or should they have tried having him home longer?

Here we see the father's denial of the seriousness of the illness and the mothers fear, concern and guilt. The therapist has to take care of both parents on their different levels of insight. He has to take seriously the father's concern of his son's academic career, giving him realistic hopes and giving him

time to adjust to the new situation. The mother is concerned about whether they have done the right thing taking him to the hospital, and the therapist can feel her concern and pressing guilt for other subjects in her mind. He also senses that the mother sees a fuller picture of the situation than the father. At this early phase it is often more important for the therapist to receive and contain than give information. The patient in the beginning of the illness often has enough with his or her symptoms and how to survive from day to day. Perhaps he struggles with the strangeness he feels, and the anxiety that goes with it. He often is skeptical to the health systems explanations and looks for other ways to understand the symptoms. He may not describe the psychosis as an illness, but sees it as an influence from outer factors. He may be confused and losing grip on reality. In this phase the therapist tries to deal with the acute situation and the crisis. The therapist meets the patient and is interested to learn his views, concerns, and his way of seeing things. He tries to explain to him that he sees the patient is trying to explain what is happening to him and that his confusion can be a result of much inner stress and a kind of overload.

Case: family

Anna's parents had followed Anna to the hospital for the seventh admission in 9 years. At the therapist's office they looked a bit lost and gray. They had not been given many opportunities to talk to therapists before and did not know what to think when they were given this appointment. Had they done something wrong? When the opening question was how they felt, tears ran into Anna's mothers eyes. Never had they been asked the question before during the 9 years of Anna's illness. This opened up a well of grief and sorrow, and when the hour had passed they were not halfway through their story. They were given new appointments knowing that dealing with their guilt, shame, and fear would improve the climate at home providing a better environment for Anna on her return. It is important for the therapist to give their guilt attention without blaming, to see their sorrow and still give hope.

Hallucinating in the deficit stage
Case

Jim and his parent are joining a multifamily group for the first year. Multifamily groups allow carers and patients to meet in a supportive and nonstigmatizing manner in which improved understanding and coping can be facilitated. Jim is staying at home spending most of the days in his bed. He takes his time trying to answer his mothers questions and demands, and sometimes she has a hard time getting contact with him. He wants to listen to heavy music played loud, but the rest of the family sets limits to that. In this group meeting the mother brings this up and the group leaders in cooperation with Jim decide this is the problem to address in this group meeting. To see what the problem really is about the therapist has to get a clear understanding of it and go deeper into what makes Jim lie in bed all day. At first Jim could not give an answer. He said he was tired, had no energy and did not want to get up. There was too much noise in the house and it turned out that he often got up to eat after the others had gone to bed. Asking him why he took more to eat in the night he said that the house was quiet and that there was not so much noise and disturbing sounds. The mother commented that he was not afraid of disturbing sounds when he put his music into action. But that is to get peace from all the demands, Jim answered. The demands? Yes, from inside my head. Now it became clear that Jim suffered from auditory hallucinations, and the therapist could ask him more about that. 'What did they say. . . how many voices? 'Other sounds as well... did he know them. . . were they angry?

It turned out Jim had a lot of hallucinations during the day, mostly two voices arguing. They grew worse when he tried to talk to others and demanded him not to listen to his parents. He found that so painful that he tried to avoid such situations where the voices were provoked.

Now the therapist knew what Jim's real problem was and could with the help of the group try to problem solve that, without interpretation of the contents of the voices or psychologically go into what situations provoked them. Medication, walkman, fight back the voices, try to talk to the family about them, just stay in bed or move away from home, were some of the suggestions the group offered for Jim to look into. It was up to him, and his family, which one they wanted to test out prior to the next group meeting.

Hallucinations in a traumatic case

Case

Tina had several flashbacks after a brutal rape. She had suffered from depression with incongruent delusions and commenting voices for years and came from a family with hereditary psychosis. She was raped on her way home from being at the cinema with friends. They had taken a couple of beers before they parted, something very unusual for Tina. The rapist was a total stranger, and had he not been observed from a flat, he would probably have managed to kill her. By the time the police came, Tina was unconscious.

Her mother whom she was living with had by that time a bad period herself and urged Tina to forget all about it as soon as she could. Tina tried. She was offered some help from the health system before the case was on trial, but refused.

After some months the flashbacks, the smell, and the noises came back to her, stronger and stronger. Voices called her whore and drunk. She could not concentrate at work nor sleep at night and had to take sick leave.

At last she agreed to receive help and was together with her parent offered to join a family group. The mother still believed that the best way do deal with it was to forget, and the father believed that Tina should pull herself together and get back to work. Otherwise she would become like her mother, sitting home smoking all day. During the group meeting when Tina's problem was dealt with it turned out the father very much liked to watch crime and action films on TV. This triggered Tina's memories and did not give her peace. The group offered the family many solutions from banning action and crime programs on TV to encouraging Tina to move out. The suggestion the family agreed upon was that the father should watch TV with earphones and turn the TV a bit away from the sofa where Tina used to sit and knit. This was a suggestion where both Tina and the father had to take and give a little and there was an acceptance from the father, which apart from the practical matter of symptomatic improvement also meant a lot symbolically for her.

Delusion within the deficit state

Case

Peter stayed all day in bed looking at the roof. He did not seem either happy or depressed he just lay there. He knew for certain that he was one of the best computer specialists in the world and that both the Pentagon and Israel were looking to employ him. He believed that they sometimes sent messages to the room, messages only he could understand. He had a computer but had not touched it for weeks. Last time he tried everything got mixed up and he took that as a secret sign that he communicated with the outside world in a special way.

He was the youngest in a family of famous academics, and was the only one without an academic career. His parents had always loved him the way he was, even though they did not always understand him. One could not deny that much of the discussion in the family was about the different academic careers.

In the group meeting mother complained about Peter just laying there. Peter said he did not care to get up. Both parents were sitting at their computers anyway, and when his brothers visited they only talked work. Mother admitted that this was true, and so they started problem solving that situation to see if there was anything the family could do to make it more attractive for Peter to join them, without dealing directly with Peters feeling of inferiority and sorrow that made him develop his grandiose delusions.

Paranoid delusions in a normal personality

Case

Luke was a perfectly normal engineer or so most people believed. He was clever at work, likeable, and good humored. He was always working at inventing new machines, and now he was trying to take out a patent on his latest invention, a machine that could create energy from earth. 'Just dig a hole put it in and there will be no need of the electricity or oil industry anymore'. Because of his background and seemingly healthy personality he managed to get publicity about his work

seeking for investors. Those who looked further into the project discovered lots of things that did not go together. Dealing with this problem psychoeducationally would address how he could get a channel for his creativity and wish for fame and money that came from his day dreams, which helped him to survive his extremely deprived childhood.

Very seldom do patients like Luke agree to treatment in a psychoeducative family setting. They usually manage so well in so many fields in their life that very seldom the whole family get engaged in a treatment program. Very often the patient himself will not attend.

Key practice principles of cognitive-behavioral therapy in schizophrenia

Beck (1952) on the cusp of moving from his psychoanalytic practice to his description of cognitive therapy described some of the key practice principles in a seminal case of the psychological treatment of paranoid schizophrenia. In this case reality testing homework experiments were linked to the generation of a psychodynamic case formulation. This was developed following an examination of the antecedents of the psychotic breakdown. The delusion in question was linked to underlying repressed guilt at the schema level 'I am responsible for my father's misdemeanors' and' I should be punished for my weakness' and Beck's patient was helped to understand the formulation and systematically work with the delusion until it eventually receded. This is a classical description of a Type II delusion within an anxiety psychosis.

In terms of CBT the development of a trusting relationship in which collaborative empiricism can flourish is paramount. The pace should be slow to allow for cognitive deficits and ongoing symptomatology, such as hallucinations or delusional preoccupation. There should only be one target problem with one linked homework exercise per session. Patients, except those who are very paranoid, usually appreciate audiotapes of sessions in order that the session can be replayed at home. Indeed, much of the early progress from CBT sessions can arise while trust is developing within sessions through a gradual increase in understanding and gentle realty testing as described in the audiotapes. Therapists should maintain an open mind as they enter these early sessions and be prepared to disclose their own beliefs in relation to a wide variety of subjects from hypnosis and witchcraft to alien abduction and kundalini (chakra energy centers) phenomena. Often the therapist will have to say quite honestly 'I don't know much about this' 'let me go and photocopy some articles which we can discuss next week'. Sessions should be variable in length depending on levels of concentration, stage of therapy, and level of symptomatology. The agenda needs to be carefully set and it is usually necessary to work with the patient's model or explanation for their symptoms before working up other possible explanations for testing. Avoidance of confrontation or collusion along with strategic withdrawal in the case of any exacerbation of symptoms are important strategies. The therapist should be honest, open, clear, and empathic and should be prepared to share their own views and opinions. Humor often helps improve the quality of the therapeutic alliance and makes sessions memorable. Both therapist and patient should be prepared to undertake homework for the next session. A key strategy is to use normalizing to decatastrophize and destigmatize schizophrenic symptoms. Often the cognition surrounding the label of schizophrenia is so anxiogenic that the primary symptoms of schizophrenia, for example hallucinations and paranoid delusions, are exacerbated. Such anxiogenic automatic thoughts might include 'I will be a danger to others' or 'I am a psycho' and 'I will be locked up'. Normalizing stresses the fact that voice hearing is very common in the general community for example in sleep deprivation (Oswald, 1974) or in hostage situations (Keenan, 1992). Normalizing is extremely useful in not only making the patient feel less stigmatized and less alienated but can also actually improve their ability to cope with their hallucinations as they begin to take a less catastrophic view of them. Once the therapeutic alliance is established with viable joint working and the development of trust develops then examination of the antecedents of the psychotic symptoms can begin in order for the patient to develop insight into their vulnerabilities and the stressors that tipped them in to these particular psychotic symptoms. Further exploration of childhood experiences can allow a full case formulation to be developed and shared with clarification of underlying schemas.

For example,

Therapist: 'the Christ thing' . . . how did this happen? how did you come to hold this belief'

Patient: I lost my job then the wife left. . . .

Therapist: How did you feel? it sounds like a really rough time for you?

Patient: I was really low and then really nervy and upset . . . .

Therapist: What happened next?

Patient: I was trying to read the bible to get some answers but kept getting more anxious about it all . . .

Therapist: What then?

Patient: I had not slept for two nights and then I started to feel kind of strange (*delusional mood*) and then I saw a cross of clouds in the sky and realized that my problems were linked to the fact that I was the second coming of Christ.

Explanation of this man's childhood revealed that he had always believed that he was a failure (due partly to the critical comments of his perfectionist father) and throughout life he had striven to cope with this by striving for success. The invalidation of his achievement schema due to a series of life events led to increasing anxiety, delusional mood, and the eventual crystallization of a grandiose delusion to protect against the underlying core maladaptive schema, i.e., 'I am a failure'. Armed with the above formulation a direction of therapy becomes apparent with the possibility of the emergence of depression in due course. Once a formulation has been agreed and developed in homework sessions symptom management is then the next step. Within the deficit syndrome (sensitivity disorder) hallucinations are usually dealt with throughout the following series of steps.

Critical collaborative analysis of voice origin

Usually such patients presume that others can hear their voices and have not checked out on their geographical location. This is usually linked to avoidance of engagement with the voices and impaired coping. If the voice is active during the session this should be seen as a great opportunity and the therapist and patient can search the immediate vicinity of the consulting room to look for the source of the voice. Thereafter a list of possible explanations for the phenomenon can be constructed together. Audiotaping during the session when the voice is being heard by the patient should lead to a negative result when the tape is replayed, which can be greatly reassuring to the patient who is often embarrassed by the voices' content. The next step would be to take a baseline recording of voice activity using a simple voice diary to detect any fluctuations of the voice hearing experience. Such a recording is usually a mater of some interest to patients and they are usually agreeable to write down the various fluctuations in the intensity of the voices. Review of the diary usually shows times of silence or greatly reduced voice intensity linked to certain affects and behaviors. Continuing to use the voice diary combined with an activity schedule can allow a coping strategy, for example, increase socialization to be tested during the following week.

Therapist: It looks like the voices are more in the background at certain times . . .

Patient: Yes when I was playing the computer game it was easier to ignore them . . . they went right down when I was playing pool in the pub with my friend . . . when I was bored and sitting on my own at home they were a real pest.

Therapist: Okay so lets give the voices a score out of 10 for how much of a pest they are and lets do 1 hour of the computer game each afternoon and 30 minutes of sitting being bored each day at night and lets see what happens.

Voices that are not traumatic in origin usually show some benefit from these simple techniques and lead to an increase in perceived control and self-efficacy. The affect linked to the voice hearing is often a potent reinforcer.

Therapist: When you were in the corner shop and the voice was talking about you, what were you doing and how did you feel?

Patient: I was trying not to look at anybody and I felt annoyed and embarrassed . . . .

Therapist: What was going through your mind?

Patient: I was thinking 'how dare they why pick on me' and 'its not fair what if somebody else hears that'.

Therapist: So you normally run out when this happens

Patient: Yes

Therapist: Can you remember when we tried to tape the voice? There was nothing to be heard on the tape and I know that you have asked your GP and he said that he could not hear them . . . is that right?

Patient: Yes no one seems to say that they can hear them.

Therapist: So maybe they are really caused and worsened by stress and if you get angry then you are more stressed. Lets try and see if we can stay in the shop a bit longer and talk ourselves through it and bring the anger down. What could you say to yourself to make yourself less angry?

Patient: I could say, 'it is just me being stressed' and 'no one else can actually hear them' and 'I will stay in the shop and see if they start to settle down a bit'.

Usually a normalizing explanation linked to behavioral experiments in cognitive homework as described will often show clear benefit. Voices, however, can be linked to underlying schemas and then it is helpful to use rational responding linked to schema level work.

Therapist: You came to believe early on in life that you were different from other children is that right?

Patient: Yes at school I was bullied . . . .they said I had 'the touch' if any of them touched me they ran away screaming and tried to touch somebody else to get rid of 'the touch'

Therapist: When did this all start?

Patient: I was in hospital with really bad measles and my skin was marked for a number of months thereafter . . .

Therapist: So what do these voices say?

Patient: They say 'she is ugly', 'don't go near her keep away'

Therapist: We know how cruel children can be but the voices sound like they were from that very early time of your life . . .

Patient: Yes the voices are children's voices . . .

Therapist: This is obviously a painful subject would you like to do some work on this?

Patient: Yes okay (*upset*)

Therapist: In terms of how different you believe yourself to be from others where would you place yourself on this scale from completely different to completely the same as others? (*use of the continuum*)

Patient: Points to the extreme different end of the scale and also places the Elephant Man and Pinocchio at that end of the scale.

Therapist: Why not over the next week answer the voices gently back by talking to them, for example, 'I have left that time of my life behind' 'I am not so different really anymore'. Also let's write down in this log how often it actually happens in the course of a week that one of your friends or relatives says or indicates to you in some way that you are very different from others (*positive log*)

The techniques as described above work from superficial to deep and usually will achieve some degree of improved control and reduced distress linked to the voice hearing experience.

Traumatic hallucinosis

The voice-hearing situation is complicated further when there is an underlying trauma, which is congruent with the voice content and with linked schemas. Here there are other maintaining factors, including increased arousal and prominent avoidance of linked stimuli. There can also be abuse congruent visual imagery or even visual hallucinations linked to the voice hearing. If the patient is psychologically robust enough and agreeable to a reliving approach based on imagery linked cognitive work then the trauma can be tackled directly as in posttraumatic stress disorder. Otherwise the core trauma should be left and linked schemas worked with. Such schemas usually include 'I deserved it', 'I am guilty', 'I am bad', or 'I am unclean'.

Type I delusions

These are those in which there is a jump into delusional knowing during the psychotic prodrome often linked to cognitive deficits and negative symptoms. In sensitivity disorder there is a gradual slide into social withdrawal, magical thinking, affective blunting, alogia, and depersonalization with sleep deprivation. In such a state patients will often jump to an explanation of this bizarre change in themselves based on current media topics, which are prominent in newspaper and television reporting in relation to phenomena, which are not fully understood. Religious delusions and witchcraft used to be very common in delusional content but they are now much less so. They have been replace by microchips, satellites and aliens as the subject matter for Type I delusions. Type I delusions have much less of the typical features as described by Jaspers (1963) they are also more straightforward to treat. The patient should be engaged in an open and interested manner and a model of the delusion gently explored and tested out gradually with reality testing both within and out with the session. At times the help of a key worker or carer can be crucial to help the testing out process during the early stages. Guided discovery using Socratic questioning on the basis of the evidence produced will lead to the elucidation of other possible explanations. Confrontation and collusion need to be avoided but the therapist should try to be consistent in their opinions and express word perfect accuracy.

Patient: The republicans have my house under surveillance, there are CIA agents outside in cars . . .

Therapist: You seem very upset there must be a reason for this.

Patient: The CIA have bugged my phone, I am absolutely sick of it.

Therapist: You could be right . . . the CIA are certainly well resourced and do work undercover but how do you know it is the CIA rather than some other organization or some other explanation altogether?

Patient: I just presumed it had to be the CIA.

Therapist: Well let's do some homework on this . . . could you have a think of any reason why you might be under surveillance by the CIA? Also could you check three times a day to see if a car with people in it is actually parked in your street somewhere? I will check in the newspapers to see if the CIA are involved in this neighborhood just now and we can discuss it again at our next session.

Beck (1952) explained the importance of focusing the patient's reality testing on specific areas of enquiry. Examples might be as to what kind of car would they be using, what would they be wearing, what would their facial expressions be like? In relation to Type II delusions, which are rarely linked to negative symptoms, the above approaches are of much less effect and work with the underlying linked schema seems crucial. The delusion in such a case is often a systematized persecutory or grandiose delusion and is usually protective of a strongly emotionally invested underlying schema (Turkington and Siddle, 1998).

Patient: I am in charge of all NATO forces.

Therapist: What might that mean to you (*interested*)

Patient: I can put things right . . . there is so much that has gone wrong. (*entitlement schema*)

Therapist: Why would that be so important?

Patient: I was always the black sheep of the family, dad never gave me a fair deal (*anger and distress*)

Here the inference chain has led very quickly to an underlying core maladaptive schema of being the black sheep of the family and a compensatory schema of a demand for entitlement. This man's systematized grandiose delusion emerged in his mid-forties after he was dismissed from his rank as a Corporal in the US air force. He had devoted his working life to the air force and he had stood up against what he believed was unfair treatment of a colleague who had died in the course of service. He believed this was due to the negligence of his superiors and after he had attempted to prove this by writing and publishing a report saying so he gradually developed increasing anxiety and the emergence of the grandiose delusion when his claims were denied by superior officers. Here work on entitlement would allow the grandiose delusional system to start to become less prominent with the emergence of depression over the underlying core schema of being the black sheep of the family.

Thought disorder sessions

These need to be briefer as they are hard work for both therapist and patient. The intermingled themes can often to a degree be disentangled on review of a videotape of the CBT session. A videotape analysis also allows a review of body language at times of increased arousal in relation to certain themes. It can usually be discovered that there is one key theme that is driving the thought disorder (Turkington and Kingdon, 1991). Thereafter the sessions are organized using focus linked to explanation, education, and rapid responding to reduce the key driving affect behind the thought disorder. Thereafter, whenever the patient jumps from 'x' to 'z' as in a knight's move jump the therapist brings the patient back to clarify the link by asking him to explain the links between 'x' and 'z', i.e., to put in the 'y'. Patients can usually do this. Work is focused thereafter on the main driving theme along with thought linkage and this usually allows a thought disorder to become more comprehensible and for progress to be made towards a formulation and symptom management.

Difficult situations and solutions

Capgras syndrome

Certain delusions such as Capgras and Cotard can have either functional or organic origins. A full neuropsychological assessment is often necessary to rule out cognitive deficits. In the case of Capgras, which is linked to neurocognitive deficit, a combination of cognitive remediation and CBT techniques may be the most effective. In those cases where the delusion is assessed to be more determined by its psychological function, suitability will be assessed in a similar way to other functional psychotic problems.

Folie a deux

This is a situation in which both parties will change at different rates if they are separated and treated individually. Here the partner who through separation is released from the pressure of the dominating psychosis in the other can in time be of a great help to the psychotic partner in gradually testing out the key psychotic material during homework assignments. Both partners should be included in therapy.

Othello syndrome or the delusion of morbid jealousy

This dangerous delusion often arises in the setting of alcohol dependence or as a psychotic deterioration in a personality disorder where jealousy or envy has been a central feature whether manifest or latent. The alcohol condition would need to be treated as much as possible either before or alongside engaging or on the underlying belief of inadequacy at the schema level.

Schizoaffective disorders

These require a combination of the approaches that are so well described for CBT of bipolar disorder (Scott, 2002) and that described for schizophrenia (Kingdon and Turkington, 1994; Fowler *et al.*, 1995). Schema vulnerability can include schemas of specialness, which can underpin mania, and schemas of worthlessness, which can underpin depression. A number of schizoaffective patients hold core beliefs about specialness and worthlessness simultaneously. Therefore, both coping strategies, relapse prevention, and formulation work leading to schema level work are all pertinent to schizoaffective disorder. The coexistence of specialness and worthlessness schemas fits in with psychodynamic views of their dynamic relation to one another and indicates that self-esteem would be a central focus if longer-term psychodynamic work proves to be possible once the more extreme psychotic manifestations have settled.

Somatic delusions are often linked to somatic hallucinations and to trauma

Patient: I have a snake in my abdomen

Therapist: How do you know that it is a snake?

Patient: I feel it moving in my lower tummy I also feel it trying to get out (*somatic hallucination*) and there is a vague pain in that area of that body . . .

Therapist: Do you experience anything else when this happens?

Patient: Yes I smell the oil from my uncle's clothes he used to baby-sit regularly when I was younger . . . . (*disclosure*)

Here the symptom complex is linked to sexual trauma, which is worked with as under traumatic psychosis as described above.

Command hallucinations

These behave like obsessional thoughts both in terms of content (sexuality, violence, religion) and in terms of the patient's response with anxiety distress and avoidance.

Patient: The voice tells me to pick up a fork and stab the man beside me at dinner whenever I am trying to eat in the kitchen in the hostel

Therapist: How do you feel when that happens?

Patient: I feel very tense and I very quickly run out of the kitchen area

Therapist: Would you like to attempt to work with this to cope better with the voice?

Patient: Okay

Therapist: Let's look at the situation in your imagination now and see if we can cope with it a bit better. Everybody gets the odd violent thought (*normalizing*). These are obsessional thoughts and people hardly ever actually do these things. Having the thought is not the same thing as doing the action. Why not say to yourself that the voice is like one of these obsessional thoughts . . . it is just a thought caused by stress. If you stick with it then it will gradually settle down and pass over.

Patient: I have tried it in imagination and after a few extra minutes it did start to settle down

Therapist: Okay lets repeat the imagination exercise for 10 minutes every day and see how it feels by the end of the week.

Specific indications for particular therapies

Early intervention

The most viable early intervention approach seems to involve (McGorry *et al.*, 1996) individual and group support with normalizing and use of basic CBT reality testing techniques as described above. The family should be kept fully informed of the strategies being used. The needs-adapted model incorporates psychodynamically informed supportive psychotherapy along with family therapy with a prominent emphasis on continuity of care.

The need-adapted model was developed by psychoanalysts. The central psychoanalytic components are (1) the ongoing detailed assessment of the unconscious psychodynamics of the case, on the basis that most psychotic breakdowns are the result of an overwhelming of the mind by unbearable affects from trauma, loss, and/or developmental strains, sometimes in a biologically vulnerable individual, and (2) establishing long-term therapeutic relationships are central to the treatment method. The psychoanalytic concepts of containment and countertransference are a central component of sophisticated therapeutic ego support until the patient is ready to take back projected aspects of the self. Other aspects of the need-adapted approach are not strictly psychoanalytic—but the essence of the overall approach is: (1) that there is a full complement of treatment resources available so that the most relevant intervention is offered at a particular phase of the therapy—need adapted; (2) low-dose medication is used as an aid when necessary in order to maintain the capacity for psychotherapeutic work; (3) the purpose of therapy is to go beyond psychotic manifestations and help the person (with assistance from the families where indicated) to attend to developmental impasses, disturbances in self and interpersonal relations and manage as full a range of affects as he or she can using the most appropriate interventions; and (4) a realistically hopeful attitude is essential and this includes an expectation that many normal aspects of living will be achieved including a capacity to work. Further details are in Alanen (1997).

This form of early intervention has given rise to the most robust medium-term durability results. For example, Alanen's latest reported cohort treated in Turku by the need-adapted method found that at 5 years 82% were without sickness benefits, 57% were in active work, and 61% were without psychotic symptoms (Alanen, 1997).

Acute relapse

The jury remains out as to which are the most appropriate psychological strategies in relation to working with those patients with acute relapse in schizophrenia. The excellent results of Drury *et al.* (1996) in terms of treatment of emerging psychotic symptoms were not replicated in the more powerful and well designed Socrates study where CBT was compared with supportive counseling and treatment as usual (Lewis *et al.*, 2002). In this study the end of therapy results showed that supportive counseling and CBT were both more effective than treatment as usual in reducing overall symptoms and that CBT was significantly more benefit in reducing hallucinations. It would certainly seem clear that a psychological treatment is crucial in the management of acute relapse to improve symptomatic scores at time of discharge. Further research should be undertaken to elucidate further the most effective psychological treatment modality in the setting of acute relapse. In many cities inpatient wards have lost their therapeutic potential and are highly disturbing environments when tranquillity and friendly unhurried environments are essential. It is to be hoped that low stimulus temporary accommodation in the community suited to the age of the patient will be more available, but much will depend on the quality of staffing (Barker, 2000).

Pitfalls and therapy

Patients who are extremely psychotic and insightless often drop out of therapy early on. As many as 12–15% of patients with schizophrenia drop out in this way and psychological treatments cannot be further considered until a period of stabilization is achieved often requiring intensive home treatment and the use of antipsychotic medication or a period of inpatient care. Sudden jumps in insight can also lead to periods of increased depression often due to catastrophic cognition sometimes linked to the label of schizophrenia or to awareness of traumatic events leading up to the psychosis. Such cognitions need to be adequately dealt with in session or drop out may ensue. Sessions need to be tailored to individual needs working from superficial to deep and with the use of appropriate homework exercises. The use of techniques both in terms of homework or reality testing, which are too penetrating, can also lead to disengagement. It would also appear likely that certain ethnic groups have greater difficulty in working psychologically than do others. Within the brief CBT in the community study, Turkington *et al.* (2002) described that black African and African Caribbean patients were much more likely to drop out of the therapy than were the Caucasian patients. There is also evidence that Chinese schizophrenic patients for cultural reasons find talking therapies to be more difficult (Chan, 2003). Many patients are also very sensitive to loss and every effort needs to be made to ensure the stability of the teams and of the key staff involved that patients have the best relationship with.

Conclusions

It would seem therefore that psychological treatment in schizophrenia has a viable evidence base across the spectrum of schizophrenic symptoms. Certain modalities of psychological treatment alone and in combination would also appear to be viable at different stages from the prodrome all the way through to treatment resistance. We would now appear to need more carefully designed trials to get more reliable indicators as to which patients will most benefit most from which approaches, for example, psychodynamic psychotherapy and/or cognitive behavioral therapy compared with treatment as usual in chronic schizophrenia. These trials would need to reach agreement on outcome criteria and be able to identify therapist variables, including the important nonspecific components that are part of all psychotherapeutic endeavors (Paley and Shapiro, 2002). We also need to test combinations of treatment that include cognitive remediation and family therapy to find the most effective combinations. In terms of trial design there is a great need for much more in the way of pragmatic trials such as that of the Parachute Project (Cullberg *et al.*, 2002) and the Finnish multicenter trial (Lehtinen *et al.*, 2000), which would allow results to be more generalizable into the general clinical population of schizophrenic patients in the community. The Cullberg study is a large multicenter one that indicates that even after only 1 year the need-adapted model led to a reduction in use of inpatient beds and neuroleptics compared with a high-quality control group. The Finnish study indicated good treatment outcomes at 2 years for a whole population of first episode psychosis patients using the need-adapted approach and little more than half the patients needing antipsychotic medication at any time.

Wider implementation of these psychological treatments will require changes in the education programs for all mental health professionals and the development of robust local supervision systems and whole system management. The advances described in this chapter in relation to psychological treatments for schizophrenia have been paralleled by improvements in antipsychotic medication and by some understanding of the biological substrates involved in schizophrenia. These rapid advances herald an era of renewed hope to these patients with this most feared psychiatric diagnosis.

References

Alanen, Y., *et al.* (1991). Need-adapted treatment of new schizophrenic patients. Experiences and results of the Turku Project. *Acta Psychiatrica Scandinavica*, **83**, 363–72.

Alanen, Y. (1997). *Schizophrenia. Its origins and need-adapted treatment*. London: Karnac Books.

Barbato, A. and D'Avanzo, B. (2000). Family interventions in schizophrenia and related disorders: a critical review of clinical trials. *Acta Psychiatrica Scandinavica*, **102**, 81–97.

Barker, D. (2000). *Environmentally friendly? Patients' views of conditions on psychiatric wards*. London: Mind.

Barrowclough, C., *et al.* (2001). Randomized controlled trial of motivational interviewing, cognitive behaviour therapy and family intervention for patients with comorbid schizophrenia and substance use disorders. *American Journal of Psychiatry*, **158**, 1706–13.

Bateson, G., *et al.* (1956). Towards a theory of schizophrenia. *Behavioural Science*, **1**, 251.

Beck, A. T. (1952). Successful outpatient psychotherapy of a chronic schizophrenic with a delusion based on borrowed guilt. *Psychiatry*, **15**, 305–12.

Bion, W. (1957). Differentiation of the psychotic from the non-psychotic personalities. *International Journal of Psychoanalysis*, **38**(Parts 3/4), 266–75.

Bion, W. (1959). Attacks on linking. *International Journal of Psychoanalysis*, **40**(Part 5/6), 308–15.

Birchwood, M., McGorry, P., and Jackson, H. (1997). Early intervention in schizophrenia. *British Journal of Psychiatry*, **170**, 2–5.

Bleuler, E. (1911). *Dementia praecox or the group of schizophrenias*. New York: International University Press.

Bookhammer, R. S., Myers, R. W., Schober, C. C., and Piotrowski, Z. A. (1966). A five-year clinical follow-up study of schizophrenics treated by Rosen's 'direct analysis' compared with controls. *American Journal of Psychiatry*, **123**, 602–4.

Brown, G. W. and Birley, J. L. T. (1968). Crisis and life changes and the onset of schizophrenia. *Journal of Health and Social Behaviour*, **9**, 203–14.

Brown, G. W., Birley, J. L. T., and Wing, J. H. (1972). The influence of family life on the course of schizophrenic disorders: a replication. *British Journal of Psychology*, **121**, 241–58.

Carpenter, W. T., Heinrichs D. W., and Wagman, A. M. (1988). Deficit and nondeficit forms of schizophrenia: the concept. *American Journal of Psychiatry*, **145**, 578–83.

Carroll, Z., *et al.* (1998). The effect of an educational intervention on insight and suicidal ideation in schizophrenia. *Schizophrenia Research*, **29**(1–2), 28–9.

Chan, S. W. (2003). Brief cognitive behavioural therapy intervention delivered by nurses reduces overall symptoms in schizophrenia. Commentary. *Evidence Based Mental Health*, **6**, 26.

Crow, T. J. (1980). Molecular pathology of schizophrenia: more than one disease process? *British Medical Journal*, **280**, 66–8.

Cullberg, J., *et al.* (2002). One-year outcome in first episode psychosis patients in the Swedish Parachute project. *Acta Psychiatrica Scandinavica*, **106**, 276–85.

Davies, L. M. and Drummond, M. F. (1994). Economics and schizophrenia: the real cost. *British Journal of Psychiatry*, **165**, (Suppl. 25), 18–21.

Dixon, L. B. and Lehman, A. F. (1995). Family interventions for schizophrenia. *Schizophrenia Bulletin*, **21**, 631–43.

Drury, V., *et al.* (1996). Cognitive therapy and recovery from acute psychosis: a controlled trial: 1. Impact on psychotic symptoms. *British Journal of Psychiatry*, **169**, 593–601.

Ehlers, A. and Clark, D. (2000). A model of persistent P.T.S.D. *Behaviour Research and Therapy*, **38**, 319–45.

Esquirol, J. E. D. (1838). On mental diseases. On hallucinations. Reprinted (1999). In: F.-R. Cousin, J. Garrabé, and D. Morozov, ed. *Anthology of French language psychiatric texts*. Institut Sanofi-Synthélabo.

Falloon, I. R. H., *et al.* (1985). Family management in the prevention of morbidity of schizophrenia: clinical outcome of a two-year longitudinal study. *Archives of General Psychiatry*, **42**, 887–96.

Fowler, D., Garety, P., and Kuipers, E. (1995). *Cognitive behaviour therapy for people with psychosis: a clinical handbook*. Chichester: Wiley.

Freud, S. (1895). *Extracts from the Fleiss Papers Draft H. Paranoia*. In: J. Strachey, ed. *The standard edition of the complete psychological works of Sigmund Freud*, Vol. 1. London: Hogarth Press.

Freud, S. (1911). *Psycho-analytical notes on an auto-biographical account of a case of paranoia*. In: J. Strachey, ed. *The standard edition of the complete psychological works of Sigmund Freud*, Vol. 12. London: Hogarth Press.

Fromm-Reichmann, F. (1950). *Principles of intensive psychotherapy*. Chicago: University of Chicago Press.

Garety, P., *et al.* (2001). Cognitive model of the positive symptoms of psychosis. *Psychological Medicine*, **31**(2), 189–95.

Gould, R. A., *et al.* (2001). Cognitive therapy for psychosis in schizophrenia: an effect size analysis. *Schizophrenia Research*, **48**, 335–42.

Grinspoon, L., Ewalt, J. R., and Shader, R. I. (1972). *Schizophrenia, pharmacotherapy, and psychotherapy*. Baltimore, MD: Williams and Wilkins.

Grotstein, J. S. (1995). Orphans of the 'Real'. 1. Some modern and postmodern perspectives on the neurobiological and psychosocial dimensions of psychosis and other mental disorders. *Bulletin of the Menninger Clinic*, **59**(3), 287–311.

Gunderson, J. G., *et al.* (1984). Effects of psychotherapy in schizophrenia: 11: comparative outcome of two forms of treatment. *Schizophrenia Bulletin*, **10**, 564–98.

Heins, T., Gray, A., and Tennant, M. (1990). Persisting hallucinations following childhood sexual abuse. *Australian and New Zealand Journal of Psychiatry*, **24**, 561–5.

Hinshelwood, R. D. (1989). *Dictionary of Kleinian thought*. London: Karnac Books.

Holmes, J. (2001). *The search for the secure base. Attachment theory and psychotherapy*. Hove: Brunner Routledge.

Jackson, M. (2001). *Weathering the storms. Psychotherapy for psychosis*. London: Karnac Books.

Jaspers, K. (1963). *General psychopathology* (J. Hoenig and M. N. Hamilton, trans.). Manchester: Manchester University Press.

Johannessen, J. O., *et al.* (2001). Early detection strategies for untreated first-episode psychosis. *Schizophrenia Research*, **51**, 39–46.

Jones, C., *et al.* (2000). *Cognitive behaviour therapy for schizophrenia (Cochrane review on CD-rom)* (Version Update software, Issue 4). Oxford: Cochrane Library.

Karon, B. P. (1989). Psychotherapy versus medication for schizophrenia: empirical comparisons. In: S. Fisher and R. P. Greenberg, ed. *The Limits of biological treatments for psychological distress. Comparisons with placebo*. Hillsdale, NJ: Lawrence Erlbaum Associates.

Karon, B. P. and Vandenbos, G. R. (1981). *Psychotherapy of schizophrenia: the treatment of choice*. New York: Aronson.

Keenan, B. (1992). *An evil cradling*. London: Arrow.

Kemp, R., *et al.* (1996). Compliance therapy in psychotic patients: randomised controlled trial. *British Medical Journal*, **312**, 345–9.

Kemp, R., *et al.* (1998). A randomised controlled trial of compliance therapy: 18-month follow-up. *British Journal of Psychiatry*, **172**, 413–19.

Kingdon, D. and Turkington, D. (1994). *Cognitive-behavioural therapy of schizophrenia*. Hillsdale, NJ: Lawrence A. Earlbaum Associates.

Kingdon, D. and Turkington, D. (1998). Cognitive behavioural therapy of schizophrenia: styles and methods. In: T. Wykes, N. Tarrier, and S. Lewis, ed. *Outcome and innovation in psychological treatment of schizophrenia*. Chichester: Wiley.

Kirkpatrick, B., Amador, X. F., and Yale, S. A. (1996). The deficit syndrome in the DSM IV field trial, II: depressive episodes and persecutory beliefs. *Schizophrenia Research*, **20**, 79–90.

Kuipers, E., *et al.* (1997). London-East Anglia randomised controlled trial of cognitive-behavioural therapy for psychosis, 1: effects of the treatment phase. *British Journal of Psychiatry*, **171**, 319–27.

Leff, J. P. (2000). Role of the community psychiatric nurse in the management of schizophrenia. Commentary. *Advances in Psychiatric Treatment*, **6**(4), 250–1.

Leff, J. P. and Vaughn, C. E. (1985). *Expressed emotion in families: its significance for mental illness*. New York: Guilford Press.

Leff, J. P. and Wing, J. K. (1971). Trial of maintenance therapy in schizophrenia. *British Medical Journal*, **3**, 599.

Lehtinen, V., Aaltonen, J., Koffert, T., Räkköläinen, V., and Syvälahti, E. (2000). Two-year outcome in first episode psychosis treated according to an integrated model. Is immediate neuroleptisation always needed? *European Psychiatry*, **15**, 312–20.

Lewis, S., *et al.* (2002). Randomised controlled trial of cognitive-behavioural therapy in early schizophrenia: acute phase outcomes. *British Journal of Psychiatry*, **181**, S91–7.

Lidz, T., *et al.* (1957). The interfamilial environment of schizophrenic patients II: marital schism and marital skew. *American Journal of Psychiatry*, **114**, 241.

Martindale, B. V., Bateman, A., Crowe, M., and Margison, F., ed. (2000). *Psychosis: psychological approaches and their effectiveness*. London: Gaskell.

May, P. R. A. (1968). *Treatment of schizophrenia: a comparative study of five treatment methods*. New York: Science House.

McCreadie, R. G. and Robinson, A. D. (1987). The Nithsdale Schizophrenia Survey VI, relatives' expressed emotion: prevalence, patterns, and clinical assessment. *British Journal of Psychiatry*, **150**, 640–4.

McGorry, P., *et al.* (1996). EPPIC: an evolving system of early detection and optimal management. *Schizophrenia Bulletin*, **22**, 305–26.

McGorry, P., *et al.* (2002). Randomized controlled trial of interventions designed to reduce the risk of progression to first-episode psychosis in a clinical sample with subthreshold symptoms. *Archives of General Psychiatry*, **59**, 921–8.

Meyer, A. (1950). *The collected papers of Adolf Meyer*. Baltimore: Johns Hopkins University Press.

Migone, P. (1995). Expressed emotion and projective identification: a bridge between psychiatric and psychoanalytic concepts? *Contemporary Psychoanalysis*, **31**, 617–40.

Morrison, A. P. (1998). A cognitive analysis of the maintenance of auditory hallucinations: are voices to schizophrenia what bodily sensations are to panic? *Behavioural and Cognitive Psychotherapy*, **26**, 289–302.

Mueser, K. T. and Berenbaum, H. (1990). Psychodynamic treatment of schizophrenia: is there a future? *Psychological Medicine*, **20**, 253–62.

National Institute for Clinical Excellence (2002). *Clinical guideline 1: schizophrenia. Core interventions in the treatment and management of schizophrenia in primary and secondary care*. London: National Institute for Clinical Excellence.

Ogden, T. (1979). On projective identification. *International Journal of Psychoanalysis*, **60**, 357–73.

Oswald, I. (1974). *Sleep*. Harmondsworth: Penguin.

Padesky, C. A. (1994). Schema change processes in cognitive therapy. *Clinical Psychology and Psychotherapy*, **1**(5), 267–78.

Paley, G. and Shapiro, D. A. (2002). Lessons from psychotherapy research for psychological interventions for people with schizophrenia. *Psychology and Psychotherapy: Theory, Research and Practice*, **75**(Part 1), 5–17.

Pestalozzi, J. (2003). The symbolic and the concrete. Psychotic adolescents in psychoanalytic psychotherapy. *International Journal of Psychoanalysis*, **84**(3), 733–55.

Pitschel-Walz, G., *et al.* (2001). The effect of family interventions on relapse and rehospitalisation in schizophrenia: a meta-analysis. *Schizophrenia Bulletin*, **27**, 73–92.

Robbins, M. (1993). *Experiences of schizophrenia: an integration of the personal, scientific and therapeutic*. New York: Guilford Press.

Rogers, C. R., Gendlin, E. T., Kiesler, D. J., and Truax, C. B. (1967). *The therapeutic relationship and its impact: a study of psychotherapy with schizophrenics*. Madison, WI: University of Wisconsin.

Scott, J. (2002). Cognitive therapy for clients with bipolar disorder. In A. P. Morrison, ed. *A casebook of cognitive therapy for psychosis*. Hove: Brunner Routledge.

Sensky, T., *et al.* (2000). A randomised controlled trial of cognitive-behavioural therapy for persistent symptoms in schizophrenia resistant to medication. *Archives of General Psychiatry*, **57**, 165–72.

Sullivan, H. S. (1962). *Schizophrenia as a human process*. New York: Norton.

Tarrier, N., *et al.* (1998). Randomised controlled trial of intensive cognitive behaviour therapy for patients with chronic schizophrenia. *British Medical Journal*, **317**, 303–7.

Tienari, P., *et al.* (1994). The Finnish adoptive family study of schizophrenia. Implications for family research. *British Journal of Psychiatry*, **164**(23), 20–6.

Tuke, J. B. (1889). Lunatics as patients not prisoners. *Nineteenth Century*, **25**, 595–609.

Turkington, D. and Kingdon, D. G. (1991). Ordering thoughts in thought disorder. *British Journal of Psychiatry*, **158**, 160–1.

Turkington, D. and Siddle, R. (1998). Cognitive therapy for the treatment of delusions. *Advances in Psychiatric Treatment*, **4**, 235–42.

Turkington, D., *et al.* (2002). Effectiveness of a brief cognitive-behavioural therapy intervention in the treatment of schizophrenia. *British Journal of Psychiatry*, **180**, 523–7.

Wallerstein, R. S. (1995). *The talking cures*, pp. 139–42. New Haven, CT: Yale.

Wilcox, J. A. and Nasrallah, H. A. (1987). Perinatal insult as a risk factor in paranoid and non-paranoid schizophrenia. *Psychopathology*, **20**, 285–7.

Wykes, T., *et al.* (2002). Effects on the brain of a psychological treatment: cognitive remediation therapy: functional magnetic resonance imaging in schizophrenia. *British Journal of Psychiatry*, **181**, 144–52.

Zubin, J. and Spring, B. (1977). Vulnerability—a new view on schizophrenia. *Journal of Abnormal Psychology*, **86**, 103–26.

15 Eating disorders

Kelly M. Vitousek* and Jennifer A. Gray

Introduction

The kindred disorders of anorexia nervosa and bulimia nervosa present a number of common problems to the psychotherapist. Both: (1) are organized around a characteristic set of beliefs about the importance of weight as an index of personal worth; (2) lead to stereotyped behaviors designed to manipulate food intake and energy expenditure; and (3) disrupt normal physiology, with predictable and sometimes profound effects on psychological and social functioning as well as physical health. The central ideas about eating and weight are often highly resistant to modification, especially in individuals with anorexia nervosa; at the same time, the physical consequences that result from the belief-consistent behaviors of undereating, overexercising, and purging require close attention and sometimes prompt intervention on the part of clinicians.

The distribution of these disorders is approximately parallel, and markedly skewed by sex, age, culture, and perhaps era. Females are disproportionately vulnerable to both conditions, with males seldom representing more than 5% of identified cases. (Because the great majority of individuals with anorexia nervosa and bulimia nervosa are female, feminine pronouns are used throughout the chapter to refer to individuals with these disorders.) Anorexia nervosa usually develops between the prepubertal period and the beginning of adulthood; onset for bulimia nervosa is slightly later, with symptoms commonly emerging in late adolescence through young adulthood. Prevalence rates are low for both disorders, with anorexia affecting up to 0.5% of young females and bulimia present in 1–2%. These conditions are rare in underdeveloped countries, often appearing for the first time during periods of rapid social change associated with exposure to Western culture.

Controversy persists regarding the nature and degree of the relationship between these conditions. The two symptom clusters often overlap concurrently or sequentially. Approximately half of low-weight anorexic patients also binge and/or purge, and substantial proportions cross diagnostic boundaries over the course of their disorder, most often from anorexia to bulimia. The picture is further obscured by the fact that many individuals develop persistent eating disturbances that share features with one or both of these disorders, but fail to match the specifications for either and are consigned to the residual category of 'eating disorder not otherwise specified' (ED-NOS). Some experts argue that the high percentage of unclassifiable cases, the frequent migration of patients across categories, the similarity of symptoms and distribution patterns, and the evidence of cross-transmission of familial risk suggest the operation of common mechanisms (Holmgren *et al.*, 1983; Beumont *et al.*, 1994; Palmer, 2000; Fairburn *et al.*, 2003; Fairburn and Harrison, 2003). To better reflect this reality, Fairburn *et al.* (2003) have proposed a 'transdiagnostic' approach to conceptualizing and treating the eating disorders.

On the other hand, a number of features suggest meaningful distinctions between anorexia nervosa and bulimia nervosa. The disorders are differentially associated with a variety of background characteristics and personality features. In anorexic patients, low weight status dominates the presenting picture and early phases of intervention. Throughout therapy, the disorders are distinguished by the extent to which symptom resolution is desired, attempted, achieved, and maintained. Anorexic individuals are much less likely to seek treatment, to persevere in efforts to change, and to obtain benefit even if they remain engaged. One follow-up of 246 cases treated an average of 7.5 years earlier found that 74% of patients with bulimia nervosa achieved a full recovery at some point during the follow-up period, compared with 33% of those with anorexia nervosa (Herzog *et al.*, 1999). A prospective naturalistic study of 220 eating-disordered individuals found similarly high rates of symptom remission for those diagnosed 5 years earlier with bulimia or ED-NOS, while a substantially greater proportion of anorexic participants retained eating disorder and/or other psychiatric symptoms (Ben-Tovim *et al.*, 2001).

Another distinction that will be evident throughout this review is that the study of these disorders has followed markedly different developmental sequences. Although anorexia nervosa has been the subject of intensive investigation for more than half a century, only a handful of controlled studies of psychotherapy have been conducted. In contrast, treatment research was initiated soon after the designation of bulimia nervosa as a psychiatric disorder in 1980, and has continued to accumulate at an impressive rate.

In the next sections, we will outline three treatment modalities for bulimia nervosa [cognitive-behavioral therapy (CBT), interpersonal psychotherapy (IPT), and pharmacotherapy] and four for anorexia nervosa (family therapy, psychodynamic therapy, CBT, and pharmacotherapy). These were selected on the basis of their prominence in the field and degree of empirical support. Space limitations prevent a more exhaustive review of the full range of approaches proposed, including behavior therapy (BT; e.g., Rosen and Leitenberg, 1982, 1985), feminist therapy (e.g., Orbach, 1985; Fallon *et al.*, 1994; Kearney-Cooke and Striegel-Moore, 1997), nonverbal expressive approaches such as art and movement therapy (e.g., Hornyak and Baker, 1989; Maclagan, 1998), narrative therapy (e.g., Madigan and Goldner, 1999), and solution-focused therapy (e.g., McFarland, 1995). We omit a number of these with regret; however, on balance it seems preferable to include more detailed information about several approaches than to offer thumbnail sketches of all.

Treatment approaches for bulimia nervosa

The central feature of bulimia nervosa is the presence of recurrent episodes of binge eating, defined as uncontrolled consumption of objectively large amounts of food, accompanied by compensatory behaviors intended to prevent weight gain (American Psychiatric Association, 2000). Compensatory methods include self-induced vomiting, laxatives, diuretics, enemas, fasting, and excessive exercise. Bulimia nervosa is subdivided into purging and non-purging types on the basis of the strategies employed. Initially, individuals with this disorder may not view their behavior as problematic, in that the advantage of being able to eat freely without gaining weight overshadows

* The former name of the first author is Kelly Bemis.

concern about the negative ramifications of binge eating and purging. Over time, this perspective is likely to change, as episodes become more frequent and adverse consequences begin to accumulate.

As the following case examples illustrate, bulimia nervosa varies widely in severity and can occur in patients with vastly different levels of global adjustment. For some individuals, the pattern is experienced as an isolated symptom cluster in the context of relatively successful overall functioning; in other cases, life is dominated by the disorder and additional severe psychiatric problems may be present.

Case examples

Sharon is a 24-year-old graphics designer with a 5-year history of bulimia nervosa. She started dieting and exercising rigorously after gaining 12 pounds during her first year in college. Although these efforts initially resulted in the desired weight loss, her success began to erode as she developed a pattern of eating larger and larger quantities of food late at night. After reading a personal account of bulimia in connection with a psychology course, Sharon experimented with self-induced vomiting. At first the act was difficult and painful, and she attempted it only when extremely distressed by the amount she had eaten. Over time, she found the reflex easier to elicit, and binge–purge episodes increased in frequency to their present level of three to five times per week. Although Sharon sought counseling for stress and mild depression while in college, she did not disclose her disordered eating behavior to her therapist. Sharon is now motivated to seek professional help for her bulimia because she plans to move in with her fiancé and fears that she will be unable to conceal her pattern once they are living together.

Emily is a 38-year-old woman with severe, unremitting bulimia nervosa dating back to mid-adolescence. It is probable that Emily briefly met criteria for anorexia when she was 15; however, she received no treatment for her eating disorder at that time, and soon shifted into a pattern of bulimic behavior. She has been hospitalized twice for treatment of her bulimia, excessive drinking, self-injury, and suicidal ideation. At present, her life is dominated by nearly continuous cycles of binge eating and purging, with vomiting induced five to 10 times daily. Emily is separated from her abusive husband and estranged from her divorced parents and two sisters. She is currently subsisting on disability payments and occasional temporary work as a data entry clerk. Emily has seen several therapists on an outpatient basis, but frequently fails to attend scheduled sessions and has never remained engaged in treatment for more than several months. Her present weight is at the low end of the normal range, and she is reluctant to gain for fear of becoming overweight, as she was during childhood and early adolescence; however, she believes that the principal determinant of her bulimic behavior is the need to blunt the pain of her empty existence.

Cognitive-behavioral therapy

Theoretical base

Fairburn's cognitive-behavioral model of bulimia nervosa proposes that the disorder arises from excessive reliance on weight and shape as bases for self-evaluation (Fairburn, 1981, 1997a; Fairburn et al., 1986, 1993b). Extreme concerns about the size and shape of the body, in combination with low self-esteem, lead to increasingly determined attempts to limit the quantity and type of foods consumed. These persistent efforts create physiological and psychological vulnerability to episodes of binge eating. Individuals try to undo these lapses in restraint by vomiting, taking laxatives, and imposing still more stringent exercise regimens and dietary rules; however, resort to these behaviors reinforces the bulimic cycle by triggering distress, diminishing self-esteem, renewing concern about weight and shape, and increasing deprivation. CBT is designed to address each of the principal elements in the model.

Support for the cognitive-behavioral analysis of bulimia nervosa comes from a number of sources, including risk factor research, correlational studies, and some experimental investigations (Vitousek, 1996; Cooper, 1997; Fairburn, 1997a; Byrne and McLean, 2002; Fairburn et al., 2003). In addition, patterns of treatment response are consistent with this model of symptom maintenance. Across therapeutic modalities, the reduction of dietary restraint mediates decreases in bingeing and purging (Wilson et al., 2002). The central role assigned to cognitive factors is affirmed by two findings: dismantled versions of CBT that retain its behavioral components but omit direct work on beliefs are less effective than the full treatment package (Fairburn et al., 1991, 1993a; Thackwray et al., 1993; Cooper and Steere, 1995), and the persistence of distorted attitudes at posttreatment predicts relapse (Fairburn et al., 1993a).

Description

The standard intervention is a structured, manual-based approach that includes 19 individual sessions spanning 5 months (Fairburn et al., 1993b; Wilson et al., 1997). Treatment is divided into three stages, which are characterized by distinct therapeutic goals.

The first phase begins by establishing a therapeutic relationship and presenting the CBT model and treatment rationale. The clinician emphasizes that therapy will address all facets of the eating disorder, with particular stress in the beginning on the importance of reducing dietary restraint. Many individuals with bulimia nervosa hope that therapy will help them excise the unwanted behaviors of bingeing and purging so that they can diet more effectively and achieve a lower preferred weight. The message delivered at the inception of CBT contains both good news and bad news from these patients' perspective. They have not become trapped in their current pattern of behavior because they are greedy or crazy or lack self-control, but because they are attempting to impose unreasonable and counterproductive standards of dietary restraint. Overeating is the normal response to food deprivation in humans and animals alike; indeed, it should not be construed as 'overeating' at all, but as a lawful reaction to conditions of deficit or irregular supply. The unwelcome corollary is that the two goals of eliminating bulimic behavior and achieving a higher level of dietary restraint are incompatible. In order to gain freedom from binge-eating, bulimic individuals must adopt a pattern of regular eating.

Accordingly, the intervention begins with a strong emphasis on consuming (and retaining) the regular, spaced meals and snacks that reduce susceptibility to bulimic episodes. A number of behavioral techniques are introduced during the first stage, including self-monitoring and the scheduling of alternative activities to replace binge-eating and purging (see section on Attention to eating and weight). Patients are also provided with psycho-educational material about dietary restraint, nutrition, weight regulation, and the consequences of bulimia. Some of this information is intended to correct erroneous beliefs about specific bulimic behaviors. For example, laxative abuse is usually based on the assumption that cathartics prevent weight gain by shooting food so rapidly through the intestinal tract that calories cannot be absorbed. In fact, even massive doses of laxatives eliminate only a small fraction of the calories consumed during binges (Bo-Linn et al., 1983). Other psychoeducational material is helpful in underscoring the CBT model or decreasing concern about the consequences of giving up bulimic behavior. For example, while most patients fear that the lessening of dietary restraint will cause substantial weight gain, the evidence shows that the great majority of patients gain little or no weight after a successful course of CBT (Fairburn, 1993, 1995; Fairburn et al., 1993a).

In the second stage, the emphasis on regular eating patterns continues; in addition, patients are asked to start reintroducing excluded foods into their diets and to resume eating in settings (such as restaurants) and social situations that they may have been avoiding. Cognitive restructuring techniques are used to analyze thinking patterns that help sustain symptoms, including dichotomous judgments about eating, weight, and personal performance. Patients are encouraged to review the evidence for and against their beliefs in order to reach reasoned conclusions that can be used to guide their behavior.

The final stage focuses on relapse prevention strategies. The patient reviews the tactics that she has found especially helpful during treatment, anticipates high-risk situations, and outlines an individualized 'maintenance plan.'

Consistent with general CBT principles, therapists combine a directive, problem-solving focus with a collaborative style throughout therapy.

Clients must take an active role in achieving symptom control through collecting data, generating solutions, and practicing new behaviors. An important goal is for patients to develop the skills and self-confidence that allow them to 'become their own therapists' during and after the time-limited course of CBT (Wilson et al., 1997).

Empirical evidence, indications for use, and unresolved questions

The empirical examination of CBT for bulimia nervosa has followed a thoughtful and systematic sequence of investigation. The approach was developed through clinical experimentation with some of the first bulimic cases reported in the literature, and was guided by a clear, concise model of symptom maintenance. It was translated into a manualized intervention and tested in more than 25 controlled trials in a variety of settings against a number of well-chosen alternative modalities. Within 15 years of the time the approach was proposed (Fairburn, 1981), research had begun to examine therapeutic mechanisms, combined and sequential treatment approaches, generality of effects across different patient populations and providers, and dissemination strategies. On the basis of this impressive body of evidence, CBT has earned the status of treatment of choice for bulimia nervosa (Wilson, 1996; Agras, 1997; Compas et al., 1998; Wilson and Fairburn, 1998; American Psychiatric Association, 2000; Cochrane Depression Anxiety and Neurosis Group, 2000; Fairburn and Harrison, 2003).

In the reduction of both core and associated symptoms, CBT is clearly superior to wait-list control conditions, and matches or exceeds all other examined psychological interventions, including psychodynamic therapy, supportive treatment, IPT, BT, stress management, exposure and response prevention, and nutritional counseling. Reviews indicate that CBT results in mean reductions of 73–93% for binge eating and 77–94% for purging; total remission of symptoms is attained by one-third to one-half of CBT-treated patients when results are analyzed on an intent-to-treat basis (Craighead and Agras, 1991; Wilson et al., 1997; Wilson and Fairburn, 1998; Fairburn and Harrison, 2003; Thompson-Brenner et al., 2003). Consistent with the theoretical model that informs the treatment approach, CBT has also been shown to reduce dietary restraint, decrease depression, enhance self-esteem, and produce positive changes on global measures of adjustment and social functioning (Fairburn et al., 1991; Garner et al., 1993; Wilson et al., 1997; Wilson and Fairburn, 1998).

One clear advantage is that CBT works quickly in comparison with other psychotherapies (Wilson and Fairburn, 1998). For example, Wilson et al. (1999) determined that CBT had already produced most of the improvement evident at posttest by the third week of treatment. The rapid gains associated with CBT are also enduring. Reductions in binge eating and purging are characteristically maintained at 6–12-month follow-up assessments (Wilson et al., 1997). In the longest follow-up reported to date, 71% of the participants who had achieved full symptom remission by the end of the active treatment period remained symptom-free an average of 5.8 years later (Fairburn et al., 1995).

Although the positive effects of CBT are robust and stable, it is also well-established that no more than 50% of patients recover completely, while a substantial minority obtain minimal symptom relief from participation in this mode of therapy. Across studies, the half or more of patients who do not attain full recovery through CBT continue to binge an average of 2.6 times per week and to purge 3.3 times per week at treatment termination (Thompson-Brenner et al., 2003). Little is known about the factors that influence response to CBT, as the few variables that appear to be associated with outcome in individual studies are seldom replicated across them (Wilson and Fairburn, 1998). The most consistent predictors of poor response are comorbid personality disorder and high baseline frequency of bingeing and purging. In addition, the strong relationship between symptom reduction during the first few weeks of CBT and eventual outcome provides some rational basis for continuing the standard approach or considering modified, supplementary, or alternative interventions (Wilson et al., 1999; Agras et al., 2000). Unfortunately, there is scant empirical basis for

anticipating that patients who fail to respond to CBT will derive greater benefit from a different treatment approach (Wilson et al., 2000).

Clinical lore holds that CBT is appropriate only for relatively 'simple' cases of bulimia nervosa such as that represented by Sharon, but contraindicated for complex, severe, and/or comorbid symptom pictures, exemplified by the description of Emily. Certainly, Sharon is far more likely than Emily to be symptom-free after 19 sessions of CBT; however, it is a fallacy to conclude that CBT is therefore the wrong treatment for a patient with Emily's symptom profile. Such reasoning holds only if an alternative approach is known to support superior outcomes in comparable patients (Hollon and Kriss, 1984; Wilson, 1995, 1996). No such evidence exists in the treatment of bulimia. A reasonable course for Emily's case might be clinical experimentation with modifying CBT by increasing its intensity and/or duration, and by including additional components to address difficulties with affect regulation (e.g., Segal et al., 2002), self-harm (e.g., Linehan, 1993), and substance abuse (e.g., A. T. Beck et al., 2001; Parks et al., 2001) (see discussions in Wilson, 1996; Wilson et al., 1997 and Fairburn et al., 2003).

More generally, commentators from both within and outside the CBT orientation have suggested that modifications to the basic approach might provide greater benefit to a broader range of patients. Critiques of CBT for bulimia nervosa usually highlight three overlapping limitations. First, the standard intervention is narrowly focused on specific eating disorder symptoms, paying minimal attention to interpersonal issues or generic concerns about self-worth (Hollon and Beck, 1994; Vitousek, 1996; Garner et al., 1997). CBT for other disorders characteristically extends to a wider range of topics as relevant to individual cases, and there is no obvious clinical justification for restricting the scope of CBT for bulimic patients. Second, the manual-based approach relies predominantly on behavioral tactics, with fairly cursory attention paid to the exploration of beliefs and less to the role of affect (Hollon and Beck, 1994; Meyer et al., 1998; Ainsworth et al., 2002). A third and related concern is that CBT appears less effective in reducing patients' focus on weight and shape than in eliminating the behavioral symptoms of bingeing and purging (Wilson, 1999). Greater change might be obtained through more emphasis on cognitive work; in addition, closer focus on body image issues through therapist-assisted exposure and other targeted CBT techniques could be beneficial (Tuschen and Bent, 1995; Rosen, 1996; Fairburn, 1997a; Wilson et al., 1997; Wilson, 1999; Fairburn et al., 2003).

On the basis of these observations, Fairburn et al. (2003) recently proposed a revised model of the maintenance of bulimia nervosa and outlined a broader approach to its treatment. The new formulation is intended to supplement rather than replace the original model, principally through the inclusion of four additional foci, if indicated for individual patients: perfectionism, low self-esteem, mood intolerance, and interpersonal difficulties.

If the standard course of manual-based CBT is not sufficient for all patients, the full treatment may be unnecessary for some (Wilson, 1995; Wilson et al., 1997). The pressures of cost containment and the scarcity of trained specialists have stimulated efforts to find economical, readily disseminable treatments for bulimic patients. Several streamlined interventions consistent with the CBT approach have been evaluated. One of these involves self-help manuals (Schmidt and Treasure, 1993; Cooper, 1995; Fairburn, 1995) designed for direct use by bulimic individuals with or without guidance by a professional or paraprofessional (Fairburn and Carter, 1997; Birchall and Palmer, 2002; Carter, 2002). Another possibility is an abbreviated CBT intervention that can be applied in primary care settings (Waller et al., 1996). Additional alternatives are group CBT that includes all components of the standard model but can be delivered economically to multiple patients (Agras, 2003; Chen et al., 2003) or a shorter group series that presents the psychoeducational content covered in the full approach (Olmsted and Kaplan, 1995).

Each of these approaches has been examined, and the same general conclusion appears to apply across all: truncated and/or group-administered variants of CBT provide substantial benefit to a subgroup of patients, but typically yield lower rates of improvement and remission than the complete individual approach (e.g., Olmsted *et al.*, 1991; Treasure *et al.*, 1994, 1996; Thiels *et al.*, 1998; Mitchell *et al.*, 2001; Palmer *et al.*, 2002; Chen *et al.*, 2003). The appropriate use of self-help and/or group psychoeducation may be as initial interventions in a stepped-care model, with individuals who fail to respond offered a subsequent course of the full treatment; conclusions about brief CBT and a group version of standard CBT are more tentative pending the accumulation of additional data.

Interpersonal psychotherapy

Theoretical base

In contrast to CBT, the use of IPT in the treatment of bulimia nervosa is not predicated on an elegant, disorder-specific model of symptom maintenance. The approach was first applied to this population because it suited the purposes of clinical researchers who needed a short-term, well-specified modality that had minimal conceptual or procedural overlap with CBT. IPT fulfilled these specifications admirably, and was initially selected for comparison with CBT and BT in a trial conducted by Fairburn *et al.* (1991).

Although IPT was in some senses chosen as a foil, it would be unjust to both the researchers and IPT itself to assume that it was meant to be a 'straw treatment' that would make the results of CBT appear more impressive by contrast. IPT was already established as an effective therapy for depressed outpatients (Weissman *et al.*, 1979; Elkin *et al.*, 1989), and would have been a poor bet for investigators seeking an attention-placebo condition. Moreover, if there is no elaborated 'interpersonal theory' of bulimia nervosa, there is substantial evidence that interpersonal issues are implicated in the disorder. Family problems, sensitivity to criticism, conflict avoidance, and concern about social presentation are all prominent in bulimic patients, and binge episodes are often precipitated by interpersonal stress. Therefore, IPT offered a credible alternative treatment that was manual based and approximately matched to CBT in format, yet focused on different issues, employed different techniques, and presumably worked through different mechanisms.

In its original formulation for depressed patients, IPT was also designed as a 'research treatment' that gave structure to the emphasis many clinicians place on their clients' relationships (Klerman *et al.*, 1984). Drawing on Sullivan's (1953) interpersonal approach, IPT makes few assumptions about the variables that produce specific symptom patterns. The rationale for its use across diagnostic categories and clients is that all psychiatric disorders develop and persist in a social context, and are often ameliorated by resolving interpersonal problems. IPT focuses on patients' current social relationships rather than attempting to address childhood issues or enduring personality characteristics (Weissman and Markowitz, 1994).

Description

The adaptation of IPT for bulimia is outlined in several descriptive articles (Fairburn, 1993, 1997b, 2002b; Apple, 1999; Wilfley *et al.*, 2003). Therapy is delivered in 19 sessions over 18–20 weeks, scheduled twice weekly in the first month, weekly for the subsequent 2 months, then in alternate weeks. This represents a slight reduction and rearrangement of the sessions specified for work with depressed patients, in order to align the format more precisely with CBT and BT. With a few exceptions, the intervention for bulimia is otherwise identical to the approach detailed in the IPT manual for depression (Klerman *et al.*, 1984; Weissman *et al.*, 2000). Two changes in content are prescribed: the initial sessions involve an analysis of the chronology and context of eating disorder symptoms; thereafter, discussion of disorder-specific material is actively discouraged to maintain the focus on interpersonal issues. The first of these modifications is entirely consistent with the principles of IPT for depression; however, the second represents a departure that was intended to sharpen the distinction between IPT and CBT/BT (Palmer, 2000). In other applications, IPT does not exclude direct work on current symptoms. As reformulated for bulimia, IPT avoids any reference to eating patterns, compensatory behaviors, and weight concern between the first and last few sessions of the treatment course. If these topics are raised by patients, therapists are instructed to try to 'limit patients' discussion of their disordered eating behaviors to 10 seconds or less' (Apple, 1999, p. 717).

The first phase of IPT is completed in three or four sessions, which are devoted to a thorough assessment of the interpersonal context surrounding bulimic symptoms. Therapist and patient trace the historical association between significant events, relationships, mood, self-esteem, and changes in eating patterns and weight. This review is used to create a 'life chart' that illustrates the connection between experiences and symptoms. The assessment also includes identification of interpersonal triggers for episodes of binge-eating (Fairburn, 2002b).

On the basis of the information collected and organized during this initial phase, therapist and patient identify one or more problem areas that will become the focus of the next stage of treatment. Paralleling IPT for depression, these are drawn from four categories: grief reactions, interpersonal role disputes, difficulties arising from role transitions (such as moving out of the parental home or starting work), and interpersonal deficits. For bulimic patients, the most common targets are role disputes (relevant for 64% of clients) and role transitions (identified in 36%); issues related to grief (12%) or interpersonal deficits (16%) are less often implicated for this population (Fairburn, 1997b).

With reference to the case examples outlined earlier, a natural focus of IPT for Sharon might be her impending transition from living alone to forming a new household with her fiancé. In view of Emily's profound social isolation, therapy might focus on her interpersonal deficits or unresolved issues in her conflicted relationships with her estranged husband and family. Unfortunately, just as the standard CBT intervention may not be effective in Emily's case, patients presenting with longstanding interpersonal deficits are difficult to help through IPT as well (Fairburn, 1997b).

In the final phase of treatment, the patient and therapist review progress to date, discuss remaining difficulties, and anticipate and plan for possible future problems. At this point, patients are encouraged to identify any changes in eating-disordered symptoms over the course of therapy, and to note their linkage to improvements in relationship patterns (Apple, 1999).

Empirical evidence, indications for use, and unresolved questions

In the study that prompted the adaptation of IPT for bulimia nervosa, the approach appeared moderately effective when status was assessed at the end of the treatment period (Fairburn *et al.*, 1991). IPT and CBT were associated with comparable reductions in binge frequency and depression, as well as equivalent improvements in social functioning; however, CBT was more effective than IPT (or BT) in modifying attitudes about weight and shape, and produced greater reductions in dietary restraint and vomiting frequency. Data collected after a 1-year closed follow-up period revealed some surprising trends (Fairburn *et al.*, 1993a). While participants in the BT condition were doing quite poorly, those who had received IPT had caught up to the CBT-treated patients so that the groups had become statistically indistinguishable across all indices of outcome. A similar pattern of results was obtained in a subsequent multisite study (Agras *et al.*, 2000). CBT again outperformed IPT at posttreatment assessment; once more, no differences were discernible by follow-up as a function of continuing improvement in participants previously treated with IPT.

The unanticipated efficacy of IPT at follow-up seemed to raise important questions for models of bulimia nervosa. Clearly, some individuals were able to accomplish significant (if slightly delayed) changes in their eating-disordered behavior even when therapy paid little or no attention to the specific symptoms that prompted them to seek treatment. The different temporal pattern of change also supported the view that these modalities worked through alternative mechanisms. Fairburn speculated that IPT might facilitate change by increasing patients' feelings of self-worth, indirectly lessening their tendency to evaluate themselves on the basis of body shape and weight (Fairburn, 1988, 1997b; Fairburn *et al.*, 1991). This hypothesis appeared consistent with the lag between the active treatment phase and the achievement of symptom control—perhaps it simply took more time for individuals to translate improvements in self-esteem into modifications of their eating behavior.

The intriguing intimation of a delayed treatment response or 'sleeper effect,' however, was disconfirmed by further analyses of data from the second study (Wilson *et al.*, 2002). In fact, the same proportion of patients who remained symptomatic after IPT *or* CBT continued to improve during the follow-up period; thus, IPT appeared to 'catch up' to CBT simply because there were more symptomatic patients left at the end of IPT who were still eligible for a late shift toward recovery. The conjecture that the two treatments work through different mechanisms was contradicted as well. The mediators believed to account for improvement in IPT—improved self-esteem and interpersonal functioning—showed no relationship to symptom changes in either IPT or CBT. Instead, both treatments decreased bingeing and purging through reductions in dietary restraint, with CBT appearing more effective than IPT at posttest because it accomplished this objective more rapidly.

Although it remains unclear how IPT works, the equivalence of IPT and CBT by follow-up supports the conclusion that these modalities are comparably effective (Fairburn, 1993). On that basis, either treatment is a defensible first-choice alternative for bulimia nervosa, with the selection between them influenced by patient and therapist preference, availability of expertise, and the importance of prompt symptom control. Another possibility is that IPT might be reserved as a second-line treatment for patients who do not achieve satisfactory results through CBT. The sole study that has investigated the merits of such sequential treatment, however, was not supportive (Mitchell *et al.*, 2002).

Pharmacotherapy

An eclectic assortment of drugs has been proposed and tested for the treatment of bulimia nervosa, often on the basis of short-lived theories about the nature of the disorder. It was reasoned variously that opiate antagonists might work if patients are 'addicted' to bulimic behavior, anticonvulsants if their 'trance-like' state during binges reflects seizure activity, and appetite suppressants if they are responding to faulty signals of hunger and satiety. Whatever the merits of these models, the medications they recommended proved unhelpful. Only one group of agents, the antidepressant drugs, outlasted the abandoned model that first suggested its use. Although the view that bulimia nervosa represents a variant form of affective disorder (Pope and Hudson, 1984) is no longer tenable, antidepressants make a moderate contribution to its treatment.

Most classes of antidepressant medication have been examined, including tricyclics, monoamine oxidase inhibitors, SSRIs, and atypical antidepressants (Walsh, 2002a). In virtually all trials, these medications have been superior to placebo, yielding consistent and approximately equivalent reductions in symptom frequency and associated features (for reviews, see Craighead and Agras, 1991; Mitchell and de Zwaan, 1993; Compas *et al.*, 1998; Mayer and Walsh, 1998; Wilson and Fairburn, 1998; Peterson and Mitchell, 1999; Walsh, 2002a). In the short-term, binge–purge episodes are reduced by an average of approximately 60% and suppressed completely in about one-third of patients (Compas *et al.*, 1998; Wilson and Fairburn, 1998); however, relapse rates appear to be substantial if drugs are administered on a long-term basis, and astronomical if they are discontinued (Pope *et al.*, 1985; Pyle *et al.*, 1990; Walsh *et al.*, 1991). Although all tested antidepressants offer comparable benefits, fluoxetine is generally favored for its low side-effect profile (Wilson and Fairburn, 1998; Walsh, 2002a).

Interestingly, it has been established that antidepressants do not decrease bulimic behavior through the alleviation of depressed mood. Neither the presence nor the severity of mood disturbance predicts response to medication, and positive effects on bingeing and purging often precede changes in depressive symptoms (Johnson *et al.*, 1996; Walsh, 2002a). Moreover, higher doses of fluoxetine (60 mg/day) are required for the control of bulimic behavior than the levels typically indicated (20 mg/day) for the management of depression (Fluoxetine Bulimia Nervosa Collaborative Study Group, 1992).

Direct comparisons of antidepressants and CBT consistently favor the latter. A meta-analysis indicated that CBT is significantly more effective in reducing binge–purge frequency, modifying attitudes toward shape and weight, and decreasing depression (Whittal *et al.*, 1999). CBT is also associated with lower rates of attrition, greater reduction of dietary restraint, and better

preservation of treatment gains. Only one investigation has suggested modest incremental benefit for simultaneous treatment with CBT and antidepressants (Walsh *et al.*, 1997). Leading researchers in pharmacotherapy for eating disorders conclude that in most cases antidepressants should be used as a second-line treatment for patients who fail to respond to an adequate trial of CBT (Mitchell *et al.*, 2001; Walsh, 2002a). The only two studies that have examined the use of medication as a follow-up treatment reached differing conclusions about its incremental advantage (Walsh *et al.*, 2000; Mitchell *et al.*, 2002).

Treatment approaches for anorexia nervosa

Anorexia nervosa is defined by the assiduous pursuit of thinness through dietary restriction and other weight-control measures, resulting in a body mass index (BMI) substantially below the normal range. As patients' weights decline, their fear of gaining weight paradoxically increases, so that the prospect of going from 89 to 90 pounds may seem almost as intolerable as reaching 150 pounds. Their attitudes toward their current dimensions are complex. On the one hand, many describe feeling overweight even while emaciated; simultaneously, most take pride in their exemplary thinness and may be offended if it is not recognized by others (Bruch, 1978; Vitousek, 2005). The cardinal features of the disorder are ego-syntonic—indeed, they are often fiercely and assertively so. Low weight and restrictive eating are not merely accepted as consistent with the 'real self,' but valued as accomplishments of the 'best self.' Many patients keep this dynamic to themselves; those who discuss it use striking imagery to describe the appeal of semistarvation:

> When I eventually weighed under 80 pounds and looked at myself in the mirror . . . I saw someone beautiful: I saw myself. . . . The clearer the outline of my skeleton became, the more I felt my true self to be emerging. . . . I was, literally and metaphorically, in perfect shape . . . I was so superior that I considered myself to be virtually beyond criticism.
>
> MacLeod (1982, pp. 69–70)

> For me—this is really sick—it's like winning the Nobel Prize or something. It's like you get a kingdom or become a goddess . . . I felt it was to *be* someone, like I was becoming a unique person, creating my own identity. You feel that you are nobody before, and when you starve, you're getting yourself down to the bones: 'This is really me. This is what I am.'
>
> Patient quoted in Way (1993, p. 69)

The ego-syntonic quality of symptoms seems to account for much of the variance in explaining why anorexia nervosa is so distinctively difficult to treat. In most disorders, lack of motivation is considered a 'special problem' in psychotherapy. In anorexia nervosa, however, attachment to symptoms and reluctance to change are not special problems but expected features that affect almost every aspect of treatment with virtually all patients. Without some understanding of this central issue, it is difficult to appreciate why controlled trials of psychotherapy are so rare, attrition rates so high, and results so unsatisfactory. Awareness of the phenomenon also provides essential context for the treatment modalities outlined below, illuminating why family therapy favors external control by parents, why dynamic therapy is usually supplemented with symptom-focused treatment, why CBT expects little attitude change from cognitive restructuring techniques, and why pharmacotherapy has failed to identify any medications (at least to date) that influence the core psychopathology of this disorder.

The achievement of restraint and thinness, however, comes at substantial cost. Patients are haunted by anxiety about the risk of losing control and increasingly constrained by self-imposed rules about what, when, where, and how to eat. These distressing concerns are accompanied by other characteristic symptoms, including depression, irritability, social withdrawal, and sexual disinterest, as well as a host of major and minor physiological disturbances. Most of these symptoms are secondary to semistarvation; all are exacerbated by undereating and weight loss. The pattern that most consistently precedes anorexia nervosa and survives its resolution is a cluster of obsessional and perfectionistic traits (Vitousek and Manke, 1994; Fairburn *et al.*, 1999a; Serpell *et al.*, 2002; Shafran *et al.*, 2002; Anderluh *et al.*, 2003). There is evidence that these features have a genetic basis (Lilenfeld *et al.*, 1998), and some experts believe that they help to account for both the appeal of a narrowed focus on weight control and the capacity to persevere in the demanding routines required.

Data on the course of anorexia nervosa indicate that it can be a persistent, disabling, and sometimes lethal condition. Rapid weight gain can be accomplished in the hospital through operant programs or skilled nursing care, without resort to nasogastric feeding; however, patients often begin losing weight immediately after discharge. When outcomes are averaged across follow-up studies of varying lengths, it is typically reported that somewhat fewer than half of anorexic patients have recovered, while a third are improved but still manifest significant eating disorder symptoms and a fourth remain severely ill or have died of the disorder (Pike, 1998; Steinhausen, 2002; Sullivan, 2002).

These aggregate statistics, however, obscure considerable heterogeneity in the odds for recovery in the individual case (Fairburn and Harrison, 2003). One variable that contributes to the prediction of outcome in anorexia (but less consistently in bulimia) is the duration of illness at intake (Steinhausen, 2002; Keel *et al.*, 2003). In some young patients with a short symptom history, the disorder appears to be either self-limiting or responsive to brief, low-intensity interventions; after the disorder is well-established, it is often highly resistant to change efforts (Wilson and Fairburn, 1998; Fairburn and Harrison, 2003). Comparisons of outcome figures across treatment trials are uninformative without reference to the age and duration of illness of the samples treated—even if the current severity of symptoms appears approximately equivalent, as in the two cases outlined below.

Case examples

Chloe is a 16-year-old high school sophomore who began dieting after her track coach suggested that her performance might be enhanced if she lost 5 or 10 pounds. She immediately reduced her food intake during the day to a single carton of yogurt and an apple, and did her best to avoid eating 'fattening' foods during family dinners. In addition to her track practice, she also began running for an hour each morning before school and doing calisthenics in her room at night. Within several months, she had lost 20 pounds. Chloe was elated by her weight loss (as well as her improved race times), and felt confused and angry when her coach suspended her from the team and contacted her parents after she fainted during practice. On the advice of the family physician, Chloe was initially seen by a counselor who worked with adolescent (but rarely eating-disordered) clients. When Chloe's weight continued to decline, her physician prescribed an antidepressant and referred her to a dietitian for nutritional counseling, to no apparent effect. At that point, she was briefly hospitalized on a pediatric unit for medical stabilization and an attempt at weight restoration. By the time her increasingly desperate parents brought Chloe (figuratively kicking and screaming) to a specialty eating disorder program, she had reached a BMI of 14.5, just over 1 year after the onset of her anorexia nervosa.

Amanda is a 29-year-old English instructor in a community college who has a long history of restricting anorexia nervosa. She was hospitalized for 6 months when she was 20, but lost weight soon after discharge. Amanda maintained a BMI between 15 and 17 for the remainder of her years in college and graduate school. She was in therapy on and off during this period, but studiously avoided any form of treatment in which she would be expected to gain weight. At present, Amanda follows a highly restrictive vegetarian diet, and exercises 2 hours per day. Her life centers around her disorder and her teaching. She lives alone but remains close to her parents, who are resigned to their inability to affect her eating behavior. She has few social contacts outside of work, and rarely dates. After Amanda's weight recently drifted down an additional 7 pounds, her co-workers and physician began urging her to seek help.

Family therapy

Theoretical base

Dominant schools of family therapy have taken a keen interest in anorexia nervosa and had considerable impact on the field (e.g., Minuchin *et al.*, 1978;

Selvini-Palazzoli, 1978; Dare, 1985; Dare and Eisler, 1992). Minuchin's structural model identified anorexia as the prototype 'psychosomatic' disorder, in which family dysfunction (including enmeshment, overprotectiveness, rigidity, and conflict avoidance) is expressed by the symptom-bearing child. The treatment approach featured 'family lunch sessions,' during which the therapist observed family dynamics and carried out on-the-spot interventions. Parents were urged to unite and force their anorexic child to eat—in some instances by holding her down and pushing food into her mouth with the therapist's encouragement and support. The method was widely publicized through the distribution of filmed sessions, which for a time were shown routinely in abnormal psychology classes throughout the United States. Many undergraduates found these disturbing to view—as did most eating disorder specialists. The results Minuchin claimed to have achieved, however, were every bit as dramatic as the sample sessions: nearly 90% of patients were said to be doing well at follow-up (Rosman *et al.*, 1978). Critics have questioned the rigor, representativeness, and even the veracity of these data; many experts also dispute the assumption that family dynamics are uniform or causal in anorexia nervosa (e.g., Yager, 1982; Rakoff, 1983; Vandereycken, 1987).

The most influential contemporary form of family therapy for anorexia nervosa is the 'Maudsley model,' which combines elements from both structural and strategic approaches (Dare and Eisler, 1995, 1997; Lock *et al.*, 2001). Following Minuchin, therapists direct parents to assume control over the anorexic child's eating behavior and orchestrate crises during meal sessions to empower them in this role. The Maudsley approach is more closely aligned with strategic family therapy, however, in favoring an 'agnostic' view of etiology. Family members are charged with responsibility for the anorexic individual's recovery, but explicitly exonerated from blame for her disorder.

Description

As applied to adolescent patients, the Maudsley approach involves 10–20 family sessions spaced over 6–12 months. The 'conjoint' format specifies that all family members—siblings as well as parents and the anorexic child—should be seen together. A recently published manual (Lock *et al.*, 2001) describes the implementation of conjoint family therapy (CFT) in detail. As discussed below, a form of 'separated' family therapy has also been devised and tested.

CFT is divided into three phases, with transition from one to the next dependent on the achievement of specific objectives. The approach is highly structured—indeed, almost scripted, particularly in the early sessions. The key therapeutic maneuver in Phase I is to reestablish parental authority in the family system, with particular reference to asserting control over the anorexic child's eating and weight. Several tactics are adopted to further this goal. Using a sympathetic but authoritative style, the therapist works to heighten the parents' level of anxiety by underscoring the severity of their daughter's condition. In an 'almost ritualistic' fashion (Lask, 1992), clinicians are advised to assume a 'portentous, brooding, and grave manner' (Lock *et al.*, 2001, p. 208) when they greet parents; in the first session, they should 'concentrate on the horror of this life-threatening illness,' (p. 52) warning parents that 'something very drastic has to happen for you to save [your child's] life' (p. 47).

Another recommended technique is the externalization of anorexic symptoms. The disorder is construed as an alien force that has overtaken the patient so completely that she is incapable of controlling her own behavior—and therefore critically in need of her parents' forceful intervention. This 'benevolent dissociation' is intended to assuage parents' guilt about using strong measures to combat the illness, as well as to convey support for the patient as an individual distinct from her disorder (Lock *et al.*, 2001; Russell, 2001).

Parents are asked to bring food to the second treatment session, and coached by the therapist to find ways of compelling their daughter to eat. Outside of therapy, they are advised to keep her under parental supervision 24 hours a day during the first few weeks, temporarily arranging leaves of absence from school and work to accomplish the task of refeeding. External control tactics are also applied to other eating-disordered behaviors; for example, parents are told to lock the refrigerator and cupboard doors if necessary to prevent binge-eating, and to inform neighborhood pharmacies that their daughter must not be allowed to purchase laxatives.

Phase II begins when the patient is surrendering relatively consistently to the demand to increase her intake and weight, typically after 3–5 months of weekly family sessions (Lock *et al.*, 2001). During this stage, the therapist encourages a gradual fading of close supervision and reinforces the patient's return to age-appropriate activities and levels of autonomy. The message is that anorexia nervosa deprived her of the right to make her own choices, as she had functionally regressed to a child-like incompetence and dependency; now that she is beginning to improve, she is entitled to reclaim more control over her life in this and other domains. Parents are asked to focus their attention on strengthening the marital relationship; all members of the family are enlisted in reestablishing 'intergenerational boundaries' between the parental dyad and the children.

Phase III is initiated after the patient demonstrates her capacity to maintain a stable weight without high levels of external control. This stage involves several sessions spaced 4–6 weeks apart. Parents are provided with information about normal adolescent development, and the emphasis on fostering independence continues; however, the therapist also works to instill fear about the possibility that symptoms could resurface, in order to ensure continued parental vigilance to the risk of relapse.

A modified form of family therapy is recommended for adult patients. It is inappropriate (as well as impossible) for the family or partner of an adult patient to seize control of her eating behavior—clearly, the 29-year-old Amanda's parents cannot be advised to hold her down and push food into her mouth. Instead, CFT for older patients focuses on restructuring family relationships so that the eating disorder no longer dominates the picture. This application has not been described in the same detail as family therapy for adolescents and, as discussed below, appears to be much less effective. It should also be noted that in the case of adult patients, a decision to implement CFT does imply certain assumptions about the significance of family dynamics in the maintenance of symptoms. It may well be possible to take an 'agnostic' view of etiology when using the approach with adolescents, as the tactic of enlisting parents as treatment agents can be justified on purely pragmatic grounds. Because adults necessarily retain principal responsibility for the management of their own symptoms, however, a preference for working with such individuals through a family unit that may no longer reside together requires a theory-based explanation. Many individual therapists might schedule a few sessions with the spouse, parents, or friends of an older anorexic patient (generally because she requests it); however, a therapist who elects to see her primarily or exclusively with her family members present is making a much stronger statement about *why* she became or remains ill.

Empirical evidence, indications for use, and unresolved questions

Family therapy is the most extensively researched treatment for anorexia nervosa, contributing at least one cell to half of all controlled trials of psychotherapy. Only one of these studies found family therapy clearly superior to a comparison treatment, and the effect was restricted to patients who carried particularly favorable prognoses by virtue of their young age and brief duration of illness. At least for this subgroup, however, no alternative treatments have been demonstrated to work *better* than some version of family therapy. On the basis of the accumulated evidence, family therapy is the sole intervention that currently meets the standard of an 'empirically supported treatment' for adolescent anorexia nervosa.

The strong association between recency of onset and the likelihood of positive response to family therapy was evident in the first trial conducted by the originators of the Maudsley approach (Russell *et al.*, 1987). In that study, CFT was much more effective than a supportive, dynamically oriented individual therapy with a subset of patients who had become anorexic before the age of 19 and been symptomatic for less than 3 years. The effects of initial treatment were still discernible at 5-year follow-up: 90% of those who had received CFT were classified as 'recovered,' while 45% of the patients originally allocated to individual therapy remained anorexic or bulimic (Eisler *et al.*, 1997). In contrast, family therapy was neither effective nor differentially effective for other subsets of patients who had a longer history or a later onset; in fact, there was a tendency for the latter group to do better in individual therapy, although few patients responded well to either treatment.

Subsequent research has confirmed the importance of short duration as a predictor of response to CFT. Indeed, the data suggest that the window for successful intervention is even narrower than the 3-year period used to form subgroups in the Russell *et al.* (1987) study. In a project carried out by the same investigators, all participants had been anorexic for just 2–36 months, with an average duration of 12.9 months and a mean age of 15.5 years (Eisler *et al.*, 2000). Even within this extremely restricted range, there was a significant correlation between how very recent onset had been and treatment outcome in either of two forms of family therapy. Patients who were doing well at 1 year had been anorexic for a mean of 8 months at the inception of treatment, compared with 16 months for those with intermediate or poor outcomes. Another historical variable was also linked to treatment response. When patients who had received repeated prior treatment on an inpatient or outpatient basis were compared with those obtaining therapy for the first time, the contrast was again sharp: 73% of the treatment veterans did poorly in family therapy, while only 19% of the novices failed to improve.

The significance of these data is underscored when we consider their implications for the sample cases of Chloe and Amanda. There is no reason to anticipate that 29-year-old Amanda would respond to family therapy; indeed, she falls into the category of adult patients for whom individual therapy appeared slightly—if rarely—more effective in the initial study. Chloe, however, seems to match all specifications for the empirically supported treatment of CFT: the onset of her disorder was squarely in the middle of adolescence, she has been anorexic for just over a year, and she is still living at home in an intact (and concerned) family. If we try to extrapolate her prognosis from the figures provided by Eisler *et al.* (2000), however, Chloe's outlook appears less sanguine. At a duration of 13 months, she falls right in between the group of patients for whom family therapy was found to be effective and those for whom it was not. The fact that she has already been a treatment failure elsewhere is ominous as well. Even though the nonspecific therapy, nutritional counseling, drug treatment, and brief hospitalization to which she has been exposed may not represent particularly promising interventions for her disorder, their presence on her treatment record consigns her to the category from which only one-fourth of patients will emerge as successful responders to family therapy.

This pattern could have a number of plausible explanations, and the alternative possibilities hold different implications for how we should view the results of family therapy. In the early stages of anorexia nervosa, patients may not yet have crystallized their identities around the disorder, and it is conceivable that it is easier and more efficacious to exercise external control over the expression of symptoms in such cases. It is also possible that early intervention appears to work better in part because we end up counting among our 'treatment successes' the subset of patients whose disorders would be self-limiting with or without professional (or parental) intervention.

Although it is clear that family therapy is effective principally for briefly ill anorexic patients, it has not been established that it differs from other forms of treatment in this regard. It may well be that alternative approaches are comparably constrained. Certainly, the general pattern of correlation between duration and outcome obtains across most of the treatment trials and uncontrolled follow-up studies reported in this field; however, few have analyzed data with sufficient precision to confirm or disconfirm the stark association between months of symptom persistence and treatment response evident in Eisler *et al.* (2000).

The view that family therapy is *preferentially* indicated for the treatment of recent-onset anorexia nervosa depends on the demonstration that it resolves such cases faster or more completely or in a higher proportion of patients than alternative therapies. The answers to those questions are less clear than the wide disparity found by Russell *et al.* (1987) suggested. The pronounced superiority of family over individual treatment in that initial study—evident even with samples of 10 and 11 patients per cell—certainly offered a compelling basis for further investigation. Commendably, proponents of family therapy did continue to examine the method they advocate; inexplicably, however, they stopped comparing it with anything else. The Maudsley group never tried to replicate their remarkable finding with larger samples or alternative forms of individual therapy. Instead, they embarked on a series of intramural studies comparing different formats and intensities of family therapy (le Grange et al., 1992; Lock, 1999; Eisler et al., 2000), as if the case for its superiority over other modalities were already amply documented.

Three different teams of investigators did take up some of the basic questions bypassed by the Maudsley group, with mixed results. Two studies revisited the question of family versus individual treatment. When individual therapy was operationalized in the form of an 'ego-oriented' approach in one trial, family therapy (combined with some CBT elements) appeared slightly but not durably more effective with a sample of adolescent patients who had been ill for less than a year (Robin et al., 1994, 1995). When the individual treatment condition was CBT, both modalities yielded equivalent and fairly positive results with adolescent and young adult patients, with no trends favoring either approach for any subgroup (Ball, 1999). A third study found no differences between eight sessions of family therapy and eight sessions of group family psychoeducation when these were provided adjunctively in connection with inpatient treatment for adolescents (Geist et al., 2000).

Interestingly, the intramural research to which the Maudsley investigators turned did identify one mode of treatment that appears superior to CFT: an alternative format for delivering the same Maudsley message. In two studies, the standard 'conjoint' approach was compared with 'separated' family therapy (SFT), in which parents and the anorexic child were counseled in different sessions (le Grange et al., 1992; Eisler et al., 2000). In parent meetings, the therapist provided advice consistent with the parental control strategies of CFT, while anorexic patients received supportive individual therapy that could include discussion of both family and eating/weight issues. On theoretical and clinical grounds, SFT was clearly expected to prove weaker than CFT, as it offered no direct opportunities to observe and intervene in family dynamics, did not include meal sessions, and did not involve siblings.

Across both trials, however, there was a trend favoring SFT over CFT. In the second and larger project (Eisler et al., 2000), nearly twice as many patients achieved a 'good' outcome through SFT (48% versus 26%), while fewer than half as many patients did poorly (24% versus 53%). This effect was accounted for by the subset of families in which parents frequently directed critical remarks toward the anorexic child. When subgroups of cases high and low in expressed emotion (EE) were compared, SFT was significantly and strikingly more effective than CFT with high EE families, benefiting 80% versus 29% of the patients treated; for low EE families, no trend favored either format.

It is commendable that the Maudsley investigators put themselves in a position to learn that their assumptions about what works best for anorexia nervosa were mistaken. To date, however, their response to these unusually decisive results has been disappointing—both for this specialty area and the evidence-based treatment movement as a whole. Their own findings indicate that SFT is a slightly better treatment option overall and a dramatically better one for patients with the misfortune to come from contentious families. Yet the Maudsley group recently published a manual that strongly advocates the less effective conjoint format (Lock et al., 2001), and is using that approach rather than SFT in ongoing research (Lock, 1999). At present, then, a curious anomaly attaches to the empirical standing of family therapy for anorexia nervosa. CFT is at once the best-supported treatment for recent-onset adolescent patients—and one of the very few 'active' modalities in the field that has been found inferior to an alternative approach. A therapist who was committed to practicing validated treatments should indeed adopt the Maudsley model for cases matching the profile of Chloe; ironically, however, he or she should not adhere to the manual written to

disseminate the approach, as it describes a version of family therapy that has been shown to disadvantage a sizeable subgroup of the patients to whom it is applied.

More broadly, it should be noted that no study has yet examined the merits of the specific type of family intervention espoused in the Maudsley model. Across orientations, most specialists advocate working with parents when treating individuals in the young-to-mid-adolescent age group, sometimes using principles and techniques quite different from those associated with the Maudsley model. Only direct comparisons can illuminate which of these should be preferred. At present, all that can be stated with some confidence is that seeing family members together does not contribute to positive outcomes, and is contraindicated for a subgroup of particularly vulnerable patients.

Psychodynamic therapy

Theoretical bases and treatment descriptions

Psychodynamic approaches do not fit comfortably into the format used to profile other modalities in this chapter. The difficulty is that there are too many alternatives to cover, none of which is dominant in the eating disorder field. They differ so markedly that there would be multiple 'theories' and 'treatment descriptions' to summarize under the section subheadings, while the 'empirical evidence' that has been collected bears only on the specific variants tested.

In this specialty area, the designation of a treatment approach as 'psychodynamic' conveys little information about the conceptual model that guides it or the techniques it subsumes. Drive-conflict, object relations, and self-psychological models disagree about why people become anorexic and how they should be helped to recover (Goodsitt, 1997). According to different accounts, self-starvation is a defense against oral impregnation or aggressive fantasies (Waller et al., 1940/1964; Masserman, 1941; Freud, 1958; Szyrynski, 1973), a reaction to maternal impingement and/or hostility (Masterson, 1977; Selvini-Palazzoli, 1978), or a desperate attempt to organize and empower the self (Bruch, 1973; Casper, 1982; Goodsitt, 1985, 1997; Geist, 1989; Strober, 1991). Therapists may be advised to interpret the meaning of the patient's symptoms (Thoma, 1967; Sours, 1974, 1980; Crisp, 1980, 1997) or to offer her a healing relationship with a caring adult (Goodsitt, 1997); alternatively, both of these prescriptions may be misguided and perhaps downright dangerous (Bruch, 1988). Depending on the source consulted, eating and weight issues should be addressed, ignored, or delegated to someone other than the therapist. Some treatment proposals specify a 25-session course of outpatient psychotherapy (Treasure and Ward, 1997a), while others advocate 6–24 months of residential care (Story, 1982; Strober and Yager, 1985). Clearly, any attempt to generalize across such diverse models, methods, and formats would be uninformative.

Only a few characteristics help to distinguish psychodynamic approaches from alternative methods (although none is universal across or exclusive to this group of therapies). Psychodynamic therapists are more likely to endorse the view that 'it's not about eating and weight,' to explore the origin of symptoms, to focus on longstanding conflicts or deficits, to encourage the expression of emotion, and to highlight the therapeutic relationship. They are, in general, less likely to emphasize the provision of facts about the disorder, to give advice about the management of eating and weight, to examine disorder-specific beliefs, to suggest extra-therapy activities, or to use an active, directive style during sessions.

Another factor complicating the review of psychodynamic models is that they are routinely combined with other approaches in the treatment of anorexia nervosa. Virtually all therapists find their accustomed modes of practice challenged by the distinctive features of this disorder, and many venture outside familiar frameworks in search of better alternatives (Garner and Bemis, 1982; Casper, 1987; Tobin and Johnson, 1991; Palmer, 2000). The identity crisis seems especially acute, however, for those who practice nondirective forms of therapy. To a greater extent than family therapists or CBT therapists, clinicians whose primary affiliation is psychodynamic tend to favor a 'hyphenated' approach when working with anorexic patients, borrowing elements from family systems, CBT, interpersonal, experiential, and medical models. Most are (commendably) reluctant to overlook patients' current health, weight, eating behavior, and patently false beliefs, while tracing the origins of their difficulties to early developmental deficits. In response, some adopt a pragmatic eclectic approach, importing symptom management strategies from other orientations to put alongside the techniques they prefer. Others modify psychodynamic therapy itself to suit the distinctive features of patients with this disorder.

For example, the influential theorist and therapist Hilde Bruch (1973, 1978, 1988) outlined a causal model of anorexia nervosa consonant with her psychoanalytic training, yet cautioned that traditional psychodynamic therapy was 'singularly ineffective' and 'potentially harmful, even fatal' when applied to these patients. She recommended using a more direct 'fact-finding treatment' that enlisted the patient as a 'true collaborator' in the effort to identify and challenge specific 'false assumptions or illogical deductions' (Bruch, 1962, 1978, 1985). The therapeutic style that Bruch described as more effective with this population bears a striking resemblance to Aaron Beck's cognitive therapy (A. T. Beck, 1976; A. T. Beck et al., 1979; J. S. Beck, 1995; Greenberger and Padesky, 1995) and adapted versions designed for use with anorexic patients (Garner and Bemis, 1982, 1985; see subsequent section on CBT).

Only a few psychodynamic interventions for anorexia nervosa have been outlined in detail, including the hybrid approaches labeled 'feminist psychoanalytic therapy' (which also incorporates elements of CBT; Bloom et al., 1994) and cognitive analytical therapy (CAT; Treasure and Ward, 1997a). Still fewer have been both specified and examined in controlled trials, including CAT and focal psychoanalytic psychotherapy (FPP; Dare and Crowther, 1995).

CAT is a time-limited dynamic therapy (Ryle, 1990) that is described as 'uniquely positioned between [the] extremes' of symptom focus and insight orientation (Bell, 1999, p. 36). As applied to anorexic patients, the format involves 20 weekly sessions followed by 3–5 monthly follow-up visits (Treasure and Ward, 1997a; Dare et al., 2001; Tanner and Connan, 2003). Working collaboratively, the therapist and patient identify target problems and analyze the 'traps,' 'snags,' and 'dilemmas' through which these are maintained. Therapy also examines interpersonal patterns, termed 'reciprocal roles,' which are traceable to early relationships and form the background for the patient's present experience. This information is mapped on to a visual schematic called the 'sequential diagrammatic reformulation' that depicts connections between the individual's symptoms and her relationships and self-concept, and becomes the basis for ongoing monitoring and discussion in therapy.

FPP is a more traditional approach based on Malan's work (1976, 1979) and adapted for anorexia nervosa by Dare and Crowther (1995). In the context of research, treatment is delivered weekly for 1 year. Therapy is organized around a 'focal hypothesis' that links the patient's internalized representation of significant people in her past to her evolving feelings for the therapist and the function of her symptom in current personal relations. Anorexia nervosa is viewed as a means of gaining a spurious sense of control, in an effort to manage patients' central fear of the vulnerability experienced through closeness, and as a powerful method of soliciting care from others. Analysis of transference and countertransference phenomena is prominent in this mode of treatment. Weight is monitored by a nurse and reported to the therapist, who charts and discusses weight changes with the patient in connection with other developments as they unfold in psychotherapy.

Empirical evidence, indications for use, and unresolved questions

Six controlled trials have included at least one cell of psychodynamic therapy. Unfortunately, three of these describe the modalities in minimalist terms, saying little more than that one treatment condition was 'psychodynamically oriented.' In view of the diversity of models, such brevity means that we have no way to determine which treatment principles are being supported or invalidated by the results. One of these investigations found

a psychodynamic condition inferior to dietary counseling (Hall and Crisp, 1987), one inferior to family therapy for adolescent but not late-onset cases (Russell et al., 1987), and one equivalent to inpatient care and superior to treatment as usual (Crisp et al., 1991).

The remaining three trials, two of which included CAT, provide more interpretable information. As noted in the section on family therapy, Robin et al. (1994) reported that ego-oriented individual therapy was slightly less effective than family therapy with young, recent-onset anorexic patients. A pilot study comparing CAT to an 'educational behavioral' treatment found no differences between conditions at 1-year follow-up (Treasure et al., 1995). Most patients in both groups gained weight but only about a third of each achieved a good outcome.

A subsequent study compared CAT, FPP, family therapy, and low-contact routine treatment (Dare et al., 2001). All interventions were provided on an outpatient basis to a sample of adult patients who would be expected to carry a poor prognosis as a function of their average age (26 years), extended duration of illness (6 years), low weight (BMI of 15.4), and history of prior treatment (79% overall, 43% inpatient). When reassessed a year after treatment initiation, most patients in all conditions remained underweight, with an average BMI of 16.5. A few group differences attained significance: patients assigned to routine treatment were more likely to require hospitalization than those in any of the three specialized therapies, and gained less weight than patients in focal psychoanalytic or family therapy (but not CAT). On an intent-to-treat basis, 28–37% of those allocated to the specialized treatments had recovered or significantly improved, versus 5% of those getting routine care; however, half to two-thirds of the former and three-fourths of the latter were still doing quite poorly. Moreover, because of design inequities, even the obtained differences between the specialized therapies and routine treatment are not clearly interpretable as support for any one (or all three) of these specific modalities. Widely varying lengths and densities of therapy were used across conditions; routine treatment was delivered by psychiatric trainees with less overall and disorder-specific experience, who transferred their anorexic patients/subjects to another therapist when rotated to a new service every 6 months. As a result of these discrepancies, differences in outcome cannot be attributed to particular models versus the general advantages of treatment amount, continuity, and expertise.

While the available evidence is not strongly supportive of any form of psychodynamic treatment, it should be stressed again that no intervention of any kind has so far yielded satisfactory results with the patient group most often included in these trials: older adolescents or adults with established anorexia nervosa. Psychodynamic models have been highly influential, however, in shaping the ways therapists conceptualize and treat eating disorders. Although few clinicians practice therapy precisely as specified by CAT or FPP, psychodynamic principles inform the work of most. Bruch's characterization of symptoms as a desperate struggle for a self-respecting identity, Crisp's depiction of flight from psychobiological maturity, and Goodsitt's emphasis on the importance of a healing relationship have all been incorporated into dominant clinical views of the disorder. Above all, psychodynamic approaches underscore that the eating and weight symptoms that command our attention do not define the scope of problems faced in the treatment of anorexia nervosa.

Cognitive-behavioral therapy

Theoretical base

A cognitive-behavioral framework for understanding and treating anorexia nervosa was initially described by Garner and Vitousek (Garner and Bemis, 1982, 1985; Garner et al., 1997). The model overlaps substantially with Fairburn's (1981, 1985) analysis of bulimia nervosa, reflecting the CBT perspective that these disorders share many core features and maintaining variables. At the center of both is the premise that personal worth is dependent on the size and shape of the body. This dominant idea spins off a host of specific irrational beliefs, conditions a characteristic set of fears, and prompts stereotyped avoidance behaviors. Over time, anorexic and bulimic individuals begin to process information in accordance with predictable cognitive biases and respond to increasingly eccentric reinforcement contingencies. In addition, anorexic individuals incur the hard-wired consequences of semistarvation, which also contribute to the entrenchment of the pattern (Garner and Bemis, 1982).

To a greater extent than other models, cognitive accounts stress the positively reinforced and 'organizing' functions of anorexia nervosa, postulating that these explain its most unusual features better than the avoidance-based functions that are also present and influential (Garner and Bemis, 1982; Slade, 1982; Bemis, 1983; Vitousek and Hollon, 1990; Vitousek and Ewald, 1993; Wolff and Serpell, 1998; Fairburn et al., 1999b; Vitousek, 2005). These distinctive features include a sense of 'specialness,' moral certitude, competitiveness, and positive identification with the disorder (Vitousek, 2003). Because the sum of these distinctive elements seems to explain the distinctive resistance to change in this disorder, CBT for anorexia nervosa is organized around efforts to address them.

Description

The CBT approach has been outlined in a series of papers that describe different components of the treatment package (Garner and Bemis, 1982, 1985; Garner, 1986, 1997; Orimoto and Vitousek, 1992; Pike et al., 1996; Garner et al., 1997; Vitousek et al., 1998; Wilson and Vitousek, 1999); however, no treatment manual combining this material is available. The format specifies an extended course (1–2 years) of individual therapy, supplemented with family sessions if indicated. One-to-one therapy is considered essential to the delicate work of addressing motivational issues and idiosyncratic beliefs. The long duration reflects the time required to engage reluctant patients as active participants in the change process, as well as to help them reach normal weight and recover from the persistent after-effects of semistarvation.

The CBT model has a strong bias toward accomplishing weight restoration on an outpatient basis whenever possible, to maximize patients' sense of responsibility for decision making and minimize the risk of reactance to external control. In some cases, inpatient or partial hospital treatment may be essential; guidelines are available for using CBT principles in such settings (Bowers et al., 1997).

Treatment phases parallel the three-stage sequence common to CBT and IPT for bulimia (and to some extent, family therapy for anorexia): an initial phase for engagement, provision of rationale, and beginning steps toward change; a middle phase for focused work on identified maintaining variables; and a concluding phase for consolidation and relapse prevention (Garner et al., 1997). In practice, however, the progression of CBT for anorexia nervosa is less fixed than these divisions imply. The general movement is from developing motivation to modifying eating and weight to examining disorder-specific beliefs to focusing on broader aspects of self-concept; however, all of these issues are necessarily addressed throughout therapy, and many CBT techniques target multiple areas simultaneously.

In descriptions of CBT for anorexia nervosa, considerable space is devoted to suggested strategies for engaging patients' interest in the prospect of change and then translating that interest into action. Four emphases are identified as crucial to the promotion of change (Vitousek et al., 1998). The first involves the nonconfrontational use of *psychoeducational* information to help the patient reassess the perceived risks and benefits of her symptoms and reconstrue their meaning. The second is an affirmation of the *experimental* method of CBT, which casts each proposed step in therapy as an opportunity to gather information rather than an irrevocable commitment to change. A third key theme is an emphasis on exploring the *functional* effects of patients' choices, rather than challenging their rationality or validity. A substantial portion of the first few sessions of therapy is typically devoted to helping the patient develop a list of the advantages and disadvantages of her eating disorder, phrased in her own terms (Vitousek and Orimoto, 1993). Samples of the kinds of material provided by patients such as Chloe and Amanda are included in Table 15.1 (see discussion in the subsequent section on Attention to motivational issues). The serious attention given to the perceived advantages of symptoms can be disarming to patients

Table 15.1 Advantages and disadvantages of anorexia nervosa

Advantages	Disadvantages
Chloe	
I just like being skinny	My parents fight over this
I can wear tiny sizes and cute clothes	I don't like to upset my mom
It makes me feel strong when I don't need to eat	I'm not allowed to run track
I'm really good at this	Everyone makes a huge deal about my weight (actually, I kind of
People always ask me how I got so thin	like that and kind of don't)
I can run faster	I have no privacy
I don't get my period	I hated the hospital—it was totally
I kind of like it that people worry about me	demeaning
I have more self-confidence	My hair is falling out
I like being different from other people	I feel cold all the time
	It's hard to concentrate
	I'm getting lower grades
	I'm not as close to my friends
	I've been kind of bitchy
Amanda	
It's important to me to eat right and be healthy	I am tired much of the time
I don't like being wasteful and taking up too many resources	I seem to have lost the spirit I used to have
I like having a system for everything	I think it's superficial to worry so much about trivial matters
This is just the way I prefer to be	It's difficult to plan for social occasions
I like being self-disciplined	My family is concerned about me
I look better when I'm thin	I don't want to be doing this when I'm 40
I can't help feeling that it is somehow *better* to be this way	At times I feel lonely, and no one really understands
This is preferable to the alternatives	I believe that I would have accomplished more in my
If I gained weight, I would only feel worse about myself	professional life if this had never happened
I feel safer this way	I am weary of having to keep track of everything
I still feel good when I lose weight, even though I know I shouldn't	I miss some of the things I used to eat
If I let myself slide, I just get lazy	My bones are thinning
	It is getting more and more difficult to do this

who are accustomed to being warned about the dangers of their behavior. The therapist is advised to acknowledge these benefits without minimizing or disputing them. At the same time, she or he introduces a theme that will recur throughout treatment: the disadvantages the patient is experiencing are inextricably linked to subnormal weight; however, it may be possible to secure the positive effects at lower cost through alternative means.

The fourth theme is an exploration of *philosophical* issues that bear on patients' attachment to symptoms and fear of change (Vitousek et al., 1998; Vitousek, 2005). CBT advocates working through each patient's personal values to convince her that her anorexic way of life violates key principles that are even more fundamental to her sense of identity. For example, Amanda echoed the common anorexic view that denying herself desired foods and working out several hours a day were testimony to her strength and self-discipline—characteristics she valued highly in herself and others. In fact, after years of anorexia nervosa, adherence to these rigid, fear-driven patterns of behavior represented the path of least resistance. For Amanda, the truly brave and difficult choice would be to violate her anorexic system of rules by eating forbidden foods or defying the impulse to exercise.

Because many anorexic individuals are passionately committed to their beliefs, work with these patients can seem more analogous to the conversion of a member of the National Rifle Association to a gun control advocate, or a religious fundamentalist to Unitarianism, than it does to psychotherapy with a depressed or anxious patient. It follows that attempts to dispute anorexic beliefs logically are seldom successful—and are not advised by CBT experts in this area. The treatment approach does make use of the conventional CBT techniques of cognitive restructuring and prospective hypothesis testing; for example, the therapist and patient might collaborate in designing an experiment to check out the patient's belief that other people respond to her more favorably when she loses weight. Contrary to stereotype, however, CBT does not assume that anorexic patients will give up their symptoms once the therapist points out their 'errors in thinking' and challenges their irrational beliefs. Instead, therapists are encouraged to draw on a blend of factual, functional, and value-related material to enlist patients in reexamining the relationship between anorexic symptoms and their own goals and ideals.

The processes of dietary rehabilitation and weight restoration are not carried out in isolation from the rest of CBT but integrated with the ongoing examination of patients' beliefs. Initially, patients are encouraged to follow individualized, structured meal plans, gradually introducing larger amounts and avoided food types. Meal planning is usually incorporated into regular sessions and conducted by the primary therapist. *In vivo* therapy sessions may be used to assist patients with particularly challenging situations, such as grocery shopping, eating in restaurants, or trying on new clothes (see section on Attention to eating and weight).

During the course of therapy, attention gradually shifts from the focal symptoms of anorexia nervosa to more general aspects of self-concept and interpersonal relationships. It is not necessary to switch paradigms in order to address these issues, as CBT offers mode-consistent principles for work on this level. In the later stages, patients are encouraged to experiment with new strategies for achieving their goals, new sources of positive reinforcement, and new standards for gauging personal worth.

Empirical evidence, indications for use, and unresolved questions

Paralleling the general state of treatment research across the eating disorders, there is a vast gap between the empirical standing of CBT for anorexia nervosa and for bulimia nervosa. During the first 7 years after the approach was proposed, several case studies (Cooper and Fairburn, 1984; Garner, 1988; Peveler and Fairburn, 1989) and one small controlled trial (Channon *et al.*, 1989) were reported. Very recently, four comparative studies have been completed and others are in progress. Only a few tentative observations are warranted pending publication of these data.

Two recent controlled trials compared CBT with nutritional counseling. The first of these broke down after 100% of the 10 patients assigned to nutritional counseling dropped out of treatment and refused further contact; in contrast, 92% of the 25 patients allocated to CBT persisted to completion of the 20-session series (Serfaty *et al.*, 1999). Although statistical analyses of outcome were precluded by the mass defection of patients from nutritional counseling, it was reported that those who had received CBT showed significant changes in BMI and on measures of eating disorder and general symptoms.

Findings from a second study confirmed the pattern of differential attrition from these treatment conditions (Pike *et al.*, 2003). This investigation was designed as a 'relapse prevention' trial, with patients randomly assigned to 50 sessions of individual CBT or nutritional counseling and medical management after completing inpatient weight restoration. The study included a severe sample of 33 adult patients (average age 25 years) with longstanding anorexia nervosa (7.5 years). Fewer patients in the CBT condition terminated prematurely (27% for CBT versus 53% for nutritional counseling) and more met criteria for 'good' outcome at the end of treatment (44% versus 7%).

Another trial compared CBT, fluoxetine, and combined treatment conditions with a sample of 108 partially weight-restored anorexic patients (Halmi, 2000). Final results have not been reported, but the interim data suggested that CBT, alone or in combination with medication, also conferred some protection against premature termination compared with medication alone. The extremely high dropout rates already evident for all conditions

at mid-treatment are troubling, however, and inconsistent with the patterns seen in other investigations.

Collectively, these findings support the tentative conclusion that CBT does further at least two of the goals it was expressly designed to fulfill: higher rates of initial engagement and treatment persistence in these notoriously 'resistant' patients. While it is tempting to attribute these desired effects to the collaborative style and motivational emphasis of CBT, such inferences are premature. Because each of these studies compared CBT with a non-psychological intervention, they suggest only that *psychotherapy*—perhaps, but not necessarily, in the specific form of CBT—produces better outcomes than nutritional counseling and/or drug treatment alone (Vitousek, 2002). Ironically, the choice of weak comparison treatments has made it difficult to gauge the efficacy of CBT. In order to determine whether CBT confers any benefits beyond its apparently greater capacity to retain patients, researchers must identify comparison treatments that serve the same objective at least equally well, so that sufficient numbers of patients are willing to remain in the alternative condition.

To date, only two investigations have examined the effects of CBT relative to other forms of psychotherapy. Both used abbreviated versions of CBT (20–25 sessions) with patients who were underweight or partially weight restored. One of these found CBT equal to BT and treatment-as-usual with adult patients (Channon *et al.*, 1989); a second obtained positive and equivalent results using CBT or family therapy with adolescents and young adults (Ball, 1999).

In view of the fact that no form of psychotherapy has been shown to work better than any other form of psychotherapy for adult anorexic patients, how should clinicians evaluate the merits of CBT relative to other treatment options, pending the availability of more instructive data? Several considerations recommend the approach as a defensible interim choice (Vitousek, 2002; Fairburn and Harrison, 2003). One argument is the documented success of a related approach for bulimia nervosa. Because anorexic and bulimic patients share many beliefs and behaviors, it seems likely that at least some of the same strategies will prove effective in treating them. Another putative benefit of CBT is its integration of direct work on eating and weight with attention to motivational issues—a characteristic that may become increasingly appealing as outpatient services are forced to take on more responsibility for the weight restoration phase of treatment.

A disadvantage of CBT is the fact that this complex intervention requires considerable training to deliver. In addition, all CBT experts concur that the treatment must be lengthy—not the 18–25 sessions used in most trials to date, but something on the order of 40–60 sessions in the usual case of established anorexia nervosa (Garner *et al.*, 1997; Fairburn *et al.*, 2003; Pike *et al.*, 2003). Such extended outpatient treatment clearly requires justification through data showing that it reduces the need for expensive inpatient care and subsequent services to a greater extent than brief interventions.

Recently, this area has been invigorated by new proposals for shifts in emphasis in the basic CBT model, offered both by its originators and other CBT experts in the eating disorder field. Like the initial approach, however, these suggested revisions are based on clinical experience rather than accumulated evidence about the strengths or weaknesses of existing models. As we know very little about how well the 'traditional' CBT approach to anorexia nervosa works, it remains a matter of conjecture how it might be improved (Vitousek, 2002). Some specialists have suggested that the 'traditional' model is too narrow, paying insufficient attention to interpersonal issues and 'deep' aspects of the self (Leung *et al.*, 1999); others have speculated that the model is too broad, allocating unnecessary attention to interpersonal issues and 'deep' aspects of the self (Fairburn *et al.*, 1999b). Specific aspects of the approach have also been recommended for closer focus, notably work on the extreme need for self-control (Fairburn *et al.*, 1999) and the connection between symptoms and values (Vitousek, 2005). Because the few data available already indicate that many anorexic patients will fail to achieve full recovery with CBT (or any other tested modalities), thoughtful modifications to the existing approach should be examined through systematic case study or small group designs.

Pharmacotherapy

If the length of this section were proportionate to the number of medications tested, it would dominate a review of alternative treatments for anorexia nervosa. According to a leading specialist (Walsh, 2002b), however, the list of agents that have proven beneficial can be summarized succinctly: none. Paradoxically, the most important contribution of pharmacotherapy research may be the repeated demonstration that drugs are ineffective in the resolution of this disorder.

In other specialty areas, pharmacotherapists are sometimes suspected of overstating the merits of drug treatment relative to psychotherapy. In contrast, their counterparts in this field consistently emphasize the limits on what they have to offer (e.g., Garfinkel and Walsh, 1997; Mayer and Walsh, 1998; Garfinkel, 2002b; Walsh, 2002a,b; Bruna and Fogteloo, 2003). Reviews summarize the evidence in bleak (if honorable) terms: 'no psychopharmacological treatment for anorexia nervosa has ever proved satisfactory' (Andersen, 1995, p. 373); 'to date, no medication has been shown to change eating behavior reliably, assist weight gain . . . or alter body image disturbance' (Johnson *et al.*, 1996); 'to date, medications have added little to overall management' (Garfinkel, 2002b, p. 225). The recurrence of the phrase 'to date' holds out some hope for the future; after all, as one specialist notes, 'there are always new medications appearing' (Garfinkel, 2002b, p. 225), and it is conceivable that one will break the string of failures being reviewed. Yet the same phrase reappears in summaries written many years apart, as each promising debut is followed inexorably—at least, 'to date'—by the accumulation of more discouraging data.

In some instances, drugs are prescribed for anorexia nervosa simply because they carry side-effects that promote weight gain (Walsh, 2002b). As in the case of pharmacotherapy for bulimia nervosa, however, most candidate drugs are linked to specific models about what has gone awry and why the proposed medication should help put it right. Most of these conjectures are plausible, because anorexia nervosa subsumes a variety of psychiatric and medical symptoms for which useful drug treatments have been identified (Walsh, 2002a). For example, the ubiquity of depression and prominence of obsessive-compulsive patterns in anorexic patients support the use of antidepressants, while the near-delusional quality of their distorted thinking warrants trials of antipsychotic medication.

Antidepressants seem to provide little benefit in promoting weight gain, but one study has reported that fluoxetine may help forestall relapse after weight restoration (Kaye *et al.*, 1997; Ferguson *et al.*, 1999), and additional investigations are currently in progress. In one of these, however, the dropout rate from the medication condition had already reached two-thirds by treatment midpoint (Halmi, 2000). Case reports suggest some benefit from the atypical neuroleptic olanzapine (La Via *et al.*, 2000; Boachie *et al.*, 2003; Malina *et al.*, 2003). In view of the long record of dashed hopes in this area, however, even cautious optimism should be deferred until results are replicated. (Curiously, the lack of evidence supporting the efficacy of medication has done little to discourage its use; if Chloe had not been placed on antidepressants by her family physician, there is a good chance that they would have been prescribed at the time of her referral to a specialty clinic.)

From one perspective, it may be unreasonable to expect medication to be particularly effective for the purpose of dismantling organized, coherent, highly valued systems of belief. Few pharmacotherapists would be chagrined by their failure to identify a drug that could change the attitudes of political extremists, religious fanatics, or extreme high altitude mountain climbers. Biological factors might well be involved in the development of such patterns; once established, however, they may become inaccessible to modification even if the underlying vulnerability is correctly identified and treated. The same may hold for anorexia nervosa.

Key practice principles

Specialized expertise

Clinicians with minimal background in the eating disorder field are often wary of treating anorexic or bulimic patients. Their reluctance is warranted: in most circumstances, competent care involves referral to specialized services. The treatment of these conditions puts a premium on specific expertise for a number of reasons.

First, semistarvation and the binge–purge cycle have profound effects on physiology and psychology. These consequences are predictable to experts, but can be obscure, alarming, and/or misleading to inexperienced practitioners. For example, chronic caloric deprivation produces an array of symptoms, including depression, anxiety, irritability, impulsivity, social withdrawal, and sexual disinterest, as well as characteristic peculiarities in food-related attitudes and behaviors. Therapists who are not aware that these patterns emerge in well-adjusted individuals undergoing semi-starvation (Keys *et al.*, 1950) are prone to make up case-specific explanations and complicated treatment plans for general phenomena with a parsimonious cause.

Second, as noted earlier, the provision of psychoeducational material is a prominent component of treatment for anorexia and bulimia across most modalities (Olmsted and Kaplan, 1995; Garner, 1997). Clinicians cannot impart such information credibly and persuasively unless they have acquired a solid background in a wide range of relevant topics. It is unrealistic to expect that nonspecialists will have the time to acquire and update the necessary knowledge base; even clinicians who devote their practice to this population have difficulty keeping current across these rapidly developing fields.

Mastery of such material is especially crucial because many patients are themselves amateur experts on dieting, weight, and exercise. They tend to be keen consumers of the jumble of accurate and inaccurate information that is disseminated in popular culture, and often cite specific sources in support of their symptoms. For example, Amanda had audited several nutrition classes at the college where she taught, and justified her abstemious eating in part by referring to solid evidence on the retardation of aging through caloric restriction (Weindruch, 1996; Vitousek *et al.*, 2004). At the same time, she quoted freely from pamphlets picked up at health food stores, attributing her avoidance of specific foods (which happened to be high in calories or fat) to concerns about allergens or toxic build-up in her gastrointestinal tract. In order to help her disentangle the true and false bits of input that she has muddled together, her therapist should know more than Amanda—and more than the average physician or dietitian—about factual matters that affect her willingness to change.

Finally, familiarity with the phenomenology of anorexia and bulimia helps the clinician ask crucial questions, evaluate the plausibility of answers, and establish credibility as someone who understands the private and often protected experience of individuals with eating disorders (Vitousek *et al.*, 1998).

In circumstances where specialized expertise is not available, therapists may find it valuable to act as 'guides' for the use of self-help manuals by their clients—a process that can facilitate the acquisition of knowledge and skill by both parties (Birchall and Palmer, 2002). Supervision through teleconferencing may also be beneficial for clinicians who work in sparsely populated areas (Mitchell *et al.*, 2003).

Attention to eating and weight

Most experts consider direct work on eating disorder symptoms essential for patients with anorexia nervosa and desirable for those with bulimia nervosa. There is some disagreement, however, about the degree of emphasis such work should be given and whether it should occur within or outside the context of psychotherapy.

As discussed in the section on bulimia, at least one modality that does not address specific symptoms (IPT) can yield benefits approximately equal to the 'treatment of choice' that does (CBT), while therapy focusing exclusively on behavior (BT) may be contraindicated (Fairburn *et al.*, 1993a). Even if bulimic symptoms can be eliminated without specific assistance, however, it is not clear why therapists would choose to withhold it. We know that dietary restraint is a risk factor for bingeing and that its reduction mediates improvement during treatment (Wilson *et al.*, 2002)—and we know that bulimic patients get better faster when clinicians give them direct help in changing these patterns.

In the case of anorexia nervosa, we lack the evidence for data-based conclusions about the relative merits of treatments that pay considerable attention, some attention, and no attention to eating and weight; once again, purely symptom-focused treatment in the form of dietary counseling seems to be associated with particularly abysmal results. In practice, however, few specialists are willing to let anorexic symptoms take care of themselves while psychological issues are addressed. There are obvious medical and ethical reasons for a more active approach, and some compelling clinical grounds as well. The heart of the matter is that professionals must attempt to modify undereating and low weight because anorexic patients probably *won't*, left to their own devices. Unlike bulimic patients who want to stop bingeing and purging, they are not disposed to translate any improvements in overall functioning into symptom control. Moreover, there are much sharper constraints on the extent to which general improvements *can* occur while semistarvation persists.

The field includes instructive examples of what can happen when therapists focus on 'deeper' issues in preference to eating and weight. One disturbing case report describes narrative therapy with a 29-year-old anorexic patient whose BMI was approximately 10 (Lemberg, 1999). The therapist— who apparently persisted in the same approach for 7 years, while the patient's weight remained critically low—wrote that this brilliant young woman 'deserved much more' out of life than enslavement by anorexia nervosa. Most experts would agree: At a minimum, she deserved a form of therapy that would not continue discussing her dilemma from alternative perspectives while her life remained on hold and potentially in jeopardy. Another account details the consequences of a day-hospital program that focused on the 'difficulties underlying [patients'] eating problems'—but elected not to attend to the eating problems themselves (Thornton and Russell, 1995, cited in Zipfel *et al.*, 2002, p. 114). Of the 23 anorexic patients treated with this approach, 95% lost weight while in the program, and 64% required readmission to the hospital.

Some therapists who agree that direct intervention is necessary would prefer that the battles be waged in someone else's office. In many programs, eating and weight issues are managed by dietitians, physicians, and/or nursing staff. The rationale for separating symptom-focused work from psychotherapy is sometimes that sessions should be reserved for matters more significant than what brand of breakfast cereal the patient selects and whether or not a 2-ounce change really constitutes weight gain; it is also argued that the therapeutic relationship should be shielded from the unpleasantness that often surrounds such discussions (e.g., Rampling, 1978; Powers and Powers, 1984). Others simply see dietitians as better prepared for this work (Beumont *et al.*, 1997); certainly, they are less likely to let it slide.

The alternative position has been stated most forcefully by CBT experts, who maintain that dietary counseling and weight management should be incorporated into regular therapy sessions (Garner *et al.*, 1982, 1997; Garner and Bemis, 1985; Wilson and Agras, 2001). Meal planning is not simply a matter of imparting information and issuing instructions, but a persuasive and essentially 'therapeutic' undertaking best handled by a clinician who is familiar with all aspects of the patient's situation (Wilson and Agras, 2001). Work on eating and weight invariably provides access to important beliefs and intense emotions, and offers numerous opportunities to take on motivational issues and explore 'deeper' concerns. The obvious interdependence of these variables in patients' own experience should be reflected in the structure of treatment.

Guidelines for conducting this work are available in basic CBT articles (e.g., Garner and Bemis, 1985; Fairburn *et al.*, 1993b; Garner *et al.*, 1997; Wilson *et al.*, 1997; Wilson and Vitousek, 1999) and materials on nutritional counseling (e.g., Beumont *et al.*, 1987, 1997; Rock and Yager, 1987; Reiff and Reiff, 1997). Specific controversies persist about matters such as how rapidly weight gain should proceed and whether or not calories should be monitored, patients informed of their exact weights, and vegetarian diets accepted. The invariant principle is that highly restrictive eating and extremely low weight are incompatible with progress in therapy. A continued trend toward improvement in these areas is a marker of effective outpatient treatment. In general, a different pace of change would be expected for subgroups

of patients matching the profiles in the section on anorexia nervosa. For individuals such as Chloe, whose weight loss was recent and precipitate, a fairly assertive program of weight restoration might be appropriate. For patients such as Amanda, whose low weight has been relatively stable for years, more gradual increments are usually indicated—in part because they are often all that these patients can be persuaded to consider.

One basic strategy used in CBT, BT, and adjunctive nutritional counseling is self-monitoring of food intake. For both bulimic and anorexic patients, self-monitoring provides a means of assessing the temporal pattern, quantity, and quality of dietary intake, and can yield information about the precipitants and consequences of targeted events such as binge-eating. A sample record from the bulimic patient Sharon is shown in Figure 15.1. The form is similar to that recommended by Fairburn (1995), and can be adapted to suit the specific needs of individual patients. Typically, such forms include columns for recording the timing and context of eating episodes, the type and amount of foods consumed, the patient's subjective judgment about whether the event constituted a binge, the occurrence of purging, and the type and duration of exercise. CBT therapists usually encourage patients to record food quantities in approximate and colloquial terms (such as 'a large bowl of cereal' or 'half a piece'), avoiding the precise measuring or weighing of food and the counting of calories or fat grams (Fairburn, 1995; Wilson and Vitousek, 1999). In addition, patients may be asked to summarize their thoughts and emotions during different phases of the binge–purge cycle, or to write down a brief analysis of the factors contributing to its occurrence. It can also be useful for patients to identify the point at which they made a decision to initiate an episode or to designate eating that was already underway as a 'binge.' In Figure 15.1, Sharon has used an asterisk to mark when this occurred.

Review of Sharon's daily record suggests several themes that may contribute to maintaining her disorder and triggering specific incidents of binge eating, including erratic meals, long periods of deprivation, fatigue, isolation, and interpersonal disappointment. These linkages can help Sharon and her therapist identify and change patterns that increase her vulnerability to overeating and purging. For example, one obvious goal for Sharon would be to include breakfast in her regular routine, in part to lessen the likelihood that she will eat unplanned foods on a haphazard basis (such as the chocolate doughnut she encountered at work), and then interpret her 'lapse' as proof that she cannot exercise self-control. If the association between feelings of loneliness and/or abandonment and symptomatic behavior recurs in a number of situations, it would also become an important focus for work in psychotherapy.

Some behavioral changes are so challenging that they may not be attempted without more direct assistance from the therapist. In these instances, *in vivo* sessions can be an invaluable addition to discussions in psychotherapy. Although therapist-assisted exposure is a common component of BT and CBT for other anxiety-related disorders, this strategy has been surprisingly neglected in the eating disorder field—except in the form of office-based sessions for exposure and response prevention (ERP) to bingeing and/or purging cues (e.g., Rosen and Leitenberg, 1985; Wilson *et al.*, 1986; Agras *et al.*, 1989; Jansen *et al.*, 1992; Carter *et al.*, 2003) and, more recently, body size in the mirror (e.g., Tuschen and Bent, 1995; Rosen, 1996; Wilson, 1999). In addition to these applications, exposure principles can be applied flexibly to a wide range of issues that hamper progress in recovery.

In the very early stages of therapy, *in vivo* sessions can take the form of supervised meals with patients who are eating infrequently or extremely poorly, or who are unable to interrupt the binge–purge cycle without external structure and support. For example, for a patient such as Emily, who induces vomiting almost every time she eats, the therapist might arrange several extended sessions that involve eating a regular meal, then assisting with anxiety management until the high-risk period for self-induced vomiting has elapsed. Clearly, sessions of this kind cannot be scheduled with sufficient frequency to replicate the meal supervision available in day hospital or inpatient settings, and should not be used for more than brief periods of intensive support. In our experience, however, such interventions sometimes help patients surmount barriers to change that they cannot negotiate on their own between therapy sessions, allowing them to accomplish the initial

Day of the Week: Monday

Time	Food Intake	Situation	Binge?	Purge?	Exercise	Thoughts
5:30am		Skipped breakfast because binged and purged last night			30 minute run	Still feel bloated from night before
8:00am	2 c. black coffee					
10:30am	1/2 chocolate donut	Work—donut left over from a morning meeting	No	No		Should have tried to resist eating this—feel incredibly guilty for my lack of control
2:30pm	salad with vegetables and chicken with fat-free Italian dressing	Work—grabbed a late lunch due to meeting with my boss	No	No		Meeting with boss took longer than expected—had to eat quickly—feel unsatisfied
6:00pm	1/2 bag pretzels	Car—stuck in traffic on the drive home	No	No		Too tired to think
7:15pm	1/2 bag pretzels diet coke	Home—watching TV	No	No		Anticipating phone call from Mark
8:30pm	1/4 box cereal *3 cookies 2 pieces cold pizza 1 pint ice cream handful cheese crackers	Home—alone—Mark did not call when he said he would	Yes	Yes		Feel very lonely—no one really cares about me

Fig. 15.1 Food record.

steps toward symptom control without the cost or disruption of inpatient treatment.

In vivo eating sessions can also be focused on the reintroduction of especially distressing 'forbidden foods,' exposure to avoided situations (such as fast-food restaurants), and modification of specific eating rituals (such as eating slowly or 'dissecting' food). Other kinds of sessions can be devised to target a variety of problems related to food, weight, and exercise. For example, the long-term anorexic patient Amanda adhered to a highly restrictive vegetarian diet, limiting her selection to just eight specific food items (e.g., defatted tofu, a single brand of plain yogurt, one type of bran cereal) that she was willing to consume, in addition to fruits and vegetables she deemed 'safe.' During meal planning sessions, Amanda was unable to come up with any alternatives she might consider sampling, and rejected each suggestion offered by her therapist as unappealing, inconvenient, or 'unhealthy.' Rather than debating the merits of each candidate in the office, the therapist suggested spending a session in a health food store (and subsequently in a regular supermarket) reviewing and selecting additional choices. To some clinicians, this kind of intervention may seem superficial and 'nonpsychological,' in that it takes expressed concerns at face value and addresses them as practical problems to be solved. As emphasized above, however, direct work on these issues usually elicits valuable material that may be less accessible through verbal reconstructions. When patients are assisted in taking active steps to live differently, rather than simply encouraged to talk about their inability to do so, both parties get a much clearer view of the attitudes and fears that support eating disorder symptoms.

More 'advanced' *in vivo* sessions can be organized around creative scenarios that often include elements of role-play. For example, after making substantial progress in therapy, the adolescent patient Chloe came to a session distraught over a comment a friend had made about Chloe's increased weight and more normal eating behavior. Chloe recognized that the remark had been intended as a compliment, but felt humiliated that her weight gain was obvious to others and ambivalent about losing her identity as 'the anorexic' in her school. Chloe also said that she found it distressing to be around other girls who made disparaging comments about their own body

size and talked about their diet regimens, at a time when she was trying to reduce the salience of these concerns in her own self-evaluation.

After affirming the difficulty of change in the context of conflicting messages, the therapist helped Chloe consider the relative merits of coping through attempted avoidance of such events versus building her confidence that she could handle their inevitable occurrence. Chloe and her therapist decided to set up an *in vivo* lunch session in which the therapist would play the role of a friend who repeatedly talked about feeling fat, asked for advice about dieting, and expressed surprise about the nonrestrictive food choices Chloe was making. During that session, Chloe tried out a variety of different responses to the scenarios presented, and gained on-the-spot assistance in working through her own reactions. She subsequently reported that similar events were much less upsetting, noting that 'instead of walking around wondering when the next hurtful thing is going to happen, I get kind of curious about which way I'll decide to handle it when it does.'

Across all *in vivo* experiences—particularly those designed to elicit anxiety in a sensitive domain—it is crucial that the patient view the exercise as *chosen* rather than imposed. Each session should be worked out collaboratively on an individual basis, with the parameters negotiated and fixed in advance. If a patient becomes distressed and reluctant to continue during an exercise, the therapist should be in a position to refer her back to her own decision to take on the problem through this experiment, rather than pressuring her to comply with an external demand for change.

Attention to motivational issues

Until quite recently, specialists have agreed that anorexic symptoms are ego-syntonic without making much effort to find out *why*—at least from the perspective of the patients themselves. Belatedly, the field has become more curious, setting out to explore patients' opinions through questionnaires (e.g., Vitousek *et al.*, 1995; Ward *et al.*, 1996; Blake *et al.*, 1997; Rieger *et al.*, 2000), structured interviews (e.g., Geller and Drab, 1999; Geller, 2002b), and a bit of qualitative research (e.g., Serpell *et al.*, 1999; Surgenor *et al.*, 2003). The results of the assessment research confirm the view that anorexic patients are more invested in retaining their symptoms than bulimic individuals—or patients with most other psychiatric disorders. Strategies for enhancing motivation have been proposed (e.g., Goldner *et al.*, 1997; Treasure and Ward, 1997b; Vitousek *et al.*, 1998; Kaplan and Garfinkel, 1999; Treasure and Bauer, 2003) and a few related interventions examined (e.g., Treasure *et al.*, 1999; Feld *et al.*, 2001). Most importantly, many clinicians are beginning to reconceptualize their task in therapy, accepting patients' views as the necessary starting point for any efforts at change, rather than a particularly vexing byproduct of their psychopathology.

Of necessity, all existing treatment approaches for anorexia nervosa have adopted methods for handling resistance to change. The modalities outlined in preceding sections propose different—and sometimes opposite—tactics for accomplishing the shared goal of helping anorexics recover in spite of their reservations. There are basically three ways to go: (1) clinicians can try to override the desire to retain symptoms by making it difficult or impossible for symptoms to continue; (2) they can attempt to decrease the attachment indirectly by addressing the underlying problems it is presumed to reflect; and (3) they can make direct efforts to change patients' attitudes about symptoms and recovery (Vitousek, 2005). Most modalities include some components fitting each of these descriptions; however, it may be useful to divide methods according to where they invest most of their therapeutic capital.

The 'overriding' approach is characteristic of inpatient weight restoration, parental control models of family therapy, and pharmacotherapy (when prescribing drugs for their weight gain side-effects). Indirect efforts to reduce the investment in symptoms are favored by psychodynamic therapy, IPT, narrative therapy, feminist therapy, and pharmacotherapy (when using medication to treat depression, anxiety, and/or obsessionality). Direct work on motivation is featured in CBT and to some extent in the psychodynamic variants that resemble it most closely, such as CAT and Bruch's ego-oriented approach. Again, it should be stressed that these divisions are not absolute; indeed, they cannot be. 'Overriding' methods must still enlist a degree of cooperation from the patient, unless she is very young or in imminent danger. Drugs can't work if the pharmacotherapist fails to convince the patient to take them. CBT and most (but not all) of the 'indirect' modalities agree that some forms of external control are indicated with some patients at some times, although they may work assiduously to keep the number of patients limited, the touch light, and the duration brief.

As noted in the review of modalities, there is still insufficient information to conclude which of these treatment packages works best with what subgroups of patients. At present, clinical decisions about how to address motivational issues must be based on some combination of each therapist's preferences and each patient's characteristics and circumstances. In the past, most clinicians opted for a blend of 'overriding' and 'indirect' methods when treating anorexia nervosa. In recent years, for a variety of philosophical and pragmatic reasons, there has been a clear trend toward the 'direct' approach. Increasingly, therapists are seeking ways to affect patients' own views of their symptoms and the prospect of change—and discovering an unusual convergence of opinion about the strategies that further these goals. For 'direct' work on motivation, the same basic principles are recommended with reassuring reliability across different orientations and populations (Vitousek *et al.*, 1998).

Notably, the eating disorder field has been influenced by exposure to motivational interviewing (MI; Miller and Rollnick, 1991, 2002). This approach was initially developed as an alternative to confrontational tactics for inducing alcoholic individuals to enter treatment. Miller and Rollnick argue that traditional methods of breaking down denial (such as highlighting the irrationality and danger of the symptomatic behavior, urging acceptance of the label 'alcoholic,' and insisting on the need for treatment) tend to backfire, paradoxically increasing the individual's investment in defending the *status quo*. MI uses a variety of strategies to heighten the salience of the patient's own concerns about the problem behavior, including reflection, affirmation of the patient's experience, emphasis on individual choice and control, exploration of personal values, amplification of discrepancies, and sharing of psychoeducational information. Most of all, the approach describes a stance toward treatment that is based on respect for the patient's

perspective (Geller, 2002a)—along with the pragmatic recognition that in the end, the patient's opinions about the merits of change are the only ones that will determine the success or failure of attempted interventions.

The discovery of MI struck many in the eating disorder field with the force of revelation. Applications of the approach for anorexic and bulimic patients were outlined (e.g., Killick and Allen, 1997; Treasure and Ward, 1997b; Tantillo *et al.*, 2001; Treasure and Schmidt, 2001), scores of training workshops delivered, and pretherapy motivational sessions added to treatment protocols in many specialty clinics. Therapists with a CBT background have welcomed the approach not because it represents a paradigm shift, but because its popularity has contributed to the wider dissemination of shared principles. MI is essentially a focused application of the Socratic style advocated in both general and disorder-specific models of CBT, usefully elaborated for the achievement of a particular objective during the initial phase of treatment. Many of the same strategies are featured in both approaches; for example, MI and CBT would be equally disposed to focus on exploring the 'pros and cons' of change (see Table 15.1), and outline precisely the same principles for using this technique (Miller and Rollnick, 1991, 2002; Vitousek and Orimoto, 1993; Vitousek *et al.*, 1998).

In both approaches, review of the material shown in Table 15.1 is often the principal focus of initial sessions with a new patient. On one level, the exercise is transparent and straightforward: the therapist encourages the patient to share her views about the advantages and disadvantages of her disorder. Yet the simple exercise of reviewing perceived benefits and costs embodies many of the most central assumptions that these approaches share—and, when implemented correctly, offers a highly economical means of conveying them in the first hour of contact. By paying serious, sustained attention to what the *patient* thinks about being anorexic, the therapist communicates a number of important messages: her opinions are respected and her goals are important; she won't be forced to defend or to denounce her disorder; she will be treated as an individual rather than a predictable case of anorexia nervosa; she has the capacity to make active choices about her behavior; therapy is a collaborative process intended to help her find more rewarding ways to live in future.

Therapists should begin by asking patients what they *like* or *value* about their symptoms. By the time they enter treatment, individuals with anorexia nervosa are accustomed to being told what is wrong with what they are doing. Clinicians who depart from the script by asking them what feels right about anorexia are likely to learn considerably more about *both* sets of consequences, as experienced by the patients themselves. For example, Chloe started the first session by declaring that she was happy, healthy, and symptom-free, insisting that 'everything would be totally *fine* if people would just stay out of my business.' Rather than confronting Chloe with evidence that she was manifestly not 'fine' or enumerating the dangers she faced, her therapist encouraged her to describe what felt so good about anorexia that it counterbalanced the problems caused by outside interference. Chloe expounded eagerly on the rewards of thinness—and then, with little prompting from the therapist, began to divulge some of its drawbacks. By maintaining a curious, nonjudgmental tone about both sides of Chloe's experience, the therapist disinhibited much more self-disclosure of Chloe's own ambivalence than she had shared with other professionals.

The diversity of concerns expressed by anorexic patients is evident in the two examples charted in Table 15.1. Chloe's lists feature interpersonal considerations on both sides of the question: She values her thinness in part because it makes her attractive, enhances her status, elicits caretaking, and provides a distinctive identity—but it also troubles her that her disorder causes dissension, distresses her mother, decreases her privacy, and isolates her from friends. Amanda's concerns are more abstract and evaluative: Her ascetic life-style is virtuous, self-disciplined, productive, and safe—yet it seems to her simultaneously trivial, enervating, and, she fears, ultimately futile. These themes may (or may not) presage important issues to address in ongoing therapy; for the moment, they suggest ways to engage the patient's interest in getting it underway.

Throughout the process of reviewing pros and cons, it is crucial to remember the premise for the inquiry. The patient has been asked to share *her own perspective* on the rewards and costs of her symptoms. If the therapist asserts that a declared advantage is invalid, superficial, short-sighted, or 'typically anorexic,' the terms under which the patient chose to reveal her experience are violated. Any intimation that stated motives are not the 'real' reason for the disorder is also contrary to the spirit of the inquiry. At this stage of therapy, the patient's beliefs about her disorder are more important than its actual origins and effects (Miller and Rollnick, 1991). Her personal causal model may be inaccurate, and is always incomplete; however, its influence on her decision to stick with the *status quo* or experiment with change is not constrained by its validity (Vitousek *et al.*, 1998).

While taking care not to dictate or dismiss patients' views, the skilled MI or CBT therapist does much more than simply reflect and record them. Review of pros and cons often provides opportunities to insert psychoeducational material naturally and gracefully, so that didactic elements are less intrusive in the early phase of therapy. For example, when Chloe admitted that she felt cold all the time, her therapist took a minute to explain the phenomenon of starvation hypothermia—noting that one implication of this effect is that fewer calories are required to maintain weight. Common complications not mentioned by the patient can be introduced through the 'hippocket patient' technique: 'I don't know whether you've experienced this at all, but another thing sometimes reported by people who have lost a lot of weight is that their hair begins to fall out—have you noticed that happening?' This angle of approach is especially valuable for content that might be seen as unsympathetic, blameworthy, or bizarre. For example, if the therapist suspects a reluctance to admit to competitive motives, he or she might raise the topic as follows: 'Some people say that they get a private sense of satisfaction out of knowing they can do something really tough that other folks don't have the will power to accomplish. Does that sound similar to how you've felt at times, or has your experience been different?' It should be noted that in all instances the patient is offered the opportunity to endorse, reject, or modify the possibility proposed. Even if the content is acknowledged, its meaning and importance for the individual should be assessed rather than assumed.

Taking the patient's slate of perceived costs and benefits as a whole, one obvious question is whether the disorder seems like a good package deal. The calculations that determine the balance are not always logical—and certainly not additive, as a single powerful incentive may trump numerous liabilities (Miller and Rollnick, 1991). Clearly, it would be an error to conclude that as Chloe has listed more costs than benefits while Amanda identified an equal number of each, the former has become disaffected from her disorder and the latter is poised between two evenly weighted options.

If the patient attests that the *status quo* is preferable to the possibility of change, several lines of inquiry may be useful. While the balance of costs and benefits may be acceptable in the present, does she anticipate that it will remain so 5 or 10 years in the future? In her experience, has the ratio of advantages and disadvantages stayed constant over the course of her disorder, or has she noticed a trend toward diminishing returns? What plans has she considered for mitigating the costs she finds difficult to bear? If her eating disorder is working well, would she be pleased if her own daughter adopted the same strategy some day?

One of the most consistently helpful techniques is to frame the patient's dilemma by juxtaposing specific pros and cons she has identified. Almost without exception, lists such as those charted in Table 15.1 are full of internal inconsistencies. Chloe likes the attention she receives for her thinness, but hates it when people make a fuss about her weight and feels increasingly estranged from her friends. Amanda maintains that her disorder keeps her disciplined and diligent, but believes she would have accomplished more in her professional life in its absence; she prides herself on 'eating right and being healthy,' but has developed osteoporosis as a direct consequence of her diet; she believes that restriction makes her a 'better person' in moral terms, but recognizes that it has constricted and trivialized her concerns. Without going outside the patient's own system of goals and values, the therapist can highlight discrepancies between the objectives she hopes to fulfill through anorexia and her own assessment of its net effects: 'So one

reason that you value being thin is that it attracts a lot of attention from other people—yet on the other hand, you've noticed that you are lonelier and more isolated than you were before this started. That sounds like a real bind . . . What are your thoughts about why that might be happening?' The patient is encouraged to begin exploring the possibility that different coping mechanisms might yield the desired outcomes at a substantially lower price. Most of the goals she seeks—such as self-control, emotional stability, and respect from others—are separable from the means she has relied on to achieve them; it is the means of food restriction and low weight that cannot be detached from their unwelcome consequences.

While the current enthusiasm for MI reflects an encouraging trend in the eating disorder field, two caveats are in order. The first is that clinicians who expect too little from the approach are unlikely to receive much more. Motivational work is often misconstrued as a nondirective form of counseling designed to help the patient sort through her options in a warm, accepting environment, so that she can pick the one that best suits her current stage of 'readiness.' Miller and Rollnick (1991, 2002) emphasize that MI is not simply empathic listening and reflection. It is, rather, a biased, systematic effort to accomplish a specific objective: a decision on the part of the patient to change the problematic behavior, followed by action consistent with that resolve. Both MI and CBT are trying to *influence*; the fact that they proceed more subtly than many other persuasive efforts simply increases the odds that they will succeed.

The other concern is that some therapists may expect more from brief, first-phase work on motivation than it can reasonably deliver. MI is usually conceptualized as a discrete intervention, delivered in one to five sessions preceding treatment proper. In contrast, CBT regards the emphasis on motivation as an integral, ongoing part of all treatment efforts. Particularly in the case of anorexia nervosa, resistance to change is not an initial barrier that is cleared as soon as patients are persuaded to enter treatment and begin the 'real work' of psychotherapy. In many ways, dealing with motivational issues *is* the real work of psychotherapy for this population, and should be considered in designing all of its elements (Vitousek, 2002).

Although attention to motivational issues is especially crucial in the treatment of anorexia nervosa, the same strategies can be extended to work with any clients in whom ambivalence is marked, including bulimic patients who are desperate to stop bingeing but reluctant to stop dieting and those who fear giving up a pattern that has provided some relief from negative self-awareness. In fact, these principles represent good therapeutic practice for all individuals with eating and weight concerns, with the need to implement them systematically increasing in proportion to patients' investment in the *status quo*.

Stepped-care treatment models

The ideal system would be one in which patients could be referred to the type and intensity of treatment that maximized their probability of success while minimizing the financial and personal costs of exposure to too much, too little, or the wrong sort of care. Unfortunately, even in the well-studied case of bulimia nervosa, the use of such a 'matching' strategy has been thwarted by the failure to find consistent predictors of treatment response (Wilson *et al.*, 2000). A less elegant alternative is the stepped-care model, in which interventions of increasing cost, complexity, and/or intensity are delivered sequentially. In a pure stepped-care protocol, all patients are started off with the least expensive and intrusive treatment that is known to provide some benefit, even if it does not offer the best statistical chance for improvement (Garner and Needleman, 1997; Wilson *et al.*, 2000). If patients do not respond, they are provided with progressively more intensive and specialized interventions until a successful result is achieved (or until the optimism or resources of the individual and/or treatment agency are depleted).

For several reasons, a stepped-care approach of some kind seems indicated for bulimia nervosa (Fairburn and Peveler, 1990; Fairburn *et al.*, 1992; Carter and Fairburn, 1997; Garner and Needleman, 1997; Wilson *et al.*, 2000; Birchall and Palmer, 2002; Fairburn, 2002a; Fairburn and Harrison, 2003).

The two forms of psychotherapy (CBT and IPT) that have demonstrated effectiveness for this disorder are both complex treatments that specify 19 hours of individual contact time and require specialized training to deliver. The necessary expertise is unavailable in many locations; in other settings, cost containment measures discourage routine use of the full course of treatment. Moreover, in the case of bulimia nervosa, there is no clear empirical basis for advocating rapid, maximally intensive treatment at the moment of case detection, as duration may not influence the odds of recovery.

As noted in the section on CBT, several economical and readily disseminable alternatives have demonstrated effectiveness with some bulimic patients, including CBT-based self-help and brief psychoeducational group treatment. The low cost and widespread availability of these approaches make them appealing first steps on the treatment hierarchy, with patients who do not achieve a satisfactory response moving on to the 'gold standard' treatment of full CBT (or perhaps IPT). It should be noted, however, that the moderately encouraging data on abbreviated treatments do not provide direct support for a stepped-care strategy. Most of the studies have delivered a single brief treatment, such as self-help or group therapy, without following nonresponders through subsequent rounds of higher-level intervention to gauge the cumulative effect of successive treatments. Although symptom duration alone does not predict treatment response, it is certainly conceivable that repeated failures in less potent treatments might discourage some patients from persisting to forms of therapy that could have been helpful if provided from the outset (Garner and Needleman, 1997; Palmer, 2000).

In practice, few specialists would advocate the use of a stepped-care model that automatically initiated treatment at the lowest level for every patient. Guided self-help might be an excellent opening move in the case of Sharon, the 24-year-old woman with bulimia nervosa who is bingeing and purging at fairly low frequency, shows no significant psychopathology, has a strong support system, and is highly motivated to recover. Indeed, Sharon might well appreciate an intervention that imposed few demands on her work schedule and maximized her sense of autonomy and self-efficacy. In contrast, even in the absence of data to support a matching strategy, most clinicians would reject the option of low-level modalities for patients such as Emily. The severity of her bulimic symptoms suggests that such treatments would be futile—and interventions that are unlikely to work are not cost-effective if they are simply unnecessary preludes to further treatment. In addition, a number of clinical considerations discourage the use of self-help or minimal group treatment in Emily's case, including her social isolation, fluctuating motivation, and suicidal risk.

The field is many more years away from accumulating data of the kind and quality that would permit evidence-based stepped-care protocols for anorexia nervosa. At present, there is no 'gold standard' treatment to recommend, much less an empirically supported 'first step' or 'follow-up' intervention. Some features of anorexia do provide a rational basis for eliminating the lower levels of stepped-care models from consideration (Wilson et al., 2000). Self-help manuals are inappropriate for this population; indeed, programs written for other eating disorders typically caution underweight individuals *not* to 'try this at home' without professional assistance (Cooper, 1993; Fairburn, 1995). Group and psychoeducational strategies are seldom recommended as stand-alone treatments, and medication offers little or no benefit (Walsh, 2002a). In contrast to bulimia nervosa, there is a strong relationship between treatment delay and poor response (Eisler et al., 2000; Steinhausen, 2002); moreover, the medical complications associated with low weight status are clear contraindications for postponing effective treatment. In addition, these patients' lack of motivation for change creates a different context for stepped-care decision making (Wilson et al., 2000).

There is no clinical or ethical basis for deferring research on the higher levels of the stepped-care hierarchy, however, and some compelling reasons to proceed. The most crucial priority is study of the indications for inpatient care. Some experts consider hospitalization the standard approach for the management of anorexia nervosa, exempting only mild cases of recent onset. Although inpatient refeeding is clearly indicated for patients who are medically compromised, there is little evidence that it confers long-term advantages that justify its routine or extended use. Moreover, some correlational evidence suggests that hospitalization may actually contribute to negative outcomes (Gowers et al., 2000; Ben-Tovim et al., 2001; Meads et al., 2001). Studies that randomly assign eligible patients to different levels and lengths of treatment are long overdue.

Special issues
Chronicity

In spite of repeated attempts at treatment, eating disorders prove refractory in a substantial minority of patients. Few data are available on long-term outcome in bulimia nervosa. In anorexia nervosa, 20–25% of surviving patients still meet criteria for an eating disorder when reassessed one to two decades after the index treatment episode, while another sizeable subgroup is improved but symptomatic (Steinhausen et al., 1991; Strober et al., 1997; Zipfel et al., 2000; Steinhausen et al., 2002). Several studies have suggested that chronic patients reach a point of no return—or at least extremely rare return—approximately 10–15 years after the initial treatment contact (Theander, 1985; Strober et al., 1997; Lowe et al., 2001), with virtually none of those still unrecovered by that point crossing over to complete remission when reexamined years later.

No treatment studies have been designed exclusively for individuals with long histories of anorexia nervosa, although some projects include a high proportion of chronic patients (e.g., Dare et al., 2001; Pike et al., 2003). Thoughtful (and generally convergent) clinical recommendations are available for work with this population (e.g., Hall, 1982; Kalucy et al., 1985; Yager, 1995, 2002; Goldner et al., 1997; Geller et al., 2001a; Noordenbos et al., 2002). Most experts stress the importance of 'steering a balance between expecting too much and too little' (Yager, 2002, p. 346) from these individuals, who are often disheartened by previous treatment failures yet unwilling to take the behavioral steps essential to recovery. Many writers caution against coercive or overzealous interventions (Goldner et al., 1997; Rathner, 1998; Yager, 2002), warning that aggressive treatment may precipitate severe depression and suicide attempts (Kalucy et al., 1985; Garfinkel, 2002b) or drive patients away from the longer-term, slower-paced therapy from which they might be more likely to benefit. Moreover, even when treatment is successful in producing weight gain, the loss of anorexia nervosa can leave these isolated, constricted individuals feeling bereft, unable to find another organizing principle or sense of purpose to replace their disorder (Hall, 1982).

With some patients, the most helpful approach is the harm reduction model advised for resistant or intractable cases of substance abuse (Marlatt and Tapert, 1993). Using the empathic, collaborative style favored by MI and CBT, the therapist can encourage the patient to set and achieve more modest goals, such as stabilization at a low but safer weight, selection of a restrictive but balanced diet, and elimination of the most dangerous practices of laxative abuse, fluid restriction, frequent vomiting, and extreme exercise. Principles may also be drawn from the rehabilitative model used to support patients with other severe mental illnesses, which focuses on minimizing inpatient care and fostering participation in social and occupational activities (Goldner et al., 1997).

A harm abatement approach may be indicated as well for severe cases of bulimia nervosa that are unresponsive to sustained trials of high-quality, individually tailored treatment. Again, duration is less likely to be a relevant consideration, but extraordinarily high frequency and atypical reluctance to give up the bulimic pattern may contribute. In such instances, it might be reasonable to target eating small retained meals during the day and postponing binge episodes, working simultaneously on other treatment goals such as coping with negative affect and strengthening interpersonal connections.

The decision to use a management model should be reached slowly, reluctantly, and above all tentatively (Vitousek et al., 1998). Certainly, just as with the constructs of 'readiness' and 'stages of change,' there is a risk that clinicians may use 'chronicity' to give both themselves and their patients a pass, abandoning active treatment efforts in cases that are not intractable but merely difficult. In view of the early age of onset in anorexia nervosa, most persistently ill patients will qualify for 'chronic' status while still in their 20s—which leaves a lot of years ahead consigned to a very limited, very hungry, and very tired life. That is a steep price to pay for unwarranted therapeutic pessimism. Even in truly refractory cases, the hope of transformational change should never be extinguished (Palmer, 2000; Yager, 2002). Anecdotal accounts describe instances of recovery in patients who have been anorexic for more than 25 years—in one case, accomplishing symptom remission at the age of 67, after half a century of life as an anorexic (Noordenbos *et al.*, 1998).

Comorbidity

On one level, the treatment of eating disorder patients with a comorbid Axis I or II condition should not be considered a 'special problem.' Like the issue of resistance to change in anorexia nervosa, it is an expected rather than exceptional complication of work in this area. Anorexia and bulimia often co-occur with affective disorders, anxiety disorders, substance use disorders, and personality disorders (for reviews, see Wonderlich and Mitchell, 1997; Pearlstein, 2002 and O'Brien and Vincent, 2003). Specific rates vary widely across studies as a function of referral and recruitment patterns, assessment procedures, and changes in diagnostic criteria over time (Grilo *et al.*, 2003; O'Brien and Vincent, 2003). It is clear, however, that in the majority of cases clinicians treating anorexic and bulimic patients will confront psychiatric profiles that include more than one symptom cluster. It is far less clear how treatments should be adapted to address those diverse clinical pictures.

An obvious point to underscore is that not all comorbidities are equally meaningful or problematic. In a sense, comorbidity with depression is built into severe eating disorders. Any individual who ate less than 1000 calories per day at a BMI of 14, like the chronically anorexic Amanda, would be depressed; no one who matched the behavioral pattern of the severely bulimic Emily could maintain a normal mood state. From that perspective, it is nonsensical to speak of treating depression before taking on the eating disorder—or even alongside management of the eating disorder. We treat depression *by* alleviating the eating disorder, and wait to discover what vestiges remain after it is resolved.

Other kinds of problems are less inevitably linked to eating and weight pathology, even though they frequently co-occur with such symptoms and are usually exacerbated by them. These may (or may not) need to be addressed directly. In some instances, such interventions should precede close focus on the eating disorder, as in the case of serious substance abuse or active psychosis. In general, however, it is preferable to defer the treatment of extraneous psychopathology unless it poses a significant barrier to work on the eating disorder, as anxiety, depression, and even maladaptive 'personality' patterns all tend to improve with amelioration of anorexia or bulimia (Wilson *et al.*, 1997).

Comorbidity figures prominently in the current debate about the value of empirically supported treatments (e.g., Seligman, 1995). Clinicians often hold that research findings are of limited relevance to their own practice (Haas and Clopton, 2003), which includes complex, treatment-resistant cases not represented in the tidy samples selected for study in controlled trials. Wilson (1995, 1996, 1998a,b) makes a persuasive case that the opposite is true in the eating disorder field. Anorexic and bulimic patients referred to specialty services and treated in the context of research tend to be especially challenging cases, with severe eating disorder pathology, high levels of comorbidity, and a record of repeated failures in previous treatment attempts. For example, in one trial comparing CBT and IPT for bulimia nervosa, 37% of participants had at least one Axis II disorder and 22% currently met criteria for major depressive disorder (Agras *et al.*, 2000). In addition, the record of lifetime psychiatric illness included rates of 53% for major depression, 23% for substance abuse or dependence, and 24% for anorexia nervosa.

Therapists are correct, however, that the research literature offers little guidance about how to assist patients with so much compound psychopathology that their eating disorder symptoms may rank second, third, or fourth on a list of priority treatment targets. The sample case of Emily matches this profile. Whether or not she would be accepted into a controlled trial would probably depend on the level of her fluctuating substance use and suicide risk at the time she is evaluated. If she does make it into a study, she is fairly likely to drop out before completion (just as she has dropped out of nonresearch treatments in the past); if she did persist, she is fairly unlikely to obtain full symptom control (just as she has failed to respond to a variety of previous interventions). As discussed in the section on CBT for bulimia, the fallacy arises when we assume that because patients like Emily do poorly in research treatments, they can only profit from different (and usually 'deeper') treatments guided by clinical judgment rather than empirical data (Wilson, 1995, 1996, 1998a,b). In fact, patients who fare poorly tend to do so across modalities, and there is no evidence that they do better when treated outside the context of research or with untested approaches.

Clearly, the field needs to experiment with more effective ways to help these severely impaired patients. One clinical approach is based on the assumption that individuals similar to Emily have a subtype of eating disorder termed 'multi-impulsive bulimia,' in which binge–purge behavior is associated with other patterns such as substance abuse, self-harm, sexual disinhibition, and shoplifting (Lacey and Evans, 1986; Lacey, 1993). An eclectic treatment program has been proposed for such cases, but has not yet been examined in controlled trials. Most experts construe this profile as a not-uncommon overlap between Axis I and Axis II pathology, and recommend combining treatments that have been validated for each. Recently, several specialists have described adaptations of dialectical BT (DBT; Linehan, 1993) for bulimia (Wiser and Telch, 1999; Safer *et al.*, 2001a,b; Palmer and Birchall, 2003; Palmer *et al.*, 2003). A clinical case series reported encouraging results using the full DBT program for treatment-resistant bulimic patients with comorbid borderline personality disorder (Palmer *et al.*, 2003).

Attitudes of clinicians

We have been reviewing features of the eating disorders and individual patients that make change difficult to accomplish; for balance, it is important to note that the attitudes and behaviors of clinicians can prove equally resistant to modification. Some persistent problems in this area include: (1) rejecting, patronizing, and punitive responses to eating disordered individuals; (2) denial of key dynamics that are theoretically inconvenient or clinically unsympathetic; (3) resort to the extremes of aggression or passivity; (4) stereotyping of anorexia and bulimia; (5) insensitivity to sociocultural context; (6) personal issues with eating and weight that interfere with optimal treatment; and (7) reluctance to change accustomed therapeutic practices.

Traditionally, the therapist–patient relationship is abysmal in anorexia nervosa (Garner and Bemis, 1982, 1985; Garner, 1985; Goldner *et al.*, 1997; Beumont and Vandereycken, 1998; Kaplan and Garfinkel, 1999). A former anorexic patient wrote: 'It is difficult not to gain the impression from the literature [on anorexia nervosa] that individual therapy has been devalued because (among other reasons) psychotherapists do not like anorexics, and anorexics do not like psychotherapists' (MacLeod, 1982, p. 122).

MacLeod's impression of the antipathy aroused by people who share her diagnosis has been confirmed in surveys of therapists, physicians, and nurses (e.g., Brotman *et al.*, 1984; Fleming and Szmukler, 1992; Burket and Schramm, 1995). Few symptom patterns evoke stronger negative reactions from professionals or create more dissension among treatment teams (Tinker and Ramer, 1983; Hamburg and Herzog, 1990).

A number of factors appear to contribute to the unsavory clinical reputation of anorexic patients, including the views that they are deceptive, manipulative, defiant, rigid, suspicious, and ungrateful for the efforts clinicians make on their behalf. Perhaps the most provocative element is the perception that these patients' suffering is self-inflicted. Like individuals who abuse drugs or commit acts of self-harm, they become ineligible for compassion by taking part in the manufacture of pathology. The eating disorders are often regarded as 'diseases of the will' (Halleck, 1988), in which symptoms arise 'because of stubbornness (anorexia) or lack of willpower (bulimia)' (Beumont and Vandereycken, 1998). Across mental and physical illnesses, people who are considered able but unwilling to recover are viewed as having less 'respectable' and more blameworthy disorders (Halleck, 1988). These attitudes undoubtedly contribute to the occasional use of punitive interventions in this specialty area (Garner, 1985), and the much higher rate of contentious and controlling ones.

Ironically, some of the most impassioned pleas for more sensitive treatment are based on the same judgmental premise. Apparently sharing the view that patients would be culpable if they *did* contribute to their own pathology, many clinicians insist that they do *not*, casting anorexic patients as unwilling victims of an unwelcome disease. Although this construction is perhaps the most economical way for professionals to sustain 'therapeutic' attitudes toward difficult patients, it should not be confused with genuine empathy. Our goal must be to understand the complex experience of anorexia nervosa, not to distort it for the purpose of getting around the constraints on our own compassion.

Problems also arise from the fact that many eating-disordered beliefs are exaggerated versions of *culturally*-syntonic ideas (Garner and Bemis, 1985). Some clinicians (often, but not exclusively, male clinicians) are insensitive to the social context in which their patients are immersed; other therapists (often, but not exclusively, female therapists) run into trouble because they are susceptible to the same pressures—or have rejected those influences on political grounds and are frustrated that their clients succumb (Gutwill, 1994; Garner *et al.*, 1997). There are numerous discussions in this area of the relative assets and handicaps of female and male therapists (e.g., Frankenburg, 1984; Wooley, 1991; Kopp, 1994; Stockwell and Dolan, 1994; Katzman and Waller, 1998; McVoy, 1998) and of clinicians with or without eating disorder histories (e.g., Kalucy *et al.*, 1985; Jasper, 1993; Johnson, 2000). Whatever the therapist's sex, politics, personal background, or current weight, it is crucial that she or he is both attuned to the sociocultural environment that surrounds the eating disorders and sufficiently distanced from it to avoid transmitting mixed messages (Garner *et al.*, 1997).

Like virtually every eating-disordered individual, all four patients profiled in this chapter could enumerate troubling encounters with professionals who seemed to endorse elements of their pathology. For example, a physician told the weight-suppressed bulimic patient Emily that her low BMI would be ideal if she could only manage to sustain it without vomiting five to 10 times per day; the dietitian to whom the young anorexic patient Chloe was sent applauded her avoidance of 'junk food' while suggesting that she increment her caloric intake with additional 'healthy' choices. In our view, whether or not therapists have had a clinical eating disorder in the past, it is also unacceptable for highly restrained or weight-conscious clinicians to work with bulimic or anorexic patients—not least because it is hypocritical.

Conclusions

After 20 years of treatment research, efforts to help individuals with bulimia nervosa can now be guided by information about what works best, fastest, and most reliably. Two very different forms of psychotherapy (CBT and IPT), as well as antidepressant medication, have been shown to benefit these patients. CBT is by far the most examined, supported, and endorsed approach. This treatment produces greater symptom reduction more rapidly in a higher percentage of patients than any other modality, and its effects have proven stable over time and robust across settings. Although CBT is by no means universally accepted (or even widely practiced, at least in its specified form), its influence can be gauged by the fact that CBT is a party to almost all of the active debates in this specialty area. Critics generally contend that we would do better in the treatment of bulimia if we shifted the focus of standard CBT or included additional elements; rarely, however, do they propose jettisoning the model in favor of a radically different approach. Similarly, the key questions in pharmacotherapy concern whether drugs can add to CBT or benefit the subset of CBT nonresponders.

There is still substantial room for improvement in the results obtained through CBT, and the next logical stages of research are proceeding with efforts to streamline the approach for patients who respond well and to broaden or supplement it for those who do not. At present, however, CBT stands not only as the best validated treatment for bulimia nervosa, but as one of the most thoughtfully investigated and strongly supported interventions across the psychological disorders. In many ways, progress in this relatively new specialty area is a model for how systematic research can enhance our understanding and treatment of psychopathology.

At the same time, the status of CBT for bulimia also illustrates a persistent problem in our discipline. Relatively few patients receive this effective treatment because most practitioners are neither inclined nor trained to use it (Wilson, 1998b; Crow *et al.*, 1999; Fairburn, 2002a). One of the highest immediate priorities must be the development of more successful strategies for disseminating both information about the approach and the skills required to deliver it.

The situation is quite different in the case of anorexia nervosa, where no single treatment model is preeminent in either the empirical literature or clinical practice. The most discouraging commentary on the state of psychotherapy research is that there is remarkably little evidence to summarize. Few controlled trials have been attempted; some have broken down after a majority of patients dropped out or failed in treatment. Sample sizes are uniformly small, and results seldom replicated. As a result, the field sometimes draws unwarranted conclusions about what treatments work best for which patients on the basis of single studies that included eight to 10 participants per cell.

Unfortunately, the meager data we possess confirm the clinical impression that no known treatments work especially well, rapidly, or consistently for established cases of anorexia nervosa. Although it is clear that many anorexic individuals do recover and most improve, we have yet to identify psychological or pharmacological interventions that clearly contribute to the likelihood of a favorable outcome. Only a few conclusions are justified at present—and offer more guidance about treatments to avoid (dietary counseling alone, medication alone, methods that concentrate solely on underlying issues) than what approaches to adopt. In the persistent absence of data, 'best practice' standards for the treatment of anorexia nervosa continue to be defined by the 'best guess' opinions of experts rather than the 'best evidence' criteria of research.

While there are grounds for pessimism, it is much too soon for hopelessness. Because many individuals do overcome anorexia nervosa—and seem responsive to environmental factors rather than solely influenced by intrinsic disease processes—it is reasonable to surmise that we might be able to speed up recovery and perhaps change ultimate outcomes by varying what we do in treatment. A few dimensions that seem to make a difference have been identified. For example, it is desirable to intervene as soon as possible after onset; if patients are still adolescent, it is probably important to work with family members as well as the anorexic individual, although the optimal methods for doing so have yet to be identified; it appears preferable to see parents and patients separately, at least if a parental control model of therapy is used.

With older patients or those with a longer history of illness, the parameters of effective treatment are unclear, and the results likely to remain less satisfactory. In a backwards sort of way, however, the accumulation of data about the difficulty of modifying established anorexia nervosa should contribute to the design and delivery of more promising treatments. For example, in view of what we know about the nature of this disorder, it was not reasonable to anticipate that the minimalist 20-session treatments provided in some controlled trials would transform the attitudes and behavior of ambivalent patients with longstanding anorexia nervosa. Future studies should offer interventions that are better matched to the well-studied features of the disorder than the short-term and/or crisis-driven models of care often used. There is also increasing recognition that it is crucial to attend to the patient's own views about her symptoms and the prospect of change, and foolish to neglect either specific eating/weight-related behaviors or the broader context that makes them meaningful for the anorexic individual. Just as most psychodynamic therapists perceive a need for direct attention to symptoms, most CBT experts stress the importance of exploring their meaning and function. At least to some extent, anorexia nervosa seems to impose a degree of convergence on the factional field of psychotherapy. The high levels of agreement on a number of practice principles increase the confidence with which these can be recommended until more conclusive evidence is available.

References

Agras, W. S. (1997). The treatment of bulimia nervosa. *Drugs of Today*, **33**, 405–11.

Agras, W. S. (2003). Commentary. *International Journal of Eating Disorders*, **33**, 255–6.

Agras, W. S., *et al.* (2000). Outcome predictors for the cognitive behavior treatment of bulimia nervosa: data from a multisite study. *American Journal of Psychiatry*, **157**, 1302–8.

Agras, W. S., Schneider, J. A., Arnow, B., Raeburn, S. D., and Telch, C. (1989). Cognitive-behavioral and response-prevention treatments for bulimia nervosa. *Journal of Consulting and Clinical Psychology*, **57**, 215–21.

Agras, W. S., Walsh, T., Fairburn, C. G., Wilson, G. T., and Kraemer, H. C. (2000). A multicenter comparison of cognitive-behavioral therapy and interpersonal therapy for bulimia nervosa. *Archives of General Psychiatry*, **57**, 459–66.

Ainsworth, C., Waller, G., and Kennedy, F. (2002). Threat processing in women with bulimia. *Clinical Psychology Review*, **22**, 1155–78.

American Psychiatric Association (2000). *Diagnostic and statistical manual of mental disorders* (text revision). Washington, DC: American Psychiatric Association.

Anderluh, M. B., Tchanturia, K., Rabe-Hesketh, S., and Treasure, J. (2003). Childhood obsessive-compulsive personality traits in adult women with eating disorders: defining a broader eating disorder phenotype. *American Journal of Psychiatry*, **160**, 242–7.

Andersen, A. E. (1995). Sequencing treatment decisions: cooperation or conflict between therapist and patient. In: G. Szmukler, C. Dare, and J. Treasure, ed. *Handbook of eating disorders: theory, treatment, and research*, pp. 363–79. Chichester: Wiley.

Apple, R. F. (1999). Interpersonal therapy for bulimia nervosa. *Journal of Clinical Psychology, In Session*, **55**, 715–25.

Ball, J. (1999). A controlled evaluation of cognitive-behavioural therapy for anorexia nervosa: results of a four year outpatient trial. Paper presented at the meeting of the International Conference on Eating Disorders, London, UK.

Beck, A. T. (1976). *Cognitive therapy and the emotional disorders*. New York: International Universities Press.

Beck, A. T., Rush, A. J., Shaw, B. F., and Emery, G. (1979). *Cognitive therapy of depression*. New York: Guilford Press.

Beck, A. T., Wright, F. D., Newman, C. F., and Liese, B. S. (2001). *Cognitive therapy of substance abuse*. New York: Guilford Press.

Beck, J. S. (1995). *Cognitive therapy: basics and beyond*. New York: Guilford Press.

Bell, L. (1999). The spectrum of psychological problems in people with eating disorders: an analysis of 30 eating disordered patients treated with cognitive analytic therapy. *Clinical Psychology and Psychotherapy*, **6**, 29–38.

Bemis, K. M. (1983). A comparison of functional relationships in anorexia nervosa and phobia. In: P. L. Darby, P. E. Garfinkel, D. M. Garner, and D. V. Coscina, ed. *Anorexia nervosa: recent developments in research*, pp. 403–15. New York: Alan R. Liss.

Ben-Tovim, D. I., *et al.* (2001). Outcome in patients with eating disorders: a 5 year study. *The Lancet*, **357**, 1254–7.

Beumont, P. J. V. and Vandereycken, W. (1998). Challenges and risks for health care professionals. In: W. Vandereycken and P. J. V. Beumont, ed. *Treating eating disorders: ethical, legal and personal issues*, pp. 1–29. New York: New York University Press.

Beumont, P. J. V., O'Connor, M., Touyz, S. W., and Williams, H. (1987). Nutritional counselling in the treatment of anorexia and bulimia nervosa. In: P. J. V. Beumont, G. D. Burrows, and R. C. Casper, ed. *Handbook of eating disorders: Part 1: anorexia and bulimia nervosa*, pp. 349–59. New York: Elsevier.

Beumont, P. J. V., Garner, D. M., and Touyz, S. W. (1994). Diagnoses of eating or dieting disorders: what may we learn from past mistakes? *International Journal of Eating Disorders*, **16**, 349–62.

Beumont, P. J. V., Beumont, C. C., Touyz, S. W., and Williams, H. (1997). Nutritional counseling and supervised exercise. In: D. M. Garner and P. E. Garfinkel, ed. *Handbook of treatment of eating disorders*, pp. 178–87. New York: Guilford Press.

Birchall, H. and Palmer, B. (2002). Doing it by the book: what place for guided self-help for bulimic disorders? *European Eating Disorders Review*, **10**, 379–85.

Blake, W., Turnbull, S., and Treasure, J. (1997). Stages and processes of change in eating disorders: implications for therapy. *Clinical Psychology and Psychotherapy*, **4**, 186–91.

Bloom, C., Gitter, A., Gutwill, S., Kogel, L., and Zaphiropoulos, L. (1994). *Eating problems: a feminist psychoanalytic treatment model*. New York: Basic Books.

Blouin, J. H., *et al.* (1994). Prognostic indicators in bulimia nervosa treated with cognitive-behavioral group therapy. *International Journal of Eating Disorders*, **15**, 113–24.

Boachie, A., Goldfield, G. S., and Spettigue, W. (2003). Olanzapine use as an adjunctive treatment for hospitalized children with anorexia nervosa: case reports. *International Journal of Eating Disorders*, **33**, 98–103.

Bo-Linn, G., Santa-Ana, C. A., Morawski, S. G., and Fordtran, J. S. (1983). Purging and calorie absorption in bulimic patients and normal women. *Annals of Internal Medicine*, **99**, 14–17.

Bowers, W. A., Evans, K., and Anderson, A. E. (1997). Inpatient treatment of eating disorders: a cognitive therapy milieu. *Cognitive and Behavioral Practice*, **4**, 291–323.

Brotman, A. W., Stern, T. A., and Herzog, D. B. (1984). Emotional reactions of house officers to patients with anorexia nervosa, diabetes, and obesity. *International Journal of Eating Disorders*, **3**, 71–7.

Bruch, H. (1962). Perceptual and conceptual disturbances in anorexia nervosa. *Psychosomatic Medicine*, **24**, 187–94.

Bruch, H. (1973). *Eating disorders: obesity, anorexia nervosa, and the person within*. New York: Basic Books.

Bruch, H. (1978). *The golden cage: the enigma of anorexia nervosa*. Harvard University Press, Cambridge, MA.

Bruch, H. (1985). Four decades of eating disorders. In: D. M. Garner and P. E. Garfinkel, ed. *Handbook of psychotherapy for anorexia nervosa and bulimia*, pp. 7–18. New York: Guilford Press.

Bruch, H. (1988). *Conversations with anorexics*. New York: Basic Books.

Bruna, T. and Fogteloo, J. (2003). Drug treatments. In: J. Treasure, U. Schmidt, and E. van Furth, ed. *Handbook of eating disorders*, 2nd edn, pp. 311–24. Chichester: Wiley.

Burket, R. C. and Schramm, L. L. (1995). Therapists' attitudes about treating patients with eating disorders. *Southern Medical Journal*, **88**, 813–18.

Byrne, S. M. and McLean, N. J. (2002). The cognitive-behavioral model of bulimia nervosa: a direct evaluation. *International Journal of Eating Disorders*, **31**, 17–31.

Carter, F. A., McIntosh, V. V., Joyce, P. R., Sullivan, P. F., and Bulik, C. M. (2003). Role of exposure with response prevention in cognitive-behavioral therapy for bulimia nervosa: three-year follow-up results. *International Journal of Eating Disorders*, **33**, 127–35.

Carter, J. C. (2002). Self-help books in the treatment of eating disorders. In: C. G. Fairburn and K. D. Brownell, ed. *Eating disorders and obesity: a comprehensive handbook*, 2nd edn, pp. 358–61. New York: Guilford Press.

Carter, J. C. and Fairburn, C. G. (1997). Cognitive-behavioral self help for binge eating disorder: a controlled effectiveness study. *Journal of Consulting and Clinical Psychology*, **66**, 616–23.

Casper, R. C. (1982). Treatment principles in anorexia nervosa. In: S. C. Feinstein, J. G. Looney, A. Z. Schwatzenberg, and A. D. Sorosky, ed. *Adolescent psychiatry*, Vol. 10, pp. 431–54. Chicago: University of Chicago Press.

Casper, R. C. (1987). The psychopathology of anorexia nervosa: the pathological psychodynamic processes. In: P. J. V. Beumont, G. D. Burrows, and R. C. Casper, ed. *Handbook of eating disorders: Part 1: anorexia and bulimia nervosa*, pp. 159–69. New York: Elsevier.

Channon, S., de Silva, P., Hemsley, D., and Perkins, R. (1989). A controlled trial of cognitive-behavioural and behavioural treatment of anorexia nervosa. *Behaviour Research and Therapy*, **27**, 529–35.

Chen, E., *et al.* (2003). Comparison of group and individual cognitive-behavioral therapy for patients with bulimia nervosa. *International Journal of Eating Disorders*, **33**, 241–54.

Cochrane Depression Anxiety and Neurosis Group (2000). Psychotherapy for bulimia nervosa and bingeing. The Cochrane database of systematic reviews [on-line serial]. Available: Issue 2.

Compas, B. E., Haaga, D. A. F., Keefe, F. J., Leitenberg, H., and Williams, D. A. (1998). Sampling of empirically supported psychological treatments from health psychology: smoking, chronic pain, cancer, and bulimia nervosa. *Journal of Clinical and Consulting Psychology*, **66**, 89–112.

Cooper, M. (1997). Cognitive theory in anorexia nervosa and bulimia nervosa: a review. *Behavioural and Cognitive Psychotherapy*, **25**, 113–45.

Cooper, P. (1993). *Bulimia nervosa: a guide to recovery.* London: Robinson Publishing.

Cooper, P. J. (1995). *Bulimia nervosa and binge eating: a guide to recovery.* New York: New York University Press.

Cooper, P. J. and Fairburn, C. G. (1984). Cognitive behaviour therapy for anorexia nervosa: some preliminary findings. *Journal of Psychosomatic Research*, **28**, 493–9.

Cooper, P. J. and Steere, J. (1995). A comparison of two psychological treatments for bulimia nervosa: implications for models of maintenance. *Behaviour Research and Therapy*, **33**, 875–85.

Craighead, L. W. and Agras, W. S. (1991). Mechanisms of action in cognitive-behavioral and pharmacological interventions for obesity and bulimia nervosa. *Journal of Consulting and Clinical Psychology*, **59**, 115–25.

Crisp, A. H. (1980). *Anorexia nervosa: let me be.* London: Academic Press.

Crisp, A. H. (1997). Anorexia nervosa as flight from growth: assessment and treatment based on the model. In: D. M. Garner and P. E. Garfinkel, ed. *Handbook of treatment for eating disorders*, 2nd edn, pp. 248–77. New York: Guilford Press.

Crisp, A. H., *et al.* (1991). A controlled study of the effect of therapies aimed at adolescent and family psychopathology in anorexia nervosa. *British Journal of Psychiatry*, **159**, 325–33.

Crow, S. J., Mussell, M. P., Peterson, C. B., Knopke, A., and Mitchell, J. E. (1999). Prior treatment received by patients with bulimia nervosa. *International Journal of Eating Disorders*, **25**, 39–44.

Dare, C. (1985). The family therapy of anorexia nervosa. *Journal of Psychiatric Research*, **19**, 435–43.

Dare, C. and Crowther, C. (1995). Psychodynamic models of eating disorders. In: G. Szmukler, C. Dare, and J. Treasure, ed. *Handbook of eating disorders: theory, treatment, and research*, pp. 125–39. Chichester: Wiley.

Dare, C. and Eisler, I. (1992). Family therapy for anorexia nervosa. In: P. J. Cooper and A. Stein, ed. *Feeding problems and eating disorders in children and adolescents*, pp. 147–60. Chur, Switzerland: Harwood Academic Publishers.

Dare, C. and Eisler, I. (1995). Family therapy. In: G. I. Szmukler, C. Dare, and J. L. Treasure, ed. *Handbook of eating disorders: theory, treatment, and research*, pp. 333–49. Chichester: Wiley.

Dare, C. and Eisler, I. (1997). Family therapy for anorexia nervosa. In: D. Garner and P. E. Garfinkel, ed. *Handbook of treatment for eating disorders*, 2nd edn, pp. 307–24. New York: Guilford Press.

Dare, C., Eisler, I., Russell, G., Treasure, J., and Dodge, L. (2001). Psychological therapies for adults with anorexia nervosa: randomised controlled trial of out–patient treatments. *British Journal of Psychiatry*, **178**, 216–21.

Elkin, I., *et al.* (1989). National Institute of Mental Health treatment of depression collaborative research program: general effectiveness of treatments. *Archives of General Psychiatry*, **46**, 971–82.

Eisler, I., *et al.* (1997). Family and individual therapy in anorexia nervosa. *Archives of General Psychiatry*, **54**, 1025–30.

Eisler, I., *et al.* (2000). Family therapy for adolescent anorexia nervosa: the results of a controlled comparison of two family interventions. *Journal of Child Psychology and Psychiatry and Allied Disciplines*, **41**, 727–36.

Fairburn, C. G. (1981). A cognitive behavioural approach to the management of bulimia. *Psychological Medicine*, **11**, 707–11.

Fairburn, C. G. (1985). Cognitive-behavioral treatment for bulimia. In: D. M. Garner and P. E. Garfinkel, ed. *Handbook of psychotherapy for anorexia nervosa and bulimia*, pp. 160–92. New York: Guilford Press.

Fairburn, C. G. (1988). The current status of psychological treatments for bulimia nervosa. *Journal of Psychosomatic Research*, **32**, 635–45.

Fairburn, C. G. (1993). Interpersonal psychotherapy for bulimia nervosa. In: G. L. Klerman and M. M. Weissman, ed. *New applications of interpersonal psychotherapy*, pp. 353–78. Washington, DC: American Psychiatric Association.

Fairburn, C. G. (1995). *Overcoming binge eating.* New York: Guilford Press.

Fairburn, C. G. (1997a). Eating disorders. In: D. M. Clark and C. G. Fairburn, ed. *Cognitive behaviour therapy: science and practice*, pp. 209–41. Oxford: Oxford University Press.

Fairburn, C. G. (1997b). Interpersonal psychotherapy for bulimia nervosa. In: D. M. Garner and P. E. Garfinkel, ed. *Handbook of treatment for eating disorders*, 2nd edn, pp. 278–94. New York: Guilford Press.

Fairburn, C. G. (2002a). Cognitive-behavioral therapy for bulimia nervosa. In: C. G. Fairburn and K. D. Brownell, ed. *Eating disorders and obesity: a comprehensive handbook*, 2nd edn, pp. 302–7. New York: Guilford Press.

Fairburn, C. G. (2002b). Interpersonal psychotherapy for eating disorders. In: C. G. Fairburn and K. D. Brownell, ed. *Eating disorders and obesity: a comprehensive handbook*, 2nd edn, pp. 320–4. New York: Guilford Press.

Fairburn, C. G. and Carter, J. C. (1997). Self-help and guided self-help for binge-eating problems. In: D. M. Garner and P. E. Garfinkel, ed. *Handbook of treatment for eating disorders*, 2nd edn, pp. 494–99. New York: Guilford Press.

Fairburn, C. G. and Harrison, P. J. (2003). Eating disorders. *The Lancet*, **361**, 407–16.

Fairburn, C. G. and Peveler, R. C. (1990). Bulimia nervosa and a stepped care approach to management. *Gut*, **31**, 1220–2.

Fairburn, C. G., Cooper, Z., and Cooper, P. J. (1986). The clinical features and maintenance of bulimia nervosa. In: K. D. Brownell and J. P. Foreyt, ed. *Handbook of eating disorders: Physiology, psychology, and treatment of obesity, anorexia, and bulimia*, pp. 389–404. New York: Basic Books.

Fairburn, C. G., *et al.* (1991). Three psychological treatments for bulimia nervosa: a comparative trial. *Archives of General Psychiatry*, **48**, 463–9.

Fairburn, C. G., Agras, W. S., and Wilson, G. T. (1992). The research on the treatment of bulimia nervosa: practical and theoretical implications. In: G. H. Anderson and S. H. Kennedy, ed. *The biology of feast and famine: the relevance to eating disorders*, pp. 353–78. Academic Press, New York.

Fairburn, C. G., Jones, R., Peveler, R. C., Hope, R. A., and O'Connor, M. (1993a). Psychotherapy and bulimia nervosa: longer-term effects of interpersonal psychotherapy, behavior therapy, and cognitive-behavior therapy. *Archives of General Psychiatry*, **50**, 419–28.

Fairburn, C. G., Marcus, M. D., and Wilson, G. T. (1993b). Cognitive-behavioral treatment for binge eating and bulimia nervosa: a comprehensive treatment manual. In: C. G. Fairburn and G. T. Wilson, ed. *Binge eating: nature, assessment, and treatment*, pp. 361–404. New York: Guilford Press.

Fairburn, C. G., *et al.* (1995). A prospective study of outcome in bulimia nervosa and the long-term effects of three psychological treatments. *Archives of General Psychiatry*, **52**, 304–12.

Fairburn, C. G., Cooper, Z., Doll, H. A., and Welch, S. L. (1999a). Risk factors for anorexia nervosa: three integrated case-control comparisons. *Archives of General Psychiatry*, **56**, 468–76.

Fairburn, C. G., Shafran R., and Cooper, Z. (1999b). A cognitive behavioural theory of anorexia nervosa. *Behaviour Research and Therapy*, **37**, 1–13.

Fairburn, C. G., Cooper, Z., and Shafran, R. (2003). Cognitive behaviour therapy for eating disorders: a 'transdiagnostic' theory and treatment. *Behaviour Research and Therapy*, **41**, 509–28.

Fallon, P., Katzman, M. A., and Wooley, S. C., ed. (1994). *Feminist perspectives on eating disorders.* New York: Guilford Press.

Feld, R., Woodside, D. B., Kaplan, A. S., Olmsted, M. P., and Carter, J. (2001). Pretreatment motivational enhancement therapy for eating disorders: a pilot study. *International Journal of Eating Disorders*, **29**, 393–400.

Ferguson, C. P., La Via, M. C., Crossan, P. J., and Kaye, W. H. (1999). Are selective serotonin reuptake inhibitors effective in underweight anorexia nervosa? *International Journal of Eating Disorders*, **25**, 11–17.

Fleming, J. and Szmukler, G. I. (1992). Attitudes of medical professionals towards patients with eating disorders. *Australian and New Zealand Journal of Psychiatry*, **26**, 436–43.

Fluoxetine Bulimia Nervosa Collaborative Study Group (1992). Fluoxetine in the treatment of bulimia nervosa. A multicenter placebo controlled double-blind trial. *Archives of General Psychiatry*, **49**, 139–47.

Frankenburg, F. R. (1984). Female therapists in the management of anorexia nervosa. *International Journal of Eating Disorders*, **3**, 25–33.

Freud, A. (1958). Adolescence. *The Psychoanalytic Study of the Child*, **13**, 255–78.

Garfinkel, P. E. (2002a). Classification and diagnosis of eating disorders. In: C. G. Fairburn and K. D. Brownell, ed. *Eating disorders and obesity: a comprehensive handbook*, 2nd edn, pp. 226–30. New York: Guilford Press.

Garfinkel, P. E. (2002b). Eating disorders. *The Canadian Journal of Psychiatry*, **47**, 225–6.

Garfinkel, P. E. and Walsh, B. T. (1997). Drug therapies. In: D. M. Garner and P. E. Garfinkel, ed. *Handbook of treatment for eating disorders*, 2nd edn, pp. 372–80. New York: Guilford Press.

Garner, D. M. (1985). Iatrogenesis in anorexia nervosa and bulimia nervosa. *International Journal of Eating Disorders*, **4**, 701–26.

Garner, D. M. (1986). Cognitive therapy for anorexia nervosa. In: K. D. Brownell and J. P. Foreyt, ed. *Handbook of eating disorders*, pp. 301–27. New York: Basic Books.

Garner, D. M. (1988). Anorexia nervosa. In: M. Hersen and C. G. Last, ed. *Child behavior therapy casebook*, pp. 263–76. New York: Plenum Press.

Garner, D. M. (1997). Psychoeducational principles. In: D. M. Garner and P. E. Garfinkel, ed. *Handbook of treatment for eating disorders*, 2nd edn, pp. 145–77. New York: Guilford Press.

Garner, D. M. and Bemis, K. M. (1982). A cognitive-behavioral approach to anorexia nervosa. *Cognitive Therapy and Research*, **6**, 123–50.

Garner, D. M. and Bemis, K. M. (1985). Cognitive therapy for anorexia nervosa. In: D. M. Garner and P. E. Garfinkel, ed. *Handbook of psychotherapy for anorexia nervosa and bulimia*, pp. 107–46. New York: Guilford Press.

Garner, D. M. and Needleman, L. D. (1997). Sequencing and integration of treatments. In: D. M. Garner and P. E. Garfinkel, ed. *Handbook of treatment for eating disorders*, 2nd edn, pp. 50–63. New York: Guilford Press.

Garner, D. M., Garfinkel, P. E., and Bemis, K. M. (1982). A multidimensional psychotherapy for anorexia nervosa. *International Journal of Eating Disorders*, **1**, 3–46.

Garner, D. M., et al. (1993). Comparison of cognitive-behavioral and supportive–expressive therapy for bulimia nervosa. *American Journal of Psychiatry*, **150**, 37–46.

Garner, D. M., Vitousek, K., and Pike, K. M. (1997). Cognitive behavioral therapy for anorexia nervosa. In: D. M. Garner and P. E. Garfinkel, ed. *Handbook of treatment for eating disorders*, 2nd edn, pp. 91–144. New York: Guilford Press.

Geist, R. (1989). Self psychological reflections on the origins of eating disorders. *Journal of the American Academy of Psychoanalysis*, **17**, 5–27.

Geist, R., Heinmaa, M., Stephens, D., Davis, R., and Katzman, D. K. (2000). Comparison of family therapy and family group psychoeducation in adolescents with anorexia nervosa. *Canadian Journal of Psychiatry*, **45**, 173–8.

Geller, J. (2002a). What a motivational approach is and what a motivational approach isn't: reflections and responses. *European Eating Disorders Review*, **10**, 155–60.

Geller, J. (2002b). Estimating readiness for change in anorexia nervosa: comparing clients, clinicians, and research assessors. *International Journal of Eating Disorders*, **31**, 251–60.

Geller, J. and Drab, D. L. (1999). The readiness and motivation interview: a symptom-specific measure of readiness to change in the eating disorders. *European Eating Disorder Review*, **7**, 259–78.

Geller, J., Cockell, S. J., and Drab, D. L. (2001a). Assessing readiness for change in the eating disorders: the psychometric properties of the readiness and motivation interview. *Psychological Assessment*, **13**, 189–198.

Geller, J., Williams, K. D., and Srikameswaran, S. (2001b). Clinician stance in the treatment of chronic eating disorders. *European Eating Disorder Review*, **9**, 365–73.

Goldner, E. M., Birmingham, C. L., and Smye, V. (1997). Addressing treatment refusal in anorexia nervosa: clinical, ethical, and legal considerations. In: D. M. Garner and P. E. Garfinkel, ed. *Handbook of treatment for eating disorders*, 2nd edn, pp. 450–61. New York: Guilford Press.

Goodsitt, A. (1985). Self psychology and the treatment of anorexia nervosa. In: D. M. Garner and P. E. Garfinkel, ed. *Handbook of psychotherapy for anorexia nervosa and bulimia*, pp. 55–82. New York: Guilford Press.

Goodsitt, A. (1997). Eating disorders: a self-psychological perspective. In: D. M. Garner and P. E. Garfinkel, ed. *Handbook of treatment for eating disorders*, 2nd edn, pp. 205–28. New York: Guilford Press.

Gowers, S. G., Weetman, J., Shore, A., Hossain, F., and Elvins, R. (2000). Impact of hospitalisation on the outcome of adolescent anorexia nervosa. *British Journal of Psychiatry*, **176**, 138–41.

le Grange, D., Eisler, I., Dare, C., and Russell, G. F. M. (1992). Evaluation of family treatments in adolescent anorexia nervosa: a pilot study. *International Journal of Eating Disorders*, **12**, 347–57.

Greenberger, D. and Padesky, C. A. (1995). *Mind over mood: change how you feel by changing the way you think*. New York: Guilford Press.

Grilo, C. M., et al. (2003). Do eating disorders co-occur with personality disorders? Comparison groups matter. *International Journal of Eating Disorders*, **33**, 155–64.

Gutwill, S. (1994). Transference and countertransference issues: the impact of social pressures on body image and consciousness. In: C. Bloom, A. Gitter, S. Gutwill, L. Kogel, and L. Zaphiropoulos, ed. *Eating problems: a feminist psychoanalytic treatment model*, pp. 144–71. New York: Basic Books.

Haas, H. L. and Clopton, J. R. (2003). Comparing clinical and research treatments for eating disorders. *International Journal of Eating Disorders*, **33**, 412–20.

Hall, A. (1982). Deciding to stay an anorectic. *Postgraduate Medical Journal*, **58**, 641–7.

Hall, A. and Crisp, A. H. (1987). Brief psychotherapy in the treatment of anorexia nervosa: outcome at one year. *British Journal of Psychiatry*, **151**, 185–91.

Halleck, S. L. (1988). Which patients are responsible for their illnesses? *American Journal of Psychotherapy*, **42**, 338–53.

Halmi, K. A. (2000). Collaborative anorexia nervosa study: 6 months results. Paper presented at the meeting of the International Conference on Eating Disorders, New York, NY.

Hamburg, P. and Herzog, D. (1990). Supervising the therapy of patients with eating disorders. *American Journal of Psychotherapy*, **44**, 369–80.

Herzog, D. B., et al. (1999). Recovery and relapse in anorexia and bulimia nervosa: a 7.5-year follow-up study. *Journal of the American Academy of Child and Adolescent Psychiatry*, **38**, 829–37.

Hollon, S. D. and Beck, A. T. (1994). Cognitive and cognitive-behavioral therapies. In: A. E. Bergin and S. L. Garfield, ed. *Handbook of psychotherapy and behavior change: an empirical analysis*, 4th edn, pp. 428–66. New York: Wiley.

Hollon, S. D. and Kriss, M. R. (1984). Cognitive factors in clinical research and practice. *Clinical Psychology Review*, **4**, 35–76.

Holmgren, S., Humble, K., Norring, C., and Roos, B. (1983). The anorectic bulimic conflict: an alternative diagnostic approach to anorexia nervosa and bulimia. *International Journal of Eating Disorders*, **2**, 3–14.

Hornyak, L. M. and Baker, E. K. (1989). *Experiential therapies for the eating disorders*. New York: Guilford Press.

Jansen, A., Broekmate, J., and Heymans, M. (1992). Cue-exposure vs. self-control in the treatment of binge eating: a pilot study. *Behaviour Research and Therapy*, **30**, 235–41.

Jasper, K. (1993). Out from under body-image disparagement. In: C Brown and K Jasper, ed. *Consuming passions: feminist approaches to weight preoccupation and eating disorders*, pp. 195–218. Toronto: Second Story Press.

Johnson, C. L. (2000). Been there, done that: the use of clinicians with personal recovery in the treatment of eating disorders. *The Renfrew Center Foundation Perspective*, **5**, 1–4.

Johnson, W. G., Tsoh, J. Y., and Varnado, P. J. (1996). Eating disorders: efficacy of pharmacological and psychological interventions. *Clinical Psychology Review*, **16**, 457–78.

Kalucy, R. S., Gilchrist, P. N., McFarlane, C. M., and McFarlane, A. C. (1985). The evolution of a multitherapy approach. In: D. M. Garner and P. E. Garfinkel, ed. *Handbook of psychotherapy for anorexia nervosa and bulimia*, pp. 458–87. New York: Guilford Press.

Kaplan, A. S. and Garfinkel, P. E. (1999). Difficulties in treating patients with eating disorders: a review of patient and clinician variables. *Canadian Journal of Psychiatry*, **44**, 665–70.

Katzman, M. A. and Waller, G. (1998). Gender of the therapist: daring to ask the questions. In: W. Vandereycken and P. J. V. Beumont, ed. *Treating eating disorders: ethical, legal and personal issues*, pp. 56–79. New York: New York University Press.

Kaye, W. H., *et al.* (1997). Relapse prevention with fluoxetine in anorexia nervosa: a blind-placebo-controlled study. Paper presented at the meeting of the American Psychiatric Association, San Diego, CA.

Kearney-Cooke, A. and Striegel-Moore, R. (1997). The etiology and treatment of body image disturbance. In: D. M. Garner and P. E. Garfinkel, ed. *Handbook of treatment for eating disorders*, 2nd edn, pp. 295–306. New York: Guilford Press.

Keel, P. K., *et al.* (2003). Predictors of treatment utilization among women with anorexia and bulimia nervosa. *American Journal of Psychiatry*, **159**, 140–42.

Keys, A., Brozek, J., Henschel, A., Mickelson, O., and Taylor, H. L. (1950). *The biology of human starvation* (2 vols). Minneapolis, MN: University of Minnesota Press.

Killick, S. and Allen, C. (1997). 'Shifting the balance'—Motivational interviewing to help behaviour change in people with bulimia nervosa. *European Eating Disorders Review*, **5**, 33–41.

Klerman, G. L., Weissman, M. M., Rounsaville, B. J., and Chevron, E. S. (1984). *Interpersonal psychotherapy of depression*, pp. 1–22. New York: Basic Books.

Koepp, W. (1994). Can women with eating disorders benefit from a male therapist? In B. Dolan and I. Gitzinger, ed. *Why women? Gender issues and eating disorders*, pp. 65–71. Atlantic Highlands, NJ: Athlone Press.

La Via, M. C., Gray, N., and Kaye, W. H. (2000). Case reports of olanzapine treatment of anorexia nervosa. *International Journal of Eating Disorders*, **27**, 363–6.

Lacey, J. H. (1993). Self-damaging and addictive behavior in bulimia nervosa: a catchment area study. *British Journal of Psychiatry*, **163**, 190–4.

Lacey, J. H. and Evans, C. D. H. (1986). The impulsivist: a multi-impulsive personality disorder. *British Journal of Addiction*, **81**, 641–9.

Lask, B. (1992). Management of pre-pubertal anorexia nervosa. In: P. J. Cooper and A. Stein, ed. *Feeding problems and eating disorders in children and adolescents*, pp. 113–22. Chur, Switzerland: Harwood Academic Publishers.

Lemberg, R. (1999). Narrative therapy: introduction to 'Death of a Scalesman': in her own voice. In: R. Lemberg and L. Cohn, ed. *Eating disorders: a reference sourcebook*, pp. 147–53. Phoenix, AZ: Oryx Press.

Leung, N., Waller, G., and Thomas, G. (1999). Group cognitive-behavioural therapy for anorexia nervosa: a case for treatment? *European Eating Disorders Review*, **7**, 351–61.

Lilenfeld, L. R., *et al.* (1998). A controlled family study of anorexia nervosa and bulimia nervosa: psychiatric disorders in first-degree relatives and effects of proband comorbidity. *Archives of General Psychiatry*, **55**, 603–10.

Linehan, M. M. (1993). *Cognitive-behavioral treatment of borderline personality disorder*. New York: Guilford Press.

Lock, J. (1999). Manualized family-based therapy for adolescents with anorexia nervosa. Paper presented at the meeting of the Eating Disorders Research Society, San Diego, CA.

Lock, J., le Grange, D., Agras, W. S., and Dare, C. (2001). *Treatment manual for anorexia nervosa: a family-based approach*. New York: Guilford Press.

Lowe, B., *et al.* (2001). Long-term outcome of anorexia nervosa in a prospective 21-year follow-up study. *Psychological Medicine*, **31**, 881–90.

Maclagan, D. (1998). Anorexia: the struggle with incarnation and the negative sublime. In: D. Sandle, ed. *Development and diversity: new applications in art therapy*, pp. 78–91. New York: Free Association Books Limited.

MacLeod, S. (1982). *The art of starvation: a story of anorexia and survival*. New York: Schocken Books.

Madigan, S. P. and Goldner, E. M. (1999). A narrative approach to anorexia: discourse, reflexivity, and questions. In: M. F. Hoyt, ed. *The handbook of constructive therapies: innovative approaches from leading practitioners*. San Francisco, CA: Jossey-Bass.

Malan, D. M. (1976). *The Frontier of brief psychotherapy*. New York: Plenum.

Malan, D. M. (1979). *Individual psychotherapy and the science of psychodynamics*. London: Butterworth.

Malina, A., *et al.* (2003). Olanzapine treatment in anorexia nervosa: a retrospective study. *International Journal of Eating Disorders*, **33**, 234–7.

Marlatt, G. A. and Tapert, S. F. (1993). Harm reduction: reducing the risks of addictive behaviors. In: J. S. Baer, G. A. Marlatt, and R. J. McMahon, ed. *Addictive behaviors across the lifespan: prevention, treatment, and policy issues*, pp. 243–73. Newbury Park, CA: Sage.

Masserman, J. H. (1941). Psychodynamisms in manic-depressive psychoses. *Psychoanalytic Review*, **28**, 466–78.

Masterson, J. F. (1977). Eating disorders. In: S. C. Feinstein and P. L. Govaccini, ed. *Adolescent Psychiatry*, vol. 6, pp. 344–59. Chicago: University of Chicago Press.

Mayer, L. E. S. and Walsh, B. T. (1998). Eating disorders. In: B. T. Walsh, ed. *Child Psychopharmacology*, pp. 149–74. Washington, DC: American Psychiatric Association.

McFarland, B. (1995). *Brief therapy and eating disorders: a practical guide to solution-focused work with clients*. San Francisco, CA: Jossey-Bass Publishers.

McVoy, J. (1998). Personal experiences of a male therapist. In: W. Vandereycken and P. J. V. Beumont, ed. *Treating eating disorders: ethical, legal and personal issues*, pp. 80–105. New York: New York University Press.

Meads, C., Gold, L., and Burls, A. (2001). How effective is outpatient care compared to inpatient care for the treatment of anorexia nervosa? A systematic review. *European Eating Disorders Review*, **9**, 229–41.

Meyer, C., Waller, G., and Waters, A. (1998). Emotional states and bulimic psychopathology. In: H. W. Hoek, J. L. Treasure, and M. A. Katzman, ed. *Neurobiology in the treatment of eating disorders*, pp. 271–87. Chichester: Wiley.

Miller, W. R. and Rollnick, S. (1991). *Motivational interviewing*. New York: Guilford Press.

Miller, W. R. and Rollnick, S. (2002). *Motivational interviewing*, 2nd edn. New York: Guilford Press.

Minuchin, S., Rosman, B. L., and Baker, L. (1978). *Psychosomatic families: anorexia nervosa in context*. Cambridge, MA: Harvard University Press.

Mitchell, J. E. and de Zwaan, M. (1993). Pharmacological treatment of binge eating. In: C. G. Fairburn and G. T. Wilson, ed. *Binge eating: nature, assessment and treatment*, pp. 250–69. New York: Guilford Press.

Mitchell, J. E., Peterson, C. B., Meyers, T., and Wonderlich, S. (2001). Combining pharmacotherapy and psychotherapy in the treatment of patients with eating disorders. *The Psychiatric Clinics of North America*, **24**, 315–23.

Mitchell, J. E., *et al.* (2002). A randomized secondary treatment study of women with bulimia nervosa who fail to respond to CBT. *International Journal of Eating Disorders*, **32**, 271–81.

Mitchell, J. E., Myers, T., Swan-Kremeier, L., and Wonderlich, S. (2003). Psychotherapy for bulimia nervosa delivered via telemedicine. *European Eating Disorders Review*, **11**, 222–30.

Noordenbos, G., Jacobs, M. E., and Hertzberger, E. (1998). Chronic eating disorders: the patients' view of their treatment history. *Eating Disorders: The Journal of Treatment and Prevention*, **6**, 217–23.

Noordenbos, G., Oldenhave, A., Muschter, J., and Terpstra, N. (2002). Characteristics and treatment of patients with chronic eating disorders. *Eating Disorders: The Journal of Treatment and Prevention*, **10**, 15–29.

O'Brien, K. M. and Vincent, N. K. (2003). Psychiatric comorbidity in anorexia and bulimia nervosa: Nature, prevalence and causal relationships. *Clinical Psychology Review*, **23**, 57–74.

Olmsted, M. P. and Kaplan, A. S. (1995). Psychoeducation in the treatment of eating disorders. In: K. D. Brownell and C. G. Fairburn, ed. *Eating Disorders and obesity: a comprehensive handbook*, pp. 299–305. New York: Guilford Press.

Olmsted, M. P., *et al.* (1991). Efficacy of a brief group psychoeducational intervention for bulimia nervosa. *Behaviour Research and Therapy*, **29**, 71–83.

Orbach, S. (1985). Accepting the symptom: a feminist psychoanalytic treatment of anorexia nervosa. In: D. M. Garner and P. E. Garfinkel, ed. *Handbook of psychotherapy for anorexia nervosa and bulimia*, pp. 83–104. New York: Guilford Press.

Orimoto, L. and Vitousek, K. (1992). Anorexia nervosa and bulimia nervosa. In: P. W. Wilson, ed. *Principles and practices of relapse prevention*, pp. 85–127. New York: Guilford Press.

Palmer, R. L. (2000). Helping people with eating disorders: a clinical guide to assessment and treatment. Chichester: Wiley.

Palmer, R. L. and Birchall, H. (2003). Dialectical behaviour therapy. In: J. Treasure, U. Schmidt, and E. van Furth, ed. *Handbook of eating disorders*, 2nd edn, pp. 271–7. Chichester: Wiley.

Palmer, R. L., Birchall, H., McGrain, L., and Sullivan, V. (2002). Self-help for bulimic disorders: a randomised controlled trial comparing minimal guidance with face-to-face or telephone guidance. *British Journal of Psychiatry*, 181, 230–5.

Palmer, R. L., et al. (2003). A dialectical behavior therapy program for people with an eating disorder and borderline personality disorder—description and outcome. *International Journal of Eating Disorders*, 33, 281–6.

Parks, G. A., Marlatt, G. A., and Anderson, B. K. (2001). Cognitive behavioral alcohol treatment. In: N. Heather and T. J. Peters, ed. *International handbook of alcohol dependence and problems*, pp. 557–73. New York: John Wiley and Sons.

Pearlstein, T. (2002). Eating disorders and comorbidity. *Archives of Women's Mental Health*, 4, 67–78.

Peterson, C. B. and Mitchell, J. E. (1999). Psychosocial and pharmacological treatment of eating disorders: a review of research findings. *Journal of Clinical Psychology, In Session*, 55, 685–97.

Peveler, R. C. and Fairburn, C. G. (1989). Anorexia nervosa in association with diabetes mellitus: a cognitive-behavioural approach to treatment. *Behaviour Research and Therapy*, 27, 95–9.

Pike, K. M. (1998). Long-term course of anorexia nervosa: response, relapse, remission, and recovery. *Clinical Psychology Review*, 18, 447–75.

Pike, K. M., Loeb, K., and Vitousek, K. (1996). Cognitive-behavioral therapy for anorexia nervosa and bulimia nervosa. In: J. K. Thompson, ed. *Body image, eating disorders, and obesity: an integrative guide for assessment and treatment*, pp. 253–302. Washington, DC: American Psychological Association.

Pike, K. M., Walsh, B. T., Vitousek, K., Wilson, G. T., and Bauer, J. (2003). Cognitive behavior therapy in the posthospitalization treatment of anorexia nervosa. *American Journal of Psychiatry*, 160, 2046–9.

Pope, H. G. Jr and Hudson, J. I. (1984). *New hope for binge eaters: advances in the understanding and treatment of bulimia*. New York: Harper & Row.

Pope, H. G. Jr, Hudson, J. I., Jonas, J. M., and Yurgelun-Todd, D. (1985). Antidepressant treatment of bulimia: a 2-year follow up study. *Journal of Psychopharmacology*, 5, 320–7.

Powers, P. S. and Powers, H. P. (1984). Inpatient treatment of anorexia nervosa. *Psychosomatics: Journal of Consultation Liaison Psychiatry*, 25, 512–27.

Pyle, R. L., et al. (1990). Maintenance treatment and 6-month outcome for bulimic patients who respond to initial treatment. *American Journal of Psychiatry*, 147, 871–5.

Rakoff, V. M. (1983). Multiple determinants of family dynamics in anorexia nervosa. In: P. L. Darby, P. E. Garfinkel, D. M. Garner and D. V. Coscina, ed. *Anorexia nervosa: recent developments in research*, pp. 29–40. New York: Alan R. Liss.

Rampling, D. (1978). Anorexia nervosa: reflections on theory and practice. *Psychiatry*, 41, 296–301.

Rathner, G. (1998). A plea against compulsory treatment of anorexia nervosa patients. In: W. Vandereycken and P. J. V. Beumont, ed. *Treating eating disorders: ethical, legal and personal issues*, pp. 179–215. New York: New York University Press.

Reiff, D. W. and Reiff, K. K. L. (1997). Eating disorders: nutrition therapy in the recovery process. Mercer Island WA: Life Enterprises.

Rieger, E., et al. (2000). Development of an instrument to assess readiness to recover in anorexia nervosa. *International Journal of Eating Disorders*, 28, 387–96.

Robin, A. L., Siegel, P. T., Koepke, T., Moye, A. W., and Tice, S. (1994). Family therapy versus individual therapy for adolescent females with anorexia nervosa. *Developmental and Behavioral Pediatrics*, 15, 111–16.

Robin, A. L., Siegel, P. T., and Moye, A. (1995). Family versus individual therapy for anorexia: impact on family conflict. *International Journal of Eating Disorders*, 17, 313–22.

Rock, C. L. and Yager, J. (1987). Nutrition and eating disorders: a primer for clinicians. *International Journal of Eating Disorders*, 6, 267–80.

Rosen, J. C. (1996). Body image assessment and treatment in controlled studies of eating disorders. *International Journal of Eating Disorders*, 20, 331–43.

Rosen, J. C. and Leitenberg, H. (1982). Bulimia nervosa: treatment with exposure and response prevention. *Behavior Therapy*, 13, 117–24.

Rosen, J. C. and Leitenberg, H. (1985). Exposure plus response prevention treatment of bulimia. In: D. M. Garner and P. E. Garfinkel, ed. *Handbook of psychotherapy for anorexia nervosa and bulimia*, pp. 193–209. New York: Guilford Press.

Rosman, B. L., Minuchin, S., Liebman, R., and Baker, L. (1978). Input and outcome of family therapy in anorexia nervosa. *Adolescent Psychiatry*, Vol. 5. New York: Jason-Aronson.

Russell, G. F. M. (2001). Foreword. In: J. Lock, D. le Grange, W. S. Agras, and C. Dare, ed. *Treatment manual for anorexia nervosa: a family-based approach*. New York: Guilford Press.

Russell, G. F. M., Szmukler, G. I., Dare, C., and Eisler, I. (1987). An evaluation of family therapy in anorexia nervosa and bulimia nervosa. *Archives of General Psychiatry*, 44, 1047–56.

Ryle, A. (1990). *Cognitive analytical therapy: active participation in change. A new integration in brief psychotherapy*. Chichester: Wiley.

Safer, D. L., Telch, C. F., and Agras, W. S. (2001a). Dialectical behavior therapy adapted for bulimia nervosa: a case report. *International Journal of Eating Disorders*, 30, 101–6.

Safer, D. L., Telch, C. F., and Agras, W. S. (2001b). Dialectical behavior therapy for bulimia nervosa. *American Journal of Psychiatry*, 158, 632–4.

Schmidt, U. and Treasure, J. (1993). *Getting better bit(e) by bit(e)*. London: Lawrence Erlbaum Associates.

Segal, Z. V., Williams, J. M. G., and Teasdale, J. D. (2002). *Mindfulness-based cognitive therapy for depression: a new approach to preventing relapse*. New York: Guilford Press.

Seligman, M. E. (1995). The effectiveness of psychotherapy: the Consumer Reports study. *American Psychologist*, 12, 965–74.

Selvini-Palazzoli, M. (1978). *Self-starvation: from individual to family therapy in the treatment of anorexia nervosa*. New York: Jason Aronson.

Serfaty, M. A., Turkington, D., Heap, M., Ledsham, L., and Jolley, E. (1999). Cognitive therapy versus dietary counselling in the outpatient treatment of anorexia nervosa: effects of the treatment phase. *European Eating Disorders Review*, 7, 334–50.

Serpell, L., Treasure, J., Teasdale, J., and Sullivan, V. (1999). Anorexia nervosa: friend or foe? *International Journal of Eating Disorders*, 25, 177–86.

Serpell, L., Livingstone, A., Neiderman, M., and Lask, B. (2002). Anorexia nervosa: obsessive compulsive disorder, obsessive compulsive personality disorder or neither? *Clinical Psychology Review*, 22, 647–69.

Shafran, R., Cooper, Z., and Fairburn, C. G. (2002). Clinical perfectionism: a cognitive-behavioural analysis. *Behaviour Research and Therapy*, 40, 773–91.

Slade, P. (1982). Towards a functional analysis of anorexia nervosa and bulimia nervosa. *British Journal of Clinical Psychology*, 21, 167–79.

Sours, J. A. (1974). The anorexia nervosa syndrome. *International Journal of Psycho-Analysis*, 55, 567–76.

Sours, J. A. (1980). *Starving to death in a sea of objects: the anorexia nervosa syndrome*. New York: Jason Aronson.

Steinhausen, H.-C. (2002). The outcome of anorexia nervosa in the 20th century. *American Journal of Psychiatry*, 159, 1284–93.

Steinhausen, H.-C., Rauss-Mason, C., and Seidel, R. (1991). Follow-up studies of anorexia nervosa: a review of four decades of outcome research. *Psychological Medicine*, 21, 447–54.

Steinhausen, H.-C., Siedel, R., and Metzke, C. W. (2000). Evaluation of treatment and intermediate and long-term outcome of adolescent eating disorders. *Psychological Medicine*, 30, 1089–98.

Stockwell, R. and Dolan, B. (1994). Women therapists for women patients? In: B. Dolan and I. Gitzinger, ed. *Why women? Gender issues and eating disorders*, pp. 57–64. Atlantic Highlands NJ: Athlone Press.

Story, I. (1982). Anorexia nervosa and the psychotherapeutic hospital. *International Journal of Psychoanalytic Psychotherapy*, 9, 267–302.

Strober, M. (1991). Disorders of the self in anorexia nervosa: an organismic-developmental perspective. In: C. Johnson, ed. *Psychodynamic treatment of anorexia nervosa and bulimia*, pp. 354–73. New York: Guilford Press.

Strober, M. and Yager, J. (1985). A developmental perspective on the treatment of anorexia nervosa in adolescents. In: D. M. Garner and P. E. Garfinkel, ed. *Handbook of psychotherapy for anorexia nervosa and bulimia*, pp. 363–90. New York: Guilford Press.

Strober, M., Freeman, R., and Morrell, W. (1997). The long-term course of severe anorexia nervosa in adolescents: survival analysis of recovery, relapse, and outcome predictors over 10–15 years in a prospective study. *International Journal of Eating Disorders*, **22**, 339–60.

Sullivan, H. S. (1953). *The interpersonal theory of psychiatry*. New York: Norton.

Sullivan, P. F. (2002). Course and outcome of anorexia nervosa and bulimia nervosa. In: C. G. Fairburn and K. D. Brownell, ed. *Eating disorders and obesity: a comprehensive handbook*, 2nd edn, pp. 226–30. New York: Guilford Press.

Szyrynski, V. (1973). Anorexia nervosa and psychotherapy. *American Journal of Psychotherapy*, **27**, 492–505.

Tanner, C. and Connan, F. (2003). Cognitive analytic therapy. In: J. Treasure, U. Schmidt, and E. van Furth, ed. *Handbook of eating disorders*, 2nd edn, pp. 279–90. Chichester: Wiley.

Tantillo, M., Bitter, C. N., and Adams, B. (2001). Enhancing readiness for eating disorder treatment: a relational/motivational group model for change. *Eating Disorders: The Journal of Treatment and Prevention*, **9**, 203–16.

Thackwray, D. E., Smith, M. C., Bodfish, J. W., and Myers, A. W. (1993). A comparison of behavioral and cognitive-behavioral interventions for bulimia nervosa. *Journal of Consulting and Clinical Psychology*, **61**, 639–45.

Theander, S. (1985). Outcome and prognosis in anorexia nervosa and bulimia: some results of previous investigations compared with those of a Swedish long-term study. *Journal of Psychiatric Research*, **19**, 493–508.

Thiels, C., Schmidt, U., Treasure, J., Garthe, R., and Troop, N. (1998). Guided self-change for bulimia nervosa incorporating use of a self-care manual. *American Journal of Psychiatry*, **155**, 947–53.

Thoma, H. (1967). *Anorexia nervosa*. New York: International Universities Press.

Thompson-Brenner, H., Glass, S., and Westen, D. (2003). A multidimensional meta-analysis of psychotherapy for bulimia nervosa. *Clinical Psychology Science and Practice*, **10**, 269–87.

Thornton, C. E. and Russell, J. D. (1995). Evaluation of an integrated eating disorders day program. Paper presented at the meeting of the International Conference on Eating Disorders, London, UK.

Tinker, D. E. and Ramer, J. C. (1983). Anorexia nervosa: staff subversion of therapy. *Journal of Adolescent Health Care*, **4**, 35–9.

Tobin, D. L. and Johnson, C. L. (1991). The integration of psychodynamic and behavior therapy in the treatment of eating disorders: clinical issues versus theoretical mystique. In: C. Johnson, ed. *Psychodynamic treatment of anorexia nervosa and bulimia*, pp. 374–97. New York: Guilford Press.

Treasure, J. and Bauer, B. (2003). Assessment and motivation. In: J. Treasure, U. Schmidt, and E. van Furth, ed. *Handbook of eating disorders*, 2nd edn, pp. 219–31. Chichester: Wiley.

Treasure, J. and Schmidt, U. (2001). Ready, willing, and able to change: motivational aspects of the assessment and treatment of eating disorders. *European Eating Disorders Review*, **9**, 4–18.

Treasure, J. and Ward, A. (1997a). Cognitive analytical therapy in the treatment of anorexia nervosa. *Clinical Psychology and Psychotherapy*, **4**, 62–71.

Treasure, J. and Ward, A. (1997b). A practical guide to the use of motivational interviewing in anorexia nervosa. *European Eating Disorders Review*, **5**, 102–14.

Treasure, J., *et al.* (1994). First step in managing bulimia nervosa: controlled trial of a therapeutic manual. *British Medical Journal*, **308**, 686–9.

Treasure, J., Todd, G., Brolly, J., Nehmed, A., and Denman, F. (1995). A pilot study of a randomised trial of cognitive analytical therapy vs. educational behavioral therapy for adult anorexia nervosa. *Behaviour Research and Therapy*, **33**, 363–7.

Treasure, J., *et al.* (1996). Sequential treatment for bulimia nervosa incorporating a self-help manual. *British Journal of Psychiatry*, **168**, 94–8.

Treasure, J., *et al.* (1999). Engagement and outcome in the treatment of bulimia nervosa: first phase of a sequential design comparing motivation enhancement therapy and cognitive behavioural therapy. *Behaviour Research and Therapy*, **37**, 405–18.

Tuschen, B. and Bent, H. (1995). Intensive brief inpatient treatment of bulimia nervosa. In: K. D. Brownell and C. G. Fairburn, ed. *Comprehensive textbook of eating disorders and obesity*, pp. 354–60. New York: Guilford Press.

Vandereycken, W. (1987). The constructive family approach to eating disorders: critical remarks on the use of family therapy in anorexia nervosa and bulimia. *International Journal of Eating Disorders*, **6**, 455–67.

Vitousek, K. M. (1996). The current status of cognitive-behavioral models of anorexia nervosa and bulimia nervosa. In: P. M. Salkovskis, ed. *Frontiers of cognitive therapy*. New York: Guilford Press.

Vitousek, K. (2002). Cognitive-behavioral therapy for anorexia nervosa. In: C. G. Fairburn and K. D. Brownell, *Eating disorders and obesity: a comprehensive handbook*, 2nd edn, pp. 308–13. New York: Guilford Press.

Vitousek, K. M. (2005). *Working through anorexia nervosa*. New York: Guilford Press.

Vitousek, K. B. and Ewald, L. S. (1993). Self-representation in eating disorders: a cognitive perspective. In: Z. Segal and S. Blatt, ed. *The self in emotional disorders: cognitive and psychodynamic perspectives*, pp. 221–57. New York: Guilford Press.

Vitousek, K. B. and Hollon, S. D. (1990). The investigation of schematic content and processing in eating disorders. *Cognitive Therapy and Research*, **14**, 191–214.

Vitousek, K. and Manke, F. (1994). Personality variables and disorders in anorexia nervosa and bulimia nervosa. *Journal of Abnormal Psychology*, **103**, 137–47.

Vitousek, K. B. and Orimoto, L. (1993). Cognitive-behavioral models of anorexia nervosa, bulimia nervosa, and obesity. In: K. S. Dobson and P. C. Kendall, ed. *Psychopathology and cognition. Personality, psychopathology, and psychotherapy series*, pp. 191–243. San Diego, CA: Academic Press Inc.

Vitousek, K., DeViva, J., Slay, J., and Manke, F. M. (1995). Concerns about change in eating and anxiety disorders. Paper presented at the meeting of the American Psychological Association, New York, NY.

Vitousek, K., Watson, S., and Wilson, G. T. (1998). Enhancing motivation for change in treatment-resistant eating disorders. *Clinical Psychology Review*, **18**, 391–420.

Vitousek, K. M., Gray, J. A., and Grubbs, K. M. (2004). Caloric restriction for longevity: I. Paradigm, protocols, and physiological findings in animal research. *European Eating Disorders Review*, **12**, 279–99.

Waller, D., *et al.* (1996). Treating bulimia nervosa in primary care: a pilot study. *International Journal of Eating Disorders*, **19**, 99–103.

Waller, J., Kaufman, M. R., and Deutsch, F. (1940/1964). Anorexia nervosa: a psychosomatic entity. In: M. R. Kaufman and M. Heiman, ed. *Evolution of psychosomatic concepts: anorexia nervosa, a paradigm*. New York: International Universities Press. (Reprinted from *Psychosomatic Medicine*, **2**, 3–16.)

Walsh, B. T. (2002a). Pharmacological treatment of anorexia nervosa and bulimia nervosa. In: C. G. Fairburn and K. D. Brownell, ed. *Eating disorders and obesity: a comprehensive handbook*, 2nd edn, pp. 325–9. New York: Guilford Press.

Walsh, B. T. (2002b). Pharmacotherapy for anorexia nervosa. Paper presented at the Workshop on Overcoming Barriers to Treatment Research on Anorexia Nervosa, National Institutes of Health, Rockville, MD.

Walsh, B. T., Hadigan, C. M., Devlin, M. J., Gladis, M., and Roose, S. P. (1991). Long-term outcome of antidepressant treatment for bulimia nervosa. *American Journal of Psychiatry*, **148**, 1206–12.

Walsh, B. T., *et al.* (1997). Medication and psychotherapy in the treatment of bulimia nervosa. *American Journal of Psychiatry*, **154**, 523–31.

Walsh, B. T., *et al.* (2000). Fluoxetine for bulimia nervosa following poor response to psychotherapy. *American Journal of Psychiatry*, **157**, 1332–4.

Ward, A., Troop, N., Todd, G., and Treasure, J. (1996). To change or not to change—'how' is the question? *British Journal of Medical Psychology*, **69**, 139–46.

Way, K. (1993). *Anorexia nervosa and recovery: a hunger for meaning*. Binghamton, NY: Harrington Park Press.

Weindruch, R. (1996). Caloric restriction and aging. *Scientific American*, **274**, 46–52.

Weissman, M. M. and Markowitz, J. C. (1994). Interpersonal psychotherapy: current status. *Archives of General Psychiatry*, **51**, 599–606.

Weissman, M. M., *et al.* (1979). The efficacy of drugs and psychotherapy in the treatment of acute depressive episodes. *American Journal of Psychiatry*, **136**, 555–8.

Weissman, M. M., Markowitz, J. C., and Klerman, G. L. (2000). *Comprehensive guide to interpersonal psychotherapy*. New York: Basic Books.

Whittal, M. L., Agras, W. S., and Gould, R. A. (1999). Bulimia nervosa: a meta-analysis of psychosocial and pharmacological treatments. *Behavior Therapy*, **30**, 117–35.

Wilfley, D., Stein, R., and Welch, R. (2003). Interpersonal psychotherapy. In: J. Treasure, U. Schmidt, and E. van Furth, ed. *Handbook of eating disorders*, 2nd edn, pp. 253–70. Chichester: Wiley.

Wilson, G. T. (1995). Empirically validated treatments as a basis for clinical practice: problems and prospects. In: S. C. Hayes, V. M. Follette, R. D. Dawes, and K. Grady, ed. *Scientific standards of psychological practice: issues and recommendations*, pp. 163–96. Reno, NV: Context Press.

Wilson, G. T. (1996). Treatment of bulimia nervosa: when CBT fails. *Behaviour Research and Therapy*, **34**, 197–212.

Wilson, G. T. (1998a). The clinical utility of randomized controlled trials. *International Journal of Eating Disorders*, **24**, 13–29.

Wilson, G. T. (1998b). Manual-based treatment and clinical practice. *Clinical Psychology: Science & Practice*, **5**, 363–75.

Wilson, G. T. (1999). Treatment of bulimia nervosa: the next decade. *European Eating Disorders Review*, **7**, 77–83.

Wilson, G. T. and Agras, W. S. (2001). Practice guidelines for eating disorders. *Behavior Therapy*, **32**, 219–34.

Wilson, G. T. and Fairburn, C. G. (1998). Treatments for eating disorders. In: P. E. Nathan and J. M. Gorman, ed. *A guide to treatments that work*, pp. 501–30. New York: Oxford University Press.

Wilson, G. T. and Vitousek, K. M. (1999). Self-monitoring in the assessment of eating disorders. *Psychological Assessment*, **11**, 480–9.

Wilson, G. T., Rossiter, E., Kleifield, E. I., and Lindholm, L. (1986). Cognitive-behavioral treatment of bulimia nervosa: a controlled evaluation. *Behaviour Research and Therapy*, **24**, 277–88.

Wilson, G. T., Eldredge, K. L., Smith, D., and Niles, B. (1991). Cognitive-behavioural treatment with and without response prevention for bulimia. *Behavioral Research and Therapy*, **29**, 575–83.

Wilson, G. T., Fairburn, C. G., and Agras, W. S. (1997). Cognitive-behavioral therapy for bulimia nervosa. In: D. M. Garner, and P. E. Garfinkel, ed. *Handbook of treatment for eating disorders*, 2nd edn, pp. 67–93. New York: Guilford Press.

Wilson, G. T., *et al.* (1999). Psychological versus pharmacological treatments of bulimia nervosa: predictors and processes of change. *Journal of Clinical and Consulting Psychology*, **67**, 451–9.

Wilson, G. T., Vitousek, K. M., and Loeb, K. L. (2000). Stepped care treatment for eating disorders. *Journal of Consulting and Clinical Psychology*, **68**, 564–72.

Wilson, G. T., Fairburn, C. G., Agras, W. S., Walsh, B. T., and Kraemer, H. (2002). Cognitive-behavioral therapy to bulimia nervosa: time course and mechanisms of change. *Journal of Consulting and Clinical Psychology*, **70**, 267–74.

Wiser, S. and Telch, C. F. (1999). Dialectical behavior therapy for binge eating disorder. *Journal of Clinical Psychology*, **55**, 755–68.

Wolff, G. and Serpell, L. (1998). A cognitive model and treatment strategies for anorexia nervosa. In: H. W. Hoek, J. L. Treasure, and M. A. Katzman, ed. *Neurobiology in the treatment of eating disorders. Wiley series on Clinical and Neurobiological Advances in Psychiatry*, pp. 407–29. Chichester: Wiley.

Wonderlich, S. A. and Mitchell, J. E. (1997). Eating disorders and comorbidity: empirical, conceptual, and clinical implications. *Psychopharmacology Bulletin. Special Issue: Research Priorities in Eating Disorders*, **33**, 381–90.

Wooley, S. (1991). Uses of countertransference in the treatment of eating disorders: a gender perspective. In: C. L. Johnson, ed. *Psychodynamic treatment of anorexia nervosa and bulimia*, pp. 245–94. New York: Guilford Press.

Yager, J. (1982). Family issues in the pathogenesis of anorexia nervosa. *Psychosomatic Medicine*, **44**, 43–60.

Yager, J. (1995). The management of patients with intractable eating disorders. In: K. D. Brownell and C. G. Fairburn, ed. *Eating disorders and obesity: a comprehensive handbook*, pp. 374–8. New York: Guilford Press.

Yager, J. (2002). Management of patients with intractable eating disorders. In: C. G. Fairburn and K. D. Brownell, ed. *Eating disorders and obesity: a comprehensive handbook*, 2nd edn, pp. 345–9. New York: Guilford Press.

Zipfel, S., Löwe, B., Reas, D. L., Deter, H.-C., and Herzog, W. (2000). Long-term prognosis in anorexia nervosa: lessons from a 21-year follow-up study. *The Lancet*, **2355**, 721–2.

Zipfel, S., *et al.* (2002). Day hospitalization programs for eating disorders: a systematic review of the literature. *International Journal of Eating Disorders*, **31**, 105–17.

16 Dissociative disorders

Giovanni Liotti, Phil Mollon, and Giuseppe Miti

Introduction

After decades of relative neglect, due mostly to the concurrent neglect of the effects of real-life traumatic experiences in psychopathology and psychotherapy, there has been an upsurge of interest in the dissociative disorders (DDs). The introduction of this diagnostic category in the third edition of the *Diagnostic and statistical manual of mental disorders* (DSM), has been instrumental, since 1980, in calling attention to disturbances in the integrative functions of memory, consciousness, and identity. This renewed interest notwithstanding, the nosology of the DDs remains a problematic issue (Dell, 2001). Arguments supporting the clear differentiation of the DDs from other disorders—e.g., personality disorders of the dramatic cluster (especially borderline personality disorder, BPD), conversion disorders, chronic posttraumatic stress disorders, and trauma-related psychotic states (as described by Kingdon and Turkington, 2002)—are not compelling. The prototypic disorder in the category, dissociative identity disorder (DID, formerly known as multiple personality disorder), is the subject of particular controversy. While many psychotherapists, especially in North America, diagnose it with an impressive frequency, others, mainly in Europe, doubt the real existence or the prevalence of DID, and regard many published clinical cases of DID as artifacts. Moreover, current DSM-IV nosology, while it focuses on the presence of alternate personalities (*alters*) for the diagnosis of DID, does not provide clear guidance with regard to the phenomenology of alters. The possibility of clinical syndromes in which ego states are only partially dissociated (and therefore cannot be considered full-blown alters) is acknowledged by DSM-IV in the subcategory of 'dissociative disorders not otherwise specified' (DDNOS). This possibility adds to the difficulty of identifying patients suffering from DID insofar as it is not always easy to decide when an ego state is fully rather than only partially dissociated. As a result, whereas most papers on the psychotherapy of the DDs are concerned with DID, reliable information on the prevalence of this disorder, on the boundaries between it and related DDs, and on the treatment of DDs different from DID, is scarce.

The unsatisfactory status of the nosology and the epidemiology of the DDs, and the paucity of controlled outcome studies of their treatment, requires a particularly careful consideration of what we know about their etiology in order to understand the logic and the potentialities of their psychotherapy.

Conceptualization

The DDs can be regarded as very complex and long-term types of posttraumatic stress disorder, beginning acutely during childhood and becoming chronic throughout adolescence and adulthood. As trauma has repeatedly impinged during crucial years of development, many different dimensions of the experience of self are affected (Mollon, 1996). Childhood sexual abuse, often perpetrated by family members, is particularly prominent among the traumatic memories of patients suffering from DDs (Allen, 2001). Other types of traumas (e.g., neglect, physical violence, severe humiliations) also play a part in the etiology of the DDs.

Trauma elicits dissociation, which is a discontinuity of experience (consciousness) and memory. Allen (2001) suggests there are broadly two components to this—*detachment* from the overwhelming experience, and *compartmentalization* of the experience. Dissociation may serve initially as an adaptive function of making fear and psychological pain accompanying trauma more tolerable. Over time, however, dissociation distorts personality development and the ongoing integration of memories, self-perception, and perception of emotions in other people. It also acts as a fragmented representation of the original traumatic experiences through the perpetuation of hyperarousal in response to stimuli reminiscent of trauma, as well as through its other manifestations in numbing, intrusive flashbacks, and nightmares. Dis-integrated perceptions of self and the environment may give way to depersonalization and derealization. To these reverberating echoes of the traumatic experience, patients may react with panic and the deepest discouragement. Thus the flashbacks create secondary trauma. Greater discontinuities of memory (amnesia) and even of identity (fugue) may grow out of the dissociative defenses against the original traumas. Reciprocally dissociated ego states (alters) may form, giving rise to the experience of internal conflict and sometimes resulting in different ego states and identities taking executive control at different times. Understandably, when personality development takes place in such a traumatic-dissociative climate, the ability to regulate emotions and to control aggressive impulses (both toward oneself and toward others) is usually underdeveloped. Also undermined is the development of those metacognitive abilities that allow for critical reflection on one's own or other people's states of mind ('theory of mind' and mentalization: Fonagy *et al.*, 2002). Interpersonal relationships, as a consequence, become often stormy or otherwise very difficult.

It may be noted that this description of the DDs may widely apply also to BPD: high rates of childhood trauma are reported by BPD patients, dissociation of mental states is among the clinical features required for diagnosing BPD, and the comorbidity between DID and BPD is very frequent. Some psychoanalysts hold that different defense mechanisms (dissociation and splitting, respectively) are responsible for the different features of DID and BPD. Other clinicians, however (Ross, 1989; Blizard, 2001) deny any substantial difference between DID and BPD. It is therefore debatable whether the conceptualization of psychotherapy interventions in cases of DID and of BPD should differ significantly or not.

However important the role of traumatic experiences in the genesis of the DDs, it should be noted that other risk factors concur in their development, the understanding of which is important in treatment conceptualization. These other risk factors explain the existence of cases, although comparatively rare, of DDs where no history of childhood trauma can be reconstructed, and of cases of severe childhood trauma associated with other disorders (anxiety disorders and mood disorders). Temperamental traits (e.g., susceptibility to hypnosis, linked to the genetic make-up of the individual: Bliss, 1986) may increase the tendency to react to trauma with dissociation. Unbearable loneliness may also contribute to the development of imaginary friends and alternative 'realities'. These factors may allow for the possibility that a DD develops as the consequence only of subtle relational traumas in the absence of obvious child maltreatment. Particular types of early attachment relationship (attachment disorganization: see below) seem to exert an adverse influence, since the earliest phases of life, on the integrative functions of memory, consciousness, and identity (Main and Morgan, 1996; Liotti, 1999; Lyons-Ruth and Jacobvitz, 1999; Schore, 2001): they may therefore constitute risk factors in the development of disorders implying dissociation.

It should also be emphasized that, very often, the perpetrator of the abuses reported by the wide majority of dissociative patients is a caregiver. Therefore, most dissociative patients had to face, as children, a series of relational dilemmas whose core is that, in order to maintain attachment to the caregiver, the abuse must be denied, forgotten, and dissociated (Freyd, 1996), while at the same time, in order to protect themselves from abuse, attachment wishes must be disavowed (Blizard, 2001). These relational dilemmas and the related defensive strategies (usually taking place within previously disorganized attachment relationships), rather than traumas as such, set the stage for the development of dissociated ego states.

From this consensus view of the etiology and pathogenesis of the DDs, follows the conceptualization of the psychotherapy. The goals to be pursued are:

- the stabilization and reduction of symptoms of anxiety, depression, or impulse dyscontrol;
- the processing of traumatic experience;
- the integration of memory, consciousness, and identity;
- the development of the capacity of trusting interpersonal relationships and of the relational skills necessary to both self-protection and secure attachment.

Although the restoration of the integrative functions of memory, consciousness, and identity requires the processing of trauma, the emphasis is not, as in some earlier recommendations, on abreaction (i.e., on the supposedly cathartic 'reliving' of the original painful experience within the therapeutic dialog). Rather, it requires attention to developmental, relational, and self-regulation issues.

Research

The importance, for the efficacy of psychotherapy in the DDs, of achieving integration (of traumatic memories, ego states, or alters), is asserted by two follow-up studies (Ellason and Ross, 1997; Coons and Bowman, 2001). However, methodological limits of these studies mean they can only be regarded as preliminary findings.

Despite the paucity of methodologically satisfactory outcome studies, three areas of research have provided reliable findings that are of great relevance in the psychotherapy of the DDs. The first is concerned with the strong links between early childhood trauma (sexual abuse and notably incest, physical and emotional abuse, especially intrafamilial) and dissociation in adolescence and adulthood (Ross *et al.*, 1989; Coons, 1994; Simeon *et al.*, 2001; Pasquini *et al.*, 2002). The second has to do with the reliability of traumatic childhood memories, as they may be retrieved during adult psychotherapy. The third deals with the developmental consequences of attachment disorganization in increasing the risk for abnormal dissociative reactions to trauma.

Reliability of traumatic childhood memories

Extensive and diverse research findings show that autobiographical memory is an active process of reconstruction, liable to influence by suggestion and the incorporation of information from various sources, rather than an accurate and stable registration/retrieval of events (Loftus, 1993; Mollon, 2002a). Moreover, trauma can differentially affect explicit and implicit memory. The nonverbal (nondeclarative) aspects of the experience, such as the fear response, may be encoded as implicit memory, while the verbal aspects (i.e., the comments of the perpetrator, the victim's inner dialog during the experience, the narrative of the experience) may not be encoded. According to recent neuropsychological findings, the fact that the declarative or narrative aspects of the traumatic experience *may* not be encoded as

explicit memory is due to disruption of the functions of the hippocampus in the brain. This hippocampal dysfunction, in turn, is linked to the high levels of stress neurohormones produced during serious traumas. At the same time, the perceptual, physiological, emotional, and motor aspects of the traumatic experience, and particularly the fear response, are recorded in other neural maps involving the amygdala (which, unlike the hippocampus, is not affected by the stress neurohormones). Therefore, the traumatic experience cannot be retrieved in any narrative form during verbal interchanges concerning the patient's memories. While the body memory of the trauma persists in the form of phobias and psychosomatic disturbances, the traumatic experience may never become part of autobiographical memory (Allen *et al.*, 1999; Allen, 2001; Mollon, 2002a).

Because of the complex interplay between declarative and nondeclarative memory, traumatic memories verbally reported by patients in psychotherapy may combine confabulation and accurate recall (Mollon, 2002a). The psychotherapist should therefore be alert to the dangers of suggesting (either explicitly or inadvertently) that the patient may have been abused as a child if this has not already been reported, and should be tolerant of uncertainty regarding the accuracy of traumatic memories emerging during the treatment of dissociative patients (see below, particularly 'Middle phase: processing trauma and beginning integration', for details on what such 'tolerance of uncertainty' may mean in clinical practice).

Attachment disorganization

Infants are said to be disorganized in their attachments when they show a mixture of approach and avoidance behaviors toward the caregiver during a standard sequence of brief episodes of separation from and reunion to the caregiver, known as *Strange Situation* (Main and Hesse, 1990; Lyons-Ruth and Jacobvitz, 1999). Disorganized attachment may also show as disoriented attitudes of the infant toward the caregiver (e.g., trance-like states during the interactions with the caregiver in the *Strange Situation*).

Disorganized attachment patterns develop in infants as the consequence of caregiving parental behaviors that are frightening to the child, either because they are violent or because they express fear and/or dissociative experience in the parent (Schuengel *et al.*, 1999). These frightened/frightening parental attitudes, in turn, are linked to unresolved losses and/or traumas (Main and Hesse, 1990; Lyons-Ruth and Jacobvitz, 1999).

The relevance of such studies for an understanding of dissociation is suggested by certain similarities between the experiences and behavior of dissociative patients, the behavior of infants showing disorganized attachment, and the mental states of these infants' parents (Liotti, 1992, 1999; Main and Morgan, 1996). Furthermore, the early, implicit representations of self-with-others (or internal working model, IWM) stemming from disorganized attachment are very likely to be multiple, incoherent, and dissociated. This is at striking variance with the IWM of the organized patterns of early attachment (secure, insecure-avoidant, and insecure-resistant), that are single and coherent (Main and Hesse, 1990; Liotti, 1999). The IWM of disorganized attachment conveys dramatic emotions that quickly shift from rage to fear to hopelessness, closely mimicking the mutable dramatic interpersonal emotions so easily observed in dissociative and borderline patients. Moreover, the implicit memory structures composing this type of IWM convey information that facilitates the later construction of dissociated representations of self and others according to the three stereotypes of the 'drama triangle': persecutor, rescuer, and victim (Liotti, 1999). These three stereotypes correspond to the basic structure of the most common dissociated ego states, or alternate personalities, which have been observed in DID (protective alters, persecutor alters, and victim alters that often rehearse the traumatic memories).

Controlled studies, both longitudinal (Ogawa *et al.*, 1997; Carlson, 1998) and correlational (Liotti *et al.*, 2000; Pasquini *et al.*, 2002), support the hypothesis that early disorganized attachment is linked, throughout development, to propensities toward dissociation, DDs and BPD. These studies not only contribute to clarifying the etiology of the DDs; they also suggest how the knowledge of attachment disorganization helps in dealing with the complex dramatic type of therapeutic relationship these patients tend to establish (Liotti, 1995; Liotti and Intreccialagli, 1998; Fonagy, 1999; Blizard, 2001; Steele *et al.*, 2001).

Key practice points

Over the past 20 years, clinicians treating dissociative patients and other adult survivors of childhood abuse have achieved, according to informed reviewers (Courtois, 1997; Chu and Bowman, 2000), wide consensus as to the treatment of these disorders. This consensus model is based on the idea that the psychotherapy should be phase oriented, with attention to the therapeutic relationship, belief systems, and the structure and experience of self taking precedence over the exploration of trauma (see, e.g., Putnam, 1989; Herman, 1992; Davies and Frawley, 1994; Courtois, 1997; Fine, 1999; Kluft, 1999; Blizard, 2001; Gold *et al.*, 2001; Steele *et al.*, 2001). The preliminary phase of the treatment, according to the consensus model, is devoted to alliance building and safety. The intermediate one is focused on processing traumatic memories. The late phase aims at personality integration and relational rehabilitation (i.e., further integration of dissociated mental functions and development of self-care and relational skills). This sequence is not strictly linear; although phase oriented, the treatment alternates as a spiral between the themes of the three stages. Knowledge of disorganized attachment, as it will argued below ('Preliminary phase: alliance building and safety operations' and especially 'Middle phase: processing trauma and beginning integration'), may usefully guide the psychotherapist in deciding the individualized timing and manner of such alternations.

It should be noticed that, while the consensus model provides a schematic conceptualization of the therapeutic process, some (e.g., Mollon, 2002a,b) are less impressed with the idea of a clearly sequential approach in practice, and emphasize extreme caution regarding therapeutic goals.

Preliminary phase: alliance building and safety operations

Dissociative patients are prone to expect dramatic shifts in the attitudes of the caregivers, reflecting their experience of being abused or neglected by the primary caretakers. In more traditional psychodynamic terms, these expectations have been linked to the simultaneous operations of sadistic and masochistic defenses (Blizard, 2001). In terms of attachment theory, these expectations, reflecting the patients' early experiences, make them unconsciously prone, *whenever their attachment system becomes active*, to shift or switch between reciprocally dissociated implicit mental structures (IWMs) for organizing experience and behavior. Liotti (1999) has suggested that these switches can be captured by the model of the drama triangle, where three basic narrative templates for representing self-with-others alternate with each other. The first template has, as a theme, the helplessness of self and/or others (theme of the victim). The second narrative template is defined by the theme of the persecutor, and the third by the theme of the rescuer. Whenever this drama triangle regulates the inner narrative and the emotional experience, the integrative functions of the mind (metacognitive capacity, theory of mind, self-reflection) are seriously hindered.

The therapeutic relationship is particularly apt to facilitate the activation of the attachment system among the various motivational systems of which human beings are endowed (e.g., the competitive system, the cooperative system, the sexual system, and the exploratory system: Gilbert, 1989; Lichtenberg, 1989). This means that during psychotherapy it is very likely that the patients will come to represent self and the psychotherapist according to the drama triangle, with consequent hindrance to metacognitive ability (metacognition is the capacity to monitor one's own mental states, and to reflect critically upon them). Patients (and their therapists) are often confronted during psychotherapy with a relational dilemma, in which it seems impossible to achieve both self-protection and protective closeness (Blizard, 2001). Because of the hindrance to metacognitive abilities, it is difficult to deal with this dilemma by critically reflecting upon it. In these situations, the patient may oscillate between abnormal dependence on the therapist (construed as the rescuer) and equally abnormal independence (e.g., when the therapist is perceived as a potential persecutor: Steele *et al.*, 2001).

Thus, the too early, too frequent, or too intense activation of the attachment system could create a situation that exceeds the capacity of the patient to regulate interpersonal emotions and reflect on interpersonal experience. It is therefore vital that the therapeutic relationship is so structured as to titrate the activation of the patients' attachment system. In order to avoid the risk of too strong an activation of the attachment system, the treatment guidelines of the International Society for the Study of Dissociation (2000) suggest as optimal the frequency of two or three sessions each week; more than three sessions should be considered only after having carefully evaluated the risk of fostering excessive dependence. For the same reason, at the beginning of treatment, dealing too closely on traumatic memories should be avoided; the painful experience of retrieving such memories would bring with itself the powerful activation of the attachment system (see Bowlby, 1982, for an account of how the activation of the attachment system may relate to the experience of either physical or emotional pain). Rather, the therapist should strive to facilitate the activation of the patients' cooperative system, that corresponds to the building of a therapeutic alliance in which both patient and therapist explicitly perceive themselves as sharing a common goal.

In order to build up the therapeutic alliance at the beginning of psychotherapy, some clinicians ask the patient what his or her goals for the treatment are, and accept them explicitly as a preliminary aim (provided, of course, that they are reasonable and ethically acceptable). Patients who may often have experienced being powerless at the hand of an abusing caretaker, or being unheeded by a neglecting caregiver, are thus empowered within the therapeutic relationship (Courtois, 1997). Mollon (2002a,b) emphasizes the importance of seeking an internal consensus among dissociative parts concerning whether to proceed or not with psychotherapy; to go ahead only on the basis of the wishes of one dissociative part is to risk an internal 'civil war'.

In this phase of treatment, when the patient may ask for relief from anxiety symptoms or depression, the therapist may reply with standard cognitive-behavioral techniques for anxiety and mood disorders (Kennerley, 1996), and/or with the prescription of serotonergic or mood-stabilizer drugs. Thus, while aiming at symptom reduction and stabilization, it may become clear to the patient that the therapist not only listens empathically to him/her, but actively and efficiently cares for his/her well-being. In so doing, it is important to avoid any violation of therapeutic boundaries (e.g., through protective overinvolvement, or collusion with the patients' fantasies of having met a loving rescuer from their sufferings). Boundary violation, always a great danger in psychotherapy, is particularly harmful to dissociative patients, as it subtly repeats and confirms structurally similar violations in the relationship with abusive parents. The therapist should never attempt through physical contact (of any variety) to meet the dissociative patient's often desperate quest for affection and comfort. Similarly, the therapist should also avoid acting upon the often powerful countertransferential wishes to offer reparation for what may have been the patient's extreme childhood experiences of pain and betrayal. While offering professional protection and understanding, they should be wary of the risk of overprotecting their patients (see also below, 'Difficult situations and their solution').

While boundary *violation* should never be allowed, sporadic, prudent boundary *crossing* for therapeutic purposes may be beneficial to dissociative patients (Dalenberg, 2000).

Lisa, suffering from a DDNOS that could be described as an incomplete multiple personality (she had partially dissociated 'parts of herself', rather than fully dissociated 'alters'), came to a session with a large bandage on her upper arm and forearm. She reported having cut herself with a lancet she had previously stolen from her husband (a surgeon). Her comments and her tone of voice on reporting the episode expressed only contempt toward the 'cowardly' and 'bitchy' part of herself ('That little bitch, what a coward . . . unable to stand even this little pain . . . and she had deserved quite a bigger one . . .'). While listening to Lisa's cruel report of how she had cut herself, the therapist—who was supervised by G.L.—was aware of the extremely brutal and sadistic sexual abuse which she, when only 4, had suffered from her father (Lisa's older brother had witnessed the abuse and reported it to the therapist). He felt moved at the idea of the little victim Lisa had been, now again victimized by herself. He decided not to conceal his feelings from the patient, and let a tear run through his face. On the next session, Lisa commented that the therapist's tears had been a topic on which she had reflected. Her insight may be summarized as follows: 'Maybe I needed that somebody else could cry over my pain, to become able to cry over it myself. Nobody ever cried or was moved when I suffered as a child'.

Another instance of rather courageous therapeutic boundary crossing is reported by Brenner (1996, p. 791), when he describes his reaction to an assaultive and suicidal patient, suffering from DID, who revealed during a session that she was hiding a blade. While realizing that she could have easily cut him or herself, the therapist offered his outstretched hand asking for the blade, which the patient, after a menacing look, carefully handed over to him. The patient was much relieved by this interaction and 'the incident became a nodal point in the treatment' (Brenner, 1996, p. 791).*

Brenner's clinical vignette illustrates also the second main theme of the preliminary phase of psychotherapy: together with the building of alliance, it is of vital importance that dissociative patients experience, quite explicitly and from the beginning of treatment, that the therapist regards their safety as a primary goal. Whenever the patient, verbally or behaviorally, raises an issue concerning any type of self-harm (e.g., grossly abnormal eating behavior, self-mutilation, promiscuous sexuality without prevention of infection, threats of suicide), the therapist should immediately and primarily focus attention on it, suspending any other type of therapeutic work. In addition to exploring the meaning and function of the behavior, safety contracting, along the lines so profitably suggested by Linehan (1993) for the cognitive-behavioral therapy of borderline patients, may be instrumental in conveying, without emotional overinvolvement, that the therapist wants the patient alive and well. This creates the condition for a type of corrective relational experience that is much needed by dissociative patients. As their previous attachment relationships may have been with caregivers who were abusive in the extreme, as well as neglecting—and who were themselves extraordinarily vulnerable, being traumatized and dissociative—these patients usually hold, consciously or not, the belief that nobody cares for their life and well-being. The experience of a secure attachment to a therapist who, within the boundaries of a cooperative therapeutic relationship, explicitly and coherently values the patient's life, safety, and well-being, challenges this pathogenic belief. In the mind of the patient, this ongoing experience of cooperation and secure attachment presents an alternative to the IWM of previous disorganized attachments.

The interpersonal meanings associated with disorganized attachment (drama triangle) are thus mobilized within the therapeutic relationship in a context of relative safety, enabling a test of the validity of the new interpersonal information as against the old IWM (cf. Weiss, 1993). Patients can act on the assumption that they are evil, guilty, and not deserving of care (self in the 'persecutor' role of the drama triangle); that they are hopelessly deemed to suffering and no type of care could ever heal them (the 'victim' role); that they have finally found in the now idealized therapist an omnipotent rescuer who will heal them without any effort on their part (therapist in the 'rescuer' role); or that the therapist is only concealing his real, evil intentions under the mask of a faked protective attitude only to exploit, disillusion, and perhaps abuse them later on (therapist in the 'persecutor' role of the drama triangle). Within a group of sessions or even within the same session, the patient's attitudes may shift between these roles, in such a quick manner as to deserve the label 'kaleidoscopic'. In DID, these shifts may correspond to one or more alternate personalities entering the stage of therapeutic dialog. In DDNOS and in other DDs, they may

correspond to ego states that are less 'autonomous' and less reciprocally dissociated. Also, previously avoided images or narratives of abuse may begin to surface. This opens up the second phase of the treatment, as in the following clinical illustration.

Tina had been in psychotherapy for about a year when she had the first, and only, occurrence of generalized dissociative amnesia (acute and total loss of autobiographic memory). She woke up one morning having forgotten her name, her history, and the identities of her husband and her child. In a panic, speaking with a childlike voice that was unfamiliar to her frightened husband, she stated that she did not recognize anybody in the house, nor the house as her home, and was unable to remember anything of her past.

At the beginning of treatment, she had been severely depressed. Her recurrent depressive episodes were further complicated by dissociative experiences, in the form of prolonged trance-like states (that had been mistaken, by her GP, for the apathy of depression). Her clinical history revealed, since adolescence, a mild and atypical anorexia nervosa, orgasmic dysfunction, and somatoform symptoms suggestive of childhood traumatic experiences. The daughter of an alcoholic man, she had reported severe emotional abuse from her mother during the first phase of treatment, but not from her father.

Tina felt much helped by her psychotherapist (G.L.) during the first months of treatment. Soon thereafter, she begun to report feelings of sexual arousal during the sessions, and became explicitly seductive toward the therapist. He politely refused her advances, stating that the only relevant thing in their relationship was the pursuing, through joint reflections on her experiences, of the therapeutic goals they had agreed upon during the very first session. After a brief phase of resentment for the refusal, Tina seemed relieved, as if she now felt safer in the relationship. At the same time, she started having dreams concerning apparent memories of incest with her father when she was about 7. She was bewildered by the veracity of these dream memories, and begun to wonder with the therapist whether or not they could reflect actual, until then forgotten events of her late childhood. The episode of dissociative amnesia took place in this context.

The therapist responded to the crisis by accepting the necessity of crossing the boundaries of psychotherapy. He responded to the request of Tina's frightened husband, to visit her at home as soon as possible (she was obviously unable to go anywhere on her own, and she refused to be accompanied by him, whom she now saw as a stranger). When the therapist arrived at Tina's home, a few hours from the beginning of the generalized amnesia, she did not recognize him, and asked 'Who are you?'. He replied: 'I am a doctor. Could I help you?' She then expressed her extreme fear at finding herself in that unknown place, and at having 'totally lost memory'. The therapist empathically said that he, too, would have felt frightened if he had lost his memory and awoke in a place he was unable to *remember*, thereby reframing Tina's way of constructing her experience (while 'being in an unknown place together with strangers' and 'having lost memory' were separate issues to her, the therapist indirectly suggested that, *as* she had lost her memory, she may not remember her home and her own family). Tina looked at him perplexedly for perhaps a minute, than she cried 'Now I remember! You are my psychotherapist! I have told you that I have been abused by my father!'

The subsequent phase of the treatment was devoted to exploring both her emerging memories of incest, their veracity, and the meaning that remembering them had to her. This exploration was guided by the principles outlined in the following section.

Middle phase: processing trauma and beginning integration

The processing of traumatic memories and of their meanings is the core of the treatment of DDs. In DID, this exploration of painful childhood memories is intertwined with the need to deal with alternate personalities that show up in the therapeutic dialog.

Some psychotherapists advocate a careful exploration of the alternate identity system once the first alter has spontaneously established direct contact with the therapist *and* the patient has been stabilized and strengthened (e.g., Kluft, 1996; Fine, 1999). They thus ask (most of them nowadays avoiding hypnosis during this exploration) if there are other identities willing to share their issues and concerns besides the one

* The reader should notice that the two therapists in these clinical vignettes, although taking a risk and crossing the boundaries of the therapeutic relationship, did not violate them (e.g., by touching the patient or by expressing any affect that should be illegitimate to express within a therapeutic dialog).

that had already established contact with the therapist. Other therapists fear that this clinical choice may encourage confabulation and iatrogenic expansion of the number of alters, and prefer to dialog only with those that may spontaneously enter the stage of psychotherapy. There is, however, wide consensus that, if an ego state does not present him/herself as a separate identity with a different name, therapists should be wary not to reify it (e.g., asking for his/her name or speaking as if they believed in the existence of different persons sharing the same body with the patient's host—i.e., primary— personality). Whenever possible without invalidating the patient's experience of switching to an alternate and separate identity, the therapist should address dissociated mental structures and behaviors (such as Tina's speaking with the voice of a child) as 'parts' or 'states' of the patient's self. That there is a unitary self for each human body may be an illusion, as has been argued by authoritative philosophers and psychologists (see, e.g., Dennett, 1991), but then it is a necessary and universal illusion. Equally, the idea that disorganized parts are separate 'individuals' is an illusion—a pretence that has structured the personality—as all are part of the overall holonomic mind (Mollon, 1996, 2002a,b).

Even wider is the consensus on the need, in order to achieve the integration of hitherto dissociated mental structures, to deal carefully in this phase of the treatment with the patients' traumatic memories (whether they be of frank abuse or of more subtle relational traumas in the early attachments). Courtois (1997) has described three main scenarios concerning the status of traumatic memories in dissociative patients. In the first, traumatic memories are accessible to the patient from the beginning of treatment, but not divulged because of shame, guilt, and family loyalty. In the second scenario, they are not known to the patient at the beginning of treatment. In the third scenario, they are not known with certainty but are suspected by the patient. Moreover, the position is complicated by processes of dissociation, which mean that what may be known in one state of mind is not known in another.

In the first phase of treatment, even if strongly suspecting the existence of traumas, therapists must tolerate the patients' not knowing or not disclosing, and avoid any pressure toward remembering or disclosure. In the second phase, therapists not only empathically listen to the patients' spontaneous report of traumatic memories, but should also actively inquire on them. Hypnosis should be avoided in this exploration of past traumatic experiences, because of the risk of creating false memories. The exploration should not aim at mere abreaction, but at meaning: the therapist should empathically inquire on the meaning that both the remembered experiences and the experience of remembering has to the patient (Mollon, 2002a,b).

Sally, an intelligent but very troubled woman of 19, was hospitalized after becoming very disturbed following a sexual assault. She appeared at times disoriented to time and place, and displayed signs of extreme fear. In the calm ambiance of psychotherapy she began to settle. However, she would still sometimes express anxieties that the therapist (P.M.) would attack her physically. Gradually she disclosed more about an internal image that had begun to haunt her. It was of a little girl alone in a room. At times she spoke of hatred and fear of this little child. On other occasions she would deny that there was such a child in her mind. In lucid moments she would speak of her realization that the image was of her child self—the child who had been extensively abused by the 'uncle' she had been sent to live with after her mother became ill when Sally was age 3. She described a process whereby she had believed she could omnipotently repudiate her abused child self and create a new version of herself; she would 'pretend' that the bad experiences had not happened—but then found that she was confused about what was pretence and what was real. This process was spontaneously enacted within the therapy, in that she would speak of her uncle's terrifying behavior towards her, but then a moment later would state that none of what she had just said was true, that there was no little girl, and that there was nothing wrong with her. She would say she had just pretended there was a little girl—but might then express confusion about whether she was pretending to pretend. Repudiating what she had just said became a recurrent pattern in the therapy. There were periods when she would appear extremely child-like, but these episodes were associated with considerable anxiety. Overall, Sally seemed to become more relaxed and trusting as she discovered that the therapist

remained calm, interested, and inquiring, while not reaching for premature conclusions about the content and meaning of her memories and fantasies.

The above vignette illustrates how, during trauma work, considerable uncertainty must sometimes be tolerated both by patient and therapist. When patients ask for the therapist's assurance that their traumatic memories are totally real, honesty in the therapist's reply is particularly important. The therapist should acknowledge that there is no method to distinguish with absolute certainty accurate memories from inaccurate ones, and help the patient in accepting this fact. Empathy for the anguish with which patients reflect on their uncertainty about the real occurrence of traumas is essential. Therapists should be clear and explicit that they consider the painful *meaning* of the uncertainly surfacing memories absolutely real and dramatically important in the patients' life, even if they cannot confirm or disconfirm the reality of their *content*.

Therapeutic techniques such as 'eye movement desensitization and reprocessing' (EMDR: Shapiro, 2001), which have been promisingly used in the treatment of posttraumatic stress disorder (see Chapter 13 for a description of the technique), have also been advocated for working with the traumatic childhood memories of adult dissociative patients. This method, involving bilateral stimulation of the two hemispheres, through eye movements or auditory stimulation alternating in either ear, can be viewed as a method of accelerated processing of emotional information (Mollon, 2001b). It has been argued that incorporating EMDR in the trauma work with dissociative patients may provide a protective format for the processing of otherwise overwhelmingly painful memories, by reducing the risk of negative transferences during trauma work (Twombly, 2000). Extreme caution, however, should be exercised in the use of EMDR with patients who have suffered extensive trauma in childhood (Mollon, 2002a), because of the danger of 'opening the floodgates' to unmanageable levels of dissociated memory and affect.

The therapeutic work on memories of abuse is a phase, often unavoidably long, of mourning and resolution of the traumas. It is also a phase of psychotherapy in which integration begins. The exploration of traumatic experiences allows for the joint understanding, by patient and therapist, of the coping reactions that have led to dissociative experiences (e.g., numbing, trance-like states, amnesia, depersonalization) and dissociated ego states, which thus begin to be integrated in the patients' explicit self-knowledge. The function of alternate personalities, if present, becomes intelligible when matched with the experience of abuse and with the dramatic status of attachment relationships. For instance, protective personalities may have had the function of coping with aspects of reality that exceeded the coping capacity of the traumatized host personality. Persecutor personalities may have been created in order to express both overwhelming rage and guilt (linked to the belief of being responsible for the abuse or of having deserved it). Victim personalities may had the function of preserving both the memory of the abuse and the associated meaning of being totally helpless at the hand of the perpetrator.

As a primary attachment figure may have been the perpetrator of abuse or may have been neglecting, or may have been perceived as exceedingly fragile and unable to protect the patient from the abuse, the therapist's close attention to the dynamics of attachment is usually rewarding. In this phase, the patient may begin to share with the therapist and understand the simultaneous presence of utterly incompatible and dramatically strong feelings toward, for instance, a parent who was at times frightening, abusive, and deeply emotionally ill, while at other times offered them at least some protection and comfort (otherwise they, as children, would not have survived). The therapist's awareness of the dynamics of disorganized attachment assists in expecting and understanding the patients' dramatically shifting transferences. This understanding is invaluable in protecting therapists from untoward countertransferential reactions and from misunderstanding of the meaning of a patient's shifts, say, from gratitude and hope to expressed hopelessness, fear, suspicion, or even hatred toward the therapist—and it must be recognized that at certain points in the vicissitudes of the transference the therapist will be perceived as being as bad as the original abuser. The therapist is offering empathy and support to a deeply suffering patient who is mourning over very painful memories. This interpersonal situation—a therapist offering empathic understanding to a deeply suffering patient—unavoidably activates the patient's attachment system within the therapeutic relationship (the attachment system is activated when one's suffering is met by a person perceived as 'stronger and wiser than the self': Bowlby, 1979, p. 129). As the patient's IWM of attachment is disorganized, it is likely that he/she will be prone to construe the therapist's role, alternately, as that of the rescuer, the perpetrator of abuses, and even the victim of the patient's alleged evilness.

When changes of ego state in the transference are understood as shifting aspects of the relational dilemmas of attachment disorganization, therapeutic exploration of their meaning begins to center on a unitary meaning. Patients, while beginning to experience a secure attachment to the therapist (an important emotional corrective experience), may understand that a unitary motive—the wish to be understood and of having their suffering soothed by another person—is at the base of their manifold shifts from idealizing to devaluing or attacking self and others. This corrective emotional experience and these reflections foster integration at the level of the patient's basic meaning structures of self-with-other.

In cases of DID, reciprocally dissociated protective, persecuting, and victim 'personalities' alternate during the sessions. Attachment theory, in these cases, offers to the therapist a way to conceive the basic, unitary psychic structure of self-with-other from which the alters are created out of reciprocally incompatible and disowned memories, expectations, beliefs, affects, and wishes. Bearing in mind this structure (however, it is conceived within different theoretical frameworks) it becomes easier to establish moments of dialog with the patient in which the attitudes of two or more alters are considered together as different ways to deal, in the same traumatic interaction with the caregiver, with the needs for both attachment and self-protection. Two or more 'alters', so to speak, 'sit together with the therapist' and become able to consider their common origin.

In this therapeutic interaction lies the integrative power of psychotherapy in the DDS, common to different types of theoretical approaches. To it, some therapists add 'fusion rituals', often utilizing hypnosis, aimed at further facilitating the blending of alters in a unitary sense of self (Kluft, 1993). Others instruct patients to bring the alters together in their mind, in a sort of imagined group meeting, in order to develop 'group thinking' and 'group feeling' as a preliminary to a unitary sense of self (Fine, 1999). Outcome studies evaluating the specific advantages of these techniques are needed.

There is, however, an integrative flow inherent in the psychotherapeutic process. This follows from the point that, although the shifting mental and behavioral states are dissociated within the patient's mind, they are not dissociated within the therapist's mind. Thus, integration takes place first within the therapist, who hears about and observes many different aspects of the patient. The therapist can reflect upon (mentalize) these multiple experiences, behaviors, narratives, and affects—and, indeed, multiple transferences—and gradually communicate the emerging meanings and perspectives to the patient.

Late phase: self-care and relational development

Over the course of treatment, a sense of self less encumbered by intrusions of traumatic memories and dissociative experiences is developed. Many patients, in the late phase of treatment, express the wish for a more thorough mastery of what they now understand as a tendency to dissociate in response to specific situations, e.g., attachment-related feelings of anger or anxiety. Cognitive techniques of journal-keeping, through which patients may more carefully assess the external contingencies, the emotions and the thoughts related to the tendency to dissociate, may be useful at this juncture. Patients may also benefit from repeating mentally simple verbal formulas, such as 'I am here now', as an instrument for keeping attention on ongoing experiences and thus countering the tendency to dissociate (Kennerley, 1996).

> Mario had achieved many insights on the childhood, traumatic origins of his shifting ego states (besides having been brutally beaten by his father, he had been the

victim of extreme neglect by both his parents). He had also achieved a good capacity for metacognitive monitoring of his tendency to enter into dissociative mental states. In an advanced phase of his treatment, he had been instructed by his therapist (G.M.) to register in a journal information concerning where he was, what he was feeling and what he was thinking every time he noticed in himself the tendency to dissociate. Here is a page of his journal:

> *Context in which the dissociative experience tend to emerge*: 'I am traveling by train, and I am alone in the compartment'.

> *Feelings*: 'Loneliness, anxiety, wish to have Anna (wife) here.'

> *Thoughts*: 'That curtain . . . the door for another world . . . I do not want to enter it . . . I'd rather stay here . . . maybe have a coffee . . .'

> On that occasion, then, Mario had been able to resist the temptation to absorb his attention in the swinging rhythmical movements of the curtain, and to enter thereby in the trance-like state that was so easily accessible to him whenever he felt afraid, distressed, or lonely. It was in this state that most of his shifts between different ego states took place, as he had learned during psychotherapy. Keeping the journal was instrumental in reminding him of his decision—one that he had painfully reached during a long therapeutic work—to give up his dissociative defenses. The journal also made it increasingly clear that most of his dissociative tendencies emerged concurrently with his attachment wishes (e.g., in situations of loneliness, mental pain, threatened losses).

Cognitive-behavioral techniques of self-control and self-regulation may be used in the late phase of psychotherapy also for problems (e.g., sexual dysfunctions, abnormal eating patterns, addictions, and compulsions) that were not amenable to therapeutic influence before the resolution of core traumatic issues. The relational message implicit in the use of such techniques is that the therapist considers the patient as both potentially able and wholly entitled to take care of themselves. Before using these techniques, trauma-related pathogenic beliefs of not deserving care or of utter helplessness should therefore have been corrected. Patients should also have been able to modulate the emotions of guilt, shame, and abnormal dependency (abnormal anxiety at separations) accompanying such beliefs. The completion of such therapeutic accomplishments could be the task of the late phase.

Another task of the late phase is to clarify the difference between self-care and compulsive self-sufficiency. Issues of expected separation from the therapist may set the stage for completing the therapeutic work on this distinction. The prospect of ending the therapy may facilitate comments on normal emotional reactions to separation, on the difference between separation and loss, and on how to aspire, in other relationships, to the standards of secure attachment and mutual cooperation now experienced in the therapeutic relationship. The dramatic past relational experiences of dissociative patients may induce them to search for support to these reflections by testing the therapist's availability after having agreed upon ending treatment. Follow-up or booster sessions (e.g., once every 2–3 months), scheduled for two or more years, may be instrumental in passing this test successfully. Patients should, as the outcome of treatment, become able to rebalance their old relationship and to select/build up new ones according to the normal needs for relational safety, mutuality, and respect.

Most therapists agree that the more severe forms of DD require at least 3–5 years of intensive individual psychotherapy to reach these goals (International Society for the Study of Dissociation, 2000).

Difficult situations and their solution

Dissociative patients are prone to harm themselves in various ways, and many of them are at risk of suicide. Some of them may also severely harm other people. These harming tendencies may be particularly difficult to deal with in the usual outpatient setting when they are menaced by persecutor alters emerging in the therapeutic dialogs. When hospitalization needs be considered to cope with these risks, it should be planned so that inpatient treatment aims at achieving specific goals of the psychotherapy. An instance is the planned processing of traumatic material (to clarify the meaning of the aggressive tendencies and regulate them), resorting to the protective hospital setting during such a planned exploration.

Particularly during trauma work, dissociative patients may feel utterly destabilized and disoriented by the surfacing memories and their meaning. Even when the risk of harming themselves or others in such moments of destabilization is not so serious as to require hospitalization, particular interventions should be considered that may assist in soothing the patients and reorienting them. Some therapists find hypnosis useful in this respect, as a context in which patients may more easily accept useful suggestions, e.g., to terminate spontaneous flashbacks and reorient themselves to present reality, or to momentarily 'put to sleep' a particularly troublesome alter.

When shame or family loyalties or overwhelming emotions prohibit trauma work in the individual setting, participation in group therapy involving other survivors of childhood abuse may be of great value (Buchele, 1993)—although some authors caution that this may provoke vicarious traumatization and provide suggestive stimuli for confabulated memories (Mollon, 2002a,b). While pharmacotherapy is not a primary treatment for the DDs, it may help in managing the destabilizing features of trauma work, or in dealing with comorbid mood or anxiety disorders. Group interventions and pharmacotherapy should preferably be the responsibility of a different clinician, with whom the individual psychotherapist keeps constant cooperative dialog. In this way, having a relationship with two different but communicating therapeutic attachment figures, the activation of the patients' attachment system toward the individual psychotherapist becomes usually less intense and more easily manageable (because of the concurrent lessening of the dissociating influences of the disorganized IWM).

Another instance in which the individual psychotherapists may usefully cooperate with another clinician is when a family therapist is consulted (e.g., because of risk of repeated abuse in the patients' new family, or because of sexual problems in the patient's conjugal couple: Porter et al., 1993). The cooperation between two different therapists in the treatment of particularly difficult cases of dissociative pathology is so potentially useful that even the simultaneity of two individual psychotherapies has been advocated (Wine and Carter, 1999).

Therapists of patients reporting memories of childhood intrafamilial abuse should also be aware of two major legal problems that can complicate the treatment: the risk of being accused by family members of having induced false memories and the possible request by the patient to be supported in suing an abusive family member. Every care should be taken in order to avoid the risk of inducing false memories, or of sanctioning any memory as *certainly* factual rather than reconstructive and therefore potentially fallible. As to actively assisting patients in taking legal actions against family members, this possibility is appropriate only when the adult patient's *present* safety is threatened, i.e., in the face of ongoing abuse. In all other cases, the patient should be aware that therapy's task is concerned with meaning and the exploration of memory, feeling, thought, intention, wish, or behavior pattern, but not with assistance in (nor dissuasion from) claiming legal acknowledgment of any past injustice the patient may have suffered.

Finally, it cannot be emphasized enough that psychotherapeutic work with dissociative patients, while frequently rewarding, can be extremely difficult and hazardous. Perhaps more than with any other patients, considerable clinical skill and experience are required—to understand and manage such aspects as the complexity of the presented material, the shifting self states, the enactments in the consulting room, the multiple transferences, the extent of anxiety and overwhelming affect held within the dissociative structure, and the profound ambivalence that the patient will feel about allowing the therapist access to the secrets of their internal world. Although the hope may be that the patient can surrender the dissociative mode of being and achieve greater integration, the reality in some cases may be that instead of improving through therapy he or she deteriorates. Instead of gratitude for hard therapeutic work, the patient feels hatred for the therapist who has undone the dissociative defenses against unbearable annihilatory pain—and now it may be the therapist that has to be both

clung to and annihilated. This is the danger of malignant regression. It is not exclusive to DDs, but is a hazard in all cases where a patient has experienced severe emotional deprivation and interpersonal trauma in childhood; the combination of rage, envy, and intense need may mean that the therapist becomes ultimately the patient's victim. In a state of manic triumph, the 'bad' or vulnerable self is projectively located in the therapist—and there it is condemned and persecuted.

> A young female clinical psychologist, working in relative isolation from colleagues with more psychotherapeutic experience, found herself working with a woman with DID. She felt fortunate to have such an interesting case, finding the patient's shifting self states fascinating, and soon the therapy sessions were becoming more and more frequent and longer in duration—these and other boundary violations being rationalized as adaptation to what she viewed as the patient's obvious need for 'special' conditions. Child alter states began to emerge and the psychologist allowed the patient, in these states, to sit on her knee cuddling her for long periods. She felt shock and deep compassion at the narratives of severe childhood abuse—and felt she must work extra hard for such a damaged and deserving patient. However, the psychologist became increasingly alarmed when angry and very demanding states were presented. As she attempted to withdraw and limit her 'therapeutic' involvement, the patient became increasingly agitated, alternating between threatening and pathetic pleading modes. The psychologist experienced rage, fear, and bewilderment. She felt guilty about her own hatred towards the patient, resulting in attempts to compensate by trying even harder to meet the patient's 'needs'—thus alternating between being overly gratifying and rejecting. Steadily the psychologist became more and more exhausted—and her judgment increasingly impaired. She was herself suffering traumatic stress, as a result both of hearing terrible narratives of childhood abuse, and also through the enactments in their interaction. Her feelings of shame at the unorthodox position she found herself in, with many deviations from the normal boundaries of therapy, meant that she did not feel able to seek supervisory consultation. The patient assumed greater and greater power over the psychologist, even succeeding in getting the latter to agree to social meetings. Four years after the therapy began, the patient made an official complaint about the psychologist, alleging that that she had encouraged the development of a multiple personality and made her worse as a result of malpractice.

On the other hand, with appropriate caution, modesty of therapeutic aims, and continual attention to pacing of the work, in such a way that the patient can feel some degree of control over the process while also experiencing the reassurance of a secure frame, the psychotherapist may enjoy the privilege and grace of witnessing moments of true healing.

Conclusions

Individual outpatient psychotherapy is the treatment of choice for DDs. The most commonly cited treatment orientation is psychodynamic-eclectic, focused on relational themes, and often incorporating cognitive therapy techniques and/or hypnosis (for soothing and containment, not for abreaction of traumatic memories). Pharmacotherapy, group, and family interventions may be of great but ancillary value with respect to the individual therapy. It is essential to establish the therapeutic alliance and to fortify the patient before working on traumatic memories. Trauma work, in turn, is necessary to achieve integration. Although conclusive evidence is still lacking, integration seems both a possibility and a necessity for the successful treatment of these disorders.

References

Allen, J. G. (2001). *Traumatic relationships and serious mental disorders*. Chichester: Wiley.

Allen, J. G., Console, D. A., and Lewis, L. (1999). Dissociative detachment and memory impairment: reversible amnesia or encoding failure? *Comprehensive Psychiatry*, **40**, 160–71.

Bliss, E. (1986). *Multiple personality, allied disorders and hypnosis*. Oxford: Oxford University Press.

Blizard, R. A. (2001). Masochistic and sadistic ego states: dissociative solutions to the dilemma of attachment to an abusive caregiver. *Journal of Trauma and Dissociation*, **2**, 37–58.

Bowlby, J. (1979). *The making and breaking of affectional bonds*. London: Tavistock Publications.

Bowlby, J. (1982). *Attachment and loss. Vol. 1: attachment*, 2nd edn. London: Hogarth Press.

Brenner, I. (1996). On trauma, perversion and multiple personality. *Journal of the American Psychoanalytic Association*, **44**, 785–814.

Buchele, B. J. (1993). Group psychotherapy for persons with multiple personality and dissociative disorders. *Bulletin of the Menninger Clinic*, **57**, 362–70.

Carlson, E. A. (1998). A prospective longitudinal study of disorganized/disoriented attachment. *Child Development*, **69**, 1970–9.

Chu, J. A. and Bowman, E. S. (2000). Trauma and dissociation: 20 years of study and lessons learned along the way. *Journal of Trauma and Dissociation*, **1**, 5–20.

Coons, P. M. (1994). Confirmation of childhood abuse in children and adolescents cases of multiple personality disorder and dissociative disorder not otherwise specified. *Journal of Nervous and Mental Disease*, **182**, 461–4.

Coons, P. M. and Bowman, E. S. (2001). Ten years follow-up of patients with dissociative identity disorder. *Journal of Trauma and Dissociation*, **2**, 73–90.

Courtois, C. A. (1997). Healing the incest wound: a treatment update with attention to the recovered-memory issue. *American Journal of Psychotherapy*, **51**, 464–96.

Dalenberg, C. J. (2000). *Countertransference and the treatment of trauma*. Washington, DC: American Psychological Association.

Davies, J. M. and Frawley, M. G. (1994). *Treating the adult survivor of childhood sexual abuse: a psychoanalytic perspective*. New York: Basic Books.

Dell, P. F. (2001). Why the diagnostic criteria for dissociative identity disorder should be changed. *Journal of Trauma and Dissociation*, **2**, 7–37.

Dennett, D. (1991). *Consciousness explained*. Boston: Little Brown.

Ellason, J. W. and Ross, C. A. (1997). Two years follow-up of inpatients with dissociative identity disorder. *American Journal of Psychiatry*, **154**, 832–9.

Fine, C. G. (1999). The tactical-integration model for the treatment of dissociative identity disorder and allied dissociative disorders. *Journal of Trauma and Dissociation*, **1**, 361–76.

Fonagy, P. (1999). The transgenerational transmission of holocaust trauma: Lessons learned from the analysis of an adolescent with obsessive-compulsive disorder. *Attachment and Human Development*, **1**, 92–114.

Fonagy, P., Gergely, G., Jurist, E. L., and Target, M. (2002). *Affect regulation, mentalization and the development of the Self*. New York: Other Press.

Freyd, J. J. (1996). *Betrayal trauma: the logic of forgetting child abuse*. Cambridge, MA: Harvard University Press.

Gilbert, P. (1989). *Human nature and suffering*. London: LEA.

Gold, S. N., *et al.* (2001). Contextual treatment of dissociative identity disorder: three case studies. *Journal of Trauma and Dissociation*, **2**, 5–35.

Herman, J. L. (1992). *Trauma and recovery*. New York: Basic Books.

International Society for the Study of Dissociation (2000). Guidelines for treating dissociative identity disorder (multiple personality) in adults (1997). *Journal of Trauma and Dissociation*, **2**, 117–34.

Kennerley, H. (1996). Cognitive therapy of dissociative symptoms associated with trauma. *British Journal of Clinical Psychology*, **35**, 325–40.

Kingdon, D. and Turkington, D. (2002). *The case study guide to cognitive behaviour therapy of psychosis*. Chichester: Wiley.

Kluft, R. P. (1993). Clinical approaches to the integration of personalities. In: R. P. Kluft and C. G. Fine, ed. *Clinical perspectives on multiple personality disorder*, pp. 101–33. Washington, DC: American Psychiatric Press.

Kluft, R. P. (1996). Treating the traumatic memories of patients with dissociative identity disorder. *American Journal of Psychiatry*, **153**, 103–10.

Kluft, R. P. (1999). An overview of the psychotherapy of dissociative identity disorder. *American Journal of Psychotherapy*, **53**, 289–319.

Lichtenberg, J. D. (1989). *Psychoanalysis and motivation*. Hillsdale, NJ: Analytic Press.

Linehan, M. M. (1993). *Cognitive-behavioral treatment of borderline personality disorder*. New York: Guilford Press.

Liotti, G. (1992). Disorganized/disoriented attachment in the etiology of the dissociative disorders. *Dissociation*, **5**, 196–204.

Liotti, G. (1995). Disorganized/disoriented attachment in the psychotherapy of the dissociative disorders. In: S. Goldberg, R. Muir, and J. Kerr, ed. *Attachment theory: social, developmental and clinical perspectives*, pp. 343–63. Hillsdale, NJ: Analytic Press.

Liotti, G. (1999). Disorganized attachment as a model for the understanding of dissociative psychopathology. In: J. Solomon and C. George, ed. *Attachment disorganization*, pp. 291–317. New York: Guilford Press.

Liotti, G. and Intreccialagli, B. (2003). Disorganized attachment, motivational systems and metacognitive monitoring in the treatment of a patient with borderline syndrome. In: M. Cortina and M. Marrone, ed. *Attachment theory and the psychoanalytic process psychotherapy of psychotic and personality disorders*, pp. 356–81. London: Whurr Publishers.

Liotti, G., Pasquini, P. and The Italian Group for the Study of Dissociation. (2000). Predictive factors for borderline personality disorder: patients' early traumatic experiences and losses suffered by the attachment figure. *Acta Psychiatrica Scandinavica*, **102**, 282–9.

Lyons-Ruth, K. and Jacobvitz, D. (1999). Attachment disorganization: unresolved loss, relational violence and lapses in behavioral and attentional strategies. In: J. Cassidy and P. R. Shaver, ed. *Handbook of attachment*, pp. 520–54. New York: Guilford Press.

Main, M. and Hesse, E. (1990). Parents' unresolved traumatic experiences are related to infant disorganized attachment status: Is frightened and/or frightening parental behavior the linking mechanism? In M. T. Greenberg, D. Cicchetti, and E. M. Cummings, ed. *Attachment in the preschool years*, pp. 161–82. Chicago: Chicago University Press.

Main, M. and Morgan, H. (1996). Disorganization and disorientation in infant Strange Situation behavior: phenotypic resemblance to dissociative states? In: L. Michelson and W. Ray, ed. *Handbook of dissociation*, pp. 107–37. New York: Plenum Press.

Mollon, P. (1996). *Multiple selves, multiple voices. working with trauma, violation and dissociation*. Chichester: Wiley.

Mollon, P. (2001a). *Releasing the Self. The healing legacy of Heinz Kohut*. London: Whurr Publishers.

Mollon, P. (2001b). Psychoanalytic perspectives on accelerated information processing (EMDR). *British Journal of Psychotherapy*, **17**(4), 448–64.

Mollon, P. (2002a). *Remembering trauma. A psychotherapist's guide to memory and illusion*, 2nd edn. London: Whurr Publishers.

Mollon, P. (2002b). Dark dimensions of multiple personality. In: V. Sinason, ed. *Attachment, trauma and multiplicity*, pp. 177–94. London: Routledge.

Ogawa, J. R., Sroufe, L. A., Weinfield, N. S., Carlson, E. A., and Egeland, B. (1997). Development and the fragmented self: longitudinal study of dissociative symptomatology in a nonclinical sample. *Development and Psychopathology*, **9**, 855–79.

Pasquini, P., Liotti, G., and The Italian Group for the Study of Dissociation (2002). Risk factors in the early family life of patients suffering from dissociative disorders. *Acta Psychiatrica Scandinavica*, **105**, 110–16.

Porter, S., Kelly, K. A., and Grame, C. J. (1993). Family treatment of spouses and children of patients with multiple personality disorder. *Bulletin of the Menninger Clinic*, **57**, 371–9.

Putnam, F. W. (1989). *Diagnosis and treatment of multiple personality disorder*. New York: Guilford Press.

Ross, C. A. (1989). *Multiple personality disorder: diagnosis, clinical features and treatment*. New York: John Wiley.

Ross, C. A., Norton, G. R., and Wozney, K. (1989). Multiple personality disorder: an analysis of 236 cases. *Canadian Journal of Psychiatry*, **34**, 413–18.

Schore, A. N. (2001). The effects of early relational trauma on right brain development, affect regulation and infant mental health. *Infant Mental Health Journal*, **22**, 201–69.

Schuengel, C., Bakermans-Kranenburg, M. J., and VanIJzendoorn, M. (1999). Frightening maternal behavior linking unresolved loss and disorganized infant attachment. *Journal of Consulting and Clinical Psychology*, **67**, 54–63.

Shapiro, F. (2001). *Eye movement desensitization and reprocessing. Basic principles, protocols and procedures*, 2nd edn. New York: Guilford Press.

Simeon, D., Guralnik, O., Schmeidler, J., Sirof, B., and Knutelska, M. (2001). The role of childhood interpersonal trauma in depersonalization disorder. *American Journal of Psychiatry*, **158**, 1027–33.

Steele, K., Van der Hart, O., and Nijenhuis, E. R. (2001). Dependency in the treatment of complex posttraumatic stress disorder and dissociative disorders. *Journal of Trauma and Dissociation*, **2**, 79–115.

Twombly, J. H. (2000). Incorporating EMDR and EMDR adaptations into the treatment of clients with dissociative identity disorders. *Journal of Trauma and Dissociation*, **1**, 61–81.

Weiss, J. (1993). *How psychotherapy works: process and technique*. New York: Guilford Press.

Wine, B. and Carter, J. (1999). Parallel individual therapy: a treatment model for the seriously disturbed. *Voices*, **35**, 22–38.

17 Paraphilias

Peter J. Fagan, Gregory Lehne, Julia G. Strand, and Fred S. Berlin

Introduction

Individuals with paraphilia entering psychotherapy often have led a very secret sexual life for many years. Therapy may be their first opportunity to speak with another about impulses, urges, and behaviors that may have been at best a curiosity and at worst a torment. Therapy can be rewarding as therapist and patient speak about thoughts, feelings, and behaviors that have heretofore been shrouded in secrecy, often regarded with shame, a source of pleasure as well as a possible source of suffering for the self or others.

Paraphilias are psychosexual disorders in which the individual experiences recurrent, intense sexual fantasies or urges to engage in unusual or unacceptable sexual behavior. To qualify as a psychiatric disorder according to the diagnostic criteria of DSM-IV-TR (*Diagnostic and statistical manual of mental disorders*, 4th edn, text revision edn), the behaviors, sexual urges, or fantasies must 'cause clinically significant distress or impairment in social, occupational, or other important areas of functioning' (American Psychiatric Association, 2000, p. 566). Although paraphilic behavior may be episodic, the sexual content of paraphilic disorders is generally relatively fixed and stable for any given individual, being significantly present for at least 6 months rather than situational, transitory, or experimental. Paraphilias have traditionally been classified and discussed based upon the content of the sexual fantasies or behaviors. The most commonly diagnosed paraphilias listed in alphabetic order in DSM-IV-TR are: exhibitionism, fetishism, frotteurism, pedophilia, sexual masochism, sexual sadism, transvestic fetishism, and voyeurism. These categories largely reflect historical, forensic, or social concerns with behavior that causes problems for others, rather than being based upon the distress or dysfunction for the affected individual.

More than 40 different paraphilias have been identified (Money, 1986, 1999), and perusal of recent publications and the Internet suggests that the number of paraphilias defined by their unusual sexual content may be much larger (Love, 1992; Francoeur *et al.*, 1995). Individuals who have symptoms of one paraphilia may also have symptoms of other paraphilias (Abel *et al.*, 1988; Kafka and Prentky, 1994). Symptoms of different paraphilias may be combined in an individual's life history as a multiplex paraphilia (Lehne and Money, 2000, 2003). Human sexuality is diverse and complicated. Practitioners must always remember that many individuals with unusual sexual fantasies, interests, or practices do not experience significant distress or impairment, and must be careful not to pathologize the diversity of human sexuality.

The diagnosis of a paraphilia does not preclude diagnosis of any other comorbid conditions. Mood and anxiety disorders, as well as alcohol and substance abuse problems, are prevalent among men with paraphilia (Allnutt *et al.*, 1996; McElroy *et al.*, 1999; Raymond *et al.*, 1999). No personality disorder (including antisocial) is particularly associated with paraphilia. However, any and all of the personality disorders may be found in individuals with paraphilia (Raymond *et al.*, 1999). Paraphilias can be associated with organic, degenerative, or traumatic brain damage (Simpson *et al.*, 1999; Mendez *et al.*, 2000).

Clearly, comorbid disorders must be diagnosed and treated along with the paraphilia for treatment to be maximally effective. Paraphilias may be found with higher frequencies than in the general population in males who suffer from schizophrenia, mental retardation, autism, pervasive developmental disorder, and attention deficit hyperactivity disorder (Kafka and Prentky, 1994, 1998). These groups may be at risk for the development of paraphilia for multiple reasons, as yet not fully determined. Most apparently, however, their deficits in interpersonal relationships skills are likely to limit their negotiating interpersonal sex with age appropriate partners (Ousley and Mesibov, 1991; Van Bourgodien *et al.*, 1997; Kohn *et al.*, 1998; Realmuto and Ruble, 1999). After completing a comprehensive evaluation of both the cognitive assets and vulnerabilities of these patients with special needs, the therapist should tailor the social learning interventions to the level of the patient. For example, group experience is recommended for patients with these conditions.

Conceptualization of the disorder

There are three components of human sexuality that may be disordered in individuals with paraphilia: *sexual urge* (the physiological motivation or sex drive), *sexual fantasy* (recurrent mental imagery), and *sexual behavior* (which is often the product of the first two). These components function in an interrelated feedback loop, and thus disorder in any area can affect the others. The basic disorder in paraphilia is that any or all of these three components operate in an excitable state that the affected individual has difficulty regulating. Thus paraphilias may be better thought of as *hyperphilias*, i.e., an abnormally high degree of sexual responsiveness (in contrast to the *hypophilias*, which are considered sexual dysfunctions).

This conceptualization allows us to identify the aspects of paraphilia that cause distress or impairment for patients and so become the focus of treatment. *Sexual urges* can be preoccupying and difficult to control (hypersexuality), causing the individual to feel frustration and distress. Sexual urges can energize and intensify both sexual fantasies and behavioral enactment. *Sexual fantasies* may be so frequent or intrusive that they make it difficult for the individual to concentrate, in a way similar to the interference of other types of obsessional thinking. The content of sexual fantasies may be upsetting to individuals when the content is not congruent with their self-concept or is incompatible with the types of sexual activity available for them. Cognitive distortions and justifications of paraphilic sexual fantasies may develop in an attempt to reconcile paraphilic fantasies with self-concept. Incompatible sexual fantasies can be associated with difficulties in sexual performance (sexual dysfunction) or interfere with intimacy or pair bonding with an available partner. A high frequency or intensity of sexual fantasies may fuel uncomfortably high levels of sexual urges or behavior.

Sexual behavior may be associated with the most intense distress and the greatest social consequences for an individual with a paraphilia. Sexual behavior problems include high frequencies of masturbation, long periods of time spent in masturbation rituals, intense preoccupying search for a sexual outlet, or engaging in sexual activity in situations that ultimately are associated with harm to the self or others. Uncomfortably high levels of autonomic arousal and dissociative or fugue-like states may be part of paraphilic behavioral enactment. Sexual behavior can be so focused and ritualistic that it causes difficulties in developing mutually satisfying sexual relations with a partner. Because of the overdetermined nature of paraphilic sexual interests and associated behavior, the presence of a paraphilic disorder can introduce distortions in development and lifestyle. For example, persons with pedophilia may become excessively involved in activities that appeal to children, while neglecting the development of more adult-oriented interests.

Considerable time and money can be spent in behavior associated with the paraphilia, such as collecting paraphernalia, viewing or acquiring or producing materials associated with the content of the paraphilia, going on to the Internet in the workplace or library to view paraphilia-related sites, as well participating in paid sexual activities. Participation in sexual behavior temporarily assuages sexual fantasies and urges, but in the long run may ultimately fuel and increase them. Behavior can lead to physical, emotional, and financial risk to the self and others. Some paraphilic sexual behaviors are illegal and may result in arrest and incarceration.

Referral patterns

Sex offenses and paraphilia

While many of the commonly diagnosed paraphilias may be associated with sex-offending behavior, most paraphilias primarily cause distress for the affected individual without resulting in sex offenses. Conversely, most sex offenses are not the expression of a paraphilia. For example, most heterosexual incest offenders are not pedophilic because their objects are not prepubescent. Most acts of rape are not perpetuated by men suffering from a paraphilia, for example date rape and a rape 'of convenience' committed during incarceration. However, the diagnostic presence of a sex-offending paraphilia is the single best prognostic indicator for repeated sex offenses (Hanson and Bussiere, 1998). The content of sex-offending behavior may suggest the presence of a paraphilia, but is not diagnostically definitive. A differential diagnosis is always required as the basis of treatment where the presenting behavior problem is a sex offense.

Allegations of sex-offending behavior may be the most common reason for an individual with a paraphilia to present for evaluation or treatment. Many paraphilias, therefore, are treated in the same settings, or by the same practitioners, that treat sex offenders. As a result, the larger-sample treatment literature frequently mixes together paraphilic and nonparaphilic sex offenders, often causing marked limitations in the generalizability of the findings. Indeed, almost all of the treatment effectiveness research has been done with paraphilias associated with sexual offenders. Generally the outcome research has been with psychotherapy models described as 'cognitive-behavioral'. For a variety of reasons, there have been few well-designed studies comparing treatment and nontreatment control groups.

Relationships and paraphilia

After forensic referrals, relationship problems are the second most common reason for an individual with a paraphilia to seek treatment. For example, when an individual is discovered by his partner engaging in paraphilic behavior the discovery usually results in a sense of betrayal and a crisis in the stability of the relationship. In other situations, the individual with a paraphilia comes to treatment because of a long-standing inability to initiate or sustain a romantic relationship. These individuals and couples are treated in a variety of clinical settings and as a result there are only occasional case studies about the effectiveness of the treatment techniques employed. We shall comment further about the treatment of paraphilia as it pertains to the relationship.

General practice principles

Research-practitioners have often discussed and documented treatment outcomes according to the specific paraphilic diagnosis (Langevin, 1983;

Laws and O'Donohue, 1997). Although there are differing theories of etiology and some different approaches to treatment related to the specific content of the paraphilias, in general there is a great overlap in treatment methodologies across all of the paraphilias. The trend is toward looking at treatment approaches that can be used with any type of sexual behavioral problem, rather than treatments targeted toward a specific paraphilia (Lehne et al., 2000; Carich and Mussack, 2001). The effectiveness of treatments may vary in different studies based upon the paraphilia and the type of treatment (Greenberg, 1998; Hanson and Bussiere, 1998; Alexander, 1999; Grossman et al., 1999). Review studies have generally suggested that treatment of paraphilias can be effective, although results have varied among studies. Most treatment programs incorporate several treatment modalities (Weiss, 1989). We are not yet able to document that any one specific type of psychological treatment is uniquely effective for any paraphilia or for all types of paraphilia, although cognitive-behavioral group therapy seems to have the greatest acceptance in the published outcome studies.

Thus the current state of the art for treatment of the paraphilias is that there are a variety of distinctly different focuses and goals of treatment. While some of these can be combined in one treatment setting, others are fundamentally incompatible. Different techniques vary in their utility in different settings, such as voluntary compared with involuntary treatment settings.

In the conceptualization of the treatment of paraphilia, we recommend distinctions among the constructs of *content*, *form*, and *function* of the activity. The *content* is the *what* of the paraphilia: what is seen, done, or imagined by the person; for example, a man peeking in a bedroom window of an unsuspecting woman. The *form* is the *quality* of the behavior, particularly encompassing aspects of volition and range: Is the voyeurism a driven behavior or it is one with a significant degree of voluntary agency? Is it thought about during the day and then acted upon or does it appear to happen spontaneously? Is it restricted to mental life or is it acted upon? Can the man be sexually aroused in other situations or is voyeurism the obligatory means of sexual arousal? The *function* is the *purpose* the paraphilia may have in the individual's life or the meanings that are attributed to it. For example, the voyeur fears physical contact with his sexual object and so the behavior is a compromise solution that allows sexual arousal while avoiding personal contact. Content and function have typically been the constructs that were the focus of treatment efforts, especially those that were psychoanalytically informed. We suggest that it may be time to give due attention to the form of paraphilia in designing treatment interventions (Fagan, 2003).

Others have suggested a parallel between paraphilia and anxiety disorders, more specifically with the forms of phobias or obsessive-compulsive disorders (McConaghy, 1993; Bradford, 1999). Early evaluation and treatment of phobias was preoccupied with the many specific types of phobias of individuals. But eventually the content of any phobia was recognized as less important than the extent to which it causes distress or impairment for the individual. In general, the treatment of all phobias follows a similar process, although there may sometimes be specific adjustments based upon the content of the phobia(s) being treated. In the treatment of paraphilia, especially in the treatments that are not psychodynamic, more attention might be paid to the form of the paraphilia than the content and function. Especially as individuals present with multiple concurrent paraphilia or a sequence of paraphilia over years, one thinks, as with phobia, that the form should be given more salience than it has been in the past when determining treatment.

The psychotherapeutic treatment of an individual with a paraphilia raises other issues unique to the disorder that the potential psychotherapist should consider prior to entering into, or remaining in, the psychotherapeutic relationship. As we shall discuss in this chapter, a paraphilia may be associated with the commission of a sexual offense, opening the question of the relationship of the psychotherapy to forensic and legal systems.

Regarding therapist factors, the paraphilic behaviors may represent actions that are personally challenging to the psychotherapist, or behavior that the therapist has never encountered in therapy before. In instances such as these, the therapist should be either well trained in issues of transference and countertransference or be competently supervised in the course of the therapy. 'First do no harm' applies not only to the individual patient, but as we shall suggest, to those whose lives are affected by the patient's paraphilic behaviors.

With these caveats and before entering into a course of therapy with an individual who has a paraphilia, there are two sets of pretreatment questions that both patient and therapist should have reached agreement on. The first set should involve questions such as: Do you want to treat the paraphilia? Is the paraphilia the central focus of treatment? Answering such questions is necessary for all therapeutic modalities. Even in a psychoanalytically informed therapy in which presumably all intrapsychic conflicts are potential material for the therapy hour, the therapist should be clear about the extent to which the expectation of therapy is the control or elimination of the paraphilia. A person with an egosyntonic paraphilia that is not illegal, e.g., transvestitic fetishism, may wish to address other matters in therapy, such as life situations that are causing him to be reactively depressed or anxious. The therapist must decide if treatment can begin with the paraphilia itself excluded from treatment goals.

Given a positive response to the first set of questions, the second set revolves around the question: What is the purpose of the therapy regarding the paraphilic behavior or fantasies? This may range from accepting the *status quo* by assisting the patient to accept the paraphilia as an integral part of his sexuality to making rigorous interventions to help the patient resist any behavioral expression of the paraphilia. While it may be necessary to meet with the patient several times to explore these questions in a 'pre-therapy' period, mutual resolution is foundational for the therapeutic alliance. Similarly it is the right of the patient to give informed consent about the risks and goals of therapy, and consent can be meaningful only when the therapist and patient have similar responses to these two sorts of pretreatment questions.

The purpose of this chapter, then, is to describe psychotherapeutic modalities used to treat—usually to control—paraphilic behaviors. When at all possible we shall report treatment effectiveness, though in this area, as in most areas involving psychotherapy efficacy, studies according to specific treatment modality are few. Lastly, we shall employ the male pronoun because it is the male gender that is far more at risk for paraphilic disorders.

Psychodynamic therapy

Conceptualization

When the origin of the paraphilia is the focus of treatment, the goal of treatment is usually the elimination or cure of the paraphilia. There are two main therapeutic approaches that attempt to identify an etiological cause in history of the patient: psychodynamic and trauma theories. Our focus here is on psychodynamic, although many of the psychodynamic formulations and interventions are applicable to trauma theories. According to psychodynamic theories, the origin of the paraphilia is to be found in the failure to resolve successfully early life developmental issues. The therapeutic treatment is long-term individual psychotherapy to assist the individual in resolving these issues through the therapeutic relationship.

Trauma theory holds that paraphilia may result from being psychologically stuck in the content of an unresolved, and usually sexual, trauma, which generally occurred before the age of 8. Treatment involves reprocessing and working through the trauma through the use of short-term, intensive techniques such as actual or imagined desensitization or implosion of the traumatic content.

According to the psychodynamic view, the paraphilic internal script and sexual behavior are manifestations of an underlying pathological state that derives from developmental failures. Etiological formulations have shifted somewhat across the history of psychodynamic theories, moving from internal drive formulations to object relation formulations, from failure to resolve conflicts of the pre-oedipal and oedipal stages to failure of internal object representations in the separation/individuation phase. In general,

the paraphilia is seen as an instance of personality pathology (in contrast to their classification as a DSM-IV-TR Axis I disorder). The recommended treatment is nonspecific in the sense that it would be appropriate to any symptomatic pattern of a character disorder, of which deviant sexual behavior is only one of many possible symptom sets.

The etiology of deviant sexuality has been described by Freud (1905), first as the residue of unresolved infantile polymorphous perversity, in which there is a failure to suppress and channel the wide range of sexual desires that characterize infantile sexuality. Freud postulates a continuum from perversion (which is evident in both childhood sexuality and in the unconscious mental life of 'ordinary neurotics') through neurotics to normal adult sexuality. In this view, the neurotic symptom is seen as a better solution to the universal problem of sexual and aggressive drives than is the more disturbed symptom of deviant sexuality. Freud later (1919) revised this formulation to describe paraphilia as a defense against castration anxiety.

Classical psychodynamic case formulation was based on hypotheses regarding the individual's internal state, which were drawn from interpretation of symbolic matter, such as dreams, and from theoretically based assumptions regarding internal drives and structures. Character pathology—typically narcissistic or borderline—was invoked to describe the individual's deficits (for example, Kahn, 1969 and Joseph, 1971).

Subsequent formulations by Stoller (1975), Kernberg (1991), and McDougall (1995), among others, have stressed the self in relation to objects, both internal and external. The individual's sexual symptoms are secondary to the failure to establish adequately internal object representations, which results in an inability to tolerate the otherness of the external object (Parsons, 2000). Here the intrapsychic problem to be solved may include as well the failure of the external world, particularly parental figures, and may range from actual abuse of the developing child to interactions that interfere more subtly with the child's ability to make sense of his experience. The deviant sexual behavior is now seen as a defense against object relations, that is, against the experience of the other as real, as complex, and as different from the self. It is also seen as a way of maintaining the self in face of distressing psychological states. In Stoller's formulation, the perverse behavior transforms an earlier traumatic experience into one of mastery; while in McDougall's the 'neo-sexuality' permits a sexual experience in the context of a threatening psychological environment.

At this point we do not know specific developmental causes of paraphilia that can be addressed in a psychoanalytic or psychodynamic modality. The most we can assert is that childhood sexual abuse is a risk factor for the development of pedophilia. Emotional abuse and family of origin dysfunction resulting in lack of emotional attachment may also be risk factors in pedophilia, exhibitionism, rape, and multiple paraphilia (Hanson and Slater, 1988; Freund and Kuban, 1994; Dhawan and Marshall, 1996; Lee *et al.*, 2002). Such risk factors are obviously more than minor vicissitudes of growing up. Why some individuals who experience them have paraphilic sexual behaviors as adults, and why others develop sexually without paraphilia remains to be understood.

Key practice principles

As this brief summary makes clear, psychodynamic treatment of paraphilia focuses on constructs such as self, integrity, and object relations. Behavior is decidedly secondary and of interest only as symbolic of internal states. Therapy is verbally mediated, reliant on insight, and employs the relationship with the therapist, real and transferential, as central. Change is sought at the internal level (some would say inferential level) of the unconscious drives and object relations. Not only are the paraphilias regarded as simply one possible symptom of an underlying pathology, the similarities between paraphilias are regarded as more significant than the differences, although gradations in object relatedness are acknowledged (Meyer, 1995). Thus, treatment proceeds similarly regardless of the specific deviant behavior. Treatment, as with any character disorder, must be long-term. For those with a paraphilia who are deemed to have sufficient ego strength, psychoanalysis would be recommended. For those who are unable to tolerate, afford, or benefit from analysis, psychodynamically informed therapy would be recommended. Given the psychological limitations of many of these patients, the value of 12-step concurrent support groups is not ruled out (McDougall, 1995).

As with other psychodynamic treatment models, there are no large-scale empirical studies of treatment outcome of psychodynamic treatment of paraphilias. The constructs of psychodynamic theory are difficult to operationalize and the course of therapy is extended and difficult to predict. Published work in support of the model is in the form of case histories, usually of individual cases, sometimes of groups (Carigan, 1999; Lothstein, 2001). Case histories are formulated around a careful reading of the individual's past, inferences regarding the individual's internal state, and interpretations of the individual's relationship with the therapist. The sexual behavior is regarded as a symptomatic solution to an intrapsychic or interpersonal problem, which must be reformulated and reworked in the therapy. One aspect of this model, which is embodied in the rich narrative form of the case history, is its emphasis on the complexity of the individual in the context of a particular life. This representation of personhood can be a useful corrective to the current tendency to demonize people who engage in deviant sexual behaviors. In summary, psychodynamic theories have proposed elaborate formulations regarding the etiology of deviant sexual behavior, but they have not generated a therapeutic strategy specific to the treatment of paraphilias.

Case example: psychodynamic therapy

Glenmullen (1993) published a case study that exemplifies many of the psychoanalytic techniques, although it relies less on formulations regarding drives and dream analysis than did earlier works (Kahn, 1969; Joseph, 1971). Glenmullen's case is too long to reproduce here, representing months (perhaps years) of therapy, so we shall summarize.

The patient was a young man who presented with a pervasive 'numbness.' He had also withdrawn sexually from his female partner. In the early phase of therapy, the patient revealed that his father had abandoned the family when the patient was in his early teens, leaving the family destitute. The father was discovered dead several months later, under suspicious circumstances. After this revelation, the therapist began to 'articulate the repressed emotions' of the patient, but the patient pulled back into a narrow focus of repetitive and detailed description of his 'numbness.' This withdrawal had a deadening effect on the sessions, and the therapist had to attend to his own internal response (countertransference) and manage it in order to avoid subverting the therapy. This stalemate was eventually infused with the patient's discontent with progress, which created a heightened emotional tone in the sessions.

At this point, the patient referred to his habit of taking late-night walks, which he described as both urgent and dangerous. The therapist guessed that the walks led to the acquisition of pornography for masturbation, and the patient, relieved, described a long-term pattern of compulsive use of pornography. This use was marked by, first, the intensity of the pursuit ('pounding the pavement' for hours) and, second, by the patient's awareness of interactions with other men (fellow customers, who may have just leafed through the same magazine, or the clerk, who must be handed money). The patient declared that he could masturbate to orgasm only with the use of pornography, and he denied that he had any sexual fantasies of his own or any sexual dreams.

Although he initially denied being drawn to any particular scene, he subsequently acknowledged that he was particularly aroused by 'threesomes,' in which he imagined the two male figures were friends. The therapist, having formulated that these 'purchased fantasies' functioned as a defense against the patient's inner life, asked the patient to resist his impulse to use pornography, a request the patient found difficult to fulfill. However, the patient ultimately achieved 'sobriety' and, in this state, his response to his experience became more emotional. In particular, he burst into tears after being corrected by an older man at work, whom he admired.

At one point, the therapist inquired regarding his earliest experience of pornography, and the patient described finding a stash of pornography in

his father's study. The patient's first masturbatory experiences employed the same images his father was using. The stash disappeared when his father abandoned the family. In the months after the father's disappearance, the patient started riding his bike for miles along rural highways. During the rides he would find abandoned pornographic magazines along the roadside. With the therapist's formulation that pornography represented a connection with other men and, ultimately, with the lost father, the patient displayed a strong affective response. The therapy then turned to working on his unresolved grief for his father. 'Stripped of its purpose, [the] pornography addiction gradually fell away' (Glenmullen, 1993, p. 29).

Cognitive-behavioral therapy

Conceptualization

Clinical practice targeting the *cognitive control of behavior* utilizes individual and group treatment to assist patients in controlling thoughts and behavior so they can minimize the impact of the paraphilia upon themselves or others. While the patient generally assumes that the paraphilic behavior is solely the result of his heightened sex drive, cognitive-behavioral therapy identifies the cognitive assumptions and rationalizations that facilitate the sexual behaviors. Once identified, the therapeutic task is to replace the facilitative assumptions with cognitive formulations that recognize both the motivating and stimulating antecedents as well as the personal and relational consequences of the paraphilic behaviors.

Group therapy comprised of members with sexual disorders (not dysfunctions) is a highly recommended modality for cognitive-behavioral interventions in the treatment of paraphilic disorders. For the treatment of those individuals whose paraphilia are sexual offenses or are coercive, the group therapy modality serves to use the social force of peers and therapist to confront the cognitive distortions and offer more appropriate assumptions to group members about their sexual relationships and behaviors.

The most widely accepted treatments for paraphilia involve helping patients better control and manage their sexualized thinking and behavior. These individual and group therapies work to help the motivated patient achieve better *cognitive control of sexual behavior*. The practice principles described here are similar to those used in the treatment of different addictions, and reflect the underlying assumption that the paraphilia cannot be eliminated but can be controlled. Individual therapies utilize cognitive-behavioral techniques, while group training and management techniques are also prevalent.

Key practice principles

Many current treatment protocols of paraphilia have as a major modality those interventions that have been developed out of the cognitive-behavioral therapy tradition. What follows are brief descriptions of various interventions that should be viewed as complementary components in a cognitive-behavioral treatment plan. Their principal contribution to treatment is to control the cognitions, including sexual fantasies, which lead to paraphilic behaviors or to the affects that trigger them.

Restructuring cognitive distortions

Based on the seminal work of Yochelson and Samenow (1977) on criminal behavior, restructuring cognitive distortions for paraphilia has a twofold task. The first is to identify the denials and distortions surrounding the sexual behavior, e.g., the man who exposes himself saying, 'I didn't touch anyone, therefore there were no victims . . . there was no harm done.' The second and more challenging task is to assist the patient to employ more expansive and empathic assumptions about his behaviors, e.g., 'While there was only confusion on the faces of the women, later they will likely be quite disturbed and frightened about the incident . . . it may cause them to have severe emotional reactions.' The patient needs to generalize the assumptive world developed in the therapy hour to the real world in which he lives and may have been expressing his paraphilic behaviors.

Empathy training

In spite of the absence of clear evidence that the development of empathy leads to long-term behavioral change, it makes clinical sense to have this as a treatment goal when deficits are apparent. Applied to the treatment of a patient with a paraphilia, it involves the development of empathic understanding of the effects of his behaviors on the lives his victims, if any, and on the lives of the people in his life. Interventions include the therapist's basic Socratic exploration of the patient's ideas about the emotional lives of the others and repeated narration of statements or videos in which others talk about how his or similar sexual behaviors have affected them and their families. The hope is that by such means the patient's empathic understanding of others can be developed. In group therapy, role-playing in which the victims and family members or victims are enacted may sometimes be helpful.

A common prejudice is that men with paraphilia are so personality disordered such that empathy is almost impossible for them. A recent study found that, indeed, among a select group of incarcerated pedophiles 60% had a personality disorder (Raymond et al., 1999). What the authors of the study pointed out, however, was that narcissistic and antisocial personality disorders accounted for only 20% and 22.5% of the subjects, respectively. Thus while many may have deficits in their ability to empathize with others, even among those men with a pedophilic paraphilia, there are many who do not have personality vulnerabilities that would prevent them from developing a sincere understanding of the feelings and reactions of others to their behaviors. For those who are unable to develop an empathic understanding, especially for their victims, it may be necessary to appeal to their self-interest, such as avoiding incarceration, as a reason to control their sexually offensive paraphilic behaviors (Fagan et al., 1991).

Social learning

Most would agree that human sexuality has as its goal the bonding of individuals in a union that is consensual, pleasurable, and for many, emotionally intimate. Paraphilic sexual behaviors may be coercive, partial in their object, secretive, and constrained by the elaboration of a fantasy, e.g., in bondage and dominance. To the extent that the paraphilic fantasy or behavior is necessary for sexual arousal, to that same extent the individual is at risk for difficulties engaging in sex as an aid to pleasurable, consensual, and intimate bonding with another nonparaphilic individual. To put this in terms of cognitive-behavioral therapy, the paraphilic individual has sexual scripts that are, under many circumstances, likely to exclude or severely restrict mutually pleasurable, consensual, and intimate sexual bonding with another (Gagnon, 1990).

Social learning interventions seek to assist the individual in developing the social skills necessary to master the interpersonal situations of his or her life. Applied to the treatment of paraphilia, social learning targets both the development of skills to interact effectively socially and sexually. The goal of the therapy is to promote a competence in age-appropriate interactions with persons who have the potential to become partners in nonparaphilic sex. Because relationships do not begin with sex, many of the skills will involve reading and responding appropriately to social cues (Gagnon and Simon, 1973).

Assertiveness training

There has been some speculation that men with paraphilia have a weakened self-concept regarding their sense of being an adequate man (Levine et al., 1990). Regardless of whether this cognitive hypothesis is valid or not, or whether any sense of inadequacy is the cause or result of the paraphilia, if there is a clear deficit in appropriate assertiveness in the patient, this should be addressed. From a cognitive-behavioral perspective, the normal assertiveness connected with interpersonal sexual activity has become highly ritualized and/or expressed in a solipsistic fantasy in men with paraphilia. To the extent that this is generalized in the interpersonal social and sexual contexts of his life, appropriate interpersonal assertiveness may be distorted in either direction: social-sexual passivity or social-sexual aggression.

In cognitive assertiveness training, the therapist asks the patient to identify those interpersonal situations in his occupational, social, familial,

and sexual life in which he is called upon to play an active and responsible role. An examination of his faulty assumptions and his fears is followed by the development of cognitive assumptions that are more adaptive and appropriately assertive. A behavioral component usually follows in which the patient attempts to employ the cognitions in the in vivo situation. Although assertiveness training may be helpful to some patients, there are no controlled studies establishing the therapeutic effectiveness in treating paraphilia, and conceivably in some cases greater assertiveness could be counterproductive.

Sexual boundaries training

Related to assertiveness training is sexual boundary training. In essence, the goal is a knowledge of and respect for the personal integrity of the other so as not to violate the emotional and physical boundaries that are proper to the relationship. In this case, 'relationship' is used in the broadest way: two individuals (even strangers) interacting with each other. For those with pedophilia, exhibitionism, voyeurism, frotteurism, and other sexual disorders, sexual boundaries training aims to instill in the patient the cognitive set that his paraphilic behaviors violate the personal and sexual boundaries of others. A secondary aim is an empathic understanding of the effects of the violation on the victim, as discussed previously. Not all persons with a paraphilic disorder necessarily require such training.

Stress and anger management

The expression of paraphilic behavior may be facilitated by the autonomic arousal caused by anxiety or anger. Confronted by a situation in which he subjectively perceives the need of 'fight or flight', the paraphilia can offer the escape that brings some anxiolytic relief. This is clearly seen in those men with transvestic fetishism who describe their cross-dressing behaviors as an 'island of repose' and who often continue to cross-dress for relaxation long after it has been an occasion of sexual arousal and orgasm in their lives.

Cognitive techniques to control stress and anger have their place, then, in the treatment of paraphilia. Similar to the assertiveness training, the therapeutic task is to identify the stress and anger triggers and to develop more adaptive ways of dealing with these situations. If trigger situations can be avoided, they should be avoided, as in the case of a man with pedophilia not volunteering to be a youth leader. If trigger situations cannot be avoided entirely, e.g., interactions with an irritable colleague at work, then strategies such as limiting contact to only that which is necessary and having verbal 'exit strategies' in the presence of the first sign of testiness should be developed.

Impulse control training

Impulse control training has as its goal bringing the sexual impulses that are connected with the paraphilia under control. The training involves both cognitive and behavioral components. In some patients whose sexual impulses and urges are not in control or whose expression would result in harm to self or other, the impulse control training should be augmented by medication as will be described later in this chapter.

The cognitive-behavioral interventions for the control of sexual impulses are similar to those connected with anger and stress management and relapse prevention (as will be described subsequently): early detection of sexual impulses and the redirection or substitution of these impulses with the aid of cognitions. The cognitions can inhibit the further elaboration of the impulses by recalling the injurious results of the impulse driven behaviors. They can also play a reinforcing role to nonparaphilic adaptive behavior by providing substitute thoughts or behavioral plans. For example, if a man is attempting to stop compulsive use of Internet pornography while at work, it may be helpful to have his computer screen turned toward the open door of his office or workstation and thus visible to the casual passer-by.

Relapse prevention

Relapse prevention is an adaptation of an addictions approach that has become the dominant treatment technique used in the treatment of paraphilia. It was first developed by George and Marlatt (1989), and popularized by Marshall and Pithers (Laws, 1989). They sought to simplify the complex cognitive-behavioral interventions with a stimulus control system that the patient could employ independently. Relapse prevention assumes that the patient is highly motivated to avoid sexual acting out, and has as its primary focus the maintenance of sexual sobriety. In practice, relapse prevention has become a series of cognitive strategies to be used by individuals seeking to avoid paraphilic and sexually offensive behaviors by avoiding stimuli that promote the behavior (Laws, 1989). Although it is widely used in group treatment programs, it was actually devised as an individualized treatment program.

Relapse prevention starts with the examination of what occurred in past history. The idea is that history repeats itself, and so the individual must reexamine every specific detail associated with sexual acting out in the past. Each patient develops his own specific relapse prevention plan (RPP), which should be written down and reviewed and revised. Relapses occur in high-risk situations (HRS), which are either internal negative emotional states or external situations. The negative emotional states of boredom, depression, and anger have been found in addictions research to be frequently associated with relapses. Situations of interpersonal conflict and social pressure (including sexualized environments) are also frequently associated with relapse. So the patient starts developing his own RPP by identifying those conditions that were associated with sexual acting out in the past, and develops a specific plan to handle these conditions differently.

Stimulus control procedures are the first group of techniques to remove, eliminate, or avoid any conditions associated with the paraphilic behavior. Then the patient must rehearse coping responses, including role-playing and covert modeling. He should develop escape strategies to remove himself from unexpected HRS. He may develop self-talk statements and techniques of thought stopping to help him cope with urges or negative emotional states. He may engage in a variety of educational and treatment activities to improve any skill areas where he may be deficient, as has been discussed, such as stress management or anger management, or social skills training. Relapse rehearsal is a key technique—imagining himself in different HRS, and imaging his positive responses.

When the patient manages HRS well, there is increased self-efficacy and decreased relapse probability. When he does not cope as well, there may be a lapse, which is the first small step toward relapse, such as giving in to sexual fantasy. The 'abstinence violation effect' (AVE) occurs when individuals become discouraged by a lapse or relapse and lose their sense of personal efficacy and self-control. It is important to recognize and discuss this condition, with an emphasis on learning from slips and mistakes.

Antecedents of relapses include lifestyle imbalance, and the desire to feel good, seeking indulgence and immediate gratification. This is called the 'problem of immediate gratification' (PIG). 'Apparently irrelevant decisions' (AIDs) are those little decisions that lead to an individual placing himself in a HRS. These need to be identified and challenged by the therapist. There are also 'seemingly unimportant behaviors that lead to errors' (SUBTLE), similar to AIDs but with a component of not being conscious decisions.

Relapse prevention cognitive techniques are employed both in the course of treatment and, as the words might suggest, as strategies to be used following therapy for a permanent strategy to avoid the unwanted paraphilic behaviors. In some clinical settings, relapse prevention groups meet on a regular basis and participants are expected to be in the group for a period of 18–24 months following treatment to consolidate treatment gains.

Counseling for acceptance

In practice, some paraphilias remain impervious to traditional cognitive-behavioral approaches. One method of cognitive therapy has as its goal the informed acceptance of the behavior and uses educational techniques and couple's counseling to help individuals cope with the chronic paraphilic condition (LoPiccolo, 1994; Paul et al., 1999). Acknowledgment and acceptance of the inevitability of some paraphilic behavior, especially in those paraphilias that have proven resistant to treatment and are not sexual offenses, for example transvestic fetishism, may be helpful for some

partnered relationships. This intervention assists both partners to accept the fixity of the condition and helps eliminate the secrecy and deception in the relationship. Provisions may be made for the limited indulgence of paraphilic activity. Special care should be taken by the therapist in couple counseling to respect the freedom of choice of the nonparaphilic partner. This requires that the therapist carefully avoid colluding with the paraphilic partner in pressuring the other to accept or participate in any paraphilic behavior that may be contrary to the partner's morals or sexual aesthetics.

Acceptance of the paraphilia is facilitated by the cultural support that websites, chat rooms, and peer support groups provide. Individuals who formerly might have sought help to eliminate paraphilic interests are now seeking assistance in coming to terms with their own different sexuality. Whether these peer support groups and the Internet chat rooms assist in controlled acceptance or whether they further the frequency, focus, and intensity of the paraphilia, resulting in increased social and occupational dysfunction, is disputed.

Cognitive-behavioral treatment outcome studies

Most of the studies of the outcome of cognitive-behavioral treatment for paraphilia had sexual offenders as their subjects. While concerns about this population may provide motivation for assessing treatment outcome, the studies have methodological limitations, particularly dealing with the randomization of treatment groups and how to handle data of subjects who drop out of treatment. Generalization of the results of treatment to nonsexually offensive paraphilias is also tenuous. Partly based upon his assessment of these methodological concerns, McConaghy concludes that relapse prevention treatment sometimes may be less effective than no treatment, and therefore have a negative effect (McConaghy, 1997, 1999a). He thinks there may be a trend that relapse prevention treatment may be more effective with married and mentally healthy men, and that more research is required regarding assignment of patients to this form of treatment (McConaghy, 1999a).

In general, however, cognitive-behavioral treatment has shown itself to be effective when compared with nontreatment. In a 25-year follow-up of cognitive-behavioral therapy with 7275 sexual offenders, Maletzky and Steinhauser (2002, p. 143) concluded, 'Within the limitations of this methodology, the treatment techniques employed in a cognitive/behavioral program generated long-lasting, positive results reducing recidivism and risk to the community'. The groups were studied in 5-year cohorts, and the authors found that there was a tendency for a reduction in the failure rates with time, suggesting that the treatment methods may have become more effective with time.

Two major reviews of cognitive-behavioral treatments for sexual offenders reported a significant treatment effect (Hall, 1995; Gallagher et al., 1999). Recently, a meta-analysis report of 43 studies of the psychological (largely cognitive-behavioral) treatment for sex offenders (Hanson et al., 2002) found that sexual offense recidivism was significantly lower for the treatment groups (12.3%) than the untreated comparison groups (16.8%) over an average 46-month follow-up period (Hanson et al., 2002). Certainly the case can be made that the threat of incarceration confounds generalizing the cognitive-behavioral treatment effect to the treatment of nonsexually offensive paraphilias. On the other hand, these results give encouragement to further testing of the hypothesis in nonsexual offense treatment settings.

Case example: relapse prevention

Tom was a 32-year-old attorney whose marriage had recently been jeopardized by his wife, Joan, after finding several inexplicable charges to their credit cards totaling $480. She confronted him with the bills. At first he said that there must be some mistake and that someone must be using his credit card number. But his wife persisted and eventually Tom admitted that he had been visiting the website 'babe-in-arms.com' and also a local massage parlor for the past 6 months and using them for sexual gratification. It did not help that during these 6 months Joan was caring for their newborn daughter, their first child. Tears flowed from both.

Upon his wife's insistence, but with agreement from him in order to save the marriage, Tom began both individual and group therapy. Tom acknowledged in treatment that the name of the website was double entendre: the men could either imagine the grown female 'babes' in their arms, or they could be the infantile babes in the arms of the women. Tom admitted that he longed to be treated like a baby by his sexual partners and had in fact visited massage parlors that catered to this desire. He found it very arousing to imagine being cleaned and diapered by a woman. His experience *in vivo* was limited to being in diapers: being verbally scolded for soiling them, and then engaging in noncoital cuddling. Apparently the scene of his wife changing the diapers of their daughter brought back sexual fantasies that had long lay dormant. The admission of this paraphilic arousal pattern was very embarrassing to Tom, but he also admitted relief that his secret was now shared with others who he had found on the Internet. The group responded with support and, to the best of their abilities, understanding.

The methods used in both Tom's individual and group therapies were cognitive-behavioral. Especially helpful was his recognition of the envy he felt at the attention his wife gave to their newborn. He replaced thoughts of sibling envy with the correct thought that this was his daughter and she was entirely dependent upon him. Behaviorally, he countered this envy by helping his wife care for their daughter. What Tom was surprised to learn was that the more he cared for his daughter, including changing her diapers, the more he felt love for his daughter and a grateful love from his wife for sharing the child-care.

With treatment and the threat of divorce, the behaviors of utilizing the website and going to the massage parlors ceased immediately. After 9 months of treatment, even the infantilism fantasies had decreased in frequency and intensity. For 6 months he had not masturbated to the thought of his being cared for like a baby. Tom considered his problem a sexual addiction, and in addition to therapy, attended group meetings of Sex and Love Addicts Anonymous (SLAA). He felt that when therapy was concluded, he would continue to attend the 12-step group for the support and program it gave to his 'sobriety'.

Tom recognized that it was important for him to establish a RPP to employ for the posttherapy future. In therapy Tom had described his pattern of behavior, his behavioral chain, and alternative thoughts and behaviors that he could use to maintain control of his desire to use the Internet and massage parlors to gratify his sexual desires. In his individual psychotherapy he worked to develop his RPP, using many of the techniques described in publications available from the Safer Society Foundation (http://www.safersociety.org; for example, Steen, 2001).

This is the RPP that Tom and his therapist developed:

1. *Identify risk states before sexually acting out*: negative emotions, like being ignored by my wife; being criticized by partners or clients at work; feeling ineffective or lonely; being bored. Feeling that I deserve a reward and to be cared for.

    (a) *What can I do instead*: use the David Burns (*Feeling Good Handbook*, 1999) Daily Mood Log and Cognitive Distortions Checklist. Do something positive and fun for myself—rent a DVD, buy a CD, take my wife out to dinner; get more involved in caring for and playing with my daughter. Don't be a PIG (Problem of Immediate Gratification)!

2. *Recognize Seemingly Unimportant Decisions (SUDS) that place in HRS*: carrying extra cash beyond what I would need; driving by areas where there are massage parlors; leaving work early for 'unaccounted for' time; being in a private area at home with the computer.

    (a) *What can I do instead*: never carry more than 15 dollars. Do not carry an ATM card; carry only one credit card, which wife pays the bill for each month. Post picture of wife and child in prominent place on car dashboard. Work out on map alternative routes so that never have to drive by high-risk areas. Call wife before leave to establish time record if feeling tempted to drive by risky areas. Look at relapse prevention card (carry in wallet). Move the computer to a room into which privacy is not a given and face the screen toward the entrance door of the room.

3. *Avoid lapse in thoughts or behavior*: thinking about past experiences with massage parlor women or images and chats on the Internet. Masturbating. Driving near areas where massage parlors are located. Reading the ads for sexual services in the newspaper.

    (a) *What can I do instead*: talk to SLAA sponsor, attend extra meetings. Call therapist to discuss. Substitute a positive activity such as a regular exercise program.

4. *Relapse*: surf on Internet for sexual sites. Go to massage parlor.

    (a) *What can I do*: remember that it is not the end of the world. I can be sober. Don't give up hope!! Go to SLAA meetings and therapy sessions.

Two years following treatment, Tom continues to employ the RPP that he developed. He and his wife were in marital therapy for 6 months, which helped to clarify the expectations each had of the other in areas such as domestic chores, sex and affection, and leisure activities together. He had one 'relapse' within the first 3 months of ending therapy in which he went into a massage parlor. He immediately felt guilty and remorseful and left without having sexual contact. Tom called his SLAA sponsor and reported the incident. They agreed he would increase the frequency of meetings to three times a week. Tom also had a consultation with his therapist. The therapist helped Tom to recognize how he had allowed risk states and SUDS to creep back into his life. They agreed that he would return every 6 months for a 'check-up' consultation.

Behavioral modification

Conceptualization

Paraphilias by definition incorporate patterns of physiological sexual arousal that are different in content from mainstream sexuality. Some behaviorists believe that the atypical association between the sexual content and arousal was acquired through a conditioning process, and can be alleviated by reconditioning. *Sexual arousal modification* focuses treatment on changing the physiological pattern of sexual arousal through the use of behavioral techniques, most commonly by modifying masturbation or physiological arousal in the presence of real or imagined paraphilic content.

Men who seek treatment for paraphilia almost always report a history of being sexually aroused and masturbating to fantasies that embody paraphilic imagery. Disordered sexual arousal is the key diagnostic criterion for the diagnosis of paraphilia, and is the factor most associated with repeated sexual misconduct or sex offending (Murphy and Barbaree, 1994; Hanson and Bussiere, 1998).

According to behavioral theories, paraphilic arousal has been conditioned by the association of paraphilic practices with reinforcement (typically pleasurable sexual arousal or orgasm, or anxiety reduction). Behavioral treatment attempts to modify this pattern by linking paraphilic arousal with aversive stimuli, or not having paraphilic arousal associated with positive stimuli. In some cases alternative patterns of arousal and behavior are conditioned.

Behavioral techniques were developed to modify the pattern of sexual arousal, and were the prevalent treatment approach for paraphilia from the 1960s to the early 1990s (Quinsey and Earls, 1990; Knopp *et al.*, 1992). There has been little research on the effectiveness of these techniques in the past 20 years, but they have a seemingly common sense validity that appeals to therapists and patients. Thus, these techniques continue to be incorporated into treatment programs of varying theoretical orientations (McGrath, 2001) and are strongly recommended by some expert practitioners specializing in the treatment of exhibitionism (Maletzky, 1997) and fetishism (Junginger, 1997).

Practice principles

Sexual arousal modification as a practice principle typically uses behavioral conditioning techniques to try to modify the pattern of physical sexual arousal.

Treatment starts with the assessment of the patient's arousal pattern, and the effectiveness of treatment is confirmed when the patient does not show (typically penile) arousal to the previously arousing stimuli. There are three different behavioral approaches to sexual arousal modification—aversive conditioning, covert sensitization, and positive conditioning—as well as mixed models of reconditioning techniques.

Assessment of sexual arousal

Disordered sexual arousal can be physiologically measured using phallometric, eye scan, or reaction time assessment. In phallometric assessment using the penile plethysmograph, a strain gauge is placed around the penis to measure change in penile circumference response (PCR) or the penis is placed in a sheath device to measure change in penile volume response (PVR). For eye scan assessments, the patient's eye movements or pupil dilations are measured during exposure to sexual stimuli. While he is connected to and monitored by the assessment equipment, the patient is shown slides or videotapes or, more commonly now, listens to audiotaped stories of different sexual scenarios. These physiological assessment techniques have face validity of providing clear and direct measures of sexual arousal. In behavioral treatment programs, they could be used as pretests and posttests to assess the effectiveness of the intervention in modifying sexual arousal, at least in a laboratory setting (Laws and Osborn, 1983; Roys and Roys, 1994; Howes, 1995). These assessment techniques may be used to determine the stimuli for the behavioral treatment. They can also be used for biofeedback during behavioral treatment.

There are, however, a number of practical problems with the use of PCR, PVR, and eye-scan methodologies. One area of concern involves the types of sexual stimuli that are used, especially the use of clothed compared with nude photographs (which could be a violation of child pornography laws, for example) in the assessment of interest in children (Miner and Coleman, 2001). Some paraphilias are better described through language, while others are more visual so comparable assessment across paraphilias can be difficult. Phallometric techniques are also vulnerable to attempts at deception, and have high false positive or false negative rates in certain situations. Thus there is disagreement about whether they provide consistently valid measures of sexual arousal or interest (McConaghy, 1993, 1999b; Murphy and Barbaree, 1994). Convincing evidence is also lacking that any treatment programs for paraphilia produce long-lasting changes in the pattern of sexual arousal (Murphy and Barbaree, 1994; McConaghy, 1999a). This is not to say that sexual arousal modification treatments are either effective or ineffective in producing changes in sexual behavior. Such treatments may increase patients' ability to control their sexual behavior, but unfortunately that is still uncertain.

In many behavioral treatment programs targeting sexual arousal modification, there is no physiological assessment of sexual arousal either before or after treatment. Some behaviorally oriented programs use self-report of sexual arousal or behavior (in a variety of situations), attempting to validate self-report through the use of polygraph methodologies. The presumed treatment goal of these programs is better control or change of the larger sequence of sexual behavior rather than eliminating the actual sexual arousal to the paraphilic stimuli, even though the treatment employed focuses more specifically upon the arousal itself.

Recently, a less intrusive behavioral assessment technique, the *Abel Assessment for Sexual Interest*™ has been developed employing a questionnaire that collects admissions of inappropriate sexual behavior and a visual reaction time (VTR) measurement (Abel *et al.*, 1998). This system assesses and classifies 'child molesters' with an abiding sexual interest in children versus 'nonchild molesters' and has shown some evidence of discriminating child molesters who deny molesting children (Abel *et al.*, 2001).

Aversive conditioning

In aversive classical conditioning the patient is exposed to the types of paraphilic stimuli that he finds arousing through slides, videotapes, auditory stories, printed stories, or self-generated fantasy. The stimulus is then immediately paired with an aversive stimulus such as electric shock, a noxious smell or taste. These techniques are reportedly effective in reducing paraphilic arousal (Maletzky, 1991) and recidivism (Maletzky, 1993). Maletzky cites evidence that nauseating odors are more effective than aversive odors (such as ammonia) and are easier to use than electric shock (Maletzky, 1997). In a variation of this technique, the patient's arousal to the stimulus is measured in real time (following exposure to the stimulus) with a penile plethysmograph, and the aversive stimulus is administered at the first sign of increased tumescence (signaled punishment or biofeedback). However, there are questions about the generalizability and stability over time of these aversive conditioning approaches. Aversive techniques, particularly those using electric shock, have become socially controversial and are ethically dubious. It is little wonder, then, that they have high patient refusal and dropout rates.

Aversive behavior rehearsal has the patient act out the paraphilic behavior to consenting treatment staff members, who give no response. Although Maletzky (1993, 1997) found this technique to be effective with exhibitionists, it is controversial and infrequently used because it can be too aversive to patients and involved staff.

Covert sensitization

Covert sensitization has largely replaced the use of physically aversive conditioning techniques. Covert sensitization uses the patient's own imagery of paraphilic scenarios. The patient stops the imagined scenario just before the offending behavior. The patient then imagines aversive consequences that can be associated with the scenario. In another variation, this may also be followed up with imagining a nonoffending escape or positive outcome. These scenario sequences may be written down or tape-recorded and rehearsed while in a relaxed state. The scenarios should always be prepared using first-person present tense ('I am . . .') that put the patient in the scene. This behavioral technique is easily incorporated into cognitive-behavioral treatment programs, and is widely used (Knopp *et al.*, 1992). This technique has not been demonstrated to be effective in producing change in arousal, but it may help some patients better control their behavior even though there are few actual data on its effectiveness (Maletzky, 1991; McConaghy, 1993).

Assisted covert sensitization augments the patient's imagery of the paraphilic scene by pairing it with a nauseating odor, and then the odor is withdrawn during the escape imagery (Maletzky, 1991).

Satiation and positive conditioning

Satiation therapies attempt to reduce paraphilic sexual arousal by having the patient masturbate to paraphilic imagery for long periods of time (until it becomes very boring), without the reinforcement of sexual arousal and ejaculation. First, the patient masturbates to orgasm using appropriate imagery immediately prior to beginning the satiation training, if possible. If this is not possible, the patient masturbates to orgasm using the most benign paraphilic imagery. The patient continues masturbating for another 30–90 minutes while reading out loud the different paraphilic imagery scenarios he has written, or listens repeatedly to a tape he previously made of this imagery. This masturbation continues without high levels of arousal or orgasm. The therapeutic goal is to disassociate paraphilic imagery from the reinforcing consequence of sexual arousal and orgasm, and to associate orgasm with more acceptable imagery.

In a verbal satiation model, the patient repeatedly reads the sexual scenarios without masturbating. Verbal satiation may be used with patients who are unable or unwilling to masturbate, but it takes much longer and has less face validity of being effective.

For satiation therapies, the therapist works with the patient in developing the practice scenarios, but the patient carries out the actual practice in privacy at home. The home practice sessions may be tape-recorded and spot-checked by the therapist for compliance. Practice sessions may be 60 minutes or longer and should occur several times a week or more often when the patient has a higher frequency of masturbation.

Orgasmic reconditioning uses positive conditioning by having the patient masturbate to orgasm while imagining or experiencing by viewing, hearing, or reading an arousing, nonparaphilic sexual fantasy. This is usually combined with a prohibition on masturbation or achieving orgasm associated with paraphilic fantasy or experience. In another variation for patients who have only weak arousal to conventional imagery, the patient masturbates using paraphilic imagery and then changes to conventional imagery prior to orgasm.

The evidence concerning the effectiveness of orgasmic reconditioning is inconclusive (Laws and Marshall, 1991). In addition, not all paraphilic patients are able to use these techniques, as they require that some arousal be associated with more conventional imagery or that the patient has the ability to readily achieve orgasm through purely physical stimulation. Some paraphilic patients have no history and little evident potential for acquiring sexual arousal to conventional sexual scenarios. Furthermore, masturbatory reconditioning techniques cannot be easily combined with pharmacological treatments that reduce sexual arousal or interfere with orgasm.

Alternative behavioral completion

Alternative behavioral completion is a positive conditioning variation of imaginal desensitization developed by McConaghy (1993) to help patients control their sexual urges, while not necessarily changing sexual arousal patterns. In a relaxed state the patient is asked to imagine a situation where he would have acted out the sexual behavior, except that he imagines an alternative ending to the episode instead of the paraphilic sexual behavior. The patient is given training in relaxation, and a strict rehearsal protocol is followed so that each imagery session ends with a relaxed state being associated with the alternative behavioral completion.

Case example: Alternative Behavioral Completion

This case example illustrates treatment of a man with exhibitionism employing Alternative Behavioral Completion according to McConaghy's protocol (McConaghy, 1993). The patient was a 26-year-old, never-married male with a history since age 16 of exposing to adult women in public parks and woods. First he was trained in progressive muscular relaxation, tensing and then releasing muscle groups starting with his feet and progressing to his head. He had written down a number of his typical exposing scenarios, which had been carefully constructed with the help of the therapist. The scenarios were composed in first-person present tense and were broken down into discrete segments. One example is:

1. I am feeling the urge to expose, I can't get the idea out of my head.

2. I go to Indian Creek Park and stand next to a tree like I am going to urinate.

3. I see an attractive woman jogging on the path.

4. I have an urge to unzip my fly and expose my penis.

   (The Alternative Behavioral Completion sequence begins.)

5. Then I realize the urge is not so strong.

6. I can control it.

7. I notice how nice the park is, the beauty of the trees, the smell of the outdoors, the sounds of the birds.

8. The woman jogs by while I stand there enjoying the park.

9. I leave the park feeling good about myself.

Treatment sessions consisted of progressive muscle relaxation, then the patient imagining the paraphilic scenario. The therapist led him through each segment (numbers 1–9) of the scenario. The patient signaled with his finger when he had successfully imagined each segment, and then he proceeded to imagine the next segment. Each of the different scenarios had first been practiced in sessions with the therapist. After the initial training sessions, the patient could audiotape the scenarios and practice them at home.

After treatment with Alternative Behavioral Completion, this patient continued to have times when he felt the urge to expose, usually on nice days in the summer. Before treatment, he reported that he felt so uncomfortable and stressed out that he would go to the park to expose to get relief. After treatment, he was able to imagine going to the park and felt more relaxed.

He reported that he did not have difficulty controlling his urges to expose. Consistent with his general relapse prevention treatment, however, he also did not allow himself to get in his car and drive to the park. Instead he would take his dog for a walk around the block where he lived, a situation where he was unlikely to encounter a situation conducive to exposing and where he had never exposed in the past.

Biological treatment

Conceptualization

The biological treatment of paraphilia involves the direct reduction of the sex drive, and is usually adjunctive to one of the 'talking' therapies. It typically involves pharmacological treatment, and rarely surgical, to reduce the intensity and frequency of sexual urges, thus reducing sexual fantasies, preoccupation, and the pressure to engage in the paraphilic behavior. Sex-drive reduction takes a direct physiological approach to the modification of sexual arousal. The sex drive, mental sexual arousal, and genital arousal are parts of a psychobiological process that frequently cause a state of uncomfortably high arousability for some individuals with paraphilia.

A large body of scientific data in both animals and men documents the association between lowered testosterone and a significant diminution in the frequency of sexually motivated behaviors. In addition, data show low rates of criminal recidivism among paraphilic patients who have undergone therapeutic sex-drive reduction (Freund, 1980). For example, in one study of surgical castration involving more than 900 sex-offending men followed for periods as long as 30 years, the sexual recidivism rate was less than 3% (Sturup, 1968). Although in the past surgical removal of the testes had been the primary means of testosterone reduction, today that same result can be accomplished via the administration of a variety of medications. Those most commonly used are Cyproterone Acetate, Depo-Provera, Depo-Lupron, or Triptorelin (Berlin et al., 1995; Rosler and Witztum, 1998). In adequate dosages, each is capable of significantly lowering testosterone levels.

Some psychotropic medications, such as selective serotonin reducing inhibitors (SSRIs) also have a side-effect of reducing the sex drive or performance, although they do not necessarily reduce testosterone levels (Greenberg and Bradford, 1997). For some individuals with paraphilia, these treatments effectively reduce paraphilic arousal so long as they are being taken, but do not provide a permanent cure for the disorder.

In the past, some theorists have minimized the role of sexual drive *per se* in attempting to understand a variety of interpersonal sexual behaviors, particularly those that involved either adult–child interactions or were coercive in nature. Often the root of such conduct was thought to be motivated more by a need for power and control than either by lust or by a desire for sexual intimacy. However, reportedly even Freud had once observed that sometimes a cigar is just a cigar. Often behaviors that appear to be sexually motivated are indeed so motivated, albeit in some instances by pathological rather than healthy sexual needs.

Not enough is known presently about qualitative biological differences in sexual makeup to cure a paraphilic disorder. For example, there is no currently known medical or surgical procedure that can erase a pedophilic sexual orientation that is directed exclusively towards children, replacing it instead with an orientation that is directed exclusively towards adults. On the other hand, much is known about the quantitative, intensity dimension of sexual desire, especially in males. Thus, for example, if one is, in effect, hungering sexually for children, the intensity of that hunger can be significantly reduced by interventions that lower testosterone, the hormone that energizes sexual drive (Berlin and Krout, 1986). Although not a cure or a replacement for psychotherapy, such an intervention can represent a useful adjunct to other modalities of treatment.

Practice principles

A metaphor helps to explain to the patient the rationale for biological treatment as part of therapy. Many patients understandably worry that lowering their sexual drive, although helpful in decreasing paraphilic urges, will also interfere with their capacity to engage in acceptable and healthy sexual interactions. Thus, it may be important to explain to them that when the appetite of a would-be dieter is pharmacologically suppressed, it makes it easier for him to diet but not impossible for him to eat. Similarly, lowering the sexual drive is intended to enable the patient to maintain proper self-control, but it is not intended to make sexual performance impossible or inordinately difficult in the context of a healthy and loving adult relationship. In instances where lowering the sexual drive has nonetheless interfered with the ability to perform sexually, such performance can be enhanced without at the same time increasing the intensity of the patient's sexual cravings, by prescribing an oral medication for arousal such as sildenafil (Viagra™).

When engaging in psychotherapy with patients receiving such medications, it is essential to evaluate the intensity and frequency of their paraphilic urges and fantasies in an ongoing fashion. It is also important to assess for any medication side-effects. Even though the sexual drive has been lowered through the use of the antiandrogen medication, it is still important to discuss with the patient strategies for minimizing exposure to unacceptable temptations, the development of a positive social support system, and to confront any denial and rationalizations that may still be present. Given the stigma associated with many of the paraphilias, it is also often important to try to provide ancillary emotional support and comfort. All of these psychological interventions are offered within the context of treatment designed to stop any paraphilic acts that could represent a threat to the well being of either the patient himself or others.

Case example: biological treatment

Roger was a 28-year-old man who had been in treatment for exhibitionism for 4 years. He was handsome, with good social skills. As a young teenager, he would masturbate from a window inside his house, watching women walking or driving by. Then he progressed to masturbating in his car while driving around, spending hours some days driving around before he was seen by a woman and finally ejaculated. He also waited in mall parking lots, positioning himself by his car door so that a woman might see his penis. This led to his first legal charge at age 16, which was eventually dropped. His parents wanted him to see a therapist, but he persuaded them that he did not do anything, his penis just slipped out of his shorts as he was getting out of his car. He continued to spend hours planning and engaging in exposing, and more hours recalling the looks on women's faces during masturbation. He could masturbate to orgasm more than four times a day.

He then started exposing himself in stores in malls, leading him to be excluded from some stores and malls and also resulting in a number of legal charges that usually did not progress to conviction because he was a juvenile with an otherwise exemplary life. Finally he was convicted as an adult, placed on probation, and participated in some general psychotherapy with a therapist who did not specialize in sexual disorders. He got involved in a relationship, with satisfying and frequent sexual intercourse. He thought his problem was over. He was discharged from therapy and completed probation without additional charges.

Despite no difficulty finding girlfriends and satisfactory sexual relations, he found himself returning to exhibitionistic practices. On some weekends, he would have sex with his girlfriend in the morning, and then spend the afternoon exposing himself in malls. He usually targeted women in their twenties or thirties. He never approached the women or even attempted to talk with them. He said that he was looking for an expression on their faces of shock and interest. Although he believed that women found him attractive and were interested in seeing his penis, no woman ever approached him when he exposed. He accumulated three adult convictions for exposing, but he was never incarcerated. Then he exposed to a female who turned out to be 15, and her family was adamant in seeking incarceration. This led him to be evaluated by a program specializing in the treatment of sexual disorders, and he enrolled in treatment. He was 24 years old, involved in a relationship for 6 months, and employed in a very good sales job.

The results of the evaluation showed that he clearly met DSM-IV diagnostic criteria for exhibitionism and apparently did not suffer from any other psychological problems. He did not give any evidence suggestive of mood or personality disorder. He did have a history of drinking alcohol at times to excess, with some binge drinking, but consumption of alcohol was not associated with his exposing. His testosterone levels were in the high end of the typical male range, and he did not have any medical problems. He was hypersexual, continuing to masturbate several times a day in addition to sexual intercourse with his girlfriend. His masturbation imagery was based upon his past episodes of exposing himself. Despite his arrests, he had never been able to go more than several months without exposing.

He participated in weekly group psychotherapy. The therapy focused on getting him to acknowledge the problem, challenging his denial and rationalization. He was able to learn from the examples of other men with similar problems. But he still found that he could not totally stop himself from exposing. In group he saw the example of other men who received weekly injections of Depo-Provera to help them control their sexual behavior by reducing their paraphilic sex drive. Upon the recommendation of his doctors, he agreed to a trial of treatment with Depo-Provera. He was started on a dose of 350 mg per week. His testosterone level dropped from 550 ng/ml to 70 ng/ml. He experienced an increase in appetite, and gained 15 pounds in the first 6 months of treatment. He was able to engage in sexual relations with his girlfriend, without sexual dysfunction, although he had a lower sex drive and lower frequency of intercourse. He reported that his sexual relationship with his girlfriend was actually more satisfying than before.

While on Depo-Provera, he had occasional thoughts of exposing. However, he was able to use the techniques he learned in the group therapy to control his behavior. He felt good about himself and his life. He kept pressing his psychiatrist to cut back on the Provera, or go off it. Near the end of his first year of treatment, he was scheduled to take a 2-week vacation, and he missed the Depo-Provera injection before this vacation as well as the medication during his vacation. While on vacation with his girlfriend, he exposed himself several times. On his return, he resumed weekly injections without further problems.

After the second year of treatment, he attended group therapy every other week, and received Depo-Provera injections biweekly. He continued to do well. During the third year, he cut back on group therapy to monthly visits and continued to receive Depo-Provera every other week. He also went to Sexaholics Anonymous meeting several times a month. In the fourth year of therapy, he continued monthly sessions of group therapy, and discontinued Depo-Provera. He married his girlfriend and seemed to settle down. When his probation was completed, he dropped out of treatment citing problems of cost and difficulty attending the sessions regularly because of his work responsibilities, which increasingly took him out of the area.

He knows that he can re-enter treatment should his problems return. We know that exhibitionism has a tendency to decrease in intensity as the individual gets older, in many cases going into remission in the late thirties or forties. However, this patient is much younger. While we cannot compel him to continue in treatment, we do not consider that he poses a great risk to the public.

Challenges in treatment

The 'correct' responses

In treating men with paraphilia, especially sexual offenders, initial training in personal and sexual boundaries may become little more than a cerebral exercise, in which 'the correct words' are dutifully provided by the patient to the cue of the therapist's question. These empty exercises are marked by such exchanges as: 'Was anyone hurt by your behaviors? ('Yes') How were they hurt? ('I violated their personal boundary space'). The questions are not improper, but the answers can be devoid of a real understanding on the part of the patient, who may be simply responding to the therapist's expectations or the pressures of the forensic system. After all, when one is talking about personal and sexual boundaries, one is talking about a somewhat abstract construct. Even among those of higher intelligence this may be difficult to grasp when confounded by intense sexual urges and the pressure of a legal or therapeutic system that is seeking 'proper' responses.

One strategy that has proved helpful in assisting others to appreciate the meaning of 'personal boundaries' is to start with any subjective experience in which their personal or sexual boundaries have been violated. Childhood sexual abuse is a risk factor for the development of pedophilia and the elaboration of the memory of the abuse can often be helpful in appreciating the meaning of the construct of personal and sexual boundaries. Even lacking such childhood parallels, there can be other interpersonal instances in which the patient may have experienced his personal or sexual boundaries trespassed. Starting with these instances and enriching them by the recall of the affective memories associated with the experience, the therapist can assist the patient to appreciate both cognitively and with affect the effects of his paraphilic behaviors upon others. This strategy can be particularly effective in group treatment.

Adolescents

Paraphilias are diagnosed and treated mostly in adolescent and adult males. Few prepubescent children or females present for evaluation or treatment of paraphilia, so there is little information available regarding these populations. Evaluation and treatment of adolescents with paraphilia is very similar to that with adults, although there are some differences. Adolescents tend to have had less sexual experience, so diagnosis can be difficult. Adolescents may also have fewer opportunities for corrective, positive sexual experiences. Therapists may be uncomfortable or have ethical objections to using treatment tasks involving masturbation or sexually explicit media with adolescents, and they are less likely to recommend medication, including testosterone-lowering antiandrogens, because of the increased possibility of harmful side-effects with long-term usage.

Forensic issues

Traditionally, when providing psychotherapy, the therapist is quite clear about the nature of his commitment that, except in rare instances, is virtually exclusively directed towards the well being of his patient. However, when treating a paraphilic disorder, such as pedophilia, treatment failure can result in an innocent victim being put at risk. This raises a host of difficult ethical and professional dilemmas, including the question of whether the therapists' primary responsibility is to the patient or to the community at large. Ideally, of course, when treatment succeeds both constituencies are well served. The dilemma arises when concerns develop that treatment may not be going so well.

In the United States, healthcare providers including mental health practitioners, are generally required by law to report suspected child abuse (sexual or otherwise) to criminal justice authorities, regardless of when the offense occurred (Berlin *et al.*, 1991). They are not required to report other prior sexual or nonsexual offenses, which are protected by rules of patient confidentiality. Thus, a patient aware of this reporting law is unlikely to self-disclose any such previously unreported criminal activities involving a child to a therapist. The result is that the therapist will not have a full rendering of the behavioral expression of the paraphilia. Treatment options such as antiandrogens may not be considered because the incidence is (falsely) judged to be low.

Another professional responsibility exists with respect to a patient's future, as opposed to prior, misconduct. For example, take the instance of a patient known to be experiencing pedophilic or coercive sexual cravings who becomes noncompliant with treatment. Under such circumstances, if the therapist has reason to believe that the patient poses an imminent threat to others, either adults or children, ethical responsibility and in many jurisdictions legal or forensic mandates regarding future dangerousness requires that the therapist take preventive measures. The therapist must either persuade his patient to accept an intervention that obviates that risk (e.g., voluntarily, or in some instances involuntary, hospitalization), or the therapist must notify the police or warn a potential victim, if he knows the person's identity.

Some patients may be in therapy as a condition of either parole or probation. Under such circumstances, hopefully the content of psychotherapy can still be kept confidential. If not, the limits on confidentiality imposed by the court or the legislature should be clarified at the outset of evaluation or treatment. In any case, noncompliance or irresponsibility by the patient must not be tolerated. Any such noncompliance should be reported to the appropriate authorities.

The management of these reporting responsibilities while maintaining a good psychotherapist/patient relationship requires clear parameters set by the therapist and a commitment by the patient to do whatever is necessary to avoid risk to others. This is the best means of trying to prevent the development of a potential conflict of interest between the therapist and patients. The patient must understand the therapist's commitment to both the patient and the community. Therapists must not knowingly allow patients to act in ways that could cause harm to others, and patients must know from the beginning that it is in everybody's best interest that this be so.

Some therapy programs use the polygraph ('lie-detector') to encourage complete candor, as well as the penile plethysmograph to assess the sorts of stimuli that elicit erotic arousal. Therapists should be aware of the limitations, as well as the strengths, of such technologies. Although the therapist should try to help the patient feel good about himself and enhance his self-esteem, the development of such positive feelings should be within the context of pride about living a healthy, productive, and fully law-abiding lifestyle. It is not the job of the therapist to assist a patient in feeling good about intentions to continue acting in a way that could cause distress or harm to others. For the patient who is working hard in therapy, helping his family and significant others to understand paraphilias as treatable psychiatric conditions, rather than as signs of moral weakness, can sometimes also be an important ancillary to treatment.

Countertransference

Finally, there are also issues of countertransference that must be examined by the therapist in the treatment of paraphilia. Perhaps the most obvious is moralizing, that is, unreflective judgment or unconscious imposition on the patient of the therapist's values regarding sexual behavior. The result may be a devaluation of the person of the patient (which the patient will feel) as well as an attempt to impose one's own values on the patient. In the United States, attitudes about sexual behavior are nearly equally divided among three camps: (1) those who see sexual behavior as recreational; (2) those who see it as part of a caring relationship; and (3) those who see it as part of a committed relationship (Laumann *et al.*, 1994). While differing value systems can and do coexist between therapist and patients, part of the work of therapy is to help the patient clarify the values inherent in his behaviors, rather than imposing the therapist's value system on the patient. One method of managing moralizing tendencies and preserving respect for the patient as a person is for the therapist to be conscious of his or her value system with all its inadequacies and his or her own behavioral inconsistencies.

The second countertransference issue in the treatment of paraphilia is the possibility of vicarious or voyeuristic excitement at the description of the sexual behaviors. Treating paraphilic patients often involves a far more detailed examination of sexual behaviors than with the nonparaphilic patient. Certainly an awareness of sexual arousal during the session is an indication that this countertransference is occurring. However, voyeuristic excitement is also likely to have occurred when the therapist speaks socially of the particulars of his or her patients with paraphilia. Even with no threat of breaking confidentiality, such casual conversation indicates that the therapist is engaged by the patient's narrative in an exciting way. The countertransference involving vicarious identification or prurient enjoyment is difficult to detect. It is usually obfuscated by conscious moralizing or joking degradation in the social gathering. The third common countertransferential issue in the treatment of paraphilia is collusion in denying or minimizing the behavior. Especially with those whose paraphilia is egosyntonic, the natural therapeutic alliance may tend to collude in the acceptability of the disordered behavior or the patient's responsibility for the behavior. As noted previously, in the early stages of treatment, there can often be a disconnection between the words of the patient describing the harmful effects of the sexual behaviors on others and his unconscious continuing acceptance of the behaviors. To the extent that this egosyntonicity remains out of the consciousness of the patient, the therapist, perhaps in projective identification with the patient, may be at risk to carry the projection of egosyntonic approval or minimization of the sexual behaviors. One method of managing this countertransference is repeatedly to imagine the patient in the gestalt of his family, colleagues, or if appropriate, victims, and to work on this gestalt with the patient in therapy. The narcissism of the disorder needs to be countered with consideration of the communitarian responsibilities of the patient.

Conclusions

Psychotherapeutic treatment of the paraphilias is challenging. In many cases the associated behaviors are deeply ingrained involving a sexual object 'preference' that is often as fixed as is sexual orientation itself. Prior to entering a course of therapy to treat an individual with a paraphilia, the therapist and patient should agree upon treatment goals and methods to reach those goals. For those cases in which there is a forensic component, the therapist should be knowledgeable about both professional responsibilities and laws of the jurisdiction.

The therapist should either be experienced in the treatment of paraphilia or be well supervised by one who is so experienced. It is necessary to evaluate for, and to treat, comorbid psychiatric and substance abuse disorders that may also be prevalent in this population. Large-scale meta-analyses have shown treatment effectiveness for cognitive-behavioral methods, although such studies have been with sexual offender samples and contain all the limitations that one might expect in studies in which the outcome measure—reported recidivism—carries subsequent negative consequences (possible incarceration). The replication of these results in the treatment of nonsexual offender paraphilia has not been made. Lastly, in the treatment of sexual offenders or patients whose paraphilia poses a serious risk of harm to self or other, the psychotherapist should consider the use of sexual drive reduction medications and the need to hospitalize some patients during periods of heightened potential risk.

References

Abel, G. G., Becker, J. V., Cunningham-Rathner, J., Mittelmen, M. S., and Rouleau J. L. (1988). Multiple paraphilic diagnoses among sex offenders. *Bulletin of the American Academy of Psychiatry and the Law*, **16**, 153–68.

Abel, G. G., Huffman, J., Warber, B. W., and Holland, C. L. (1998). Visual reaction time and plethysmography as measures of sexual interest in child molesters. *Sex Abuse*, **10**, 81–5.

Abel, G. G., Jordan, A., Hand, C. G., Holland, L. A., and Phipps, A. (2001). Classification models of child molesters utilizing the Abel Assessment for sexual interest (TM). *Child Abuse and Neglect*, **25**, 703–18.

Alexander, M. A. (1999). Sexual offender treatment efficacy revisited. *Sexual Abuse*, **11**(2), 101–16.

Allnutt, S. S., Bradford, J. M., Greenberg, D. M., and Curry, S. (1996). Co-morbidity of alcoholism and the paraphilias. *Journal of Forensic Science*, **41**(2), 234–9.

American Psychiatric Association (2000). *Diagnostic and statistical manual of mental disorders*, 4th edn (text revision edn). Washington, DC: American Psychiatric Association.

Berlin, F. S. and Krout, E. (1986). Pedophilia: diagnostic concepts, treatment and ethical considerations. *American Journal of Forensic Psychiatry*, **7**, 13–30.

Berlin, F. S., Malin, H. M., and Dean, S. (1991). Effects of statutes requiring psychiatrists to report suspected sexual abuse of children. *American Journal of Psychiatry*, **148**, 449–53.

Berlin, F. S., Malin, H. M., and Thomas, K. (1995). Nonpedophilic and nontransvestic paraphilias. In: Gabbard GO, ed. *Treatment of psychiatric disorders*. Washington, DC: American Psychiatric Press.

Bradford, J. M. (1999). The paraphilias, obsessive compulsive spectrum disorder and the treatment of sexually deviant behaviour. *Psychiatric Quarterly*, **70**, 209–19.

Burns, D. (1999). *Feeling good handbook*. London: Penguin.

Carich, M. S. and Mussack, S. E. (2001). *Handbook of sexual abuser assessment and treatment*. Brandon, VT: Safer Society Press.

Carigan, L. (1999). The secret: study of a perverse transference. *International Journal of Psycho-Analysis*, **80**, 909–28.

Dhawan, S. and Marshall, W. L. (1996). Sexual abuse histories of sexual offenders. *Sexual Abuse*, **8**, 7–15.

Fagan, P. J. (2003). *Sexual disorders: perspectives on evaluation and treatment*. Baltimore, MD: Johns Hopkins University Press.

Fagan, P. J., *et al.* (1991). A comparison of five-factor personality dimensions in males with sexual dysfunction and males with paraphilia. *Journal of Personality Assessment*, **57**, 434–48.

Francoeur, R. T., Cornog, M., Perper, T., and Scherzer, N. A. (1995). *The Complete Dictionary of Sexology*. New York: Continuum.

Freud, S. (1905, 1962). *Three essays on the theory of sexuality*. J. Strachey, trans. New York: Basic Books.

Freud, S. (1919). A child is being beaten. In: P. Rieff, ed, A. Strachey and J. Strachey, ed. and trans. *Sexuality and the psychology of love*. New York: Collier.

Freund, K. (1980). Therapeutic sex drive reduction. *Acta Psychiatrica Scandinavica*, **287**, 5–38.

Freund, K. and Kuban, M. (1994). The basis of the abused abuser theory of pedophilia: a further elaboration on an earlier study. *Archives of Sexual Behavior*, **23**(5), 553–63.

Gagnon, J. H. (1990). The explicit and implicit use of the scripting perspective in sex research. *Annual Review of Sex Research*, **1**, 1–43.

Gagnon, J. H. and Simon, W. (1973). *Sexual conduct*. Chicago, IL: Aldine.

Gallagher, C. A., Wilson, D. B., Hisschfiled, P., Coggeshall, M. B., and Mackenzie, D. L. (1999). A quantitative review of the effects of sex offender treatment on sexual reoffending. *Corrections Management Quarterly*, **3**, 19–29.

George, W. H. and Marlatt, G. A. (1989). Introduction. In: D. R. Laws, ed. *Relapse prevention with sex offenders*, pp. 1–33. New York: Guilford Press.

Glenmullen, J. (1993). *The pornographer's grief and other tales of human sexuality*. New York: HarperCollins.

Greenberg, D. M. (1998). Sexual recidivism in sex offenders. *Canadian Journal of Psychiatry*, **43**, 459–65.

Greenberg, D. M. and Bradford, J. M. (1997). Treatment of the paraphillic disorders: a review of the role of the selective serotonin reuptake inhibitors. *Sexual Abuse*, **937**, 349–61.

Grossman, L. S., Martis, B., and Fichtner, C. G. (1999). Are sex offenders treatable? A research overview. *Psychiatric Services*, **50**(3), 349–61.

Hall, G. C. (1995). Sexual offender recidivism revisited: a meta-analysis of recent treatment studies. *Journal of Consulting and Clinical Psychology*, **63**(5), 802–9.

Hanson, R. K. and Bussiere, M. T. (1998). Predicting relapse: a meta-analysis of sexual offender recidivism studies. *Journal of Consulting and Clinical Psychology*, **66**, 348–62.

Hanson, R. K. and Slater, S. (1988). Sexual victimization in the history of child sexual abusers: a review. *Annals of Sex Research*, **1**, 485–99.

Hanson, R. K., *et al.* (2002). First Report of the Collaborative Outcome Data Project on the Effectiveness of Psychological Treatment for Sex Offenders. *Sex Abuse: A Journal of Research and Treatment*, **14**(2), 169–91.

Howes, R. J. (1995). A survey of plethysmographic assessment in North America. *Sexual Abuse*, **7**, 9–24.

Joseph, B. (1971). A clinical contribution to the analysis of a perversion. *International Journal of Psycho-Analysis*, **52**, 441–9.

Junginger, J. (1997). Fetishism: assessment and treatment. In: D. R. Laws and W. O'Donohue, ed. *Sexual deviance: theory, assessment, and treatment*, pp. 92–116. New York: Guilford Press.

Kafka, M. P. and Prentky, R. A. (1994). Preliminary observations of DSM-III-R axis I comorbidity in men with paraphilia and paraphilia-related disorders. *Journal of Clinical Psychiatry*, **55**(11), 481–7.

Kafka, M. P. and Prentky, R. A. (1998). Attention-deficit/hyperactivity disorder in males with paraphilia and paraphilia-related disorders: a comorbidity study. *Journal of Clinical Psychiatry*, **59**(7), 388–96.

Kahn, M. (1969). Role of the 'collated internal object' in perversion-formulations. *International Journal of Psycho-Analysis*, **50**, 555–65.

Kernberg, O. F. (1991). Sadomasochism, sexual excitement, and perversion. *Journal of the American Psychoanalytic Association*, **39**, 333–61.

Knopp, F. H., Freeman-Longo, R. E., and Stevenson, W. F. (1992). *Nationwide survey of juvenile and adult sex-offender treatment programs and models*. Brandon, VT: Safer Society Press.

Kohn, Y., Fahum, T., Ratzoni, G., and Apter, A. (1998). Aggression and sexual offense in Asperger's syndrome. *Israel Journal of Psychiatry and Related Sciences*, **35**(4), 293–9.

Langevin, R. (1983). *Sexual strands: understanding and treating sexual anomalies in men*. Englewood Cliffs, NJ: Lawrence Erlbaum Associates.

Laumann, E. O., Gagnon, J. H., Michael, R. T., and Michaels, S. (1994). *The social organization of sexuality: sexual practices in the United States*. Chicago, IL: University of Chicago Press.

Laws, D. R. (1989). *Relapse prevention with sex offenders*. New York: Guilford Press.

Laws, D. R. and Marshall, R. D. (1991). Masturbatory reconditioning with sexual deviates: an evaluative review. *Advances in Behavior Research and Therapy*, **113**, 13–25.

Laws, D. R. and O'Donohue, W. (1997). *Sexual deviance: theory, assessment, and treatment*. New York: Guilford Press.

Laws, D. R. and Osborn, C. A. (1983). How to build and operate a behavioral laboratory to evaluate and treat sexual deviance. In: J. G. Greer and I. R. Stuart, ed. *The sexual aggressor: current perspectives on treatment*, pp. 293–335. Toronto: Van Nostrand Reinhold.

Lee, J. K., Jackson, H. J., Pattison, P., and Ward, T. (2002). Developmental risk factors for sexual offending. *Child Abuse and Neglect*, **26**, 73–92.

Lehne, G. K. and Money, J. (2000). The first case of paraphilia treated with Depo-Provera: forty-year outcome. *Journal of Sex Education and Therapy*, **25**(4), 213–20.

Lehne, G. K. and Money, J. (2003). Multiplex vs. multiple taxonomy of paraphilia: case example. *Sexual Abuse*, **15**, 61–72.

Lehne, G. K., Thomas, K., and Berlin, F. S. (2000). The treatment of sexual paraphilias: a review of the 1999–2000 literature. *Current Opinion in Psychiatry*, **13**, 569–73.

Levine, S. B., Risen, C. B., and Althof, S. E. (1990). Essay on the diagnosis and nature of paraphilia. *Journal of Sex and Marital Therapy*, **16**(2), 89–102.

LoPiccolo, L. (1994). Acceptance and broad spectrum treatment of paraphilias. In: D. J. Cox and R. J. Daitzman, ed. *Acceptance and change: content and context in psychotherapy*, pp. 149–70. Reno, NV: Context Press.

Lothstein, L. M. (2001). The treatment of non-incarcerated sexually compulsive/addictive offenders in an integrated, multimodal, and psychodynamic group therapy model. *International Journal of Group Psychotherapy*, **51**, 553–70.

Love, B. (1992). *The encyclopedia of unusual sex practices*. New York: Barricade Books.

Maletzky, B. M. (1991). *Treating the sexual offender*. Newbury Park, CA: Sage.

Maletzky, B. M. (1993). Factors associated with success and failure in he behavioral and cognitive treatment of sexual offenders. *Annals of Sex Research*, **4**, 117–29.

Maletzky, B. M. (1997). Exhibitionism: assessment and treatment. In: D. R. Laws and W. O'Donohue, ed. *Sexual deviance: theory, assessment, and treatment*, pp. 40–74. New York: Guilford Press.

Maletzky, B. M. and Steinhauser, C. (2002). A 25-year follow-up of cognitive/behavioral therapy with 7,275 sexual offenders. *Behavior Modification*, **26**(2), 123–47.

McConaghy, N. (1993). *Sexual behavior: problems and management*. New York: Plenum.

McConaghy, N. (1997). Science and the mismanagement of rapists and paedophiles. *Psychiatry, Psychology and the Law*, **4**, 109–23.

McConaghy, N. (1999a). Methodological issues concerning evaluation of treatment for sexual offenders: randomization, treatment dropouts, untreated controls, and within-treatment studies. *Sexual Abuse*, **11**(3), 183–93.

McConaghy, N. (1999b). Unresolved issues in scientific sexology. *Archives of Sexual Behavior*, **28**, 285–318.

McDougall, J. (1995). *The many faces of eros*. London: Free Association Books.

McElroy, S. L., *et al.* (1999). Psychiatric features of 36 men convicted of sexual offenses. *Journal of Clinical Psychiatry*, **60**, 414.

McGrath, R. J. (2001). Using behavioral techniques to control sexual arousal. In: M. S. Carich and S. E. Mussack, ed. *Handbook of sexual abuser assessment and treatment*, pp. 105–16. Brandon, VT: Safer Society Press.

Mendez, M. F., Chow, T., Ringman, J., Twitchell, G., and Hinkin, C. H. (2000). Pedophilia and temporal lobe disturbances. *Journal of Neuropsychiatry and Clinical Neurosciences*, **12**, 71–6.

Meyer, J. K. (1995). Paraphilias. In: H. I. Kaplan and B. J. Sadock, ed. *Comprehensive textbook of psychiatry*, 6th edn, pp. 1334–47. Philadelphia: Lippincott, William, and Wilkins.

Miner, M. H. and Coleman, E. (2001). Advances in sex offender treatment and challenges for the future. *Journal of Psychology and Human Sexuality*, **13**(3/4), 5–24.

Money, J. (1986). *Lovemaps*. New York: Irvington Publishers.

Money, J. (1999). *The lovemap guidebook: a definitive statement*. New York: Continuum.

Murphy, W. D. and Barbaree, H. E. (1994). *Assessment of sex offenders by measures of erectile response: psychometric properties and decision making*. Brandon, VT: Safer Society Press.

Ousley, O. Y. and Mesibov, G. B. (1991). Sexual attitudes and knowledge of high-functioning adolescents and adults with autism. *Journal of Autism and Developmental Disorders*, **21**(4), 471–81.

Parsons, M. (2000). Sexuality and perversions a hundred years on: discovering what Freud discovered. *International Journal of Psycho-Analysis*, **81**, 37–51.

Paul, R., Marx, B., and Orsillo, S. (1999). Acceptance-based psychotherapy in the treatment of an adjudicated exhibitionist: a case example. *Behavioral Therapy*, **30**, 149–62.

Quinsey, V. L. and Earls, C. M. (1990). The modification of sexual preferences. In: R. D. Marshall, D. R. Laws, and H. E. Barbaree, ed. *Handbook of sexual assault*, pp. 279–95. New York: Plenum.

Raymond, N. C., Coleman, E., Ohlerking, F., Christensen, G. A., and Miner, M. (1999). Psychiatric comorbidity in pedophilic sex offenders. *American Journal of Psychiatry*, **156**(5), 786–8.

Realmuto, G. M. and Ruble, L. A. (1999). Sexual behaviors in autism: problems of definition and management. *Journal of Autism and Developmental Disorders*, **29**(2), 121–7.

Rosler, A. and Witztum, E. (1998). Treatment of men with paraphilia with a long-acting analogue of gonadotropin-releasing hormone. *New England Journal of Medicine*, **338**(7), 416–22.

Roys, D. T. and Roys, P. (1994). *Protocol for phallometric assessment: a clinician's guide*. Brandon, VT: Safer Society Press.

Simpson, G., Blaszczynski, A., and Hodgkinson, A. (1999). Sex offending as a psychosocial sequela of traumatic brain injury. *Journal of Head Trauma Rehabilitation*, **14**, 567–80.

Steen, C. (2001). *The adult relapse prevention workbook*. Brandon, VT: Safer Society Foundation.

Stoller, R. J. (1975). *Perversion: the erotic form of hatred*. New York: Pantheon.

Sturup, G. K. (1968). *Treating the 'untreatable' chronic criminals at Herstedvester*. Baltimore, MD: Johns Hopkins Press.

Van Bourgodien, M. E., Reichle, N. C., and Palmer, A. (1997). Sexual behavior in adults with autism. *Journal of Autism and Developmental Disorders*, **27**(2), 113–25.

Weiss, P. (1989). [Psychological predictors of recidivism in sex offenders][Article in Czech]. *Ceskoslovenska Psychiatrie*, **85**(4), 250–5.

Yochelson, S. and Samenow, S. E. (1977). *The criminal personality: Vol. II. The change process*. New York: Jason Aronson.

18 Sexual disorders

Michelle Jeffcott and Joseph LoPiccolo

All psychological disorders present challenges to therapists, and sexual dysfunction is no exception. However, it is unique because of the variety of the disorders that are encompassed by the term and the prevalence rates of the disorders. A recent epidemiological study found overall rates for sexual dysfunction in men and women were 31% and 43%, respectively (Laumann *et al.*, 1999), highlighting a need for effective treatments for sexual problems. This chapter will focus on the evolution of theory and practice in sex therapy. Each sexual dysfunction will be addressed separately, with a specific focus on the most current and empirically supported treatments available to remedy each problem.

General information about sexual dysfunction

Each sexual dysfunction is characterized by the stage of the sexual response cycle that is affected and is defined by a change in sexual functioning that causes distress to the individual and interpersonal difficulties (American Psychiatric Association, 1994). William Masters and Virginia Johnson (1966) first described the stages of the sexual response cycle. These stages consist of the desire phase where one feels the urge to have sex, the arousal phase where one has increased physiological excitement such as higher heart rate and blood pressure, the orgasm phase where reflexive muscle contractions occur in the pelvis, and finally the resolution phase where the body returns to its pre-arousal state. Sexual dysfunction can occur in any of the first three stages of the sexual response cycle but does not occur in the latter phase.

Desire disorders consist of hypoactive sexual desire and sexual aversion (American Psychiatric Association, 1994). Hypoactive sexual desire results from a person having little or no interest in sex or in engaging in sexual activity. However, when sexual activity does occur, the person does not experience emotional distress. Contrarily, people who experience sexual aversion feel negative emotions, such as disgust or fear, when they engage in sexual activity at the insistence of a partner.

Disorders that occur during the arousal phase of the sexual response cycle are female sexual arousal disorder and male erectile dysfunction (American Psychiatric Association, 1994). Sexual arousal disorder is diagnosed in women when there is an inability to maintain lubrication of the vagina or genital swelling. Erectile disorder is diagnosed when there is a failure to obtain or maintain an erection until completion of sexual activity.

Finally, disorders that occur during the orgasm phase of the sexual response cycle are female orgasmic disorder, male orgasmic disorder, and male premature ejaculation (American Psychiatric Association, 1994). Female and male orgasmic disorders are described as a complete absence of orgasm or a delay in the experience of an orgasm during sexual activity. However, though female orgasmic disorder is relatively common, it should be noted that male orgasmic disorder is quite rare among cases seen for sexual dysfunction. It is much more common for a man to present for sex therapy due to premature ejaculation. This disorder is difficult to define, but it is generally classified as a male reaching orgasm with minimal stimulation and before

he or his partner want it to occur usually prior to or shortly after entry of the penis into the vagina.

There are two sexual disorders that cannot be defined by the stage of the sexual response cycle in which they occur. These problems are labeled as sexual pain disorders. Dyspareunia is genital pain that is experienced during sexual intercourse, and vaginismus is defined by involuntary contractions of the outer third of the vagina so that entry of the penis or another object such as the finger cannot take place (American Psychiatric Association, 1994).

Conceptualization of the disorders

Psychoanalytic therapy

There are certain overarching themes that each treatment approach supports when explaining the causes of sexual dysfunction. The manner in which sexual dysfunction is addressed in psychoanalytic theory dates back to Sigmund Freud's (1905/1965) writings on personality development. These writings stressed that sexual dysfunction results from a person failing to progress through the oral, anal, and phallic stages of psychosexual development into the genital stage by not resolving the oedipal complex. A healthy transition through these stages occurs when the child is able to progress through the oedipal conflict by behaving like and identifying with the same sex parent. If a person did not progress through the stages and resolve the oedipal conflict, s/he would experience sexual dysfunction in some form in adulthood. Therapy that was insight oriented was recommended in order to aid the client in resolving past issues regarding sexuality.

Current psychodynamic therapy incorporates both Freud's early ideas as well as more modern ideas. Some psychodynamic therapists focus treatment on making unconscious inhibitors of sexual functioning conscious through the course of therapy, while stressing that it is not only important to understand the sexual functioning problem but also the individual's personality development and defense mechanisms that may inhibit change (Rosen, 1982). This treatment relies on the patient to be the motivating person behind change without relying on specific behavioral training techniques. Other psychodynamic therapists use not only psychodynamic techniques, such as working through transference, but apply behavioral or pharmacotherapeutic techniques to best aid the client (Gabbard, 2000). This approach to diagnosing and treating sexual dysfunction relies heavily on the therapist to examine the client's presenting problem and prescribe the treatment method thought to have the best results (Gabbard, 2000). Psychodynamic therapy for the treatment of sexual dysfunction is practiced by a small percentage of psychotherapists and is not supported by the majority of research on sexual disorders.

Cognitive-behavioral therapy

Behaviorists challenged the psychoanalytic view of sexual dysfunction. Early behaviorists believed that sexual dysfunction resulted from anxiety (Wolpe, 1958). Behaviorists stressed that anxiety inhibited sexual arousal in some way, or was, at the very least, incompatible with arousal. They used systematic desensitization to remedy the problem. The client would be taught relaxation therapy techniques. While practicing these techniques, the client would visualize a self-made hierarchy of sexual behavior. When this process was mastered, the client would then engage in the sexual behaviors while still practicing the relaxation techniques. Although this technique provided help for some clients experiencing sexual dysfunction, it was unsatisfactory for solving many sexual disorders.

Masters and Johnson (1970) expanded the behavioral focus to include early experiences as contributors to sexual dysfunction. They stressed the need for anxiety reducing therapeutic techniques as well as helping the client to learn sexual stimulation procedures. Specific sexual behavior training came in the form of sensate focus, which outlines certain techniques to aid the couple in overcoming anxiety that contributes to sexual dysfunction.

With the advent of the cognitive-behavioral approach, therapy for those with sexual dysfunction was expanded to include a client's cognitions regarding sexuality. Albert Ellis (1962) introduced the idea, but it was expanded upon by later theorists and researchers. Some cognitive factors that may contribute to sexual dysfunction are gender identity conflicts, fears of having children, depression, or religious orthodoxy.

Couples therapy

One final general area that has contributed to the current state of knowledge about treating sexual dysfunction is the research on systemic couples therapy. Couples therapists believe that sexual dysfunction experienced by one partner is the result of or is perpetuated by the interactions of the couple. It was first stressed by systemic therapists that sexual dysfunction caused great distress to both members of the couple. More recently, theorists propose that the disorder may also serve some helpful functions within the couple's relationship (LoPiccolo, 2002). According to this perspective, the sexual dysfunction exists in the relationship because it serves a purpose, and helping the partner to overcome his or her problem serves to change the balance in the relationship. This shift, if not monitored by the therapist, can contribute to other problems in the marital dyad. Certain systemic problems that can serve to maintain a sexual disorder are lack of trust, fear of intimacy, power imbalance in the relationship, and an inability to reconcile feelings of love and sexual desire (LoPiccolo, 2002).

Female arousal and orgasmic disorders

Female sexual arousal disorder is often seen in conjunction with orgasm or desire problems. One study showed that 14% of women in the general population report lubrication difficulty (Laumann et al., 1999), but this problem is known to increase in postmenopausal women (Rosen et al., 1993). There is more information available about female orgasmic disorder, and as many as 24% of women experience orgasm difficulty at some time (Laumann et al., 1999). Women can experience either primary (global and lifelong) or secondary (situational and/or not lifelong) orgasmic dysfunction. The former term refers to women who have never had an orgasm, while the latter term refers to women who have infrequent orgasms or can have orgasms only in certain conditions. It should be noted that in order to achieve orgasm, a woman must be able to sustain arousal over time. Because the specific etiology of female sexual arousal disorder is linked so closely with orgasmic dysfunction, the conceptualizations for the disorders will be combined.

Early psychoanalysts believed that a woman who had successfully entered the genital stage would have vaginal orgasms (Freud, 1905/1965). Present psychodynamic therapists believe in order to best address female orgasmic disorder, the issues of anxiety and conflict within the relationship must be reconciled (Rosen, 1982). It is not necessary that the woman be able to progress to the vaginal orgasm, but it is important that she understands herself in relation to her partner in order to be able to attain orgasm. For example, this woman, through examining her feelings about her partner and past relationships, can learn important insight into why she is unable to reach orgasm with her husband. It may be that she internalized negative

feelings associated with being close to people for fear that they will hurt her and is now acting these feelings out with her husband.

Present day cognitive-behavioral therapists apply the general ideas of the theory in order to address sexual functioning. The cognitive-behavioral therapist will interview the client to find out the cognitions that may be interfering with her ability to achieve orgasm. The therapist then prescribes cognitive techniques to change these problematic thoughts as well as behavioral techniques to aid the woman in becoming orgasmic (LoPiccolo and Lobitz, 1972).

Systemic couples therapists traditionally view sexual dysfunction as a reflection, cause, or effect of other nonsexual issues that are problematic in the couple's relationship (Whitaker and Keith, 1981). All couples therapy relies upon both members of the couple dyad to participate in therapy. Masters and Johnson (1970) were two of the first researchers to rely upon both members of the marital dyad for changing a sexual dysfunction. Others (e.g., Schnarch, 1991) expanded this idea giving both members of the couple specific duties to perform to help the woman achieve orgasm.

Although all the therapies described have been utilized to treat female arousal and orgasmic disorders, the most support for treating this problem is an integrated approach to therapy. This integrated approach looks to tenets of cognitive-behavioral and systemic therapy as well as any physiological or medical factors that may contribute to the problem (LoPiccolo and Lobitz, 1972; Heiman and LoPiccolo, 1988). In order to best assess the client's problems in any or all of these areas, the initial interview is paramount. The therapist who practices integrative therapy will meet with the couple together and then each member of the couple separately to ensure that all the information relevant to treatment is gathered.

The case conceptualization would continue by getting a thorough orgasmic history. The couple should be asked questions about what they have tried to aid the woman to have an orgasm. It is important to find out information about their expectations about sex and how often or during what activities a woman 'should' have an orgasm. The therapist should gather information on areas of family of origin learning history, cognitive factors, relationship factors, and any operant issues in daily life, such as day to day stress, that may contribute to the problem. The therapist should also make sure that the woman has had a gynecological exam to rule out or diagnose any problems that may interfere with her ability to achieve orgasm.

Vaginismus

The spastic contractions associated with vaginismus are reported by as many as 12–17% of women who present for treatment at sex therapy clinics (Spector and Carey, 1990). Women presenting with vaginismus can have primary vaginismus where the spasms occur in any type of situation or secondary vaginismus where the spasms may occur only when penetration of some type may occur (Rosen and Leiblum, 1995). Some psychodynamic therapists view vaginismus as a means women use to either reject their role in a relationship with a man or as a physical manifestation of a fear of being violated by a male (Kaplan, 1974). Others stress the importance of factors that coincide with the beliefs of many cognitive-behavioral and systemic couples therapists (Gabbard, 2000). For example, problems such as sexual fears or a history of sexual abuse are thought to contribute to vaginismus. Therapists who adhere to this modern view of the problems contributing to vaginismus will use not only dynamic techniques to aid the client but also behavioral techniques deemed relevant (Gabbard, 2000).

Cognitive-behavioral therapists associate the spastic contractions with a fear response that may be caused by a real or imagined instance where vaginal penetration could occur (Masters and Johnson, 1970). It has been found that sexual fears and phobias as well as a history of sexual abuse are associated with vaginismus (Leiblum, 2000). Vaginismus, in this view, is due not to physical problems but due to psychological problems experienced by the woman. The cognitive-behavioral therapist helps the woman to deal with these negative associations and teaches her other techniques to stop the vaginismus.

Couples therapists conceptualize the disorder similarly to the cognitive-behavioral therapists. Couples therapists believe, as in other sexual disorders, that both partners are crucial for success. As in female orgasmic dysfunction, it is thought that the vaginismus may serve to take the focus from another problematic area of the couple's relationship (Whitaker and Keith, 1981). Couples therapists would then conceptualize the problem as not only the vaginismus but the couple's relationship, and they look to the couple's relationship as a whole in order to find where to best intervene.

An approach that integrates some aspects of all of these therapies is most often used for understanding the contributing factors to vaginismus. A thorough history should be taken and vaginal exam given to ensure that the problem is vaginismus and not related to a physical problem (LoPiccolo and Stock, 1986). Once this has been established, the therapist identifies which factors contribute the most to the present problem. The therapist will often combine tenets from cognitive-behavioral therapy, such as relaxation techniques, to help the woman to gain control over the spasms. Leiblum notes that in most cases of vaginismus, some therapy must be performed to have the couples discuss any fears about penetration or any problems that have arisen due to the couples inability to have intercourse. She goes on to describe some cognitive contributors to vaginismus. These include erroneous ideas about the size of the vagina and the changes that the woman's body undergoes during arousal that differentiate it from the normal unaroused state. Because this process can be very difficult, especially for the woman with primary vaginismus, it is important that the therapist be flexible with the prescribed techniques. Helping the client to relax and trust the therapist is essential in aiding the woman to be able to address her vaginismus.

Dyspareunia

The diagnosis of dyspareunia is given to women who describe pain during intercourse. It is often difficult to differentiate from vaginismus because many women who complain of vaginismus also complain of pain (Leiblum, 2000). Pain during intercourse has been shown to be experienced by 7% of women in one national sample (Laumann et al., 1999) and as many as 10–15% of women reporting for outpatient treatment (Rosen et al., 1993). This makes dyspareunia a likely problem for a sex therapist to treat.

Psychoanalytic writings do not address the idea of dyspareunia in great depth. However, it is thought that the same types of factors that can contribute to any sexual dysfunction are relevant for dyspareunia. These include the failure to progress through the stages of the sexual response cycle adequately, unresolved feelings about sexuality, guilt about sexuality, or any sexual traumas (Rosen, 1982). Additionally, treatment will consist of dynamic as well as possibly behavioral interventions (Gabbard, 2000).

Cognitive-behavioral therapists take a similar view to dyspareunia as they do to vaginismus. Although the presence of a physical problem contributing to the pain the woman is experiencing is recognized (Steege and Ling, 1993), it is believed that much of the problem can be dealt with by using standard cognitive-behavioral techniques. As it is the case that many women who are treated for dyspareunia by surgical means have some lingering problems (Schover et al., 1992), cognitive-behavioral techniques are very useful to aid in completely remedying the problem. Therapists using these techniques believe that the client's fears about pain during intercourse can continue even when there is no more physical problem. The therapist will use specific behavioral and cognitive techniques in order to help the woman overcome any lingering problems associated with the dyspareunia.

Couples therapy addresses dyspareunia in much of the same way it addresses other sexual dysfunction. Couples therapists will rely on both members of the dyad to be present for therapy. They conceptualize the problem as being sustained by the interactions of the couple and look to change these interaction patterns to help aid the woman in overcoming the pain she experiences during genital contact.

A modern integrated approach to understanding dyspareunia takes into account multiple factors that can contribute to dyspareunia. A thorough history taking is again prescribed where the client's pain is described by the location, quality, types of activities that elicit the pain and the length of time the pain lasts, as well as other factors; furthermore, it is important to understand what brought the woman to treatment as well as her coping strategies for dealing with the pain over time (Binik et al., 2000). Because cases of purely psychogenic dyspareunia are rare, there are not specific therapies outlined for this. However, there is reported success in using tenets of cognitive-behavioral therapy outlined for arousal and orgasmic dysfunctions to treat women with dyspareunia (Bergeron et al., 2001).

Male erectile disorder

Males who present with erectile disorder have problems obtaining or maintaining an erection. This problem has been found to affect 5% of the general population in one epidemiologic study (Laumann et al., 1999) and is most common in older men. Psychodynamic therapists currently view erectile disorder as resulting from a variety of conflicts and anxieties about intimacy and sexuality. It is also thought that the erectile problem may stem from arousal toward or guilt about some deviant sexual fantasy (Rosen, 1982). In each case, the unique convergence of this set of anxieties and conflicts must be understood along with behavioral and pharmacologic interventions in order to best aid the client.

Cognitive-behavioral therapists look to help the client uncover what ideas he possesses that can serve to perpetuate the erectile problem and look to behavioral techniques that will help to restore functioning. Some general cognitive distortions that are common to erectile failure have to do with unrealistic expectations about the man's sexual abilities. Also, a lack of knowledge about the changes that take place in older men regarding erectile response (i.e., slower response, need of more direct stimulation, longer refractory period after ejaculation, and an inability to ejaculate during intercourse every time) occurs (Schover, 1984). This may lead to added distress and anxiety experienced by the male, which also contribute to erectile failure (LoPiccolo, 1992). It is also important to gauge the amount of sexual stimulation the man is currently getting as well as the woman's preferences for sexual gratification as it may not depend on the man obtaining an erection.

Couples therapists rely on many methods used by the aforementioned therapies. They too would take a thorough history encompassing the couple's views about sexuality and the male's sexual response. They would focus on issues pertinent to how the couple is affected by the erectile problem, what has been tried to remedy the problem, and what the couple's expectations about sexual functioning are.

The most common treatment for male erectile disorder involves an integrative approach combining pieces of the cognitive, behavioral, and couples therapy models as well as treatment with Sildenafil citrate (i.e., Viagra). Current therapists stress the importance of the potential for both psychological and physiological problems that contribute to erectile dysfunction (Carson et al., 1999). For this reason, even when it seems that the problem is due mainly to psychogenic factors, it is necessary for the client to have a physical examination. As indicated in the section on cognitive-behavioral therapy, there are many cognitive factors that can contribute to erectile problems and exacerbate prior problems that have occurred with erectile functioning. It is also important to take a thorough history to gauge any individual, relationship, family of origin, or operant factors that may contribute to the erectile dysfunction (LoPiccolo, in press). Some indications that organic causes may be contributing to the erectile disorder include the presence of adequate manual or oral stimulation that do not help to produce an erection and no serious relationship factors accompanying the problem. The assessment of erectile dysfunction can be measured by self-report inventories or by physiological measures such as the recording of nocturnal penile tumescence.

Premature ejaculation

Premature ejaculation is the most commonly reported sexual dysfunction in males. One study reported 21% of men in the general population had rapid ejaculation problems (Laumann et al., 1999). Psychoanalytic therapists do not believe there is necessarily one explanation for rapid ejaculation (Kaplan, 1974). However, it has been suggested that premature ejaculation could be due to problematic masturbation practices combined with sexual fears such as being overwhelmed by sexual excitement (Rosen, 1982). Most psychodynamic therapists today view an integrated approach that includes psychodynamic understanding and behavioral intervention as optimal (Gabbard, 2000).

Cognitive-behavioral therapy views rapid ejaculation as a problem that can be solved with behavioral training. In fact, the most successful therapy used for premature ejaculation was devised by Semans (1956) and modified by Masters and Johnson (1970). This therapy is based upon the idea that the man who is rapidly ejaculating can control this process by learning certain behavioral techniques that monitor his sexual excitement as well as by increasing his orgasm threshold.

Couples therapists believe that the partner of the man who is experiencing premature ejaculation plays an important role in helping the man to stop or limit his rapid ejaculation. The integrative postmodern model illustrates this idea well (LoPiccolo, 2002). Because the woman has been frustrated by her partner's rapid ejaculation and has often been silently suffering, it is important to include her in therapy. The integrative model suggests that the woman will more happily participate in the behavioral techniques outlined by Semans (1956) and Masters and Johnson (1970) if she is receiving immediate returns on her hard work. That is, the man and his partner should agree upon a time when she will also be able to experience sexual pleasure apart from the time when she is helping him with his therapy. As always, it is important to include in therapy the systemic couple issues that may serve to impede therapeutic progress.

Male orgasmic disorder

Males who experience inhibited ejaculation are rare in clinical populations. However, the problem of inhibited ejaculation is more often seen in homosexual men (Wilinsky and Myers, 1987). Psychoanalytic therapists believe that inhibited ejaculators are stopping themselves from having an orgasm for reasons ranging from a hatred of or disgust for women (Kaplan, 1974) to early childhood conflicts that were not fully resolved and inhibit the man from fully letting go and experiencing orgasm (Rosen, 1982). Whatever the reason for the presenting problem, it is thought that this dysfunction can be difficult to treat due to the many confounding factors that contribute to the disorder.

Cognitive-behavioral therapists view male orgasmic disorder similarly to female orgasmic disorder (LoPiccolo and Stock, 1986). The aim of treatment is to decrease anxiety, increase arousal or desire, and help the client to deal with any conditioning factors that may have contributed to the current problem.

Couples therapists would look to the relationship to see what factors may be contributing the orgasmic disorder. This is best illustrated by the integrative model that includes systemic issues in the treatment of inhibited ejaculation. The model treats male orgasmic disorder by reducing performance anxiety and ensuring adequate stimulation (LoPiccolo and Stock, 1986). The integrative model also notes that in certain cases, neurological disorders may be contributing to the dysfunction. It is important that all possible contributing factors be taken into consideration when devising the best treatment for the client.

Low sexual desire and aversion to sex

Both men and women can experience low sexual desire and aversion to sex. Although women report both disorders at greater rates than men, it has been found that 22% of women and 5% of men endorse low desire in the general population (Laumann et al., 1999). Low sexual desire and aversion to sex are viewed by psychoanalytic therapists as resulting from unresolved sexual issues as well as issues of anxiety about the relationship and what it would mean to the person to have sexual desire. Cognitive-behavioral therapists believe that it is important to help the client identify any negative thoughts they have about sex or sexuality that contribute to their desire to not have sex (LoPiccolo and Friedman, 1988). The cognitive-behavioral therapist will then use this information in structured cognitive exercises as well as behavioral techniques.

Lastly, systemic couples therapists stress the importance of identifying that the client presenting for therapy may be reluctant to overcome the problem if s/he feels as though s/he is being treated as the bad person or there are systemic issues contributing to the problem (LoPiccolo, 2002). For this reason, it is important to identify these issues and use them to help therapy rather than hinder it. Systemic therapists also stress the importance of recognizing the disorder as a way in which the relationship functions rather than focusing on the aspect of the sexual dysfunction (Schnarch, 2000).

As in the other sexual disorders described, the most common treatment for either disorder is an integrated approach. It combines the use of the cognitive and behavioral techniques as well as the systemic issues that serve to keep the disorder present in the relationship. It relies on education about sexual desire and the fact that all humans do have a sex drive. LoPiccolo (2002) notes that therapy should stress that this is a loss to the person to not have a sex drive and that it is not a choice that the person consciously made. It should be stressed to the client that therapy can help to remedy the situation. However, in cases of sexual aversion, it is very important to deal completely with the cause of the aversion. In some cases the aversion may be due to sexual assault as a child or adult. In these cases, it is recommended that using techniques described by Courtois (1988) for survivors of child sexual abuse or Foa (1997) for survivors of rape be used. Therapy for the desire disorder or aversion to sex should follow treatment for the sexual abuse. Courtois outlines a therapy that includes traumatic stress, feminist, and family systems models to address the incest directly. She uses cathartic exercises such as body awareness and saying goodbye, cognitive restructuring, and many other techniques that allow for the client to progress through treatment. Foa utilizes cognitive-behavioral techniques such as cognitive restructuring and in vivo exposure to address the client's problems stemming from rape.

Research supporting sex therapy
Female arousal and orgasmic disorders

There is no controlled outcome research that examines female arousal disorder specifically, but the research on orgasmic disorder can also be applied to female arousal disorder because of the closely linked nature of the disorders. Early research showed that masturbation provided the best method for helping women achieve orgasm (Masters and Johnson, 1966). Research also supported the notion that the more the vaginal muscles are used and strengthened by exercises, the more likely it is that a woman has increased genital sensation and orgasm (Kegel, 1952). These findings helped contribute to the integrative approach in dealing with female orgasmic disorder (LoPiccolo and Lobitz, 1972). This treatment method can be used in an individual or couples therapy format. Using this treatment method, one study showed that 95% of 150 women were able to reach orgasm due to their own masturbation, 85% were able to reach orgasm due to partner stimulation, and 40% were able to reach orgasm during intercourse (LoPiccolo and Stock, 1986). Another study showed that when compared with sensate focus (Masters and Johnson, 1970) combined with supportive therapy, the integrative approach helped more women to attain orgasm (Riley and Riley, 1978). The self-help book that outlines the same integrative approach (Heiman and LoPiccolo, 1988) has also been shown to be effective in aiding women to overcome orgasmic disorder (Morokoff and LoPiccolo, 1986).

The above research supports the idea of an integrated approach for treating female orgasmic disorder. Treating women with secondary orgasmic dysfunction can be more difficult. One study found that using the integrative approach with secondary inorgasmic women did not significantly help the woman to increase her experience of orgasm with genital caressing by a partner or during intercourse (McGovern et al., 1975). It is suggested from this and other research that a treatment method focusing more on general marital difficulties combined with sex therapy is more appropriate for these women.

Group therapy is another treatment modality that has been used to treat women with orgasmic dysfunction. Research has supported that directed masturbation training in a group therapy format resulted in a 100% success rate of women being able to achieve orgasm (Wallace and Barbach, 1974). Another study found that group therapy worked better for women under 35, but partner understanding and cooperation was a key factor in aiding the women in achieving orgasm (Schniedman and McGuire, 1976).

Vaginismus

Research on vaginismus is not as prevalent as research on orgasmic dysfunction in women. A recent review found that there are few studies that compare the available treatments for vaginismus (Heiman, 2002). However, there is some research available on the efficacy of treating women with vaginismus. In a review of the literature on sexual dysfunction, LoPiccolo and Stock (1986) concluded that research on using dilator insertion to aid the woman in overcoming her vaginismus is equally effective whether it is performed by the client or a gynecologist.

Outcome research has shown support for both dilator insertion techniques as well as general sex therapy techniques. Specifically, Hawton and Catalan (1986) used sex therapy techniques derived from Masters and Johnson (1970) as well as dilator insertion to aid women with a diagnosis of vaginismus. Treatment included both the woman and her partner. The findings supported an 80% success rate for those women who completed therapy. Success was aided by the couples' motivation to be in therapy and relationship before therapy. Future research should focus on comparison studies to test the efficacy of different treatment models for overcoming vaginismus. To date, there are no such studies.

Dyspareunia

Unlike other sexual disorders, dyspareunia involves a definite physical problem that is contributing to the pain. The most common problem associated with dyspareunia is vulvar vestibulitis (i.e., inflammation of the area between the labia minora) but other conditions such as poor lubrication and vulvar atrophy can contribute to dyspareunia (Binik et al., 2000). Treatment for dyspareunia often involves a medical procedure (i.e. usually vestibulectomy), but research supports therapeutic techniques whether they are delivered with or without the surgical procedure (Bergeron et al., 2001).

A recent study has the best evidence for treatment efficacy. Bergeron et al. (2001) assigned clients to one of three treatment conditions, including group cognitive-behavioral therapy, surface electromyographic feedback (sEMG), and vestibulectomy. Treatment success was measured by less pain, better sexual functioning, and good psychosocial adjustment. For those who participated in the cognitive-behavioral therapy, 40% of the women showed significant improvement. The women who underwent vestibulectomy had a 65% success rate, and 30% of women in the sEMG condition showed significant improvement. This study shows some support for the success of different treatments of dyspareunia, but more research, including randomized controlled studies, is needed to gauge effectively the best types of treatment for women presenting with pain disorders.

Male erectile disorder

Although Viagra has become a prevalent treatment for erectile dysfunction, psychotherapeutic techniques are often important to best aid treatment outcomes. However, research involving psychotherapeutic techniques for erectile dysfunction is mixed. Most therapy involves the man and his partner, but there has been some research on men who present for treatment without a partner. Using a group therapy format focusing on sexual attitude change, masturbation exercises, and social skills training, it was found that the men showed improved self-esteem and sexual satisfaction when compared with a wait-list control group; however, there was only a trend toward improvement in erectile functioning (Price et al., 1981). Another study using different group therapy techniques showed significant improvement in erectile functioning for those who participated in therapy as opposed to the wait-list control group (Kilmann et al., 1987).

Research on therapy involving couples is more prevalent. Educational procedures for older men with erectile disorder have been shown to help improve sexual knowledge as well as frequency and satisfaction of sex (Goldman and Carroll, 1990). In another study, general sex therapy techniques outlined by Masters and Johnson (1970), helped 68% of males presenting with erectile disorder showed some improvement during therapy (Hawton and Catalan, 1986). This same study also supported factors such as good communication by the couple and high motivation for therapy to be helpful in achieving and maintaining change. Other research has suggested contributing factors to erectile dysfunction, but there are no controlled studies evaluating the efficacy of these ideas for treating clients. Specifically, it has been suggested that anxiety is not the main contributor to psychogenic erectile problems but cognitive distortions or performance demands may be more important (Rosen, 2000). It has also been suggested that support from the client's partner surrounding issues of sexuality is an important factor in effecting change (LoPiccolo, in press). However, no research to date has examined these factors in the influence of erectile dysfunction.

Premature ejaculation

The standard treatment procedures for premature ejaculation are outlined by Semans (1956) and Masters and Johnson (1970). In his initial research, Semans (1956) reported long-term gains for 15 men he had treated with the pause technique. Masters and Johnson (1970) reported success rates of 90% for men treated with the pause and squeeze combined procedure. Other research has shown improvements in premature ejaculation for men participating in cognitive-behavioral as well as retraining programs (Kilmann and Auerbach, 1979). Another study, using standard treatment for premature ejaculation, including partners, found that 65% of men who completed treatment showed some improvement in increasing time to ejaculation (Hawton and Catalan, 1986). However, it has also been shown that the long-term benefits of the pause and squeeze technique are not as good as the initial outcomes (D'Amicis et al., 1985).

Male orgasmic disorder

Research is lacking on the efficacy and effectiveness for treating male orgasmic disorder. Masters and Johnson (1970) reported that when using their standard sex therapy techniques, 14 of 17 men treated for orgasm difficulties were able to attain orgasm during some form of stimulation. Hawton and Catalan (1986) used these same therapeutic techniques and were able to achieve some success with one of five men being able to mostly overcome his orgasmic dysfunction.

Other research has presented case studies outlining successful treatment for male orgasmic dysfunction. One study combining play therapy (e.g., using paradox, reframing, assigning games for homework between the man and his partner) with cognitive restructuring techniques showed improvement in men's ability to attain orgasm due to partner stimulation (Shaw, 1990). LoPiccolo and Stock (1986) suggest that male orgasmic disorder should be treated similarly to female orgasmic disorder. Because it is thought that male orgasmic disorder may stem from medical or surgical conditions complicating the ejaculatory response (LoPiccolo and Stock, 1986), research involving medical interventions is also important for understanding what types of treatment are effective for this disorder. However, to date, there have been no randomized controlled studies examining the efficacy of the procedures outlined for treating male orgasmic disorder.

Low sexual desire and aversion to sex

The disorders of low sexual desire and aversion to sex are treated similarly. Studies that have examined treatment efficacy have focused on cases of low sexual desire. However, there are no randomized control studies that provide definitive evidence for the efficacy of any specific treatment. There is support for treatment approaches that include cognitive, behavioral, and systemic interventions.

One study, using a general sex therapy format outlined by Masters and Johnson (1970), supported the use of the treatment for women with low desire (Hawton and Catalan, 1986). Specifically, they found that 56% of women who completed treatment were able to overcome or mostly overcome their desire problems. Another study evaluated the efficacy of the treatment model that is outlined by LoPiccolo and Friedman (1988). Specifically, the research supported the use of the model for increasing the frequency of sex and marital and sexual satisfaction (Schover and LoPiccolo, 1982). Other research involving low sexual desire involves case studies and techniques that have not been empirically validated.

Key practice principles for sex therapy

Female arousal and orgasmic disorders

The standard treatment used for women with female arousal and orgasmic disorder was first described by LoPiccolo and Lobitz (1972) and was later made into a guided self-help book (Heiman and LoPiccolo, 1988). A video is also available that was produced by The Sinclair Institute in consultation with LoPiccolo (1993) that goes through the treatment step by step. The treatment program follows a nine-step model. In the first step, the woman is taught to examine her genitals with a mirror. The goal is for the woman to not only become more familiar with her genitals, but to also become more familiar and accepting of all aspects of her body.

The second step follows with exploring the whole body not just visually but with touch. Women who have global lifelong anorgasmia may experience touching their genitalia for the first time during this step. The third step involves touching the erogenous zones that are present in the body. The woman is encouraged to use lotion or oils to increase the pleasurable sensations. Step 4 involves focusing on those areas of pleasure that were uncovered in step 3. These areas often include the breasts, labia, inner thighs, and clitoris. Step 5 continues this process by encouraging the woman to continue with her pleasurable exploration but to focus on intensely stimulating these areas while using erotic fantasies, explicit literature or photographs.

A woman may reach orgasm during step 5. However, if she does not, step 6 often helps the woman to overcome other inhibitions she has about attaining orgasm. A first task prescribed during step 6 involves role-playing what the woman thinks it would be like to have an orgasm. The therapist should encourage the woman to greatly exaggerate achieving orgasm. It is thought that by doing the role-play the woman will no longer feel inhibited to actually achieve an orgasm.

A second task that is prescribed during this step is to educate the woman about orgasm triggers. It should be noted that these are helpful if performed during a high state of arousal, but can actually serve to hinder the arousal level if performed prematurely. The most effective of these triggers involves taking a breath, tipping the head far back, and pushing down with the diaphragm without letting any air escape. A final technique that is introduced to the woman at this time is the use of a vibrator.

In step 7 the woman demonstrates to her partner how she can bring herself to orgasm. In order to make this step more comfortable for the woman, it is encouraged that the partner first demonstrates how he likes to touch himself. Step 8 follows with the woman teaching her partner how to stimulate her. She should guide his hand and talk to him about what feels good to her. In step 9, the woman and her partner are encouraged to try different positions for intercourse, which allow for direct stimulation of the woman's clitoris to help in achieving orgasm.

While this is the standard program for women who experience global lifelong anorgasmia, the treatment must at times be modified to aid women who have situational orgasmic dysfunction. In the example that follows, the treatment is described in a modified manner for a woman who experiences situational orgasmic dysfunction.

Case example

LoPiccolo (in press) describes the case of Helen. Helen and Bob appeared for therapy after 14 years of marriage. Helen is 37 years old. Her presenting complaint was that she is unable to experience orgasm with Bob. She further explained that she does have orgasm when she masturbates alone. Helen began to masturbate at about age 9. Initially, this masturbation was just pressing her thighs together and squeezing her nipples. By her early teenage

years, Helen began to lie face down, with her ankles crossed. One hand squeezed and caressed her nipples, while the other caressed her stomach. She pressed her thighs together while she rocked and arched her body on the bed. Helen and Bob explained that they tried caressing her clitoris, without effect. They also tried having him present while she masturbated, which effectively prevented her from becoming aroused. They even tried including her masturbation into their lovemaking. Helen had been masturbating in this way, at a frequency of one to as much as three times per week, for more than 20 years at the time that therapy began.

As a first step in achieving stimulus generalization, Helen was asked to masturbate in the same way as usual except uncross her ankles. Once orgasm was occurring easily in this way, a second change was made. This was to have Helen turn over and lie face up rather than face down while masturbating. Once Helen was able to achieve orgasm in this position, Helen was told to place her fingers on her clitoris and labia as she performed her thigh pressure. At first Helen reported that this caused her to lose arousal, so she was instructed to switch back to thigh pressure only to regain her arousal. After a few sessions using this procedure, she was able to reach an orgasm.

Next, Helen was asked to caress her genitals while using her thigh pressure masturbation. She was again instructed to switch back and forth between thigh pressure only and caressing if she began to lose her arousal. After orgasm was achieved in this manner, Helen was asked to spread her legs apart. She was to alternate between caressing her genitals only and adding thigh pressure when necessary to the genital caressing. When she was about to achieve orgasm, Helen was instructed to spread her legs and use the orgasm triggers without thigh pressure. Helen was able eventually to achieve orgasm by clitoral stimulation without any thigh pressure.

The next steps involved Bob. Assessment had not revealed any couple systemic issues in this case, but having Bob in the room while Helen was trying to achieve orgasm was difficult for her. Bob showed Helen how he was able to masturbate to orgasm, but each time Helen masturbated with Bob present, she was able to experience arousal but not orgasm. Because a new pattern of orgasmic response had already been established for Helen, switching back to thigh pressure masturbation was not recommended. Instead, first Bob then Helen role-played the exaggerated orgasm response. However, Helen still did not achieve an orgasm.

At this point Helen made a suggestion. Helen stated that she would like to masturbate using genital caressing only with Bob holding and kissing her as they had been doing. However, after she was aroused she wanted Bob to leave the room to allow her to masturbate alone. Once she began to have the orgasm, she would call out to Bob, and he would be able to enter the room, and for the first time ever be able to see her having a real orgasm. This procedure worked, and Helen and Bob were able successfully to overcome Helen's orgasmic dysfunction.

As was illustrated in the case example, the client and the therapist must work together to achieve the best treatment protocol. Because Helen and Bob had tried clitoral stimulation to no avail on their own, it was important for the therapist to not re-prescribe a treatment approach that was destined to fail. The standard protocol for orgasmic dysfunction was modified so that Helen gradually switched from her thigh pressure masturbation to masturbation while stimulating her clitoris. This resulted in successful treatment for Helen's situational orgasmic dysfunction.

Vaginismus

The standard treatment for vaginismus involves the insertion of dilators of increasing size into the vagina (LoPiccolo and Stock, 1986; Leiblum, 2000). The treatment described here also involves gaining control of the pelvic muscles through practice procedures (LoPiccolo, 1984). Treatment focuses on the goal of helping the couple to be able to have intercourse.

It is first recommended that a thorough history is taken to best diagnose from where the vaginismus stems. The woman begins treatment by learning to gain control of all of her muscles. However, the most relevant muscle for treating vaginismus is the pubococcygeal muscle. Deep muscle relaxation is taught to the client. This is followed by exercises that contract and relax the pubococcygeal muscle. These exercises aid in the insertion of the dilators.

The woman is then given dilators that progress in size to insert into her vagina. The woman is asked to spend 30 minutes or more a night practicing the insertion of the dilator. Once a dilator has been successfully inserted and feels comfortable to the woman, she is allowed to move to the next sized dilator. Once the woman has successfully inserted all the dilators, her partner is encouraged progressively to insert the dilators into her vagina. The final stage of treatment involves intercourse. First, the woman's partner lies passively on his back while the woman kneels above him and gradually inserts his penis. The therapist should stress the need for effective stimulation of the woman in order to encourage the connection between sex and pleasure. Once the woman is able to insert the penis fully, she is encouraged to move while she is on top. Later he can move too, and finally they can try different positions when the woman is comfortable with the change.

Dyspareunia

The treatment for dyspareunia often involves both medical and psychological aspects. It is often the case that women with dyspareunia undergo a surgical procedure called a vestibulectomy, which corrects the vulvar vestibulitis responsible for the pain the woman is experiencing (Binik *et al.*, 2000). However, therapy is often a necessary follow-up to aid the woman in overcoming any residual problems (Schover *et al.*, 1992).

The therapy that is recommended combines treatment procedures specified for female arousal and orgasmic disorders (Bergeron *et al.*, 2001) as well as vaginismus. After diagnosing the contributing factors, techniques involving relaxation, focusing specifically on the pubococcygeal muscle, as well as education about the woman's body are used. Other procedures involve identifying factors that contribute to arousal and dilator insertion to achieve successful intercourse. For specific procedures see the sections on female arousal and orgasmic disorders and vaginismus.

Male erectile disorder

Male erectile disorder can involve psychological, neurological, vascular, and hormonal problems (Carson *et al.*, 1999). Because there are a multitude of factors that can contribute to the problem, both psychotherapeutic and medical interventions are used to treat the problem. Medical procedures used to address erectile disorder are implantation of a penile prosthesis, use of a vacuum erection device, injection with medication, vascular surgery to remove blocked arteries or remedy other problems, and the use of Sildenafil citrate (i.e., Viagra). For a review of these procedures see LoPiccolo (1998) and Rosen (2000); however, the use of Viagra in conjunction with therapy for erectile dysfunction will be addressed.

The introduction of Viagra for the treatment of erectile disorder has significantly affected therapeutic procedures. Viagra was introduced to the public in 1998. Since then, it has become widely prescribed in the treatment of erectile dysfunction. It is highly effective in men with organic, psychogenic, or mixed impairments resulting in significantly better effects than a placebo (Shabsigh, 1999). Because Viagra works by physiologically aiding the man to get an erection when there is sexual stimulation present, the man is more easily able to overcome his performance anxiety. Viagra is a highly effective treatment for erectile disorder when the assessment indicates its use.

It is often the case that psychotherapy is used along with Viagra to best aid men with erectile dysfunction. The standard psychotherapeutic treatment for erectile disorder involves reducing anxiety and increasing the amount of sexual stimulation the man is receiving. It is indicated for couples who have cognitive, behavioral, or systemic problems that contribute to the erectile disorder. During the first phase of treatment, the anxiety the couple or individual feels about sexual intercourse is discussed. A standard treatment for helping to reduce the anxiety felt by the male is sensate focus (Masters and Johnson, 1970). Sensate focus consists of instructing the client to relax, enjoy the sensual massage, and not to expect to get an erection. LoPiccolo (in press) points out that in this day of 'pop' psychology procedures, sensate focus does not always work to reduce anxiety because the man then gets anxious about not feeling relaxed enough to get an erection.

An alternative way to help the man to reduce his anxiety comes from his partner reassuring him that her sexual gratification is not dependent upon him having an erection. If the partner can stress to the man that she enjoys the orgasms she receives due to his manual or oral stimulation of her genitals, this will greatly reduce his performance anxiety. Sometimes, however, it is not as easy for the woman to make this statement. It is important to examine the woman's reasons for her sexual gratification being so dependent upon her husband's erection, and, if possible, resolve these therapeutically to aid the man's performance anxiety. Some reasons that a woman may not be satisfied by sexual acts other than intercourse may include age-related stereotypes about a male's role, lack of experience with other manners of love-making, or religious 'taboos'.

Increasing the amount of direct stimulation of the penis is often another important factor in remedying erectile disorder. If a man has some organic impairment, simply reducing his anxiety about getting an erection will not result in an erection. Also, as erectile disorder is more common in aging men, and the erection response is more dependent upon direct stimulation as a man gets older, it is important to educate the client and his partner about appropriate stimulation of the penis. If couples have used direct stimulation before, it is stressed that it needs to take place for a longer period of time in order for the man to maintain an erection. For couples who are reluctant to use direct penile stimulation, this issue needs to be dealt with therapeutically looking at any relationship or history variables that may contribute to the reluctance.

Premature ejaculation

The standard treatment for premature ejaculation involves techniques developed by Semans (1956) and Masters and Johnson (1970). Treatment begins by using the pause and squeeze technique during manual stimulation of the penis. If the man masturbates regularly or does not have a partner, he can do the technique by himself. However, the procedure is also recommended with a partner. First, the man's partner is instructed to stimulate his penis manually. The man is instructed to gauge his sexual arousal during this process. When he reaches a high level of arousal, about a 6–8 on a scale of 10, he is to instruct his partner to stop. They wait until the man's level of arousal has decreased and repeat the procedure up to four more times before allowing the man to ejaculate.

Masters and Johnson (1970) added to this procedure the squeeze technique. Directly after the couple pauses from stimulating the man, the penis is to be squeezed firmly at the point where the head of the penis joins the shaft. This technique helps in reducing sexual arousal at a quicker rate and should then be followed by the pause. When the pause and squeeze technique results in less rapid ejaculation for the man, the couple is instructed to do the procedure during intercourse.

There are some special factors to keep in mind during treatment. If a man has a low frequency of sex and/or masturbation, it can be helpful to increase the frequency of either in order to help decrease time to ejaculation. Also, it is sometimes found that the partners of men presenting with premature ejaculation are reluctant to participate in therapy. In these instances, it is helpful to set aside times when the man is in charge of performing pleasurable activities for his partner to increase her desire to participate in therapy (LoPiccolo, in press). This usually results in the woman cooperatively participating in therapy.

Male orgasmic disorder

Although men presenting with male orgasmic disorder often have a neurological or physiological problem associated with their inability to attain orgasm (Rosen, 1991), there are psychological treatments available. Generally, male inorgasmia is treated similarly to female inorgasmia (LoPiccolo and Stock, 1986). Treatment procedures involve, first, addressing cognitive issues that may contribute to inorgasmia. Some common issues include anxiety about performing, fear of having children, not being sexually attracted to a partner, or issues of power and control in the relationship.

Next, it is important to address the amount and type of stimulation that the man is getting during sexual activity. It is often necessary to increase the types of stimulation applied directly to the penis. Manual or oral stimulation can be added during foreplay to increase the man's arousal level. Also, as many men presenting with male orgasmic disorder have some neurological or physiological complicating factors, men are taught orgasms triggers, such as bearing down while holding their breath and throwing their head backwards. Another treatment factor that can aid in orgasm is the use of a vibrator, specifically used around the scrotum or perianal area.

Low sexual desire and aversion to sex

The disorders of low sexual desire and aversion to sex can be especially hard to treat. They rely on the therapist's skill to engage the client so that he or she does not feel that therapy is only for the benefit of the partner's sex life. One way to begin to engage the client and his or her partner at the start of therapy is to have them make two lists of possible gains and losses if therapy is successful, one pertaining to the relationship and one pertaining to the individual (LoPiccolo, in press). It may also be necessary to help the client redefine the problem and educate the client on the sexual drive (LoPiccolo, in press).

Therapy can then begin with the program for low sexual desire outlined by LoPiccolo and Friedman (1988). The model is a four-stage program. The first stage, affectual awareness, focuses on the emotions involved with having sex. As most clients deny that they have any negative feelings toward sex, the therapist disputes this stressing the biological evidence for a sex drive and reasons that can interfere with being aware of this drive. The lists the clients made of gains and losses of acquiring a sex drive can be helpful during this stage of therapy.

The second stage, insight, involves the client gaining an understanding of what first contributed to the low sex drive and what has maintained this condition. The third stage of therapy involves different cognitive and systemic techniques to help the client deal with the initial contributing factors and negative emotions associated with sex. Systemic techniques are then used to help the client and his or her partner deal with the maintaining or current causes of the low drive.

The final stage of therapy, drive induction, involves behavioral interventions. The client is asked to start noticing external cues to become aware of his or her sex drive. At first, the person may be asked to keep a 'desire diary' where s/he keeps track of instances when they notice sexually relevant clues (e.g., movie scenes). As therapy progresses the person may be asked to write erotic fantasies. Furthermore, tasks to enable the low drive client to become aware of and enjoy sensual rather than sexual pleasure are important. Both partners must agree that any sexual activity initiation must be verbal. Once that is agreed upon, the low drive client is asked to identify sensual activities (e.g., kissing, dancing) that s/he would like to do with his or her partner. Once these activities have been identified, the low drive person is encouraged to take the lead in initiating any of the sensual behaviors.

The clients are then trained to initiate sexual activity in different ways than before. First the low drive patient role-plays how his or her partner had initiated sex in the past that resulted in a negative or hurtful emotional response. Next the client demonstrates how s/he would prefer the partner to initiate sex. The partner is then asked to role-play the client refusing to make love in a way that was hurtful in the past. Next, the partner is to role-play an acceptable way for the partner to turn down an invitation to make love.

The sexual activities being participated in by the couple up to this point depend on the couple. However, for clients who experience sexual aversion, therapy tends to take more time. Often clients who feel an aversion to sex know what this emotion stems from. More time is spent, often, during stages 2 and 3 of therapy to work through these negative emotions and thoughts. In the most severe cases, the aversion is the result of sexual abuse either as a child or adult. If this is the case, the therapies outlined by Courtois (1988) for child sexual abuse survivors or Foa (1997) for rape survivors are recommended.

Challenges in treating sexual dysfunction

Two challenges that are relevant to all sexual disorders are an unwillingness of one member of the couple to work on the problem or an ongoing affair.

If, during the initial interview, it is brought forth that one member of the couple is unwilling to work toward remedying the problem or one member is having an affair, this must be dealt immediately. If one member of the couple does not want to put forth the effort to work on the problem, the therapist should stress that this may not be the best time for the couple to be in therapy. If it is revealed that one member of the couple is having an affair, the spouse that is having the affair must be told that s/he must stop the affair or at least stop it for the duration of therapy. If the spouse will not agree, the therapist must reconvene with both spouses and explain that therapy cannot continue to address the sexual dysfunction because, it seems to the therapist, there are other marital problems that need to be addressed before the therapy can be helpful (LoPiccolo, in press).

Female arousal and orgasmic disorders

Some clients present with special cases of orgasmic dysfunction that rely on the therapist to be able to change subtly the treatment model to best aid the client and her partner. These special cases include reaching orgasm only through the use of a vibrator or through some form of thigh pressure masturbation. Modification of the model for women who use thigh pressure masturbation was demonstrated in the case of Helen and Bob. For those women who can obtain an orgasm only through the use of a vibrator, they are encouraged to stop the use of a vibrator completely and start the treatment protocol beginning with the first step.

Another challenge to the therapist treating orgasmic dysfunction and arousal disorders is the notion that all women must have an orgasm during intercourse. In fact, many women do not have orgasms during intercourse, and this failure to achieve orgasm is often due to a lack of direct stimulation of the clitoris during coitus. If orgasm can be achieved during manual or oral stimulation and is satisfactory to the woman, this should be regarded as a therapeutic success.

Vaginismus and dyspareunia

A main challenge to the therapist treating vaginismus and/or dyspareunia is the differential diagnosis of the disorders. Because the disorders are so similar, it is often hard for the treating therapist to ensure that s/he is following the best procedure to aid the client. It is also difficult to ensure that clients are getting the best treatment available because there seem to be both psychological and physiological factors that complicate the situation. It has been suggested that to understand better the pain disorders described by women, the disorders should be reconceptualized as genital pain disorders that can interfere not only with sexual activity but also any penetration that affects the genitalia (Binik et al., 2000). Because there are no controlled outcome studies examining the effectiveness of any medical or psychological interventions for the disorders, therapists must use the current classification system that is available to best treat their clients.

Male erectile disorder

Two main challenges in treating erectile dysfunction come from age related issues and the increased medicalization of treatment. Many people who present for treatment of erectile dysfunction are older. Engaging the partner in treatment can be especially hard in an older couple. It is often seen that the women in these relationships were raised with the idea that real men do not need help to get an erection. It is important to spend time thoroughly educating the clients about the erection response and what can be expected now and as the man continues to age.

Another challenge to the therapist treating erectile dysfunction can come from Viagra. One problem occurs if the man has low sexual desire. If he does not want to be having sex, but the pill makes him get an erection, he will avoid taking the pill. This can then lead to other marital problems, including fights about him not taking his pill. Another contraindication for the use of Viagra occurs when the systemic problems of the couple's relationship are the only problems contributing to the erectile failure. It is important for the therapist treating erectile disorder to take all of these factors into consideration when recommending treatment for the client.

Premature ejaculation and male orgasmic disorder

The main challenge for the therapist treating premature ejaculation presents in the form of maintaining long-term treatment effects. Research has shown that the immediate benefits of treatment are helpful, but over time, many men return to their pretreatment conditions (D'Amicis *et al.*, 1985). One way to remedy this problem is to ensure that during therapy the clients return to their previous frequency of sexual activity while continuing with the therapeutic techniques (LoPiccolo, in press). This helps to ensure that when the clients leave therapy, the results that were shown were not just artifacts of the higher frequency of sexual activity initiated during treatment.

Male orgasmic disorder is so rarely seen in sex therapy clinics, that having a client with this disorder is a challenge in itself. There are many recommendations about how to treat this problem, but there is no clear research on what works with these clients. As with erectile dysfunction, the partners of these men may challenge the need for the client to have different forms of stimulation to aid in the ejaculation response. It is important to work with the clients in educating them about what is currently known of the dysfunction, and trying different techniques in order to find what will best help the client to reach orgasm.

Low sexual desire and aversion to sex

The main challenge to the therapist treating low sexual desire and aversion to sex is the complex psychological issues that accompany these problems. Treatment is usually longer term than most other sex therapy (LoPiccolo, in press). It often takes a long amount of time to work with the client on the negative feelings s/he associates with sexual activity. It is also hard to engage the client in therapy because these clients do not necessarily want to regain or gain a desire for sexual activity. They may believe that their partners will be the ones mainly benefiting from the therapy because the end result will be them getting what they want (i.e., sex). For these reasons, the initial stage of therapy, affectual awareness, is paramount in order to identify potential issues that the client may use to later hinder therapy.

Conclusions

The field of sex therapy continues to be encroached upon by the many medical treatments. There is often more funding available to study the effects of different drugs on sexual problems than on therapy for sexual problems. However, researchers are cautioning the increased medicalization of treatment for sexual dysfunction (e.g., Bancroft, 2002). This chapter illustrates that for all sexual dysfunctions, a therapeutic component helps to remedy the problem. Psychotherapy for sexual disorders utilizing cognitive, behavioral, and systemic techniques is most effective. Therapies for female orgasmic disorder and premature ejaculation are well established in the literature. Therapies for desire disorders, erectile disorder, male orgasmic disorder, and pain disorders all show support for remedying the existing problems. In the future, it will be important for researchers and therapists to focus on what types of treatment work best for clients. As some disorders have greater influence from physiological factors and some have greater influence from psychological factors, treatment could be matched to best aid the client.

References

American Psychiatric Association (1994). *Diagnostic and statistical manual of mental disorders*, 4th edn. Washington, DC: American Psychiatric Association.

Bancroft, J. (2002). The medicalization of female sexual dysfunction: the need for caution. *Archives of Sexual Behavior*, **31**, 451–5.

Bergeron, S., *et al.* (2001). A randomized comparison of group cognitive-behavioral therapy, surface electromyographic feedback, and vestibulectomy in the treatment of dyspareunia resulting from vulvar vestibulitis. *Pain*, **91**, 297–306.

Binik, Y., Bergeron, S., and Khalife, S. (2000). Dyspareunia. In: S. R. Leiblum and R. C. Rosen, ed. *Principles and practices of sex therapy*, 3rd edn. New York: Guilford Press.

Carson, C. C., Kirby, R. S., and Goldstein, I., ed. (1999). *Textbook of male erectile dysfunction*. Oxford: Isis Media Ltd.

Courtois, C. (1988). *Healing the incest wound: adult survivors of therapy*. New York: Norton.

D'Amicis, L., Goldberg, D., Lopiccolo, J., Friedman, J., and Davies, L. (1985). Clinical follow-up of couples treated for sexual dysfunction. *Archives of Sexual Behavior*, **14**, 467–89.

Ellis, A. (1962). *Reason and emotion in psychotherapy*. New York: Lyle Stewart.

Foa, E. B. (1997). *Treating the trauma of rape*. New York: Guilford Press.

Freud, S. (1905/1965). *Three essays on the theory of female sexuality*. New York: Avon.

Gabbard, G. O. (2000). *Psychodynamic psychiatry in clinical practice*, 3rd edn. Washington, DC: American Psychiatric Press, Inc.

Goldman, A. and Carroll, J. (1990). Educational intervention as an adjunct to treatment of erectile dysfunction in older couples. *Journal of Sex and Marital Therapy*, **16**, 127–41.

Hawton, K. and Catalan, J. (1986). Prognostic factors in sex therapy. *Behavior Research and Therapy*, **24**, 377–85.

Heiman, J. R. (2002). Psychologic treatments for female sexual dysfunction: are they effective and do we need them? *Archives of Sexual Behavior*, **31**, 445–50.

Heiman, J. R. and LoPiccolo, J. (1988). *Becoming orgasmic: a personal and sexual growth program for women*. Englewood Cliffs, NJ: Prentice-Hall Press.

Kaplan, H. (1974). *The new sex therapy*. New York: Brunner/Mazel.

Kegel, A. H. (1952). Sexual functions of the pubococcygeus muscle. *Western Journal of Surgery in Obstetrics and Gynaecology*, **60**, 521–4.

Kilmann, P. and Auerbach, R. (1979). Treatments for premature ejaculation and psychogenic impotence: a critical review of the literature. *Archives of Sexual Behavior*, **8**, 81–100.

Kilmann, P., *et al.* (1987). Group treatment of secondary erectile dysfunction. *Journal of Sex and Marital Therapy*, **13**, 168–82.

Laumnann, E. O., Paik, A., and Rosen, R. C. (1999). Sexual dysfunction in the United States: prevalence and predictors. *Journal of the American Medical Association*, **281**, 537–44.

Leiblum, S. R. (2000). Vaginismus: a most perplexing problem. In: S. R. Leiblum and R. C. Rosen, ed. *Principles and practices of sex therapy*, 3rd edn. New York: Guilford Press.

LoPiccolo, J. (1984). *Treating vaginismus* (video). New York: Multifocus.

LoPiccolo, J. (1992). Post-modern sex therapy for erectile failure. In: R. C. Rosen and S. R. Leiblum, ed. *Erectile failure: assessment and treatment*, pp. 171–97. New York: Guilford Press.

LoPiccolo, J. (1993). *Becoming orgasmic: a personal and sexual growth program for women* (video). Chapel Hill, NC: The Sinclair Institute.

LoPiccolo, J. (2002). Post-modern sex therapy. In: F. Kaslow, editor in chief. *Comprehensive handbook of psychotherapy*, Vol. 4. New York: John Wiley and Sons.

LoPiccolo, J. and Friedman, J. (1988). Broad spectrum treatment of low sexual desire: integration of cognitive, behavioral and systemic therapy. In: S. Leiblum and R. Rosen, ed. *Assessment and treatment of desire disorders*, pp. 107–44. New York: Guilford Press.

LoPiccolo, J. and Lobitz, W. C. (1972). The role of masturbation in the treatment of orgasmic dysfunction. *Archives of Sexual Behavior*, **2**, 163–71.

LoPiccolo, J. and Stock, W. E. (1986). Treatment of sexual dysfunction. *Journal of Consulting and Clinical Psychology*, **54**, 158–67.

Masters, W. H. and Johnson, V. E. (1966). *Human sexual response*. Boston: Little Brown.

Masters, W. H. and Johnson, V. E. (1970). *Human sexual inadequacy*. Boston: Little Brown.

McGovern, K., Stewart, R., and LoPiccolo, J. (1975). Secondary orgasmic dysfunction: Analysis and strategies for treatment. *Archives of Sexual Behavior*, **4**, 265.

Morokoff, P. J. and LoPiccolo, J. (1986). A comparative evaluation of minimal therapist contact and 15 session treatment for female orgasmic dysfunction. *Journal of Consulting and Clinical Psychology*, **54**, 294–300.

Price, S. C., Reynolds, B., Cohen, B., Anderson, A., and Schochet, B. (1981). Group treatment of erectile dysfunction for men without partners: a controlled evaluation. *Archives of Sexual Behavior*, **10**, 253–68.

Riley, A. J. and Riley, E. J. (1978). A controlled study to evaluate directed masturbation in the management of primary orgasmic failure in women. *British Journal of Psychiatry*, **135**, 404–9.

Rosen, I. (1982). The psychoanalytical approach. *British Journal of Psychiatry*, **140**, 85–93.

Rosen, R. (2000). Medical and psychological interventions for erectile dysfunction: toward a combined treatment approach. In: S. R. Leiblum and R. C. Rosen, ed. *Principles and practices of sex therapy*, 3rd edn. New York: Guilford Press.

Rosen, R. C. and Leiblum, S. R. (1995). Treatment of sexual disorders in the 1990s: an integrated approach. *Journal of Consulting and Clinical Psychology*, **63**, 877–90.

Rosen, R. C., Taylor, J. F., Leiblum, S. R., and Bachman, G. A. (1993). Prevalence of sexual dysfunction in women: results of a survey of 329 women in an outpatient gynecological clinic. *Journal of Sex and Marital Therapy*, **19**, 171–88.

Schnarch, D. M. (1991). *Constructing the sexual crucible: an integration of sexual and marital therapy*. New York: Norton.

Schnarch, L. R. (2000). Desire problems: a systemic perspective. In: S. R. Leiblum and R. C. Rosen, ed. *Principles and practices of sex therapy*, 3rd edn. New York: Guilford Press.

Schneidman, B. and McGuire, L. (1976). Group therapy for nonorgasmic women: two age levels. *Archives of Sexual Behavior*, **5**, 239–48.

Schover, L. R. (1984). *Prime time: sexual health for men over fifty*. New York: Holt Rhinehart, and Winston.

Schover, L. R. and LoPiccolo, J. (1982). Treatment effectiveness for dysfunctions of sexual desire. *Journal of Sex and Marital Therapy*, **8**, 179–97.

Schover, L. R., Youngs, D. D., and Cannata, R. (1992). Psychosexual aspects of the evaluation and management of vulvar vestibulitis. *American Journal of Obstetrics and Gynecology*, **167**, 630–8.

Semans, J. H. (1956). Premature ejaculation: a new approach. *Southern Medical Journal*, **49**, 355–7.

Shabsigh, R. (1999). Efficacy of Sildenafil citrate (Viagra) is not affected by aetiology of erectile dysfunction. *International Journal of Clinical Practice, Supplement*, **102**, 19–20.

Shaw, J. (1990). Play therapy with the sexual workhorse: successful treatment with twelve cases of inhibited ejaculation. *Journal of Sex and Marital Therapy*, **16**, 159–64.

Spector, I. and Carey, M. (1990). Incidence and prevalence of the sexual dysfunctions: a critical review of the empirical literature. *Archives of Sexual Behavior*, **19**, 389–96.

Steege, J. F. and Ling, F. W. (1993). Dyspareunia: a special type of chronic pelvic pain. *Obstetrics and Gynecology Clinics of North America*, **20**, 750–9.

Wallace, O. and Barbach, L. (1974). Preorgasmic group treatment. *Journal of Sex and Marital Therapy*, **1**, 146–54.

Whitaker, C. A. and Keith, D. V. (1981). Symbolic experiential family therapy. In: S. Gurman and D. P. Kniskern, ed. *Handbook of family therapy*, pp. 187–225. New York: Brunner/Mazel.

Wilinsky, M. and Myers, M. F. (1987). Retarded ejaculation in homosexual patients: a report of nine cases. *Journal of Sex Research*, **23**, 85–91.

Wolpe, J. (1958). *Psychotherapy by reciprocal inhibition*. Stanford, CA: Stanford University Press.

19 Individual psychotherapy and counseling for addiction

Delinda Mercer and George E. Woody

Counseling and psychotherapy are critical components of effective treatments for addictions and have been among the most widely used types of interventions for treatment of addiction. Previously, psychosocial interventions often comprised the entire program (Onken and Blaine, 1990); however, the introduction of new medications and other new types of interventions have led to a more multimodality treatment approach that can simultaneously address the biochemical, psychological, and behavioral aspects of addiction.

As addiction to substances is a very heterogeneous disorder, there are many different approaches to using psychotherapy and/or counseling in its treatment, and thus no single treatment would be expected to be appropriate for all individuals. For example, there are numerous types of addictive drugs: stimulants, narcotics, hallucinogens, and nicotine, to name a few. In addition, the demographic, psychosocial, and personality characteristics patients vary as does the severity of their addiction. People also have a variety of co-occurring mental or physical health problems. Common psychiatric problems are anxiety and depression. Some drug-related physical ailments include poor nutrition, liver problems, and chronic pain. Among injection drug users, the blood-borne infections, hepatitis B and C and HIV are concerns.

Increased recognition of the magnitude of addiction as a public health problem has led to increased interest in effective treatments among all who are involved in the provision of health care. Among these have been studies on a wide range of psychosocial treatments including psychotherapy and counseling, as well as studies on their use in combination with pharmacotherapies. This chapter will review studies on individual psychotherapy and counseling for addictions and will include comments on the relative benefits of each approach, the rationale for using psychotherapy, the pharmacology of abused drugs, 12-step programs, treatment settings, duration, frequency and intensity of treatment, family involvement, therapeutic alliance, HIV risk reduction, major models of psychotherapy, and research on treatment for specific drugs, research implications for treatment, and key practice principles. We will conclude by illustrating some examples of treatment challenges and what to do about them through clinical vignettes.

Psychotherapy versus counseling

The term, 'psychotherapy,' describes a psychological treatment that aims to change problematic thoughts, feelings, and behaviors by creating a new understanding of the thoughts and feelings that appear to be causally related to the problem(s). The patient is led to ask, 'Why do I use drugs?' The psychotherapy addresses the underlying addictive behaviors and the thoughts and feelings that appear to promote, maintain, or occur as a result. A goal is to help the patient resolve some of the associated problems so that he/she will no longer need to self-medicate to feel relief. Along with the goal of ceasing drug self-administration, psychotherapy addresses issues related to other problematic aspects of patients' lives, both past and present, whether these problems contribute to drug abuse or not.

Addiction counseling, rather than psychotherapy, is the most widely used psychosocial intervention in substance abuse treatment. It differs from psychotherapy by being fairly directive and focusing on managing current problems related to drug use rather than exploring internal, intrapsychic processes. The client would ask, 'Which people, places, and things make me feel like using drugs?' 'How can I avoid those people, places, and things?' 'How can I change my life so that I reduce the urge to use drugs?' 'Who can I turn to when I feel the need to use drugs?' 'Addiction counseling' is the management of addiction, by giving support, structure, monitoring behavior, encouraging abstinence, and providing concrete services such as referrals for job counseling, medical services, or legal aid. This approach often uses the language and concepts of the 12-step program developed by Alcoholics Anon-ymous.

Increasingly, some methods used in addiction counseling and psychotherapy have merged in the actual practice of treatment. Effective therapists and counselors employ similar basic counseling skills, regardless of therapeutic orientation. These would include among other things active listening, empathy, and support. In addition to basic counseling skills, there are strategies or tools that are associated with specific theories of therapy. For example, identifying the precipitants to relapse is basically a cognitive intervention, while practicing refusing an offer of drugs is skill building, which is a behavioral intervention yet each of these techniques is often used in both psychotherapy and counseling.

Rationale for using psychotherapy to treat addiction

Many addicts will self-administer drugs to reduce stress. This same constellation of symptoms can be more appropriately addressed with psychotherapy. For example, opioids have potent sedative and analgesic effects, stimulants can enhance mood and benzodiazepines reduce anxiety. In this sense, psychological factors such as anxiety, anger, and depression may encourage drug use as an attempt to escape from painful subjective experiences (Khantzian and Khantzian, 1984; Khantzian, 1985).

Studies have consistently shown that high levels of comorbidity exist between substance use and a wide range of other psychiatric problems, many of which meet symptomatic and duration criteria for DSM (*Diagnostic and statistical manual of mental disorders*)-III-R or DSM-IV diagnoses (American Psychiatric Association, 1987, 1994) (Rounsaville *et al.*, 1982, 1991; Woody *et al.*, 1983, 1990a,b; Khantzian and Treece, 1985; Weiss *et al.*, 1986; Kessler *et al.*, 1996). Major depression, dysthymia, posttraumatic stress disorder, and generalized anxiety disorder commonly co-occur with addiction. Because chronic use of most abused drugs (with the possible exception of opioids and nicotine) will magnify or even produce psychiatric symptoms, it is often difficult to determine which symptoms represent independent psychiatric disorders and represent substance-induced conditions.

However, whether emotional symptoms are drug related or represent independent disorders, studies have shown that they have prognostic significance (Woody *et al.*, 1985, 1990a,b; Carroll *et al.*, 1995). This finding is especially relevant to psychotherapeutic approaches for treating substance use disorders, because the psychotherapies were developed specifically to address such emotional symptoms. When viewed in this way, the presence of psychiatric symptoms in the context of a substance use disorder identifies a subgroup of patients that may benefit from a combination approach that includes a drug-focused intervention such as methadone maintenance, and psychotherapy.

Familiarity with the pharmacology of abused drugs

Knowledge of the pharmacological effects of the various drugs of abuse is basic to treating addiction, regardless of the therapeutic approach or orientation. Nonmedically trained clinicians need to become aware of these effects, their routes of administration, drug combinations that are commonly used, and the typical patterns of use. Clinicians need to recognize the clinical presentations of intoxication and the withdrawal syndromes for the major categories of abused drugs. They also need to know the effects of common drug combinations such as 'speedballing', which is taking an opiate with cocaine or amphetamines, or the popular pairing of cocaine with alcohol. Clinicians also need to know the potential health consequences, both emotional and physical, of using the different drugs of abuse. For example, clinicians should recognize the risk for paranoia and depression among cocaine users, the heightened risk of HIV among injection drug users from sharing injection equipment, and the increased risk for HIV among users of cocaine or amphetamines that is associated with their tendency to engage in high levels of unprotected sex.

Twelve-step programs

Studies have shown that 12-step participation is associated with improved outcomes. Twelve-step programs, such as Alcoholics Anon-ymous and Narcotics Anon-ymous, are abstinence oriented and foster a network of healthy social support. In addition, their philosophy imparts ideas that many recovering persons find helpful in dealing with everyday life and that appear to help establish and maintain a sober life-style. Also, they are widely available and free of charge.

Key aspects of the 12-step philosophy for therapists treating addiction are: (1) the belief that addiction is a disease, rather than bad behavior; (2) addiction damages the whole person, physically, mentally, and spiritually and that recovery must address all of those domains; (3) healing or recovery comes from connecting to something larger than oneself; (4) the paradox of surrendering power in order to ultimately be empowered to attain sobriety; (5) the idea that interpersonal support is critical for recovery; and (6) the belief that recovery is a lifelong process that encompasses continued personal growth.

Research has shown that frequency of attendance (Hoffman et al., 1983; Etheridge et al., 1999) and degree of participation (Weiss et al., 1996) in 12-step meetings is positively associated with treatment outcome, including preventing relapse (Fiorentine, 1999). As a result, these programs are strongly recommended by most addiction treatment programs (Fiorentine and Anglin, 1996). Furthermore these programs can easily be combined with psychotherapy or counseling, which seems to have an additive effect on enhancing outcomes (Fiorentine and Hillhouse, 2000). A recent study found that belief in the philosophy of the 12-step program improved drug use outcomes for patients receiving addiction counseling (Crits-Christoph et al., in press). There are other models of self-help programs, such as Rational Recovery and Women for Sobriety, but these tend to be less widely available and less well known. However, they also appear to foster continued recovery, and they may be a better 'fit' for some people than the 12-step programs.

Treatment settings

There are six common settings for the provision of substance abuse treatment, and any one can use psychotherapy or counseling. These are: (1) inpatient (within psychiatric or general hospitals); (2) penal institutions; (3) outpatient (clinics or private practice settings); (4) intensive outpatient programs (IOPs); (5) halfway houses; and (6) therapeutic communities. The philosophy of treatment varies by setting, and particular psychotherapeutic approaches may fit better into some programs than others but drug counseling would likely be part of the program in each setting. Some programs would also integrate psychotherapy, particularly for patients with additional psychiatric problems.

Urine drug testing, is traditionally associated with drug counseling but not with psychotherapy; however, it is recommended by most addiction treatment programs because it appears to increase program effectiveness, regardless of the setting. Urinalysis encourages honesty, and it helps hold the patient accountable for his or her behavior. It may also lead the recalcitrant patient to seek ways to evade detection of drug use and thus should be observed or monitored for urine temperature to ensure compliance. Prompt results and feedback on drug-positive and drug-negative urine samples often help the patient feel that the therapist is knowledgeable and concerned with his or her progress in recovery. Positive feedback given for negative urine samples reinforces continuing abstinence and recovery. In the case of a positive test or self-report, analysis of what led to the drug use combined with ways to avoid it in the future can be an important component of psychotherapy or counseling.

Drug treatment programs vary greatly in basic aspects of service delivery such as availability of psychiatric and medical services, control of behavior problems, level of illicit drug use, type of physical facilities, use of psychotropic drugs, level of staff morale, educational level of staff, and types of patients receiving treatment (Ball et al., 1986). These programmatic qualities may play a major part in the feasibility, efficacy, or relative importance that psychotherapy may have in different settings.

Duration, frequency, and intensity of psychotherapy

The 'dose' of psychotherapy or counseling necessary to produce improvement is unclear. Research looking at three different levels of counseling in methadone-maintained opiate addicts found that when the standard methadone maintenance was combined with enhanced psychosocial treatment, patients maintained a greater reduction in drug use (McLellan et al., 1993). Furthermore, the results showed a stepwise effect, such that the more psychosocial services provided, the greater the reduction in drug use. In other words, more treatment equated to a better result provided that the treatment was not just all the same (for example, 6 hours a day of just drug counseling) and that the services were useful and addressed specific, identified problem areas such as family interventions, vocational services, or psychiatric services delivered on site.

According to research on psychotherapy for methadone-maintained patients addicted to opioids has typically been offered once a week, but patients attend, on average, only once every 2 weeks (Woody et al., 1983). However, patients also received daily doses of methadone, so the intensity of the combined pharmacotherapy plus psychotherapy treatment was quite high involving daily or near daily visits.

For cocaine-dependent patients, Kleinman et al. (1990) attempted once-a-week outpatient treatment, of several different modalities, and found that attrition was high and there was no evidence of any treatment effect for any of the modalities implying that once a week therapy was insufficient for these cocaine users. Hoffman et al. (1991) combined individual, family, and group therapies at different frequencies for treatment of cocaine dependence. The results showed a better outcome with group and individual conditions, which provided intensive day treatment compared with weekly outpatient therapy. The NIDA Cocaine Collaborative study (Crits-Christoph et al., 1999) looked at outpatient treatments and found that the combination of group and individual therapy or counseling, with group offered once-a-week and individual offered twice-a-week to start and tapering down to once-a-week was successful in assisting cocaine addicts to reduce or eliminate their cocaine use. Alterman (1990) reported a 50–60% abstinence rate at 6-month follow-up among cocaine-abusing patients receiving 12-step-oriented drug counseling in either inpatient or intensive day treatment (5 days per week) for 1 month, followed by twice-weekly therapy. These studies suggest that for cocaine-dependent patients, participation in drug treatment should be relatively intense, at least initially, and can decrease over time as the patient progresses.

Two controlled trials of psychotherapy for marijuana dependence showed benefits from once a week counseling. One study on group treatment (Stephens et al., 1994) and another on individual treatment (Grenyer et al., 1996) found substantial reduction in marijuana use and related problems with once-weekly therapy in the individual treatment study, as well as reductions in the group therapy condition that began with once-weekly therapy and decreased to once every other week.

For treating alcohol dependence, Project MATCH, found once a month motivational enhancement therapy as effective as other more intensive interventions, thus suggesting that certain therapeutic approaches can be effective at relatively low doses, at least for some types of addictions (Project MATCH Research Group, 1997).

Overall, these data suggest that the intensity of treatment needed varies with the specific drug, the severity of the dependence, and the nature of the patient's associated problems, particularly psychiatric conditions. For most patients, opioid or cocaine dependence appears to require more intense treatment than marijuana or alcohol dependence. In Woody and colleagues' methadone studies, psychotherapy was most useful for patients who had moderate to high levels of psychiatric symptoms in addition to their substance use disorders. However, in the two largest studies for other substance dependence (Project MATCH Research Group, 1997; Crits-Christoph et al., 1999), psychotherapy provided no advantage over drug counseling, even for patients with high levels of psychiatric symptoms. Reasons for this disparate finding might be that the methadone maintenance patients were receiving an effective pharmacotherapy in combination with psychotherapy and counseling while the alcohol and cocaine studies did not have this advantage. The therapists in the methadone program may have been better able to focus on the co-occurring psychiatric symptoms and behavioral problems rather than focusing entirely on stopping drug use because the methadone was doing much of that work for them.

Other studies have shown that the mix of drug-focused treatments versus treatments that address associated problems may be important. These studies show that it is helpful to provide services that address associated concerns, such as family, employment, and psychiatric, in addition to drug-focused treatments, and these services are especially important for patients with difficulties in these areas (McLellan et al., 1993, 1997).

Family involvement

Family member involvement is generally felt to be associated with better outcomes, and programs usually try to involve other family members or significant others in treatment. This may be through individual family therapy, a multifamily group or occasional family workshops, which are psychoeducational rather than psychotherapeutic in nature. Through these interventions family members can be informed of the nature and consequences of addiction and the treatment process with the intent that it will enable families to more effectively support their addicted member through the process of recovery. Also, family involvement allows the therapist to explore historical or relationship factors in the family that can undermine and frustrate treatment. Such factors might include addiction in other family members, codependency and enabling behaviors, or the development of family crises in response to the patient's improvement. Lastly, family involvement in treatment may help family members access treatment and/or the support that they need to reduce adverse effects of the addiction on other family members.

One newer intervention model, behavioral couples counseling or behavioral family counseling, has been used in combination with individual counseling for drug-addicted men and their spouses or other family members. This approach is demonstrating positive outcomes in two dimensions. One is reduction of spousal abuse in abusive relationships (Fals-Stewart et al., 2002); the other has been better attendance, greater compliance with naltrexone and more days abstinent, and fewer legal and family problems as compared with individual treatment alone for opioid-dependent men (Fals-Stewart and O'Farrell, 2003).

Therapeutic alliance

Therapist qualities appear to have an effect on success in therapy (Luborsky et al., 1985, 1986). Three qualities appear to be generally predictive of outcome in psychotherapy: overall adjustment, skill, and interest in helping patients (Luborsky et al., 1985). For crack- and cocaine-abusing patients, Kleinman et al. (1990) found some therapists reliably retained patients better, and retention is a generally a critical measure of success in addiction treatment. Presumably this relates to the qualities of the therapists, although specific qualities were not explored in this study. Despite the apparent significance of therapist differences in treatment effectiveness, research has not identified which 'types' of therapists tend to be more or less effective in treating addiction (Crits-Christoph et al., 1990). Thus, there may not be specific 'types' of therapists who will be more effective. Rather, there appears to be something in the therapist–patient relationship that is related to outcome. This is often referred to as the therapeutic alliance or the helping alliance and scales have been developed to measure it.

These measures have found that therapists who can establish a positive connection with patients and are perceived by the patient as 'helpful' are more likely to achieve successful outcomes (Luborsky et al., 1985). This therapeutic alliance to outcome relationship holds across different therapeutic modalities (Horvath and Symonds, 1991) and a variety of psychiatric problems, including substance abuse (Conners et al., 1997). Patients' and therapists' ratings of the therapeutic alliance tend to be consistent, but where there are differences, patients' ratings are better predictors of outcome than therapists' ratings (Horvath and Symonds, 1991). In addiction treatment, these outcomes translate to better retention and greater reduction in drug use.

According to Project MATCH data, a national multisite study of psychosocial treatments of alcoholism, in an outpatient sample ($n = 952$) rating of the alliance by the therapist or the patient predicted treatment participation, days abstinent, and drinks per drinking day (Conners et al., 1997). These changes were all in the expected direction, that is, a positive alliance predicted greater participation in treatment and greater reduction in alcohol use. However, the study also looked at patients after discharge from inpatient rehabilitation and found that client's ratings of the aftercare therapist were not significant predictors of treatment participation or drinking-related outcomes. The lack of a correlation between alliance and outcome for the aftercare group following an inpatient stay could be because these patients had already achieved some degree of abstinence, and were compliant and/or motivated enough to continue treatment. Also, aftercare patients may have established a positive alliance with members of the inpatient treatment staff, and it was the strength of this alliance (which was not studied) that promoted their continued treatment participation and recovery.

Therapists' emotional reactions to substance abusers may be important determinants of outcome as well. While true to some extent in all psychotherapy, these emotional reactions are considered to be particularly significant in the treatment of substance abuse because they are presumed to be more intense and negative (Imhof, 1991). Negative feelings can be particularly problematic because many addicts have feelings of shame and guilt over the addiction and its associated behaviors. Thus, we might expect addicted patients to be particularly sensitive to negative therapist reactions. In one early study of alcoholism treatment (Milmoe et al., 1967), the more anger and anxiety in the clinician's voice in the initial session, the less likely the patient was to follow through on getting treatment.

A good general principle for psychotherapy or counseling is that the therapist should be interested in and comfortable with addiction-related problems and behaviors. These include the manipulative, impulsive, or demanding behaviors that are sometimes observed, and the self-abusing aspect of the condition that may create negative countertransference feelings. An ability to accept the patient where they are, not pass judgment, and convey respect for the individual and the severity of his/her problem can strengthen the therapeutic alliance. Along these lines, Washton and Stone-Washton (1990) recommended that therapists working with addicted patients have a high degree of empathy, confidence, and hope, and a low wish to control the patient.

To promote a positive alliance, therapists should refrain from being judgmental and should occasionally extend themselves a little more with addicted patients than with other types of psychiatric patients. The dependency needs of addicted patients often express themselves in the therapist–patient relationship, and occasional appropriate, concrete, supportive responses are probably useful, especially in the early phases of treatment. This therapeutic posture may involve greeting the patient in a friendly manner on entering the office, actively seeking to reestablish contact when an appointment is missed, being generous with reinforcement for abstinence, and agreeing to see or speak with the patient occasionally at unscheduled times if necessary.

HIV risk reduction

Drug users are at increased risk of HIV infection as well as other infections transmitted by blood and body fluids such as hepatitis B and C. Drug treatment has been found to be associated with sustained reductions in HIV risk and a lower incidence of HIV infection among drug users. This is true for methadone maintenance (Metzger et al., 1998) and cocaine treatment (Shoptaw et al., 1997). In the National Institute on Drug Abuse (NIDA) cocaine collaborative treatment study, in which treatment consisted entirely of psychotherapy and counseling, treatment was associated with a 49% decrease in HIV risk across all treatment, gender, and ethnic groups, due mainly to fewer sexual partners and less unprotected sex (Woody et al., 2003). Shoptaw and Frosch also reviewed a number of studies of treatment and its relationship to HIV risk among men who have sex with men and concluded that substance abuse treatment has significant value as an HIV risk reduction intervention to reduce sexual risk among men who have sex with men. Motivational interviewing (Yahne et al., 2002) used in an outreach approach successfully encouraged high-risk women sex workers who were using drugs to reduce their drug use and HIV risk behaviors and increase lawful employment. This underscores the role of counseling and psychotherapy in substance abuse treatment to reduce HIV risk.

Major models of psychotherapy for addiction

NIDA has sponsored research testing a number of individual psychotherapy and counseling approaches for efficacy. The key concepts of the approaches that currently appear most promising are seen in the following.

Cognitive-behavioral therapy and relapse prevention therapy

Cognitive-behavioral therapy (Carroll et al., 1991) and *relapse prevention* therapy (Marlatt and Gordon, 1985) are related and are based on the theory that learning processes play a crucial part in the development of addiction, similar to other maladaptive behavior patterns. These approaches involve strategies and techniques to enhance self-control and foster abstinence. They include self-monitoring to recognize false beliefs and drug cravings, identification of high-risk situations for use, and development of strategies for avoiding or coping with affects of situations that stimulate drug craving without resorting to use. A central element of this approach is learning to anticipate the problems one may meet in recovery and developing effective coping strategies prior to the occurrence of the problem.

Individual drug counseling

Individual drug counseling helps the client by setting present-oriented, behavioral goals and focusing directly on reducing or stopping the illicit drug use. It also addresses related areas of impaired functioning such as employment, illegal activity, and social and family relations, and the structure and content of the personal recovery program. Addiction counseling helps the patient develop behavioral tools and some very basic cognitive coping strategies to abstain from drug use and maintain abstinence. It employs the philosophy of the 12-step program and encourages 12-step participation.

Supportive-expressive psychotherapy

Supportive-expressive psychotherapy (Luborsky, 1984) derives from psychoanalytic theory and has been modified to address substance use disorders, specifically opioid and cocaine dependence (Luborsky, 1985; Luborsky et al., 1995). It has two main components: supportive techniques to help patients feel comfortable, and expressive or interpretive techniques to help patients identify and work through problematic interpersonal issues. Special attention is paid to the role of drugs in relation to feelings and behaviors and how problems may be solved without resorting to drug use. Interpersonal psychotherapy is another supportive/dynamic treatment that has been effective in some studies. It focuses on resolving interpersonal problems and has been adapted for use in treating both opioid and cocaine dependence (Rounsaville et al., 1983, 1991).

Motivational enhancement therapy

Motivational enhancement therapy (Miller et al., 1992) is a client-centered counseling approach that has demonstrated efficacy in a number of studies. Motivational enhancement therapy attempts to facilitate reduction or cessation of drug use by assisting patients to resolve ambivalence about engaging in treatment and stopping drug use. This model attempts to create rapid, internally motivated change in the client by encouraging the client to explore their own ambivalence while simultaneously helping the client to move toward greater motivation reduce or stop drug use. Motivational enhancement therapy is usually brief, often involving only one to four sessions. In practice, it is sometimes conducted as a single session intervention, when a drug abuse problem is first recognized. This may occur in an emergency room, for example, when a patient comes in with recent drug use. Its purpose then is to help the patient resolve ambivalence and agree to get into drug treatment. Motivational enhancement therapy has also been adapted to a longer therapeutic intervention.

Contingency management

Contingency management (Higgins et al., 1993; Silverman et al., 1996; Budney et al., 2000) is a behavioral intervention that directly rewards the desired behavior (usually abstinence but it can be attendance) by giving vouchers that can be exchanged for retail goods or services as incentives for either drug-negative urines or another desired behavior. It is essentially giving positive reinforcement via vouchers for desired behaviors. The positive reinforcement occurs within the context of a more comprehensive psychosocial program, sometimes referred to as community reinforcement. This approach has been used with alcoholics, methadone-maintained cocaine users, and for cocaine- and marijuana-dependent patients and has been highly successful. While this model has been shown to be efficacious in research programs there are two possible limitations regarding its utility in clinical treatment. One is that providing vouchers for abstinence is not consistent with how most clinicians want to treat addiction because clinicians want abstinence and sobriety to be a choice that is internally reinforcing. Related to this is the problem that transferring reinforcement from external to internal when the period of rewarding abstinence with vouchers ends can be difficult and is sometimes associated with an increase in relapse. A third problem has been getting funds to pay for vouchers and another has been the resistance of some clinicians to reward patients for abstaining from doing something they were not supposed to be doing in the first place. The NIDA Clinical Trials Network has developed protocols to avoid many of these problems and results from clinical trials in community-based programs should be available within the next year.

Research on treatment for specific drugs

Psychosocial components of drug abuse treatment have been the subject of formal research only in the past two decades. Most research has concluded that psychotherapy can be an effective treatment for substance use disorders (Resnick et al., 1981; Woody et al., 1983; Carroll et al., 1991, 1994, 1999; Stephens et al., 1994; Grenyer et al., 1996) though it has not outperformed standard drug counseling except for a few studies done in methadone programs. These studies and reviews have examined individual and group psychotherapies in the treatment of opioid, cocaine, alcohol, and marijuana dependence. The comparison of specific models of therapy for substance use disorders has become the focus of much interest.

Treatment of opioid dependence

Early experience with psychotherapy for opioid dependence showed that in the absence of methadone-maintenance, psychotherapy was not effective (Nyswander et al., 1958). Dropout rates were extremely high, and few patients improved. The introduction of methadone reduced opioid use and kept patients in treatment, and this changed the results significantly.

One early study compared supportive-expressive psychotherapy and cognitive-behavioral therapy plus drug counseling with drug counseling alone for opioid-addicted methadone maintenance patients in a Veterans Affairs treatment program (Woody et al., 1983). All patients showed improvement but the addition of professional psychotherapies to the drug counseling benefited patients more who had higher levels of psychopathology than drug counseling alone. Both drug counseling and the combined treatment were equally helpful for patients with low levels of psychopathology. A parallel study did not find a beneficial psychotherapy effect (Rounsaville et al., 1983). The differing outcomes may be the result of the low enrollment in the Rounsaville et al. study and other programmatic differences (Woody et al., 1998). A follow-up study in three community-based methadone programs also showed that patients with high levels of psychiatric symptoms did better with counseling plus psychotherapy than with counseling alone (Woody et al., 1995). Other investigators have found evidence for the efficacy of psychotherapy for opioid dependence when it is used in conjunction with methadone maintenance or naltrexone (Resnick et al., 1981).

A recent study of naltrexone for opioid dependence found that contingency management improved naltrexone compliance and opioid use outcome relative to standard naltrexone treatment (Carroll et al., 2001). Unlike methadone, which is an opioid agonist and thus creates effects that are similar to heroin, naltrexone is an opiate antagonist, produces no physiologic dependence, and has no opioid effects. Naltrexone makes it very difficult, if not impossible, to get the desired effects of ingested opiates. Consequently, many patients do not like to take naltrexone as much as they like methadone or other substitution drugs, so medication compliance can be problematic. In the Carroll et al. study, 127 opioid-dependent patients who completed outpatient detoxification were randomized to three conditions: standard naltrexone treatment, naltrexone treatment plus voucher-based contingency management, or naltrexone treatment plus voucher-based contingency management and significant other involvement. It was found that contingency management enhanced the outcomes of treatment retention, medication compliance and reduction in drug use when compared with standard naltrexone treatment. Significant other involvement did not improve outcomes over contingency management.

Another study of naltrexone treatment for opioid-dependent patients showed that a manualized psychosocial intervention designed to enhance the clinical value of naltrexone treatment showed greater retention with the more naltrexone taken, the more psychosocial services received, and the greater reduction in opioid use (Rawson et al., 2001). This study, like several mentioned earlier that were done in methadone programs, showed that pharmacological and behavioral treatments can be effectively combined to provide improved outcomes.

Treatment of cocaine use disorders

A NIDA multisite study investigated the efficacy of four psychosocial treatments when delivered in outpatient settings: (1) cognitive therapy plus group drug counseling; (2) supportive-expressive therapy plus group drug counseling; (3) individual drug counseling plus group drug counseling; and (4) group drug counseling alone (Crits-Christoph et al., 1997). All groups showed substantial reductions in cocaine use; however, patients in the individual drug counseling plus group drug counseling condition had a greater reduction than those in the other three groups. Patients with higher levels of psychiatric symptoms had poorer outcomes, but unlike the methadone studies and like the findings of Project MATCH, psychotherapy did not provide additional benefits to this more psychiatrically symptomatic group.

In another study, relapse prevention (a cognitive-behavioral model) showed better results than interpersonal psychotherapy, provided once per week for 12 weeks, in the treatment of cocaine abuse in ambulatory patients (Carroll et al., 1991). Fifty-seven percent of the relapse prevention subjects achieved greater than 3 weeks of abstinence during the 12 weeks, whereas only 33% of the interpersonal psychotherapy subjects met the same criterion. Also, relapse prevention appeared to be slightly more effective than interpersonal psychotherapy among patients with severe levels of cocaine dependence, although this finding was not statistically significant.

Higgins et al. (1993) compared community reinforcement with standard drug counseling. Community reinforcement, sometimes referred to as contingency management, involves positively reinforcing abstinence with a tangible reward that is usually given in the form of a voucher within the context of a psychosocial intervention. Sixty-eight percent of patients in the community reinforcement condition achieved 8 weeks of abstinence compared with 11% of the standard drug counseling patients. Research examining treatments for cocaine dependence in methadone maintenance patients has also shown support for voucher-based reinforcement for abstinence (Silverman et al., 1996; Rawson et al., 2001) or for treatment plan-related tasks (Iguchi et al., 1997).

Although psychotherapy and counseling alone have shown moderate efficacy, their dropout rates have often been high. This has fostered interest in developing combined psychotherapeutic and pharmacotherapeutic approaches to the treatment of cocaine dependence. One study compared relapse prevention plus desipramine, clinical management plus desipramine, relapse prevention plus placebo, and clinical management plus placebo to treat cocaine abuse in ambulatory patients (Carroll et al., 1994). All groups showed improvement, but there were no main effects for medication or psychotherapy. However, there was a significant interaction effect in that relapse prevention was associated with better outcomes for higher-severity cocaine users than was clinical management. Further analysis of these data (Carroll et al., 1995) suggests differential symptom reduction in depressed versus nondepressed cocaine patients. The depressed patients tended to have better retention and better cocaine outcomes than did the nondepressed patients. Desipramine was effective to reduce depressive symptoms, but not to reduce cocaine use. This points to the importance of comprehensive evaluation of drug-dependent patients and psychiatric problems, with the need for psychiatric treatment in drug treatment for those with dual diagnoses.

Treatment of alcohol use disorders

Project MATCH found no significant difference in outcome by type of treatment when comparing cognitive-behavioral therapy, to 12-step facilitation therapy (Nowinski et al., 1992), and motivational enhancement therapy (Miller et al., 1992) for the treatment of alcohol dependence. Patients decreased their alcohol use significantly and maintained improvement at 1-year posttreatment in all treatment conditions. Although higher levels of psychiatric severity were associated with worse outcome, the psychiatrically focused treatments did not alter this relationship.

Treatment of marijuana use disorders

Several studies have examined psychotherapy for marijuana abuse and dependence. Grenyer *et al.* (1996) compared a modification of supportive-expressive therapy (Grenyer *et al.*, 1995) with a brief (one-session) intervention for treatment of marijuana dependence. The supportive-expressive therapy was offered for 16 weeks. At 16 weeks, the supportive-expressive group showed significantly larger decreases in marijuana use, depression, and anxiety and significantly larger increases in psychological health than did the brief intervention group.

In a study of group treatment of marijuana dependence (Stephens *et al.*, 1994), patients were randomly assigned to either a relapse prevention (Marlatt and Gordon, 1985) group or a social support group. All groups were conducted weekly for the first 8 weeks, and then biweekly for the next 4 weeks for a total of ten 2-hour sessions. Patients in both treatments achieved and maintained reductions in marijuana use and related problems; however, outcomes did not differ between the two treatments.

Adding vouchers to behavioral therapies improved outcomes among heavy marijuana users (Budney *et al.*, 2000). Sixty heavy marijuana users were randomly assigned to one of three treatments: motivational enhancement therapy, motivational enhancement plus behavioral coping skills therapy, or motivational enhancement plus behavioral coping skills therapy plus voucher-based incentives. During the 14-week study, 40% of patients in the incentives group achieved at least 7 weeks of continuous abstinence from marijuana compared with 5% of patients in each of the other groups. At the end of the 14-week treatment, 35% of the incentives group had stopped using marijuana, as compared with 10% of the motivational enhancement plus coping skills group, and 5% of the group receiving motivational enhancement alone.

Research implications for treatment

Although the relative benefits of psychotherapy versus counseling vary in the studies reviewed here, most agree that psychotherapy and counseling can be effective in the treatment of substance abuse and addiction (Resnick *et al.*, 1981; Woody *et al.*, 1983; Carroll *et al.*, 1991; Crits-Christoph and Siqueland, 1997) and moreover that some type of psychosocial intervention is a necessary component of substance abuse treatment. However, it appears that other conditions must be met in order for positive outcomes to occur.

The chemically dependent patient usually requires more structure and greater frequency of visits than traditional psychotherapy provides. An intensive treatment program, with sessions twice a week to everyday depending on the patient and the drug, is usually needed in the beginning. Then the intensity can be decreased as progress is achieved. Psychotherapy appears to be most effective when combined with drug-focused treatment services, either within the context of a structured addiction treatment program or when organized as needed by the individual psychotherapist. Additional services, such as vocational counseling, are very helpful for patients who have employment problems. Family involvement tends to support retention and compliance in treatment. In the case of outpatient treatment for opioid dependence, methadone maintenance or some other type of substitution therapy is essential for psychotherapy or counseling to have an effect. This combined approach, offering both psychotherapy and/or counseling and medication for addictive disorders for which an appropriate medication exists is probably the optimal treatment in many cases. The more traditional psychotherapies, such as cognitive-behavioral, supportive-expressive, and interpersonal, may be more helpful for patients experiencing clinically significant psychiatric symptoms, but this interaction has only been shown to exist in the context of methadone maintenance (Woody *et al.*, 1985).

Research has not clearly indicated that one kind of psychotherapy is superior to any other for the treatment of addiction. However, among psychosocial approaches, the current frontrunners are probably cognitive-behavioral therapy, individual addiction counseling, contingency management, and motivational enhancement. It is important to recognize that we are in a dynamic period in this field and new approaches are developed all the time that improve upon previous work. There is much current interest to combine psychosocial and pharmacological treatments as it appears to be a valuable approach for many addictions. This approach recognizes the value of self-help participation, whether it be 12-step or another model. It is also important to view treatment of addiction as a long-term process that extends well beyond the end of formal treatment and involves continuing personal commitment and growth on the part of the patient.

Practice principles

The following guidelines may be helpful for the clinician treating chemical dependence with psychotherapy.

- Be familiar with the pharmacology of abused drugs. One should know the pharmacological effects of specific drugs of abuse (including their adverse and dangerous effects), the common drug combinations used and why addicts prefer these combinations, the signs and symptoms of intoxication and withdrawal from the various drugs of abuse, and the medical complications associated with various drug classes (including interactions that may occur with other medications that the patient is taking for medical or psychiatric problems). Much of this information can be found in the Treatment Improvement Protocols that are published by the Substance Abuse and Mental Health Administration.

- Be knowledgeable about the subculture of addiction in your area. This includes such information as which drugs are easily available, how they are typically ingested, if there are common combinations, how they are purchased and what they cost the buyer.

- Be knowledgeable about places the patient can go to receive help for the addiction and its associated problems, including 12-step programs, other self-help groups, vocational training and educational programs, legal assistance, and public assistance programs.

- Be prepared to provide education on the nature of addiction and the process of recovery. It is not recommended that the therapist do more talking than listening, but it is usually helpful to educate the patient about important aspects of the disease.

- Form clear goals (a treatment plan) early in treatment. Initially, these goals should be simple and should include abstinence from all nonprescribed drugs and alcohol, attendance in treatment, compliance with prescribed medications as appropriate, and participation in a program of self-help. Keep abreast of the patient's progress with these goals but review them, however briefly, in each session.

- Establish a positive, supportive alliance with the patient. Sometimes addicted patients may transfer some of their dependency needs on to the therapist so it can be helpful to offer more concrete support if necessary, such as calling to follow-up if a session is missed and being willing to schedule an extra session for the patient if they are feeling as if they might relapse.

- Incorporate direct, drug-focused interventions into the treatment program. Such interventions include advising patients to attend a self-help program and monitoring abstinence by self-report and urine drug screens or breathalyzer, preferably at each visit. Provide prompt feedback on drug screens regarding the presence or absence of drugs.

- Explore pharmacotherapeutic options, when they are available, in combination with psychotherapy and other behavioral treatments.

- Recognize that because the recovering addicted patient usually requires structure in addition to psychotherapy or counseling.

- Be prepared to refer the patient to other services as needed.

- Communicate to the patient that you appreciate the difficulty involved in abstaining and breaking the addictive cycle. Be accepting of where they have been and where they are now and be generous with positive reinforcement for gains.

- Be prepared to work with the patient on areas of their life adversely impacted by addiction. These may include financial problems, employment problems, relationship, and parenting difficulties, etc.

- Target the mental health interventions to patients with high levels of associated psychiatric or psychological problems, and address those difficulties simultaneously in the treatment.

Treatment challenges and what to do about them

This section describes some common difficulties the clinician treating addiction will most likely face: addressing ambivalence, dealing with relapse after a period of abstinence, and depression.

Addressing ambivalence

Mr X is a 38-year-old, successful business executive who entered treatment for cocaine dependence at the insistence of his wife. His pattern of use was that he would binge about once every 2 weeks, spend $500–1000, and stay out all night. At these times he was often unfaithful to his wife with women he met while using the cocaine. He realized that this secret life was risky but he was excited by the risks and had not yet experienced significant consequences. His wife knew he was using but was not aware of the extent of his use and the associated expenses and infidelities. Mr X was aware that he was at risk of HIV infection and of being robbed or perhaps even killed for his money. Thus, Mr X realized the risks involved, and did not want to harm his family, his employment situation, or himself. However, he had not personally experienced any negative consequences yet and also he sought the excitement of this life-style. He was very ambivalent about giving up or even reducing his drug use.

The therapist employed a motivational enhancement approach in treatment. This approach involves actively listening to the patient and helping the patient evaluate and clarify his or her goals in treatment, while simultaneously promoting the goal of cessation of drug use. The therapist asked Mr X what he wanted from treatment and listened as he described his ambivalence. Mr X was able to state that he wanted to abstain from cocaine use because he knew the risks he was taking. He did not want to damage his career or financial resources. Moreover, he liked being married and loved his wife, although he found it unexciting and he loved his children and wanted to have his family intact. Also he recognized the risk of personal harm, either through unsafe sexual contact or by harmful effects of the cocaine or by being the victim of drug-related crime. On the other hand, he had a sensation-seeking aspect to his personality. He loved the excitement of the risks and had never experienced any severe consequences. The therapist was able to listen actively and to refrain from giving advice and this created an environment in which the patient was able to explore his ambivalence, identify the pros and cons of his drug use, and choose to abstain. Through acknowledgment of where the patient was in his own decision-making process, followed by questions and discussion, the therapist was able to help Mr X see the value of stopping cocaine use because that was best for him and his family. The therapist's approach created internal motivation in the patient by assisting him to identify what was truly in his best interests.

Motivational enhancement is usually brief, often involving only one to four sessions. In some situations, one to four sessions is enough to help the patient change problematic behavior but in other situations this type of intervention is used to get the patient into treatment and committed to working on the problem. In this case, the motivational enhancement intervention helped Mr X decide to stop using cocaine and commit to a course of outpatient treatment that then continued with regular sessions for a period of 6 months. During this time, he was able to achieve and maintain abstinence.

Recommitting to recovery after relapse

Ms Y was a 32-year-old, employed, single woman. She was in treatment for cocaine and alcohol dependence. Her addiction was quite severe and she felt that she had hit a personal bottom and was ready to surrender and get into recovery. She was committed to treatment and worked very hard to achieve abstinence. She attended individual and group sessions regularly, was engaged and diligent in therapy, and submitted urines for drug screens regularly. She also attended frequent 12-step meetings, had a sponsor, and was working the 12 steps. She was supported in her efforts by her family and her employment situation.

After almost a year of sobriety, she relapsed. She went to a neighborhood bar, where she used to drink and buy cocaine, had several drinks saw a person she used to use with and picked up cocaine. She used cocaine through one evening and the following day before she felt exhausted enough to want to stop. Fortunately, she was engaged enough in therapy that she told her therapist and returned to treatment immediately. Her therapist analyzed the relapse with Ms Y. Together they identified what seemed to trigger the relapse, which in retrospect appeared to have been worries and dysphoric feelings about approaching the end of treatment. They also reviewed, in detail, the process leading up to the actual drug use.

In addiction counseling it is said that a relapse is a process that begins long before the actual drug use. The relapse process usually begins with negative, subtle changes in thoughts, feelings, and/or behaviors where the patient moves away from things associated with remission. Relapse analysis seeks to make the patient aware of these subtle changes. The next step in treatment is to develop strategies for how the patient could more effectively manage the events that triggered the relapse. Strategies or tools provide the patient with healthier alternatives that could be done if the same or similar events occurred again. Strategies are developed by the patient or suggested by the therapist and may include things such as increasing attendance at 12-step meetings or therapy sessions, avoiding unhealthy people, places, and things that could remind one of using, and enlisting the support of healthy others. Next the therapist has to persuade the patient to recommit to recovery. This can be quite difficult because patients often feel like they lost everything in the relapse and may also feel guilty and ashamed. Negative feelings, such as guilt and shame tend to promote continued drug use because the person feels so bad about their behavior that they may try to avoid feeling bad by further drug use. The therapist would want to reduce the recovering person's feelings of shame, guilt, or frustration by accepting the patient where he or she is, acknowledging that relapse is part of the process and helping the patient to get back on course. The relapse should be viewed as an opportunity, albeit painful, to learn more about one's personal process of recovery.

Ms Y was able to recommit to recovery and she and her therapist were able to deal with her impending termination (which was several months delayed by the relapse). She was able to generalize from this particular situation to other potential situations that would involve dysphoric feelings that could trigger a relapse. In therapy, Ms Y developed strategies to use the social support of her extended family, continue to work on her 12 steps and begin to volunteer at her 12-step meetings when she again achieved enough clean time. These strategies were helpful and Ms Y was able to become abstinent and stable in her recovery.

Addiction and depression

Mr Z, a 17-year-old male high school junior was referred to treatment for substance abuse after experiencing chest pain and having problems breathing following heavy use of amphetamine and cocaine together. Young people often come to treatment when their drug use has been discovered by others, which are usually parents, law enforcement, or the local emergency department. This man was no exception. He came for treatment at the insistence of his mother, but did not identify drug use as a problem. He was using crystal methamphetamine, cocaine, and alcohol; mostly because where he lived, and in his peer group, these drugs were available. He reported a history of drug use including: alcohol since age 14, methamphetamine use several times/week for the last 6 months, and cocaine use on this single occasion.

A clinical interview revealed that he had a number of stressors including his parents' divorce 2 years earlier, the death of a peer in a car accident about a year ago, and a breakup with his girlfriend 8 months ago. Asking about school performance indicated that he had been a better than average student, but his grades started slipping after his parents' divorce and continued downward. He reported not liking school and often skipping classes. His social interactions were reasonably good, but his mother reported that he had become distant from her and had only limited interactions with his father. He reported little interest in school or extracurricular activities and feelings of low self-esteem. He denied that the event that brought him into treatment was a suicide attempt, but acknowledged feeling indifferent toward life, with occasional suicidal thoughts, which he would describe as having a way out, if life got too hard.

It appeared that this patient was suffering from depression as well as amphetamine dependence and other substance abuse. The therapist treated the substance dependence with many drug counseling techniques, including teaching about the cycle of addiction and the recovery process, identifying triggers and strategies to avoid them, encouraging self-help participation, and monitoring drug use with urine drug screens. Simultaneously, the therapist addressed the depression with cognitive therapy and a psychiatric referral for antidepressant medication. With psychotherapy and medication, the depression lifted and with addiction counseling, the patient was able to stop using amphetamines and cocaine, although he would still drink infrequently with his peers. Fortunately within his peer group, which was mostly his extended family, there was no strong pressure to use. His school performance improved, self-esteem increased, and he no longer had suicidal thoughts. He began to think about what he would like to do after high school, which was a significant developmental step.

A common mistake made with dual diagnosis patients is to try to treat one or the other of the problems first (often whichever one the therapist feels more competent with), while for the patient they are not two disorders but one interconnected problem. Another common error is to essentially blame one of the disorders on the other. Addiction counselors may attribute the depressive symptoms to protracted withdrawal and assume they will clear up spontaneously with time in recovery, and this is sometimes true, but not always. Patients may insist that they are using to self-medicate their depression and if the depression lifts they won't feel compelled to use. The first assertion may well be true, but the later assertion is almost certainly not true. Treating the depression is very unlikely to solve a substance abuse problem. The key to treating dual diagnosis conditions is having an appreciation of the whole interconnected problem and giving appropriate concern and treatment for both elements.

To determine if a patient's depression is a substance-related temporary phenomenon or a separate syndrome, the simplest way is to take a careful history and find out if the psychological problem pre-dated the substance abuse or occurred in periods when the patient was not using. If the depression preexisted the addiction or occurred when the patient was not using, the therapist should certainly think of the condition as a dual diagnosis and treat accordingly. Even if that is not true, severe depressive symptoms (such as frequent suicidal thoughts) or a number of significant symptoms warrant using a dual diagnosis approach in treatment.

These vignettes illustrate just a few of the common clinical challenges faced by clinicians treating addiction and provide some pointers for how to handle them. Our hope is that readers will gain a better understanding of these common clinical issues in addiction treatment.

References

Alterman, A. I. (1990). Day hospital versus inpatient cocaine dependence rehabilitation: an interim report. In: L. Harris, ed. *Problems of drug dependence 1990*, pp. 363–4. NIDA Research Monograph 105. Rockville, MD: US Department of Health and Human Services.

American Psychiatric Association (1987). *Diagnostic and statistical manual of mental disorders*, 3rd edn (revised). Washington, DC: American Psychiatric Association.

American Psychiatric Association (1994). *Diagnostic and statistical manual of mental disorders*, 4th edn. Washington, DC: American Psychiatric Association.

Ball, J. C., *et al.* (1986). Medical services provided to 2394 patients at methadone programs in three states. *Journal of Substance Abuse Treatment*, 3, 203–9.

Budney, A., Higgins, S., Radonovich, K. J., and Novy, P. L. (2000). Adding voucher-based incentives to coping skills and motivational enhancement improves outcomes during treatment for marijuana dependence. *Journal of Consulting and Clinical Psychology*, 68, 1051–61.

Carroll, K. M., Rounsaville, B. J., and Treece, F. H. (1991). A comparative trial of psychotherapies for ambulatory cocaine abusers: relapse prevention and interpersonal psychotherapy. *American Journal of Drug and Alcohol Abuse*, 17, 229–47.

Carroll, K. M., *et al.* (1994). Psychotherapy and pharmacotherapy for ambulatory cocaine abusers. *Archives of General Psychiatry*, 51, 177–87.

Carroll, K. M., Niche, C., and Rounsaville, B. J. (1995). Differential symptom reduction in depressed cocaine abusers treated with psychotherapy and pharmacotherapy. *Journal of Nervous and Mental Disease*, 183, 251–9.

Carroll, K. M., *et al.* (2001). Targeting behavioral therapies to enhance naltrexone treatment of opioid dependence. *Archives of General Psychiatry*, 58, 755–61.

Conners, G. J., Carroll, K. M., and DiClemente, C. C. (1997). The therapeutic alliance and its relationship to alcoholism treatment participation and outcome. *Journal of Consulting and Clinical Psychology*, 65, 588–98.

Crits-Christoph, P., Beebe, K. L., and Connolly, M. B. (1990). Therapist effects in the treatment of drug dependence: implications for conducting comparative treatment studies. In: L. S. Onken and J. D. Blaine, ed. *Psychotherapy and counseling in the treatment of drug abuse*, pp. 39–48. NIDA Research Monograph 104. Rockville, MD: US Department of Health and Human Services.

Crits-Christoph, P., *et al.* (1997). The National Institute on Drug Abuse Collaborative Cocaine Treatment Study: rationale and methods. *Archives of General Psychiatry*, 54, 721–6.

Crits-Christoph, P., *et al.* (1999). Psychosocial treatments for cocaine dependence: results of the NIDA Cocaine Collaborative Study. *Archives of General Psychiatry*, 56, 493–502.

Crits-Christoph, P., *et al.* Mediators of outcome for psychosocial treatment for cocaine dependence. *Journal of Consulting and Clinical Psychology* (in press).

Etheridge, R. M., Craddock, S. G., Hubbard, R. L., and Rounds-Bryant, J. L. (1999). The relationship of counseling and self-help participation to patient outcomes in DATOS. *Drug and Alcohol Dependence*, 57, 99–112.

Fals-Stewart, W. and O'Farrell, T. (2003). Behavioral family counseling and Naltrexone for male opioid dependent patients. *Journal of Consulting and Clinical Psychology*, 71, 432–42.

Fals-Stewart, W., Kashdan, T. B., O'Farrell, T., and Birchler, G. R. (2002). Behavioral couples therapy for drug-abusing patients: effects on partner violence. *Journal of Substance Abuse Treatment*, 22, 87–96.

Fiorentine, R. (1999). After drug treatment. Are 12-step programs effective in maintaining abstinence? *American Journal of Drug and Alcohol Abuse*, 25, 93–116.

Fiorentine, R. and Anglin, M. D. (1996). More is better: counseling participation and the effectiveness of outpatient drug treatment. *Journal of Substance Abuse Treatment*, 13, 341–8.

Fiorentine, R. and Hillhouse, M. P. (2000). Drug treatment and 12-step participation. The additive effects of integrated recovery activities. *Journal of Substance Abuse Treatment*, 18, 65–74.

Grenyer, B. F. S., Luborsky, L., and Solowij, N. (1995). *Treatment manual for supportive-expressive dynamic therapy: special adaptation for treatment of cannabis (marijuana) dependence*. Technical Report 26. Sydney, Australia: National Drug and Alcohol Research Centre.

Grenyer, B. F. S., Solowij, N., and Peters, R. (1996). Psychotherapy for marijuana addiction: a randomized controlled trial of brief versus intensive treatment. Presentation given at the Society for Psychotherapy Research, Amelia Island, FL, June 19–23, 1996.

Higgins, S. T., *et al.* (1993). Achieving cocaine abstinence with a behavioral approach. *American Journal of Psychiatry*, 150, 763–9.

Hoffman, N. G., Harrison, P. A., and Belille, C. A. (1983). Alcoholics Anonymous after treatment: attendance and abstinence. *International Journal of Addictions*, 18, 311–18.

Hoffman, J. A., *et al.* (1991). Effective treatments for cocaine abuse and HIV risk. the cocaine abuse treatment strategies (CATS) project. Plenary lecture given at 5th International Congress on Drug Abuse, 'The Global Village' Research, Policies, and Community Action, Jerusalem, Israel, September 1–6, 1991.

Horvath, A. O. and Symonds, B. D. (1991). Relation between working alliance and outcome in psychotherapy: a meta-analysis. *Journal of Counseling Psychology*, **38**, 139–49

Iguchi, M. Y., *et al.* (1997). Reinforcing operants other than abstinence in drug abuse treatment: an effective alternative for reducing drug use. *Journal of Consulting and Clinical Psychology*, **65**, 421–8.

Imhof, J. (1991). Countertransference issues in alcohol and drug addiction. *Psychiatric Annals*, **21**, 292–306.

Kessler, R. C., *et al.* (1996). The epidemiology of co-occurring addictive and mental disorders: implications for prevention and service utilization. *American Journal of Orthopsychiatry*, **66**, 17–31.

Khantzian, E. J. (1985). The self-medication hypothesis of addictive disorders: focus on heroin and cocaine dependence. *American Journal of Psychiatry*, **142**, 1259–64.

Khantzian, E. J. and Khantzian, N. J. (1984). Cocaine addiction: is there a psychological predisposition? *Psychiatric Annals*, **14**, 753–9.

Khantzian, E. J. and Treece, C. (1985). DSM-III psychiatric diagnosis of narcotic addicts. *Archives of General Psychiatry*, **42**, 1067–71.

Kleinman, P. H., *et al.* (1990). Crack and cocaine abusers in outpatient psychotherapy. In: L. S. Onken and J. D. Blaine, ed. *Psychotherapy and counseling in the treatment of drug abuse*, pp. 24–34. NIDA Research Monograph 104. Rockville, MD: US Department of Health and Human Services.

Luborsky, L., *et al.* (1985). Therapist success and its determinants. *Archives of General Psychiatry*, **42**, 602–11.

Luborsky, L., Crits-Christoph, P., and McLellan, A. T. (1986). Do therapists vary in their effectiveness? Findings from four outcome studies. *American Journal of Orthopsychiatry*, **66**, 501–12.

Luborsky, L., *et al.* (1995). Supportive-expressive dynamic psychotherapy for opiate drug dependence. In: J. Barber and P. Crits-Christoph, ed. *Dynamic therapies for psychiatric disorders*, pp. 131–60. New York: Basic Books.

Marlatt, G. A. and Gordon, J., ed. (1985). *Relapse prevention: maintenance strategies in the treatment of addictive behaviors*. New York, Guilford.

McLellan, A. T., *et al.* (1993). Are psychosocial services necessary in substance abuse treatment? *Journal of the American Medical Association*, **269**, 1953–9.

McLellan, A. T., *et al.* (1997). Similarity of outcome predictors across opiate, cocaine, and alcohol treatments. role of treatment services. *Journal of Consulting and Clinical Psychology*, **62**, 1141–58.

Metzger, D. S., Navaline, H., and Woody, G. E. (1998). Drug abuse treatment as AIDS prevention. *Public Health Reports*, **113** (Suppl. 1), 97–106.

Miller, W. R., *et al.* (1992). *Motivational enhancement therapy manual. A clinical research guide for therapists treating individuals with alcohol abuse and dependence*. NIAAA Project MATCH Monograph, Vol. 2 (DHHS Publication No. ADM-92-1894). Washington, DC: US Government Printing Office.

Milmoe, S., *et al.* (1967). The doctor's voice: postdictor of successful referral of alcohol patients. *Journal of Abnormal Psychology*, **72**, 78–84.

Nowinski, J., Baker, S., and Carroll, K. (1992). *Twelve-step facilitation therapy manual: a clinical research guide for therapists treating individuals with alcohol abuse and dependence*. NIAAA Project MATCH Monograph, Vol. 1. (DHHS Publ No ADM-92-1893). Washington, DC: US Government Printing Office.

Nyswander, M., *et al.* (1958). The treatment of drug addicts as voluntary outpatients: a progress report. *American Journal of Orthopsychiatry*, **28**, 714–29.

Onken, L. S. and Blaine, J. D. (1990). Psychotherapy and counseling research in drug abuse treatment: questions, problems, and solutions. In: L. S. Onken and J. D. Blaine, ed. *Psychotherapy and counseling in the treatment of drug abuse*, pp. 1–5. NIDA Research Monograph 104. Rockville, MD: US Department of Health and Human Services.

Project MATCH Research Group (1997). Matching alcoholism treatments to client heterogeneity: Project MATCH posttreatment drinking outcomes. *Journal of Studies on Alcohol*, **58**, 7–29.

Rawson, R. A., *et al.* (2001). Naltrexone for opioid dependence: evaluation of a manualized psychosocial protocol to enhance treatment response. *Drug and Alcohol Review*, **20**, 67–78.

Resnick, R. B., *et al.* (1981). Psychotherapy and naltrexone in opioid dependence. In: L. S. Harris, ed. *Problems of drug dependence*, pp. 109–15. NIDA Research Monograph 34. Rockville, MD: US Department of Health and Human Services.

Rounsaville, B. J., *et al.* (1982). Heterogeneity of psychiatric diagnoses in treated opiate addicts. *Archives of General Psychiatry*, **39**, 161–6.

Rounsaville, B. J., *et al.* (1983). Short-term interpersonal psychotherapy in methadone maintained opiate addicts. *Archives of General Psychiatry*, **40**, 629–36.

Rounsaville, B. J., *et al.* (1991). Psychiatric diagnoses of treatment-seeking cocaine abusers. *Archives of General Psychiatry*, **48**, 43–51.

Shoptaw, S. and Frosch, D. (2000). Substance abuse treatment as HIV prevention for men who have sex with men. *AIDS & Behavior*, **4**, 193–203.

Shoptaw, S., Frosch, D., Rawson, R. A., and Ling, W. (1997). Cocaine abuse counseling as HIV prevention. *AIDS Education and Prevention*, **9**, 511–20.

Silverman, K., *et al.* (1996). Sustained cocaine abstinence in methadone maintenance patients through voucher-based reinforcement therapy. *Archives of General Psychiatry*, **53**, 409–15.

Stephens, R. S., Roffman, R. A., and Simpson, E. E. (1994). Treating adult marijuana dependence: a test of the relapse prevention model. *Journal of Consulting and Clinical Psychology*, **62**, 92–9.

Washton, A. and Stone-Washton, N. (1990). Abstinence and relapse in cocaine addicts. *Journal of Psychoactive Drugs*, **22**, 135–47.

Weiss, R. D., *et al.* (1986). Psychopathology in chronic cocaine abusers. *American Journal of Drug and Alcohol Abuse*, **12**, 17–29.

Weiss, R. D., *et al.* (1996). Self-help activities in cocaine dependent patients entering treatment. Results from the NIDA CCTS. *Drug and Alcohol Dependence*, **43**, 79–86.

Woody, G. E., *et al.* (1983). Psychotherapy for opiate addicts: does it help? *Archives of General Psychiatry*, **40**, 639–45.

Woody, G. E., *et al.* (1985). Psychiatric severity as a predictor of benefits from psychotherapy. *American Journal of Psychiatry*, **141**, 1172–7.

Woody, G. E., *et al.* (1990a). In: L. S. Onken and J. D. Blaine, ed. *Psychotherapy and counseling for methadone maintained opiate addicts. Results of research studies*, pp. 9–23. NIDA Research Monograph 104. Rockville, MD: US Department of Health and Human Services.

Woody, G. E., McLellan, A. T., and O'Brien, C. P. (1990b). Research on psychopathology and addiction: treatment implications. *Drug and Alcohol Dependence*, **25**, 121–3.

Woody, G. E., *et al.* (1995). Psychotherapy in community methadone programs: a validation study. *American Journal of Psychiatry*, **152**, 1302–8.

Woody, G. E., *et al.* (1998). Psychotherapy with opioid-dependent patients. *Psychiatric Times*, November.

Woody, G. E., *et al.* and the Cocaine Psychotherapy Study Group (2003). HIV risk reduction in the NIDA cocaine collaborative treatment study. *Journal of Acquired Immune Deficiency Syndromes*, **33**, 82–7.

Yahne, C. E., Miller, W. R., Irvin-Vitela, L., and Tonigan, J. S. (2002). Magdalena pilot project: motivational outreach to substance abusing women street sex workers. *Journal of Substance Abuse Treatment*, **23**, 49–53.

20 Psychotherapy of somatoform disorders

Don R. Lipsitt and Javier Escobar

Since medicine's earliest beginnings, physicians have been perplexed and vexed by patients whose symptoms seem medically unexplainable and who respond poorly to treatment. In 1927, the legendary Francis W. Peabody, Harvard Professor of Medicine at Boston City Hospital, wrote that teachers and students are at risk of '. . . serious error in their attitude toward a large group of patients who do not show objective, organic pathologic conditions, and who are generally spoken of as having "nothing the matter with them" ' (Peabody, 1927). Peabody identifies these patients as having conditions under the broad heading of 'psychoneuroses,' with the 'ultimate causes . . . to be found, not in any gross structural changes in the organs involved, but rather in nervous influences emanating from the emotional and intellectual life which, directly or indirectly, affect in one way or another organs that are under either voluntary or involuntary control' (Peabody, 1927, p. 878). Treatment, he said, is most appreciably the responsibility of the internist and general practitioner, and its effectiveness is most attributable to the quality of a caring patient–doctor relationship. He is most famously quoted for his concluding statement that '. . . the secret of the care of the patient is in caring for the patient' (Peabody, 1927, p. 882).

How far have we come regarding diagnosis and treatment of these 'difficult patients' since these perceptive words were written? Because organized medicine has had little success with these patients and perhaps because of the prickly relationships they have with their physicians, understanding of their illness behavior, diagnosis, and treatment have, over the years, moved from medicine into psychiatry's domain under the current rubric of 'somatoform disorders,' disorders that present in the form of physical distress but are believed to have a significant emotional (psychological) dimension. The treatment literature consists largely of cumulative experience and clinical wisdom but disappointingly few reliable well-controlled studies. With few research studies and attempts at classification that have been beset with confusion, controversy, and inconsistency, we are left confronted with uncertain treatments for uncertain disorders. But there are new advances appearing on the horizon.

This chapter reviews what is known about the psychotherapeutic interventions that have succeeded or failed with these disorders and the challenges they present to healthcare professionals. Matters of diagnosis, clinical description, prevalence, and etiology are covered sufficiently in other texts and will be touched on only briefly here. Similarly, detailed elements of psychopharmacotherapy remain beyond the scope of this chapter. Our focus will be on key practice principles of psychosocial treatments of the entire group of somatoform disorders. Each disorder will be discussed in terms of unique therapeutic requirements or specific pertinent research, concluding with a general therapeutic formulation appropriate to the entire group.

Conceptualization

Detailed inspection of functional somatic syndromes reveals that all include common elements.

1. No gold standard to confirm or rule out the diagnosis.

2. Presence of multiple unexplained symptoms originating in several organ systems.

3. High levels of psychiatric comorbidity.

4. No clear pathophysiology; while a number of pathophysiological mechanisms have been invoked to explain many of these syndromes (e.g., symptom amplification, muscle contraction, catecholamine release, persistent neurobiological dysfunction, neurological hyperreactivity, elevated cortisol) no clear pathophysiological knowledge has emerged for any of them.

5. No consistent explanation emanating from physical and laboratory assessments.

6. No good fit with rules of allopathic medicine.

7. Comparable responses with certain psychological [e.g., cognitive-behavior therapy (CBT)] and pharmacological (e.g., antidepressants) interventions.

8. The presence of emotionally charged, highly politicized groups of patients/advocates. Indeed, patients with functional somatic syndromes such as 'chronic fatigue,' 'fibromyalgia', and in general, many of those who prefer other 'medicalized' labels such as Lyme disease, or 'environmental disorders,' have been forming highly passionate groups.

Research

In 1991 excellent reviews of this topic appeared almost simultaneously on both sides of the Atlantic (Barsky and Borus, 1999; Wessely *et al.*, 1999). These reviews underlined the many common epidemiological, clinical, and psychopathological aspects of these 'functional' syndromes in efforts to set the stage for much-needed collaborative research in this area.

Barring more convincing research evidence, it is ultimately one's personal definition of somatization that influences the selection of treatment: thus, therapists favoring the concept of a learned dysfunction may prefer cognitive-behavioral approaches while those theorizing a developmental failure in mothering, for example, may prefer more dynamic and supportive techniques, and so on.

While descriptive accounts of somatization abound, theoretical or causal explanations are scarce. In this context, and despite its dualism, we find the developmental schema of Max Schur (a psychoanalyst and Freud's personal physician) appealing as a well-rounded theory supported by experience. Schur (1955) posited that the infant is born with a capacity for only undifferentiated physical expression and it is not until the development of motor control, neural structures, and language ('ego development') that the child has the capacity for direct emotional expression.

According to Schur, the child passes from a totally somatized state to one that is gradually *de*-somatized. In the face of trauma, deprivation, developmental failure, and other debilitating factors, the child may revert ('regress') to *re*-somatizing states. Henceforth, somatization may be resorted to for the expression of 'unspeakable' emotional distress. Such a theory has some endorsement from studies that have shown a high correlation between medically unexplained symptoms and early childhood sexual and/or physical abuse (E. A. Walker *et al.*, 1999; Newman *et al.*, 2000). It is also supported by findings that suggest a correlation between physical symptom reporting and alexithymia (Sifneos, 1973). Further theoretical elaboration by Scheidt and Waller (1999) emphasizes the importance of the quality of early maternal attachment in determining later (adult) predisposition to somatization.

Another body of research, particularly within the last 5 years, has examined the efficacy of CBT for somatization. According to the research, CBT seems to help patients modify thoughts and behaviors that are associated with somatization and recognize the role of 'stress' in physical dysfunctions, such as sleep disturbance, fatigue, pain, and so on. Patients are subsequently helped to combat this effect via numerous behavioral techniques, including relaxation training and graded increases in activities. From a cognitive perspective, CBT helps these patients identify thoughts that contribute to increased stress, inactivity, and health concern. Often, these patients think catastrophically about their physical symptoms, leading to conclusions that one is sick and that one must limit physical activity, contributing to a cycle that perpetuates the somatic process.

A number of studies support the use of CBT for patients suffering from somatization. Allen and associates (Allen et al., 2001) showed that CBT helped patients with full DSM (*Diagnostic and statistical manual of mental disorders*) somatization disorder (SD) significantly reduce their physical discomfort, anxiety, and depression, as well as increase their physical functioning. Other investigators have conducted CBT in the primary care setting with patients presenting unexplained physical symptoms (Lidbeck, 1997; McLeod et al., 1997; Sumathipala et al., 2000). These studies have demonstrated reductions not only in physical and emotional symptoms, but also in physical impairments and medical utilization.

Although CBT has been typically administered in mental health specialty settings, there seem to be a number of advantages to providing CBT in primary care, when working with somatizing patients. First, because these patients preferentially use medical services, providing CBT in primary care helps to match treatment to the somatizing patients' expectations; somatizing patients are apt to feel more comfortable in the primary care environment. Second, patients suffering from medically unexplained symptoms often receive signals from others that their symptoms are less than genuine. For this reason, referral to mental health settings often conveys more stigma, and the perception that referral to a mental health facility invalidates their physical distress by suggesting that it is 'all in their heads.' As a result, patients often do not follow through with mental health referral and frequently switch physicians (Lipsitt, 1964; Lipsitt, 1968; Lin et al., 1991). Moreover, providing CBT in the primary care setting has the obvious benefit of maximizing coordination between the mental health provider and the primary care physician.

As almost all individuals experience one or another physical symptom in a period of a week or two (Kellner and Sheffield, 1973; Pennebaker et al., 1977) it should be obvious that it is only when such symptoms exceed a threshold prompting medical help-seeking that the label 'somatization' is typically warranted.

It is the primary care physician, not the psychiatrist, who most often sees patients with somatizing conditions. Moreover, the multiple definitions for these syndromes that exist in psychiatry and medicine, make prevalence data very difficult to gather, and the frequent changes in the nomenclatures add to the confusion. Because most somatoform disorders are seen in outpatient practices, little is known about the prevalence of somatoform disorders in the general or psychiatric hospital. And because patients with somatizing conditions do not usually identify themselves as having psychiatric illness and will commonly reject referral to a psychiatrist if it is offered, the prevalence in psychiatric practice is probably less than in primary care.

In medical practice, somatization is tied to the issue of the 'frequent consulters.' These patients present with symptoms that change over time. They receive more medical diagnoses, have unhealthy lifestyles (in terms of diet and use of alcohol and tobacco), and a high frequency of mental disorders (over 50% reported psychological 'distress'). However, despite their high levels of psychological symptoms these patients are very unlikely to see themselves as 'psychiatric' patients, even though about one-fourth of them meet diagnostic criteria for major depression, 22% for anxiety disorders, 17% for dysthymia, and up to 20% for full DSM criteria for SD (Gill and Sharpe, 1999).

Although little is understood about the precise way in which the somatization process is mediated, some have suggested a central nervous system elaboration of stimuli, with 'amplified' perception (Barsky, 1992). Others have posited some kind of physiological reactivity or hypersensitivity (Miller, 1984; Sharpe and Bass, 1992; Rief and Auer, 2001). James and associates (James et al., 1989) suggest that attentional processes of somatizing patients are affected by some fundamental neuronal and physical dysfunction. EEG studies showed that somatizers responded to both relevant and irrelevant stimuli in the same way, suggesting that some filter mechanism may be missing, making it difficult or impossible for the somatizer to ignore irrelevant stimuli. Psychological studies have demonstrated this 'blocking' action to occur more often in individuals who have either high or low hypnotizability as well as high scores on the Marlowe-Crowne Social Desirability Scale (Wickramasekera, 1998). PET scan studies (Garcia Campayo et al., 2001) have shown changes in somatizing patients that resemble those found in depressed patients. Other studies suggest that biological and pathophysiological changes may contribute to somatizing conditions (Fink et al., 2002).

In spite of their shared characteristics, each somatoform disorder shows variations in history, conceptualization, and treatment as described separately below. Pain disorder will be omitted as the psychotherapy of these patients is comprehensively discussed in Chapter 33 (Medical patients).

Somatization disorder

SD has been defined as a complex, usually chronic condition primarily of females with a history of multiple unintentionally produced physical complaints beginning at a young age and always before 30. Briquet's virtual encyclopedia of physical symptoms was reduced in DSM-III to 14 physical symptoms for women and 12 for men of a possible 37 to reach diagnostic threshold (quite arbitrarily, some have said), changed in DSM-IIIR to 13 total, and finally, in DSM-IV, modified to eight physical complaints referable to four pain sites or functions (e.g., back, chest, urination), two nonpain gastrointestinal symptoms (e.g., nausea, bloating), one nonpain sexual or reproductive system symptom (e.g., menstrual irregularity, loss of libido), and one pseudoneurological symptom (e.g., urinary retention, aphonia, blindness). Although symptoms are unaccounted for by known general organic pathology or substance abuse, they may nevertheless be 'exaggerations' of ordinarily expected symptoms of coexisting physical disease. Symptoms generally occur over a period of several years accompanied by significant impairment of social and occupational function and high utilization of medical resources, usually resulting in either ineffective and/or unnecessary medical/surgical treatments. Many encounters of these patients with physicians generally evoke frustration in both parties of the relationship.

Several researchers, responding to an expressed need for a diagnosis of subtypes seen in primary care in the range between full-fledged SD and the undifferentiated form, have offered suggestions of 'somatization syndrome,' 'abridged SD' (Escobar et al., 1989), 'polymorphous,' 'multisomatoform' (Kroenke et al., 1997), or 'polysomatoform' (Rief and Hiller, 1999) disorder. Because of the difficulty in applying the unwieldy diagnostic criteria in primary care practice, Escobar et al. (1989) devised an abridged somatization construct, called a Somatic Symptom Index (SSI), requiring only four symptoms for males and six for females to reach diagnostic significance. When the full criteria are not met for SD, patients with multiple unexplained somatic complaints lasting at least 6 months are usually given the diagnosis undifferentiated somatoform disorder. This classification may include such entities as fibromyalgia, irritable bowel syndrome, chronic fatigue syndrome, and others. DSM-IV criteria were designed primarily for adult populations, but may have applicability to child and adolescent patients.

Conceptualization

Freud's first patients were somatizers. As a clinical neurologist beginning practice, his patients comprised essentially other physicians' failures, not dissimilar to what is experienced by new young physicians today. His meticulous study of his patients' symptoms and histories culminated in his theories of psychoanalysis, the significance of symptoms as derivatives of early life experience and even the concept of negative therapeutic reaction in which patients 'resist' symptomatic improvement. Freud's famous descriptions of his earliest 'hysterical' patients might well be considered to have SD if seen today. While a specific etiology is unknown, the origins of SD share many features with other somatoform disorders. Some have suggested that patients with SD have an intensified sensitivity to normal physiologic events and may also exhibit 'masked depression' in response to trauma, loss, deprivation, and rejection.

Various descriptions of SD rely on psychodynamic principles to understand the symptom profile and the behavior of patients so diagnosed. Treatment may depend upon whether that conceptualization focuses on developmental failure, disturbances in the infant–mother or infant–caretaker relationship, affective deficits, alexithymia, object relations problems, homeostasis disruption, selectively learned dysfunction, or faulty developmental regulation (Knapp, 1989). Emphasis on learned behaviors may lead more commonly to cognitive-behavioral or group interventions, while other conceptualizations may encourage more relational, interpersonal, or psychodynamic approaches. Psychopharmacological approaches may be independent or combined with other interventions.

No preferred treatment has been established for SD. A search of the Cochrane Library databases for research into the psychotherapy of SD reveals no relevant findings. Most researchers indicate that the best therapeutic achievements, as modest as they may be, are the result of an ongoing empathic relationship with a consistent caregiver. Research on interventions with SD patients is hampered by a variety of problems: patients are usually seen in primary care settings, where therapists may be poorly prepared to work with demanding, frustrating patients; comorbid physical disease often is a major confounder. Studies have shown a 60% comorbidity with medical disease, 55–94% with depression, 26–45% with panic disorder, and 17–31% with alcohol abuse or dependence in SD patients (Bass and Murphy, 1991); and there is a relatively high rate of personality disorder in patients with SD, the most frequent types being avoidant, paranoid, and self-defeating, not borderline or histrionic as previous observers have reported (Rost et al., 1992).

Counteracting the prevailing rather nihilistic attitude about treatment of SD, one study showed improvement over a period of 2 years in 30 patients treated in an inpatient psychosomatic hospital in Germany (Rief et al., 1995); treatment utilized an 'integrative behavioral medicine approach' consisting of individual psychotherapy, assertiveness training, problem-solving training, progressive muscle relaxation, and 'other cognitive-behavioral, emotional and movement therapies.' Patients showing most improvement had fewer symptoms and less psychiatric comorbidity.

It is generally acknowledged that to treat effectively patients with SD, primary physicians must be recruited as participants. A groundbreaking controlled study by Smith et al. (1986) demonstrated the effectiveness of a 'consultation letter' to primary physicians instructing them on a few key management techniques to use with their patients. Although patients did not show great change diagnostically or symptomatically, they did improve in function, decreased their overutilization of resources and generated significant cost-savings.

While no adequately controlled studies of psychotherapeutic intervention existed prior to the study by Smith and colleagues, a number of studies of undifferentiated forms of somatoform disorder suggest therapeutic benefits from an accepting attitude in the therapist (Rost et al., 1994), cautious efforts to shift the patient's attention from somatic to emotional features (Morriss and Gask, 2002), or the use of groups that focus on explanation, support, relaxation, and cognitive-behavioral approaches to emphasize adaptation to chronic somatic distress (Ford and Long, 1977; Melson and Rynearson, 1986; Hellman et al., 1990; Kaplan et al., 1993; Guthrie et al., 1993; Payne and Blanchard, 1995; Speckens et al., 1995). More recently, brief psychodynamic therapy of unexplained somatic symptoms proved superior in both controlled randomized and uncontrolled studies (Nielsen et al., 1988) compared with regular medical treatment alone. An uncontrolled

intensive inpatient treatment program for chronic severe somatizing patients described a 33% improvement rate in 92 patients treated with combinations of relaxation training, physical activation, and pharmacotherapy (Shorter et al., 1992).

Key practice principles

SD embodies virtually all the characteristics that make somatizing patients very refractory to attempts at therapeutic intervention: multiplicity of symptoms; chronicity; imperviousness to traditional types of reassurance; rigidity of adherence to belief in the presence of physical disease; high and usually inappropriate utilization of medical resources; unresponsiveness to pharmacologic treatment trials; alexithymia; risk of 'occult' comorbidities; sensitivity to rejection; and frequent dysfunctional patient–physician relationships. Such a context represents a profound challenge to the most well-intentioned, dedicated physician. With this realization, first attempts at establishing a therapeutic setting must begin with a caring rather than curing orientation, one that conveys acceptance, sincerity, and flexibility to the patient.

Therapeutic 'triumphs' may be measured in reduced overutilization of resources, limitations on unrealistic expectations, a commitment to a single primary care physician, and minimalization of 'furor therapeuticus' that may result in useless procedures, tests, and surgeries. The physician must be prepared for a long-term commitment to patients with SD. Restraint must be exercised in the urge to refer for specialist consultation, unless there is reasonable evidence to suggest specific comorbid conditions and thorough preparation of the patient for such referral. Wishful expectations in findings and outcome should be curtailed and the patient must be assured of the continuing interest of and appointments with the primary physician. Helping patients to correct distortions about symptom relevance and meaning or to perceive somatic distress as a common response to life stresses may be a slow protracted process that, if pushed too abruptly, may mistakenly convey to the patient the physician's distrust, disbelief, or outright rejection of the patient's complaints. Families of patients with SD commonly have already registered disbelief in the patient's illness, perhaps even accusing them of malingering; the advocacy of the physician in such circumstances becomes an even more essential ingredient for management.

Some of the elements of CBT may be incorporated conveniently into the primary care physician's treatment strategy. For example, diary-keeping by the patient, activity prescriptions such as exercise and yoga, and ancillary 'somatic' treatments such as acupuncture, relaxation, meditation, massage, and so on are more easily accepted by these somatizing patients than attempts at 'mental' recommendations. When SD patients request medications, as they frequently do, it is necessary to review the patient's (usually) previous negative experience, the failure of medications to offer relief, and the variety of side-effects that usually accompany trials of any new drug. Adhering to the low- or no-drug treatment approach may be difficult for the physician, but in time can demonstrate to the patient greater interest in the patient herself, with a deflection of exclusive focus on the symptom(s) alone. The presence of well-defined comorbid states such as anxiety, depression, panic disorder, or psychosis may, of course, call for the judicious prescription of specifically targeted pharmacologic agents. In time, the physician and patient may both be rewarded with a dampened 'organ recital,' decreased agitation, improved functional capacity, and more appropriate, beneficial and less costly use of health resources.

Case examples

Case 1

The following case vignette illustrates a supportive, psychodynamic approach.

Mrs N's first visit as a new patient to a medical clinic was at the age of 45 with a complaint of varicose veins, 4 years after a hysterectomy in another hospital, where she had been seen for many years with multiple physical complaints. In this first visit she revealed that her husband had died 2 years before her hysterectomy and her father died of a stroke at age 72 several months before her visit to the new clinic. In the next 12 years she had had surgery for hemorrhoids, varicose veins, adhesions, and scar reconstruction. Her medical record noted many visits to specialty clinics as well as the emergency room for a variety of major and minor complaints. In Skin Clinic alone, she was treated for eczema, varicose dermatitis, fibrous polyp of the vulva, contact dermatitis of the ears, seborrheic dermatitis, and contact neuro-dermatitis. She had had several minor accidents, dental problems and repeatedly lost her eyeglasses. It was not until 12 years later that 'emotional difficulty' was noted in her chart when she was seen in Neurology Clinic with 'intense pain that could not be accounted for on the basis of her vascular disease.' However, she was returned to Medical Clinic where she 'complained excessively of joint pain' thought by her doctor to be 'out of proportion to physical findings.' Finally, an entry of 'neurasthenia' was made in the record and she was referred for psychiatric evaluation. At first reluctant to see the psychiatrist, she ultimately accepted and in addition to current complaints she said that she had been sick 'all my life' but that things had gotten worse after her father died. She was now experiencing fatigue, abdominal and chest pain, and difficulty sleeping. She said she can usually 'take things on the chin and come up fighting,' but things had become more than she could handle. Accustomed to doing things for others, she found satisfaction in work as a saleslady, although she had stopped working because of her ailments. Other doctors, she said, had tried many drugs but they either did not help or she developed side-effects. Complaining of her prior treatment, she said that she could take better care of herself than some doctors could. A plan was presented to see Mrs N once a month for a half hour. Because many medications had already failed to help her, a decision was made not to prescribe anything, but rather to appeal to her inherent strength to help herself. She was praised for her strength and her ability to 'come up fighting.' Her 'organ recital' was listened to patiently and frequently (a major aspect of each session) with the 'reassurance' that these things had bothered her for a long time and that it surely must have been frustrating, as was the failure of previous treatments to help; the physician expressed his awe that she was 'able to survive all these stresses and strains and still be able to manage.' She was informed that her symptoms might, in fact, not get better, although she may be able to fight them to some degree. Because she always felt better doing for others rather than for herself, she was encouraged to resume her work as a saleslady and found satisfaction and distraction in that endeavor. Furthermore, because she said she was sympathetic with those who are unhappy and neglected, she was advised also to offer part-time volunteer work in a neighborhood nursing home, work that she found very satisfying (masochistic characteristics of her personality were constructively satisfied). Although symptoms did not remit, in time she reduced her visits to specialty clinics, discontinued her use of the emergency room, and began to talk more about her family relationships than her physical complaints. In time (that is, 2 years or a total of 24 half-hour visits), the patient requested lengthening the time between visits as she felt she was functioning better and wanted to 'try it myself.' Although this was granted, she was advised that she could always return to the old schedule if she felt it necessary, but that she did seem ready to use her own strong resources. Eventually she was seen every 4–6 months, with only an occasional phone call in between. She continued to see her primary doctor at 6-month intervals; this physician was given suggestions about how to work with a person with Mrs N's character traits and psychological defenses. He was encouraged to avoid the use of medications as she seemed to experience them as the physician's wish to be rid of her.

Case 2

The following case vignette illustrates the application of CBT principles to SD.

Ms J, a 48-year-old female, raised in Mexico, with a very difficult and impoverished childhood, emigrated to the United States 6 years prior to treatment in search of a 'better life,' planning on earning enough money to return to Mexico and live more comfortably. Married at a very early age, and with three children, she had separated from her husband 1 year previously due to 'domestic violence' that had started early in the marriage and worsened after her grown children left the house.

Ms J was referred by the social worker at her primary care center after she complained to her physician about multiple somatic symptoms. At the time of the referral, she was living with her oldest son, his wife, and children, serving as the children's caretaker. Symptoms included stomach aches, back pain, joint pain, arm pain, chest pain, headaches, menstrual irregularities, urinary pain and problems, burning in her genitals, vomiting, nausea, diarrhea, excess gas, difficulty digesting certain foods, difficulties with her sight and hearing, difficulties with balance, fatigue, throat pain/problems, and sexual dysfunction, all of them medically unexplained.

The psychologist's evaluation revealed that Ms J met full criteria for SD. She also had significant depression and anxiety symptoms. Therapy consisted of a 10-week CBT program at the primary care clinic as part of an ongoing study. At the first session, the patient discussed her physical symptoms and her thoughts about causes of her symptoms. She thought many of her pain symptoms were related to 'exposure to hot and cold temperatures.' She did acknowledge that the stress of leaving her husband and adjusting to life without him may have precipitated many of her symptoms. She was able to connect stressors with symptoms. She welcomed the use of diaphragmatic breathing and was able to utilize the exercise as a way of lowering stress levels as well as creating time for herself.

Because of her past history of abuse and deprivations, encouraging pleasurable activities as well as utilizing distraction techniques was important. As treatment progressed, Ms J was able to exercise on a daily basis, walking approximately 15 minutes a day. Furthermore, she listened to music as a form of distraction from her physical symptoms, allowing the accompanying relaxation to lower her stress levels and decrease physical symptoms.

Sleep hygiene was another focus of treatment. Ms J did not have a routine for sleeping. She complained of fatigue and awakening with bodily pain. Setting a routine of at least 7–8 hours of sleep per night helped to structure her day, changing her perception of pain upon awakening and decreasing feelings of fatigue throughout the day.

The final focus of treatment was to challenge dysfunctional thoughts. Ms J's pessimistic outlook of her life included conviction that: her symptoms would never get better; she would die young; and she was a burden on her children (even though she helped them raise their own children by caring for them while the parents worked). By helping her look at her thought processes and teaching her the skills necessary to question and change them, she was able to decrease her symptoms and improve her quality of life. This included assertiveness training to address her inability to express her own needs and her low self-esteem.

During the last session, Ms J and her psychotherapist discussed a plan to continue to examine dysfunctional thinking, to exercise, to adhere to a sleep routine and engage in pleasurable activity to help maintain the acquired behavioral and cognitive techniques that had significantly decreased her physical symptoms, including cessation of headaches and leg pains.

Hypochondriasis

Clinical descriptions of hypochondriasis today are impressively consistent with those of earliest times and have been distilled and formalized in DSM-IV as follows: preoccupation with fears of having, or the idea that one has, a serious disease based on the person's misinterpretation of bodily symptoms, with duration of at least 6 months; the preoccupation persists despite appropriate medical evaluation and reassurance; the belief is not of delusional intensity and is not restricted to a circumscribed concern about appearance; the preoccupation causes clinically significant distress or impairment in social, occupational, or other important areas of functioning; the preoccupation is not better accounted for by generalized anxiety disorder, panic disorder, a major depressive episode, separation anxiety, or another somatoform disorder.

Conceptualization

While there is general agreement that hypochondriasis is a 'mental' disorder categorically distinct from others, some subscribe to a dimensional concept in which hypochondriacal symptoms exist on a continuum from heightened awareness of bodily function to extreme delusional bodily preoccupation. Some consider distinctions between health anxiety, disease phobia, and disease conviction (Barsky and Wyshak, 1989); panic (Furer et al., 1997); a variant of obsessive-compulsive disorder (OCD) (Hollender, 1993) or a personality disorder (Tyrer et al., 1990). Psychoanalytic concepts are retained in the view that hypochondriasis is a defensive reaction against the guilt of aggressive impulses and overwhelming fear of 'annihilation' (Vaillant, 1977; Lipsitt, 2001a).

As with other somatoform disorders, clinicians who subscribe to the conceptualization of hypochondriasis as a learned behavior will lean towards CBT approaches, while believers in the primacy of developmental, interpersonal, or character structure as explanations of hypochondriasis will favor psychoanalytic/psychodynamic approaches. Differentiating the disorder as primary or secondary will influence treatment (Speckens, 2001), especially with a preference for psychopharmacologic treatment for accompanying diagnoses of anxiety or affective disorders. In spite of a wide choice of therapies, controlled studies showing therapeutic superiority of one over another have been rare.

Research

There has been a paucity of controlled studies of the treatment of hypochondriasis, but past reports of several case series of cognitive-behavioral psychotherapy had suggested benefits (Kellner, 1982; Salkovskis and Warwick, 1986; Warwick, 1989; Logsdail et al., 1991; Visser and Bouman, 1992). Kellner's study demonstrated improvement in 36 patients with behavioral interventions that corrected misinformation and distortions and demonstrated to patients how these factors contributed to misattribution and persistent fearful beliefs.

More recently, several controlled studies have confirmed the earlier suggestions of the effectiveness of cognitive-behavioral interventions. A recent review (Kroenke and Swindle, 2000) from 1966 to 1999 identified 31 controlled studies, 29 of which were randomized in the treatment of a variety of somatizing syndromes. In this survey, CBT-treated patients improved significantly more than control subjects in 71% of studies, with a trend of improvement in an additional 11% of studies. In one such controlled study, hypochondriacal patients were randomly assigned to either individual CBT or a no-treatment waiting-list. After 4 months of weekly treatment, 76% of treated patients showed significant improvement, sustained in 3-month follow-up (Warwick et al., 1996). This finding has been replicated in other randomized controlled trials (Speckens et al., 1995). One such study (Clark et al., 1998) compared treatment of 48 patients with cognitive therapy to behavioral stress management and a no-treatment wait-list control group. Both therapeutic groups were effective, maintaining improvement after 1 year, with cognitive treatment showing more improvement in hypochondriacal measures than on general mood disturbance at 3 months follow-up. A recent controlled study (Barsky, 2004) randomizing patients to individual CBT or 'standard' medical care appears to have shown 'significant beneficial effects' at one year follow-up with CBT. The distinction in many studies between cognitive and behavioral treatment is not always clear.

One study (Bouman and Visser, 1998) evaluated the effectiveness of 'pure' time-limited cognitive or behavioral interventions in 17 patients in 12 one-hour sessions. Patients in both treatment groups showed equivalent improvement over controls on specific measures of hypochondriasis and depression. However, nonspecific factors such as patient motivation, therapist attitudes, and the therapeutic relationship could not be ruled out as contributing factors (studies of these important nonspecific dimensions of treatment in somatizing disorders are conspicuously lacking in the research literature). Treatment preference by patients may also influence outcome (J. Walker et al., 1999).

Group therapy using cognitive-educational methods has had reported success in several studies (Barsky et al. 1988; Stern and Fernandez, 1991; Avia et al., 1996). With an 'educational' focus, studies showed significant reductions in illness fears and attitudes, fewer somatic symptoms and long-term benefits in dysphoric mood and wellbeing. A study of 96 patients receiving combined individual and group 'intensive' inpatient CBT showed 'substantial improvements or recovery' from hypochondriacal symptomatology (Hiller et al., 2002). Predictors of poor outcome and course of illness were higher degree of pretreatment hypochondriasis, more somatized symptoms and general psychopathology (as measured on Symptom Checklist-90R), greater dysfunctional cognition, higher levels of psychosocial disability, and more extensive utilization of healthcare resources. Treatment was administered on a daily basis individually and in groups according to a therapy manual (Rief and Hiller, 1998). Goals of treatment were defined according to customary CBT principles: identification and modification of dysfunctional perceptions and thoughts; improved interpersonal and occupational function; and decreased dependency on healthcare resources. Educational and explanatory interventions, physical exercise, assertiveness training, progressive relaxation, and biofeedback were included in the manualized treatment.

Most studies involve patients already utilizing either mental or physical healthcare systems and not the community at large. In order to tap this resource and to assess effectiveness of interventions on 'lower-level' hypochondriasis, one study invited, by advertisement, 'participants' to apply for an 'educational course' called 'Coping with Illness Anxiety' (Bouman, 2002). Six 2-hour sessions, each dedicated to specific themes about hypochondriasis, were held for 21 participants in four groups of five to six, facilitated (not 'treated') by two graduate students of clinical psychology trained in individual cognitive-behavioral techniques, using a detailed manual. Parameters for hypochondriasis and depression (on selected pre- and posttest measures) showed improvement at 4 weeks and 6 months following the 'course,' suggesting that this is an acceptable, effective, and probably low-cost way to reduce hypochondriacal psychopathology, potentially applicable to nonhospital, nonclinic general medical practice. Other uncontrolled studies have shown benefits of brief explanatory therapy (Kellner, 1986; Barsky et al., 1988; Avia et al., 1997; Lloyd et al., 1998; Papageorgiou and Wells, 1998). A more recent study of 20 patients randomly assigned to a treatment group and a wait-list group confirmed the benefits of explanatory therapy on helping patients 'maintain control' of symptoms but with little change in symptomatology (Fava et al., 2000). Exposure, imaginal, and response-prevention therapies are also said to help correct misinformation or misperception, but no controlled studies are reported (Logsdail et al., 1991; Sisti, 1997).

Very few psychoanalytic studies exist. One Spanish study reports effectiveness of group psychoanalytic treatment (Garcia Campayo and Sanz Carrillo, 2000). The few reports on psychodynamic or psychoanalytic treatment of hypochondriasis generally warn of the negative consequences of 'uncovering' or 'interpretive' therapies that have a high risk of promoting 'quasi autistic withdrawal,' 'tormenting self-observation', and other regressive behaviors (Nissen, 2000). This is not to say that psychoanalytic and psychodynamic precepts do not have applicability in establishing and enhancing appropriate therapeutic relationships and treatment approaches in the management of hypochondriacal patients (Lipsitt, 2001a,b).

The role of reassurance in hypochondriasis has been a controversial one. While DSM-IV has made inability to reassure hypochondriacal patients a criterion of diagnosis, virtually all therapy reports include reassurance as one of many interventions. The ease with which somatizers can successfully be reassured varies with the chronicity and intensity of symptoms, personality variables in the patient, attitudes, and treatment style of the therapist (Kathol, 1997). Starcevic has provided a thoughtful and comprehensive overview of the varieties, pitfalls, and uses of reassurance in the treatment of hypochondriasis (Moene et al., 2000; Starcevic, 2001). Reassurance is regarded by cognitive-behavior therapists as a safety behavior for patients that interferes with progress and therefore should be avoided.

Key practice principles

Although there have been suggestive case series reports that pharmacotherapy may be helpful in some cases of hypochondriasis (Fallon, 2001), there are insufficient controls to suggest that drug treatment has any significant advantage over long-term supportive therapy. It would appear that psychotherapeutic interventions work in the context of an interested, accepting, and concerned relationship. Suggestions for enhancing this relationship are similar to those for managing SD. However, most hypochondriacal patients do not manifest the same intensity or demandingness seen in patients with SD. Some may even respond to judicious attempts at reassurance. If hypochondriacal patients can be systematically maintained over an extended period of time, opportunity for insight development may arise, along with lessening of symptoms and improved functional adaptation.

Patients rarely appear with 'pure' forms of hypochondriasis but may present with hypochondriacal reactions to established physical disease. For example:

A 58-year-old married woman with an obsessive-compulsive personality style, following a mild myocardial infarction, became hypochondriacally preoccupied with every minor physical sensation, certain that it was evidence of a fatal outcome. Accompanying depression was successfully treated with antidepressants, but fearful reaction to physical symptoms was chronically unreassureable. The patient was seen in supportive psychotherapy, with measured reassurance over time a major intervention, in half-hour sessions monthly for a year before she began to trust and accept her physicians' optimistic reports. In each session, she anxiously reviewed medication directions to be sure she was meticulously following medical orders. By the end of a year, she was able to be more flexible and less fearful, with little insight but increasing trust in the reassuring comments of psychiatrist and cardiologist, who coordinated their treatment.

In other approaches, cognitive-behavioral techniques show promise of hastening improvement. The following case vignette illustrates a CBT approach to treating combined hypochondriasis and abridged somatization.

Ms E is a 44-year-old married former history teacher who stopped working to care for her son and ailing mother. Five years previously, she presented with symptoms of chest pain and heart palpitations which, she feared, indicated cardiovascular disease. A cardiologist found no organic pathology and prescribed alprazolam, which she took only 'once or twice' before discontinuing it because it made her 'drowsy and spaced out.' About 6 months later, Ms E again presented to her primary physician with new complaints, describing severe headaches of several months' duration and worry that she had a brain tumor. Her physician had been trained in identifying somatization, and with Ms E could identify several recent 'stressors' in her life. He referred her for a stress management program, being careful to schedule a follow-up appointment with himself. Ms E hesitantly accepted and scheduled an appointment for the following week with a psychologist who worked in her primary physician's practice.

A diagnostic evaluation included questionnaires to assess her psychological health. The evaluation revealed that Ms E met criteria for abridged somatization and hypochondriasis. She reported a history of irregular and painful menstruation, diarrhea, abdominal bloating, as well as the chest pain, palpitations, and headaches described earlier, that remained medically unexplained. For the next week, the patient was asked to complete a daily diary recording the type and severity of physical discomfort, recorded as very high (average daily diary score = 3.0 on a 1–5-point Likert scale). She also endorsed significant hypochondriacal beliefs (Whiteley Index = 11), and anxiety symptoms (Beck Anxiety Inventory score = 21).

Ms E began a 10-session CBT. Although she expressed doubts about the potential benefits of this treatment, she agreed 'to give it a try.' Treatment began by teaching her to monitor her physical symptoms and related thoughts and emotions. She quickly recognized that she often experienced headaches and chest pain after difficult interactions with her son and mother. She was instructed in the daily practice of progressive muscle relaxation and diaphragmatic breathing. Over time, she began taking three relaxation breaks per day in order to eliminate muscular tension and to soothe herself. She also began to use relaxation techniques when she felt angry at her son or mother.

The next focus of treatment was teaching Ms E sleep hygiene skills, including regulation of her sleep schedule and restriction of her time in bed to sleeping. She said that even though she felt exhausted at the end of the day, she experienced early insomnia (at least 1 hour) every night. She used her relaxation skills just prior to bedtime. After a few weeks, on most nights she began falling asleep within 30 minutes.

Ms E's daily activities were also addressed. Spending her days working so hard to take care of her son, mother, and doing the housework, she was too tired to do anything in the evenings except rest on the couch. She and her therapist 'problem-solved' about reducing her responsibilities and increasing her pleasurable activities. The advantages and disadvantages of enrolling her mother in a day treatment program were reviewed with Ms E, after which she decided the potential benefits outweighed the costs. Once she had freed up a part of each day, she began taking increasingly long walks with a friend in the afternoons. Also, she and her husband began scheduling a night out once every week.

At the sixth session, Ms E and her therapist began discussing some of her hypochondriacal beliefs. She learned to look for evidence supporting and contradicting

her beliefs about having cardiovascular disease and a brain tumor. Substantial improvement in her chest pain and headaches was convincing enough for her to accept the possibility she may not have a progressive fatal disease. In addition, she could remind herself that her physicians had found no sign of organic pathology. Learning to create the symptoms on her own by running up a staircase to create palpitations and grinding her teeth to create headaches was further evidence that the existence of physical symptoms was not sufficient proof of the existence of a serious illness.

In the final sessions, Ms E and her therapist delineated a relapse prevention plan. She agreed to continue using each of her newly acquired skills, i.e., relaxation exercises, engaging in pleasurable activities/exercise, sleep hygiene, and challenging distorted thinking. In addition, she continued to meet with her primary physician every 2 months for a check-up. She reported that these brief physical exams helped remind her that she was physically healthy. At the final session with the therapist, Ms E reported significant improvement in her headaches and chest pain. Her post-treatment questionnaires showed improvements in her daily diary scores (average = 1.3 on a 1–5 point Likert scale), hypochondriacal beliefs (Whiteley Index = 5), and anxiety (Beck Anxiety Inventory score = 10).

A final report to Ms E's primary physician described her progress and encouraged him to continue seeing her every 2 months for brief physical exams and to discuss her relapse prevention plan with her.

Body dysmorphic disorder

Background

This particular somatizing condition has only recently (American Psychiatric Association, 1987) been included under the rubric of somatoform disorders and is usually considered a subtype of hypochondriasis because of the presence of intense fear of and belief in bodily defect, usually experienced subjectively as ugliness. It is defined as a distressing preoccupation with imagined defects of appearance or excessive concern over minor physical anomalies, unaccounted for by other mental disorders. Complaints may focus on the head and face, but may involve any part of the body. With onset in adolescence, many adults seek 'corrective' surgery from plastic surgeons and dermatologists (Phillips, 1996).

Conceptualization

Poorly understood, it had previously been considered a delusional aspect of other psychiatric disorders. Psychodynamic authors have ascribed it to a defense against more overwhelming anxiety, with displacement from other emotional concerns to dissatisfaction with appearance or body configuration (Fisher, 1986). Others consider early experience and learning of greatest importance in affecting self-image, self-esteem, and bodily self-approval (Phillips, 1996). More contemporary thought regards dysmorphophobia as part of a physiological spectrum disorder that includes eating disorders, affective disorders, and OCD (Hollander et al., 1992), with its manifestation a function of culture and environment (Pope et al., 1997). Perhaps the disorder can best be conceptualized as a body image disorder with social, psychological, and possibly biological influences (Cororve and Gleaves, 2001).

Research

Until recently, treatment recommendations were fairly pessimistic, with major intervention consisting of warnings to cosmetic surgeons to screen carefully patients requesting surgery for body changes, keeping in mind the fairly high incidence of disappointment with outcomes (Phillips et al., 2001). While early case reports indicated successful outcomes with exposure, systematic desensitization, self-confrontation, and response prevention, more recent therapeutic trials have stressed the promise of CBT (Cororve and Gleaves, 2001). An open case series of patients treated in small groups with CBT for 12 weekly 90-minute sessions, showed significant improvement in both body dysmorphic disorder (BDD) and depressive symptoms (Wilhelm et al., 1999). A 2-year follow-up of behaviorally treated patients followed with 6-month maintenance programs prevented symptom relapse and assisted in patient self-management of lapses typically associated with BDD (McKay, 1999).

A randomized trial of CBT combined with exposure and response prevention in 35 women for eight 2-hour sessions found significant improvement in self-image, self-esteem, and psychological distress compared with the untreated wait-list control group (Rosen *et al.*, 1995). Another study (Veale *et al.*, 1996) of 19 patients randomly assigned to CBT or wait-list control group for 12 weeks showed significant improvement (77%) on specific measures of BDD and depressed mood. BDD patients were found to be different from those with 'real' disfigurement who sought cosmetic surgery or were emotionally well-adjusted, as well as from healthy controls without defect.

Studies have noted that BDD shares many features in common with OCD, including responsiveness to CBT, medication, and psychosocial rehabilitation. Ninety-six patients with OCD were compared with 11 BDD patients in a 6-week intensive partial hospitalization program assessed with rating scales for depression, anxiety, and global symptomatology (Saxena *et al.*, 2002). The two groups showed similar direction of responses to SSRIs and antipsychotics in depressive, anxiety, and obsessive-compulsive symptoms, although BDD showed greater improvement in depression and anxiety. It was concluded that BDD can respond to intensive, multimodal treatment. CBT, with or without medication, appears to be favored as the treatment of choice for BDD.

Key practice principles

The importance of establishing a good therapeutic alliance has special salience with BDD patients as they are often reluctant to accept psychiatric or psychological care, being strongly attached to the idea that their 'defects' require surgical or medical 'correction.' History-taking should follow the usual recommendations for somatizing patients, with special attention to questions about self-image, self-esteem, previous forms of help-seeking, experience with surgical or dermatologic treatment, age of onset, avoidance of occupational or social situations or personal/sexual relationships (because of self-consciousness), and levels of perceived distress. Special attention must be paid to comorbidities of anxiety and/or depression, as it has been reported that as many as 29% of BDD patients attempt suicide (especially women concerned about perceived facial defects). In the context of a therapeutic relationship, SSRIs appear to be the first line of treatment, but require doses in excess of those for treatment of depression (e.g., fluoxetine 40–80 mg/day and fluvoxamine 200–300 mg/day). Concurrent CBT is recommended, including exposure and desensitization techniques, imagery, and self-confrontation. Long-term maintenance on therapeutic level doses of medication is advised because of high incidence of relapse. Meetings with family members, spouse, or significant others can help inform, educate, and provide understanding supportive assistance for the patient.

Conversion disorder

Background

Clinical interest in hysteria very likely set the stage for subsequent psychoanalytic thought, for of all the somatizing disorders, it was clearly the one most associated with psychological conflict. Some say it is the most common of all the somatoform disorders (Schwartz *et al.*, 2001).

Patients usually present with complaints of weakness, gait disturbance, blindness, aphonia, deafness, convulsions (pseudoseizures), or tremors. Of patients entering a clinical setting with complaints of motor disability and diagnosed conversion disorder, 33% may be expected to have other Axis I diagnoses, and 50% Axis II diagnoses (Binzer *et al.*, 1997). Characteristics of 'la belle indifference' (bland emotional reaction to presence of otherwise alarming symptoms), hysterical or histrionic personality and secondary gain, often associated in older literature with conversion disorder, appear to have no predictive diagnostic significance. Physical illness and conversion disorder are not mutually exclusive.

Conceptualization

In addition to the psychoanalytic model of conversion alluded to above, others have suggested physiological and behavioral models. The neurophysiological conceptualization proposes an inherent defect in poorly identified brain functions, especially of the dominant hemisphere (Drake, 1993), interfering with verbal associations, while the behavioral theory suggests faulty childhood learning, with the child exercising learned helplessness utilized for secondary gain and control of interpersonal relationships (Barr and Abernathy, 1977). The psychoanalytic theory, on the other hand, describes symptoms as compromise formations with primary gain of conflict resolution through partial expression of the conflict without conscious awareness of its significance (Barsky, 1995).

Some have suggested a strong relationship between childhood traumatization by sexual or physical abuse and a later propensity for conversion disorder (Roelofs *et al.*, 2002). However, one study of 30 patients with motor conversion disorder, with high degrees of parental rejection and low levels of affection and warmth as perceived by the patients, did not confirm an association of childhood physical and/or sexual abuse with conversion disorder (Binzer and Eisemann, 1998).

Research

Although a variety of explanations and treatments have been reported in the literature, there is little systematic research available. Using hypnotherapy, one of the oldest reported treatments, a comprehensive treatment program of 85 patients suffering motor conversion symptoms reported unusual and unexpected responses in 16 patients during hypnosis (Moene and Hoogduin, 1999). While raising caution about this intervention, the authors also suggest that such events may offer opportunities to help patients enhance understanding and gain better control over symptoms. One of few randomized controlled trials (Moene *et al.*, 2002), treating 45 inpatients comprehensively with symptom-oriented as well as expression- and insight-oriented techniques, found significant improvement in all subjects, whether hypnosis was used or not. Furthermore, hypnotizability was not predictive of treatment outcome.

A retrospective case series of eight children ages 9–18 with conversion disorder involving motor disturbance of gait, treated with inpatient behavioral management using a reward system, reported that all patients attained normal gait and improved activities of daily living (Gooch *et al.*, 1997). To maintain improvement after discharge, instruction of the patient and family in pain and stress management appeared essential. Lacking controlled trials, other case reports include effectiveness of negative reinforcement (Campo and Negrini, 2000), culturally-relevant (shamanistic) treatment (Razali, 1999) showing the benefits of 'indigenous psychotherapy,' and rehabilitative inpatient treatment (Watanabe *et al.*, 1998) using functional and behavioral therapies and extensive psychosocial support to produce rapid improvement in hysterical hemiparesis (mean length of stay 11 days). One study of psychological defense constellations comparing 19 patients diagnosed with conversion disorder to 32 healthy nonpatients showed nonpatients better able to perceive and express affective response to a stimulus picture, supporting the psychoanalytic hypothesis that conversion symptoms are nonverbal communications replacing perception and verbal expression of emotion (Sundbom *et al.*, 1999). A recent report highlights the benefits of a multidimensional treatment approach that utilizes inpatient, partial hospitalization, and outpatient treatment employing psychodynamic, behavioral, psychosocial, hypnotic, pharmacologic, and culture- and religion-focused techniques (Schwartz *et al.*, 2001).

To test the clinical theory that conversion disorder is promoted or perpetuated through questioning by parents and physicians, one study compared the interrogative suggestibility of 12 patients diagnosed with conversion disorder with a matched group with confirmed neurological disease, concluding that interrogative suggestibility was of no significant importance in the etiology of conversion disorder (Foong *et al.*, 1997). Clinicians often caution that conversion disorder sometimes reveals subsequent organic disease in long-term follow-up. To assess this potential, 73 patients with medically unexplained motor symptoms were assessed and followed for 6 years, with only three patients manifesting new organic neurological disorders, in contrast to the 1965 classic study of Slater and Glithero (1965) showing 50% new neurological or psychiatric disorders in 10 years (Crimlisk et al., 1998). Others have also confirmed a decrease in percentage of patients initially diagnosed with conversion disorder who later are identified as having an organic (neurological) disorder (Mace and Trimble, 1996; Moene et al., 2000). Long-term chronic patients were at risk to develop SD in the absence of diagnosis of another disease.

Key practice principles

Without adequate controlled studies providing evidence-based direction, treatment choice will depend largely on therapist preference and experience. The usual caveats on history-taking prevail, with special attention to history of trauma, sexual and physical abuse, and family history of conversion symptoms. Physical examination must pay particular attention to ruling out neurological diseases, such as multiple sclerosis and other peripheral and central nervous system disorders. Routine laboratory studies are indicated as well as EEG (to distinguish between epilepsy and pseudoseizures) and other special studies (e.g., MRI, X-rays, spinal tap, etc.) to rule out possible organic etiology. Many conversion syndromes will remit spontaneously with understanding and support, but early intervention can forestall potential chronicity and development of entrenched SD. Once chronicity has developed, intensive treatment may make use of all treatment modalities, including hospitalization, individual or group therapy, insight-oriented therapies, behavioral techniques, negative reinforcement, hypnosis, sodium amytal interview, physical therapy, biofeedback, relaxation training, and medication (primarily for comorbid anxiety, depression or other somatoform disorders). The therapeutic value of a trusting ongoing relationship is illustrated in the following case:

> A 54-year-old married man was being treated pharmacologically and monitored monthly with supportive half-hour visits for chronic recurring depression. One day he paid a rare visit to his hated mother residing in a nursing home following a serious stroke. He found himself physically distressed in her presence, with nausea and a concern he might vomit and hastily had to leave. One day later he developed a left-sided hemiparesis. He had virtually no capacity for insight or appreciation of the possible connection between his mother's ailment and his acute physical reaction. His therapist, a consultation-liaison psychiatrist based in a general hospital, obtained the minimum essential tests and consults to rule out bona fide neurological disease. The therapist interpreted the completely normal studies to the patient, not that 'nothing was the matter,' but rather that ' the tests are reassuring that this is a completely reversible illness.' Because of the therapist's acquaintance with hospital medical and nursing staff, arrangements could be made by a team effort for a brief medical hospitalization for this patient, during which time he was treated very much as a true stroke patient would be, with rehabilitation, physical therapy, respiratory therapy, and the like. Within approximately 3 weeks, with virtually no psychotherapeutic intervention except regular supportive visits by his therapist, his illness had completely and 'miraculously' remitted, with neither physical residual nor understanding by him of how his feelings about his mother may have influenced his physical response. His depression continued.

Offering psychological interpretations/explanations or reassurance too early may subvert treatment efforts; on the other hand, reassuring patients that critical tests are normal and that symptoms will eventually improve may hasten improvement. Because repression is very strong in some conversions, patients will be initially reluctant to divulge or explore early contributing conflicts or experience. This may have to wait on a comforting/comfortable, trusting and safe relationship before there can be progress, especially true for children and adolescents where the support and participation of family, teachers, and physicians may be required in a team effort; often the pediatrician, with psychiatric or psychological backup consultation, may be the best option to assume the role of therapist. Any implication of malingering will be very counterproductive. Accompanying comorbid depression, anxiety, and behavior problems may respond to accepted pharmacologic ministrations. Use of hypnotic or narcoleptic techniques, if utilized, must be

tentatively offered to patients whose fear of passivity or loss of control may induce overwhelming anxiety. Behavioral interventions should focus on improving self-esteem, capacity for emotional expression and assertiveness, and ability to communicate comfortably with others.

Factitious disorder
Background

Originally known only by its most extreme clinical presentation in Munchausen's syndrome, the category of factitious disorders has only recently (and perhaps arguably) been included in the domain of somatoform disorders (DSM-IV).

Clinical presentations meet diagnostic criteria for factitious disorder if they: (1) intentionally feign physical or psychological signs and symptoms; (2) appear motivated only to assume the sick role; and (3) reveal no incentives characteristic of malingering. Psychological and physical signs and symptoms may present separately or in combination. Patients are often very intelligent, with a good grasp of medical knowledge and language, and frequently occupied in some aspect of medicine or related fields. They are persuasive and 'creative' in their medical narratives, capable of defying easy diagnosis. They may be male or female, although earliest reports are almost entirely of men; it is now reported that most patients with factitious disorder are women between ages 20 and 40. They have histories of multiple hospitalizations, frequently in various locations ('peregrinating'), and may display multiple surgical scars (establishing the 'veracity' of their stories). Presentations may be of actual self-induced symptoms, of factitious medical history, embellishment of naturally-occurring anatomical anomalies, or the offering of (usually forged) documentation of previous treatment. They are generally very receptive (unlike malingerers) to invasive procedures, often at high risk of morbidity or mortality. Being confronted with the possibility of their deception often evokes denial, hostility, and/or flight. Rarely will patients with physical factitia accept referral for psychiatric treatment.

Conceptualization

Understanding why anyone would intentionally wish to be sick has challenged the best clinical and theoretical minds. Psychoanalytic hypotheses posit the need (both conscious and unconscious) to master the anxiety that accompanies fear of real illness with repetitive reenactment of the child's 'doctor game,' playing both active and passive sexualized roles as victim (masochistic) and victimizer (sadistic). Others hold that it is a manifestation of borderline personality disorder in which identity problems and conflicts over control and authority are acted out in the theatre of medicine, with rage projected on to the 'inept, humiliated, snookered' physician. Still other suggestions include a stress response to having been thwarted in the ambition to become a physician, to a reaction to serious loss, or a history of illness, abuse, or hospitalization of oneself or other meaningful figures. Presumed histories of neglect, abandonment, or abuse support the notion that factitious patients seek nurturance and dependence, albeit in faulty ways. The idea that patients are merely seeking attention seems unconvincing as there are so many other ways to behaviorally satisfy this wish (Lipsitt, 1982). Factitious illness by proxy invokes similar explanations in a mother (rarely a father) who vicariously fulfills psychological needs through illness perpetrated on a child.

Research

The paucity of reliable findings in factitious illness arises from the elusiveness of these patients as well as their fabricated histories. Furthermore, their inability to form genuine relationships with staff and physicians who are often biased and resent patients' deception reduces opportunities for meaningful cooperative study. In this context, it is not surprising that no controlled studies exist and it would appear unlikely that they will be possible in the future. Reports of therapeutic trials consist almost entirely of individual case reports (Fras and Coughlin, 1971; Earle and Folks, 1986; Merrin et al., 1986), some of which report variable success with treatment. In one reported series of 24 patients, 10 agreed to engage in psychodynamic psychotherapy for up to 4 years, with 'favorable progress,' according to the author (Plassman, 1994). Another treatment effort was reported to have modified reliance on the sick role in two patients in an inpatient behaviorally oriented program designed to avoid confrontation (Solyom and Solyom, 1990).

Key practice principles

For reasons stated above, difficulty in forming an alliance with factitious patients is a major impediment to treatment. Early distinction between malingering and factitia may be possible if the seeking of secondary gain in the former is detectable. Willingness to undergo risky or painful procedures is more apparent in factitious disorder. Occasionally, it is possible, especially with the less severe cases, to establish a relationship that facilitates gathering a more or less accurate history and making a psychiatric referral for continuing management. If there is a hint of a therapeutic alliance, one may try to interest the patient in explanations of illness as related to stress or to help find alternative ways other than the sick role to obtain gratification. Early detection is encouraged by verifying elements of history either by noting inconsistencies in early background or by checking with other sources regarding previous hospitalizations and treatments. This latter endeavor, when exercised without the patient's consent, raises ethical questions without decisive answers. Laboratory studies can help to rule out impostured diseases.

Customary medical treatment is necessary for any self-induced pathological conditions. Working with hospital staff to control impulses of angry retribution may help to gain patients' trust and confidence, in anticipation of further contact. Direct or especially insensitive confrontation of deception in these patients usually results in heated denial, outbursts of rage, or elopement, with potential further regressive and self-destructive behavior. If attempted treatment intervention is successful, it will likely be for the long term. Collaborative care between psychiatrist or psychologist and primary care physician may have more long-term success in containing factitious patients than psychotherapy alone, in hopes that the patient may ultimately accept and develop a trusting relationship with a primary physician. Pharmacotherapy can be offered for accompanying comorbid Axis I disorders. When factitious illness by proxy involves child abuse, it is essential to notify proper child care agencies. Offering protective care and perhaps therapy to the afflicted child and family therapy to the parents and child may be useful. It should be kept in mind that, although rare, factitious patients may occasionally launch malpractice suits (Lipsitt, 1986). Other isolated and occasional idiosyncratic interventions have been extensively reviewed elsewhere (Eisendrath, 2001). There are no controlled treatment studies.

Summary of general guidelines for treatment of somatoform disorders

Historically, the treatment of somatizing patients has been considered difficult and frustrating (Lipsitt, 1970, 1992). These patients tend to be dissatisfied with their medical care and may complain when their symptoms do not quickly resolve. Patients with multiple unexplained physical symptoms report high rates of disability. These patients also have a propensity for remaining idle, avoiding productive and meaningful activities (Katon et al., 1991). They tend to overutilize primary care and specialty services; it has been estimated that their expenditures are two to nine times the average of nonsomatizing patients (Smith et al., 1986; Barsky et al., 2001).

In our review of psychotherapy of somatoform disorders, it appears that available studies, both controlled and uncontrolled, fail to establish definitively any individual psychotherapy as clearly superior to any other. In this, there is confirmation of earlier reports of psychotherapy research (Bergin, 1971; Smith and Glass, 1977; Hartley, 1985; Lin et al., 1991). While case reports suggest that cognitive-behavioral approaches may be preferred in this era of urgent demand, reduced funding, and stringent regulations, adequate studies have yet to be performed that establish long-term benefits with this approach as superior to that of others. We are led to the conclusion that it is very likely that the ultimate efficacy of any therapeutic intervention with 'difficult' somatizing patients is realized as much (or more) through the nature of the patient–therapist relationship as through any other specific intervention. If this is indeed the case, then we must emphasize aspects of the therapeutic relationship that would appear to enhance an optimal outcome with this large group of patients. We therefore conclude with a summary of the challenges presented by patients who suffer from somatoform disorders and suggestions to deal with those challenges. Such an alliance will depend upon the respective contributions of patient and therapist to the relationship they establish between themselves.

Challenges

Building a trusting alliance

Chronically somatizing patients approach each new medical encounter with both magical expectations and great pessimism and distrust, based on previous experiences with doctors who convey disinterest or disbelief in the patient's complaints and suffering. Building a trusting alliance in this context must begin with respect for the patient's symptoms and acknowledgment of their validity; a tolerance for repetition; an attitude of active, receptive listening; and a neutral approach that is neither dismissive, confrontational, nor overly reassuring. It is only with time, consistency, and continuing trustworthiness that a relationship will ripen into a trusting potentially therapeutic partnership. Promoting a certain level of dependence will fulfill a requirement for a 'working alliance,' while reminders to the patient of areas of strength, 'survivorship,' and courage will support optimal self-regard and autonomy while avoiding regressive tendencies.

The manner in which the clinician takes a history as part of a psychotherapeutic evaluation may pave the way for a therapeutic alliance. Somatizing patients come to a new encounter not only with a string of disappointments and thinly veiled anger, but also with a rich history of many previous encounters, multiple tests, and procedures (often redundant and without clear rationale). They are designated the 'thick chart' cases of medical practice. The prospect of reviewing their medical records is a daunting challenge, often establishing a negative 'mind-set' in the busy physician on first acquaintance. When patients' response to opening questions is 'It's all in the record,' it is helpful to remind them that it is preferable to hear directly from the patient, to get a better sense of who that person really is, rather than read some impersonal remarks by others. Notations or forewarnings of 'crocky patient' (or other pejorative labelings) should be ignored in favor of the physician's own assessment of the patient's illness behavior and pattern of interacting. A good *medical* history should not be short-cut on the basis of preformed expectations. Attempts to hastily rush to *psychological* history-taking or 'explanations' will fall on deaf ears, as this is rarely the somatizing patient's language or conceptualization of illness. Likewise, premature reassurance, while seeming appropriate to the physician, may be perceived by the patient hungering for connectedness as the physician's disinterest or dismissiveness. The timing and degree of reassurance must be based on adequacy of data and the trust and security of the relationship.

Somatizing patients will be most 'comfortable' revealing historical details in physical or somatic terms, but this should not deter an exploration of significant events (e.g., losses, trauma, disappointments, deprivation, and so on) surrounding earliest onset of symptoms. However, patients who do not acknowledge, recognize, or describe emotional reactions ('alexithymia') may respond more readily to questions about 'physical symptoms' than about 'depression' or 'grief' as responses to stressful events. Some historical details may not be revealed until the patient feels assured that a trustworthy relationship exists; the more chronic and disappointing the patient's prior medical experience has been, the longer it will be before the patient reveals important historical information.

As the history evolves, attitudes, beliefs, and attributions may become clearer, as well as certain patterns of interaction and illness behavior, that is, the ways that the patient fulfills the 'sick role.' Distorted beliefs, contradictory ideas, and fears can be addressed at moments during the gathering of historical data when the patient appears receptive.

Management

Because of the refractoriness of somatized symptoms to general interventions, physicians and therapists will be more successful with somatizing patients by adopting a 'caring' rather than a 'curing' approach to these patients. Therapeutic zeal often is met with increased resistance to change. 'Rescue fantasies' with these patients are usually thwarted, heightening the would-be rescuer's frustration. Such frustration often fosters intensified efforts at (usually inappropriate) treatment, on the one hand, or specialty referral or dismissal on the other. Restraint in the use of medication is advised, although when positively indicated for comorbid affective and anxiety states, it is best administered with an expression of modest expectations.

Clear assignment of appointment times at fairly regular (but infrequent: approximately monthly) intervals is more effective than random appointments based on fluctuations in symptoms. Gentle limit-setting can be accomplished by spelling out a treatment plan from the beginning and then reminding the patient of the policy when 'testing-out' of the therapist's commitment occurs. In time, with increasing trust and comfort, the patient's repertoire will expand beyond the confines of symptom complaints. Inquiring about the 'disappearing' symptoms is unnecessary and may only suggest to the patient a greater interest in the patient's complaints than in his or her social world and family relationships.

When a solid working relationship is in evidence, therapists may fulfill their pedagogical function by explaining the causal connection between external stressors, physiological repercussions, and the experience of somatic symptoms. Although insight may be slow to develop, sufficient awareness of an emotional component may suffice to enhance receptivity to referral for specialized behavioral intervention. Discussion of the variety of treatment programs and enlisting the patient's preferences will help to ensure acceptance of referral and follow-through in treatment. If referral is successful, contact with the primary care physician should be maintained with the patient to avoid a sensitive reaction to intimations of rejection.

Whichever form of treatment the patient selects, it is likely that a good outcome will be greatly enhanced by a strong relationship of the patient with a primary care physician. Collaboration between the mental health professional and primary physician will strengthen the patient's belief and trust in the interest of his or her treaters. In this context, patients are likely to respond positively whether treatment is behaviorally, psychodynamically, or psychosocially oriented.

Acknowledgments

Drs Lesley Allen and Angelica Diaz-Martinez provided CBT clinical vignettes. Carole Berney, M.A., assisted with references. This work was supported in part by NIMH grant RO1 NH60265 (Dr Escobar).

References

Allen, L. A., Woolfolk, R. L., Lehrer, P. M., Gara, M. A., and Escobar, J. I. (2001). Cognitive behavioral therapy for somatization disorder: a preliminary investigation. *Journal of Behaviour Therapy and Experimental Psychiatry*, **32**, 53–62.

American Psychiatric Association (1987). *Diagnostic and statistical manual of mental disorders*, 3rd edn (revised). Washington DC: American Psychiatric Association.

Avia, M. D., Ruiz, M. A., and Olivares, M. E. (1996). The meaning of psychological symptoms: effectiveness of a group intervention with hypochondriacal patients. *Behavioural Research and Therapy*, **34**, 23–31.

Avia, M. D., *et al.* (1997). Educating the 'worried well': description of a structured programme and implications for treatment and prevention. *Clinical Psychology and Psychotherapy*, **4**, 136–44.

Barr, R. and Abernathy, V. (1977). Conversion reaction. Differential diagnoses in the light of biofeedback research. *Journal of Nervous and Mental Disease*, **164**, 287–92.

Barsky, A. J. (1992). Amplification, somatization, and the somatoform disorders. *Psychosomatics*, **33**, 28–34.

Barsky, A. J. (1995). Somatoform disorders. In: H. I. Kaplan and B. J. Sadock, ed. *Comprehensive textbook of psychiatry*, 5th edn, Vol. 1, pp. 1009–27. Baltimore, MD: Williams and Wilkins.

Barsky, A. J. and Ahern, D. K. (2004). Cognitive behavior therapy for hypochondriasis: a randomized controlled trial. *JAMA*, **291**, 1464–70.

Barsky, A. J. and Borus, J. F. (1999). Functional somatic syndromes. *Annals of Internal Medicine*, **130**, 910–21.

Barsky, A. J. and Wyshak, G. (1989). Hypochondriasis and related health attitudes. *Psychosomatics*, **30**, 412–20.

Barsky, A. J., Geringer, E., and Wool, C. A. A. (1988). Cognitive-educational treatment for hypochondriasis. *General Hospital Psychiatry*, **10**, 322–7.

Barsky, A. J., Ettner, S. L., Horsky, J., and Bates, D. W. (2001). Resource utilization of patients with hypochondriacal health anxiety and somatization. *Medical Care*, **39**, 705–15.

Bass, C. and Murphy, M. (1991). Somatization disorder in a British teaching hospital. *British Journal of Clinical Practice*, **45**, 237–44.

Binzer, M. and Eisemann, M. (1998). Childhood experience and personality traits in patients with motor conversion symptoms. *Acta Psychiatrica Scandinavica*, **98**, 288–95.

Binzer, M., Andersen, P. M., and Kullgren, G. (1997). Clinical characteristics of patients with motor disability due to conversion disorder: a prospective control group study. *Journal of Neurology, Neurosurgery and Psychiatry*, **63**, 83–8.

Bouman, T. K. (2002). A community-based psychoeducational group approach to hypochondriasis. *Psychotherapy and Psychosomatics*, **71**, 326–32.

Bouman, T. K. and Visser, S. (1998). Cognitive and behavioral treatment of hypochondriasis. *Psychotherapy and Psychosomatics*, **67**, 214–21.

Campo, J. V. and Negrini, B. J. (2000). Case study: negative reinforcement and behavioral management of conversion disorder. *Journal of the American Academy of Child and Adolescent Psychiatry*, **39**, 787–90.

Clark, D. M., *et al.* (1998). Two psychological treatments for hypochondriasis. A randomized controlled trial. *British Journal of Psychiatry*, **173**, 367–8.

Cororve, M. B. and Gleaves, D. N. (2001). Body dysmorphic disorder: a review of conceptualizations, assessment, and treatment strategies. *Clinical Psychology Review*, **21**, 949–70.

Crimlisk, H. L., *et al.* (1998). Slater revisited: 6 year follow up study of patients with medically unexplained motor symptoms. *British Medical Journal*, **316**, 582–6.

Drake, M. E. Jr. (1993). Conversion hysteria and dominant hemisphere lesions. *Psychosomatics*, **34**, 524–30.

Earle, J. R. and Folks, D. G. (1986). Factitious disorder and coexisting depression: a report of successful psychiatric consultation and case management. *General Hospital Psychiatry*, **8**, 448–50.

Eisendrath, S. J. (2001). Factitious disorders and malingering. In: G. Gabbard, ed. *Treatments of psychiatric disorders*, 3rd edn, Vol. 2, pp. 1825–42. Washington DC: American Psychiatric Publishing Inc.

Escobar, J. I., Rubio-Stipec, M., Canino, G., and Karno, M. (1989). Somatic symptom index (SSI): a new and abridged somatization construct. Prevalence and epidemiological correlates in two large community samples. *Journal of Nervous and Mental Disease*, **177**, 140–6.

Fallon, B. A. (2001). Pharmacologic strategies for hypochondraiasis. In: V. Starcevic and D. R. Lipsitt, ed. *Hypochondriasis: modern perspectives on an ancient malady*, pp. 329–51. New York: Oxford University Press.

Fava, G. A., Grandi, S., Rafanelli, C., Fabbri, S., and Cazzaro, M. (2000). Explanatory therapy in hypochondriasis. *Journal of Clinical Psychiatry*, 2000, **61**, 317–22.

Fink, P., Rosendal, M., and Toft, T. (2002). Assessment and treatment of functional disorders in general practice: the extended reattribution and management model—an advanced educational program for nonpsychiatric doctors. *Psychosomatics*, **43**, 93–131.

Fisher, S. (1986). *Development and structure of the body image*. Hillsdale, NJ: Lawrence Erlbaum.

Foong, J., Lucas, P. A., and Ron, M. A. (1997). Interrogative suggestibility in patients with conversion disorder. *Journal of Psychosomatic Research*, **43**, 317–21.

Ford, C. and Long, K. D. (1977). Group psychotherapy of somatizing patients. *Psychotherapy and Psychsomatics*, **28**, 295–304.

Fras, I. and Coughlin, B. E. (1971). Treatment of factitious disease. *Psychosomatics*, **12**, 117–22.

Furer, P., Walker, J. R., Chartier, M. J., and Stein, M. B. (1997). Hypochondriacal concerns and somatization in panic disorder. *Depression and Anxiety*, **6**, 78–85.

Garcia Campayo, J. and Sanz Carrillo, C. (2000). Effectiveness of group psychoanalytic therapy in somatizing patients (Spanish). *Actas Espanolas Psiquiatria*, **28**, 105–14.

Garcia Campayo, J., Sanz Carrillo, C., Baringo, T., and Ceballos, C. (2001). SPECT scan in somatization disorder patients: an exploratory study of eleven cases. *Australian and New Zealand Journal of Psychiatry*, **35**, 359–63.

Gill, D. and Sharpe, M. (1999). Frequent consulters in general practice: a systematic review of studies of prevalence, associations and outcome. *Journal of Psychosomatic Research*, **47**, 115–30.

Gooch, J. L., Wolcott, R., and Speed, J. (1997). Behavioral management of conversion disorder in children. *Archives of Physical Medicine and Rehabilitation*, **78**, 264–8.

Guthrie, E., Creed, F., Dawson, D., and Towenson, B. (1993). A randomized controlled trial of psychotherapy in patients with refractory irritable bowel syndrome. *British Journal of Psychiatry*, **163**, 315–21.

Hartley, D. E. (1985). Research on the therapeutic alliance in psychotherapy. In: R. E. Hales and A. J. Frances, ed. *Psychiatry update, American Psychiatric Association annual review*, Vol. 4, pp. 532–49. Washington DC: American Psychiatric Press Inc.

Hellman, C., Budd, M., Borysenko, J., McClelland, D. C., and Benson, H. (1990). A study of the effectiveness of two group behavioral interventions for patients with psychosomatic complaints. *Behavioral Medicine*, **16**, 165–73.

Hiller, W., Leibbrand, R., Rief, W., and Fichter, M. M. (2002). Predictors of course and outcome in hypochondriasis after cognitive-behavioral treatment. *Psychotherapy and Psychosomatics*, **71**, 318–25.

Hollender, E. (1993). Obsessive-compulsive spectrum disorders: an overview. *Psychiatric Annals*, **23**, 355–8.

Hollander, E., Neville, D., Frenkel, M., Jospehson, S., and Liebowitz, M. R. (1992). Body dysmorphic disorder. Diagnostic issues and related disorders. *Psychosomatics*, **33**, 156–65.

James, L., Gordon, E., Kraiuhin, C., Howson, A., and Meares, R. (1989). Selective attention and auditory event-related potentials in somatization disorder. *Comprehensive Psychiatry*, **30**, 84–9.

Kaplan, K., Goldenberg, D. L., and Galvin-Nadeau, M. (1993). The impact of group meditation-based stress reduction program on fibromyalgia. *General Hospital Psychiatry*, **15**, 284–9.

Kathol, R. G. (1997). Reassurance therapy: what to say to symptomatic patients with benign or non-existent medical disease. *International Journal of Psychiatry Medicine*, **27**, 173–80.

Katon, W., Lin, E., Von Korff, M., Russo, J., Lipscomb, P., and Bush, T. (1991). Somatization: a spectrum of severity. *American Journal of Psychiatry*, **148**, 34–40.

Kellner, R. (1982). Psychotherapeutic strategies in hypochondriasis: a clinical study. *American Journal of Psychotherapy*, **36**, 146–57.

Kellner, R. (1986). *Somatization and hypochondriasis*. New York: Praeger.

Kellner, R. and Sheffield, B. F. (1973). The one-week prevalence of symptoms in neurotic patients and normals. *American Journal of Psychiatry*, **130**, 102–5.

Knapp, P. (1989). Psychodynamic psychotherapy for somatizing disorders. In: S. Cheren, ed. *Psychosomatic medicine: theory, physiology and practice*, Vol. 2, pp. 813–39. Madison, CT: International Universities Press, Inc.

Kroenke, K. and Swindle, R. (2000). Cognitive-behavioral therapy for somatization and symptom syndromes: a critical review of controlled clinical trials. *Psychotherapy and Psychosomatics*, **69**, 205–15.

Kroenke, K., *et al.* (1997). Multisomatoform disorder: an alternative to undifferentiated somatoform disorder for the somatizing patient in primary care. *Archives of General Psychiatry*, **54**, 352–8.

Lidbeck, J. (1997). Group therapy for somatization disorders in general practice: effectiveness of a short cognitive-behavioural treatment model. *Acta Psychiatrica Scandinavica*, **96**, 14–24.

Lin, E. H., *et al.* (1991). Frustrating patients: physician and patient perspectives among distressed high users of medical services. *Journal of General Internal Medicine*, **6**, 241–6.

Lipsitt, D. R. (1964). Integration clinic: an approach to the teaching and practice of medical psychology in an outpatient setting. In: N. E. Zinberg, ed. *Psychiatry and medical practice in the general hospital*, pp. 231–49. New York: International Universities Press, Inc.

Lipsitt, D. R. (1968). The 'rotating' geriatric patient: challenge to psychiatrists. *Journal of Geriatric Psychiatry*, **2**, 51–61.

Lipsitt, D. R. (1970). Medial and psychological characteristics of 'crocks.' *International Journal of Psychiatry Medicine*, **1**, 15–25.

Lipsitt, D. R. (1982). The enigma of factitious illness. *Medical and health annual*, pp. 114–27. Chicago, IL: Encyclopedia Britannica.

Lipsitt, D. R. (1986). The factitious patient who sues. *American Journal of Psychiatry*, **143**, 1482. (Letter)

Lipsitt, D. R. (1992). Challenges of somatization: diagnostic, therapeutic and economic. *Psychiatric Medicine*, **10**, 1–12.

Lipsitt, D. R. (2001a). Psychodynamic perspectives on hypochondriasis. In: V. Starcevic and D. R. Lipsitt, ed. *Hypochondriasis: modern perspectives on an ancient malady*, pp. 183–201. New York: Oxford University Press.

Lipsitt, D. R. (2001b). The patient-physician relationship in the treatment of hypochondriasis In: V. Starcevic and D. R. Lipsitt,. ed. *Hypochondriasis: modern perspectives on an ancient malady*, pp. 265–90. New York: Oxford University Press.

Lloyd, K. R., *et al.* (1998). The development of the Short Expanatory Model Interview (SEMI) and its use among primary-care attenders with common mental disorders. *Psychological Medicine*, **28**, 1231–7.

Logsdail, S., Lovell, K., Warwick, H., and Marks, I. (1991). Behavioral treatment of AIDS-focused illness phobias. *British Journal of Psychiatry*, **159**, 422–5.

Mace, C. J. and Trimble, M. R. (1996). Ten-year prognosis of conversion disorder. *British Journal of Psychiatry*, **169**, 282–8.

McKay, D. (1999). Two-year follow-up of behavioral treatment and maintenance for body dysmorphic disorder. *Behavior Modification*, **23**, 620–9.

McLeod, C. C., Budd, M. A., and McClelland, D. C. (1997). Treatment of somatization in primary care. *General Hospital Psychiatry*, **19**, 251–8.

Melson, S. and Rynearson, E. K. (1986). Intensive group therapy for functional illness. *Psychiatric Annals*, **16**, 687–92.

Merrin, E. L., Van Dyke, C., Cohen, S., and Tusel, D. J. (1986). Dual factitious disorder. *General Hospital Psychiatry*, **8**, 246–50.

Miller, L. (1984). Neuropsychological concepts of somatoform disorders. *International Journal of Psychiatry Medicine*, **14**, 31–46.

Moene, F. C. and Hoogduin, K. A. (1999). The creative use of unexpected responses in the hypnotherapy of patients with conversion disorders. *International Journal of Clinical and Experimental Hypnosis*, **47**, 209–26.

Moene, F. C., *et al.* (2000). Organic syndromes diagnosed as 'conversion disorder' identification and frequency in a study of 85 patients. *Journal of Psychosomatic Research*, **49**, 7–12.

Moene, F. C., Spinhoven, P., Hoogduin, K. A., and van Dyck, R. (2002). A randomised controlled clinical trial on the additional effect of hypnosis in a comprehensive treatment programme for in-patients with conversion disorder of the motor type. *Psychotherapy and Psychosomatics*, **71**, 66–76.

Morriss, R. K. and Gask, L. (2002). Treatment of patients with somatized mental disorder: effects of reattribution training on outcomes under the direct control of the family doctor. *Psychosomatics*, **43**, 394–9.

Newman, M. G., *et al.* (2000). The relationship of childhood sexual abuse and depression with somatic symptoms and medical utilization. *Psychological Medicine*, **30**, 1063–77.

Nielsen, G., Barth, K., Brit, H., and Havik, O. (1988). Brief dynamic psychotherapy for patients presenting physical symptoms. *Psychotherapy and Psychosomatics*, **50**, 35–41.

Nissen, B. (2000). Hypochondria: a tentative approach. *International Journal of Psychoanalysis*, **81**, 651–6.

Papageorgiou, C. and Wells, A. (1998). Effects of attention training on hypochondriasis: a brief case series. *Psychological Medicine*, **28**, 193–200.

Payne, A. and Blanchard, E. B. (1995). A controlled comparison of cognitive therapy and self-help support groups in the treatment of irritable bowel syndrome. *Journal of Consulting and Clinical Psychology*, **63**, 779–86.

Peabody, F. W. (1927). The care of the patient. *Journal of the American Medical Association*, **88**, 877–82.

Pennebaker, J. W., *et al.* (1977). Lack of control as a determinant of perceived physical symptoms, *Journal of Personality and Social Psychology*, **42**, 347–51.

Phillips, K. A. (1996). Body dysmorphic disorder: diagnosis and treatment of imagined ugliness. *Journal of Clinical Psychiatry*, **57** (Suppl. 8), 61–4.

Phillips, K. A., Grant, J., Siniscalchi, J., and Albertini, R. S. (2001). Surgical and nonpsychiatric medical treatment of patients with body dysmorphic disorder. *Psychosomatics*, **42**, 504–10.

Plassman, R. (1994). Inpatient and outpatient long-term psychotherapy of patients suffering from factitious disorders. *Psychotherapy and Psychosomatics*, **62**, 96–107.

Pope, H. G. Jr., Gruber, A. J., Choi, P., Olivardia, R., and Phillips, K. A. (1997). Muscle dysmorphia. An underrecognized form of body dysmorphic disorder. *Psychosomatics*, **38**, 548–57.

Razali, S. M. (1999). Conversion disorder: a case report of treatment with the Main Puteri, a Malay shamanistic healing ceremony. *European Journal of Psychiatry*, **14**, 470–2.

Rief, W. and Auer, C. (2001). Is somatization a habituation disorder? Physiological reactivity in somatization syndrome. *Psychiatric Research*, **101**, 63–74.

Rief, W. and Hiller, W. (1998). *Somatisierungsstorung und Hypochondrie* [Somatization disorder and hypochondriasis: a treatment manual]. Gottingen, Hogrefe Publishers, 1998.

Rief, W. and Hiller, W. (1999). Toward empirically based criteria for the classification of somatoform disorders. *Journal of Psychosomatic Research*, **46**, 507–18.

Rief, W., Hiller, W., Geissner, E., and Fichter, M. M. (1995). A two-year follow-up study of patients with somatoform disorder. *Psychosomatics*, **36**, 376–86.

Roelofs, K., Keijsers, G., Hoogduin, K., Naring, G., and Moene, F. (2002). Childhood abuse in patients with conversion disorder. *American Journal of Psychiatry*, **159**, 1908–13.

Rosen, J., Reiter, P., and Orosan, P. (1995). Cognitive-behavioral body image therapy for body dysmophric disorder. *Journal of Consulting and Clinical Psychology*, **63**, 263–9.

Rost, K. M., Akins, R. N., Brown, F. W., and Smith, G. R. (1992). The comorbidity of DSM-IIIR personality disorders in somatization disorder. *General Hospital Psychiatry*, **14**, 322–6.

Rost, K., Kashner, T. M., and Smith, G. R. (1994). Effectiveness of psychiatric intervention with somatization disorder patients: improved outcomes at reduced costs. *General Hospital Psychiatry*, **16**, 381–7.

Salkovskis, P. and Warwick, H. M. (1986). Morbid preoccupations, health anxiety and reassurance: a cognitive-behavioural approach to hypochondriasis. *Behaviour Research and Therapy*, **24**, 597–602.

Saxena, S., *et al.* (2002). A retrospective review of clinical characteristics and treatment response in body dysmorphic disorder versus obsessive-compulsive disorder. *Journal of Clinical Psychiatry*, **62**, 67–72.

Scheidt, C. E. and Waller, E. (1999). Attachment representation, affect regulation and psychophysiological reactivity—Comments on the relevance of current findings in the field of attachment research for psychosomatic medicine. *Zeitschrift fur Psychosomatische Medizine und Psychotherapie*, **45**, 313–32.

Schur, M. (1955). Comments on the metapsychology of somatization. *Psychoanalytic Study of the Child*, **10**, 119–64.

Schwartz, A. C., Calhoun, A. W., Eschbach, C. L., and Seelig, B. J. (2001). Treatment of conversion disorder in an African American Christian woman: cultural and social considerations. *American Journal of Psychiatry*, **158**, 1385–91.

Sharpe, M. and Bass, C. (1992). Pathophysiological mechanisms in somatization. *International Review of Psychiatry*, **4**, 81–97.

Shorter, E., Abbey, S. E., Gillies, L. A., Singh, M., and Lipowski, Z. J. (1992). Inpatient treatment of persistent somatization. *Psychosomatics*, **33**, 295–300.

Sifneos, P. E. (1973). The prevalence of 'alexithymic' characteristics in psychosomatic patients. *Psychotherapy and Psychosomatics*, **22**, 255–62.

Sisti, M. (1997). Hypochondriasis. In: R. Leahy, ed. *Practicing cognitive therapy: a guide to interventions*, pp. 169–91. Northvale NJ: Jason Aronson.

Slater, E. and Glithero, E. (1965). A follow up of patients diagnosed suffering from 'hysteria.' *Journal of Psychosomatic Research*, **9**, 9–13.

Smith, M. L. and Glass, G. V. (1977). Meta-analysis of psychotherapy outcome studies. *American Psychologist*, **132**, 752–60.

Smith, R. G., Monson, R. A., and Ray, D. C. (1986). Psychiatric consultation in somatization disorder. *New England Journal of Medicine*, **314**, 1407–13.

Solyom, C. and Solyom, L. (1990). A treatment program for functional paraplegia/ Munchausen syndrome. *Journal of Behavior Therapy and Experimental Psychiatry*, **21**, 225–30.

Speckens, A. E. M. (2001). Assessment of hypochondriasis. In: V. Starcevic and D. R. Lipsitt, ed. *Hypochondriasis: modern perspectives on an ancient malady*. New York: Oxford University Press.

Speckens, A. E. M., *et al.* (1995). Cognitive behavioral therapy for medically unexplained physical symptoms: a randomised controlled trial. *British Medical Journal*, **311**, 1328–32.

Starcevic, V. (2001). Reassurance in the treatment of hypochondriasis. In: V. Starcevic and D. R. Lipsitt, ed. *Hypochondriasis: modern perspectives on an ancient malady*, pp. 291–313. New York: Oxford University Press.

Stern, R. and Fernandez, M. (1991). Group cognitive and behavioral treatment for hypochondriasis. *British Medical Journal*, **303**, 1229–31.

Sumathipala, A., Hewege, S., Hanwella, R., and Mann, A. H. (2000). Randomized controlled trial of cognitive behaviour therapy for repeated consultations for medically unexplained complaints: a feasibility study in Sri Lanka. *Psychological Medicine*, **30**, 747–57.

Sundbom, E., Binzer, M., and Kullgren, G. (1999). Psychological defense strategies according to the defense mechanism test among patients with severe conversion disorder. *Psychotherapy Research*, **9**, 184–98.

Tyrer, P., Fowler-Dixon, R., Ferguson, B., and Keleman, A. (1990). A plea for the diagnosis of hypochondriacal personality disorder. *Journal of Psychosomatic Research*, **34**, 637–42.

Vaillant, G. (1977). *Adaptation to life*. Boston: Little Brown.

Veale, D., *et al.* (1996). Body dysmorphic disorder: a cognitive behavioural model and pilot randomised controlled trial. *Behaviour Research Therapy*, **34**, 717–29.

Visser, S. and Bouman, T. K. (1992). Cognitive-behavioral approaches in the treatment of hypochondriasis: six single-case crossover studies. *Behaviour Research and Therapy*, **30**, 301–6.

Walker, E. A., *et al.* (1999). Adult health status of women with histories of childhood abuse and neglect. *American Journal of Medicine*, **107**, 332–9.

Walker, J., Vincent, N., Furer, P., Cox, B., and Kjernisted, K. (1999). Treatment preference in hypochondriasis. *Journal of Behavior Therapy and Experimental Psychiatry*, **30**, 251–8.

Warwick, H. (1989). A cognitive-behavioral approach to hypochondriasis and health anxiety. *Journal of Psychosomatic Research*, **33**, 705–11.

Warwick, H. M., Clark, D. M., Cobb, A. M., and Salkovskis, P. M. (1996). A controlled trial of cognitive-behavioural treatment of hypochondriasis. *British Journal of Psychiatry*, **169**, 189–95.

Watanabe, T. K., O'Dell, M. W., and Togliatti, T. J. (1998). Diagnosis and rehabilitation strategies for patients with hysterical hemiparesis: a report of four cases. *Archives of Physical Medicine and Rehabilitation*, **79**, 709–14.

Wessely, S., Nimnuan, C., and Sharpe, M. (1999). Functional somatic syndromes: one or many? *Lancet*, **354**, 936–9.

Wickramasekera, I. (1998). Secrets kept from the mind but not the body or behavior: the unsolved problems of identifying and treating somatization and psychophysiological disease. *Advances*, **14**, 81–132.

Wilhelm, S., Otto, M. W., Lohr, B., and Deckersbach, T. (1999). Cognitive behavior group therapy for body dysmorphic disorders: a case series. *Behaviour Research Therapy*, **37**, 71–5.

III

Psychotherapy of personality disorders

21 'Cluster A' personality disorders

Paul Williams
with the assistance of Rex Haigh and David Fowler

'Cluster A' comprises paranoid personality disorder (PPD), schizoid personality disorder (SPD), and schizotypal personality disorder (StPD). These disorders affect 2%, slightly less than 1%, and 4% of the Western population, respectively, and can be highly disabling. Their incidence is higher in men than in women and the conditions are characterized by odd, eccentric, or 'cold' behavior (particularly SDP and StPD). It is thought that a biological relationship may exist between the disorders and the schizophrenias, although of the three, StPD is more demonstrably linked to schizophrenia phenomenologically and genetically (McGlashan, 1983). SPD and StPD are sometimes grouped as part of a continuum, given the similarity of certain symptoms. No distinctive set of psychoanalytic, cognitive-behavioral therapy (CBT) or group theories is applicable to these conditions. More research is needed before specific psychological theories can be established. Conceptualization of Cluster A disorders tends to utilize theories developed from the study of psychosis.

Paranoid personality disorder

The main characteristic of PPD is distrust and suspiciousness. The motives of others are construed as hostile and exploitative. The PPD patient's thoughts and feeling are preoccupied by conflicts and threats *felt to emanate from outside*. They experience doubts about the loyalty of others and anticipate betrayal. Given their preoccupation with threats, they are highly vigilant. Negative stereotyping can occur and this may lead to a search for security through contact with people who share the patient's paranoid beliefs. Individuals can express PPD through hostility, sarcasm, stubbornness, or a cynical world view. A beleaguered, self-righteous attitude conceals deep sensitivity to obstacles or setbacks, an unwillingness to forgive, inflation of subjective judgment, and difficulty in accepting another's viewpoint. These defenses reflect feelings of inferiority based on low self-esteem. Humiliation, shame, and depressive feelings are underlying affective characteristics of PPD. Encounters with PPD can leave others offended and disoriented or even provoked into conflict. History-taking may indicate that in childhood the patient withdrew from relationships and became preoccupied with ruminative, conflict-based fantasies. PPD can be differentiated from psychotic illness by an absence of delusions or hallucinations (Sperry, 1995). It is advisable to differentiate symptoms of PPD from those produced by substance abuse; they can appear similar but have different origins. Medication—usually neuroleptics or SSRI antidepressants—may be given, often in combination with psychotherapy. PPD patients struggle with any treatment regimen due to their distrust.

Schizoid personality disorder

SPD is characterized by emotional detachment from social and personal relationships. Expressions of feeling towards others are limited because contact is painful and felt to lack meaning. Compelling experiences seem to pass the SPD individual by. At the same time they can feel isolated if left alone for too long. Close contact with others leads to feeling overwhelmed and a fear of loss of identity (sense of self). Hostility is rare; passive resistance and withdrawal predominate. Poor social skills and limited emotional

range compound the 'mechanical' characteristics of SPD behavior. When under threat SPD individuals detach themselves still further. Confrontational therapy techniques are inadvisable as they heighten already severe anxieties. The fantasy life of SPD individuals can be intense: the difficulty for the psychotherapist lies in accessing it but if this is achieved SPD patients may do well. SPD can be differentiated from PPD by a reduced suspiciousness of others, although paranoid ideation is sometimes present. SPD is distinguishable from StPD by its less odd, eccentric, or obviously disturbed presentation. Similarities of presentation of SPD with autistic or Asperger's syndrome can sometimes make diagnosis difficult. Psychotic illness or severe depression may occur within SPD but severe symptoms can be associated with an accompanying personality disorder (such as avoidant or paranoid). Despite their detachment, many SPD individuals become concerned about the unfulfilling lives they lead. Many do not marry or form sexual relationships and if they do, they tend to settle for nondemanding partners. Enough contact to offset loneliness may be found in the workplace or through limited socializing. There is no generally accepted treatment for SPD, although group therapy can help with socialization. Psychotherapy (which may be a combination of group and individual), perhaps with some medication, is sometimes recommended. Pharmacological treatments alone seem to have little impact on the low affectivity and deep anxieties of these patients, as their problems lie primarily with relationships. Substance abuse in SPD (and in StPD) tends to be related to attachment to fantasy experiences as part of a general avoidance of human contact.

Schizotypal personality disorder

StPD is characterized by a 'pervasive pattern of social and interpersonal deficits marked by acute discomfort with, and reduced capacity for, close relationships as well as by cognitive or perceptual distortions and eccentricities of behavior' (DSM-IV-TR, 1994; ICD-10, 1992). 'Schizotypal personality' derives from the term schizotype employed by Rado in 1953 to bring together schizophrenic and genotype into one category. 'Schizotypal' refers to a disordered personality in which there are constitutional defects similar to those underlying schizophrenia. Brief psychotic episodes due to stress may arise in StPD but these are usually transient. Some StPD individuals may go on to develop schizophrenia but they are a small minority. The principal characteristics of StPD are distortions in cognition and perception, including a disturbed view of the body, and the presence of odd, magical, or eccentric beliefs or ideas. StPD (and SDP) individuals have difficulty in experiencing pleasure (anhedonia). They may show ideas of reference and superstitions and suffer chronic social anxiety. Close relationships are felt to be threatening and social isolation is not uncommon. StPD individuals feel themselves to be at odds with, not part of, the world. Withdrawal and avoidance are used to counter feelings of confusion and conflict. Strong feelings evoke intense anxiety, and this can threaten their hold on reality. The need to avoid strong feelings leads to a tendency to overfocus on tangential issues (hence the characteristic of eccentricity). Their illusions and preoccupations defend against fragmented ego functioning and a precarious sense of identity. Social contacts, support from family and friends and engagement in therapeutic relationships are necessary to counter the tendency to remain withdrawn. Despite the genetic link with schizophrenia, StPD patients who enter psychotherapy can do better than SPD patients due to their greater affective availability. Progress may be slow and erratic and results rarely approximate to a normal life, but gradual personality integration can lead to a marked improvement in daily living. Treatment, especially in severe cases, may involve low dosages of the kind of medications used in schizophrenia. SSRIs can improve obsessive, compulsive, and depressive symptoms in StPD.

Conceptualization

Paranoid personality disorder

Psychoanalytic theory underpins *psychodynamic approaches*. Paranoia, in Freudian theory, has been defined traditionally as a defense against homosexuality (Freud, 1911/1958). Many psychoanalysts today understand this to reflect an object relations crisis in which the subject feels unable to surrender or yield to the experience of dependence upon the primary object (originally the mother/caregiver) for fear of unmanageable conflict and disintegration. Melanie Klein sought a similar foundation for the origins of paranoia, but through a slightly different route. Having located the paranoid phase within Abraham's first anal stage, she subsequently conceived of it as the earliest object relationship of the oral stage, from which evolved her concept of the paranoid-schizoid position. This concept is useful to understanding Cluster A disorders. The initial object is partial (the earliest representation being the breast, followed by the mother) and is subject to splitting into 'good' and 'bad' aspects—idealized and denigrated respectively. The ego attempts to rid itself of 'bad' object experiences using projective mechanisms. Introjection of the 'bad' part-object threatens the infant with a fear of destruction. Splitting, idealization, and disavowal contribute to a defensive, omnipotent attempt to ward off the 'bad' object, and are today accepted by the majority of psychoanalysts and psychotherapists as pivotal to understanding paranoid conditions such as PPD. Kernberg (1975), Rosenfeld (1975), Stone (1993), and Gabbard (2000) among others have noted how the PPD patient violently splits the object leading to separated 'good' and 'bad' aspects, reflecting developmental failure of mentalization in infancy (Target and Fonagy, 1996a,b). Object constancy (the internalization of a reliably available, caring other) is not established. The PPD patient expels aggressive impulses by projection: projective identification locates the impulses in others as a means of controlling fears of annihilating the object and of being annihilated in return. Beneath this defensive structure lie infantile feelings of helplessness, worthlessness, inadequacy, and depression (Rosenfeld, 1975; Meissner, 1995). Environmental failure to contain infantile feelings, above all aggression and hatred, plays a fundamental paranoiagenic role (cf. Winnicott, 1962; Balint, 1968; Kohut and Wolf, 1978).

A key assumption in *cognitive-behavioral approaches* to PPD is that the beliefs in PPD exist on a continuum between normal threat beliefs and persecutory delusions. Cognitive therapists focus on reducing distress and preoccupation with disturbing beliefs. Models of persecutory beliefs provide a basis for developing clinical formulations for people with PPD and for persecutory delusions in paranoid psychotic disorders. There are two main types of cognitive-behavioral conceptualizations of persecutory delusions. The first considers that the belief that others are persecutors may arise through processes of social learning (initially involving conditioning in threatening, humiliating, or submissive situations; cf. Carson, 1999). This evolves over the life course as an exaggerated response to threatening situations by a process of increasing vigilance and avoidance akin to a trauma or anxiety reaction (e.g., Pretzer, 1988; Beck *et al.*, 1990; Fowler, 2000; Freeman *et al.*, 2002). Depression and low self-esteem associated with paranoia are regarded as comorbid or secondary. The second conceptualization suggests that paranoid belief represents adaptation to social threat, and to the consequences of low self-esteem or depression (Colby, 1981; Turkat, 1985; Bentall *et al.*, 2001). The primary concern is a need to avoid the devastating consequences of further social threat or of social isolation

on the self-view of the subject. Persecutory beliefs are held to have arisen due to a tendency to externalize blame and project it on others, leading to paranoia. Chadwick *et al.* (1996) have described two types of paranoia arising from differing underlying processes linked to the above conceptualizations.

Schizoid personality disorder

Psychodynamic approaches emphasize the extent to which schizoid individuals have detached themselves from human relating. Schizoid patients complain of being unable to maintain close relationships. They rapidly identify with others, becoming transiently dependent, and then withdraw. They are demanding, controlling, and often devaluing of others and tend to have grandiose ideas about themselves that conceal feelings of hopelessness and helplessness. Their sexual identity is usually unstable. Psychoanalytic theory considers the schizoid to be someone who craves love but who cannot love for fear that love (not only hate) will destroy the object (Fairbairn, 1954; Guntrip, 1968). He is enclosed in a claustro-agoraphobic object relational dilemma (Rey, 1994). This dynamic can be described as a fantasy of *being trapped inside an object* (other person), or else of being threatened by psychic disintegration when outside it, as a result of belief in its total loss. The anxiety derives from the proximity or distance the individual feels from the object. Too much closeness yields claustrophobic anxiety due to the intensity of affects aroused by fears of merging and engulfment. Too much distance creates agoraphobic fears of loss and collapse. The experience of time and space may become confused due to poor secondary process functioning. The schizoid individual tends to oscillate between extremes that are the product of massively divergent views of the object created by persistent, intense splitting and fragmentation of the object, ego, and internal objects. Expelled 'bad' parts of the self are introjected and then persecute the ego. 'Good' parts of the self are also projected into others leading to ego depletion and fears of loss of the object and sense of self. Problems of identity failure due to the retreat from object relationships lie at the crux of schizoid pathology (Winnicott, 1962, 1965).

Cognitive-behavioral approaches acknowledge that SPD is the least understood or researched of Cluster A conditions. Schizoid problems may exist on a continuum of behaviors between normality and negative symptoms. From the perspective of personality theorists schizoid disorders are seen to relate to extreme introversion (Jackson, 1998), and there may also be continuities with autistic spectrum disorders (Wolff, 1998). Problems in relationships, socializing, and emotional functioning may occur because of disorders in understanding and experiencing emotions, social rules, and interpersonal behavior. In a manner akin to autistic spectrum disorders, cognitive deficits in processing other peoples' theory of mind may be crucial to the disorder (Millon, 1981). An alternative CBT conceptualization draws from psychoanalytic theory and implies that the disorder may arise from disturbed maternal relationships and compounded by failed social learning.

Schizotypal personality disorder

Psychodynamic approaches stress early fragmentation of the ego and damage to the sense of self of a type associated with schizophrenic states. Psychological functioning reveals primitive, part-object relationships (cf. Rey, 1994), impoverished mental representations, developmental deficits in terms of the capacity to mentalize and there is a potential for psychotic thinking under stress. The StPD patient's failure to internalize adequate representations of the object gives rise to a precarious sense of self. Development remains fixated at the paranoid-schizoid level (Klein, 1946) but because trauma is held to have occurred at the oral stage many psychotherapists see StPD anxieties as very primitive, requiring containment and interpretation at points when the ego is neither overwhelmed by anxiety nor paralyzed by defenses. Balint described two internal solutions to failure of the relationship between mother and baby. The 'basic fault' in the infant's personality can later be expressed as either the 'ocnophilic' or the 'philobatic' tendency. The former is a response to a chronic 'emptiness inside' and seeks to fill it by demanding more and more from others. The latter involves giving up on others and retreating into a world of fantasy (Balint, 1968). SDP and StPD patients fit the latter profile. Bowlby's 'avoidantly attached' category also characterizes these individuals who are too afraid of aversive contact to seek it (Bowlby, 1988).

Cognitive-behavioral approaches see ideas of reference, paranoid and suspicious thinking, odd beliefs, and magical ideation in StPD as part of a continuum between normality and the positive symptoms of psychosis. CBT conceptualizations of psychosis (Kingdon and Turkington, 1994; Fowler, 2000; Garety *et al.*, 2000) are applicable to the disorder. Source monitoring problems are important (i.e., confusion about the origins of thoughts) and these states may link with everyday experiences such as 'déjà vu'. Typically, the StPD patient may have little awareness of the internal origins of his or her cognitive confusion and may have succumbed to extensive irrational thinking. Development of bizarre convictions of apparently external origin, e.g., preoccupation with spirits, telepathy, hypnosis, spirits, etc., are not uncommon in StPD and are influenced and maintained, CBT theory argues, by internal emotional and reasoning biases.

Research

There is little research into Cluster A disorders compared with other personality disorders (notably borderlines) and more is needed if these conditions are to become better understood. *Psychodynamic research* notes the stability of diagnosis and treatment outcomes, e.g., Stone (1983, 1985, 1993), McGlashan (1986), Gunderson (1993), Sandell *et al.* (1997). Psychoanalytic authors tend to study intrapsychic object relationships, defenses, psychotic anxieties, and transference–countertransference phenomena related to these conditions (e.g., Rosenfeld, 1964, 1975; Segal, 1978; Meissner, 1986; Lucas, 1992; Rey, 1994; Grotstein, 1995; Sohn, 1995; Target and Fonagy, 1996a,b; Caper, 1998; Gabbard, 2000; Jackson, 2000; Robbins, 2002). Attention to 'psychotic anxieties' is of special interest to psychoanalysts: psychotic elements may occur in severe neuroses, psychosomatic disorders, sexual perversions, and personality disorders *alongside* neurotic constellations. Such patients are not psychotic *per se*, but are vulnerable to compromised ego functioning that creates confusion between internal and external realities. Research into the role of countertransference factors has confirmed the centrality of the therapist's responsiveness (particularly to psychotic anxieties) for successful treatment as well as the hazards of inattention to countertransference phenomena (Hinshelwood, 1994; Lieberz and Porsch, 1997).

Cognitive research into PPD supports a continuum model of persecutory beliefs (Peters *et al.*, 1999) and outcome studies show the benefits of CBT with persecutory beliefs through studies of schizophrenia, delusional disorder, and psychosis (Garety and Freeman, 1999; Bentall *et al.*, 2001; Pilling *et al.*, 2002; Turkington *et al.*, Chapter 14, this volume). Cuesta *et al.* (1999) found that negative symptoms were associated with premorbid SPD behavior. Tsuang *et al.* (2002) and Faraone *et al.* (2001) indicate that negative schizotypy (schizotaxia) is more common in relatives of people with schizophrenia than schizotypal features and is associated with neuropsychological deficit (this supports a continuum model between schizoid behavior and negative symptoms). Theory of mind deficits in schizophrenia (Pickup and Frith, 2001; Roncone *et al.*, 2002) are reflected in schizoid children and adults who were diagnosed as schizoid as children (Wolff and Barlow, 1979; Chick *et al.*, 1980). StPD research has focused on the transition to psychosis in high-risk schizotypal groups (Peters *et al.*, 1999, McGorry *et al.*, 2002a,b). CBT concepts and research data that are employed in the study of psychosis are applicable to the study of schizotypal states. However, all theories remain speculative.

Group and therapeutic community (TC) research traditionally addresses these fields at a descriptive level linked to case studies and qualitative data. No randomized controlled trials have been undertaken with group therapy for personality disorders. The use of validated research instruments is a relatively recent development. Roberts (1991) has described how schizoid people function in group analytic psychotherapy and makes suggestions for adjunct therapeutic measures and preparatory individual work. He concludes pessimistically that 'the sad truth is that we have no sure way of enabling release from this confinement'. Henderson Hospital research demonstrated that severe personality disorders are likely to be diagnosable with numerous single disorders in more than one cluster (Dolan *et al.*, 1995). The Henderson and units like it that offer residential treatment have yielded a reduction in personality disorder symptoms and interpersonal problems (Dolan *et al.*, 1997; Chiesa and Fonagy, 2000). Canadian and Norwegian day unit TCs confirm similar improvements on the basis of greater involvement with the patient (Piper *et al.*, 1996; Wilberg *et al.*, 1999). A Cassel Hospital study, however, showed increased improvement for those who have a shorter inpatient program of 6 months, followed by outpatient group therapy and nursing support, compared with a longer inpatient program of 1 year. Both groups improved significantly more than matched treatment-as-usual controls (Chiesa and Fonagy, 2000). A Finnish TC program yielded long-term follow-up and predictive factors for successful engagement (Isohanni and Nieminen, 1992). See also Vaglum *et al.* (1990). A review of TCs demonstrated positive findings indicating that there is accumulating evidence, albeit at a low level of research, of the effectiveness and suitability of the TC model to the treatment of personality disorder, particularly severe personality disorder (Lees *et al.*, 1999).

Key practice principles

Psychodynamic and cognitive-behavioral practice principles will be addressed first, followed by group and TC concepts and practices.

Psychodynamic approaches pay special attention to transference–countertransference phenomena in order to grasp what is taking place in the therapeutic relationship. Without careful attention to the therapeutic alliance and interpretation of the transference—particularly the negative transference—treatment can founder, above all with PPD where levels of suspicion are high. In practice, this means that the therapist must try to understand how he or she is being experienced by the patient, not least in object relations terms ('*Who am I currently representing for the patient, and in what way?*') and to how the patient is making the therapist feel [e.g. '*I am now experiencing strong feelings* (these may be boredom, sexual, aggressive feelings, etc.): *to what extent do these feelings originate in me or is the patient inducing me to feel these?*'). The effects of splitting of the patient's ego and of the object (cf. the paranoid-schizoid position, Klein, 1946) underlie these transference/countertransference issues and can make treatment confusing and erratic. At one moment the therapist may be experienced positively, even as an idealized figure; this can change dramatically into the therapist being seen as a persecuting critic or tyrant. This can take place without the therapist saying anything controversial and signifies a radical disjuncture in the patient's affective experience of others. A nondefensive, nonconfrontational approach, and willingness on the part of the therapist to tolerate being a sufficiently 'bad' (i.e., inadequate) as well as good object is essential to facilitate basic trust and reduce splitting and projection. The more a patient can express true feelings in the transference, the more therapeutic the treatment is likely to be. Avoiding malignant regression is important. Regression is a defensive reversion, under stress, to earlier forms of thinking and object-relating and is often inevitable in therapy. *Benign* regression signifies a healthy satisfying of certain infantile needs by working these through collaboratively in the therapy. *Malignant* regression denotes a situation is which the patient tries but fails to have these needs met and the situation yields a vicious cycle of demanding, addiction-like states. The analyst's technique, countertransference responses and capacity for maintaining boundaries are important in avoiding malignant regression (Balint, 1968). To achieve the trust of a Cluster A patient the therapist must tolerate difficult, even extreme countertransference feelings. These feelings are commonplace because the patient will try to rid him or herself of unacceptable feelings by projecting them on to the therapist. This activity needs to be attended to for its communications value and for its potential to derail an understanding of the patient's emotional state if the therapist reacts in an overemotional way (Heimann, 1950; Carpy, 1989; Gabbard and

Wilkinson, 1994). Negative therapeutic reactions (stubborn resistances to improvement usually following some improvement; cf. Freud, 1923; Riviere, 1936; Steiner, 1994) are to be expected and the separation anxieties, narcissistic rages, and envious impulses associated with these require interpretation. For SPD patients transference interpretation of claustro-agoraphobic anxieties is necessary (Rey, 1994). Actings-out by patients and crises over money, timings, holidays, etc. can arise and these may need to be responded to by reality-based, supportive interventions, together with interpretation of the anxieties being defended against.

An SPD patient in her 40s found that the separation anxiety evoked by gaps in the therapy (between sessions, breaks, etc.) made her want to quit. She could not 'hear' interpretations of her emotional distress, so focused was she on the concrete action of quitting. The therapist was able to say:

> I understand your wish to stop your therapy and, of course, I have no power to stop you: it is a difficult undertaking for anyone and I think that recently you have been finding it especially painful (*supportive intervention*). You feel frustrated and hurt by the comings and goings to and from our sessions and are left having to cope with a great deal on your own. I think this makes you feel resentful and you feel like sacking me. It must feel very hard to talk about these feelings—perhaps even to reach them—maybe because you are afraid that I might not be able to stand you if you complain (*interpretation of underlying anxieties*).

By working through the crisis on these lines the patient gained insight into her fantasy of the destructiveness of her feelings and was able to begin to use thinking and speech rather than action to deal with her fear.

Awareness of deficit as well as conflict models is useful in understanding the quality of patients' attachments as these can be primitive and confused. Therapeutic goals require realistic assessment and regular monitoring: progress may be slow and erratic with setbacks and perhaps limited eventual gains. Interpretation and explication together may be required to support movement from disorganized thinking towards integration of severe anxieties, especially in StPD where fragmentation of the ego may prevail. Nonetheless, StPD patients may reveal areas of reasonable ego strength; this, combined with less rigid defenses than SPD patients, may enable them to respond more readily to analytic interpretations and tolerate depressive affects. Family, psychiatric, and community support alongside therapy can improve outcome for all Cluster A patients.

Cognitive approaches tend be technically similar for all Cluster A disorders in that they target the pathological belief or system ('schema') and this helps particularly in the amelioration of maladaptive habits and in limit setting. Associated problems of depression and self-image are tackled as secondary phenomena. Establishing initial trust in the therapeutic relationship requires a flexible approach that is sensitive to changes in the patient's mental state. A neutral standpoint is maintained in relation to the patient's perspective of their problems alongside validation of the affective experience. The therapist teases out particular life circumstances and events that provide a context for the formation and maintenance of the patient's beliefs. One important difference between a psychodynamic and CBT perspective is that paranoid responses (these are common in Cluster A disorders) are not necessarily regarded as transference issues but instead as reactions to perceived threat. In CBT the patient is invited to test out their beliefs and to review evidence and alternative hypotheses. A new, more realistic model of events is constructed with the patient. The therapist and patient collaborate to examine and assess evidence for and against certain beliefs using behavioral experiments. Negative self-evaluations may be isolated and reviewed according to a more realistic appraisal of the person's circumstances. A typical intervention, in this case with a paranoid patient, is one that would be characteristic of work with Cluster A or psychotic patients (Kingdon and Turkington, 2002):

> Mary is 62 and had suffered a prolonged paranoid illness that centered around a fear that her husband was being unfaithful. The first two CBT sessions were spent with Mary gathering information about her perception of her condition. The third session included her husband to gain his perspective. A full history was taken and a formulation arrived at that took into account Mary's long-standing negative view of herself, her vulnerability, and the severity of her conviction in her beliefs. An action

plan was drawn up to consider her experiences as beliefs; to make links between her perceptions, beliefs, and affects; to test the beliefs as hypotheses; to draw up alternative hypotheses and to review evidence for both. Given Mary's high level of conviction in her beliefs it was important during the first main intervention (below) to validate their affective component and to link current feelings to previous experiences.

Therapist: So what seems to be happening now?

Mary: Well, George's daughter obviously wants the house to herself. That's why she said that. She can get all the money then, leaving me with nothing.

Therapist: How did you feel when you heard that?

Mary: Sick. Really bad. Worried. And angry.

Therapist: I can understand that. It must have been made even worse given your experiences with your mum—is that right?

Mary: Yes, that was a frightening time. Not knowing where we were going to end up that night.

Mary: George keeps stealing money from my purse. I don't know why he's doing it. He only needs to ask and I'd give it to him. I don't understand why he needs to steal.

Therapist: Any ideas as to what's going on here?

Mary: It must be because he's spending it on some other woman.

Therapist: What does George say about this?

Mary: Oh, he denies it, of course.

Therapist: Right. So money seems to be disappearing from your purse, and you believe that George is taking it?

Mary: Yes.

Therapist: And your explanation for that is that he must be spending it on another woman, otherwise he'd tell you, right?

Mary: Yes

Therapist: Does this situation remind you of any of your early experiences?

Mary: Oh yes. We were always running short of money when I was a child. And my first husband was always having affairs. We never had any money then either.

Therapist: Do you remember any feelings of insecurity around those times?

Mary: Of course!

Therapist: So is it possible that your memories of those experiences have stayed with you, and that as a result you may pay particular attention to things that are happening now that look the same?

Mary: Maybe. I hadn't really thought of it like that.

A link is being made here between Mary's current belief and her long-standing, 'schematic' beliefs in order to provide a rationale for the beliefs and relief from feelings of stigma around them. Subsequently, certain hypotheses were generated around the missing money, including that Mary may have spent it but forgotten about it. Mary was then set homework to monitor any incidents of forgetting, especially concerning money, and this proved to be fruitful. An incident of a forgotten bill she had already paid opened up a new, more questioning attitude in her towards her behavior in relation to money. As she discovered during her sessions that there were plausible, alternative explanations to a number of different situations, so her affective investment in her convictions waned and her psychotic symptoms gradually receded. Making narrative sense of symptoms and contextualizing their emergence, as in the above example, is often a crucial initial component in CBT, as a shared rationale is usually missing. The CBT therapist works collaboratively to develop a less distressing understanding of the patient's difficulties, and this can involve normalizing or destigmatizing the nature of disturbing experiences. Kingdon and Turkington cite a normalizing rationale during the interview of Sarah, a psychotic patient, which would also be applicable to a StPD patient. Sarah was asked during the initial meeting how her psychotic symptoms had arisen and she described how, at the time, she was suffering a serious physical injury, was sleep-deprived and that her husband was in serious dispute with neighbors. A distress-reducing, normalizing rationale was sought to help explain Sarah's symptoms as understandable in the context of her physical and mental stress at the time (Kingdon and Turkington, 2002, pp. 101–2). This explanation reduced Sarah's anxiety levels and allowed her to reflect upon the hypervigilance associated with her symptoms and how this might lead to misinterpretation of environmental cues. Once a more settled state was achieved the scene was set for further, systematic examination of beliefs and evidence.

Group approaches are based upon the conscious and unconscious network of relationships within groups, sometimes referred to as the 'matrix' (Blackwell, 1998). The emphasis lies on social functioning rather than individual unconscious drives ('the whole is more elementary than the parts'). The 'matrix'—or the way the group functions as a social unit—is a powerful agency. It is an object of attachment and a source of safety and containment, and these harbor therapeutic potential. Group analytic theory was developed by Foulkes, a psychoanalyst, who paved the way for understanding group relations processes (Foulkes, 1964, 1986). He identified processes in groups such as 'resonance', 'condenser phenomenon', and 'mirroring' through which unconscious activity can be described: (1) *resonance* involves shared experience of supportive identifications between group members; (2) *condenser* phenomena describe articulation of unconscious feelings through shared forms of symbolization; and (3) *mirroring* is where group members can observe and integrate split-off parts of themselves by seeing them in others and coming to understand them through engagement with the group. Nonverbal therapeutic techniques such as acceptance of silence without striving to explore or interpret (particularly for schizoid members), tolerance of oddness (for the schizotypal) and use of sympathetic eye contact can be therapeutically effective in addition to verbal interventions. Foulkes' ideas have been applied to work in TCs (Rawlinson, 1999) where the activities of daily living offer a benefit to Cluster A patients as they can be engaged in therapeutic relationship building without needing to talk. They observe what goes on before starting to benefit from meaningful verbal contact. The psychoanalyst Wilfred Bion (1961) conceived of basic assumptions operating in groups, expressed through the activities of pairing, fight/flight, or dependency. These assumptions seemed to him to be innate or instinctual and underlie, and sometimes override, the conscious communication system (Hinshelwood, 2002). The treatment objective is to transcend basic assumptions and help group members establish a capacity for sustained relationships founded on concern and respect. Cluster A patients tend to not normally seek group psychotherapy and will leave if they find it aversive. Substantial effort at engagement is required, and members of the group usually support and encourage this. For extremes of pathology, such as Cluster A, the creation of groups with more than one individual with a Cluster A presentation can provide a more understanding therapeutic environment.

TC approaches embody two main precepts: the community as the agent of change and the TC culture of self-help. Typically, TCs are residential facilities and the resident is expected to adhere to certain behavioral norms. The resident may progress through a hierarchy of increasingly more important roles, with greater privileges and responsibilities. Individual and group therapy, group sessions with peers, community-based learning, confrontation, games, and role-playing may all be utilized as part of an extensive therapeutic experience. Identifying, expressing, and managing feelings are important goals, as is heightened awareness of the impact of attitudes and behaviors on oneself and the social environment. TC members often become role models who reflect the values and teachings of the community. TC treatment varies but can be broadly divided into three major stages: (1) induction during the first month or so in order to assimilate the individual into policies and procedures; (2) systematic involvement at multiple levels of engagement—individual, group and social using the methods described above (a typical day might start at 7 a.m. and end at 11 p.m. and comprise morning and evening community groups/meetings, groups, seminars, work tasks, individual therapy, and recreation); and (3) a phased

transition into the outside world in which the values and practices of TC are carried into normal living.

Challenges

Cluster A individuals are the least likely of the personality disorder groups to undertake psychotherapy of any kind due to their reduced capacity to engage in relationships. However, it does not follow that psychotherapy is automatically contraindicated: many patients do benefit from therapy. All forms of therapy face significant challenges with Cluster A patients, although their strategies for dealing with these differ. PPD patients threaten the therapeutic relationship through their suspiciousness and distorted conviction that hostility and danger are omnipresent. Alertness to signs of mounting suspiciousness is therefore essential: this needs to be responded to by transference interpretation (psychodynamic therapists), empathic discussion, and review of evidence for beliefs (CBT) and open acknowledgement within the matrix (group therapists). Directly confronting PPD beliefs by argument can have the effect of reinforcing the belief as PPD patients use projective identification extensively to externalize hostile impulses for fear of destroying the therapeutic relationship. The following is an extract from a psychoanalytic psychotherapy session with a 40-year-old patient with PPD symptoms. She suffered an internal, superego 'voice' that advised her against relationships. This exchange took place following a session in which the patient had felt understood and closer to the therapist. A negative therapeutic reaction had ensued:

Patient: You don't understand. My mother never understood me. When my grandmother was dying, she was very old, I tried to give her the kiss of life. I was breathing into her. I was trying to get her heart going. My mother thought I was hurting her. I wasn't. I wanted to keep her alive, not die. She didn't understand, she just didn't understand. You don't understand (she cried, paused, and then resumed her complaint that I didn't understand her for several more minutes, before suddenly stopping and shouting, in alarm). You're trying to kill me. (Pause)

Therapist: 'I think you are afraid of what you could do to me if you make demands on me. When you complain about me, as you are doing now, a voice in your head warns you that I will retaliate, even want to kill you. I think that the voice is trying to stop you from telling me more of what you're really feeling.

In this example the therapist responds to both psychotic and nonpsychotic areas of mental functioning and attempts to interpret their relationship to each other, in the transference, in order to reduce the split between these different levels of anxiety. SPD patients are often unable to describe their difficulties in the way the above PPD patient does, and may remain withdrawn for long periods. This can be unrewarding, challenging, and confusing for the therapist. As disengagement from the emotional aspect of relationships is the hallmark of SPD, the task is to expand their atrophied capacity for human contact. This is not easy: for example, some SPD patients cry in sessions without realizing the fact that they are in pain. Or they may appear to regard their social isolation or interpersonal behavior as unproblematic and ignore the therapist's interventions. Long silences can be bewildering and the therapist might be tempted to make sense of the silence with intellectual interventions. These are likely to make the patient more, not less, anxious, especially if the intervention remains at a reconstructive level. Tolerating and addressing the cold, mechanical, deadening defenses of SPD is the challenge for the psychodynamic, cognitive, or group therapist. StPD, in contrast, often produces chaotic and eccentric thinking that may be mixed with paranoid and manic ideation. The patient may not be aware of the oddness of their beliefs and behavior and feel threatened if confronted. Ongoing assessment of the StPD patient's ego strength is therefore required. Containing the patient's multifarious anxieties and interpreting their fixed ideas (that sometimes resemble delusions) is necessary, as in this example:

A female StDP in her 50s presented for psychoanalytic therapy with symptoms of StPD and severe hysteria. She suffered intense, sometimes unmanageable anxiety and thought disorder; she exhibited eccentric behavior and was paranoid; her ego was fragmented and her sense of self fragile. It required a great deal of containing activity on the part of the therapist before the patient was able to begin to be able to talk about her feelings, as she was consumed by a delusional conviction that the therapist could not bear her. Containment and interpretation of terror of rejection and associated paranoid anxieties was the main therapeutic task. When she eventually did talk of her feelings, she was impeded by retching, inside and outside the sessions. This continued for some weeks: she carried a utensil/container with her and sometimes could not leave her bed for fear of dying or committing suicide. The therapist's countertransference experience was one of anxiety that she might not survive as well as frustration and resentment at her inability to speak. These countertransference responses enabled the therapist to interpret likely feelings the patient was holding at bay and to speculate as to why. Eventually the patient began to speak, little by little, of her lifelong tendency to be compliant, her frustrations and longings and an internal hatred that paralyzed her thinking.

The above is a somewhat severe but not altogether unusual StPD presentation and requires of the psychodynamic therapist patience, sensitivity, and a capacity to sustain various axes of apprehension that encompass conflict, deficit, and developmental perspectives. The cognitive therapist is likely to approach the situation differently and would focus on a more pragmatic course of assessing the patient's beliefs and ideas and their relationship to external reality. StPD patients who do manage to trust their therapist can develop a capacity to tolerate more depressive affect and anxiety than they had previously imagined. However, setting realistic goals for StPD is advisable, given the severity of the condition.

Group therapy faces its most severe obstacles in treating PPD patients who are likely to be hostile and aversive to group situations. They believe others reject them and as a result are rarely referred (Haigh, 1998). SPD patients can become responsive to group or community treatments given their long-standing failure to socialize and spirals of increasing withdrawal and isolation. Their isolation can undermine reality testing and group treatment can help to reverse this regressive trend. Individual and group treatment combined may be particularly effective for many of these patients. The excessive social anxiety in StPD that, without therapy, may not abate over time renders improved socialization difficult. However, the accessibility of these anxieties, which may at times be psychotic, can help make these patients more amenable to contact at deeper levels in group, analytic, and cognitive therapy.

Conclusions

There are serious difficulties in treating Cluster A patients whatever the therapeutic setting or modality, as these individuals have to a great extent fallen out of the orbit of normal human relations. They display defenses sometimes seen in psychosis and will not respond to a therapist who does not take seriously their loss of faith in people. This lost capacity to depend on others leaves its imprint on their internal world: failed internalization of trusting relationships generates chronic mistrust and anxiety. Because these patients tend not to present voluntarily for treatment, there is a need for more detailed research and documented clinical experience if their conditions are to be better understood. Once in treatment, a capacity in the therapist for flexibility will improve treatment prospects. A multimodal approach can be more valuable than a single therapy alone in managing multiple anxieties. For example, a period of asylum may be helpful for some patients; a combination of minimal medication with group and individual therapy has also been shown to benefit many patients (cf. Jackson and Williams, 1994). Many psychotherapists find it important to obtain psychiatric back-up during therapy to act as a support for both patient and therapist. However, it needs to be underscored that whatever the therapeutic context, insufficient research or outcome evidence is available to offer definitive conclusions regarding therapy for Cluster A patients.

Despite the difficulties and setbacks involved in treating Cluster A conditions, there can be significant rewards not least when basic trust and new forms of relating develop, often after decades of isolation and illness. Despite their cold, hostile, or bizarre behavior, Cluster A patients suffer painful, confusing feelings, and significant problems of self-esteem based on their fragmented personality structures and primitive self-representations. Therapeutic gains in these areas, although often limited, can make a considerable difference to the quality of their lives.

References

American Psychiatric Association (1994). *Diagnostic and statistical manual of mental disorders*, 4th edn. Washington DC: American Psychiatric Association.

Balint, M. (1968). *The basic fault*. London: Tavistock.

Beck, A. T., *et al.*, ed. (1990). Paranoid personality disorder. In: *Cognitive therapy of personality disorders*. New York: The Guildford Press.

Bentall, R. P., *et al.* (2001). Persecutory delusions: a review and theoretical integration. *Clinical Psychology Review Special Issue: Psychosis*, **21**(8), 1143–92.

Bion, W. R. (1961). *Experiences in groups*. London: Tavistock.

Blackwell, D. (1998). Bouded instability, group–analysis and the matrix: organizations under stress. *Journal of Group Analysis and Psychotherapy*, **31**, 4.

Bowlby, J. (1988). *A secure base: clinical applications of attachment theory*. London: Routledge.

Caper, R. (1998). Psychopathology and primitive mental states. *International Journal of Psycho-Analysis*, **79**, 539–51.

Carpy, D. V. (1989). Tolerating the countertransference: a mutative process. *International Journal of Psycho-Analysis*, **70**, 287–94.

Carson, R. C., *et al.* (1999). *Abnormal psychology and modern life*, 11th edn. Boston, MA: Allyn & Bacon.

Chadwick, P., Birchwood, M., and Trowe, P. (1996). *Cognitive therapy for delusions, voices and paranoia*. Chichester: Wiley.

Chick, J., Waterhouse, L., and Wolff, S. (1980). Psychological construing in schizoid children grown up. *Annual Progress in Child Psychiatry and Development*, pp. 386–95.

Chiesa, M. and Fonagy, P. (2000). Cassel personality disorder study— Methodology and treatment effects. *British Journal of Psychiatry*, **176**, 485–91.

Colby, K. M. (1981). Modelling a paranoid mind. *Behavioural and Brain Sciences*, **4**, 515–60.

Cuesta, M. J., Peralta, V., and Caro, F. (1999). Premorbid personality in psychoses. *Schizophrenia Bulletin*, **25**(4), 801–11.

Dolan, B., Evans, C., and Norton, K. (1995). Multiple axis-II diagnoses of personality disorder. *British Journal of Psychiatry*, **166**, 107–12.

Dolan, B., Warren, F., and Norton, K. (1997). Change in borderline symptoms one year after therapeutic community treatment for severe personality disorder. *British Journal of Psychiatry*, **171**, 274–9.

Fairbairn. W. R. D. (1954). *An object relations theory of the personality*. New York: Basic Books Inc.

Faraone, S. V., Green, A. I., Seidman, L. J., and Tsuang, M. T. (2001). 'Schizotaxia': clinical implications and new directions for research. *Schizophrenia Bulletin*, **27**, 1–18.

Foulkes, S. H. (1964). *Therapeutic group analysis*. London: Allen and Unwin.

Foulkes, S. H. (1986). *Group analytic psychotherapy. Method and principles*. London: Karnac Books.

Fowler, D. (2000). Psychological formulation of early psychosis: a cognitive model. In: M. Birchwood, D. Fowler, and C. Jackson, ed. *Early intervention in psychosis: a guide to concepts, evidence and interventions*. Chichester: John Wiley and Sons.

Fowler, D., Garety, P. A., and Kuipers, E. (1995). *Cognitive behaviour therapy of psychosis: theory and practice*. Chichester: John Wiley and Sons.

Freeman, D., Garety, P. A., Kuipers, E., Fowler, D., and Bebbington, P. (2002). A cognitive model of persecutory delusions. *British Journal of Clinical Psychology*, **41**(4), 331–47.

Freud, S. (1911/1958). Psychoanalytic notes on an autobiographical account of a case of paranoia (Dementia Paranoides). In: J. Strachey, trans. and ed. *The standard edition of the complete psychological works of Sigmund Freud*, Vol. 12, pp. 12–58. London: Hogarth Press.

Freud, S. (1923). The ego and the id. In: J. Strachey, trans. and ed. *The standard edition of the complete psychological works of Sigmund Freud*, Vol. 19, pp. 12–66. London: Hogarth Press (1961).

Gabbard, G. O. (2000). *Psychodynamic psychiatry in clinical practice*. Washington DC: American Psychiatric Press.

Gabbard, G. O. and Wilkinson, S. M. (1994). *Management of countertransference with borderline patients*. Washington, DC: American Psychiatric Press.

Garety, P. A. and Freeman, D. (1999). Cognitive approaches to delusions: a critical review of theories and evidence. *British Journal of Clinical Psychology*, **38**, 113–54.

Grotstein, J. S. (1995). Object relations theory in the treatment of the psychoses. *Bulletin of the Menninger Clinic*, **59**, 312–32.

Haigh, R. (1998). The quintessence of a therapeutic environment. In: P. Campling and R. Haigh, ed. *Therapeutic communities: past present and future*. London: Jessica Kingsley.

Heimann, P. (1950). On counter-transference. *International Journal of Psycho-Analysis*, **31**, 81–4.

Hinshelwood, R. D. (1994). *Clinical Klein: from theory to practice*. New York: HarperCollins Publishers Inc.

Hinshelwood, R. D. (2002): 'Group mentality and having a mind' http://www.psychematters.com

ICD-10 (1992). *International statistical classification of diseases and related health problems*, 10th revision. Geneva: WHO publications.

Isohanni, M. and Nieminen, P. (1992). Participation in group-psychotherapy in a therapeutic–community for acute patients. *Acta Psychiatrica Scandinavica*, **86**, 495–501.

Jackson, H. (1998). The assessment of personality disorder: selected issues and directions. In: P. McGorry and C. Perris, ed. *Cognitive psychotherapy of psychotic and personality disorders: handbook of theory and practice*. Chichester: John Wiley and Sons.

Jackson, M. (2000). *Weathering the storms*. London: Karnac Books.

Jackson, M. and Williams, P. (1994). *Unimaginable storms: a search for meaning in psychosis*. London: Karnac Books.

Kernberg, O. (1975). *Borderline personality and pathological narcissism*. New York, NJ: Jason Aronson.

Kingdon, D. and Turkington, D. (1994). *Cognitive-behavioural therapy of schizophrenia*. New York: Guilford Press.

Kingdon, D. and Turkington, D. (2002). *The case study guide to cognitive behaviour therapy of psychosis*. Chichester: John Wiley and Sons.

Klein, M. (1946). Notes on some schizoid mechanisms. *International Journal of Psycho-Analysis*, **27**, 99–110.

Kohut, H. and Wolf, E. S. (1978). The disorders of the self and their treatment: an outline. *International Journal of Psycho-Analysis*, **59**, 413–26.

Lees, J., Manning, N., and Rawlings, B. (1999). *Therapeutic community effectiveness—a systematic international review of therapeutic community treatment for people with personality disorders and mentally disordered offenders*. CRD Report 17. York: NHS Centre for Reviews and Dissemination, University of York.

Lieberz, K. and Porsch, U. (1997). Countertransference in schizoid disorders. *Psychotherapie, Psychosomatik, Medizinische Psychologie*, **47**(2), 46–51.

Lucas, R. N. (1992). The psychotic personality. A psycho-analytic theory and its application in clinical practice. *Psychoanalytic Psychotherapy*, **6**, 73–9.

McGlashan, T. (1986). The Chestnut Lodge Follow-up Study III: long-term outcome of borderline personalities. *Archives of General Psychiatry*, **43**, 20–30.

McGlashan, T. H. (1983). The borderline Syndrome. II. Is it a variant of schizophrenia or affective disorder? *Archives of General Psychiatry*, **40**(12), 1319–23.

McGorry, P. D., Yung, A., Phillips, L. J., Frances, S., and Jackson, H. (2002a). *Archives of General Psychiatry*, **59**(10), 921–8.

McGorry, P. D., Yung, A., and Philips, L. J. (2002b). 'Closing in' what features prdict the onset of first-episode psychosis within an ultra-high risk group? In: R. B. Zipursky and C. Schulz, ed. *The early stages of schizophrenia*. Washington, DC: American Psychiatric Publishing Inc.

Meissner, W. W. (1986). *Psychotherapy and the Paranoid Process*. Northvale, NJ: Jason Aronson.

Meissner. W. W. (1995). In the shadow of death. *Psychoanalytic Review*, **82**, 535–57.

Millon, T. (1981). *Disorders of personality DSM III: Axis II*. New York: Wiley.

Peters, E., Joseph, S. A., and Garety, P. A. (1999). The measurement of delusional ideation in the normal population. *Schizophrenia Bulletin*, **25**, 553–76.

Pickup, G. and Frith, C. D. (2001). Theory of mind impairments in schizophrenia: symptomatology, severity and specificity. *Psychological Medicine*, **31**(2), 207–20.

Pilling, S., Bebbington, P., Kuipers E., and Garety P. A. (2002). Psychological treatments in schizophrenia: I. Meta-analysis of family intervention and cognitive behaviour therapy. *Psychological Medicine*, **32**(5), 763–782.

Piper, W. E., Rosie, J. S., Joyce, A. S., and Azim, H. F. A. (1996). *Time-limited day treatment for personality disorders: integration of research and practice in a group program*. Washington DC: American Psychological Association.

Pretzer, J. L. (1988). Paranoid personality disorder: a cognitive view. *International Cognitive Therapy Newsletter*, **4**(4), 10–12.

Rawlinson, D. (1999). Group analytic ideas: extending the group matrix into TCs. In: P. Campling and R. Haigh, ed. *Therapeutic communities: past present and future*, pp. 50–62. London: Jessica Kingsley.

Rey, H. (1994). *Universals of psychoanalysis in the treatment of psychotic and borderline states*. London: Free Association Books.

Riviere, J. (1936). A contribution to the analysis of the negative therapeutic reaction. *International Journal of Psycho-Analysis*, **17**, 304–20.

Roberts, J. (1991). The schizoid character in groups. In: J. Roberts and M. Pines, ed. *The practice of group analysis*, pp. 120–3. London: Routledge.

Robbins, M.(2002). The language of Schizophrenia and the world of delusion. *International Journal of Psycho-Analysis*, **83**(2), 383–405.

Roncone, R., Falloon, I. R. H., and Mazza, M. (2002). Is theory of mind in schizophrenia more strongly associated with clinical and social functioning than with neurocognitive deficits? *Psychopathology*, **35**(5), 280–8.

Rosenfeld, H. (1964). On the psychopathology of narcissism: a clinical approach. *International Journal of Psycho-Analysis*, **45**, 332–7.

Rosenfeld, H. (1975). Negative therapeutic reactions. In: P. L. Giovacchini, ed. *Tactics and techniques in psychoanalytic therapy*, pp. 217–28. New York: Jason Aronson.

Sandell, R., *et al.* (1997). Findings of the Stockholm Outcome of Psychotherapy and Psychoanalysis Project (STOPPP). Paper presented at the Annual Meeting of the Society for Psychotherapy Research, Geilo, Norway.

Segal, H. (1978). On symbolism. *International Journal of Psycho-Analysis*, **59**, 315–19.

Sohn, L. (1995). Unprovoked assaults-making sense of apparently random violence. *International Journal of Psycho-Analysis*, **76**, 565–76.

Sperry. L. (1995). *Handbook of diagnosis and treatment of the DSM-IV personality disorders*. Now York: Brunner/Mazel.

Steiner, J. (1994). *Psychic retreats*. London: Routledge.

Stone, M. (1985). Schizotypal personality: psychotherapeutic aspects. *Schizophrenia Bulletin*, **11**(4), 576–89.

Stone, M. (1993). Long-term outcome in personality disorders. *British Journal of Psychiatry*, **162**, 299–313.

Target, M. and Fonagy, P. (1996a). Playing with reality II: The development of psychic reality from a theoretical perspective. *International Journal of Psycho-Analysis*, **77**, 459–79.

Target, M. and Fonagy, P. (1996b). *An outcome study of psychotherapy for patients with borderline personality disorder*. New York: International University Press.

Tsuang, M. T., Stone, W. S., Tarbox, S. I., and Faraone, S. V. (2002). An integration of schizophrenia with schizotypy: identification of schizotaxia and implications for research on treatment and prevention. *Schizophrenia Research*, **54**(1–2), 169–75.

Turkat, I. D. (1985). Formulation of paranoid personality disorder. In: I. D. Turkat, ed. *Behavioural case formulation*. New York: Plenum.

Vaglum, P., *et al.* (1990). Treatment response of severe and non-severe personality disorders in a therapeutic community day unit. *Journal of Personality Disorders*, **4**, 161–72.

Wilberg, T., *et al.* (1999). One-year follow-up of day treatment for poorly functioning patients with personality disorders. *Psychiatric Services*, **50**, 1326–30.

Winnicott, D. W. (1962). *The aims of psychoanalytic treatment, the maturational processes and the facilitating environment*, pp. 166–70. London: Hogarth Press.

Wolff, S. (1998). Schizoid personality in childhood: the links with Asperger syndrome, schizophrenia spectrum disorders and elective mutism. In: E. Schopler, *et al.*, ed. *Asperger syndrome or high functioning autism?*, pp. 123–42. New York: Plenum Press.

Wolff, S. and Barlow, A. (1979). Schizoid personality in childhood: a comparative study of schizoid, autistic and normal children. *Journal of Child Psychology and Psychiatry*, **20**, 29–46.

22 'Cluster B' antisocial disorders

Christopher Cordess, Kate Davidson, Mark Morris, and Kingsley Norton

Introduction

Antisocial personality disorder (ASPD) (DSM-IV-R, 1997), dyssocial personality disorder (ICD-10 WHO, 1992), and psychopathy are overlapping terms that are each more or less unsatisfactory in their own particular ways. The terms ASPD and dyssocial personality disorder cast their definitional net so wide as to include about half of the prison population, which limits their usefulness—i.e., they are low on 'specificity' and high on 'sensitivity'. Psychopathy for its part is variously defined and for Aubrey Lewis (1974) was a 'most elusive category'. Gunn and Robertson (1976) described five 'facts' about the term:

1. it is unreliable;

2. authors disagree about its definition;

3. it is used in the vernacular as a term of derogation;

4. it has a legal use;

5. many doctors use the term to indicate that a patient is incurable or untreatable.

Contemporary operational definitions by Hare (Psychopathy check-list, revised PCL-R, 1991) are drawn narrowly so as to exclude many who fall within the ASPD and dyssocial personality disorder definitional boundaries—thus limiting relevance; i.e., they are high on specificity and low on sensitivity.

What each of these behavioral disorders (with their attendant mental states) have in common is that they involve action against the environment, a violation—whether against human 'objects', as in violent and sexual offences, or indirectly in theft; or against material objects as in vandalism and criminal damage. When in treatment people/patients with these conditions can be expected to 'act out' as a central characteristic of the therapeutic engagement (or lack of it).

This confronts, at least the psychoanalytic psychotherapist, with a challenge if not a paradox. Charles Rycroft in *A critical dictionary of psychoanalysis* (1979) writes that 'Acting out is characteristic of Psychopathy and Behavior Disorders and reduces the accessibility of these conditions to psychoanalysis'. Further,

> a patient is said to be acting out if he engages in activity which can be interpreted as a substitute for remembering past events. The essence of the concept is the replacement of thought by action and it implies that either (a) the impulse being acted out has never acquired verbal representation, or (b) the impulse is too intense to be dischargeable in words, or (c) that the patient lacks the capacity of inhibition

by means of ego or super-ego function. 'Since psychoanalysis is a "talking or super-ego cure" carried out in a state of reflection', writes Rycroft 'acting out is anti-therapeutic'.

From a purist point of view this is correct. This chapter, then, challenges that purist view by offering considerations, techniques, and *applications* of psychoanalytic therapy, psychodynamic therapeutic community (TC), and cognitive-behavior therapy (CBT) treatment methods for the treatment and management of this type of personality and way of being, and the related behavior. While some ASPD patients are indeed, at least at a given stage in their lives, intractable, many are helpable and are often rewarding

subjects to treat. We should resist moralization in our professional attitude to a group who are, quite naturally, heavily stigmatized in their everyday lives. We aim to modify the maladaptive traits that lead to offending behavior: the aim is for some *transformation* not major *reformation*.

That we should have some creative responses to the problems presented by ASPD and overlapping categories could not be more significant, as all Western societies are challenged to find adequate or alternative responses to increasing rates of crime and violence. ASPD is broadly considered to affect about 1.5% of the populations of Western countries—i.e., approximately 3–4 million Americans and just short of 1 million Britons—in a ratio of an estimated 3:1 male to female. Any condition that is so common will necessarily occur in a great variety of guises as well as different degrees of severity.

Again, speaking generally, some 50% of the male prison population and 20% of the female prison population is estimated to suffer from this category of disorder, although, clearly there is a degree of variance one nation from another. All these figures are illustrative and subject to sociopolitical variables: For example, in the USA 686 people per 100 000 (and rising) are incarcerated in prisons, whereas in the UK the comparable figure is 'only' 139 per 100 000 (rapidly rising)—itself now the highest rate in Europe.

The main point to be made in a chapter on the *psychotherapy* of ASPD is that the diagnosis is a sociopolitical as well as a psychological construct. It seems that an increase in the prevalence of ASPD, and a massive and increasing rate of imprisonment, is largely associated with the overall material success of Western capitalist societies combined with the marginalization of large subgroups. Which particular aspects of these societies are potent in the generation of ASPD is a subject for research and for debate. The psychodynamic view encompasses failures of parenting in early (and later) childhood; leading to poor emotional development, and problems of attachment and failures of the social environment—placing more emphasis upon these factors than the indisputable effects of biological inheritance. While there is some research evidence that a small core of 'psychopaths' have biological—autonomic system—differences from 'normal' control populations, and a smaller volume prefrontal cortex, the interpretation of this finding is problematic. For example, to what degree is the former finding a *functional* variation and to what extent structural, and how is it related to previous trauma?

It is widely accepted that the concept and practice of the 'rehabilitative ideal' of reform of the antisocial personality effectively now barely exists within our contemporary overcrowded prisons, with very few exceptions (and one which in the UK is described later in this chapter). People who are sent to prison generally leave it in a worse psychological condition than when they entered; they will invariably be socially more isolated; in many instances they will have been further abused and corrupted by the system. Generally, in the USA and now in Britain the ethos of our societies have moved from those of 'welfare' to 'control' (Garland, 2001). Increasingly psychiatrists are expected to become agents of public protection and social control (Cordess, 2004). It is uncertain to what extent effective psychotherapy can survive in such cultures, especially for ASPD.

Most psychotherapists, however, do not work within this dispiriting penal system, which should, and could, be so much better. What follows are accounts of ways of thinking to enable the best possible interventions, mostly, but not exclusively, outside of the major coercive institutions. All mental health professionals working in whatever context will inevitably come up against incidents of antisocial behavior, as well as people manifesting ASPD. Although a specialist area its also one about which all practitioners need to have some knowledge.

First, some general observations about a psychoanalytic understanding and 'stance' with regard to ASPD patients in individual and group settings are provided. Accounts are then given of three specific modes of treatment for ASPD: (1) the TC; (2) the treatment of ASPD in a therapeutic (locked) prison; and (3) cognitive therapy for ASPD.

Individual and group psychotherapy of antisocial personality disorder

For Winnicott, the first necessity in the treatment of the delinquent was for clinical *management*; and the same applies for the treatment of ASPD. Only when sufficient control has been achieved, can further therapeutic intervention proceed. Thus, treatment may frequently require initial residential, possibly locked, provision, and only later may outpatient, ambulant, therapy be possible; different examples are described later. Sometimes ambulant therapy may be possible from the outset, sometimes with more or less support between therapeutic sessions, e.g., via partial hospitalization (day hospital). For milder psychopathology outpatient individual or group psychotherapy will be indicated. As all forms of 'acting out' are to be expected, there may commonly be sabotage of the therapeutic setting in a variety of ways if management is insufficient, e.g., there may be gross misuse of drugs or alcohol. Even in the best set-up this may happen from time to time and needs to be understood as part of the problem, rather than evoking a response of immediate rejection.

The mode of psychotherapy offered will depend on many factors: the degree of psychological mindedness; motivation; the extent and nature of 'denial'; the degree of subjective distress—or ulterior reasons, such as the recognition of the self-destructive consequences of the antisocial acts.

As a whole spectrum of different types of people and psychopathology are encompassed within the term ASPD, only a few general statements or guidelines, largely of a practical nature, will be offered.

What sort of psychotherapy might prove effective?

It may be useful to consider whether the antisocial actions are 'reactive', or 'impulsive' (far more common) on the one hand, or predatory, and potentially, therefore, far more complicated to manage on the other. Patients with severe borderline or psychotic states, those who rely on alcohol and drugs for their 'defenses', or those who have been grossly emotionally neglected or severely abused as children need especially careful assessment. A history of decompensations in the past—into violence or suicidal behavior—should be taken seriously. Essentially the question is 'what sort of psychotherapy might prove effective?' rather than a purist assessment that finds the subject unsuitable and is therefore likely to exclude the majority. Put another way, the assessor needs to consider positive aspects of the person that may be helpful to grow, as well as negative features.

There has been considerable work on the establishment of a therapeutic alliance with people with ASPD (see, e.g., Gerstley *et al.*, 1989); that alliance is necessary, and a significant predictor of outcome. It is also true that the creation of the therapeutic alliance depends greatly upon the skills of the therapist, and upon his correct assessment of the appropriate mode of psychotherapy. Psychodynamically, one may ask oneself, what are the ego strengths that can 'contain' the anxiety that may arise from exploratory, in-depth psychoanalytic psychotherapy? Related to this, to what extent is nonexploratory, supportive psychotherapy, which accepts and seeks to buttress defenses, preferable in a given psychologically fragile case?

One particular danger is that of the severely narcissistic, envious patient, who may initially idealize the therapist by a process of profound splitting.

He may experience the therapist, later, as withholding from him what he is certain would be his 'cure' and 'salvation'. In ordinary psychiatric practice these patients may actually engage the therapist in excessively long interviews, as idealization of the health professional—yet disappointment with the ordinariness of what they seem to offer—becomes increasingly a provocation; the longer the interview goes on the greater the perceived withholding.

These patients underline the general rule of establishing set parameters of time for each session, which may be anything up to 2 hours for assessment, and from half an hour, up to an hour, for therapeutic sessions. The frequency of sessions may also vary from the more usual pattern of once or twice weekly, to once every 2 weeks (or even less frequency) for those who are psychologically fragile and cannot cope with interpretive psychotherapy, but instead need psychological support.

Much of the published literature assumes or implies a highly defensive and suspicious posture from the therapist, which may be an 'acting out' of a paranoid countertransference—even to the stereotype or 'idea' of the patient with ASPD. Aside from this suspiciousness of 'dangerousness', the potential therapist may come with a particular, and excessive expectation of the potential (and need) for the ASPD person to deceive or lie; after all, 'deceitfulness, as indicated by repeated lying, use of aliases, or conning others for personal profit or pleasure' is one of the criteria—but, note, not a *necessary* criterion—for the DSM-4-R diagnosis of this disorder.

Frequently the apparent or real need to 'deceive' or 'lie' is actually a primitive defense at an unconscious level. Thus it may be (for example, by splitting and projection) a part of the covert psychopathology, i.e., that of the denial of psychic and actual reality, e.g., despair and bleakness too painful to experience directly, and not consciously mendacious at all. When deceit and lying do occur they need understanding and interpreting and should *not*—at least until a fair trial has been made—be assumed to be a contraindication to further therapy.

By contrast, one may be impressed by a naive honesty in some ASPD patients—itself possibly indicative of raw unsublimated id, as well as superego function—in which one may even feel, in the countertransference, they need protection from for themselves, particularly if they are in positions of potentially implicating themselves in further crime. Such patients may often be especially motivated to engage in treatment, offering the possibility of escaping from their cycle of offending. The human tendency towards repetition, in all its aspects, is however, an ever-present hazard.

The question of the psychotherapists' attitude in these matters is all important. The stereotype of the universality of deceitfulness and 'conning' in ASPD patients can lead to an attitude of nihilism, both within therapeutic services and for the individual clinician. For example, a prison medical officer said—without a hint of apparent shame and with self-satisfied confidence; 'personally I don't believe a word of any of them (*i.e., of the prisoners in his care*) say'. A more sophisticated and necessary therapeutic position is to offer a trusting and listening ear, for both conscious and subtextual (less conscious and unconscious) communications, giving the benefit of the doubt, but with part of one's mind nevertheless prepared for not always being told the entire truth. It may even be helpful to tell the patient that this is one's position. Often such an intervention is met by considerable relief and greater use of the therapeutic relationship.

In arguing for emotional openness of the therapist to the person with ASPD we are not, of course, advocating collusion with severely psychopathic manipulative patients; but the experienced (and well supervised) therapist will (ideally) be able to keep these extreme possibilities in mind without polarizing the issues. It has been commented often that meeting the personality disordered individual in a withdrawn and emotionally defensive manner is antitherapeutic and, indeed, most likely mirrors the experience that engendered his problems, and with which he is only too familiar within his day to day life.

Gabbard (1994) offered six recommendations for the therapist who wishes to work with ASPD:

1. 'He (or she) must be incorruptible, stable and persistent'—and we would add always honest dealing and speaking. Many personality disordered patients, especially those with psychotic or prepsychotic

structures, are highly attuned to factual and emotional truths or untruths by others.

2. 'He should be "willing to confront" the patients' denial or minimization'— we would use the word 'interpret'. Confrontation, while sometimes necessary, is more likely to mobilize defenses further and therefore prove counterproductive.

3. 'He should help the patient link his or her actions with his internal (emotional/attitudinal) states'.

4. He should 'confront the here and now behaviors'.

5. 'He should monitor countertransference so as to avoid "inappropriate" responses'.

6. He should 'avoid excessive expectations of improvement.'

While these recommendations are helpful, the reader will judge for him/herself whether they betray an excessive circumspection or a realistic one. The fine line between the psychotherapists' judicious caution on the one hand, and excessive suspicion and emotional withdrawal on the other is a difficult one, but is crucial.

That said, there is no place for the inexperienced, untrained, or unsupervised to take on ASPD clients in psychotherapy. Fatalities have occurred (see, for example, Travers, 1994); the emotional and psychological toll is to an extent universal.

Hypersensitivity of the ASPD personality

The sensitivity of the ASPD personality to perceived rejection or criticism cannot be overestimated. Thus, even more than usual, the therapist must work to engage the patient by his reliability, and by his sensitivity to potential causes of the patients' 'acting out', e.g., by an excessive number of missed appointments. Holidays should be flagged up well in advance; in the early stages of engagement it is best to avoid any break or interruption of sessions altogether.

For example, a man who had been in prison for 25 years (since his teens) was referred to a therapist who agreed to see him once weekly. The patient felt disappointed, wanting more frequent sessions. These were offered then—twice weekly. For the next 3 weeks the patient did not attend, but attended on the fourth. The therapist felt that he had been 'manipulated' and then rejected. He had fortunately kept the treatment sessions open, and was able to engage the patient, despite continuing 'shows' of apparent 'rejection' of treatment by the patient. In this patient was attempting to display a lack of need for a therapist and his independence, by using a 'macho' culture of self-presentation. In fact the obverse was the case; he felt particularly alone, unsupported, and generally rejected, and had communicated that by making the therapist feel these feelings of uselessness and unwantedness on his behalf. The danger is that in this situation, the therapist will 'act out' in revenge in a similar mode as the patient.

Shame and low self-esteem

Many patients with ASPD have very low self-esteem or sense of self-worth. This may be related to a highly critical attitude to self, as in the harsh and cruel super-ego of the majority of offenders. Just as Riviere (1936) pointed out the need to balance interpretations of the bad (guilty) parts of the self with interpretations of good parts and capacities, so, too, there needs to be great sensitivity accorded in addressing the patients' poor self-image. This raises the question of shame, which Gilligan (2000) considers *the* critical personality characteristic in violent offenders.

Shame is related to consequential feelings of grievance, grudge, and desire for revenge. A sense of shame and poor self-esteem makes the sufferer hypersensitive to humiliation—upon which, of course, criminal justice systems thrive. That the ASPD person is so vulnerable to humiliation reveals to us how fragile is his sense of self-worth. Whereas feelings of guilt will frequently be relieved by the opportunity for their expression, shame and the related sense of poor self-esteem seeks to hide itself and remain silent. Frequently a defensive bravura is the 'face' shown in everyday life,

and especially, for example, among prisoners. The deep sense of shame and of failure of the ASPD patient, is one of the central technical problems for the psychotherapist in the treatment of many patients suffering ASPD. The aim of treatment is partly to evoke a concept of, and a hope for, the future, which process is itself gratifying and felt to be worthwhile.

Working with shame and humiliation is a central technical problem in psychotherapy with ASPD sufferers. The very act of self-revelation implicit in psychotherapy feels shameful, and makes the sufferer feel that he will be at the mercy of a therapist, who, armed with knowledge of his innermost feelings, will then use it to exact further humiliation. Tact and timing are crucial—knowing how much the patient can 'take' at any moment, when gently to probe, when to respect necessary defensive boundaries.

Other activities, too, including the arts therapies, and artistic and occupational involvement, as part of a multidisciplinary program—usually in an inpatient or residential setting—may be helpful in boosting the patient's sense of self-worth.

Negative therapeutic reaction

Central to the psychotherapy of ASPD is an awareness of the 'negative therapeutic reaction' ('NTR'). This refers to the patients' need, unconsciously, as well sometimes as consciously, to sabotage the psychotherapy especially when he feels it is most helpful or likely to bring about desired, positive change. Such sabotage may be the consequence of a fear of change *per se*, following, as it were, a basic conservatism—which, despite appearances to the contrary, is invariably at the psychological core of such personalities. Specifically, NTR may be traced to *envy* of those (including the therapist) who have the qualities that the patient wants for himself, or *guilt* that he (of all people) does not deserve to have a different and better life. Shame, too, as described under the previous subheading, may be a factor. The 'NTR' may be mitigated, if not completely avoided, by early interpretation encompassing such thoughts as; 'it sounds as though you feel that everything is going wonderfully well at present, and all your goals are achievable, but there may come a time, quite soon, when you think that its all pointless, that I am useless and unable to help you, and you don't want to carry on'. Later, guilt or envy can be interpreted (if thought to be the active elements in a particular case). Such an interpretation would be best expressed (and repeated) in brief sentences communicating one idea at a time.

Role of the therapist

The psychological toll on the therapist is great and any therapist can only take on so many, or few, of such patients if proper intensive, transferential work is to be undertaken. There is no room for the 'tyro' who overextends himself, through some misplaced sense of omnipotence. Good and regular supervision is an absolute necessity. Many authors, e.g., Glover (1964), have recommended 'teamwork' in the treatment of ASPD, in order to dilute transferential issues, in a 'distributive transference', as Glover described. This is certainly necessary in the more extreme cases, but many psychotherapists will find themselves struggling alone with more mild cases. Generally one would advise working psychotherapeutically—whether individual or group—within a *supportive setting*, i.e., and outpatient psychotherapy building, and not in a consulting room at home. One danger that may render the psychotherapeutic experience not only useless, but actually a negative, damaging experience, is the case of therapists (who in public services may be inexperienced and out of their depth, or experienced and burnt out) who 'shut off' and disengage from the patients' often urgent emotional communications. Such an experience is likely to be a repeat of previous negative, unrewarding, and traumatic emotional encounters of the patient's past, and as such merely reinforce expectations and psychopathology.

Length of treatment

Treatment must ideally be long term: It is generally not possible to produce personality change by short-term treatments. Equally, if 'supportive' therapy only is being offered that is likely to be a long-term need. As *trust* is lacking in many of those manifesting ASPD, the longer the therapeutic relationship (in general terms) the better.

This runs counter to current fashions where short packages of just a few weeks or months are characteristically offered. Short 'treatments' may even be worse than useless, i.e., counterproductive. These patients' lives are invariably characterized by repeated rejections and loss. Too often psychological treatments are perceived by patients as repeating these experiences. Equally, as previously emphasized, endings of therapy should be prepared for (as should all breaks) and as a rule the opportunity of working through the ending over a period of at least 6 months should be offered.

Conclusions

All these considerations apply to individual and group psychotherapy, and indeed to the institutional, social, and TC settings that are described later in this chapter. It is often felt that group psychotherapy provides a matrix of social and psychological interaction that is of greater benefit for the ASPD patient than the dynamic relationship of individual psychotherapy. This is especially the case for patients with sexual offending as their most prominent characteristic. On the other hand, group psychotherapy may be too intimidating for ASPD patients with poor self-esteem, paranoid functioning, and those for whom 'sharing' is hardly possible without overwhelming feelings of rivalry, jealousy, and rage. Individual judgments have to be made, case by case.

Therapeutic community treatment for antisocial personality disorder

Introduction

The first democratic TCs in the UK were developed in the World War II from the application of psychodynamic ideas in residential settings in the treatment of shellshock victims. In these experimental settings (e.g., Bion, 1961) it was noted that the facilitation of an exploratory psychodynamic process in a group and community living structure enabled interpatient learning therapeutic intervention as well as adding a social dimension to the treatment.

TC as with ASPD is a term that does not enjoy unequivocal definition. The term TC, first coined by Tom Main in 1946, is imprecise. Experts do not agree that certain treatment settings are 'therapeutic communities proper' as opposed to 'therapeutic approaches' (Clarke, 1965). Both 'democratic' and 'hierarchical' forms exist, see below (Kennard, 2000). The democratic variety has been construed as more 'modality' than 'method' (Kennard, 1998), meaning that it is primarily a general vehicle for other more specific approaches. The opposite view has been advanced, namely, that a TC refers to an institution in which is ascribed a deliberate, therapeutic, i.e., primary, role for its own social environment (Hunt, 1983).

It should not be forgotten that other cluster B subcategories of personality disorder, i.e., borderline personality disorder, histrionic personality disorder, and narcissistic personality disorder typically exist comorbidly with ASPD especially in cases that warrant a specialist intervention such as the residential democratic TC approach. Comorbidity is the rule for those diagnosed as 'psychopathic' on the Hare PCL-R scale.

The democratic therapeutic community

For Maxwell Jones, the TC represented a potential for the pooling of *all* the human resources contained within an institution. Importantly this included both professional members and their clients (Jones, 1952). Crucial to his pioneering method was a lessening or 'flattening' of the traditional hierarchies, between staff and between staff and clients, and a redistribution of staff power via its partial delegation to clients. To achieve this, conventional staff roles were 'blurred' in the service of a more egalitarian multidisciplinary team functioning than previously. It required a restructuring of the traditional hospital or prison, with management systems needing to be sympathetic to the therapeutic model and understanding of its greater democracy and power-sharing with service users.

For Main (1946) 'treatment of the patient who suffers from a disturbance of social relationships cannot be . . . regarded as satisfactory unless it is undertaken within a framework of *social reality* which can provide him with opportunities for attaining fuller insight and for expressing and modifying his emotional drives according to the demands of *real life*.' He saw the TC as providing such a 'satisfactory' environment, through facilitating the identification and analysis of 'interpersonal barriers' that stood in the way of the individual's full participation in community life. The TC environment thus provided, for the ASPD individual, opportunities for 'interaction', 'exploration', and 'experimentation' with others, both staff and fellow patients (Whiteley, 1986). For the therapeutic potential to be realized, this work needs to be carried out within a safe environment.

Safety within the democratic TC is maintained by a number of factors, including: the selection of those most likely to benefit (i.e., rejection of poor prognosis cases, often too violent or dangerous); an informal contract to take part actively in a range of group and communal activities; an agreement to abide by the rules of the TC, in particular, those proscribing damage to persons (including the self) and property; the provision of a predictably structured program of activities, involving both verbal and nonverbal modalities; the provision of support from the peer group; preparation for joining and leaving; and adequate support, training and supervision of staff (Norton, 2002). In this way, risk assessment and risk management depend not only on the identification of relevant factors relating to 'pathology' but also to 'health' (i.e., appropriate participation in the formal therapeutic program and also in the social life of the TC), and taking into account the containing capacity of the unit at a particular time.

Delegating to clients aspects usually considered to be the exclusive preserve of staff may be central to the success of the model. Such empowerment extends to the identification of signs of distress or disturbance through rule breaking or through over- or underparticipation in the program. The daily community meeting is the regular forum for confronting of such issues, as well as for the providing of relevant human, rather than pharmacological, support. However, there are emergency meetings of the whole community that can be convened at any time of day or night so that, in certain respects, the 'therapy' is potentially 24 hours per day. The model has been adopted in many countries and in secure, as well as open, settings.

Research evidence

In the UK the democratic TC approach has been most extensively described (Norton, 1992) and intensively evaluated at Henderson Hospital (Norton and Warren, 2001). A series of outcome studies have been undertaken, though falling short of the 'gold standard' of a randomized controlled trial. The patients, referred to as 'residents', are all diagnosed as suffering from a personality disorder by the referring practitioner, usually a consultant psychiatrist. The level of personality disorder comorbidity is high with patients each qualifying for an average of six subcategory diagnoses, according to the Personality Disorder Questionnaire (PDQ; Hyler *et al.*, 1987). This instrument may be oversensitive, producing false positives, but its total score can be seen as a guide to overall severity of personality disorder and its subcategory profile as indicative of the distribution of subcategories and their morbidity (Dolan *et al.*, 1995).

In the absence of randomization to a control population, hard to achieve both practically and ethically, a rigorous statistical method has been applied to the assessment of outcome. This data analytic method identifies reliable (i.e., unlikely to have been found by chance) and clinically significant improvement through measuring the size of change pre- and posttreatment and whether the posttreatment scoring is in the normal range for the instrument used (Jacobson and Traux, 1991). Accordingly, using the SCL-90, in an uncontrolled designed of 62 treated patients, 55% at follow-up (average 8 months posttreatment) showed reliable and 32% clinically significant improvement (Dolan *et al.*, 1992). Using the Borderline Syndrome Index-BSI, 61% of admitted compared with 37% of those not admitted had improved reliably and 43% versus 18% both reliably and clinically significantly (Dolan *et al.*, 1996). (NB All subjects admitted, regardless of their actual length of stay, were included in the treated sample.) In a cost–offset study of a cohort of 29 (Dolan *et al.*, 1996), 24 of whom were traceable 1 year after discharge, a 90% reduction in the costs of service usage posttreatment were found in comparison with the 1 year before treatment (average length of stay 7 months—again including those who left or were discharged prematurely).

In a comparable study of convicted offenders, a 7-year follow-up of 700 male inmates admitted to a UK prison run along TC lines (Grendon Underwood, see below) between 1984 and 1989, found that the admitted group were less likely to reoffend than a waiting-list comparison group (Marshall *et al.*, 1997; Taylor, 2000). These authors suggest the presence of a treatment effect for those staying more than 18 months in the program.

Key practice points

♦ Management structures need to be clear, and attitudes informed and supportive, for best results to be achieved. This is important as it is easy for managers to assume that risk can be unrealistically reduced or avoided. The latter is not possible, especially with an ASPD client group. However, to maintain harmonious relationships requires the TC to demonstrate to management the robustness of its own risk assessment and management processes.

♦ Also in the interest of safety, it is desirable that the referring agency remains in contact with the TC so that in the eventuality of premature discharge, not a rare event, this can be to a sufficiently safe destination.

♦ There is a place for clear leadership within the TC. With the latter this is to maintain clarity of task in the light of blurring of traditional staff roles (for example, the therapeutic role taken on by nursing staff, usually the preserve of other professions such as medical or clinical psychology) and flattening of the hierarchy—never entirely flat.

♦ It is part of the leader's role to ensure that there is adequate support for and supervision of staff.

♦ This is needed to avoid the destructive acting out of transference–countertransference relationships and to minimize the destructive, but inevitable, effects of splitting (Gabbard, 1988). 'Victim–perpetrator' dynamics are prominent, being played out in a variety of guises: staff as victims of residents; staff as perpetrators in relation to residents; a subgroup of staff as victim of another subgroup, such as managers within the TC; whole TC as victim of hostile outside world, etc. Ideally, the situation can yield advantages from the sustaining of, rather than suppression of, such countertransference 'information' in terms of an enhanced understanding of the internal worlds of the ASPD clients.

Difficult situations and their solution

One of the main difficulties relate to problems with establishing an authentic treatment alliance or dealing with the emergence of an 'illusory alliance'. The democratic TC has inbuilt ways of dealing with these, which have been implicit in the above description of its methods. First, there is an expectation that the individual will actively participate in the formal and informal life of the TC. Second, they should refrain from violent or other destructive behavior. Paradoxically, the latter is easier than the former for those ASPD residents who are well-used to 'doing time' in prison and 'keeping their noses clean'. However, they may 'fake good', meaning that they may pretend to fit in to what they perceive expectations to be. In this case the issue is to make explicit what it is they 'fake' and why. However, this usually is associated with other 'sins of omission'. There are mechanisms for detecting not only the rule-breaking but also a lack of participation—whether it applies to the formal or the informal aspects of the program. These latter aspects are monitored closely and fed back to the whole community on a daily basis by designated residents (monthly elected to such positions of power). This can lead to the peer group challenging inauthentic engagement as well as providing support to the negotiation of a genuine therapeutic alliance. Healthy peer

group influences are optimized especially through the delegation of power to the residents to include the major say on issues of admission and discharge, usually the preserve of senior medical staff, as well as to more mundane matters. Ideally, over time, a basic trust replaces a basic mistrust in others and a sense of belonging to a more socialized group develops (Erikson, 1959).

The treatment of antisocial personality disorder in prison therapeutic communities

Introduction

In various jurisdictions, therapeutic work is carried out with ASPD clients in prisons. The advantages to the provision of such treatment in a prison setting include the presence of a captive audience—ASPD patients during prison sojourns are predictable in their location, unlike much of the rest of their lifestyle; the 'hotel' residential costs of the program (often the most expensive aspect of residential ASPD treatments) are assumed as the clients are incarcerated anyway, and because the outcome of the treatment process (greater insight and understanding of the context of the offending cycle) can be fed into the parole and pre-release risk assessment process.

Broadly there are two TC cultures in prisons. On the one hand, there are 'concept' or 'hierarchical' communities, based on a charted progression in treatment, for example away from drug use. Many prison drug TCs have this culture, with which parallels can be drawn with the self-help and 12-step movements originally pioneered for alcoholism. Patuxent Prison in Maryland and Herdstevester Prison in Denmark were among the pioneers in this type of treatment for ASPD in prisons (see De Leon, 1994). The 'Stay n' out' program was the first to run prison TCs in New York in 1977. The 'Anti-Drug Abuse Act of 1986' earmarked funding for such projects, and they were coordinated federally, frequently with built in evaluation. An evaluation of the 'Stay 'n out' program suggested a 32.4% reduction in rearrest at 3-year follow-up (Wexler *et al.*, 1990).

In the UK and Europe, a version of TCs evolved based on a more egalitarian and democratic culture, influenced in particular by the development of group psychoanalytic psychotherapy. In these 'democratic' TCs, the notion of a treatment goal was eschewed in favor of an emphasis on exploration, understanding, and insight.

Grendon Prison in the UK is an example of such treatment facility. Opened in 1962, and with 230 beds divided up into five TCs, half the men are serving a life sentence, and a similar number score above 25 on the PCL-R (Hare, 1991). The small groups meet three times per week, resulting in a psychoanalytic-like process, and 2 days per week there is a longer community meeting, which is chaired by the resident chairman that acts as the democratic and social core of the treatment. There is an expectation that people will stay in treatment for about 2 years.

Conceptualization

In the treatment of the more severe character disorders, such as ASPD, pathology is often impervious to the well-intentioned interpretative interventions of comfortably situated therapists. Effective challenge of the very entrenched and ingrained antisocial attitudes and values of the ASPD patient may often only be achieved by the verbal battery of an equally violent but slightly more insightful peer. For example, a bank robber crowing about having made 10 000 pounds 'for an afternoon's work' being aggressively challenged by a fellow bank robber pointing out that with a 10-year sentence he'd made about a thousand pounds per year; so was it worth it?

The TC and group psychotherapeutic technique enables the power, authority, and developing (hard won) insight of peers to be utilized in the treatment of newer patients, and in the formulation and delivery of insights that would be unheard if formulated by staff. The maintenance of a culture of enquiry about all aspects of living together promotes deep exploration of current behaviors as they reenact the index offending pattern and often aspects of developmental experience. Gradually, the ASPD patient can begin to integrate aspects of their personality, the often extreme levels of rage and destructiveness sparked or potentiated by developmental traumas, and the shame and loathing that can be both the precipitant and the result of the offending.

Research evidence

Methodological obstacles to the evaluation of psychotherapy for ASPD are formidable. Again, taking research on Grendon as an example, Gunn's work (1976) identified significant improvements in psychiatric status of those treated, and interesting positive changes of levels of respect for authority figures such as police and prison officers. Following this a series of papers suggested a change in reconviction rates following treatment in Grendon lasting more than 18 months (Cullen, 1994). This work was replicated by Marshall *et al.* (1997) using a cohort of 700 in a treatment group, with a combined waiting-list and risk-matched control group. A reduction in reconviction rates of 20–25% in the treated group at 4-year follow-up was found. This same group and control were reexamined at 7 years suggesting some treatment effect was sustained, and that there was a 60% reduction in recall rates for treated lifers (Taylor, 2000).

In interpreting these data it must be borne in mind that there are considerable technical difficulties in establishing meaningful control groups for these studies. Similarly, some follow-up evidence from a Canadian facility suggested that while in lower PCL-R scorers recidivism rate was reduced, higher scorers actually increased following treatment (Rice *et al.*, 1992). This study has been influential but suffered major methodological difficulties; most significantly, those subjects who wished to leave the treatment group were forced to stay in 'treatment' and in the study. Much more research is required before any general 'truths' are further promoted. The most authoritative qualitative research of such a facility was by Genders and Player (1995) who described in Grendon the evolutionary process of dismantling antisocial defensive structures and discovering, then testing out and practicing, new ways of being and behaving.

Key practice points

Psychodynamic work with this client group can be very traumatizing for staff. From a psychodynamic perspective it is held that mutative work takes place when the therapist engages in a core relational aspect of the transference. It is thus a sobering thought that for half of Grendon's client group, this core relation has previously been the lethal prelude to their action against their victim(s). In the structure of the program, large amounts of time are given over to staff supervision and time to process the clinical material that they are dealing with.

A principal element of psychology for the ASPD patient is deception and manipulation (see Introduction). An occupational hazard for staff working with these clients is that they will be deceived or duped into supporting a particular clinical decision. The best safeguard against this is a well functioning multidisciplinary team, where staff can debate and challenge such deceptions, making decisions by majority vote if necessary. The clinical pluralistic approach to decision-making enables the multiple fragments of the patient to each find a voice in the form of different staff members or disciplines, who in the staff team matrix can balance the probabilities and agree on a compromise plan that will be the least worst option.

ASPD patients found in treatment facilities such as Grendon are high-risk offenders, and a crucial and potent disciplinary contribution is made by the custodial staff. In health settings, the skills of a prison officer or warder are seldom identified, but they possess a rich skill resource in the day to day management and maintenance of ASPD patients, as well as being custodial managers having the skills to manage organizations whose function is to contain ASPD clients.

Difficult situations and their solutions summary

There is a technique adopted by ASPD clients in prisons known as 'collaring' a staff member. A large intimidatory prisoner with a history of extreme violence will 'collar' a staff member demanding some form of concession, or that they investigate something, or to complain about some aspect of their experience. The experience is similar to being mugged—the staff member often ends up agreeing to the request, not because it is necessarily reasonable, but because agreement has effectively been extorted from (him).

The solution to this problem is the mantra 'take it to your group'. All such requests are required to be discussed in the first instance in small therapy group setting, where it can be explored in terms of its reasonableness and in terms of its psychic significance. Often the intimidatory attitude with which the request is made to the individual staff member has some resentful origin that can be explored, and will diminish as a result.

In a similar vein, concern could be expressed about the risk involved in, for example, having a single female staff member in a small group of eight dangerous men, or of having a small staff complement of three of four in a large community meeting of 40 residents. In fact, the group settings are rather safe places; anecdotally, when being controlled by other residents, the order and control in the meeting has been maintained by client members of the group or the community.

The theoretical explanation of this is to be found in Foulkes' assertion that as a collective, a group will contain the norm from which the individual members deviate. So while as individuals, each member of the groups will have made unreasonable demands, 'collaring' staff; as a collective, the aggressive and unreasonable nature of this can be recognized and challenged. Likewise, while all may be capable of violence individually, the group as a collective will have a more normal aversion to violence, leading to its suppression by the majority should it emerge.

A second difficult situation is where an ASPD patient manages to split a staff group, showing to one staff subgroup a reasonable and hardworking aspect of their personality, and showing to the other a more sadistic and vicious side, such that one subgroup wish to discharge the individual, and the other subgroup argue that this attitude is perverse.

The structuring into the program of multiple opportunities for staff to discuss and review their clinical work provides opportunities to reconcile these splits and to understand the origin. Following Main (1989) the understanding is that character pathology being exhibited by the client group will become located in the staff group, following this sort of mechanism. The task for the staff group is to recognize the splits and schisms that emerge between them, and to recast these observations of their own dynamics as information about the dynamics of the client group, and the individuals comprising them, that they are holding.

Cognitive therapy for antisocial personality disorder

Introduction

The cognitive therapy model is based on the notion that attributional bias is the main problem accounting for behavioral and affective dysfunction. The way in which information is perceived, interpreted and acted upon is problematic. Schemas are a central concept in the model and can be conceptualized as cognitive structures that organize experience and behavior. Schemas are thought of as a guiding behavior in a consistent rule bound manner. Cognitive therapy focuses on the product of schemas, the patient's behavioral and interpersonal problems, and the core beliefs that underlie them.

Cognitive theory of personality disorder

There is considerable evidence that personality is at least, in part, determined by genetic mechanisms and the cognitive model of personality disorder encompasses both a genetic and evolutionary perspective (Beck and Freeman, 1990). The possession of personality traits that are useful for procreation and obtaining resources are likely to have high survival value and are therefore likely to be passed on through genes. Take the trait of aggression as an example. In a situation where resources are scarce and there is not enough food and potential mates to allow a sufficient supply for all, an aggressive male may present as a threat to his competitors and drive them off. By doing so, the male may increase his social status and he may therefore be more likely to attract the available females. The aggressive trait has therefore been adaptive in scaring off competitors and in obtaining a sexual partner and through procreation, in passing on genes to future generations. In this way, aggressive traits may be selected for their survival value.

In Beck and Freeman's (1990) cognitive model of personality disorder, some individuals may show more extreme forms of the personality types or patterns that were once adaptive but are now maladaptive in the contemporary world. For example, in ASPD, combative and explorative behavioral patterns are overdeveloped and other behavioral patterns, such as sharing, group identification, and intimacy are underdeveloped. These latter patterns also have evolutionary survival value, particularly in maintaining relationships where consideration for others, kindness, and intimacy are valued, but in ASPD these patterns are underrepresented.

Schemas in personality disorder

The concept of schema lies at the core of cognitive therapy and is of relevance to personality disorder. Schemas are unconscious stable cognitive structures through which knowledge about the world is gathered, processed, and stored. The meaning we attach to events is the result of information being processed through schemas. Schemas are stored in long-term memory and can be active or latent. They are thought of as being triggered by events that are similar to those that originally molded them. Schemas that are concerned with information processing are grouped together into constellations that are, in turn, grouped into modes of subsystems of the cognitive organization. It is these latter groupings that are considered of evolutionary survival value. They are concerned with the degree of adaptation of the organism to its environment and represent the basic underpinning of personality.

In personality disorder, several interlocking schematic subsystems will be involved in an ongoing process whereby information is perceived, interpreted, and ultimately acted upon. The schematic subsystems involved in this process are concerned with affect, cognition, motivation, action, and self-regulation. Different subschemas will have different functions. For example, the cognitive schema will be involved in the organization, interpretation, and recall of information received by an individual. In personality disorder, evaluation of self and others are dominant cognitive schemas. These schemas are hypervalent and are activated in a wide variety of situations, which results in overgeneralized of dysfunctional responses. It is the way in which these schemas are integrated and linked together with information from the environment that determines the degree of adaptation in response. Table 22.1 provides an example of a functional analysis of schemas in ASPD.

Overdeveloped and underdeveloped behavioral strategies

In personality disorder, certain types of behavioral patterns are overdeveloped and others are underdeveloped. These patterns are related to each other in that the behavioral patterns that are overdeveloped appear to be the reciprocal of the underdeveloped behavioral patterns. It is not that the various overdeveloped behavioral strategies seen in personality disorder are, in themselves, without their usefulness. The problem arises when they are applied in a pervasive, inflexible, and exaggerated manner that is inappropriate to the situation.

Application of the cognitive model to personality disorder in general

In the cognitive model, each personality disorder demonstrates prototypical overdeveloped and underdeveloped strategies. For example, in avoidant personality disorder, social ineptness will be overly developed and social competence and gregariousness will be underdeveloped strategies. These over- and underdeveloped strategies are associated with specific views of self and others. So, taking the example noted above, individuals with

Table 22.1 Functional analysis of schemas in example of ASPD

Schemas	Content
Affect	Irritable, angry
Cognition	
View of self	I should get my own way
View of others	People should do what I want
Motivation	Wants immediate gratification
Self-regulation	Impulsive, difficulty inhibiting response to stimuli
Action	Act now, consider consequences later

Table 22.2 Typical core beliefs and overdeveloped and underdeveloped strategies

Personality disorder	Typical core belief about self	Overdeveloped strategy	Underdeveloped strategy
Antisocial	I am entitled to break the rules	Exploitation	Reciprocity
Borderline	I am bad	Self-punishment	Self-nurturance
Avoidant	I am inept and incompetent	Avoidance of situations where others may observe or judge	Self-assertion
Dependent	I am helpless	Dependence on others	Autonomy

avoidant personality disorder may hold a view of self typified by the belief 'I am incompetent' or 'I will be rejected' and those who hold such beliefs will regard others as being 'critical' or 'likely to humiliate' them. Table 22.2 illustrates the relationship between typical core beliefs about self and overdeveloped and underdeveloped behavioral strategies for a number of personality disorders.

Aim of cognitive-behavior therapy

The aim of CBT for personality disorder is to identify and modify core beliefs and associated overdeveloped behavioral patterns, which are maladaptive and prevent the individual from functioning in an adaptive manner (Davidson, 2000). There are several differences between CBT for personality disorders and CBT for Axis I disorders. The length of treatment in personality disorder is one of the main differences when compared with the relatively brisk and short length of treatment for Axis I disorder. Owing to the long-standing ingrained nature of difficulties in personality disorder, an average course of therapy will require at least 30 sessions over a time period of at least a year.

Those with ASPD are often referred for treatment because other people regard them as having a problem. They seldom initiate treatment. As a result those with ASPD often require a thorough exploration of their problems, the consequences of these for them and others, how the problems arose and became ingrained before any agreement can be reached about embarking on change. This is in contrast to patients with Axis I disorders, where patients wish to get back to the state of well-being they experienced before and recognize that their current state of mind is different from how they are usually. With personality disorder, patients have usually no experience of what it could be like to behave, feel, and act differently. Patients need to recognize that they would be helped by developing new ways of thinking about themselves and other people and that changing behavioral patterns could lead to improvements in relationships and the overall quality of life.

Developing a coherent cognitive formulation of an individual's problems is therefore central to progress in therapy. As the patient's past history plays a role in the development of problems, there is a greater degree of historical information sought in cognitive therapy for personality disorder and in arriving at the formulation compared with therapy of an Axis I disorder. In an Axis I disorder, the patient's past history is usually helpful in highlighting potential vulnerability factors rather than being central to pathology.

The function of the formulation is to engage the patient in therapy by making explicit the relationship between beliefs about self and others and long-standing behavioral patterns, which in the case of those with ASPD, particularly those that are self-destructive or have a destructive effect on others. The cognitive formulation takes into account that patient's early as well as recent experience. Reaching a *formulation* is a time consuming process for the therapist but one that is essential if therapy is to remain structured and focused. It will point to the underdeveloped behavioral patterns that require to be strengthened and uncover the content of core beliefs about self and others that need to be replaced by more adaptive beliefs. Arriving at a formulation is not an intellectual exercise for the therapist as it must make sense to the patient and be readily understood in terms of his past experience. It is also the process through which the patient engages with therapy and through which the therapist demonstrates that he has been understood. A written formulation, either in narrative or diagrammatic form, is given to the patient and this becomes the springboard for discussing and agreeing the cognitive and behavioral changes that the remainder of therapy will focus on and which will help improve the patient's quality of life. Once the formulation has been agreed—at least as a working hypothesis—behavioral and cognitive change strategies are used to assist the patient in attaining his goals. Agreed goals have to be modest and achievable within the time frame of therapy. If a patient has unrealistic goals about what can be achieved in therapy, then the therapist has to be open and honest about what is likely to be possible. For example, for a homeless 50-year-old prison recidivist, with a history of alcoholism and drug addiction, getting married in the near future might be an unrealistic goal but forming a better relationship with specific individuals might be achievable.

As with all therapies with individuals with ASPD, there should be a transparent overall structure to therapy. Generally, ASPD patients are offered up to 10 sessions at the beginning of therapy to assess problems and agree a formulation. If it has been possible to agree the formulation and identify underdeveloped behavioral strategies and beliefs that are unhelpful and counterproductive to change, then the therapist negotiates the next stage of therapy focusing on change.

Cognitive therapy for those with ASPD will usually focus on developing and strengthening more adaptive behavioral strategies aimed at improving interpersonal relationships and managing conflict by learning to see the perspective of the other. Low self-esteem, a frequent problem, is often associated with negative thoughts towards others. Beliefs such as 'I must not show that I am weak' and 'I have to get the better of everyone or they will get me' need to be loosened or weakened by strengthening new more adaptive beliefs such as 'it is okay to have both strengths and weaknesses' and 'if I behave in a reasonable way with others, they may treat me better'.

ASPD patients tend to interpret interpersonal situations as being more threatening than they are in actuality. They have poor ability to interpret ambiguity and tend to rapidly jump to negative conclusions about other people's intentions leading to actions that are often impulsive and aggressive toward others. Learning to 'stop and think' before acting helps build tolerance of uncertainty, providing that skills in the interpretation of events can be acquired. Learning that there may be more than one interpretation of an interpersonal situation is often, at first, a real revelation to individuals with ASPD.

The middle phase of therapy may take place over at least 20 sessions but regular reviews are scheduled at the beginning of this phase to assess progress. If there is a lack of progress, the therapist has to review possible reasons for this with the patient and some resolution has to be agreed before therapy proceeds. The end of therapy is flagged up long before it takes place. The final phase of therapy is also structured and the aim here is to review progress, identify what has been learnt, and to develop a behavioral and

cognitive maintenance plan with the patient to increase the likelihood that change will be maintained.

Problems in engaging individuals with personality disorder in therapy are thought to be common. Those with ASPD have a tendency to view difficulties as being the responsibility and fault of others, not themselves. Most studies have treated antisocial patients with problems such as drug dependence and the focus has not been on antisocial characteristics or traits *per se*. It is, however, possible to engage ASPD patients in therapy (Davidson and Tyrer, 1996), with clear patient-oriented goals, especially if they are no longer youthful but in their thirties or older, when their dominance and prowess may be beginning to diminish and they recognize the need to develop more effective strategies to maintain their self-esteem.

Empirical validation

Single studies and case studies

Early case studies suggested a careful formulation of patient's problems in behavioral terms could be effective in some, but not all, individuals with personality disorder (Turkat and Maisto, 1985; Beck and Freeman et al., 1990). Davidson and Tyrer (1996) evaluated a cognitive therapy treatment manual for borderline personality disorder and ASPD in a pilot study of 12 patients, five of whom had a diagnosis of ASPD. Single case methodology was used to examine the impact of cognitive therapy on specific targets chosen by individual patients as being most problematic. The three ASPD patients who adhered to the treatment protocol had forensic histories, including problems with aggressiveness and histories of assault. The time series analyses designed to control type 1 errors, indicated that only one of the overall nine nominated targets had changed significantly. Clinically, however, the patients in the study appeared to benefit from therapy and their partners corroborated that there had been improvements in relationships. Having the capacity to work collaboratively with the therapist was essential in producing change. Only one patient appeared to derive no benefit from treatment, despite attending regularly. He appeared to believe he had the right to control his children and wife using punitive and bullying methods and that he did not have to comply with the law. It was not possible to reach an agreed understanding of his problems and therefore no treatment plan could be established.

Cognitive therapy for substance abuse and antisocial personality disorder

Although some studies suggest that coexisting ASPD reduces successful outcome for substance abuse treatment programs (Alterman et al., 1998; Goldstein et al., 1999; Reid and Gacono, 2000) there is some contradictory evidence from randomized controlled trials to suggest that individuals with ASPD do respond well to CBT approaches aimed at reducing substance abuse. Woody et al., (1985) suggested that it was those patients with the combination of both ASPD and depression that responded better to cognitive therapy or psychodynamic therapy than those without depression. A later controlled trial of cognitive therapy that compared CBT with a psychotherapy control condition, either alone or in combination with desipramine or placebo treatments, supported the efficacy of CBT relapse prevention treatment for cocaine abusers (Carroll et al., 1994a). The superior effect of CBT on relapse prevention only emerged at 1-year follow-up (Carroll et al., 1994b). Over 49% of patients had a diagnosis of ASPD and 65% had another personality disorder diagnosis. It would seem that those who received CBT learnt coping skills that could be generalized and implemented long after treatment had finished. Longabaugh et al. (1995) examined drinking outcome between 13 and 28 months after treatment had been initiated in 31 antisocial personality and 188 nonantisocial alcohol abusers. Patients had been given either extended CBT or relationship enhancement therapy. In general, those with ASPD who received CBT had better drinking outcomes than those in the relationship enhancement therapy. Less promising results have been found for interpersonal and psychodynamic therapy (Rounsavile et al., 1983; Kang et al., 1991).

The National Institute on Drug Abuse (NIDA) Collaborative Cocaine Treatment Study specifically tested the hypothesis that drug-dependent patients with more antisocial personality characteristics would have a better response to cognitive therapy compared with other treatment. The results were, from the perspective of psychotherapeutic approaches to ASPD, disappointing. All patients in this study received group drug counseling, and one of three additional possibilities, cognitive therapy, individual drug counseling, or supportive-expressive psychodynamic counseling. The results of the study indicated that those in the psychotherapy conditions (cognitive therapy and supportive-expressive psychodynamic counseling) did less well on most outcome measures than those who received general or individual drug counseling. Those cocaine-dependent patients with a diagnosis of ASPD did not have a better outcome with cognitive therapy, thereby challenging the notion that CBT approaches are particularly beneficial for those with ASPD.

The match between the primary outcome measure and what treatment is designed to address may be crucial in interpreting the findings of the above study. The goal of the drug abuse treatment (IDU) was to stop drug use and the treatment that focussed on this explicitly did better than the others whose aims were wider (Strain, 1999).

CBT may have a relapse preventative effect on substance abuse. The evidence is promising but not strong. Studies need to be replicated with better control for the effect of contact time with staff and a broader set of outcome measures to capture the specific effects on substance abuse and other important indicators of outcome such as social and psychological adjustment.

Children with antisocial behavior

In longitudinal studies, conduct disorder has been shown to be relatively stable over time and can result in diverse antisocial problems in adulthood (Robins and Rutter, 1999). Kazdin *et al.* (1992) examined the effects of problem-solving skills training (PSST) and parent management training (PMT) on 97 children, aged between 7 and 13 years, with severe antisocial behavior who had been referred to a psychiatric clinic. PSST combined both cognitive and behavioral techniques. Children and Families were randomized to one of the three treatment conditions, PSST, PMT, or a combination of PSST plus PMT. At the end of the treatment phase, all treatments were associated with significant improvements in overall child dysfunction, social competence and aggressiveness, antisocial and delinquent behavior. The results at 1-year follow-up showed a similar pattern. In addition these improvements in performance had generalized to several settings, home, school, and community. In comparison with either treatment on its own, the combination of PMT plus PSST resulted in more marked all round changes in antisocial behavior and social behavior in the children and reduced parental stress and dysfunction. Given the persistence of youthful antisocial behaviors over the longer term, a follow-up of five or more years would be useful in determining the impact of early intervention on adult functioning.

Summary

Cognitive therapy has been useful in providing a theoretical model to aid understanding of ASPD and in developing treatment. As a therapy, cognitive therapy may have advantages over other psychological therapies and may be more able to engage patients with ASPD than other therapies. As a therapy, it is structured, open, and aims to give patients an understanding of their difficulties that is especially helpful in engagement. By encouraging patients to experiment with new ways of thinking and behaving and to assess the usefulness of these, a truly collaborative relationship can be formed with the therapist. With only a few randomized controlled trials of CBT for ASPD, the results so far are cautiously encouraging.

Conclusions

The term ASPD is a portmanteau term that includes people with different psychopathologies and capacities. Clearly no single psychotherapeutic modality will be appropriate for all. Nevertheless people manifesting ASPD frequently present some core clinical attributes some of which have been addressed in the section 'Individual and group psychotherapy of antisocial

personality disorder'. These general comments apply to whatever treatment mode or setting is being offered. Where outpatient (ambulant) treatment is insufficient to meet the behavioral disarray, or for reasons such as imprisonment, then models of treatment via 'sociotherapy' as much as psychotherapy, as in the TCs described in the sections 'Therapeutic community treatment antisocial personality disorder' and 'The treatment of antisocial personality disorder in prison therapeutic communities', offer the best chances of success.

ASPD, as previously described, has its origins not only in individual psychological maldevelopment, but is embedded, defined by, and has it roots in the sociopolitical and social context. As such it presents a huge challenge—for psychotherapists certainly, but even more for policy makers and for the guardians of our sociocultural world.

Overall, longitudinal studies are rarely carried out nowadays—we are all in too much of a hurry to get results, and generally such study proposals are rarely funded. Elucidation of typical pathways of development, which leads to later ASPD could, however, inform possible preventative measures. For example, it seems very likely that investment in education for parenting, support for vulnerable parents, and the provision of child care where there are deficiencies; as well as pre-school provision, and major investment in child and adolescent education, welfare, and health may well have hugely beneficial effects. Whether a particular society pursues such policies is largely a question of the dominant political ethos of any given time. The main point to be made is that the 'treatment' of ASPD should be primarily preventative.

This chapter, by contrast has described some of the psychotherapeutic interventions that can be offered to ASPD sufferers, from as humane a stance as possible. Part of the therapist's task is to 'represent' such individuals, to 'get *alongside*' them, and their difficult and disruptive lives. This can be difficult within the context of societies that naturally wish to isolate, marginalize, and frequently revenge themselves upon such individuals. The 'official' view is increasingly to be seen to be condemnatory and 'tough'— or 'macho'—echoing at least the apparent characteristics of the ASPD individual. In conclusion, we are definitely not arguing for a 'soft' or sentimental approach to the massive problems posed by ASPD, but rather for more thoughtful responses from a range of disciplines in order better to prevent and ameliorate an escalating social and psychological sickness.

References

Alterman, A., Rutherford M. J., Cacciola, J. S., McKay, J. R., and Bordman, C. R. (1998). Prediction of 7 months methadone maintenance treatment response by four measures of antisociality. *Drug and Alcohol Dependence*, **49**, 217–23.

Beck, A. T., *et al.* (1990). *Cognitive therapy of personality disorders*. New York: Guilford Press.

Bion, W. R. (1961). *Experiences in groups*. London: Tavistock.

Carroll, K. M., *et al.* (1994a). Psychotherapy and pharmacotherapy for ambulatory cocaine abusers. *Archives of General Psychiatry*, **51**, 177–87.

Carroll, K. M., *et al.* (1994b). One-year follow-up of psychotherapy and pharmacotherapy for cocaine dependence: delayed emergence of psychotherapy effects. *Archives of General Psychiatry*, **51**, 989–97.

Clarke, D. H. (1965). The therapeutic community concept: present and future. *British Journal of Psychiatry*, **111**, 947–54.

Cordess, C. (2004). The law and mental illness. Commentary on part 6. *Every family in the land*, pp. 291–5. London: The Royal Society of Medicine.

Cullen, E. (1994). Grendon: the therapeutic prison that works. *Journal of Therapeutic Communities*, **15**(4), 301–10.

Davidson, K. M. (2000). *Cognitive therapy for personality disorders: a guide for clinicians*. London: Arnold (Hodder).

Davidson, K. M. and Tyrer, P. (1996). Cognitive therapy for antisocial and borderline personality disorders: single case series. *British Journal of Clinical Psychology*, **35**, 413–29.

De Leon, G. (1994). Therapeutic communities. In: M. Galanter and H. Kleiber, ed. *Textbook of substance abuse treatment*. Washington, DC: American Psychiatric Press.

Dolan, B. M., *et al.* (1992). Therapeutic community treatment for personality disordered adults: changes in neurotic symptomatology on follow-up *International Journal of Social Psychiatry*, **38**, 243–50.

Dolan, B. M., *et al.* (1995). Multiple Axis-II diagnosis of personality disorder. *British Journal of Psychiatry*, **106**, 107–12.

Dolan, B., *et al.* (1996). Cost-offset following specialist treatment of severe personality disorders. *Psychiatric Bulletin*, **20**, 413–17.

Erikson, E. H. (1959). Growth and crises of the healthy personality. *Identify and the life cycle: psychological issues*. New York: International University Press.

Gabbard, G. O. (1988). A contemporary perspective on psychoanalytically informed hospital treatment. *Hospital and Community Psychiatry*, **39**, 1291–5.

Gabbard, G. (1994). *Psychodynamic psychotherapy in clinical practice*. Washington, DC: American Psychiatric Press.

Garland, D. (2001). *The culture of control*. London: Oxford University Press.

Genders, E. and Player, E. (1995). *Grendon: a study of a therapeutic prison*. Oxford: Clarendon Press.

Gerstley, L., *et al.* (1989). Ability to form an alliance with the therapist: a possible marker of prognosis for patients with antisocial personality disorder. *American Journal of Psychiatry*, **146**, 508–12.

Gilligan, J. (2000). *Violence. Reflections on our deadliest epidemic*. London: Jessica Kingsley Publishers.

Glover, E. (1964). *The roots of crime*. Norton Publishers.

Goldstein, R. B., *et al.* (1999). Antisocial behavioural syndromes among residential drug abuse treatment clients. *Drug and Alcohol Dependences*, **53**, 171–87.

Gunn, J. and Robertson, G. (1976). Psychopathic personality: a conceptual problem. *Psychological Medicine*, **6**, 631–4.

Gunn, J. and Robertson, G. (1982). An evaluation of Grendon Prison. In: *Abnormal offenders and the criminal justice system*. Chichester: Wiley

Hare, R. D. (1991). *Manual for the Hare psychopathy check-list—revised*. Toronto: Multi Health Systems.

Hunt, R. G. (1983). Design of therapeutic milieus. In: J. Gunderson, ed. *Principles and practice of milieu therapy*. New York: Jason Aronson.

Hyler, S., *et al.* (1987). *Personality diagnostic questionnaire—revised (PDQ–R)*. New York: Psychiatric Institute.

Jacobson, N. S. and Truax, P. (1991). Clinical significance: a statistical approach to defining meaningful change in psychotherapy research. *Journal of Consulting and Clinical Psychology*, **59**, 12–19.

Jones, M. (1952). *Social psychiatry*. London: Tavistock.

Kadzin, A. E., Siegel, T. C., and Bass, D. (1992). Cognitive problem-solving skills training and parent management training in the treatment of antisocial behaviour in children. *Journal of Consulting and Clinical Psychology*, **60**, 733–47.

Kang, S. Y., *et al.* (1991). Outcomes for cocaine abusers after once a week psychosocial therapy. *American Journal of Psychiatry*, **148**, 630–5.

Kennard, D. (1998). Therapeutic communities are back—and theres something a little different about them. *Therapeutic Communties*, **19**(4), 323–30.

Kennard, D. (2000). *Introduction to therapeutic communities*. London: Jessica Kingsley.

Lewis, A. J. (1974). Psychopathic personality a most elusive category. *Psychological Medicine*, **4**, 133–40.

Longabaugh, T., *et al.* (1995). Drinking outcome of alcohol abusers diagnosed as antisocial personality disorder. *Alcoholism: Clinical and Experimental Research*, **18**, 778–85.

Main, T. F. (1946). The hospital as a therapeutic institution. *Bulletin of the Menniger Clinic*, **10**, 66–8.

Main, T. (1989). The ailment. In: *The ailment and other psychoanalytic essays*. London: Free Association Books.

Marshall, P., *et al.* (1997). *Reduction in reconviction of prisoners at HMP Grendon*. London: Home Office.

Melroy, J. R. (1988). *The psychopathic mind: origins, dynamics and treatment*. NJ: Jason Aronson Inc.

Norton, K. R. W. (1992). Personality disordered individuals: the Henderson Hospital model of treatment. *Criminal Behaviour and Mental Health*, **2**, 180–91.

Norton, K. (2002). Henderson Hospital: Greater than the sum of its subgroups. (in press).

Norton, K. and Warren, F. (2001). Assessment and outcome in therapeutic communities: challenges and achievements. In: J. Lees, N. Manning, D. Menzies, and N. Morant, ed. *Researching therapeutic communities*. London: Jessica Kingsley.

Reid, W. and Gacono, C. (2000). Treatment of antisocial personality, psychotherapy, and other characterologic antisocial syndromes. *Behavioural Science and the Law*, **18**, 647–62.

Rice, M., Harris, G., and Cormier, C. (1992). An evaluation of a maximum security therapeutic community for psychopaths and other mentally disordered offenders. *Law and Human Behaviour*, **16**, 4.

Riviere, J. (1936). A contribution to the analysis of the negative therapeutic reaction. *International Journal of Psychoanalysis*, **17**, 304–20.

Rounsaville, B. J., Glazer, W., Wilber, C. H., Weissman, M. W., and Kleber, H. D. (1983). Short-term interpersonal psychotherapy in methadone-maintained opiate addicts. *Archives of General Psychiatry*, **40**, 629–36.

Rycroft, C. (1979). *A critical dictionary of psychoanalysis*. Penguin Books.

Strain, E. (1999). Psychosocial treatments for cocaine dependence: re-thinking lessons learned. *Archives of General Psychiatry*, **56**, 503–4.

Taylor, R. (2000). A seven year reconviction study of HMP Grendon therapeutic community. In: J. Shine, ed. *HMP Grendon, a compilation of Grendon research*. Leyhill Press.

Travers, J. A. (1994). On not fearing the devil. In: *Psychotherapy and the dangerous patient*. New York: The Haworth Press, Inc.

Turkat, I. D. and Maisto, S. A. (1985). Personality disorder: application of the experimental method to the formulation of personality disorders. In: D. H. Barlow, ed. *Clinical handbook of psychological disorders: a step by step treatment manual*, pp. 502–70. New York: Guilford Press.

Wexler, H. K., Blackmore, J., and Lipton, D. S. (1990). Outcome evaluation of a prison therapeutic community for substance abuse treatment. *Criminal Justice and Behaviour*, **17**, 71–92.

Whiteley, J. S. (1986). Sociotherapy and psychotherapy in the treatment of personality disorder. Discussion paper. *Journal of the Royal Society of Medicine*, **79**, 721–5.

Woody, G. E., McLellan, A. T., Luborsky, L., and O'Brien, C. P. (1985). Sociopathy and psychotherapy outcome. *Archives of General Psychiatry*, **42**, 1081–6.

23 Psychotherapy for the narcissistic personality disorder

Theodore Millon and Seth D. Grossman

What would it really take to save Narcissus, the legendary, dazzlingly beautiful, but misguided character of Greek mythology? As legend has it, the young Narcissus, scornful of all others but his own beautiful self, was the love object of the beautiful nymph, Echo. Though Echo's beauty was extraordinary, she received nary a glance from the self-obsessed young man, and this neglect caused her to brood to such an extent that nothing remained of her but her voice. For his heartlessness, Narcissus was duped into staring into his reflection in the pool of a fountain, an image that would dissipate upon too close encroachment; his conundrum, then, was that he could never possess *his* love object! Unwittingly obsessed with this bittersweet irony, Narcissus pined away, himself, until nothing was left of him but the flower that is his namesake. With only a 'surface' reflection of his outer beauty at his disposal, the young Narcissus could only be caught up in conflicting and confusing cognitions and feelings of euphoria and frustration, not unlike the personality pattern often encountered in contemporary therapy settings.

Narcissus may have easily benefited from some very basic interventions, such as a modicum of perceived 'objectivity' that would reaffirm his outer beauty, but this would not likely do him any long-term favors. Chances are that his next encounter with a reflection pool would bear close resemblance to the legend. Indeed, were simple comfort and restored confidence the ubiquitous goals of therapy with the narcissistic personality, these could often be achieved in but a few sessions. The therapist can hold initial interest by allowing the patient exclusive self-focus, and by further encouraging discussions of past achievements the therapist may enable the narcissist to rebuild any depleted self-esteem. Not infrequently, self-confidence in narcissists is restored by talking about themselves, by recalling and elaborating their attributes and competencies in front of a knowing and accepting person.

Merely reestablishing former levels of functioning, however, especially rebuilding the narcissist's illusions of superiority, may prove over the long run to be a disservice to the narcissistic patient. Until more realistic self-evaluation is achieved, it is not likely that narcissists will be motivated to develop competencies and socially cooperative attitudes and behaviors that would lead to more gratifying and adaptive lives. If the patient's capacity to confront their weaknesses and deficiencies is strengthened, patients may be able to acquire greater self-control, to become more sensitive and aware of reality, and learn to accept the constraints and responsibilities of shared social living. In the following review, we hope to elucidate a multifaceted, integrated approach to the treatment of this personality pattern.

Conceptualization of the narcissistic personality disorder

The essential features of this personality style are an overvaluation of self-worth and a grandiose sense of self-importance and uniqueness. The irony, however, in this inflated self-concept is an inordinate need to be loved and admired by others; this would be a surprising necessity in a person whose elevated self-worth is entirely germane. Unlike the ravenous affectional needs of histrionic and dependent personalities, however, narcissists

believe that they are entitled to tribute and praise by virtue of their 'specialness.' These personalities also share the antisocial features of egocentricity, interpersonal exploitation, and exaggerated needs for power and success. Unlike the anger and vindictiveness of antisocials, however, narcissists are frequently characterized by a benign arrogance and a sense that conventions and reciprocity of societal living is something that simply does not apply to a person of their stature. There is little real empathy for others but rather, a tendency to use people for self-enhancement and for indulging their desires. Those who satisfy their needs are idealized, while others who can serve no immediate purpose are devalued and even treated contemptuously. This shifting of overvaluation and denigration may occur frequently within the same relationship. There is an expectation of preferential treatment and special favors, without assuming reciprocal responsibilities.

The narcissistic personality's cognitive expansiveness, unrealistic goal fantasies, and tendency to overestimate abilities and achievements often leave the person quite vulnerable to injuries of self-esteem and pronounced feelings of unworthiness, should these grandiose self-expectations not be met. Although characteristically imperturbable and insouciant, repeated shortcomings and social humiliations may result in uncertainty and a loss of self-confidence. Over time, with the growing recognition of dissonance between self-perception and actual performance, self-disillusionment, feelings of fraudulence, and in some cases, a chronic state of dysthymia are likely to ensue. In other instances, a psychic blow generated from a single event (e.g., a humiliating defeat or a public criticism) may precipitate a brief but severe depressive episode. Such states rarely endure for extended periods, as depression is not experienced as consonant with the narcissist's self-image. The symptomatology of the narcissistic depression may be quite variable, shifting between dramatic expressions of worthlessness and self-deprecation to irritable demandingness and criticism of others. These perceptions tend to be attributed to external, 'universal' causes rather than to personal, inner inadequacies (Abramson *et al.*, 1978). Consistent with this formulation, a narcissist may subtly accuse others of not supporting or caring for them enough. At other times, hostility may be directly expressed, as the narcissist becomes enraged at others being witness to his/her shame and humiliation.

The legend of Narcissus gives evidence that this constellation of personality patterns has been recognized throughout the existence of civilization and, though many on the international scene argue that it is a disorder found primarily in the western hemisphere, it has been found in a number of cultures. As a psychological construct, the narcissistic personality has enjoyed a rich history, with valuable contributions to its conceptualization emanating from many of the established schools of psychotherapy. As with any personality pattern, a review of these traditions is in order to fully understand the narcissistic pattern as a personologic system, and to gain a foundation for effective treatment.

As is the case with many current *Diagnostic and statistical manual of mental disorders* (DSM) constructs, the origins of narcissism as a psychological construct and mental disorder may be traced to psychoanalytically based explorations. Perhaps the first writing on the subject may be attributed to Havelock Ellis (1898/1933), who conceptualized it as autoeroticism, that is, sexual gratification without stimulation by another person. Paul Nacke

(1899), the next year, used the term to describe the perversion of being preoccupied with the sight and pleasures of one's own body in a manner usually reserved for those of the opposite sex. In 1908, J. Sadger extended the concept to other so-called perversions, notably that of homosexuality. It was in this same era that classical psychoanalysis began to recognize the construct not as a characterologic structure, but certainly as a core component of personality development.

Freud's early dream work (1900) did not use the term, 'narcissism,' but he commented on several patients who seemed to show personality traits consistent with this disorder. These were patients who reported being favored significantly by their caretakers (primarily, their mother) and, resultantly, exhibited a kind of inimitable self-regard and indefatigable optimism that often provided for actual success. His first explicit formulations of narcissism (1910, 1911) emphasized its normal aspects, being a phase of development standing midway between autoeroticism and object love. According to Freud, this transitory period was marked by initially diverse and unconnected autoerotic sensations that eventually fused into what was experienced as one's body, which then become a single, unified love object. Within a few years, he aligned narcissism with libido theory and proposed that it ultimately matured and diffused into object relationships. Shortly thereafter he reformulated his thinking on the developmental sequence and spoke of the autoerotic phase as the 'primary narcissistic condition.' This first phase became the initial repository of libido from which emerged not only the love of self but love in general. In time Freud's conception of narcissism explicated a universal developmental process that continued through life but unfolded through sequential stages.

Freud, of course, recognized that difficulties could arise in this normal, sequential progression. First, there could be failures to advance from libidinal self-love to object love, and, second, 'peculiarities' could occur in the way the person expresses narcissistic love. In his only major paper devoted exclusively to narcissism, Freud (1914/1975) suggested that in certain cases—notably among 'perverts and homosexuals'—libidinal self-centeredness stems from the child's feeling that caretakers cannot be depended upon to provide love reliably. Either rebuffed by their parents or subjected to fickle and erratic attention—seductive one moment and deprecating the next—these children 'give up' as far as trusting and investing in others as love objects. Rather than rely on the capriciousness of others or risk their rejection, these youngsters avoid the lasting attachment they achingly desire and decide instead that it is only themselves they can trust and therefore love.

It is important to note that this early reference to the term narcissism described in Freud's chapter was not intended as a formulation of a narcissistic character structure or personality type, but rather, one of several concepts that he posited as the source of libidinal self-cathexis. Freud's interest lay in exploring and elaborating variations in both the development and the nature of libidinal cathexis. Freud wrote of a narcissistic libidinal type for the first time in 1932 (p. 249), where he described this individual as follows:

> The main interest is focused on self-preservation; the type is independent and not easily over awed . . . People of this type impress others as being 'personalities'; it is on them that their fellow men are specially likely to lean; they readily assume the role of leader, give a fresh stimulus to cultural development or break down existing conditions.

Most striking in this quote is the stark contrast between Freud's characterization of the narcissist's strength and confidence, in comparison with the low self-esteem and feelings of emptiness, pain, and depression that members of the psychodynamic revival (e.g., Kohut, 1971; Forman, 1975) attribute to this personality. Disparities in characterizations such as these often arise as a consequence of shifts from one period to another in Freud's formulations. In this case, it can be traced to the fact that Freud identified several origins of narcissistic self-cathexis, only one of which is the type of parental caprice and rejection that may lead to feelings of emptiness and low self-esteem. As evident from earlier excerpts, and as later elaborated further, Freud's description of the narcissistic libidinal type, brief though it is, corresponds much more closely to the current DSM portrayal of the narcissistic personality than do several contemporary characterizations that trace its antecedents to either parental rebuff or unreliability. Relevant to

this issue is a quote of Freud's reproduced later in the chapter that suggests that narcissistic self-investment is more likely to be a product of parental overvaluation than of parental devaluation.

Contemporary modalities

The concept of the narcissistic personality has moved forward considerably from these early psychoanalytically oriented speculations. Now a well-recognized constellation of personality attributes spanning the range from normal to pathological variants, it is well ensconced in the DSM and reflects the thinking not only of psychodynamic constructs, but of cognitive, interpersonal, and learning modalities (to name but a few); its viability is quite solidly rooted throughout the clinical psychology community.

Before reviewing the various conceptualizations of the narcissistic personality disorder, it is most important to make special note of certain crucial differences between healthy and pathological narcissism; a self-image of pride, confidence, and self-valuation is not only very common across patients seen in psychotherapy in general, it is essential for the ubiquitous goal of self-esteem and positive growth. While an overvaluation of self, be it the product of overindulgence or a compensatory strategy, runs counter to most any therapeutic goal, the individual lacking in essential 'healthy narcissism' is faced with a quite different set of obstacles. For healthy self-esteem and good object relations to evolve, a child must experience unconditional love. However, an overabundance of unearned accolades or highly inaccurate and/or uncritical reflections of a child's behavior or accomplishments has the potential to catalyze an otherwise healthy constellation of traits to problematic ones. Some remarks on neuropsychological stage development as formulated by the senior author (Millon, 1996) are in order here.

Feelings of omnipotence begin shortly after birth but do not take hold in a meaningful fashion until the sensorimotor-autonomy stage. Every minor achievement of future narcissists is responded to with such favor as to give them a deluded sense of their own extraordinary self-worth. Extreme confidence in one's child need not be a disservice, if it is well earned. In the case of an evolving problematic narcissistic personality, however, a marked disparity will exist between the child's actual competence and the impression he/she has of it. Failures in parental guidance and control will play an important part during the intracortical-initiative stage. The child is encouraged to imagine, explore, and act without discipline and regulation. Unrestrained by the imposition of parental limits, the child's thoughts and behaviors may stray far beyond accepted boundaries of social reality. Untutored by parental discipline regarding the constraints of fear, guilt, and shame, the child may fail to develop those internal regulating mechanisms that result in self-control and social responsibility.

Given our dominant cultural orientation toward self-enhancement, it is often difficult to determine which self-focused traits indicate a narcissistic disorder and which are merely adaptive styles that fit societal modes. Where the line should be drawn between self-confidence and healthy self-esteem versus an artificially inflated and empty sense of self-worth is not always an easy task. The healthy narcissist should demonstrate, in addition to the usual characteristics of the personality type, social concerns, and interpersonal empathy, a genuine interest in the ideas and feelings of others, and a willingness to acknowledge one's personal role in problematic interpersonal relationships. Where the disorder is present, we see a persistent insensitivity to others, a general social exploitiveness, and lack of reciprocity in everyday relationships.

Several perspectives have been brought to bear on the concept of the narcissistic personality that deviate in major regards from classical psychoanalytic approaches. However, a review of major psychodynamic orientations to this personality is in order, as their exceptional contributions to modern formulations is integral.

The psychodynamic approach

Analytic theorists Otto Kernberg (1967, 1970) and Heinz Kohut (1966, 1968, 1971) lit the path that has prompted revitalized interest in many modern formulations of psychoanalytic theory and therapy; their conceptions of narcissism (and borderline) served as the cornerstone of this enthusiastic revival. Kernberg, in his restructuring of a diagnostic framework for characterology, de-emphasized the psychoanalytic classification schema that has traditionally been based on libidinal development. Stage sequences are referred to as a means of identifying levels of instinctual maturation (e.g., pregenital, genital). The vicissitudes of maturation give rise to the clinical features, defensive operations, level of severity, prognosis, and, most centrally, the structural integration or organization that is likely to characterize the individual's personality. Employing his framework of levels of structural organization as a model for constructing 'a psychoanalytic classification of character pathology,' Kernberg (1967, p. 655) described the features of the narcissist as follows:

> These patients present an unusual degree of self-reference in their interactions with other people, a great need to be loved and admired by others, and a curious apparent contradiction between a very inflated concept of themselves and an inordinate need for tribute from others. Their emotional life is shallow. They experience little empathy for the feelings of others, they obtain very little enjoyment from life other than from the tributes they receive from others or from their own grandiose fantasies, and they feel restless and bored when external glitter wears off and no new sources feed their self-regard. They envy others, tend to idealize some people from whom they expect narcissistic supplies, and to depreciate and treat with contempt those from whom they do not expect anything (often their former idols). In general, their relationships with other people are clearly exploitative and sometimes parasitic. It is as if they feel they have the right to control and possess others and to exploit them without guilt feelings—and behind a surface which very often is charming and engaging, one senses coldness and ruthlessness. Very often such patients are considered to be 'dependent' because they need so much tribute and adoration from others, but on a deeper level they are completely unable really to depend on anybody because of their deep distrust and depreciation of others.

Kernberg asserted that the haughty and grandiose constellation of behaviors that characterize the narcissist is a defense against the projection of 'oral' rage that, in turn, stems from the narcissist's incapacity to depend on 'internalized good objects.' In this etiologic formulation, Kernberg claimed that the experiential background of most narcissists includes chronically cold parental figures who exhibit either indifference or covert, but spitefully aggressive, attitudes toward their children. At the same time, the young, future narcissist is often found to possess some special talent or status within the family, such as playing the role of 'genius' or being the 'only child.' This quality of specialness serves as a refuge, at first only temporarily but ultimately an often returned to haven that reliably offsets the underlying feeling of having been unloved by the vengefully rejecting parent.

Kohut, on the other hand, rejects the traditional Freudian and Kernbergian thesis that narcissistic self-investment results from a defensive withdrawal of object love attachments following a pattern of chronic parental coldness or vengeful spite. This classical view contends that narcissism is a result of developmental arrests or regressions to earlier points of fixation. Thus, the future narcissist, according to standard analytic metapsychology, regresses to or fails to progress through the usual developmental sequence of initial undifferentiated libido, followed by autoeroticism, narcissism, and, finally, object love. It is not the content as such but the sequence of libidinal maturation that Kohut challenges. His clinical observations have led him to assert that the primitive narcissistic libido has its own developmental line and sequence of continuity into adulthood. That is, it does not 'fade away' by becoming transformed into object-libido, as contended by classical theorists, but unfolds into its own set of mature narcissistic processes and structures. In healthy form, for example, these processes might include behaviors such as humor and creativity; similarly, and most significantly, it is through this narcissistic developmental sequence that the cohesive psychic structure of 'self' ultimately emerges.

Kohut contended, through much of his career, that narcissistic pathology occurs as a consequence of failures to integrate one of two major spheres of self-maturation, the 'grandiose self' and the 'idealized parental imago.' Confronted by realistic shortcomings that undermine early feelings of grandiose omnipotence, or subsequently recognizing the equally illusory nature of the idealized powers they have attributed to their parents, these children must find a way to overcome their 'disappointments' so as not to 'fragment.' If disillusioned, rejected, or experiencing cold and unempathic care at the earliest stages of self-development, serious pathology, such as psychotic or borderline states, will occur. Trauma or disappointment at a latter phase will have somewhat different repercussions depending on whether the difficulty centered on the development of the grandiose self or on the parental imago. In the former, the child will fail to develop the sense of fulfillment and self-confidence that comes from feeling worthwhile and valued; as a consequence, these needs will 'split off' and result in the persistent seeking of 'narcissistic' recognition through adulthood. Along the second line of self-development, children who are unable to 'idealize' their parents because of the latter's indifference or rejection will feel devastated, depressed, and empty. Through adulthood they will seek idealized parental surrogates who, inevitably, will fail to live up to the omnipotent powers the narcissists hoped to find within them. As they desperately seek an ideal that is 'greater' than themselves, they are often led to behave in a weak and self-effacing manner, a style that will enable others to overshadow them.

Late in his career, Kohut recognized a third sphere of self-maturation; this component, which he termed the 'twinship transference' (Kohut, 1984), represented an important addition to his thinking, though this addition was only described posthumously in work completed by his students. To Kohut, this sphere represented a third opportunity for self-cohesion, and arose in his thoughts as a result of a misinterpretation made in session; he originally felt that a patient's conjured, mythical figure was a transferential representation of him as the therapist, but this notion was rejected and explained lucidly by the patient. It appeared that this patient was experiencing the figure (a 'genie in a bottle') as a twin of herself, and needed only to remain as a presence she could talk to, but who did not have to respond. Kohut recognized an association between this phenomenon and the many pronounced silences he witnessed in therapy with her as well as other patients. This twin figure represented, to the patients, an opportunity to be self-validated, that is, to be understood and accepted by an entity just like the self. Also, it served the function of acquiring self-skills through the experience of sameness or likeness.

Kohut's is a developmental theory of self and not a personality characterization. Nevertheless, it leads to a clinical picture that is at variance with those of Freud, Kernberg, and the DSM-IV. The features that emerge from Kohut's descriptions have been summarized by Forman (1975). Listed among the more prominent are: (1) low self-esteem; (2) tendencies toward periodic hypochondriasis; and (3) feelings of emptiness or deadness. To illustrate their contrasting views, for example, the episodic depression that Kohut finds so characteristic of narcissistically injured persons is not seen by Kernberg to be a true depression at all. Rather, Kernberg contends that when 'narcissists' feel seriously disappointed or abandoned they may appear depressed on superficial examination, but they are, in fact, smoldering with constrained anger and revengeful resentment.

Kohut's model encourages the therapist to assume a sympathetic and accepting stance, while addressing the objective need for the patient to accept personal limitations. Short-term methods may be especially useful for crisis intervention and to establish a bridge to more long-term treatment procedures. Binder (1979) reports on the use of a brief treatment method for increasing self-esteem, also in preparation for a longer-term program. The hope here is to increase the patient's awareness of his/her vulnerability to shame and disappointment, as well as to increase the capacity to moderate intense affects, such as irritability and rage.

The cognitive-behavioral approach

Differing significantly from the traditional views of psychoanalytically oriented concepts, the cognitive school has followed its model for treating the dysfunctional thoughts frequently seen in cases featuring clinical depression, and recognized that these cognitions regarding the self, the world, and the future also extend to the complex personality matrix beyond immediate clinical symptoms. Contributing the insightful analysis of the narcissistic personality from a cognitive point of view, Beck *et al.* (1990,

p. 50) provide the following proposals concerning this individuals' distorted belief system:

> The *core* narcissistic beliefs are as follows: 'Since I am special, I deserve special dispensations, privileges, and prerogatives,' 'I'm superior to others and they should acknowledge this,' 'I'm above the rules'.
>
> Their main strategies consist of doing whatever they can to reinforce their superior status and to expand their personal domain. Thus, they may seek glory, wealth, position, power, and prestige as a way of continuously reinforcing their 'superior' image.
>
> Their main affect is anger when other people do not accord them the admiration or respect that they believe they are entitled to, or otherwise thwart them in some way. They are prone to becoming depressed, however, if their strategies are foiled.

The narcissistic personality, according to Beck and his colleagues, can be conceptualized as stemming from a combination of dysfunctional schemas. The early foundation of these schemas is developed by direct and indirect messages from parents, siblings, and significant others, and by experiences that mold beliefs about personal uniqueness and self-importance. Narcissists regard themselves as special, exceptional, and justified in focusing exclusively on personal gratification; they expect admiration, deference, and compliance from others, and their expectations of the future focus on the realization of grandiose fantasies. At the same time, beliefs about the importance of other people's feelings are conspicuously lacking. Behavior is affected by deficits in cooperation and reciprocal social interaction, as well as by excesses in demanding, self-indulgent, and sometimes aggressive behaviors.

The various techniques of dysfunctional thought modification, cognitive reframing, and similar techniques espoused by Beck (and many other cognitively oriented thinkers, e.g., Sperry, 1999) are well-known and highly validated components of contemporary clinical practice. More recently, Young (1999) has provided insightful cognitive schema-focused inroads to the challenges of personality pathology. Young's approach represents an integration of cognitive therapy with intrapsychic and gestalt modalities, and expands significantly on traditional cognitive approaches by giving special attention to the therapeutic relationship, early experience, and affect. Although he does not explicate personality-specific treatment regimens, his approach is very much in concert with the ideals set forth in a later discussion within this chapter regarding systematic integration of differing modalities; it differs, however, in its use of a modality within the boundaries of psychology proper (that is, cognitive theory) as the central, binding construct, rather than seeking organizing principles from the overarching natural sciences.

The interpersonal communications approach

Timothy Leary (1957), a disciple of Horney and others of the social and interpersonal school of thought, pioneered what may be termed the 'interpersonal' approach to the problem of personality pathology, and extended their notions to what he terms 'adjustment through competition.' Leary (1957) spoke of this pattern as demonstrating a competitive self-confident narcissism, which he captures well in the following series of quotes:

> In its maladaptive extreme it becomes a smug, cold, selfish, exploitive social role. In this case the adaptive self-confidence and independence become exaggerated into a self-oriented rejection of others . . .
>
> These individuals feel most secure when they are independent of other people . . . The narcissist puts . . . distance between himself and others-wants to be independent of and superior to the 'other one'. Dependence is terrifying.
>
> p. 332

> The second group of . . . patients . . . are those whose self-regard has received a decent defeat. They often report the most colorful and fearful symptomatology . . . The superficial impression of depression or dependence is deceptive. Psychological testing or perceptive interviewing will reveal that the patients are not as anxious or depressed as they appear. What becomes evident is a narcissistic concern with their own reactions, their own sensitivities. The precipitating cause for their entrance to the clinic is usually a shift in their life situation, which causes frustration or a blow to their pride.
>
> p. 335

A number of interpersonally oriented theorists followed Leary's interpersonal perspective and drafted their models of various personality disorders in highly fruitful work. Perhaps most notable among this group is Lorna Benjamin (1993) who has formulated a complex analysis of the narcissistic character. In her recent work she describes this personality as follows:

> There is extreme vulnerability to criticism or being ignored, together with a strong wish for love, support, and admiring deference from others. The baseline position involves noncontingent love of self and presumptive control of others. If the support is withdrawn, or if there is any evidence of lack of perfection, the self-concept degrades to severe self-criticism. Totally lacking in empathy, these persons treat others with contempt, and hold the self above and beyond the fray.
>
> p. 147

> [The narcissist] expects to be given whatever he or she wants and needs, no matter what it might mean to others. This does not include active deception, but rather is a consequence of the belief that he or she is 'entitled'. For example, the narcissistic personality disorder would not set out to con a 'little old lady' out of her life savings; however, if she offered them, the narcissistic personality disorder would accept such a gift without reflection about its impact on her. [He/She] will expect great dedication, overwork, and heroic performance from the people associated with him or her—without giving any thought to the impact of this pattern on their lives.
>
> p. 150

Benjamin's (1993) *interpersonal* approach suggests that achieving the first crucial therapeutic objective, the patient's recognition of problematic interpersonal patterns, is particularly challenging with narcissistic patients. While the therapist's empathic understanding is necessary in facilitating this process, the form of therapist statements needs to be carefully considered to prevent encouraging narcissistic tendencies inadvertently. Benjamin provides examples of more and less therapeutically effective statements in discussing a narcissistic patient and his dissatisfied wife. An example of a response that probably encourages a narcissistic schema is 'You have been trying so hard to make things go well, and here she (your wife) just comes back with complaints.' Benjamin notes that such a therapist response would probably enhance the patient's pattern of externalizing and blaming. A preferred alternative would be, 'you have been trying so hard to make things work well, and you feel just devastated to hear that they aren't going as perfectly as you thought'. The advantage of this latter response is that it encourages the patient to examine internal processes and reaction patterns.

Present habits become clearer when their functional significance is grasped. To this end, the patient's pattern of emotional reactions such as envy and feelings of entitlement can be traced to early interactions with significant others. Internalized representations of these early figures continue to guide present functioning. As the patient comes to recognize which attitudes and behaviors are motivated by earlier 'internalizations,' he may become freer to modify them. An example provided by Benjamin considers a patient that expressed anger and envy about a friend's receipt of public acknowledgment of success. The therapist shifted the patient's focus to issues underlying the envy by asking the patient how his mother would react to such news. Further discussion helped clarify to the patient that his concern about her reaction of disappointment (real or internalized) supports his unpleasant envious feelings. Such insight can help the patient resolve to detach from internalized representations of such figures. Finally, it is noted that once the patient accepts that unattainable ambitions and maladaptive behaviors need to be given up in favor of more realistic and fruitful cognitive and interactive habits, the bulk of the therapeutic challenge may be well on its way; new learning may be a relatively easy undertaking thereafter.

A synergistic integrative model

The modalities described above are but a few of the best known and most often utilized in interventions with the narcissistic personality. All have been considered as serious contenders for 'definitive' status, and all have been criticized for various shortcomings, which may be summarized as a whole by the following: each contributes valuably by focusing on an *area* of treatment that is necessary, but each falls short in neglecting other important treatment aspects. To this we may add: efforts at using each others' techniques is by no means a new idea, but what remains lacking is a comprehensive, coherent set of principles that allows true synergistic, integrative therapy to take place. In an earlier publication, the senior author (Millon, 1999) outlined a method for addressing these shortcomings.

As stated previously, despite their undeniably brilliant contributions throughout their rich history, *no* single school of psychological thought may lay claim to a full contextual understanding and process of treating *any* personality pathology, inclusive of the narcissist. The very nature of personality precludes this; as the senior author has stated in numerous other places (e.g., Millon, 1990, 1996, 1999; Millon and Davis, 1996), personality is a naturally-occurring *system* encompassing the spectrum of modalities represented in the virtuous though unilateral psychotherapy schools. As these phenomenological, behavioral, intrapsychic, and biophysical entities bind together and reinforce one another in their perpetual and reciprocal organization, it is virtually impossible for any unidimensional school's approach to effectively modify dysfunctional personologic processes. For a therapy to be effective, it must be as tenacious as the personality system itself, approaching difficulties from a broad-based paradigm that incorporates all the modalities present in the personality.

In the last decade of the twentieth century, Millon (1990) reformulated his biosocial-learning model of personality (Millon, 1981) to align with the greater principles of natural sciences. According to Millon, only through the perspective of the naturally occurring world could principles be derived that provided for a comprehensive, synergistic science of personology. This science would include an overarching theory, a means of classification for the various phenomena found as a result of the theory, a method for objectively identifying and assessing those phenomena, and a system for intervention, or modification, that followed logically from these three prior elements. Furthermore, the science needed to address the disparate elements (e.g., cognitions, intrapsychic structures, etc.), which had, over the history of personologic intervention, presented themselves in clinical settings. Finally, this system needed to interface with and augment the extant classification methods (i.e., *DSM-IV-TR*, 2000) used by the community of contemporary research and practice-oriented clinical professionals.

The most germane and generative source for conceptualizing the constellation of patterns that comprise the Axis II personalities, according to Millon, was the established science of evolutionary biology. Here, he felt, was a sister science whose principles were closely in alignment with the expressions of personality, and were also shared with the myriad of other sciences (e.g., particle physics, organic chemistry) that were well-grounded in terms of organizing principles. In examining the tenets of evolution, Millon deduced that all organisms (and specifically, personality) were possessed of three motivating aims that may be expressed as bipolarities, as illustrated in Figure 23.1: existence (pleasure-seeking versus pain avoidance), adaptation (active modification versus passive assimilation), and reproduction (self versus other nurturing). While a full explication of the derivation of these polarities is beyond the scope of this chapter, a basic understanding is key to conceptualizing the narcissistic personality in preparation for treatment. Their primary qualities are reviewed in context with the structure of the narcissistic personality.

The first polarity, that of existence, does not suggest a strong proclivity for either pleasure seeking or pain avoidance in basic drives. These qualities may vary considerably across situations and among narcissistic individuals, especially when characteristics of other personalities are present (as is frequently the case; see discussion on subtypes in the case examples, below). What is more central in the polarity matrix of the narcissist is the primacy of both passive/accommodation and self/individuation. What this translates into is the narcissist's focus on self as the center of one's existence, with a comparable indifference to others (nurturance). According to Millon, and in contrast with many of the classic psychodynamically oriented conceptions of the narcissist, the etiology of this personality pattern is owed to an unusual developmental background in which others overvalued the narcissists' self-worth by providing attention and tribute unconditionally.

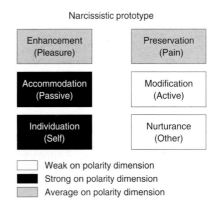

Narcissistic prototype

Fig. 23.1 Narcissistic personality disorder, in accordance with the Millon Evolutionary Model.

As a result, they fail to develop the motivation and skills ordinarily necessary to elicit these tributes. To them, merely being who they are is sufficient; one does not have to do anything, no less achieve, to elicit signs of admiration and high self-esteem. Narcissists are passive, therefore, because they expect the rest of the world to do their bidding without reciprocal efforts.

With these basic motivating aims in mind, it is now possible to examine the expression of the narcissistic personality across the various functional and structural personologic domains outlined by the theory (see Millon and Davis, 1996). As noted previously, these domains suggest representation of behavioral, phenomenological, intrapsychic, and biophysical elements of personality that coincide with a myriad of therapeutic traditions. The relative salience of these domains in the prototypal narcissistic personality, as conceived by Millon, are represented graphically in Figure 23.2.

Personologic structures and functions

Expressive behavior: haughty

This behavioral domain holds that it is not uncommon for narcissists to act in an arrogant, supercilious, and disdainful manner. There is also a tendency for them to flout conventional rules of shared social living. Viewing reciprocal social responsibilities as being inapplicable to themselves, they show and act in a manner that indicates a disregard for matters of personal integrity and an indifference to the rights of others. When not faced with humiliating or stressful situations, narcissists convey a calm and self-assured quality in their social behavior. Their seemingly untroubled and self-satisfied air is viewed, by some, as a sign of confident equanimity. Others respond to it much less favorably. To them, these behaviors reflect immodesty, presumptuousness, pretentiousness, and a haughty, snobbish, cocksure, and arrogant way of relating to people. Narcissists appear to lack humility and are overly self-centered and ungenerous. They characteristically, but usually unwittingly, exploit others, take them for granted, and expect others to serve them, without giving much in return. Their self-conceit is viewed by most as unwarranted; it smacks of being 'uppity' and superior, without the requisite substance to justify it.

Interpersonal conduct: exploitive

Also a part of the behavioral domain, but in concert with interpersonal approaches, narcissists feel entitled, expecting special favors without assuming reciprocal responsibilities. Not only are they unempathic, but they take others for granted, are shameless in the process, and use others to enhance their own personal desires. Unfortunately for them, narcissists must come to terms with the fact that they live in a world composed of others. No matter how preferred their fantasies may be, they must relate and deal with all the complications and frustrations that real relationships entail. Furthermore, and no matter how satisfying it may be to reinforce oneself, it

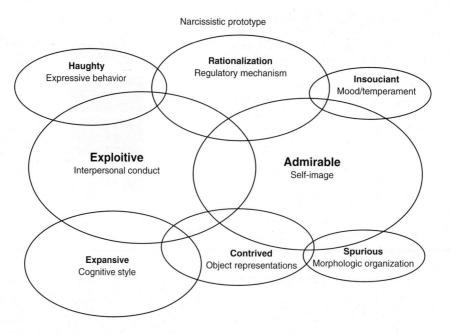

Fig. 23.2 Salience of personologic domains, narcissistic personality.

is all the more gratifying if one can arrange one's environment so that others will contribute their applause as well. Of course, true to their fashion, narcissists will seek to accomplish this with minimal effort and reciprocity on their part. In fact, some narcissists assume that others feel 'honored' in having a relationship with them, and that others receive as much pleasure in providing them with favors and attention as the narcissist experiences in accepting these tributes.

Cognitive style: expansive

This phenomenological domain notes that narcissists exhibit an undisciplined imagination, and seem preoccupied with immature and self-glorifying fantasies of success, beauty, or romance. Although nondelusional, narcissists are minimally constrained by reality. They also take liberties with facts, embellishing them, even lying, to redeem their illusions about their self-worth. Narcissists are cognitively expansive. They place few limits on either their fantasies or rationalizations, and their imagination is left to run free of the constraints of reality or the views of others. They are inclined to exaggerate their powers, to freely transform failures into successes, to construct lengthy and intricate rationalizations that inflate their self-worth or justify what they feel is their due, quickly depreciating those who refuse to accept or enhance their self-image.

Self-image: admirable

Another phenomenological domain, this one observes that the narcissist feels justified in claiming special status, and has little conception of the objectionable, even irrational nature of his or her behavior. It is the narcissists' belief that they are special, if not unique persons that deserve great admiration from others. Quite frequently they act in a grandiose and self-assured manner, often without commensurate achievements. Although they expect to be seen as meritorious, most narcissists are viewed by others as egotistic, inconsiderate, and arrogant. Their self-image is that they are superior persons, 'extraspecial' individuals who are entitled to unusual rights and privileges. This view of their self-worth is fixed so firmly in their minds that they rarely question whether it is valid. Moreover, anyone who fails to respect them is viewed with contempt and scorn.

Object representations: contrived

The final phenomenological domain holds that internalized representations of past experiences are deeply embedded and serve as a template for evaluating new life experiences. For the narcissist, these object representations

are composed far more than usual of illusory and changing memories. Problematic past relationships are readily refashioned so as to appear entirely consonant with the narcissist's high sense of self-worth. Unacceptable impulses and deprecatory evaluations are quickly transformed so as to enable this personality to maintain his preferred and contrived image of both himself and his past. Fortunately for most narcissists, they were led by their parents to believe that they were invariably lovable and perfect, regardless of what they did and what they thought. Such an idyllic existence could not long endure; the world beyond home is not likely to have been so benign and accepting. As a consequence, the narcissist must transform the less palatable aspects of his past so they are consistent with what he wishes they were, rather than what they were, in fact.

Regulatory mechanism: rationalization

This first intrapsychic domain poses the question: What happens if narcissists are not successful, if they face personal failures and social humiliations? What if realistic events topple them from their illusory world of eminence and superiority? What behaviors do they show and what mechanisms do they employ to save their wounds? While they are still confident and self-assured, narcissists are facile at the art of self-deception, devising plausible reasons to justify self-centered and socially inconsiderate behaviors. With an air of arrogance, narcissists are excellent at rationalizing their difficulties, offering alibis to put themselves in the best possible light, despite evident shortcomings or failures on their part. If rationalizations fail, dejection and feelings of emptiness are likely. Narcissists will have little recourse other than to turn for solace to their fantasies. Failing to achieve their aims and at a loss as to what they can do next, they are likely to revert to themselves to provide comfort and consolation. It is at these times that their lifelong talent for imagination takes over. These processes enable them to create a fanciful world in which they can redeem themselves and reassert their pride and status. As narcissists are unaccustomed to self-control and objective reality testing, their powers of imagination have free rein to weave intricate resolutions to their difficulties.

Morphologic organization: spurious

Narcissists hold a sanguine outlook on life that is founded on an unusual set of early intrapsychic experiences that only rarely are duplicated in later life. They suffer few conflicts; their past has supplied them, perhaps too well, with high expectations and encouragement. As a result, they are inclined to trust others and to feel confident that matters will work out well for them. Therefore, the structural organization of the narcissist's inner world for dealing with life tends to be quite flimsy and transparent, in contrast to the common misperception of a more substantial and dynamically orchestrated personality organization. Owing to the misleading nature of their early experiences, this personality has never developed the inner skills necessary to regulate impulses, to channel needs, or to acquire contingency strategies for frustrations, routine failures, and problem resolution. Consequently, even the routine demands of everyday life may be viewed as annoying incursions by narcissists. Such responsibilities are experienced as demeaning. Driven by their need to maintain their illusion of superiority in the face of conflict, some may turn against others, accusing them of their own deceptions, selfishness, and irrationalities. It is at these times that the fragility and pathology of the narcissist becomes clearly evident. 'Breakdowns' in the defensive structure of this personality, however, are not too common. More typically, the exploitive behaviors and intrapsychic maneuvers of narcissists prove highly adaptive and provide them with the means of thwarting serious or prolonged periods of dejection or decompensation.

Mood/temperament: insouciant

This last, biophysically oriented domain predicts that narcissists are generally roused by the facile workings of their imagination, and usually experience a pervasive sense of well-being, a buoyancy of mood, and an optimism of outlook—*except* when their sense of superiority has been punctured. Normally, however, affect, though based often on their semigrandiose distortions of reality, is generally relaxed, if not cheerful and carefree. There is a general air of nonchalance, an imperturbability, a feigned tranquility. Should the balloon be burst, however, there is a rapid turn to either an edgy irritability and annoyance with others or to repeated bouts of dejection that are characterized by feeling humiliated and empty. Shaken by these circumstances, one is likely to see briefly displayed a vacillation between rage, shame, and feelings of emptiness.

Key practice principles

The following represents the senior author's (T.M.) synergistic therapeutic approach for the narcissistic personality patterns that fully integrates the traditional psychotherapy schools reviewed in earlier sections.

Identifying dysfunctional domains

The most salient narcissistic dysfunctions are manifest in the self-image and interpersonal conduct domains, and are expressed in the form of an admirable self-concept and unempathic, even exploitive treatment of others. At best, the narcissist confidently displays achievements and behaves in an entitled, and occasionally grating manner. Facts are twisted and the line between fantasy and reality becomes blurred as narcissists boast of unsupportable personal successes and talent; at the same time, interpersonal behavior moves toward the inconsiderate, arrogant, and exploitive. Others may express irritation at the nonsubstantiated grandiosity of the narcissist's fantasies and at the inequitable nature of his or her social interactions. However, taking advantage of others to indulge desires and enhance his or her situation, with no consideration of reciprocal responsibilities, is considered justified owing to their sense of self-importance. As long as this self-schema is maintained, the narcissist has little chance of finding motivation to effect changes in other areas. Thus, a likely first therapeutic intervention may be a cognitive refocusing on acceptance of a realistic self-image. This may be done via reframing techniques aimed at acclimating the individual to a balanced view of self. Later techniques may include more direct cognitive disputes of the person's perceived flawlessness. As the cognitive foundation on which exploitive behavior is justified is weakened, interventions that increase empathic understanding and cooperative interactions can become the clinical focus. Synergistically speaking, this process may be enhanced by modeling an empathic and understanding stance (as suggested by Kohut, 1971, 1984) and allowing for a transference identification to take

place. The therapist should avoid being 'infallible;' rather, as the therapeutic relationship is solidified, it may be beneficial for the individual to see the therapist as a competent and respectable professional, but not as omnipotent or infallible. The benefits of these approaches—warmer receptions from others and a more solid personal sense of efficacy—can then be integrated to encourage further development.

Successful intervention in the primary domains can lead to beneficial advances within secondary domains. Furthermore, resolving secondary domain dysfunctions therapeutically can also bolster progress in the more salient areas. Behavioral interventions, including role-playing, techniques of behavioral inhibition, modeling, and systematic desensitization, which elicit nonadulating therapeutic feedback, can help extinguish haughty expressive behavior as well as exploitive interpersonal conduct. These can in turn result in more genuine interpersonal events that subsequently serve as useful counterexamples to unrealistic or contrived object representations. Such exercises and the results they generate may set the groundwork for a more searching exploration of the patient's internalized schemas and their negative consequences. Illusory ideas and memories and pretentious attitudes can eventually be replaced with reality-based experiences and object representations.

As the patient comes to grasp the nonadaptive nature of the expansive narcissistic cognitive style, preoccupation with immature fantasies may be decreased. As cognitive and behavioral dysfunctions come to be regulated, the narcissist's insouciant mood is also likely to be naturally tempered. Baseline nonchalance and buoyancy can be replaced with more context-appropriate feelings. The rages, shame, and emptiness that resulted from undeniable discrepancies between self-image and reality are often modified along with the patient's self-concept. In some cases, psychopharmacological intervention may be indicated if a resistant depression appears to be interfering with therapeutic progress.

Ultimately, therapeutic interventions in the preceding domains can have a beneficial effect on this personality's spurious morphologic organization. Flimsy defensive strategies can be replaced by stronger coping mechanisms, and the stress-reducing regulatory mechanism of rationalization can be given up for more realistic and growth-fostering inner and outer self-representations.

Establishing psychic balances

Characteristic narcissistic confidence, arrogance, and exploitive egocentricity is based on a deeply ingrained, if sometimes fragile, self-image of superior self-worth. Achievements and manifest talents are often not proportional to the narcissist's presumptions of 'specialness'. The alternative to maintaining unsustainable beliefs of personal infallibility, that is, recognition of imperfections, limitations, and flaws, however, is tantamount to reconciliation with failure and utter worthlessness. For some narcissists such unreal expectations for themselves stem from experiences in which otherwise doting parents became unsupportive or even abusive at the manifestation of 'imperfection' in their child; others simply cannot conceive of life among the 'masses.' As those around narcissists 'dare' not to notice their special uniqueness, and then behave appropriately, narcissists turn away from attempting to secure comfort from 'simple-minded' others whose place it is to tend him or her. Instead, they increasingly rely on themselves as a source of rewards. Turning inward provides opportunity to pamper and ponder the self, and to fantasize about the great recognition that will come to shine on the narcissist one day. Thus narcissists, who start out high on the self-polarity, become increasingly less other oriented with the passage of time.

In the mind of the narcissist, others are the source of all of his or her troubles and difficulties, and are responsible for any failures to achieve fantasized goals. Not only do others have to make this up to the narcissist, but their natural inferiority dictates that they should attend to all the narcissist's whims and needs. The narcissist's exploitive egocentricity is not the two-faced, contract-breaking, means-to-an-end exploitiveness of the antisocial. Rather than actively planning, the narcissists' arrogance and snobbish sense of superiority lead them to believe that others 'owe' them something, and their self-centered convictions of genuine entitlement results in the 'passive' exploitation of others. The sense of superiority often results in a lack of goal-oriented behavior in general; narcissists simply believe that good things are their due, a natural byproduct of their intrinsic 'specialness'. This nonadaptive bias toward the passive end of the active-passive dimension often results in personal, social, and professional stagnation.

A main therapeutic goal in trying to increase a narcissist's other-orientedness and active goal-directed behaviors is to help him or her accept that while human imperfections are inevitable, they are not necessarily a sign of failure or worthlessness. If narcissists can appreciate the benefits (lack of pressure, decreased fear of criticism) of not needing to be infallible, they may be able to consider their part of the responsibility for any difficulties they may be having. Active problem solving and improved interpersonal interaction is a worthy goal.

Countering perpetuations

Narcissists' characteristic difficulties almost all stem from their lack of solid contact with reality. The same disdain for objectivity prevents effective coping with subsequent troubles. The problem-perpetuating cycle begins with early experiences that provide noncontingent praise that teach narcissists to value themselves regardless of accomplishments. Their inflated sense of self-worth causes them to conclude that there is little reason to apply any systematic effort toward acquiring skills and competencies when 'it is so clear that' they already possess such obvious and valuable talents and aptitudes. Their natural gifts, they believe, are reason enough for them to achieve their goals and earn others' respect.

In time, narcissists come to realize that others, who are expending considerable effort to achieve goals, are moving ahead and receiving more recognition. Envious and resentful that the acknowledgment that is 'rightfully theirs' is being bestowed upon others, narcissists intensify their boasting and air of superiority. Eventually, the prospect of actually going out in the world and risking humiliating failure for all to witness becomes untenable in the face of the grand illusions of personal competence narcissists feed to themselves and others.

The problems posed by narcissistic illusions of competence feed into and are exacerbated by social alienation and lack of self-controls. The conviction that they are 'entitled' leads narcissists to harbor disdain for social customs and cooperative living. A lack of respect for others' opinions and feelings lead to a failure to integrate normative feedback about their behaviors and illusions. In fact, the conviction that others are simple minded and naive cause narcissists to retreat further into their illusory and isolated world of fantasy at every hint of disapproval. Self-serving rationalizations of others' lack of adulation can escalate until complementary paranoid delusions of persecution and grandiose illusions become firmly entrenched. Were narcissists to possess some self-controls, their social isolation may not have such dire consequences. Internal reality testing, however, is as neglected as are external inputs. Rathezr than working to realize ambitions, threat of failure and conceit push narcissists to retain their admirable self-image through fantasy. The regard for reality that would prevent narcissists from perpetuating their psychological and coping difficulties are notably absent.

Therapeutic intervention offers an inroad into the pathological cycle through the modification of the overblown self-image. As the self is appraised more realistically, perfection is seen as unattainable, and the need to employ self-discipline to achieve goals is understood, the narcissistic patient may come to recognize and accept his or her similarity to others. As the patient begins to make genuine efforts to improve the genuine quality of life, an appreciation for others' hard work and achievements may develop and replace chronic envy and resentment. Intervention aimed directly at increasing empathic understanding can lead to a sensitivity to other's feelings that fosters motivation to adopt cooperative interpersonal behaviors. Toward this end, the narcissist can choose to learn to tolerate and make use of constructive social feedback. Day to day successes can eventually provide the gratification that can bolster the patient's resolve not to perpetuate non-adaptive cognitive and behavioral strategies, and help control the impulse to escape into unproductive flights of fantasy. If social isolation is thus decreased, therapeutic work has led to difficult-to-realize modifications in the patient's deeply entrenched lifestyle.

Efficacious therapeutic techniques

As a general note, working with narcissists is difficult for therapists who seek change in a patient's personality. Benjamin (1993) notes that the patient's presumptions of entitlement and admiration may encourage the therapist to join the patient in mutual applause, while criticizing the rest of the world. Alternatively, the patient may maintain a stance of superiority. Neither kind of therapeutic alliance helps the patient achieve more adaptive functioning. Any confrontation of the narcissist's patterns will be experienced as criticism, however, and chances are high that the patient will choose to terminate therapy. Benjamin suggests that narcissists may consider changing their interpersonal habits if they are convinced that it will lead to a more favorable response from others. Overall, best therapeutic outcomes may come from honest interpretations presented in a tone of approval and acceptance. Good therapeutic gain will result when the patient internalizes the therapist's empathic acceptance of the patient's faults and deficits. As children, most narcissists were noncontingently praised for their 'perfection,' and may have been led to feel like utter failures when their inevitable lack of perfection was too apparent to be ignored. The therapist's attitude that faults are inevitable and perfectly human provides an opportunity for realistic self-evaluation of self-worth that were rarely provided in the typical narcissist's early learning history. Carefully timed self-disclosures of the therapist's reactions toward the patient can also potentially lead to substantial therapeutic gain. Such information can encourage the patient's insight into the negative impact of his/her habitual behaviors on others, and, if revealed with supportive skill, can foster motivation to modify these habits.

As noted previously, effective therapy must match the personality's system of interweaving domains, for unilateral approaches will lack the tenacity to effect broad-based changes. From the functional and structural domains listed in an earlier section, techniques may be suggested that interface well with the personality constellation (see Table 23.1 for an overview).

Challenges

Narcissists are not inclined to seek therapy. Their pride disposes them to reject the imperfection-confirming 'weak' role of patient. Most are convinced they can *get along* quite well on their own. Often if a narcissist does accept voluntary treatment, he or she will try to enlist the therapist to support the opinion that the patient's problems are largely the result of the imperfections and weaknesses of others. Alternatively, the narcissist may adopt a stance of superiority and discredit the therapist, or terminate treatment prematurely. In sum, narcissists will not accede to therapy willingly. Moreover, once involved, they will maintain a well-measured distance from the therapist, resist the searching probes of personal exploration, become indignant over implications of deficiencies on their part, and seek to shift responsibility for these lacks to others. The treatment setting may give witness to struggles in which narcissists seek to outwit the therapist and assert

Table 23.1 Domain-oriented tactical modalities

Expressive acts modality	counterconditioning; social skill training
Interpersonal conduct modality	group, family, and interpersonal techniques
Cognitive style modality	confrontation; cognitive-behavioral
Object representations modality	dream analysis; object relations analysis
Self-image modality	cognitive reframing; self-oriented analysis
Regulatory mechanisms modality	ego-oriented analysis; hypnotherapy
Morphologic organization modality	transference; classical psychoanalysis
Mood-temperament modality	psychopharmacologic agents

their dominance. Stone (1993) notes that much of the narcissistic patient's sarcasm, devaluation, and domination toward the therapist can been seen as a 'test' of whether the therapist will respond in kind and therefore, like the patient's parents (who may have modeled the offensive behavior), is not to be trusted. Setting limits without resorting to an accusatory or attacking stance can prove to be invaluable aids in working with these patients. Great patience and equanimity are required to establish the spirit of genuine confidence and respect without which the chances of achieving reconstructive personality change becomes even slimmer.

Cases illustrating integrative synergies

As mentioned previously, personality disorders rarely present in what may be termed 'prototypal' cases. We will not usually be confronted with a 'pure' narcissist; rather, admixtures of narcissism with other personality variants are usually seen. Experience with the Millon Clinical Multiaxial Inventory scores III (Millon *et al.*, 1997) suggest several personality blends that incorporate distinct narcissistic features. A review of the developmental background of other narcissistic personalities contributed further to the variants described in the following two cases.

Case 1: the unprincipled narcissist (narcissistic with antisocial traits)

Jules, 34, was a young hydraulics salesman who had 'risen from the plebs' to find unmitigated success in the sales field until a blatant disregard for the terms of a contract brought his actions into question, and he was asked to see a counselor through his company's employee assistance plan. Initially, he seemed to be simply a self-confident, gregarious man, but this quickly gave way to a more realistic picture of an intimidating, manipulative individual. He proudly shared the secret to his success: use unethical techniques others won't. He saw himself as separate and apart from the crowd of salesmen, as he was one who would not get 'pushed' by a customer. He also explained with a knowing grin that it was possible to butter up any deal with a little fraudulent use of the expense account. Jules viewed himself as a 'free agent,' one who didn't feel the customary rules of employment, society, and life applied to him. Consequently, this freedom allowed him to successfully pursue virtually anything he wanted. Perhaps one of the most striking moments of the interview came when Jules was describing his parents. His mother, a quiet, dutiful woman was seen by Jules as 'nothing really special;' his father, on the other hand, by virtue of his beer consumption and the ability to make his point clear (with a 'whipping') over a minor infraction, was seen as an impressive, revered figure.

Unprincipled narcissists such as Jules are seen most often these last two or three decades in drug rehabilitation programs, centers for youth offenders, and in jails and prisons. Although these individuals often are successful in society, keeping their activities just within the boundaries of the law, they enter into clinical treatment rather infrequently. Jules's behavior was characterized by an arrogant sense of self-worth, an indifference to the welfare of others, and a fraudulent and intimidating social manner. There was a desire to exploit others, to expect special recognitions and considerations without assuming reciprocal responsibilities. A deficient social conscience was evident in his tendency to flout conventions, to engage in actions that raise questions of personal integrity, and to disregard the rights of others. Achievement deficits and social irresponsibilities were justified by expansive fantasies and frank prevarications. Descriptively, we may characterize Jules as devoid of a superego, that is, evidencing an unscrupulous, amoral, and deceptive approach to his relationships with others. More than merely disloyal and exploitive, he was likely to blend in with society's con-men and charlatans, many of whom are vindictive and contemptuous of their victims. The features clearly seen in Jules support the conclusion that he was an admixture of both narcissistic and antisocial personality characteristics.

Jules evidenced a rash willingness to risk harm and was notably fearless in the face of threats and punitive action. Malicious tendencies were projected outward, precipitating frequent personal and family difficulties, as well as occasional legal entanglements. Vengeful gratification was often obtained by humiliating and dominating others. He operated as if he had no principles other than exploiting others for his personal gain. Lacking a genuine sense of guilt and possessing little social conscience, he was an opportunist who enjoyed the process of swindling others, outwitting them in a game he enjoyed playing in which others were held in contempt owing to the ease with which they can be seduced. Relationships survived only as long as he had something to gain. People were dropped with no thought to the anguish they may have experienced as a consequence of his careless and irresponsible behaviors.

Jules displayed an indifference to truth that, if brought to his attention, was likely to elicit an attitude of nonchalant indifference. He was skillful in the ways of social influence, was capable of feigning an air of justified innocence, and was adept in deceiving others with charm and glibness. Lacking any deep feelings of loyalty, he successfully schemed beneath a veneer of politeness and civility. His principal orientation was that of outwitting others, getting power, and exploiting them 'before they do it to you.' He often carried a chip-on-the shoulder attitude, a readiness to attack those who were distrusted or who could be used as scapegoats. Jules attempted to present an image of cool strength, acting tough, arrogant, and fearless. To prove his courage, he may have invited danger and punishment. But punishment only verifies his unconscious recognition that he deserves to be punished. Rather than having a deterrent effect, it only reinforces his exploitive and unprincipled behaviors.

While it would be important to garner understanding of Jules's point of view and express accurate empathy, it would be equally crucial for the therapist to maintain a steadfast posture that would remain focused on tangible interventions. It would be ill-advised to indulge in *self-image* techniques that may guide the process into digressions about his perceived grandeur. Of primary importance would be a *cognitive* reorientation that would enhance Jules's alertness to the needs of *others*, while diminishing his *self*-important illusion. On an *interpersonal* level, it would be necessary to adjust Jules's social outlook, which would include clarifying his *active-passive* conflict. One of his primary perpetuations is his tendency to actively exploit others, yet to maintain a laid-back, uncaring attitude regarding anyone or anything that doesn't immediately affect him. A major focus of behavioral therapy for Jules would be to introduce steps to overcome his deficient controls, while instilling a greater sense of empathy for others.

Short-term methods were suitable for Jules, although *environmental management*, *psychopharmacologic treatment*, and *behavior modification* could be safely disqualified. The most effective course to begin changing some of his troubling attitudes and behavior was *cognitive reorientation*. As the therapeutic relationship began to develop and a modicum of comfort was established, the therapist was able to begin confronting Jules's dysfunctional beliefs and expectations. Short-term *interpersonal* methods were also used to explore and adjust his social skills and demeanor. More expressive and time-extended techniques were not justified here, as it is more prudent in a case such as this to work at controlling Jules's illusions, rather than to foster possible grander illusions. *Group therapy* was most beneficial here, as the members provided a means for Jules to express himself without his usual arrogant front in a benevolent and noncritical environment.

While it was very important to avoid emphasizing Jules's negative attributes, the therapeutic relationship also depended upon not allowing him to assert dominance in treatment in his usual way. He fully believed himself to be perfect, and this made him notably disinclined to change any of his attitudes. He refused, initially, to commit to any amount of time investment in therapy, and early cession would have virtually guaranteed quick relapse. Throughout the early stages, he maintained a careful distance from the therapist, and would attempt to thwart any exploration of personal issues that may have implied any deficiency on his part. Cognitive confrontations arranged in graduated depths (beginning with presentation of alternatives, evolving to more direct statements challenging Jules' current mind set) were able to counter these efforts, and difficulties rooted in his evasiveness and unwillingness, though sometimes disruptive, were dealt with directly and firmly, but without emitting disapproval. With this consistently honest and confrontive stance, the treatment setting went from an environment that frequently gave witness to attempts at dominance, to one of relative cooperation and efficacious collaboration.

Jules routinely thought of others, regardless of their status, position, or intellect, as callow and stupid. Rather than ever question his viewpoint, his response to any challenge (including those he instigated) was, without question, that the other person was not only wrong, but an idiot. A direct cognitive approach confronted this habit of assuming everyone else to be wrong, and claiming superiority based on frequent arguments he could win by acumen and intimidation. Gone unchecked, this habit would have continued to encourage Jules's arrogant and presumptuous demeanor.

Jules had not sought therapy voluntarily, and was convinced that there really was no problem. After all, there were no current failures or dissatisfactions on his current 'scorecard,' so what could be wrong? Even if he had brought himself to seek help due, perhaps, to an unaccustomed loss in sales, or a declining social context, it would have been unlikely that he would conceive of any trouble as linked to his actions or demeanor. It was quite transparent that entering this office put his pride on the line, and that was not a position he was inclined to take lightly. This particularly defensive stance also called for direct, firm confrontation, while maintaining a safe but honest therapeutic environment through an empathic attitude expressed by the therapist. Jules's acceptance of this environment was questionable, and his attitude towards the process ambivalent, until he came to respect the therapist as being forthright and not easily intimidated.

Although Jules's self-esteem needed to be augmented as a result of his being placed in the role of patient, the therapist needed to maintain his authoritative therapeutic posture. Jules easily restored his self-confidence by brief visitations to his accomplishments, a process that took no more than a session or two. It was more important, however, to work with Jules to instill a sense of empathy for others through focused exploration of how he imagined their experience, and to understand and accept the 'unspoken contract' of restraint and responsibility in society. This measure, aimed at preventing recurrences, required that no deceptions were made by Jules, and that his compliance was sincere.

Case 2: the amorous narcissist (narcissist with histrionic features)

Barbara was a 27-year-old bartender who enjoyed her line of work, as it was quite agreeable with her lifestyle. There was a component of tending bar in a nightclub that allowed her to 'perform,' she explained, thereby garnering much attention and attracting multiple sexual partners. She seemed quite proud of this social life and conquests, as she spoke of her previous night's 'hook-up.' Although the majority of her experience had been with very short-term partners, she was actually once married. She described this relationship in very nonchalant terms, seeming to bestow no more importance to the arc of this 6-month relationship than to a particular afternoon's activities. When questioned regarding the ending of the marriage, she faulted her spouse's jealousy, as she still drew the attention of many men at work. Although Barbara seemed relatively content in her presentation, and was vague in her reasoning for seeking therapy, she seemed to detect some personal inadequacy that could not be fulfilled by her exploits, or a vague tinge of guilt over some of her more dishonest manipulations.

The distinctive feature of Barbara, an *amorous narcissist*, was an erotic and seductive orientation, a building up of her self-worth by engaging members of the opposite gender in the game of sexual temptation. There was an indifferent conscience, an aloofness to truth and social responsibility that, if brought to her attention, elicited an attitude of nonchalant innocence. Though highly self-oriented, she was facile in the ways of social seduction, often feigned an air of dignity and confidence, and was rather skilled in deceiving others with her clever glibness. She was skillful in enticing, bewitching, and tantalizing the needy and the naive. Although indulging her hedonistic desires, as well as pursuing numerous beguiling objects at the same time, she was strongly disinclined to become involved in genuine intimacy. Rather than investing her efforts in one appealing person, she sought to acquire a coterie of amorous objects, invariably lying and swindling as she wove from one pathological relationship to another. The qualities

just outlined are strongly suggestive of the observation that narcissistic personality types such as Barbara possess numerous characteristics that are primary among histrionic personalities, a fact clearly seen in her Millon Clinical Multiaxial Inventory scores.

Although a reasonably good capacity for sexual athletics sustains the vanity of many individuals, narcissists or not, the need to repeatedly demonstrate one's sexual prowess is a preeminent obsession among amorous subtypes. Among these personalities are those whose endless pursuit of sexual conquests is fulfilled as effectively and frequently as their bewitching style 'promises.' Others, however, talk well, place their lures and baits extremely well, that is, until they reach the bedroom door; maneuvering and seduction is done with great aplomb, but performance falls short. For the most part, the sexual exploits of the amorous narcissist are brief, lasting from one afternoon to only a few weeks.

Perhaps Barbara was actually fearful of the opposite sex, afraid that her pretensions and ambitions would be exposed and found wanting. Her sexual banter and seductive pursuits were merely empty maneuvers to overcome deeper feelings of inadequacy. Although she seemed to desire the affections of a warm and intimate relationship, when she found it (assuming her marriage appeared, at first, to provide these qualities), she undoubtedly felt restless and unsatisfied. Having won someone over, she probably needed to continue his pursuit. It is the act of exhibitionistically being seductive, and hence gaining in narcissistic stature, that compels. The achievement of ego gratification terminates for a moment, but it must be pursued again and again.

It was possible that Barbara left behind her a trail of outrageous acts such as swindling, sexual excesses, pathological lying, and fraud. Her disregard for truth and the talent for exploitation and deception was neither hostile nor malicious in intent. These characteristics appeared to derive from an attitude of narcissistic omnipotence and self-assurance, a feeling that the implicit rules of human relationships did not apply to her and that she was above the responsibilities of shared living. As with the basic narcissistic pattern, Barbara went out of her way to entice and inveigle the unwary among the opposite sex, remain coolly indifferent to the welfare of those whom she bewitched, whom she had used to enhance and indulge her hedonistic whims and erotic desires.

Caring little to shoulder genuine social responsibilities and unwilling to change her seductive ways, Barbara wouldn't 'buckle down' in a serious relationship and expend effort to prove her worth. Never having learned to control her fantasies or be concerned with matters of social integrity, Barbara maintained her bewitching ways, by deception, fraud, lying, and by charming others through craft and wit as necessary. Rather than applying her talents toward the goal of tangible achievements or genuine relationships, she devoted her energies to constructing intricate lies, to cleverly exploit others, and to slyly contrive ways to extract from others what she believed was her due. Untroubled by conscience and needing nourishment for her overinflated self-image, she fabricated stories that enhanced her worth and thereby succeeded in seducing others into supporting her excesses. Criticism and punishment were likely to prove of no avail as Barbara was likely to quickly dismiss these aspersions as products of jealous inferiors.

It was expected that Barbara would attempt to manipulate and monopolize the process of therapy, and would need to be engaged and controlled through a firm and focused attitude on the part of the therapist. *Cognitive* and *interpersonal* strategies would focus on altering her perpetuating belief of her own importance and the devaluation of (but reliance on) *others*, and would thereby serve to establish improved social skills and more genuine relationships. Concurrently, it would also be prudent to help Barbara assume a less *passive* affective stance (less nonchalant and superficial in her attitude). In addition to cognitively and interpersonally undermining Barbara's irresponsible attitudes and actions, *behavioral* interventions should be fruitful in reinforcing new habits and skills, as well as establishing responsible social actions. A *group* milieu might be a most beneficial adjunct, as well, in guiding Barbara towards reassessing her interpersonal style and self-important attitude, establishing empathy towards others, and taking on a more responsible disposition.

Cognitive reorientation seemed to be the most effective catalyst for Barbara to modify some of these attitudes about herself and her socially lamentable actions in a short-term milieu. As her more affable but trite veneer gave way to increasingly more meaningful exchanges with the therapist, Barbara was able to begin working on her erroneous assumptions regarding herself and her social context. *Interpersonal* methods also were employed to examine these assumptions and reevaluate some of her less acceptable actions. These focused interpersonal methods, most notably *group therapy*, helped her reassess herself more realistically and effectively, and provided a forum for her to experiment with more cooperative and sociable behaviors. For Barbara, the more expressive and longer-term techniques would not have been useful, as she was prone towards self-illusions too easily reinforced by the imaginative freedom these methods foster. Likewise, several other popular short-term techniques, including *environmental management*, *psychopharmacologic treatment*, and *behavior modification* would not be of value in effecting change.

In the early sessions, Barbara frequently attempted to dominate the therapeutic relationship, relying on her well-practiced and suave seductive tactics. This habit needed to be confronted, though delicately and honestly, as overemphasizing any shortcoming might have led to regression in establishing rapport. During this early stage, she navigated her way around any investigations into personal issues by using her 'charm' and jumping from one superficiality to the next, as well as casting responsibility for herself on to others. Unless dealt with directly, yet without disapproval on the part of the therapist, her evasiveness and unwillingness would have seriously interfered with short-term gains. Cognitive confrontations, which were firm but consistently honest, were effective in prompting her to examine critically her own beliefs and behaviors, avoid further attempts to win dominance, and to invest in the change process.

Cognitively based methods were effective at undermining faulty beliefs that prompted Barbara's tendency to devalue others. It was, at first, unfathomable to her that her assumptions were askew, as she had consistently assured herself that everyone else's views were inane. That is, she simply *couldn't* be wrong, as her modus operandi seemed to work well for her, yet so many others seemed to be discontent. She needed to understand the basic tenet that disparity between herself and those more sensitive (or perhaps, more accurately expressive) did not necessarily mean that her views were superior.

Generally, an illusion that calls for brief confrontive therapy with amorous narcissists is based on the fact that these patients are unlikely to seek therapy on their own. They typically believe that they will solve everything for themselves by simply being left alone. In Barbara's case where treatment was self-motivated, it may have followed an unadmitted humiliation or failure. Regardless of what her promptings were, seeking professional help harmed her pride. Though she gave lip service to accepting therapy, this attitude was rather tentative and delicate throughout the therapeutic relationship.

Although it was appropriate to help Barbara rebuild this guarded, deflated self-image, the therapist could not appear submissive lest Barbara revert rapidly to many of her older, problematic tactics. Rebuilding her self-confidence was a simple process, which merely involved indulging her in reminiscing about a few past conquests. An objective geared more at preventing recurrences was that of helping Barbara become more empathic with others, and to understand the effects of her behavior in social interactions.

Conclusions

We have attempted in this chapter to promote the view that there is not a 'singular' modality of therapy that is most indicated for a particular personality (in this case, the narcissistic personality). Rather, the therapeutic techniques that have evolved over the history of modern treatment modalities may all be useful, not in a 'grab-bag' way, but in a coherent, synergistic fashion that facilitates understanding and intervention for the multidimensional nature of the individual personality. We may learn considerably from the individual schools of thought and their evolution, and as astute clinicians, a thorough understanding of these modalities is requisite for effective therapy. We also make note that there is not one singular narcissistic personality that will easily match our preconceived notions from the DSM or psychopathology textbook. Rather, each is a unique individual,

likely expressing one of several possible admixtures of personality characteristics, and a thorough understanding of the personality matrix may prove fruitful in gaining a fuller understanding of the precise presentation of that individual.

References

Abrahamson, L., Seligman, M., and Teasdale, J. (1978). Learned helplessness in humans: critique and reformulation. *Journal of Abnormal Psychology*, **87**, 49–74.

American Psychological Association. (2000). *Diagnostic and statistical manual of mental disorders—text revision (DSM-IV-TR)*. Washington, DC: APA.

Beck, A. T., et al. (1990). *Cognitive therapy of personality disorders*. New York: Basic Books.

Benjamin, L. S. (1993). *Interpersonal and treatment of personality disorders*. New York: Guilford Press.

Binder, J. (1979). *Choosing the appropriate form of time-limited dynamic psychotherapy*. Charlottesville, VA: University of Virginia Medical Center.

Ellis, H. (1898/1933). Auto-erotism: a psychological study. *Alienist and Neurologist*, **19**, 260–99.

Forman, M. (1975). Narcissistic personality disorders and the oedipal fixations. *Annual of Psychoanalysis*, Vol. 3, pp. 65–92. New York: International Universities Press.

Freud, S. (1900). *The interpretation of dreams*. New York: Norton.

Freud, S. (1910/1957). Leonardo da Vinci and a memory of his childhood. In: J. Strachey, trans. and ed. *The standard edition of the complete psychological works of Sigmund Freud*, Vol. 2. London: Hogarth Press.

Freud, S. (1911/1925). Psychoanalytic notes upon an autobiographical account of a case of paranoia (Dementia paranoides). In: A. and J. Strachey, trans., *Collected Papers*, English translation, Vol. 3. London: Hogarth Press.

Freud, S. (1914/1925). On narcissism: an introduction. In: J. Riviere, trans., *Collected Papers*, English translation, Vol. 4. London: Hogarth Press.

Freud, S. (1932/1950). Libidinal types. In: J. Strachey, trans., *Collected Papers*, English translation, Vol. 5. London: Hogarth Press.

Kernberg, O. F. (1967). Borderline personality organization. *Journal of the American Psychoanalytic Association*, **15**, 641–85.

Kernberg, O. F. (1970). Factors in the psychoanalytic therapy of narcissistic patients. *Journal of the American Psychoanalytic Association*, **18**, 51–85.

Kohut, H. (1966). Forms and transformations of narcissism. *Journal of the American Psychoanalytic Association*, **14**, 243–72.

Kohut, H. (1968). The psychoanalytic treatment of narcissistic personality disorders. *Psychoanalytic Study of the Child*, **23**, 86–113.

Kohut, H. (1971). *The analysis of Self*. New York: International Universities Press.

Kohut, H. (1984). How does analysis cure? A. Goldberg and P. Stepansky, ed. Chicago: University of Chicago Press.

Leary, T. (1957). *Interpersonal diagnosis of personality*. New York: Ronald.

Millon, T. (1981). *Disorders of personality: DSM-III, axis II*. New York: Wiley.

Millon, T. (1990). *Toward a new personology: an evolutionary model*. New York: Wiley.

Millon, T. (1996). *Personality and psychopathology: building a clinical science*. New York: Wiley.

Millon, T. (1999). *Personality-guided therapy*. New York: Wiley.

Millon, T. and Davis, R. D. (1996). *Disorders of personality: DSM-IV and beyond*. New York: Wiley.

Millon, T., Davis, R. D., and Millon, C. (1997). *Millon Clinical Multiaxial Inventory-III*, 2nd edn. Minneapolis, MN: National Computer Systems.

Nacke, P. (1899). Die sexuellen perversitaten in der irrenansalt. *Psychiatrie en Neurologie Bladen*, **3**, 14–21.

Sadger, J. (1908). Psychiatrish-neurologisches in psychoanalytischer Beleuchtung. *Zeitschrift fuer gesamte Medizin*, **7**, 92–104.

Stone, M. H. (1993). Long-term outcome in personality disorders. In: P. Tyrer and G. Stein, ed. *Personality disorder reviewed*. London: Gaskell.

Young, J. E. (1999). *Cognitive therapy for personality disorders: a schema-focused approach*, 3rd edn. Sarasota, FL: Professional Resource Press.

24 Borderline personality disorder

Anthony W. Bateman, Sigmund Karterud, and Louisa M. C. Van Den Bosch

Introduction

The inherently ambiguous term 'borderline' on the one hand continues to evoke an ambivalent response within the psychotherapeutic and psychiatric community with many authors continuing to complain of its imprecision after two decades of research and predicting its eventual replacement by some more satisfactory formulation (Tyrer, 1999). Yet on the other hand there is an increasing acceptance of the concept and a burgeoning interest in the nature of borderline and other personality disorders (PDs), their development, and their treatment by modified psychotherapeutic methods. This is exemplified by the publication of a practice guideline for the treatment of borderline personality disorder (BPD) in the USA (American Psychiatric and Association, 2001) and a strategic review of treatment of PD by the Department of Health in the UK (DoH, 2003). Both documents highlight the importance of psychotherapy in treatment and the American guideline specifically places psychotherapy as the primary mode of treatment for BPD. Other countries are involved in similar work and are likely to respond with official guidance on the treatment of PD within their mental health services.

The irony of these developments is that research into treatment is scarce and, as this chapter will make clear, we are far from being able to state that we have an effective treatment for BPD and despite the descriptive formulations and miscellaneous theories, there is no consensus about what the core of the underlying psychological problem is in BPD. Although we will consider some of the theoretical formulations of BPD in this chapter, the zeitgeist has moved to practical treatment approaches that are required to have empirical support and this chapter will focus more on empirical evidence for the treatment of BPD than the diverse theoretical formulations.

Definition

The term 'borderline' has undergone a checkered career of multiple name changes since the early 1930s but finally emerged as the name of choice for a group of problematic patients whose original defining characteristics was being too disturbed to be treated by classical psychoanalysis. 'Borderline' patients were thought to function psychologically somewhere between neurosis and psychosis (Stern, 1938). This in-between state was later referred to variously as ambulatory schizophrenia (Zilboorg, 1941), the 'as if personality' (Deutsch, 1942), and 'pseudoneurotic schizophrenia' (Hoch and Polatin, 1949). In the 1960s and 1970s significant progress was made in understanding the disorder and findings from psychiatry and psychoanalysis were distilled over time into the nine descriptive criteria of BPD outlined in the DSM (American Psychiatric Association, 1994). Yet the definition remains problematic and the present DSM-IV does not define any 'core borderline' type. To the contrary, it has a prototype categorical design as no one of the nine criteria is necessary or jointly sufficient for the diagnosis. All that is required is five positive criteria. Accordingly there are 256 feasible combinations of criteria for a BPD diagnosis.

DSM-IV groups the PDs into Clusters A, B, and C. BPD is defined as belonging to Cluster B together with antisocial (ASPD), narcissistic (NPD), and histrionic (HPD) PDs (the flamboyant, dramatic, or help-seeking disorders). To some extent this clustering concurs with the psychoanalytic view promoted by Kernberg (see p. 292) who sees BPD as an *organization* (Kernberg, 1975a), which includes within it narcissistic and antisocial disorders and it has face validity in that comorbidity of PDs is widespread. However, diagnostic co-occurrence studies have provided mixed evidence for these associations. The best Axis II diagnostic co-occurrence study so far (McGlashan *et al.*, 2000) found a significant association between BPD and ASPD and dependent PD as well as with posttraumatic stress disorder on Axis I.

Epidemiology

BPD is a common condition with a prevalence of between 0.2 and 1.8% of the general population (Swartz *et al.*, 1990), but most studies originate from North America and the situation may be different elsewhere. The most reliable study of the prevalence of the disorder in a community sample conducted in Oslo (Torgersen *et al.*, 2001) suggested that the prevalence of BPD was not as frequent as commonly assumed with only 0.7% of patients being diagnosed as borderline from a representative community sample. But prevalence rates increase if patients within the mental health system are sampled, with the highest rates being found in those patients requiring the most intensive level of care—outpatient rates range from 8 to 11%, inpatient from 14 to 20%, and forensic services from 60 to 80%. In a Dutch forensic psychiatric hospital 80% of patients fulfilled criteria for at least one PD with paranoid, ASPD, and BPD being the most common (Ruiter and Greeven, 2000). Similar rates have been found in England and Sweden (Blackburn *et al.*, 1990) with the most common being BPD and ASPD (Dolan and Coid, 1993).

Severity

The prevalence pattern described above reflects the considerable heterogeneity among patients receiving the diagnosis BPD. The question of severity is of utmost importance for the clinician. Severity is partly dependent on which criteria the patient fulfills. Suicidality and self-mutilation are regarded as severe symptoms, often being targets of specific treatment interventions and measures of treatment effect. Grilo *et al.* (2001) found that 59% of 240 BPD patients in the American collaborative longitudinal PD study fulfilled this criterion. Severity is also related to number of BPD criteria, partly because total number is positively correlated to number of other PD criteria and other PD diagnoses.

Assessing the level of severity, including risk assessment, is of course of paramount importance for treatment planning. The more severe, the more the patient is in need of comprehensive treatment programs, while the more resourceful BPD patient can benefit from less intensive treatment.

Conceptual models

Theories are used to make sense of problems and to guide interventions. In his encounter with the borderline patient a therapist without a grounding theory will be like a boat at sea without a compass. Minimal requirements for a theory of BPD are an explanatory account of the BPD criteria, a theory of the self, of defense mechanisms, of interpersonal transactions and countertransference phenomena. Moreover, as group therapies play a crucial part in inpatient and day treatment programs, therapeutic communities, and outpatient services, a theory of BPD should optimally be compatible with the group dynamic theory that guides group therapy interventions. A good theory should have a high explanatory power, meaning that it provides a theoretical framework for a multitude of phenomena within complex interpersonal contexts. Kernberg was a pioneer in this respect. He extended his theories of borderline personality organization (BPO) to group and institutional dynamics (Kernberg, 1975b, 1993). Karterud (1990) 'translated' this theory to self psychology, and Pines (1990) and Marrone (1994) have integrated the theories of group analysis, attachment theory, and BPD. Linehan has developed a comprehensive theory and more recently cognitive-behavioral therapists, particularly Safran and Segal (1990) and Young (1990) have begun integrating cognitive and affective processes to understand BPD.

An example of how theory drives treatment intervention can be seen in differences between the combined (groups or group–individual) psychodynamic approach and dialectical behavior therapy (DBT). The DBT therapist coaches patients to develop skills, even over the telephone, while the psychodynamic group therapist observes and interprets in the here and now of the group or individual session. The borderline patient will play out his/hers internal scenarios in the group and in the group these may be generalized to external contexts. The group therapist anticipates the spontaneous unfolding of the reasons for an individual's unhappiness and has to be informed by a sophisticated theory if understanding and meaning are to be converted into containment, interpretation, and change.

Psychodynamic understanding

The psychodynamic approach to BPD is essentially a developmental view in which genetic vulnerability is unmasked as a result of disruption of the early mother–infant relationship and later environmental influences. This view has been supported by research on attachment disorders in childhood and empirical evidence demonstrating the association of childhood abuse with BPD (Johnson et al., 1999).

It was Kernberg (1967) who was the first to systematize these features using Kleinian ideas, combining classical instinct theory with object relations to define an underlying BPO, which occurs in many psychopathological situations, including BPD, NPD, HPD, psychotic disorders, some eating disorders, and in normal individuals who are exposed to extreme stress. He placed BPD between personality organizations to be found in psychotic and neurotic conditions. The four intrapsychic features pointed to by Kernberg were: (1) identity diffusion; (2) primitive defenses of projection, projective identification, splitting, and denial; (3) partially intact reality testing that is vulnerable to alterations and failures because of aggression; and (4) characteristic object relations.

Defense mechanisms

The value of characterizing defense mechanisms specific to BPD has been demonstrated in empirical studies and is relevant clinically. Patients with BPD have been shown to use the defenses of splitting and acting out more than non-BPD patients, and the defenses of suppression, sublimation, and humor less than, non-BPD patients (Bond et al., 1994). In another study, hypochondriasis, projection, acting out, and undoing were found to discriminate patients with BPD from patients with other PDs (Zanarini et al., 1990). In clinical practice the understanding of defenses enables the therapist to maintain mental closeness with the patient and allows a broader understanding of the underlying anxieties driving the patient. Through, splitting and projective identification, idealization, denial, omnipotence, and devaluation, the world in BPO is split into good and bad, black and white, friend or foe.

Object relations

According to Kernberg's structural approach the inner world in BPO is characterized by split objects. Instead of stable and smoothly integrated internal representations of people and their relationships, the self and others are experienced in chiaroscuro, or as part-objects—breasts, penises, and objects for evacuation or exploitation—and innate aggression remains unbound, leaving the mind of the borderline patient subject to severe disruption.

Kernberg relates BPO to Mahler's 'rapprochement subphase' in which the child begins to separate and to explore the world for himself, but needs to rush back to his mother for comfort and reassurance and 'narcissistic supplies'. If the mother is physically or psychologically unavailable, the child may not be able to integrate good and bad maternal imagos. The child then reacts to abandonment with an excess of aggression, which is projected outwards on to his objects and reintrojected into a split self in a way that often resists therapeutic efforts. These negative internalized object- and self-representations play havoc with the borderline patient's ability to maintain a sense of goodness and the negative introjects make them feel unworthy, shameful, and wicked. Attempts to expel them through projection and to see others as despicable may fleetingly be successful but when the projective system breaks down suicidal impulses occur.

Kernberg's object relational approach has been translated into a manualized form of treatment known as transference focused psychotherapy (TFP) and trials are underway to assess its effectiveness (see p. 295).

Self psychology

A somewhat different psychoanalytic approach arose from Heinz Kohut's reconceptualizations of narcissism (Kohut, 1966) and the self (Kohut, 1971, 1977) in which he described the developmental consequences of what he believed to be unmet mirroring needs in childhood. His contribution led to the inclusion of a NPD in DSM-III and a greater emphasis on the therapist as an empathic support for the patient.

Kohut's emphasis on empathy and his skepticism towards nonpsychoanalytical categorizations have been carried to the extreme by the intersubjectivist position advocated by (Stolorow et al., 1987). Stolorow and colleagues have questioned the very concept of BPD, arguing that it represents an objectification that mystifies the pathology and furnishes the professional community with false beliefs in disease concepts derived from the natural sciences. While this position sharpens the focus on the intersubjective transactions between patients and therapists, the price has been a neglect of empirical research.

It was Adler's (1985) understanding of the borderline patient that has had the major influence on treatment for a self-psychological perspective. Although heavily influenced by the theories of Kohut, Adler does not consider himself to be a 'Kohutian' but an eclectic who synthesizes and integrates developmental theories. Drawing on developmental ideas of Piaget and Selma Fraiberg (Fraiberg, 1969), Adler proposes that the borderline patient is unable to conjure up a soothing image of an attachment figure when under stress, resulting in a need either for the physical presence of the protector or at least a physical reminder of them. This failure of 'evocative memory' when under duress creates the panic and clinging dependency found in borderline patients and the absence of retrievable, soothing introjects leads to a 'primary inner emptiness', which leads to annihilatory panic and intense rage. Adler's approach therefore includes the therapist as support and as someone who allows selfobject transferences to flourish. The term selfobject refers to the self-regulatory function of other people (or animals or valued objects). Lacking adequate regulatory functions of the self the borderline patient is dependent on others and the therapist is encouraged to allow himself to be 'used' by the patient as a stabilizer and only later to explore the distortions and use of projective systems.

Understanding from attachment theory

To some extent the developmental views described above have gained some credence through research on attachment. Attachment theory, developed by John Bowlby (1969, 1973, 1980) postulates a universal human need to form close affectional bonds. At its core is the reciprocity of early relationships, which is a precondition of normal development probably in all mammals, including humans (Hofer, 1995). The attachment behaviors of the human infant (e.g., proximity seeking, smiling, clinging) are reciprocated by adult attachment behaviors (touching, holding, soothing) and these responses strengthen the attachment behavior of the infant toward that particular adult. The activation of attachment behaviors depends on the infant's evaluation of a range of environmental signals that results in the subjective experience of security or insecurity. The experience of security is the goal of the attachment system, which is thus first and foremost a regulator of emotional experience (Sroufe, 1996).

Although attachment theory is about proximity and the evocation of an experience of safety, it is also about the consequential development of robust, flexible, psychological processes that protect the individual from the stresses of human interaction and everyday life. Borderline patients are conceived of as failing to develop a stable sense of self because of disturbance in early attachment relationships. The experience of safety within the context of a close emotional relationship is essential for the development of an autonomous sense of self and anything that undermines the emergent self leads to anxiety and potentially an angry response as the child attempts to stabilize himself (Sroufe, 1996). The emergent self is only under serious (what might be thought of as existential) threat when it is in close emotional contact with another self—when a mind meets a mind—especially if that mind shows little understanding of the internal state of the child. Under 'good enough' conditions an agentive sense of oneself as experiencing thoughts and feelings that can effectively guide action is stabilized by a caregiver who provides an intersubjective milieu in which the self is strengthened through the interaction. Under conditions of chronic neglect and insensitivity instability of the self results first in anger and then aggression, which is evoked so frequently because of repeated parental neglect that it becomes incorporated into the self structure with the result that self-assertion, demand, wishes, and needs have to be accompanied by aggression if the self is to remain intact and stable. Such distortions to the self are not irreversible. The acquisition of the capacity to create a 'narrative' of one's thoughts and feelings, to mentalize, can overcome flaws in the organization of the self that can flow from the disorganization of early attachment. Thus the robustness of the self structure is dependent on the capacity to mentalize.

Mentalization

Mentalization is fundamentally the capacity to understand and interpret human behavior in terms of underlying mental states (for a comprehensive review of this field see Baron-Cohen et al., 2000). It develops through a process of having experienced oneself in the mind of another during childhood within an attachment context and only matures adequately within the context of a secure attachment. There is evidence from a number of sources that this is the case (Fonagy, 1997; Meins et al., 2001).

Not only does the development of mentalization depend crucially on the child's social environment, the maintenance of the capacity to think of human action in mental state terms continues to be a function of social experience. Fonagy (1991) suggested that one effect of childhood maltreatment is that, in order to cope with a caregiver who harbors malevolent intent towards the child, the child may close his mind down to minds in general, his own and that of others. It is far too painful to conceive of their attachment figures' wish to abuse them and to cause harm. Frequently, in cases of abuse, the isolation from care triggers experiences of lack of safety that in turn trigger the children's attachment system. They end up seeking proximity while closing down their mind to intersubjective interaction, resulting in the paradoxical but common observation of physical clinging but mental distance. This trap often persists and leads to profound distortions in the development of the self. If the child sees the hatred and denigration in the mind of his caregiver he is forced to experience himself as unlovable and hateful; if he exposes himself by letting his caregiver know what he experiences he will be humiliated and what he felt proud about becomes shameful; if he shows vulnerability it will be exploited or ridiculed. Stability is maintained through mental isolation, not knowing, pre-emptive acts of aggression to neutralize perceived

threats, schematic inaccurate representations of interpersonal interactions, and the dominance of projective mechanisms that force mental states on to the other and thus prevent its genuine perception, all of which are characteristic of BPD. This theoretical approach is covered extensively in Fonagy et al. (2002).

Different attachment styles in children are apparent and these have been linked to BPD. A study comparing patients with BPD with those with either ASPD or bipolar II disorder (Perry and Cooper, 1986) found greater separation-abandonment complex and greater conflict about the expression of emotional need and anger in borderline patients. Reliance on transitional objects is suggested to reflect BPD patients failed early attachment experiences (Modell, 1963), which have been suggested to be of the anxious-ambivalent subtype (Fonagy et al., 1995; Gunderson, 1996).

There are at least seven studies that have demonstrated extremely insecure attachments in patients with BPD characterized by alternating fear of involvement and intense neediness (see summaries in Bartholomew et al., 2001; Dozier et al., 1999). Variables most strongly related to BPD features are lack of expressed care and overprotection by mother and an anxious and ambivalent attachment pattern.

Cognitive-behavioral understanding

Cognitive-behavioral formulations of BPD are already as diverse as those of psychoanalysis even though it is only over the past decade that cognitive therapists have turned their attention to PDs. A clinically based approach has been proposed by a number of workers who have developed detailed conceptualizations and treatment strategies for each of the PDs. Initially these formulations built on the general view of psychopathology taken by cognitive therapy in which biased thinking patterns are considered as the core of a patient's problem and modification of these is necessary if the patient is to improve. Standard cognitive therapy focuses a great deal of attention on automatic thoughts and assumptions or beliefs. Automatic thoughts are akin to an internal running commentary, which is evoked under particular circumstances, for example when writing a chapter for a book the anxious individual may continually say to himself 'I am never going to get this done and the editors will think that I am lazy'. Assumptions function at a deeper level of cognition and are tacit rules that give rise to automatic thoughts. But it was soon apparent that this formulation was overly simplistic and inadequate and a reformulated model has been proposed to take into account the complex psychological processes and behaviors found in BPD. In a revised model, Beck and associates (Alford, 1997) define personality in terms of patterns of social, motivational, and cognitive-affective processes thereby moving away from a primary emphasis on cognitions. However, personality is considered to be determined by 'idiosyncratic structures' known as schemas whose cognitive content gives meaning to the person. But the term schemas has been used in various ways, on the one hand being considered as a structure of cognition that filters and guides the processing of information and on the other hand being suggested as the building block of latent, core beliefs. The latter is the commonest use of the term and implies basic rules that individuals apply to organize their perceptions of the world, self, and future, and to adapt to the challenges of life.

It is schemas that are the cornerstone of cognitive formulations of BPD. Patients with BPD show characteristic assumptions and dichotomous thinking. Basic assumptions in the borderline commonly include 'the world is a dangerous place', 'people cannot be trusted', and 'I am inherently unacceptable'. Dichotomous thinking is the tendency to evaluate experiences in terms of mutually exclusive categories such as good and bad, love and hate. Extreme evaluations such as these require extreme reactions and emotions, leading to abrupt changes in mood and immoderate behavior. The assumptions, dichotomous thinking and weak sense of identity are considered to form a mutually reinforcing and self-perpetuating system that governs relationships. Schemas that were once adaptive during childhood persist even after they have become seriously dysfunctional. They are maintained in the face of contradictory evidence because of distortion, discounting, seeing the evidence as an exception to the rule and extinction of the maladaptive systems does not take place as a result of negative reinforcement. In fact new experiences are filtered by the dysfunctional schemas in such a way that new experiences support existing dysfunctional beliefs and behavior patterns. Young (1990) has argued vociferously for a 'fourth level of cognition' to be added to this cognitive model of Beck, namely early maladaptive schemas (EMS). These are stable and enduring patterns of thinking and perception that begin early in life and are continually elaborated. EMS are unconditional beliefs linked together to form a core of an individual's self-image. Challenge threatens the core identity, which is defended with alacrity, guile, and yet desperation, as activation of the schemas may evoke aversive emotions. The EMS gives rise to 'schema coping behavior', which is the best adaptation to living that the borderline has found. These schemas are different conceptually from some of those discussed by Beck, which are not unconditional beliefs about the self. Beck refers to core beliefs and conditional beliefs, both of which are labeled schemas (Young, 1990). Core beliefs are more like EMS but conditional beliefs require an additional context to become active—'if he gets close to me he will find out how awful I am and then reject me'.

Safran and Segal (1990) have integrated schemas within an interpersonal context arguing that the impact of an individual's beliefs and schemas is not purely cognitive but interacts with interpersonal behavior, which in turn has a reciprocal effect on beliefs. Thus the person is seen as being in a state of dynamic balance to the extent of provoking responses from others that perpetuate underlying assumptions. The borderline patient holds poorly integrated views of relationships with early caregivers and has extreme and unrealistic expectations that determine both behavior and emotional response. This is exacerbated by problems of identity and a fragile identity leads to a lack of clear and consistent goals and results in poorly co-ordinated actions, badly controlled impulses, and unsustained achievement. Relationships become an attempt to establish a stable identity through dependency, assertiveness, and control. From this viewpoint cognitive therapy is more than just changing assumptions. It becomes much more complex, lasts longer, and requires new techniques. The therapist cannot rely on modifying beliefs through review of evidence that contradicts maladaptive or negative conclusions. Borderlines cannot be argued out of their beliefs especially when they are dissonant with their affects. This has been recognized in cognitive-behavioral therapy (CBT) and attempts are made not only to challenge maladaptive beliefs, but also to help the patient to identify, support, and develop alternative schemas.

Dialectical behavior therapy

DBT is often considered as a CBT, although its focus is primarily behavioral, but it is distinct enough to be considered in its own right. DBT is a manualized, comprehensive psychosocial treatment developed specifically for suicidal individuals with BPD. The philosophy, biosocial theory, treatment targets, structure, strategies, and protocols of standard DBT are described in two treatment manuals (Linehan, 1993a,b).

Linehan has posited that the BPD (BPD) develops as a result of a transaction between biologic dysfunction in the emotion regulation system and an 'invalidating environment.' The biological determined dysregulation of the emotion regulating system is characterized by a high sensitivity for emotional stimuli, an intense reaction to even minimal stimuli, and a slow return to baseline, in combination with the incapability to modulate the emotional condition. But studies have shown that borderline patients do not show electrodermal hyporesponsiveness, which would predispose them to stimulus-seeking and dis-inhibited, impulsive behavior (Herpertz et al., 2001) and self-report data and physiological data suggest that the intensity of affective response in BPD is no different from controls (Herpertz et al., 1999). Nevertheless the theory of dysregulation offers a perspective free from implications of manipulation and destructiveness.

Over time, this transaction between emotion vulnerability and the invalidating environment leads to pervasive emotion dysregulation that is so characteristic of BPD. As a result, individuals with BPD frequently have limited learning opportunities to develop interpersonal, self-regulation,

emotion regulation and distress tolerance skills. Furthermore, personal and environmental factors interfere with using the behavioral skills that the individual does possess and often reinforce inappropriate borderline behavior. DBT assumes that people with BPD are not at fault for having these motivational and skills deficits; they are trying their best to cope with life. DBT also assumes that people with BPD must fundamentally give up and replace dysfunctional coping behaviors (e.g., cutting, suicide attempts, abusing drugs, etc.) with functional behaviors. It logically follows that individuals with BPD need help in order to enhance their motivation and skills to develop a life worth living.

Consistent with other behavioral approaches, DBT assumes that all behavior, including dysfunctional behavior, occurs as a result of prior learning or biology. People with BPD learned to react in certain maladaptive ways to stimuli. In order to be able to change maladaptive behaviors, it is necessary to know which factors are controlling the behavior by means of a thorough behavioral assessment of the problem behavior. Following this theoretical view DBT uses a number of core methods in treatment, which are described on p. 298.

Integrative approaches

A number of integrative approaches have been developed over the past few years of which the most promising has been cognitive analytic therapy (CAT) (Ryle, 1997). The central idea of CAT formulation of BPD is that of the reciprocal role template and the procedures that secure it. It is claimed that a model of reciprocal role templates and their relations, known as the PSORM (Procedural Sequence Object Relations Model) is capable of providing a complete account of the symptoms of BPD. 'States' are described that consist of two complementary roles bound by a relationship paradigm. They are composed of attitudes to the self, and the world, which involve constellations of characteristic cognitions drives and emotions. The paired roles: caregiver–care receiver, victimizer–victim, and author–reader are all examples of states. They are learned through experience as blocks of reciprocal role pairs. Thus a child who is chastized by her mother for throwing food on the floor can often be observed to reenact this experience later with a toy and with role's reversed.

Another central CAT principle is that, in social situations, the adoption of one pole of a reciprocal role exerts a pressure on others to reciprocate and adopt a congruent pole. In any situation the role anyone adopts will be conditioned partly by the expectancies created by the situation, partly by their own state but also, to a greater or lesser extent by the roles adopted by other actors in the social setting.

In normal individuals reciprocal roles are numerous and for the most part moderated by three levels of control. Level 1 being the nature and number of the reciprocal roles and their attendant states, level 2 the command and control procedures that govern state transitions, and level 3 being the capacity for conscious self-reflection and conscious accounting for at least some of the other two structures.

In BPD often all three levels are abnormal. At level 1 the reciprocal roles are few in number and stark in nature. So that 'abusing to abused', 'contemptuous to contemptible', 'ideally caring to ideally cared for', and 'abandoning to abandoned' are all too frequently the only states in a borderline patient's reciprocal role repertoire. At level 2, states often switch rapidly following apparently minor 'insults'. This accounts for the very common experience of therapists that patients may suddenly be thrown out by an innocuous comment that the therapist has made. Level 3 disruptions are restrictions of conscious reflection. In Ryle's view these may reflect actual injunctions to secrecy by early caregivers, be the consequence of the jerky progress between states, which combined with state-dependent recall disrupts any hope of sustained reflection or be consequent on trauma-induced dissociation.

Empirical evidence for treatment

Outcome evaluation of psychotherapy of PD is hampered by the lack of specificity in psychological approaches to therapy (Roth and Fonagy, 1996) and it has been have argued that the considerable overlap between psychotherapies compromises the possibility of reaching conclusions concerning relative effectiveness (Goldfried, 1995). In the treatment of BPD, practitioners make complex choices when selecting interventions that take account of both behavioral and dynamic factors. In order to enhance specificity researchers have 'manualized' treatments and developed measures to assess the extent to which therapists are able to follow protocols outlined in these. An additional problem is the heterogeneity in severity of patients who meet criteria for BPD. There is no adequate measure of severity, although it is recognized that severity as a variable has a marked effect on outcome.

Psychodynamic therapy

For many years long-term psychoanalysis or prolonged inpatient admission was the mainstay of psychodynamic treatment of BPD. The approach, particularly inpatient treatment, has been increasingly questioned because of cost-effectiveness and absence of outcome research using randomized controlled designs even though such studies of inpatient treatment may neither be desirable nor feasible. The limited data available on cost suggests that inpatient admission may yield significant savings after completed treatment (Dolan et al., 1996), particularly in the use of criminal justice services in those with forensic histories.

Caution is suggested in ascribing benefits observed to the inpatient treatment itself by a naturalistic 5-year follow-up of individuals receiving inpatient treatment at the Cassel Hospital in London (Rosser et al., 1987). The study showed that, although patients with neurotic pathology, considerable depression, high intelligence, and lack of chronic outpatient history, did well at the end of treatment and over the follow-up period, patients with BPD had a less favorable outcome. Recent research from the same hospital has also suggested that treatment in the community following a shorter hospital treatment phase than usual is more effective than a prolonged hospital stay. Chiesa and Fonagy (2000) assessed the relative effectiveness of three treatment models for a mixed group of PDs: (1) long-term residential treatment using a therapeutic community approach; (2) briefer inpatient treatment followed by community-based dynamic therapy; and (3) general community psychiatric treatment. The results suggest that the brief inpatient therapeutic community treatment followed by outpatient dynamic therapy is more effective than both long-term residential therapeutic community treatment and general psychiatric treatment in the community on most measures, including self-harm, attempted suicide, and readmission rates to general psychiatric admission wards and is more cost-effective (Chiesa et al., 2004). However, this conclusion needs to be confirmed in a randomized study.

Marziali and Monroe-Blum have concentrated on group therapy alone without the additional milieu and social components of therapy. In a randomized controlled trial (Marziali and Monroe-Blum, 1995) they found equivalent results between group and individual therapy, concluding that on cost-effectiveness grounds group therapy is the treatment of choice. But further studies are needed to confirm their findings especially as the treatment offered was less structured than most other treatments and drop-out rates were high. Noncontrolled studies with day hospital stabilization followed by dynamic group therapy alone indicate the utility of the use of groups in BPD (Wilberg et al., 1998).

An uncontrolled study suggests that psychoanalytic psychotherapy based on ideas taken from self-psychology may be useful in BPD. Stevenson and Meares (1992) reported on 48 borderline patients treated with twice-weekly psychoanalytic psychotherapy that focused on a psychology of the self. Significant improvements were observed in the 30 patients who completed the therapy. Subjects made considerable gains in number of episodes of self-harm and violence, time away from work, number and length of hospital admissions, frequency of use of drugs, and self-report index of symptoms. Thirty percent of patients no longer fulfilled the criteria of BPD at the end of treatment. Improvement was maintained over 1 year. Further follow-up at 5 years confirmed the enduring effect of treatment and demonstrated a substantial saving associated with healthcare costs (Stevenson and Meares, 1999). The therapy concentrated early on the development of a therapeutic alliance and a relative or close friend was seen at the start of treatment. Both these factors may account for the low drop-out rate of 16%.

The most recent support for a psychoanalytically based approach has come from a randomized study examining the effectiveness of an attachment based and psychoanalytically oriented partial hospitalization program with standard psychiatric care for patients with BPD (Bateman and Fonagy, 1999, 2001). Understanding BPD as a disorder of the self resulting from a failure of mentalization (see p. 293), treatment interventions in group and individual therapy were organized to increase the reflective capacity of the patient. Thirty-eight patients with diagnosed BPD were allocated randomly to either a partially hospitalized group or to a standard psychiatric care (control) group. Treatment, which included individual and group psychoanalytic psychotherapy, was for a maximum of 18 months. On all outcome measures, including the frequency of suicide attempts and acts of self-harm, the number and duration of inpatient admissions, the use of psychotropic medication, and self-report measures of depression, anxiety, general symptom distress, interpersonal function, and social adjustment, there was significantly greater improvement in those allocated to psychotherapy. The improvement in symptoms and function were delayed by several months but were greatest by the end of treatment at 18 months. In a follow-up study, which was done on an intention-to-treat basis, gains were maintained after a further 18 months indicating that rehabilitative effects were stimulated during the treatment phase, and treatment has been found to be cost-effective (Bateman and Fonagy, 2003).

Studies of TFP are now becoming available and give promising results, although the outcome of a randomized controlled trial comparing TFP, DBT, and supportive psychotherapy is not yet known. In a cohort study (Clarkin et al., 2001) 23 female borderline patients were assessed at baseline and at the end of 12 months of treatment with diagnostic instruments, measures of suicidality, self-injurious behavior, and measures of medical and psychiatric service utilization. Compared with the year prior to treatment, the number of patients who made suicide attempts significantly decreased, as did the medical risk and severity of medical condition following self-injurious behavior. In addition patients during the treatment year had significantly fewer hospitalizations as well as number and days of psychiatric hospitalization compared with the year before. The drop-out rate was 19%.

Dialectical behavior therapy

The focus of DBT research has been on the initial stage of treatment whose aim is to help the patient to achieve behavioral control. Individual therapy in DBT first stage treatment focuses primarily on motivational issues, including the motivation to stay alive and to stay in treatment. Group therapy teaches self-regulation and change skills, and self and other acceptance skills.

In the original study (Linehan et al., 1991) 22 female patients were assigned to DBT and 22 to treatment as usual (TAU). Assessment was carried out during and at the end of therapy, and again after 1 year follow-up (Linehan et al., 1993). Control patients were significantly more likely to make suicide attempts (mean attempts in control and DBT patients, 33.5 and 6.8, respectively), spent significantly longer as inpatients over the year of treatment (mean 38.8 and 8.5 days, respectively), and were significantly more likely to drop out of those therapies they were assigned to (attrition 50% versus 16.7%, respectively). Follow-up was naturalistic, based on the proposition that the morbidity of this group precluded termination of therapy at the end of the experimental period. At 6-month follow-up DBT patients continued to show less parasuicidal behavior than controls, though at 1 year there were no between-group differences. While at 1 year DBT patients had had fewer days in hospital, at the 6-month assessment there were no between-group differences. Overall treatment with DBT for 1 year compared with TAU led to a reduction in the number and severity of suicide attempts and decreased the frequency and length of inpatient admission. However, there were no between-group differences on measures of depression, hopelessness, or reasons for living. Further, there were no differences in medically risky parasuicidal behavior between patients treated with DBT and those in alternative stable therapy suggesting that the stability of treatment may be an important factor in reducing risk.

A Dutch research project investigated standard DBT (Verheul *et al.*, 2002) in 58 women with BPD who were randomly assigned either to 12 months of DBT or TAU using a randomized controlled design. Participants were clinical referrals from both addiction treatment and psychiatric services. Outcome measures included treatment retention, and course of suicidal, self-mutilating, and self-damaging impulsive behaviors. The results showed that DBT resulted in better retention rates and greater reductions of self-mutilating and self-damaging impulsive behaviors than TAU, especially among those with histories of frequent self-mutilation. This suggests that DBT enhances treatment retention, reduces severe dysfunctional behaviors (e.g., parasuicide, substance abuse, and binge eating), and reduce psychiatric hospitalization for both substance using and nonsubstance using BPD patients.

Across studies the effect on levels of depression, hopelessness, and survival and coping beliefs, and overall life satisfaction is inconclusive. Although originally designed for the outpatient treatment of suicidal individuals with BPD, DBT has been applied to many more populations, including comorbid substance dependence and BPD, and juveniles with antisocial behaviors, and in different contexts such as inpatient wards. The studies are discussed in two reviews (Koerner and Dimeff, 2000; Koerner and Linehan, 2000). Barley *et al.* (1993) evaluated the effectiveness of DBT for treatment of BPD in an inpatient setting. They found that during and following implementation of a DBT program there was a significant fall in rates of parasuicide when compared with a period before implementation of DBT. There was no significant difference, however, between the reported rates of parasuicide on the specialized DBT unit and another unit offering the hospital's standard treatment (TAU control). The results suggest that DBT may have made a successful contribution to reducing parasuicide but it is not unique in preventing parasuicidal behavior. Confirming this argument is a study reported by (Springer *et al.*, 1996). These workers randomly assigned personality disordered patients either to a modified DBT program or to a wellness and life-styles group during a short inpatient stay. Patients in both groups improved significantly on most measures and there were no between-group differences.

Conclusions about the effectiveness of DBT as a treatment for the personality itself are premature (Levendusky, 2000; Scheel, 2000; Turner, 2000). It does seem effective for self-harm but no comparison with other potentially effective approaches have yet been reported. In addition, it is not clear which elements of DBT (psychotherapy, skills training, phone consultation, therapist consultation team) make this treatment method effective. Two process studies investigated the process of change in DBT by focusing on the possible influence of validation (Shearin and Linehan, 1992; Linehan and Heard, 1993; Linehan *et al.*, 2002), but results are inconclusive. What we know thus far is that adding a DBT skills training group to ongoing outpatient individual psychotherapy does not seem to enhance treatment outcomes. Given that DBT is described as primarily a skills-training approach (Koerner and Linehan, 1992) this finding indicates that the central skills training component of DBT may not be of primary importance.

Cognitive-behavioral therapy

Davidson and Tyrer (1996), in an open study, used cognitive therapy for the treatment of two Cluster B PDs, namely, ASPD and BPD. They evaluated a brief (10-session) cognitive therapy approach using single-case methodology, which showed improvement in target problems and is now currently being evaluated in a three-center randomized controlled trial. Another small ($n = 34$), randomized controlled trial has recently been carried out using a mixed cognitive therapy and DBT protocol for treating Cluster B personality difficulties and disorders (Evans *et al.*, 1999). Self-harm repeaters with a parasuicide attempt in the preceding 12 months were randomly allocated to Manual Assisted Cognitive Behavior Therapy (MACT) ($n = 18$), and the rest ($n = 16$) to TAU. The rate of suicide acts was lower with MACT (median 0.17/month MACT; 0.37/month TAU; $P = 0.11$) and self-rated depressive symptoms also improved ($P = 0.03$). The treatment

involved a mean of 2.7 sessions and the observed average cost of care was 46% less with MACT ($P = 0.22$). This work has now been tested further in a randomized controlled trial involving five centers comparing MACT plus a self-help manual with TAU for patients who self-harm (Tyrer *et al.*, 2003). Results are disappointing. Four hundred and eighty patients were randomized to MACT or TAU. MACT was given for five sessions with an additional two sessions later if appropriate. TAU varied across centers but consisted of psychiatric follow-up and support. Neither self-harm episodes, nor other psychometric assessment outcomes which included measures of depression and anxiety, showed any convincing differences between MACT and TAU, either at 6 or 12 months. It is possible that a longer period of treatment or greater engagement in face-to-face treatment, were this achievable in routine healthcare settings, would show more favorable results. However, a cost-effectiveness analysis suggested that there is a 90% probability that MACT is more cost-effective than TAU (Byford, 2003), although having BPD actually increased costs (Tyrer *et al.*, 2004).

Integrative psychotherapies

The paucity of robust evidence for the use of CAT in BPD is in contrast to the existence of a large number of single case reports or small uncontrolled series in CAT and to the existence of a large theoretical literature (Margison, 2000). However, Ryle and Golynkina (2000) have reported on 27 patients with BPD treated using CAT and attended a 6-month follow-up, and on 18 who also attended a follow-up at 18 months. All patients were formally diagnosed as suffering from BPD and received CAT according to strictly supervised criteria. At 6-month follow-up 14 patients no longer met formal criteria for BPD but given the instability of the diagnosis this is unlikely to have been a result of treatment itself, and in those who attended at 18 months there was a continuing decline in psychometric scores. These results need confirmation in a randomized trial and a recent comparison of CAT with TAU has suggested little benefit for the addition of CAT (personal communication), although this may be because of the small numbers in the trial.

Key practice principles

All the treatment approaches discussed above have certain common organizational features. They tend to show a high level of structure, to be consistent, to demonstrate theoretical coherence, to take into account the problem of constructive relationships, including the formation of a positive engagement with the therapist and the team, to offer flexibility, to take an individualized approach to care, and to be well-integrated with other services available to the patient. In effect, all treatments function within a similar framework irrespective of their underlying theory and clinical techniques. This unity arises because all therapies need to organize a structure within which therapeutic interventions can be delivered effectively. The characteristic behavioral and mental instability of the borderline patient interferes with this process and all therapies have to manage some specific difficulties within their own model, which include minimizing risk of suicide and self-harm or violence to others, maintaining boundaries of treatment, calming sudden crises and affect storms, and maintaining staff cohesion. In this section we will consider some of the core principles of each therapy in the treatment of BPD and how each approach tackles some of these specific problems. While this section focuses on psychotherapeutic interventions, the clinician needs to keep in mind that medication may offer considerable benefit to borderline patients. The use of medication is well-reviewed by Soloff (1998) and summarized in the APA Guidelines (American Psychiatric Association, 2001).

Psychodynamic therapy

In keeping with all other therapies used in the treatment of BPD there is general agreement that dynamic therapy should be adapted from its pure, traditional form if it is to effect personality change. It is more structured, requires an active, participating therapist (rather than the archetypal passive, unresponsive therapist), may combine individual and group therapy, and commonly agrees treatment priorities with the patient. This is illustrated by TFP. TFP relies on the techniques of clarification, confrontation, and transference interpretation within the evolving relationship between patient and therapist. The primary focus is on the dominant affect-laden themes that emerge in the therapeutic relationship in the here-and-now of the transference. At the beginning of treatment a hierarchy of issues is established: the containment of suicidal and self-destructive behaviors, the various ways of destroying the treatment, and the identification and recapitulation of dominant object relational patterns as they are experienced and expressed in the here-and-now of the transference relationship.

The initial aims in dynamic therapies are to engage the patient in treatment and to develop a 'secure enough' relationship to allow the patients inner representational world to become manifest in the relationship with the therapist. There is a continuum of intervention that moves through affirmation, advice and praise, empathic validation, encouragement to elaborate, and clarification to confrontation and interpretation (Gabbard, 1999). Only interpretation is specific to the psychodynamic approach.

Interpretation involves making conscious something that is unconscious. In order to do so the therapist focuses on the patient's experience of the therapeutic relationship from moment to moment to demonstrate to the patient her repertoire of partial internalized representations of self and other, which are represented in the interaction between patient and therapist. Overall, the goal is the resolution of primitive internalized object relations, that is, the integration of split off parts of the self and significant others into integrated conceptions. In effect the therapist shows the patient that their experience of others is not necessarily how they actually are but is a representation and helps her recognize what is hers and what is not. In doing so the self structure is strengthened and distortions are rectified.

Distortion of representations is challenged or confronted and particular emphasis is placed on defense mechanisms as they operate within the therapeutic relationship. Misrepresentation of self and other representations in BPD arises because of splitting and projective identification in which the therapist himself may be changed emotionally. For dynamic therapists it is important to understand these countertransference feelings as a communication and to analyze the role reversals within the patient and their actualization in the transference between patient and therapist. Constant monitoring of countertransference is a key therapeutic tool in dynamic therapy because of the extensive use of projective identification in BPD and the therapist will be cast as both abuser and abused, rescuer and attacker. He needs to remain equidistant from both if he is to help the patient; to do so he interprets the enforced roles in terms of the patient–therapist relationship, the patients past, and its purpose of stabilizing the self structure.

A patient arrived at his session and immediately said to the therapist 'you don't like me much do you'. Now, it happens that the therapist felt a soft spot for this particular patient and so considered the statement as a projection and asked him where that idea had come from. The patient was unclear so eventually the therapist suggested that perhaps the patient had himself felt some dislike for the therapist and was tending to see in others what was inside himself. The patient dismissed the interpretation by saying 'yeah, whatever but that doesn't help much' and carried on talking. As he talked about his contempt for his partner, the therapist gradually found himself feeling more and more dislike for the patient and somewhat angry during the session as everything he said was rejected. He considered this a development of the earlier projection into projective identification. Further content of the session was about the neglect and physical violence the patient had experienced as a child from his step-father and the therapist felt that he himself was being caste in the role of a nasty step-father so that the patient could feel justified in his dismissal of whatever the therapist said. He suggested to the patient that may be he had to see whatever the therapist said as having little importance just as he had to minimize everyone else's importance, like that of his partner, so that he could feel stable in himself and avoid confronting his own feelings of unimportance.

Containment and confrontation of anger and self-destructiveness is also a core aspect of treatment as aggression and its unmodulated expression is thought to be important as a cause of many of the borderline symptoms. The therapist should not act in the heat of the moment but analyze the underlying causes of outbursts once a crisis is over, linking feelings with actions. The aim is to make unbearable feelings bearable, the bewildering occurrence into an understandable experience, and the undigested trauma of the past into an assimilated event of the present.

Suicide and self-harm

BPD is associated with serious morbidity with nearly 10% of previously hospitalized patients eventually committing suicide and between 60 and 80% engaging in seriously damaging self-injury at some point. Effective treatment must reduce this threat to life and all treatments seek to stabilize suicidal behavior at the beginning of treatment. It is important to distinguish between suicidal acts and those of self-harm. Often they are seen as lying along a continuum but in fact they are behaviors that probably represent different psychological states albeit with some aspects in common.

There is a link between hurting yourself and getting support and treatment. It is hard to resist self-harming behavior when you know if you do it, you will get treatment
DoH (2003)

I bang my head over and over again and don't care about the blood. The more blood the better because it shows that there is something really wrong. People can see the blood but they don't see the pain when it is inside your head.

Self-harm reduces frustrations, is not an attempt to die, and may be increased by the reactions of staff who move rapidly from unconcern to concern thereby reenforcing the behavior or gratifying secondary gain. It is associated with dissociative experiences and patients report the onset of a bewildering feeling that rapidly escalates out of control, becomes unbearable, and is relieved only when cutting takes place. Dynamic therapists explore the underlying meaning to a patient to reduce the compulsion to self-harm. Episodes are placed in the transference relationship and not given undue importance and significance. The patient is encouraged to think about the episode and to talk about it in the next available session. The therapist neither takes over the responsibility of trying to stop the self-harm nor reacts by giving increasing amounts of attention to the patient. Some individuals become addicted to self-harm, integrate it into their lifestyle, and gain pleasure in a secret ritual in which they use razor blades to cut their arm, thighs, or other areas of the body, often carrying razor blades or special knives to provide reassurance wherever they go. This is understood as arising from their own recognition of the fragility of their representations that cannot be 'called forth' at times of anxiety—an Adlerian failure of evocative memory.

Suicide risk is both acute and chronic in borderline patients and can fluctuate rapidly depending on personal circumstances so predicting a lethal attempt in the context of frequent self-destructive behavior can be difficult. Therapists are advised to keep the possibility in mind at all times, to address the possibility in treatment sessions, and to be aware of any concurrent Axis I disorder such as depression, which may increase the risk.

It generally agreed that more acting out incidents occur early in treatment rather than late. Common explanations are that: (1) patients are at their worst when starting treatment; (2) particularly painful conflicts are activated during early phases; and (3) patients 'cool down' when attachment is established and treatment elements (therapist(s), fellow patients, the treatment program) are perceived as selfobjects.

In psychodynamic treatments suicide is considered from a relational and intrapsychic perspective by understanding the interpersonal context in which suicidal acts occur and identifying indicators within the transference relationship that may predict suicide attempts. The individual therapist needs to build up a picture of suicide episodes of not only by itemizing the antecedents and outcome of the episodes but also by identifying the concurrent mental experience at the time and the exact context. Clinicians are familiar with the enormous fear of physical abandonment in borderline patients. This, perhaps more than any other aspect, alerts clinicians to increased risk especially if 'the other', perhaps the therapist, is needed for self-coherence. Patients must be prepared for therapist absences and clear contingencies made if suicide risk increases. Abandonment means the reinternalization of intolerable projections and suicide represents the fantasized destruction of these projected parts within the self. Suicide attempts are often aimed at forestalling the possibility of abandonment; they seem a last ditch attempt at reestablishing a relationship. The child's experience may have been that only something extreme would bring about changes in the adult's behavior, and that their caregivers' used similarly coercive measures to influence their own behavior. This must be avoided in the therapist–patient relationship.

In TFP the therapist is asked to assure himself of his own security (physical, legal, and psychological) by seeing the family and warning of the risks right at the start of treatment. The therapist early in treatment interprets the transference implications of suicide threats in the context of the patient's past history and personality structure. A feature of suicidal acts is considered to be the activation within the patient's mind of an object representation of a sadistic and murderous quality and the complementary activation of a victim representation of that object representation. It is the hatred within the relationship of these internal object representations that leads to suicide and should be interpreted within the relationship to the therapist.

A contract depicting no suicide attempts or outlining a crisis plan may be made but the task of the therapist is to maintain a reflective stance and to provide appropriate support for the patient to access services while ensuring that his responsiveness does not feed into a cycle in which the therapists actions provide gratification to the patient thereby escalating the problem. A self psychological oriented and group-based day treatment program reported by Karterud et al. (Karterud et al., 2003) suggests a high containment function with respect to suicidality and self-harm. This approach applied neither formal contracts nor strict rules with respect to suicidality. Instead the treatment program as a whole was alerted to the significance of perceived selfobject failures and reactions to disappointments and insults were a constant focus of attention. Suicidal despair was a group concern. In a study of 1244 patients (thereof 1010 patients with PD and 356 patients with BPD) only 2% of the patients made any suicide attempt during treatment and only one patient (0.1%) actually committed suicide.

Affective instability and crises

All clinicians recognize that affective instability causes marked problems in treatment. Rapidly shifting emotional states, often triggered by apparently minor incidents, lead to sudden rejection of therapy, increasingly unreasonable demands, refusal to engage in dialog, clinging desperation, and impulsive actions. Within dynamic therapy affective instability is viewed, in part, as secondary to instability of the self so that whenever the self is threatened emotional storms persist until stability of the self is regained. Intervention therefore focuses on helping patients understand their intense emotional reactions in the context of the treatment setting and identifying aspects of interpersonal interaction that have stimulated the feelings. In transference focused work it is necessary to identify the predominant object relations active at the point of rage and to identify aggression that is seen as a problem through its effect on internal representations, which become unstable because of the borderline individual's difficulty in integrating positive and negative representations.

Certain affects are found to be particularly challenging both for patients and therapists for different reasons. These include paranoid and passive aggression, envy, idealization, hate and contempt, sexual attraction, love, and attachment. It is the interpersonal aspects of these affects that make them particularly challenging when they stimulate inappropriate responses in therapists. Situations that arouse them are the most common triggers for the disturbing symptoms of BPD, such as suicidality and self-harm and the therapist has the opportunity to reduce the likelihood of such acts if the emotions are placed in a context that is understandable to the patient.

Dialectical behavior therapy

The core strategies of DBT include: behavioral analysis, solution analysis and solution strategies, skills training (acquisition and strengthening of new skills), insight strategies, contingency management, exposure, cognitive modification, didactical interventions, orienting strategies, and the acquisition and strengthening of commitment. Because it is important that patients

show effective behavior outside the therapy, generalization of new, adaptive behaviors needs to occur. Generalization is aimed at during role-play in the group session, in homework assignments of the skills training and through the phone consultation. DBT differs from pure behavior therapy to the extent that it integrates acceptance-based approaches with cognitive-behavioral change-based procedures. Validation, mindfulness practices, reciprocity, and a focus on the patient–therapist relationship are integrated with basic behavioral procedures of skills training, exposure-based procedures, cognitive modification, contingency management, and problem solving. The concept of dialectics, with its emphasis on synthesis of these polar opposite positions, provides a fresh lens in which to envision treatment possibilities. DBT can be differentiated from other therapies by the systematic use of therapist–patient telephone consultation, and, the emphasis in DBT given to the consultation team, where therapists' capabilities and motivation to treat patients effectively are the focus. In summary, DBT is a multimodel and rather complex and comprehensive treatment strategy that is highly structured.

DBT is operationalized into five stages of treatment, although there is limited literature on treatment beyond stage 2. The goals of treatment for the first stage of DBT treatment are behavioral control, stability, and connection with treatment and care provider. Consistent with other behavioral treatments (Linehan, 1993b), has specified a pragmatic set of hierarchically arranged behavioral targets for this stage: decrease suicidal and other life-threatening behaviors, decrease therapy-interfering behaviors (e.g., not attending or coming late to therapy sessions, falling asleep during sessions, not completing therapy homework assignments), decreasing quality-of-life interfering behaviors (e.g., substance abuse, homelessness, unemployment, etc.), and increasing behavioral skills. Comprehensive DBT treatment for individuals in stage 1 includes five important functions necessary to decrease dysfunctional behaviors, to increase functionality, and to enhance quality of life. These functions include: (1) enhancing behavioral capabilities; (2) improving motivation to change; (3) assuring new capabilities generalize to the natural environment; (4) structuring the environment in the ways essential to support client and therapist capabilities; and (5) enhancing therapist capabilities and motivation to treat patients effectively.

These five functions are addressed within four different standard treatment modes of DBT lasting for 1 year: (1) weekly individual cognitive-behavioral psychotherapy sessions with the primary therapist; (2) weekly skills training groups lasting 2–2.5 hours per session; (3) weekly supervision and consultation meetings for the therapists; and (4) phone consultation, where patients are encouraged to get coaching in the appliance of new effective skills by phoning their primary therapists either during or outside office hours, for in vivo skills coaching to avert crises, facilitate skills generalization, and to repair between-session conflicts or misunderstandings between therapist and client. Individual therapy focuses primarily on motivational issues, including the motivation to stay alive and to stay in treatment. Group therapy teaches self-regulation and change skills, and self and other acceptance skills. Among its central principles is DBT's simultaneous focus on applying both acceptance and validation strategies and change (behavioral) strategies to achieve a synthetic (dialectical) balance in client functioning.

The individual advances to the second stage of treatment once behavioral control is achieved (e.g., when faced with situations that would historically trigger dysfunctional behavior, the individual is successful in applying skillful behavior to solve or withstand the problem rather instead of dysfunctional behavior). The focus during this second stage is emotional experience and processing of trauma from the past. The third stage emphasizes resolving ordinary problems in living (e.g., ordinary happiness and unhappiness). And then there is a fourth stage (transcendence) for those who desire a more meaningful existence. How change in these subsequent stages is brought about remains unclear.

Suicide and self-harm

In the pretreatment phase of DBT a global analysis is made of suicidal behaviors. This is done from a behavioral perspective by assessing the level of seriousness, in what way the suicide attempts take place, are predictive factors distinguishable, and what are the reinforcement contingencies. To some extent DBT elides suicide and self-harm into parasuicide so the treatment strategies are similar.

A suicide protocol is commonly made (what to do when your therapist is not available, who can be reached, what arrangements need to be made), based on an assumption that, although the goal is to prevent hospitalization, it can be needed to cope with a crisis situation. A contract may be set that outlines clearly the role of the patient and the therapist when suicide threats and suicide attempts occur. In DBT the primary objective is to teach patients to manage their own lives via the 'consultation-to-the-patient' principle. Rather than intervening for the patient in solving problems or getting what the patient needs or wants, the therapist teaches and coaches the patient in how to resolve problems and get what she wants and needs. A chain analysis is conducted to clarify the cognitive and emotional responses that led up to suicide attempts, alternative solutions are discussed and nonsuicidal responses are reinforced. Implicit in this approach is a belief in the patient's capabilities to learn to interact effectively. The patient is taught to actively manage the environment and her own emotions and impulses, not to submit passively to it. Yet when patients are feeling suicidal they are instructed to call for problem-solving assistance before anything happens. After a suicide attempt or self-injurious behavior (or even destructive behavior) phone contact is prohibited for 24 hours unless the situation is life threatening. DBT teaches patients how to deal with parasuicidal behavior. Patients are coached *in vivo* in managing parasuicidal behavior and crisis situations through the phone consultation with the individual therapist.

Suicide contracts have been recommended in the treatment of BPD and some clinicians seek the patient's agreement of no self-harm as part of the treatment contract, although it is of dubious value if used as an aid to reduce serious suicidal behavior (Kroll, 2000).

General treatment contracts about attendance are in common use in an attempt to limit drop-out and DBT uses some rigorous contracts about attendance. But clinicians need to be careful. BPD is a condition characterized by fear of rejection and abandonment, seriously chaotic patients find it difficult to attend consistently, and emotional expression tends to be through action. These factors suggest that confronting behavior with behavior is likely to be traumatic rather than therapeutic and the very problems that are the focus of treatment can become the same ones that result in discharge. In DBT patients are discharged from treatment if they fail to attend for 4 consecutive weeks of skills training, which may be a problem as patients who show chaotic life-styles with unstable social circumstances and antisocial traits simply see contract 'rules' as a further example of the authoritarian and coercive regimes that they have experienced either in their early lives or later, for example, when in prison.

Affective instability and crises

Borderline patients become overwhelmed by feeling and are unable to differentiate between different affective states at times of high general arousal. In the case of emotional outbursts that occur in which the patient suddenly explodes and acts, often with the therapist or other person for no obvious reason, the intervention of the therapist will be based on an understanding of the incident. For instance, when the therapist sees the behavior as an expression of 'apparent competence' (one of the dialectical dilemmas) then he will react with validation of the behavior through expressing nurturing towards the patient. When the reaction is interpreted as an expression of fear of abandonment (because the therapist has been away on holiday, or the end of treatment year is near), again validation will occur and an analysis of the fear will take place, followed by a solution analysis. If the outburst is seen as a way of avoiding exposure, validation will accompany renewed experiencing of the feared emotion. In all cases behavioral rehearsal will take place, because the patient needs to learn to express emotions in a different and more effective way. If the patient walks out shouting or just gives a barrage of insults the therapist will wait till the patient returns, or will contact the patient when she does not show up in the next session and invite her to come. Depending on the severity of the insults

made, when the patient returns the therapist will ask for change in behavior and rehearsal or will make clear that here she needs to enhance the motivation of the therapist to continue.

DBT follows the similar principles to those used in suicidal behavior during acute crises. The therapist coaches the patient in answering the question what to do. Because borderline patients often have learned to ask for help in a 'manipulative' way one of the goals in DBT is to teach the patient appropriate help-seeking skills. The use of 'irreverence' and of dialectical strategies is of the utmost importance here. Only when the therapist is convinced that the patient is literally incapable of taking action, for example because of the serious nature of the physical harm done, the therapist will take over.

Cognitive-behavioral therapy

CBT for BPDs differs from standard CBT (Davidson, 2000). Treatment is longer, there is greater emphasis on the therapeutic relationship, a focus on affects in conjunction with core beliefs, encouragement to develop new ways of behaving and thinking, and past history is explored to understand the context in which the core beliefs have developed.

Core beliefs are identified with the patient and are commonly at an extreme: 'I am no good', I am very clever', 'I am special', 'I am worthless', 'Other people cannot be trusted', 'People will abandon me'. Work on the core beliefs is combined with identification of more intricate relationships between affects, cognitions, motivation, and actions. These 'schemas' are elaborated though direct questioning of the patient. A functional analysis is performed considering the affective element, the cognition, and their effect on self-regulation, motivation, and action.

A patient identified that she always felt angry when she didn't get her own way. Underlying this was a belief that 'I should get my own way' or 'People should do what I want'. The need for immediate gratification of her wishes led to poor self-regulation with impulsivity and she had little regard for the consequences. The therapist worked with the patient to develop new schemas, for example by helping the patient ask herself 'why does this person not give me what I want'.

Information that does not fit in with core beliefs is often avoided, ignored, or distorted. Homework tasks such as using a notebook to strengthen new behaviors are given and patients asked to outline evidence for their beliefs in terms of their history and their current life.

A patient stated persistently that she had never been worthy of love saying that her mother had always criticized her, that she was bullied at school, and the teachers never said anything positive about her. On questioning it transpired that there was some evidence historically that she was lovable. Her aunt had cuddled her a lot, she had some close friends at school, and an alternative explanation for her mother's behavior was that she was unhappy not because of the patient but because her husband was constantly drunk. This was outlined by the patient in writing balancing evidence for the old belief against evidence for the new belief. The patient also kept a notebook listing the positive things that she had done during the week. This focused on her social avoidance, which was thought to arise out of her belief that she was unlovable. Between sessions she had spoken to a neighbor and chatted to someone in the supermarket and these actions were positively reinforced.

The focus on cognitive processes is combined with exploration of current relationships and examination of interpersonal difficulties, which may impact on therapy and prevent change. To this extent there is a limited use of transference, although it is not viewed as a repetition of past relationships.

Suicide and self-harm

Few specific strategies for treatment of suicide attempts and self-harm are described in CBT and the techniques are those used to tackle any problem behavior. Decreasing self-destructive behavior and behaviors that cause harm to others is an initial target of treatment and the main strategy is to understand self-harm or suicide attempts though a formulation of problems identifying the relationship between core beliefs and self-harm behaviors. The consequences of self-harm are explored while consistent attention is given to self-nurturing behaviors such as eating appropriately, sleeping, and pleasurable activities. In addition attention is paid to episodes when no self-harm takes place and yet the circumstances were similar in the hope that alternative pathways of managing the impulse can be found. The overall aim is to move the focus from negative cognitions and frustration to awareness of more adaptive coping responses.

Affective instability and crises

Once again affective outbursts are treated within a cognitive frame of identifying core beliefs, linking them to motivations and finding alternative pathways of expression. The patient's ways of coping are reviewed and any important events since the previous session are explored. The interpersonal triggers of affective outbursts or crises are detailed in order to elicit the core beliefs and schemas that were activated and may be driving the emotional volatility.

Integrative approaches: cognitive analytic therapy

CAT is offered for longer when used to treat patients with BPD than is traditional in the treatment of neurotic disorders. Twenty-four rather than 12 sessions are offered and the primary aim is to gain a developmental and social understanding of the patients problem and to share this in a clear, user-friendly way. Understanding is operationalized as defining reciprocal emotional roles that are exacerbated or perpetuated by redundant coping procedures. Many of these may have been effective solutions to childhood distress but are now outdated and inappropriate. These reciprocal roles are viewed as being enacted within the relationship to the therapist and working them through in treatment is at the heart of the therapy. The work is active and shared. Diagrams and outlines of problems are written down and emotional roles are drawn out to become tools for use within and without therapy—the practical manifestation of the PSORM. The axiom is reformulation of problems, recognition, and revision.

The initial sessions involve clarification of difficulties and completion of a psychotherapy file, which asks about typical common problems known as traps, dilemmas, and snags.

> A patient who often became aggressive in intimate relationships explained how she often felt disliked by her partner. When she experienced this she tended to avoid him and he complained that she seemed hostile a lot of the time, which made her feel even more disliked (*trap*). She then seemed to become dismissive and abusive of him on the basis that if she did not he would abuse her and be horrible to her (*dilemma*— she wanted a relationship but could not have it) and in the end she would always capitulate and apologize and blame herself for being unpleasant (*snag*). In being so self-condemning she was never able to consider whether she should leave the relationship because to do so exacerbated her sense of failure and being horrible.

The problems are explored and at around the fourth session the therapist presents the patient with a reformulation. This includes a description of the patients' life, their difficulties, and a formulation of their problems as target problem procedures that become the focus of therapy. This may also be presented as a sequential diagrammatic reformulation (SDR) and the patient is asked to reflect on it and to make modifications until a shared understanding is arrived at. The SDR is a jointly constructed diagram of a patient's interpersonal function that maps the movement of their feelings and resulting behaviors. A key task for the therapist is to avoid colluding with unhelpful aspects of the patients beliefs or being forced into specific interpersonal roles, for example becoming the victim in a victim/victimizer dynamic, an abuser in abuser/abused interaction. The different reciprocal roles and self-states are explored and towards termination the therapist writes a summary letter to the patient giving a realistic estimation of changes, an outline of further work to be done, and positive features on how the patient can be his own therapist. In general, where possible, there is a climate of therapeutic optimism and the patient is asked to write his own letter promoting self-evaluation and outlining his understanding of the achievements and disappointments of therapy.

Suicide and self-harm

No specific interventions for suicide and self-harm are described in CAT in the manual (Ryle, 1997). However, in case examples it is apparent that self-destructive actions are taken into the trajectory of therapy and form a focus for the initial reformulation and the SDR. An understanding of the emotional and relational aspects of suicide attempts may be outlined in a self-states sequential diagram.

> A patient recognized that in one 'self-state' he wanted loyal friendships and mutual care but this led him to feel he was too needy and when he felt demanding he retreated moving to a self-state of being a 'waste of space' in which he felt bad and angry. This led him to want revenge on others because he blamed them for his feelings. Not surprisingly when he enacted these feelings with his friends they avoided him leading to further feelings of hostility. This pathway had culminated in a serious suicide attempt in the past and so was drawn out in diagrammatic form so that both patient and therapist could plot where the patient was at any given time.

Special challenges

Staff responses

Supervision is of considerable importance for practitioners treating borderline patients because of the strong emotional reactions that are evoked. A distinction needs to be made between attitudinal responses to features of borderline patients, such as insatiable demand, and the emotional responses that are evoked as countertransference reactions. The more intensive the treatment and the less structured it is the more likely that problematic transference and countertransference problems will arise. All therapists have a limit to the amount of frustration, hatred, or even desire that they can tolerate without giving in to action even if these feelings are understood as arising because of the patient experiencing him as an earlier object relationship. When they are part of unresolved aspects in the therapist or overidentification and empathy with the patient treatment becomes more problematic and boundary violations can occur. It is therefore imperative that therapists obtain adequate support and supervision and are given help in structuring sessions according to the treatment model being used if they are to remain on task. The management of countertransference in borderline patients is extensively reviewed by Gabbard and Wilkinson (1994).

Boundaries

One reason that psychotherapy for BPD tends to be structured and requires supportive supervision is to counter regression in the patient, which when combined with unprocessed countertransference responses can stimulate transgression of patient–therapist boundaries. Regression in BPD remains a topic of debate following the recommendation of early practitioners that it can be therapeutic (Balint, 1968). However, expert opinion now suggests that there is no place for such actions in the treatment of borderline patients and maintenance of physical and therapeutic boundaries is as important for therapists as it is for patients, although if applied too rigorously can become antitherapeutic. A balance needs to be struck that allows some regressive process but not enough to encourage acting-out and destabilization, which in turn can lead to boundary violations.

Boundaries of therapy, for example extending the session by a few minutes, are often crossed initially without the patient or therapist understanding their potential consequences and occur under the guise of having to deal with an immediate problem such as suicidal impulses. In retrospect it can be seen that these apparently innocuous occurrences were the beginning of a slippery slope leading towards catastrophic boundary violations such as a sexual relationship between patient and therapist. In general, therapists need to be alert to any changes in their normal practice or use of techniques that are outside accepted consensus and should always seek a colleague's opinion if in doubt. With the more complex borderline patient it is important that practitioners do not work alone.

Gabbard (2003) describes a miscarriage of psychoanalytic treatment in which a suicidal borderline patient induces a belief in the analyst that only he can save her and as he becomes more frantic about her suicide risk and decides not to admit her to hospital, he agrees to allow her to spend a night at his house. Inevitably this leads to a sexual encounter and yet even though wracked with guilt the analyst continues to believe that 'at least I saved her from suicide'. Gabbard suggests that boundary transgressions such as these are directly related to the mismanagement of aggression and hatred. The analyst is determined to demonstrate that he is completely unlike abusive parents and that he can compensate the patient for her tragic past. In order to do so his analytic posture disavows any connection to an internalized representation of a bad object that torments the aggressor. He has named this 'disidentification with the aggressor' (Gabbard, 1997). While this example is from the literature on dynamic therapy there is no evidence that boundary violations by dynamic therapists are more common than by any other group and it is probable that they write about it more.

Risk, severe suicide risk, and chronic self-destructive behavior

In general borderline patients are a greater risk to themselves than they are to others and it is important to remember that they also are help seeking and therefore tend to let others know about their suicidal impulses. Assessing risk in BPD is a difficult art partly because of the fluctuating nature of symptoms but also as a result of the chronicity of suicidal ideas in many patients. It can be difficult to know when chronic ideas have tipped over into an acute suicidal crisis. All therapists have to be able to manage their own anxiety; anxiety in the patient will generate anxiety in the therapist, which, if uncontained will lead to misjudgment and mismanagement. Therapists need to be aware of factors that increase suicide risk such as previous serious attempts, use of drugs and alcohol, hopelessness, high anxiety, and lack of social support. Consultation with a colleague should occur and reasons for the severity of the suicide risk considered in the light of the prevailing relationship with the therapist. All threats of suicide should be taken seriously and explored within therapy before a decision is taken about structural intervention such as inpatient admission. Overall, it is best to allow a patient to retain responsibility for his own life and to have arranged admission pathways at the outset of therapy. Many patients are able to control their own admission and gradually learn ways of reducing risk without admission. It is at these times clinicians need to work together and to avoid the splits that arise, often with ill-considered apportionment of blame when things go wrong.

A patient had tried to kill himself on a number of occasions by hanging and by cutting his throat. This followed arguments with his mother, which were follow by drinking. He presented himself to the therapist having been drinking stating that he was going to kill himself. The therapist thanked him for coming to let her know because that meant they had a chance to do something about it. They discussed the content of his argument with his mother, which had left the patient feeling more and more angry and misunderstood. Eventually the therapist offered to help the patient admit himself to the ward. The patient agreed but before going to the ward he went out in the evening and started drinking again. When he presented himself to the ward the staff refused to admit him until he had sobered up saying that they were not having patients like him on the ward. He went home and cut his neck severely and was admitted to the general hospital. The following morning the staff phoned the therapist to say that she had not warned them of the level of risk. For her part the therapist felt let down by the inpatient staff and blamed. This split between the professionals needed to 'heal' before the patient could use the inpatient admission usefully.

Chronic self-destructive behavior takes many forms, such as drug binges, excessive promiscuity, shoplifting, self-mutilation, head banging, and should be considered within the therapy itself. It has already been mentioned that many therapists, irrespective of treatment model, set contracts, but the danger is that it then becomes the therapist rather than the patient who wants the patient to stop self-destructive behavior. This may become a countertransference enactment and is unlikely to reduce the behavior. Most clinicians move through a series of interventions that include education about the effects, understanding the triggers both internal and external, and understanding the forces behind the acts. Often chronic compulsive behavior relieves anxiety and distress and so alternative routes for reducing anxiety and emotional turmoil need to be identified.

Violence

Uncontrolled anger is a feature of BPD but violence is uncommon. Nevertheless clinicians need to consider any previous episodes and take that into account in therapy. The therapist must be able to work in safety and if risk is high someone should be outside the door during sessions or the patient seen in a safe environment. Therapists should be alert to any paranoid distortions and the possibility that they can be evoked by therapy particularly when there is an emergence of past memories associated with abuse. In seriously ill patients the therapist should beware of exploring past trauma too early in treatment or challenging core beliefs as the former may mobilize too much affect and the latter be tantamount to telling the patient that his beliefs of what happened are untrue and, implicitly he is a liar. Once a therapeutic alliance has been established these areas may be tentatively discussed.

Anger, impulsivity, and threats or outbursts of violence particularly occur when the individual feels abandoned in relationships. This may include breaks in therapy and so, as in suicidal crises, it is necessary to be sensitive about therapist absence and even to make arrangements for another practitioner to see the patient. Psychoanalytically oriented practitioners understand this in terms of the need of the patient to use others as a vehicle for intolerable self-states. Borderline patients control their relationships through crude manipulation in order to engender a self-image that they feel desperate to disown. They resort to violence at times when the independent mental existence of the other threatens this process of externalization. Dramatic and radical action is taken because the individual is terrorized by the possibility that the coherence of self achieved through control and manipulation will be destroyed by the return of what has been externalized. Clinically, the therapist must ensure that his safety is assured and address the internal terror that drives the impulse to be violent.

Conclusions

There is little doubt that individuals with BPD present a challenge to mental health professionals in terms of effective treatment but there is optimism for the future, especially for psychotherapeutic intervention. No one model is adequate to treat all patients and most therapies show elements in common. One way of interpreting these observations might be that part of the benefit that personality disordered individuals derive from treatment comes through experience of being involved in a carefully considered, well-structured, and coherent interpersonal endeavor. What may be helpful is the internalization of a thoughtfully developed structure, the understanding of the interrelationship of different reliably identifiable components, the causal interdependence of specific ideas and actions, the constructive interactions of professionals, and above all the experience of being the subject of reliable, coherent, and rational thinking. Social and personal experiences such as these are not specific to any treatment modality; however, they are correlates of the level of seriousness and the degree of commitment with which teams of professionals approach the problem of caring for this group who may be argued on empirical grounds to have been deprived of exactly such consideration and commitment during their early development and quite frequently throughout their later life (see review by Zanarini and Frankenburg, 1997).

References

Adler, G. (1985). *Borderline psychopathology and its treatment.* New York: Jason Aronson.

Alford, B. and Beck, A. (1997). *The integrative power of cognitive therapy.* New York: Guilford Press.

American Psychiatric Association. (1994). *Diagnostic and statistical manual of mental disorders (DSM-IV),* 4th edn. Washington, DC: American Psychiatric Association.

American Psychiatric Association. (2001). Practice guideline for the treatment of patients with borderline personality disorder. *American Journal of Psychiatry,* **158**, 1–52.

Balint, M. (1968). *The basic fault: therapeutic aspects of regression*. London: Tavistock.

Barley, W. D., *et al.* (1993). The development of an inpatient cognitive-behavioural treatment programme for borderline personality disorder. *Journal of Personality Disorders*, 7, 232–41.

Baron-Cohen, S., Tager-Flusberg, H., and Cohen, D. J. (2000). *Understanding other minds: perspectives from autism and developmental cognitive neuroscience*. Oxford: Oxford Universtiy Press.

Bartholomew, K., Kwong, M. J., and Hart, S. D. (2001). Attachment. In: W. J. Livesley, ed. *Handbook of personality disorders: theory, research and treatment*, pp. 196–230. New York: Guilford.

Bateman, A. and Fonagy, P. (1999). The effectiveness of partial hospitalization in the treatment of borderline personality disorder—a randomised controlled trial. *American Journal of Psychiatry*, 156, 1563–9.

Bateman, A. W. and Fonagy, P. (2001). Treatment of borderline personality disorder with psychoanalytically oriented partial hospitalisation: an 18-month follow-up. *American Journal of Psychiatry*, 158, 36–42.

Bateman, A. and Fonagy, P. (2003). Health service utilisation costs for borderline personality disorder patients treated with psychoanalytically oriented partial hospitalisation versus general psychiatric care. *American Journal of Psychiatry*, 160, 169–71.

Blackburn, R., *et al.* (1990). Prevalence of personality disorders in a special hospital population. *Journal of Forensic Psychiatry*, 1, 43–52.

Bond, M. P., Paris, J., and Zweig-Frank, H. (1994). Defense styles and borderline personality disorder. *Journal of Personality Disorders*, 8, 28–31.

Bowlby, J. (1969). *Attachment and loss*, Vol. 1: *attachment*. London: Hogarth Press and the Institute of Psycho-Analysis.

Bowlby, J. (1973). *Attachment and loss*, Vol. 2: *separation: anxiety and anger*. London: Hogarth Press and Institute of Psycho-Analysis.

Bowlby, J. (1980). *Attachment and loss*, Vol. 3: *loss: sadness and depression*. London: Hogarth Press and Institute of Psycho-Analysis.

Byford (2003). *Psychological Medicine*.

Chiesa, M. and Fonagy, P. (2000). The Cassel personality disorder study: methodology and treatment effects. *British Journal of Psychiatry*, 176, 485–91.

Chiesa, M., *et al.* (2004) Residential versus community treatment of personality disorder: a comparative study of three treatment programmes.

Clarkin, J. F., *et al.* (2001). The development of a psychodynamic treatment for patients with borderline personality disorder: a preliminary study of behavioural change. *Journal of Personality Disorders*, 15, 487–95.

Davidson, K. (2000). *Cognitive therapy for personality disorders*. Oxford: Butterworth Heinemann.

Davidson, K. and Tyrer, P. (1996). Cognitive therapy for antisocial and borderline personality disorders: single case study series. *British Journal of Clinical Psychology*, 35, 413–29.

Deutsch, H. (1942). Some forms of emotional disturbance and their relationship to schizophrenia. *Psychoanalytic Quarterly*, 11, 301–21.

DoH (2003). *Personality disorder: no longer a diagnosis of exclusion*. London: Department of Health Publications.

Dolan, B. M. and Coid, J. (1993). *Psychopathic and antisocial personality disorders: treatment and research issues*. London: Gaskell.

Dolan, B., *et al.* (1996). Cost-offset following specialist treatment of severe personality disorders. *Psychiatric Bulletin*, 20, 413–17.

Dozier, M., Stovall, K., and Albus, K. (1999). Attachment and psychopathology in adulthood. In: J. Cassidy and P. Haver, ed. *Handbook of Attachment: Theory, research and clinical applications*, pp. 497–519. New York: Guilford.

Evans, K., *et al.* (1999). Manual-assisted cognitive-behaviour therapy (MACT): a randomised controlled trial of a brief intervention with bibliotherapy in the treatment of recurrent deliberate self-harm. *Psychological Medicine*, 29, 19–25.

Fonagy, P. (1991). Thinking about thinking: Some clinical and theoretical considerations in the treatment of a borderline patient. *International Journal of Psycho-Analysis*, 72, 1–18.

Fonagy, P. (1997). Attachment and theory of mind: overlapping constructs? *Association for Child Psychology and Psychiatry Occasional Papers*, 14, 31–40.

Fonagy, P., *et al.* (1995). Attachment, borderline states and the representation of emotions and cognitions in self and other. In: D. Cicchetti and S. S. Toth, ed.

Rochester Symposium on developmental psychopathology: cognition and emotion, pp. 371–414. Rochester, NY: University of Rochester Press.

Fonagy, P., *et al.* (2002). *Affect regulation, mentalisation and the development of the Self*. London: The Other Press.

Fraiberg, S. (1969). Libidinal object constancy and mental representation. *The Psychoanalytic Study of the Child*, 24, 9–47.

Gabbard, G. (1997). Challenges in the analysis of adult patients with histories of childhood sexual abuse. *Canadian Journal of Psychoanalysis*, 5, 1–25.

Gabbard, G. (2003). Miscarriages of psychoanalytic treatment with suicidal patients. *International Journal of Psycho-Analysis*, 84, 249–61.

Gabbard, G. O. (1999). *Psychodynamic psychiatry in clinical practice*, 3rd edn. Washington, DC: American Psychiatric Press.

Gabbard, G. and Wilkinson, S. (1994). *Management of countertransference with borderline patients*. Washington, DC: American Psychiatric Press.

Goldfried, M. R. (1995). *From cognitive-behavior therapy to psychotherapy integration*. New York: Springer.

Grilo, C. M., *et al.* (2001). Internal consistency, intercriterion overlap and diagnostic efficiency of criteria sets for DSM-IV schizotypal, borderline, avoidant and obsessive-compulsive personality disorders. *Acta Psychiatrica Scandinavica*, 104, 264–72.

Gunderson, J. G. (1996). The borderline patient's intolerance of aloneness: insecure attachments and therapist availability. *American Journal of Psychiatry*, 153, 752–8.

Hellinga, G., Van Luyn, B., and Dalewijk, H. (2000). *Personalities. Master clinicians confront the treatment of borderline personality disorder*. Amsterdam: Boom.

Herpertz, S., *et al.* (1999). Affective responsiveness in borderline personality disorder: a psychophysiological approach. *American Journal of Psychiatry*, 156, 1550–6.

Herpertz, S., *et al.* (2001). Emotion in criminal offenders with psychopathy and borderline personality disorder. *Archives of General Psychiatry*, 58, 737–45.

Hoch, P. H. and Polatin, P. (1949). Pseudoneurotic forms of schizophrenia. *Psychiatric Quarterly*, 22, 248–76.

Hofer, M. A. (1995). Hidden regulators: implications for a new understanding of attachment, separation and loss. In: S. Goldberg, R. Muir, and J. Kerr, ed. *Attachment theory: social, developmental, and clinical perspectives*, pp. 203–30. Hillsdale, NJ: The Analytic Press, Inc.

Johnson, J. G., *et al.* (1999). Childhood maltreatment increases risk for personality disorders during early adulthood. *Archives of General Psychiatry*, 56, 600–5.

Karterud, S. (1990). Bion or Kohut: two paradigms of group dynamics? In: B. E. Roth, W. N. Stone, and H. D. Kibel, ed. *The difficult patient in group: group psychotherapy with borderline and narcissistic disorders*. New York: International Universities Press.

Karterud, S., *et al.* (2003). Day treatment of patients with personality disorders: Experiences from a Norwegian treatment research network. *Journal of Personality Disorders*, 17, 243–62.

Kernberg, O. F. (1967). Borderline personality organisation. *Journal of the American Psychoanalytic Association*, 15, 641–85.

Kernberg, O. F. (1975a). *Borderline conditions and pathological narcissism*. New York: Jason Aronson.

Kernberg, O. F. (1975b). A systems approach to priority setting of interventions in groups. *International Journal of Group Psychotherapy*, 25, 251–75.

Kernberg, O. F. (1993). Comprehensive group psychotherapy: paranoiagenesis in organizations. In: H. I. Kaplan and B. I. Sadock, ed. *Comprehensive Text book of psychiatry*. Baltimore, MD: Williams and Wilkins.

Koerner, K. and Dimeff, L. A. (2000). Further data on dialectical behaviour therapy. *Clinical Psychology Science and Practice*, 7, 104–12.

Koerner, K. and Linehan, M. M. (1992). Integrative therapy for borderline personality disorder: dialectical behaviour therapy. In: J. C. G. Norcross, ed. *Handbook of psychotherapy integration*, pp. 433–59. New York: Basic Books.

Koerner, K. and Linehan, M. M. (2000). Research on dialectical behavior therapy for patients with borderline personality disorder. *Psychiatric Clinics of North America*, 23, 151–67.

Kohut, H. (1966). Forms and transformations of narcissism. *Journal of the American Psychoanalytic Association*, 14, 243–72.

Kohut, H. (1971). *The analysis of the Self*. New York: International Universities Press.

Kohut, H. (1977). *The restoration of the Self*. New York: International Universities Press.

Kroll, J. (2000). Use of no-suicide contracts by psychiatrists in Minnesota. *American Journal of Psychiatry*, **157**, 1684–6.

Levendusky, P. (2000). Dialectical behavior therapy: so far so soon. *Clinical Psychology Science and Practice*, **7**, 99–100.

Linehan, M. M. (1993a). *Cognitive-behavioural treatment of borderline personality disorder*. New York: Guilford Press.

Linehan, M. M. (1993b). *The skills training manual for treating borderline personality disorder*. New York: Guilford Press.

Linehan, M. and Heard, H. (1993). Impact of treatment accessibility on clinical course of parasuicidal patients: reply. *Archives of General Psychiatry*, **50**, 157–8.

Linehan, M. M., et al. (1991). Cognitive-behavioural treatment of chronically parasuicidal borderline patients. *Archives of General Psychiatry*, **48**, 1060–64.

Linehan, M. M., Heard, H. L., and Armstrong, H. E. (1993). Naturalistic follow-up of a behavioral treatment for chronically parasuicidal borderline patients. *Archives of General Psychiatry*, **50**, 971–4.

Linehan, M., et al. (2002). Dialectical behavior therapy versus comprehensive validation therapy plus 12-step for the treatment of opioid dependent women meeting criteria for borderline personality disorder. *Drug and Alcohol Dependence*, **67**, 13–26.

Margison, F. (2000). Editorial cognitive analytic therapy: a case study in treatment development. *British Journal of Medical Psychology*, **73**, 145–9.

Marrone, M. (1994). Attachment theory and group analysis. In: D. G. Brown and L. Zinkin, ed. *The psyche and the social world*, pp. 146–62. London: Routledge.

Marziali, E. and Monroe-Blum, H. (1995). An interpersonal approach to group psychotherapy with borderline personality disorder. *Journal of Personality Disorders*, **9**, 179–89.

McGlashan, T. H., Grilo, C. M., Skodol, A. E., et al. (2000). The Collaborative Longitudinal Personality Disorders Study: baseline Axis I/II and II/II diagnostic co-occurrence. *Acta Psychiatr Scand*, **102**, 256–64.

Meins, E., et al. (2001). Rethinking maternal sensitivity: Mothers' comments on infants mental processes predict security of attachment at 12 months. *Journal of Child Psychology and Psychiatry*, **42**, 637–48.

Modell, A. (1963). Primitive object relationships and the predisposition to schizophrenia. *International Journal of Psycho-Analysis*, **44**, 282–92.

Perry, J. C. and Cooper, S. H. (1986). A preliminary report on defenses and conflicts associated with borderline personality disorder. *Journal of the American Psychoanalytic Association*, **34**, 863–93.

Pines, M. (1990). Group analytic psychotherapy and the borderline patient. In: B. E. Roth, H. D. Kibel and W. M. Stone, ed. *The difficult patient in group: group psychotherapy with borderline and narcissistic disorders*, pp. 31–44. Madison, CT: International Universities Press, Inc.

Rosser, R., et al. (1987). Five year follow-up of patients treated with in-patient psychotherapy at the Cassel Hospital for Nervous Diseases. *Journal of the Royal Society of Medicine*, **80**, 549–55.

Roth, A. and Fonagy, P. (1996). *What works for whom? A critical review of psychotherapy research*. New York: Guilford Press.

Ruiter, C. and Greeven, P. (2000). Personality disorders in a Dutch forensic psychiatric sample: convergence of interview and self-report measures. *Journal of Personality Disorders*, **14**, 162–70.

Ryle, A. (1997). *Cognitive analytic therapy and borderline personality disorder: the model and the method*. Chichester: John Wiley and Sons.

Ryle, A. and Golynkina, K. (2000). Effectiveness of time-limited cognitive analytic therapy of borderline personality disorder: factors associated with outcome. *British Journal of Medical Psychology*, **73**, 197–210.

Safran, J. D. and Segal, Z. V. (1990). *Interpersonal process in cognitive therapy*. New York: Basic Books.

Scheel, K. (2000). The empirical basis of dialectical behavior therapy: summary, critique, and implications. *Clinical Psychology Science and Practice*, **7**, 68–86.

Shearin, E. and Linehan, M. M. (1992). Patient–therapist ratings and relationship to progress in dialectical behaviour therapy for borderline personality disorder. *Behaviour Therapy*, **23**, 730–41.

Soloff, P. H. (1998). Algorithms for psychopharmacolgical treatment of personality dimensions: symptom-specific treatments for cognitive-perceptual, affective, and impulsive-behavioural dysregulation. *Bulletin of the Menninger Clinic*, **62**, 195–214.

Springer, T., et al. (1996). A preliminary report of short-term cognitive-behavioral group therapy for inpatients with personality disorders. *Journal of Psychotherapy Practice and Research*, **5**, 57–71.

Sroufe, L. A. (1996). *Emotional development: the organization of emotional life in the early years*. New York: Cambridge University Press.

Stern, A. (1938). Psychoanalytic investigation and therapy in borderline group of neuroses. *Psychoanalytic Quarterly*, **7**, 467–89.

Stevenson, J. and Meares, R. (1992). An outcome study of psychotherapy for patients with borderline personality disorder. *American Journal of Psychiatry*, **149**, 358–62.

Stevenson, J. and Meares, R. (1999). Psychotherapy with borderline patients: II. A preliminary cost benefit study. *Australian and New Zealand Journal of Psychiatry*, **33**, 473–7.

Stolorow, R., Brandchaft, B., and Atwood, G. (1987). *Psychoanalytic treatment: an intersubjective approach*. Hillsdale, NJ: Analytic Press.

Swartz, M., et al. (1990). Estimating the prevalence of borderline personality disorder in the community. *Journal of Personality Disorders*, **4**, 257–72.

Torgersen, S., Kringlen, E., and Cramer, V. (2001). The prevalence of personality disorders in a community sample. *Archives of General Psychiatry*, **58**, 590–6.

Turner, R. (2000). Understanding dialectical behaviour therapy. *Clinical Psychology Science and Practice*, **7**, 95–8.

Tyrer, P. (1999). Borderline personality disorder: a motley diagnosis in need of reform. *Lancet*, **33**, 969–76.

Tyrer, P. (2003). Randomized controlled trial of brief cognitive behaviour therapy versus treatment as usual in recurrent deliberate self-harm: the POPMACT study. *Psychological Medicine*, **33**, 969–76.

Tyrer, P., Thompson, S., Schmidt, U., et al. (2003). Randomized controlled trial of brief cognitive behaviour therapy versus treatment as usual in recurrent deliberate self-harm: the POPMACT study. *Psychological Medicine*, **33**, 969–76.

Tyrer, P., Tom, B., Byford, S., et al. (2004). Differential effects of manual assisted cognitive behaviour therapy in the treatment of recurrent deliberate self-harm and personality disturbance: the POPMACT study. *Journal of Personality Disorders*, **18**, 102–16.

Verheul, R., et al. (2003). Dialectical behaviour therapy for women with borderline personality disorder: 12-month, randomised clinical trial in The Netherlands. *British Journal of Psychiatry*, **182**, 135–40.

Wilberg, T., et al. (1998). Outpatient group psychotherapy: a valuable continuation treatment for patients with borderline personality disorder treated in a day hospital? A 3-year follow-up study. *Nordic Journal of Psychiatry*, **52**, 213–22.

Young, J. E. (1990). *Cognitive therapy for personality disorders: a schema-focused approach*. Sarasota, FL: Professional Resource Exchange.

Zanarini, M. C. and Frankenburg, F. R. (1997). Pathways to the development of borderline personality disorder. *Journal of Personality Disorders*, **11**, 93–104.

Zanarini, M., Gunderson, J. G., and Frankenburg, F. R. (1990). Discriminating borderline personality disorder from other Axis II disorders. *American Journal Psychiatry*, **147**, 161–7.

Zilboorg, G. (1941). Ambulatory schizophrenia. *Psychiatry*, **4**, 149–55.

25 Histrionic personality disorder

Arthur Freeman, Sharon Morgillo Freeman, and Bradley Rosenfield

Introduction

Histrionic personality disorder (HPD) exists along a continuum of severity, as do many other disorders. The presence of traits at one end of the continuum is critically important to the actor depending upon these characteristics to maintain the 'Hollywood' persona, while the person at the far end of the spectrum may resemble someone in a manic or hypomanic phase of bipolar disorder. Persons with a true HPD are lively, dramatic, and often charming in small doses. They crave attention, repeatedly draw the focus of conversation back to themselves, make grand entrances often at inopportune times, and are prone to exaggeration of behavior, emotion, and interpretation.

HPD patients are arousal oriented; they crave stimulation, and often respond to minor stimuli with eruptions of inappropriate laughter or irrational, angry outbursts. Their interpersonal relationships are often severely impaired; they frequently rapidly exhaust their partners with their neediness. Others generally perceive them as shallow, lacking in genuineness, demanding, and overly dependent. Rejection from others may lead to depression and suicidal ideation.

Although this chapter will focus on patients who meet the defining criteria for HPD, the concepts may also be applied to patients who demonstrate histrionic features superimposed upon another disorder, such as borderline or narcissistic personality disorders. This chapter offers models to assist clinicians in understanding the conceptualization cognitive and developing effective treatment strategies.

Background

In the early days of psychoanalytic development in Vienna, Austria, Breuer, Freud, and others conceptualized hysterical reactions as conversion disorders consisting of 'repressed' conflicts that manifested in physiological symptoms of blindness, paralysis, or seizures. Campbell's *psychiatric Dictionary* (1996) offers 24 terms related to the term 'hysteria,' a construct that is the precursor to the contemporary diagnosis of HPD. Campbell's offers the additional explanation for hysterical conversion reactions that includes the need to 'flee into illness when libidinal cathexis exceeds a certain amount' (Campbell, 1996, p. 344). The confounding factor of conversion disorder components of hysteria raises additional questions as to whether hysteria is a symptom, a disease, a personality type, or a pattern of behavior (Slavney, 1990). The only point of agreement to date is that HPD is infinitely more complicated than mere hysterical reaction.

The use of the term 'hysteria' has varied widely over its 4000-year history and has often been a source of controversy (summarized by Veith, 1963; Halleck, 1967). The Ancient Egyptians originally postulated that the womb, when not properly anchored might wander, lodge against other organs, such as the brain, and produce all manner of 'highly emotional symptoms.' By definition, therefore, hysteria became known as a disease specific to women. In the mid-nineteenth century, it was suggested that men could also manifest hysteria, as the result of psychological predispositions and psychosocial stressors (Briquet, 1859).

In studies in hysteria, Freud presented his major 'discovery' of a case of male hysteria; for Freud and the early twentieth century psychoanalytic community, the term hysteria generally referred to conversion disorders rather than a dramatic, excitable, and emotional personality style. As early as 1923, Schneider supplanted the term hysteria with 'attention-seeking' as he believed the latter was more accurate and less morally judgmental. This definition of attention-seeking behavior has become the core criteria for HPD. Histrionic individuals are viewed from a more positive frame as 'enthusiastic,' 'motivating,' and 'exciting.' Attractive individuals with these characteristics may be sought after in their younger years. As they grow older and their physical appeal fades, most adapt to the decreased amount of attention they receive. However, a person with HPD has less flexible ability to adapt to the changes associated with later life and may exhibit frantic, infantile, or indiscriminately immature behaviors in attempt to maintain youthful attention and attractiveness (Millon, 1996). Both males and females with HPD eventually develop a caricaturized facade of femininity or masculinity. This facade has been unwittingly reinforced through the positive or flattering attention of others, which is the life blood of their self-esteem (Horowitz, 1991).

Clinical presentation

The prevalence of HPD has been estimated at 2.1% of the general population with reliable diagnostic criteria and strong construct validity (Nestadt *et al.*, 1990). As is generally the case with personality disorders, people usually do not seek treatment with HPD as their presenting problem; instead they complain of periods of intense dissatisfaction, depression, or anxiety. Common comorbid conditions, in addition to depressive disorders, include the full range of anxiety disorders. These individuals are also vulnerable to substance misuse disorders, the development of somatoform disorders, and eating disorders. Because individuals with this disorder often experience periods of intense dissatisfaction and depression, they are at high risk for making dramatic suicide attempts, placing themselves at risk for accidental completion. In fact, one study found the reason for inpatient admission for 80% of HPD inpatients was related to expressions of suicidality. However, most of the attempts were not life-threatening and had generally occurred after disappointment or anger (A. T. Beck *et al.*, 2003). Owing to their dependence on the attention of other people, they are especially vulnerable to separation anxieties and may seek treatment when they become intensely upset over the breakup of a relationship.

As discussed above, the strongest indication of HPD is an overly dramatic self-presentation. These patients express emotion in an exaggerated or unconvincing manner, as if they are playing a role. In fact, when talking with these patients, the clinician may have a sense of watching a performance rather than a genuine display of emotion. Histrionic patients can appear quite warm, charming, and even seductive; yet their charm begins to seem superficial after a short period of time. This is due in part to their dramatic expression of each issue or problem with equal levels of intensity, and the use of theatrical intonation with dramatic nonverbal gestures and facial expressions. In addition, it may be noted that they present their symptoms, thoughts, and actions as if they were external entities involuntarily imposed upon them. They tend to throw up their hands (literally) and proclaim, 'These things just always seem to be happening to me!'

Histrionic patients often use strong, dramatic words, include much hyperbole in their speech, and have a proclivity for meaningless generalizations.

Persons with this disorder often dress in ways that attract attention, wearing striking or provocative styles in bright colors, exaggerated use of cosmetics, and dramatic use of hair coloring. Not surprisingly, given the desire to maintain a youthful, attractive appearance, some HPD individuals also have eating disorders (Tomotake and Ohmori, 2002).

Gender issues

The patient with HPD is often conceptualized as a female who resembles the woman in *The Perils of Pauline* from silent movie days. She is vain, shallow, self-dramatizing, immature, overly dependent, and selfish. Although less commonly diagnosed in males, this disorder is often associated with homosexuality or theatrical narcissism. These gender differentials may reflect societal expectations rather than true gender differences in the prevalence of the disorder. In fact, it has been suggested that HPD is a distortion of sex roles in general, including extreme presentations of masculinity as well as femininity (Kolb, 1968; MacKinnon and Michaels, 1971; Malmquist, 1971). Research has attempted to determine if HPD is a female variant of male-typed personality disorders, such as antisocial personality disorder, but results thus far are weak and inconsistent (Cale and Lilienfeld, 2002a).

The evolution of histrionic personality disorder through DSM

It is interesting to consider the evolution of hysteria and HPD as diagnoses in the *Diagnostic and Statistical Manual* (DSM). The DSM I (American Psychiatric Association, APA, 1952) differentiated between 'psychoneurotic' hysteria and 'personality trait disturbances' (APA, 1952, pp. 31, 32, and 34). Hysterical neurosis was further delineated into conversion reaction and dissociative reaction as opposed to hysterical personality. The criteria cited for emotionally unstable personality actually most closely resembled the eventual criteria for HPD.

It was not until DSM II that the term histrionic was first used. The criteria for hysterical personality disorder reflected clusters of behaviors and traits characterized by excitability, emotional instability, over-reactivity, and self-dramatization, attention-seeking, and often seductive behavior (APA, 1968, p. 43). Histrionic personality was officially codified with the advent of DSM III, which eliminated the diagnoses of hysteria and hysterical personality. The classification was further refined in DSM III-R (1987) with the elimination of manipulative suicidal attempts, gestures, and threats from HPD to better distinguish it from borderline personality disorder features. Finally, DSM IV (APA, 1994) and the more recent text revision, DSM IV-TR (APA, 2000) retain the criteria of a highly excitable individual who seeks attention, has global impressionistic thinking and emotional reasoning, and whose mood is labile, displaying dramatic crying spells, frightening suicidal gestures, infidelity, or even aggressive behavior.

Psychodynamic theoretical underpinnings

Early dynamic descriptions of disorders that resembled personality disorders of today emphasized unresolved oedipal conflicts as one of the primary determinants of disrupted lifelong behavior patterns. Later dynamic theorists focused on the presence of a more pervasive and primitive disturbance arising during the oral, anal, or trust building stages of development (Halleck, 1967). Other hypotheses involved theories of family triangulation: a high degree of affection from father, and a low degree of affection from mother predisposed a woman to develop oedipal conflicts and resulted in the development of a hysterical personality (Mehlman, 1997). The resultant hysterical female was fixated at the genital level and suffered from a surplus of sexual energy (Reich, 1991). The use of their sexuality was their 'armor' in the service of defending the ego. Early psychoanalysts believed that penis envy, castration anxiety, and failure to resolve the repression of oedipal conflicts generated the hysterical symptoms. Debates continued in the psychoanalytic community as to whether the primary fixation involved in the hysterical personality is oral or phallic in nature (Marmor, 1953). As recently as 1991, several theorists were differentiating between the hysterical personality and another group of 'hysteroids' who use the same behavioral mechanisms but are functioning at pregenital or psychotic levels (Easser and Lesser, 1965).

More recent psychodynamic theorists suggest three subgroups: (1) hysterical character neurosis arising from classic triadic oedipal conflicts; (2) hysterical personality disorder evolving from the initial phallic phase and related to dyadic mother–child concerns; and (3) borderline personality organization with hysterical features, employing more primitive pre-oedipal defenses, more oral than phallic in nature (Baumbacher and Amini, 1980–81). In an attempt to offer a more integrative conceptualization, Horowitz (1991), saw the patterns of the hysterical personality as a function of the individual's style of information processing. The processing is viewed as a function of the individual's schema and lack of a broader behavioral repertoire (Horowitz, 1991). Gabbard (2000), summarized the differences between *hysterical personality disorder* and *HPD*: '. . . persons who have a true hysterical personality disorder may be much more subtly dramatic and exhibitionistic, and their sexuality may be expressed more coyly and engagingly' (p. 520). He further suggests that the individual diagnosed as hysterical as opposed to those diagnosed as histrionic would be more functional by virtue of their more controlled expressions of their disorder (Gabbard, 2000).

Essentially, the psychoanalytic viewpoint today views hysterical patients as being able to assess their behavior more realistically. HPD patients find their active seductiveness as more egosyntonic and they are less able to accurately assess their behavior.

Early factor-analytical research provided some support for the psychodynamic conceptualization of the hysterical personality (Lazare *et al.*, 1970). Traits such as the tendencies to be overly emotional, sexually provocative, exhibitionistic, and egocentric strongly clustered together. Dependency fell into an intermediary position. Unexpectedly, suggestibility and fear of sexuality failed to correlate with these other variables, whereas, aggression, obstinacy, rejection of others, and oral expression did cluster with the hysterical traits (Lazare *et al.*, 1970). The authors concluded that this lent support to the notion that the hysterical personality reflected a more primitive conflict than the HPD as described by Kernberg in 1967.

Cognitive therapy formulation

A basic premise of cognitive therapy is that events are filtered through maladaptive schema, or hypothetical structures in the mind, which give rise to dysfunctional beliefs and automatic thoughts that are distorted in some predictable manner. These thoughts are presumably the precipitant of negative affective states, including sadness, anxiety, and anger. Therefore, as premised by Epictetus thousands of years ago, a situation in of itself is neither good nor bad, right nor wrong; one's perception and interpretation of the situation, however, makes it so.

Schemas govern information processing by serving as filters through which incoming information is perceived. Schemas influence what one attends to. Patients with personality disorders in particular selectively attend to information that fits with their beliefs and discount or selectively ignore information inconsistent with the same beliefs. Their interpretation of events is particularly impaired because they have significant difficulty employing metacognitive strategies to evaluate the validity of their perceptions. Others' statements and behaviors may be grossly misperceived and may go uncorrected. For example, the boyfriend of an HPD patient said, 'I need some time this weekend to get some stuff done.' The patient interpreted this statement as meaning, 'I have found someone prettier and I'm rejecting and abandoning you.'

Core beliefs about the self, world, and others may stem from early interactions in the family of origin; children glean such ideas from their parents, siblings, peers, and significant others. Beliefs are affected by early attachment and individuation difficulties. Individuals, who may have a genetic tendency toward developing histrionic traits, acquire a number of powerful, compelling dysfunctional beliefs about sexuality, masculinity, femininity, and relationships. They begin to believe that they are (and must be) exciting/excited and the center of attention. They also begin to focus unduly, and respond dysfunctionally to internal emotional events.

Millon (1981) and Millon and Davis (1996) have presented a biosocial learning theory view of personality disorders and HPD in particular. The HPD is viewed as 'The Gregarious Pattern'. The individual with HPD craves affection, attention, and the approval of others. It is not simply 'nice to be noticed,' but rather a critical component of social interaction with high focus on shifting the attention of others to themselves. Initially, others may be drawn to the HPD individual. The positive attention and affection by others is often fleeting, though, as others may quickly perceive them to be demanding, capricious, disingenuous, and dependent. Moreover, their labile affect is often perceived as insincere, exaggerated, and shallow (A. T. Beck et al., 1990).

HPD patients are typically hypervigilant for signs of rejection or disapproval, which others may or may not have actually intended or transmitted. They perceive withdrawal or uninterest as disastrous, and react with a great deal of distress. They respond to this internally driven crisis with behavioral escalation, making increasingly frantic efforts to invite or seduce others to notice and approve of them—and/or rapidly disintegrating into despair and hurt, along with righteous indignation at the perceived snub, alienating others and evoking true rejection. The activation of their schema 'I must be noticed' is most likely outside of their conscious awareness. It is the immediate cognitive affective response that is most salient at the moment.

HPD individuals typically have many dysfunctional beliefs: 'I must be noticed and admired to be happy', 'I have to be entertaining, lovable, and interesting'—they seek to be glamorous, impressive, or dramatic because at heart they believe that there is something lacking in or defective about them. This negative view of the self is reflected in their conditional assumption, 'If I can't entertain people, they will abandon me,' 'Unless I captivate people, I am nothing,' 'If others won't take care of me, I'll be helpless.' They also hold dysfunctional beliefs about others: 'People have no right to deny me,' 'If people don't respond to me in the way that I need them to, they are bad,' (A. T. Beck and Freeman, 1990, p. 50). However, because of their characteristic dissatisfaction with any single partner and lack of loyalty having once acquired the attentions of the 'desired' one with whom they had previously believed they simply could not live without, they are soon off flirting with others, leaving their partners feeling confused, frustrated, and angry.

Histrionic individuals are given to global impressionistic thinking, and make the common cognitive distortion of emotional reasoning. A common belief is, 'If I feel hurt, the other person must have intentionally mean to hurt me—and I should punish him.' Thus, simply feeling hurt becomes justification for dramatic behavior. Conversely, a mere smile from a stranger can engender a feeling of warmth that becomes justification for impulsive indiscretion (A. T. Beck et al., 2003). This maladaptive pattern is likely to make histrionic individuals interpersonal relationships rather stormy and unsatisfying. The mere perception that they are unable to attract attention may be sufficient to initiate suicidal or parasuicidal cognitions and behavior.

The overly expressive affect of HPD portrays a superficial gaiety, mirth, and carefree attitude, which belies an ominous undercurrent of anxiety and a pervasive fear of rejection. In addition, hypersensitivity to the perception of rejection leaves the HPD individual prone to extremes of emotional lability. A lifelong fundamental need to elicit attention and affection from others generally produces an individual who is acutely sensitive to the cues and to what they perceive are the feelings and desires of others. Because of their tendency to get bored easily, individuals with HPD may impulsively seek out stimulation with illegal substances and/or alcohol abuse and the type of rash sexual indiscretions that their significant others might find particularly objectionable.

Assessment

Although a dramatic portrayal of the self can serve as useful cues to the presence of HPD, a dramatic style alone certainly does not necessarily indicate that a patient has HPD. It is important to ask for details of the types of activities the patient most enjoys: Does he or she especially enjoy being the center of attention? Does he or she show a craving for activity and excitement? It is crucial to explore interpersonal relationships in depth. Details should be obtained as to how previous relationships started, what happened, and how they ended. Clinicians should be alert for women with overly romantic views of relationships, hoping or expecting that 'Prince Charming' will ride along on his white horse. Do the patients' relationships start out as idyllic and end up as disasters? How stormy are their relationships and how dramatic are the endings? How do they handle anger, fights, and disagreements? The clinician should ask for specific examples and look for signs of dramatic outbursts, temper tantrums, and the manipulative use of anger.

Many of the characteristics of histrionic personality are generally considered to be negative traits and it is certainly not productive to ask people if they are shallow, egocentric, vain, and demanding. However, it may be possible to obtain some relevant material regarding these factors by asking patients how other people tend to view them, or through information obtained directly from significant others or family members. The therapist may ask the patient what complaints other people have made about them, while exploring previous relationships that did not work out. As with any patient, clinicians should inquire about suicidal ideation or threats, and should determine whether there is currently a risk of a suicide. Histrionic patients may demonstrate a dramatic or manipulative quality to the threats or attempts.

Instruments such as the Millon's Multiaxial Clinical Inventory (Millon, Millon and Davis, 1994) or the Structured Clinical Interview for DSM III-R (SCID; Spitzer et al., 1992) can be helpful in diagnosing these patients. However, diagnosis is usually readily obtained with a thorough history taking and additional collateral interview.

The following suggestions for assessing personality disorders were suggested by Jackson (1998):

1. Take a full detailed history, including a mental status exam to rule out organic disorders that mimic personality disorders.

2. Take every precaution to ensure that an Axis I disorder is not generating a pseudopersonality disorder picture (e.g., substance misuse or mania).

3. Arrange for a single interview with a significant other who has known the patient for a period of years. This person should be reliable and know the client very well.

4. Make every effort to focus on the positive. In Adlerian terms this is referred to as determining the 'worthy purpose' of a person's symptoms as well as determining those areas of strength that will serve them in therapy.

Ongoing sessions should be used to further the therapist's understanding of the disorders as well as deepen the comprehension of the person's themes and schema (A. T. Beck et al., 1990).

Some diagnostic signs that may signal the possible presence of Axis II pathology, including HPD, include the following:

1. The patient reports the problem as being pervasive, long-standing, and dysfunctional. A significant other reports, 'Oh, he/she has always done that, since he's a little boy/girl', or the patient may report, 'I've always been this way'.

2. The patient is not compliant with the therapeutic regimen. While this noncompliance (or 'resistance') is common in many clinical problems and for many reasons, ongoing noncompliance should be used as a signal for further exploration of Axis II issues.

3. Therapy seems to have come to a sudden inexplicable stop. The clinician working with the Axis II patient can often help the patient to reduce the problems of anxiety or depression only to be blocked in further therapeutic work by the personality disorder.

4. The patient seems entirely unaware of the effect of their behavior on others. They report the responses of others, but fail to address any provocation or dysfunctional behavior that they might exhibit.

5. There is a question of the motivation of the patient to change. This problem is especially true for those patients who have 'been sent' to therapy by family members or the courts.

6. The patient gives lip service to the therapy and to the importance of change but seems to manage to avoid changing. He or she may exert more energy to avoid or avert changing than it would take to actually follow through with the recommendations.

7. The patients' personality problems appear to be acceptable and natural for them. For example, a depressed patient without an Axis II diagnosis may say, 'I just want to get rid of this depression. I know what it is like to feel good, and I want to feel that way again.' The Axis II patient may see the problems as them, perhaps stating, 'This is how I am' and 'This is who I am' (Freeman and Diefenbeck, 2005).

Case example

'The Baroness'

Robin was a 39-year-old, single, white female who was occasionally employed as a waitress in a local sports bar. Her parents divorced when she was 5 years old. She was an only child. She was referred for a psychological evaluation by her family physician after she had roller-skated into his office in a bikini and tee shirt and burst into tears claiming to be terrible depressed, needing medication, all the while lamenting a recently 'lost love.' Her physician referred Robin for therapy.

Robin breezed into her initial session 35 minutes late. She was tall, in good physical condition, and wore pigtails with shocking pink ribbons that were more appropriate at an earlier stage of her development. As she entered the office she enthusiastically proclaimed. 'I guess you are the one who is going to fix me!' Then, she abruptly burst into tears as she reported living alone for the first time in her life after her recent break up with her latest boyfriend, who had tired of her chronic infidelity. 'What will I do now? I'll just die if I'm alone.' However, almost instantaneously, she brightened and related, 'He just didn't understand that men find me so attractive and I just can't hurt their feelings! I mean, you have to admit I am pretty striking!' Then, she tearfully confided that she had recently contracted genital herpes and dreaded, not the medical consequences, but that the disease would restrict her sexual activity, but only if her partners would have to be made aware of the problem.

Although Robin's father left her and her mother when she was 5 years old, he had visited her monthly, accompanied by a series of what Robin termed 'flashy bimbos' whom she perceived to be competition for her father's attention. 'My Daddy was gorgeous. They could just stick their breasts in his face and he'd fall at their feet. How could he ever see me past them?' Robin attributed her parent's divorce to her mother's fading attractiveness. 'I can't really blame him for leaving her. I mean she really turned into a drudge.'

Robin related a series of relationships with men that began when she was 12 years old. She perceived a pattern wherein she would 'fall madly in love with the perfect guy' usually significantly older than she, until she either found someone who was even more perfect or she was caught cheating on 'Mr Perfect.' 'I feel like I make a truly spiritual connection, like I have met my soul mate. I have to follow my soul don't I?' She related how she had met a member of European royalty while working as a waitress. The gentleman was described as someone who couldn't resist her, proposed at their first meeting, and pronounced her to be 'Baroness' of some place in Europe. 'We stayed together for what seemed like forever.'

She admitted that her most recent break-up had her seriously concerned because of her age and the fact that this was the first time anyone had broken up with her ('And I wasn't even cheating on him!'), rather than the other way around. This was also the first time in her life that she had ever lived alone. Moreover, she was greatly distressed because she believed that her medical status impeded her ability to secure her next partner through the only means she could fathom, seduction. She sobbed. 'This means that I can't ever have another relationship with a man and that I will always be alone.'

Patients such as Robin may very quickly seek the therapist's approval and work to get him or her on her side. They may have more difficulty working with same-sex clinicians if they perceive their therapists as not being able to give them what they believe they need—approval by a member of the opposite sex. They may also see a same sex therapist as a competitor. Patients such as Robin may attempt to forge a special closeness with their therapists, by, for example, asking personal questions, insisting on getting direct 'advice,' asking for special favors. The therapist in this situation interrupted these behaviors each time they presented in the sessions. In addition the use of a female co-therapist on occasion as a 'consultant' was extremely beneficial in that adding the component of trust in a same sex therapist challenged the beliefs from her family of origin regarding the powerlessness and lack of intellectual ability in women.

Cognitive therapy treatment

The structure of cognitive psychotherapy for personality disorder patients is much more complex than the treatment for patients with Axis I disorders alone. Special care must be taken to evaluate and understand the underlying schematic structures as multidimensional forces pressing on the person's cognitive, behavioral, and affective interpretation of any and all stimuli. Suggested modifications of treatment include increased focus on the therapeutic relationship, increased emphasis on developmental events, individualized variations in session structure, and utilization of specialized strategies to alter dysfunctional beliefs and compensatory behavioral strategies (J. Beck, 1998).

The full range of cognitive and behavioral techniques, as outlined by J. Beck (1995) are applicable to HPD patients. In fact, using a variety of techniques will ensure that therapy remains interesting, and therefore important to the person with HPD. As with most of their patients, cognitive therapists help HPD patients collaboratively set incremental, short-term goals, which are meaningful to the patients. Encouraging the patient to write each goal to increase commitment, reduce premature termination, and produce stronger shifts in cognition (Cialdini, 2001). Generated goals are specific, measurable behavioral tasks that serve to challenge maladaptive cognitions while progressively moving the patient closer to their long-term goals (Bordin, 1979; A. T. Beck et al., 2003). Therapists also formulate in their own minds several important goals for them to work toward with their HPD patients: learning to slow down, interrupt their impulsive behavior, and modify their global emotional reasoning style.

At each session, patients and therapists collaboratively set an agenda and orient the session toward helping patients solve their problems. Behavioral skills training and cognitive restructuring are important components of the problem-solving process. A particularly useful technique is behavioral experimentation outside of the therapy office. Using a collaborative style, the therapist and the patient design experiments to test a new behavior or cognitive response. One patient, for example, experimented with trying not to be the center of attention at a party honoring another person—and with the therapist's advanced help, was able to give herself significant credit for acting in this way. HPD patients view these experiments as opportunities to 'act' and to prove that they possess the information and experience required for successful completion. If the experiment is set up correctly, that is with high possibility for a positive outcome, the patient will be excited about the results and want to share their excitement in great detail.

On the other hand, some experiments, especially if they are not well planned, can fail. The HPD patient may express significant emotion toward the therapist, including anger, devastation, and embarrassment. The patient may be quick to say 'I told you so,' and insist that the experience is further evidence of their inadequacy and helplessness. In these situations the therapist must be prepared to use techniques to de-escalate the patient and move forward without responding defensively to the display of emotion and blame from the patient. Indeed, maintaining this stable, reliable, and flexible presence with the patient is one of the most critical techniques involved in their treatment.

It is important for the therapist to use HPD patients' own words when summarizing or reflecting. HPD patients have heightened sensitivity and may perceive approximate statements as uncaring or lacking understanding and may take offense. However, patient wording and examples may not always be in good taste, and if therapists are uncomfortable with this language, they should sensitively address the issue. However, in most cases, it is appropriate and powerful to use the patient's language or metaphors as often as possible.

HPD patients bring the same distorted beliefs that they have about other people to the therapeutic experience. Therefore, therapists must always be aware of a potentially negative potential impact of their own behaviors with the patient. HPD patients may expect their therapists to be as equally impressionistic and intuitive as they are in the treatment, expecting the therapist to 'read their minds' without the patients offering the necessary objective data. They are particularly vulnerable to making false attributions of thoughts, actions, attitudes, and emotions to the therapist because of limited flexibility in their thinking and relating. These patients are frequently very sensitive to the slightest negative nuance or suggestion within the relationship, and they respond quickly and intensely when they perceive a slight, a challenge, a disagreement, or a loss. For example, if a therapist is a few minutes late for a session, the patient may think that the therapist is devaluing her, and she may become quite angry. Therefore it is essential in the process of trust establishment and maintenance that the therapist to monitor themselves and to be alert for patients' negative reactions. When therapists notice that patients have become distressed in the session, it is important for them to elicit patients' thinking and help them test and adaptively respond to it. Therapists can then help patients generalize what they learned from this therapeutic experience to experiences with other people outside of therapy.

Therapists must also be aware of their countertransference. They may feel inclined to unduly 'rescue' their distressed patients and therefore must resist the temptation to inadvertently reinforce the patient's voiced helplessness, childish pleas of incompetence, or highly sexualized style. These behaviors should be sensitively discussed and their associated underlying beliefs elicited and evaluated. It is also helpful to discuss the negative outcomes of other situations where the patient had tried to elicit rescue, parenting, or sexual responses.

Case example

Elaine was a 27-year-old woman who sought therapy for depression. She had legally changed her name to 'Elan', which she thought better suited her approach to life. Her presenting problem was that she stated that she said that she 'simply loved sex' and was 'incredibly promiscuous' and then 'felt very guilty and depressed' about her actions. She would often have sex with three different men in one evening. She reported that she would come home from work and be in her apartment and begin to feel 'jumpy.' This was a signal to go to a bar at about 6:00 p.m., pick a man up and come back to her apartment and have intercourse. She would then tell him that he had to leave before her roommate came home. (She had no roommate.) She would later feel terribly guilty, extremely depressed, and suicidal. She might, however, feel 'jumpy' once or twice more that evening and the scene would repeat itself.

She discussed with her therapist the details of her experiences. Eventually she wanted to 'thank' him for helping her stop her active sexual behavior and offered to have a romantic evening, with dinner and an implication of sex with him. When he asked her what it would mean to her if he accepted her offer, she responded that it would show her that he cared about her and would continue to help her. The therapist helped her recognize that her offer would actually have an opposite effect—he would no longer be able to help her therapeutically. The therapist and the patient worked together to further conceptualize her goals regarding sexual communication and behaviors, as well as the usual consequences that the behaviors resulted in for her. In order to respond in this adaptive way, the therapist had to examine and respond to his own countertransference and develop strategies to deal with it appropriately.

Psychodynamic components of treatment

Psychodynamic treatment goals include the gradual uncovering of the HPD patients' underlying conflicts and the development of insight into the

highly exaggerated behavior. The primary focus of therapy is to 'address the resistance before attempting to interpret the underlying content' (Gabbard, 2000, p. 529). Issues of interpersonal style, family relationships, behavioral repertoire, and schema are brought out by examining current relationship situations and exploring where the patient first learned the behavior described. It has been hypothesized that HPD families of origin are high in control, highly intellectual-cultural, and low in cohesion (Baker et al., 1996). The parents in these families were most likely self-absorbed with difficulty expressing sincere, deep, and genuine emotion. If this hypothesis holds true, uncovering the schema related to the use of superficiality, every 'man' for himself and 'I must be first, needed, etc.' would assist the patient in normalizing their development and choosing a healthier alternative.

The most useful technique for uncovering these schema is the use of Socratic questioning. Using this technique early in therapy acclimates the patient to the style and encourages self-exploration. As the therapy moves forward it is much more powerful for the patient to uncover latent or inactive schema rather than the therapist providing expert intellectual interpretation that actually reinforces the family of origin dynamic. As the patient uncovers their own dynamics the experience increases the feeling of independence, reduces dependent behavior, increases the use of problem-solving skills, reduces impulsive conclusion formation, and reinforces more adaptive thinking.

Transference and countertransference are essential components of treating the HPD patient. A particularly difficult issue is dealing with erotic transference. There are several issues involved in self-monitoring of seductive or erotic countertransference issues: (1) there is the need for therapists to examine, understand, and accept their countertransference; (2) therapists must accept the erotic transference as an important element in treatment; (3) therapists must be able to accept their own sexual reactions and feelings and not exploit the patient; (4) the sexual transference has multiple meanings and each of them must be explored as a potential source of resistance; (5) the transference will be microcosmic of the patient's relationships, both past and present, and clinicians should use this information to explore the use of seduction as a means of communication, protection, and/or avoidance; (6) therapists must be tuned in to their own reactions, and not attribute all sexual feelings as emanating from the patient; and (7) the therapist must use caution when asking the patient to describe sexual situations, being careful that there is a genuine need to know the details; only when it serves to advance the therapy—and not when it is possibly a voyeuristic opportunity (Gabbard, 2000).

Outcome research

There are few randomized controlled trials of psychotherapy for specific personality disorders. A survey of the outcome research literature suggests that most outcome studies have been conducted on samples with different types of personality disorders represented. A recent meta-analysis (Leichsenring and Leibling, 2003) indicated that both dynamic and cognitive behavior therapies are generally effective in treating personality disorders. There are no controlled trials of HPD alone. However, HPD patients were included in a study that randomized 81 patients to an average of 40 sessions of dynamic therapy, brief adaptive therapy, or a waiting-list control (Winston et al., 1994). The patients who received dynamic therapy and brief adaptive therapy, which included some with HPD, improved significantly on all measures compared with waiting-list controls. These gains were maintained at 1.5 years follow-up. Two uncontrolled studies used some behavioral techniques in treating hysteria with some fairly positive results (Kass et al., 1972; Woolson and Swanson, 1972). Individuals with HPD who were being treated with cognitive-behavioral therapy for anxiety disorders responded better than others in the frequency of panic attacks (Turner, 1987; Chambless et al., 1992).

Conclusions

The person with HPD truly suffers from the consequences of their maladaptive perceptions, behaviors, and emotional lability. While these patients desire to have others perceive themselves as friendly, fun-loving, and agreeable, they have a genuine fear of rejection that plays heavy on their psyche and reinforces their desperate attempts to avoid being thought of in a negative light. These patients have a fragile sense of self-esteem that manifests in expressions of helplessness and dependency. Given these feelings of dependency and helplessness, it is imperative that the therapist maintains a collaborative style with the patient but allow them to experience and reinforce their own ability to use adaptive problem-solving techniques. These patients tend to befriend and flatter the therapist and are often difficult when they display a seductive style or make overt sexual advances to the therapist. Therapists must be adept at self-monitoring their countertransference and avoid becoming trapped by the patient into repeating dysfunctional patterns from the family of origin.

As with most patients with personality disorders, these patients generally seek therapy for reasons other than their pervasive personality style, which is seen as egosyntonic. These patients respond well to therapists who are able to maintain a stable, flexible, and dependable therapeutic relationship. The use of techniques, such as behavioral experiments, evaluation of cognitions, Socratic dialog to uncover schema related to family of origin issues, or lessons learned early in life can be very beneficial.

References

American Psychiatric Association. (1952). *Diagnostic and statistical manual of mental disorders*. Washington, DC: American Psychiatric Association.

American Psychiatric Association. (1968). *Diagnostic and statistical manual of mental disorders*, 2nd edn. Washington, DC: American Psychiatric Association.

American Psychiatric Association. (1980). *Diagnostic and statistical manual of mental disorders*, 3rd edn. Washington, DC: American Psychiatric Association.

American Psychiatric Association. (1987). *Diagnostic and statistical manual of mental disorders*, 3rd edn (revised). Washington, DC: American Psychiatric Association.

American Psychiatric Association. (1994). *Diagnostic and statistical manual of mental disorders*, 4th edn. Washington, DC: American Psychiatric Association.

American Psychiatric Association. (2000). *Diagnostic and statistical manual of mental disorders*, 4th edn (text revised). Washington, DC: American Psychiatric Association.

Baker, J. D., Capron, E. W., and Azorlosa, J. (1996). Family environment characteristics of persons with histrionic and dependent personality disorders. *Journal of Personality Disorders*, 10, 82–7.

Baumbacher, G. and Amini, F. (1980–81). The hysterical personality disorder: a proposed clarification of a diagnostic dilemma. *International Journal of Psychoanalytic Psychotherapy*, 8, 501–32.

Beck, A. T., *et al.* (1990). *Cognitive therapy of personality disorder*. New York: Guilford Press.

Beck, A. T., *et al.* (2003). *Cognitive therapy of personality disorder*, 2nd edn. New York: Guilford Press.

Beck, J. S. (1995). *Cognitive therapy: basics and beyond*. New York: Guilford Press.

Beck, J. S. (1998). Complex cognitive therapy treatment for personality disorder patients. *Bulletin of the Menninger Clinic*, 62(2), 170–94.

Bordin, E. S. (1979). The generalizability of the psychoanalytic concept of the working alliance. *Psychotherapy: Theory, Research and Practice*, 16, 252–60.

Briquet, P. (1859). *Trait clinique de therapeutique de l'hysterie*. Paris: J. B. Baillitre.

Cale, E. M. and Lilienfeld, S. O. (2002a). Histrionic personality disorder and antisocial personality disorder: sex-differentiated manifestations of psychopathy? *Journal of Personal Disorders*, 16, 52–72.

Cale, E. M. and Lilienfeld., S. O. (2002b). Sex differences in psychopathy and antisocial personality disorder. A review and integration. *Clinical Psychology Review*, 22, 1179–207.

Campbell, R. J. (1996). *Psychiatric dictionary*, 7th edn. New York: Oxford University Press.

Chambless, D. L., Renneberg, B., Goldstein, A., and Gracely, E. J. (1992). MCMI-diagnosed personality disorders among agoraphobic outpatients: prevalence and relationship to severity and treatment outcome. *Journal of Anxiety Disorders*, 6(3), 193–211.

Cialdini, R. B. (2001). *Influence: science and practice*, 4th edn. Boston: Allyn and Bacon.

Easser, B. R. and Lesser, S. R. (1965). Hysterical personality: a re-evaluation. *Psychoanalytic Quarterly*, 34, 390–415.

Freeman, A. and Diefenbeck, C. (2005). CBT with personality disorders. In: S. Morgillo Freeman and A. Freeman, ed. *Handbook of cognitive behavior therapy in nursing practice*. New York: Springer.

Gabbard, G. O. (2000). *Psychodynamic psychiatry in clinical practice*, 3rd edn. Washington, DC: American Psychiatric Press, Inc.

Halleck, S. L. (1967). Hysterical personality traits: psychological, social, and iatrogenic determinants. *Archives of General Psychiatry*, 16, 750–7. 1967 (p. 4).

Horowitz, M. J., ed. (1991). *Person schemas. In person schemas and maladaptive interpersonal patterns*. Chicago: The University of Chicago Press.

Kass, D. J., Silvers, S. M., and Abrams, G. M. (1972). Behavioral group treatment of hysteria. *Archives of General Psychiatry*, 26, 42–50.

Kernberg, O. F. (1967). Borderline personality organization. *Journal of the American Psychoanalytic Association*, 15, 641–85.

Kolb, L. C. (1968). *Modern clinical psychiatry*, 7th edn. Philadelphia, PA: W. B. Saunders.

Lazare, A., Klerman, G. L., and Armor, D. J. (1970). Oral, obsessive and hysterical personality patterns: replication of factor analysis in an independent sample. *Journal of Psychiatric Research*, 7, 275–90.

Leichsenring, F. and Leibling, E. (2003). The effectiveness of psychodynamic therapy and cognitive behavior therapy in the treatment of personality disorders: a meta-analysis. *American Journal of Psychiatry*, 160, 1223–33.

MacKinnon, R. A. and Michaels, R. (1971). *The psychiatric interview in clinical practice*. Philadelphia, PA: W. B. Saunders.

Malmquist, C. P. (1971). Hysteria in childhood. *Postgraduate Medicine*, 50, 112–17.

Marmor, J. (1953). Orality in the hysterical personality. *Journal of the American Psychoanalytic Association*, 1, 656–75.

Mehlman, E. (1997). Hysterical personality style in women and the manifestation of oedipal issues. *Dissertation Abstracts International: Section B: The Sciences and Engineering*, 57(8B), 5378.

Millon, T. (1981). *Disorders of personality*. New York: John Wiley and Sons.

Millon, T. (1996). *Disorders of personality: DSM-IV and beyond*, 2nd edn. New York: John Wiley and Sons.

Millon, T., Millon, C., and Davis, R. (1994). Millon Clinical Multiaxial Inventory, 3rd edition (MCMI-III). Minneapolis: Pearson Assessment.

Nestadt, G., *et al.* (1990). An epidemiologic study of histrionic personality disorder. *Psychological Medicine*, 20, 413–22.

Slavney, P. (1990). *Perspectives on hysteria*. Baltimore, MD: Johns Hopkins University Press.

Spitzer, R. L., Williams, J. B., Gibbon, M., and First, M. B. (1992). The structural clinical intervierw for DSM-III-R (SCRD): history, rationale, and description. *Archives of General Psychiatry*, 151, 190–4.

Turner, R. M. (1987). The effects of personality disorder diagnosis on the outcome of social anxiety symptom reduction. *Journal of Personality Disorders*, 1, 136–43.

Veith, I. (1963). *Hysteria, the history of a disease*. Chicago: University of Chicago Press.

Winston, A., Laiken, M., and Pollack., J. (1994). Shortterm psychotherapy of personality disorders. *American Journal of Psychiatry*, 151(2), 190–4.

Woolson, A. M. and Swanson, M. G. (1972). The second time around: psychotherapy with the 'hysterical women.' *Psychotherapy: Theory, Research and Practice*, 9, 168–75.

26 Psychotherapy for avoidant personality disorder

Cory F. Newman and Randy Fingerhut

Introduction

The diagnostic category of *avoidant personality disorder* (AvPD) is among those Axis II disorders classified informally as the 'anxious and fearful' subgroup (DSM-IV; American Psychiatric Association, 1994, see Box 26.1 for standardized criteria), and is one of the more prevalent forms of personality pathology (Ekselius *et al.*, 2001; Alden *et al.*, 2002). Patients who meet criteria for this chronic condition typically demonstrate the following characteristics: (1) high vulnerability to feelings of overstimulation; (2) low tolerance for physical and emotional discomfort; (3) great sensitivity to being interpersonally judged, criticized, or rejected; and (4) a propensity for engaging in avoidance behaviors as a chief default strategy when under subjective duress. By extension, persons with AvPD have underdeveloped or underutilized coping skills, as well as a relatively limited scope of life experiences borne of neglected tasks, self-handicapping strategies, and multiple missed opportunities.

Avoidance is an important strategy that has survival value for humans (see Gilbert, 2002). When real dangers are recognized and sidestepped, people reduce their vulnerability to harm, and extend their lives. However, if engaged in excessively, avoidance can limit people's lives in insidious ways. The result is their feeling vaguely dissatisfied, low in self-efficacy, anxious and perhaps dysphoric in benign situations, and having a heightened sense that life is passing them by. To expound, when avoidance is a person's main 'coping' strategy over many years and across many situations, it can

Box 26.1 DSM-IV (APA, 1994) diagnostic criteria for avoidant personality disorder

A pervasive pattern of social inhibition, feelings of inadequacy, and hypersensitivity to negative evaluation, beginning in early adulthood and present in a variety of contexts, as indicated by four (or more) of the following:

1. avoids occupational activities that involve significant interpersonal contact, because of fears of criticism, disapproval, or rejection;

2. is unwilling to get involved with people unless certain of being liked;

3. shows restraint within intimate relationships because of the fear of being shamed or ridiculed;

4. is preoccupied with being criticized or rejected in social situations;

5. is inhibited in new interpersonal situations because of feelings of inadequacy;

6. views self as socially inept, personally unappealing, or inferior to others;

7. is unusually reluctant to take personal risks or to engage in any new activities because they may prove embarrassing.

produce the following consequences (see Newman, 1999), in which AvPD patients:

- Focus excessively on possible risks, and insufficiently on probable rewards. They play it too safe in life, limit their range of experiences, and reduce their amount of trial-and-error learning that would otherwise produce important knowledge and skills with which to navigate life.

- Do not allow themselves to habituate to feared but otherwise safe situations, thus remaining intimidated by situations over which they could develop a sense of mastery if they were to give themselves the chance.

- Miss opportunities to surprise themselves with unexpected successes such as the acceptance of respected others, and accomplishing challenging tasks that have the potential to improve self-esteem and socioeconomic standing.

- Unwittingly deny themselves the kinds of peak experiences that stem from striving, persevering through difficulties and discomfort, overcoming adversity, and ultimately succeeding.

- Become regretful, self-reproachful, and even embittered as they see their lives become consumed with strategies for self-protection at the expense of those for the pursuit of fulfillment and self-actualization.

- Sadly earn the disapproval and disappointment of important others who they have let down due to their avoidance. For example, when a person fails to attend her best friend's opening of her art exhibit owing to 'discomfort with crowds of unfamiliar people,' the avoidant person erodes that friendship by putting her need for self-protection ahead of her ethic of 'being there' to support her friend. Ironically, this brings about the very sort of interpersonal criticism and exclusion the avoidant person fears in the first place—the classic self-fulfilling prophecy.

There has been some discussion as to whether AvPD is a separate disorder from the Axis I generalized social phobia (GSP), or simply a more pronounced or extended version of it (Heimberg, 1996; Reich, 2000; Tillfors *et al.*, 2001). Indeed, the high rates of comorbidity between AvPD and GSP are well documented (e.g., Brown *et al.*, 1995; Tran and Chambless, 1995; Feske *et al.*, 1996; Rettew, 2000), and even more pronounced due to the DSM-IV's de-emphasis of nonsocial factors in the criteria for AvPD. In order to restore a useful distinction between the diagnostic categories of AvPD and GSP, Arntz (1999) suggests a reinstatement of the older conceptualization of AvPD, including such factors as intolerance of strong emotions. Indeed, in this chapter we endeavor to portray AvPD as something more than interpersonal shyness, but rather a more extensive problem of shying away from important subjective experiences (e.g., strong emotions, critical decisions), and opportunities for personal growth.

As with many Axis II disorders, AvPD often coexists with other personality disorders (Alden *et al.*, 2002). In particular, there is a highly significant overlap with dependent personality disorder (DPD), with one study finding 43% of AvPD sufferers also meeting criteria for DPD, and 59% of DPD individuals coming up positive for AvPD (Stuart *et al.*, 1998). There is also evidence that some individuals with AvPD abuse alcohol and other drugs in order to 'self-medicate' their anxiety (Stravynski *et al.*, 1986). In addition to the problem of addiction *per se*, this maladaptive strategy decreases social effectiveness, thus feeding into a vicious cycle that worsens the person's low self-confidence.

Conceptualization of the disorder

Although this section presents an overview of the major psychosocial models for AvPD, it should be acknowledged that there is ample evidence for a genetic component related to the extreme shyness, reserved temperament, and overreactivity to novel stimuli often associated with AvPD (Widiger, 2001). At the same time, the 'nurture' part of the nature–nurture interaction provides us with potentially useful ways in which to understand the development and maintenance of AvPD, as described below.

Psychodynamic-based models

Variations of a conceptual framework within which to understand AvPD have come from writers from a psychodynamic tradition. For example, the marked discomfort and ambivalence that individuals with AvPD experience in navigating close relationships is well captured by the term *anxious attachment* (Bowlby, 1973). The person who is prone to anxious attachments wants to have meaningful interpersonal ties, but simultaneously feels extremely vulnerable to the potential punishment and neglect of important others. Two subtypes of this categorization are the *anxious-avoidant* person and the *anxious-ambivalent* person. Those who are anxious-avoidant seem to correspond to those AvPD patients who demonstrate a pervasive avoidance of situations that stir up significant affect, including relationships and life tasks that require a personal investment. Those AvPD patients who seem to fit the anxious-ambivalent subtype are more likely to be those with comorbid DPD. Such individuals tend to cling to one or more significant others, all the while fearing getting too close lest they be discovered to be unlovable, leading to potential rejection and abandonment.

From a general psychodynamic perspective, persons who demonstrate AvPD are theorized to have had upbringings with primary caregivers who were inconsistent at best, and perhaps absent and/or abusive. Recipients of such treatment at early stages of development do not learn to feel at ease in 'being themselves,' as they believe that their natural behaviors will likely elicit rebuke, withdrawal of love, or other harmful shaming responses. In adulthood, many AvPD persons will be frustrated and self-reproachful as they come to realize that they are too frightened to seek and maintain the sort of relaxed, mutually accepting relationships for which they long. Even if they are fortunate enough to find a caring, accepting, mature partner, the individual with AvPD remains insecure, and the quality of the relationship may suffer.

More recently, Gabbard (2000) has similarly described maladaptive avoidance behavior as a defense mechanism against embarrassment, humiliation, rejection, and failure. Individuals who evince this clinical problem are believed to harbor a great deal of shame, evolving from early developmental interactions. For example, adults with AvPD retrospectively reported perceiving a discouraging home climate, and receiving fewer demonstrations of love and parental pride than their control group counterparts (Arbel and Stravynski, 1991). In a similar vein, Meyer and Carver (2000) reported that their college student sample of avoidant subjects reported a significantly greater incidence of childhood rejection and isolation than control subjects, even when taking current mood level into account as a covariate.

The Core Conflictual Relationship Theme (CCRT) is a defining feature of Luborsky's (1984) supportive-expressive therapy (SE). In this psychodynamic model, AvPD patients tend to have harsh superegos and subsequently project their own unrealistic expectations of themselves on to others. As a result, the AvPD patients wish to be close to others, but view them (and expect them) to be rejecting, and so they withdraw from the start so as to pre-empt the interpersonal harm they anticipate.

Another variation on this conceptualization comes from Benjamin's (1993) Structural Analysis of Social Behavior model (SASB). In her formulation, individuals who later develop AvPD are subject in childhood to relentless control directed toward creating a favorable social image. When such children reveal or demonstrate flaws and mistakes, they are responded to with shunning, humiliation, exclusion, and banishment. This results in the AvPD sufferers' choosing to remain alone rather than take further risks in interacting with others who are expected to judge and reject them. As they go through life, these individuals face an ongoing conflict between their wish for social contact and their extreme sensitivity to humiliation. Thus, they will try to minimize outward signs of disagreement with others, instead 'swallowing' their opinions and feelings. However, the resultant inauthenticity of their interpersonal encounters eventually bring about the very criticisms they fear so much. A mutual cycle of interpersonal blaming and ignoring is created, resulting (in the more severe instances) in paranoid fears of those outside the family (if not inside the family as well).

Millon's model (e.g., Millon and Martinez, 1995) similarly describes dysfunctionally avoidant persons as wanting social acceptance, but being very sensitive to perceived and anticipated social humiliation. They restrain themselves in social interactions, initially thinking that by being inconspicuous they will remain safe. However, as their desires for closeness remain unfulfilled, they no longer feel safe as much as ignored, rejected, and ostracized. Their moods are often characterized by tension, sadness, and a quiet anger (behind the facade of a smile), and they over-rely on 'numbing' and fantasy as defense mechanisms.

Cognitive-behavioral models

An overarching formulation that describes the phenomenon of anxiety disorders in general from a cognitive therapy standpoint is the *risk-resources* model (A. T. Beck *et al.*, 1985). In this framework, individuals who tend to shy away from important tasks and relationships in life are prone to magnify the *risks* of a given situation they must face, while concomitantly minimizing their sense of coping *resources*. For example, a man with AvPD who makes a date with a female neighbor and then fails to show up may have feared that the woman would find him boring and then would tell all her friends. At the same time, he may have ignored the fact that he had already made her laugh in conversation on many occasions, and that he had a number of interesting ideas about how they could spend their time together. Unfortunately, his cognitive exaggeration of the possible pitfalls and his overlooking of his strengths led to his standing up his date—the worst outcome he could have produced in terms of fostering an unfavorable public impression.

The problematic behaviors and emotions of individuals with AvPD are well described in the DSM-IV (APA, 1994). However, the *belief systems* of such persons are informative as well (see A. T. Beck *et al.*, 1990, 2001). Typical beliefs held by AvPD patients include:

♦ 'I cannot tolerate unpleasant feelings.'

♦ 'If people get close to me, they will discover the 'real' me and reject me.'

♦ 'It is better not to do anything than to try something that might fail.'

♦ 'If I ignore a problem, it will go away.'

♦ 'I am socially inept and undesirable in work or social situations.'

♦ 'If I keep my expectations low, I can never be disappointed.'

♦ 'Keeping things to myself is good, but talking things out can only lead to trouble.'

Related to the above, Young (1999) has postulated a series of *early maladaptive schemas* (henceforth to be referred to generically as *schemas*) that are related to the development of rigid, chronic mindsets (and concomitant behavioral sets and emotional patterns) that plague persons with personality disorders. Schemas that are most pertinent to those with AvPD would be *incompetence, unlovability, social undesirability, vulnerability to harm*, and (to a lesser degree perhaps) *lack of individuation*. The above beliefs and related schemas serve to perpetuate the AvPD sufferer's interpretation of the environment as demanding, hazardous, critical, and rejecting, and their own responses as inadequate and potentially shameful. Thus, their chief mode of 'coping' is to steer clear of as many situations as possible that they do not find familiar or comfortable, a strategy that negatively reinforces them by reducing their anxiety and bringing temporary relief. Unfortunately, such persons experience a long-term sense of low self-efficacy that has little chance of being modified naturally, as the individuals with AvPD continue to sidestep life situations that would potentially teach them valuable skills for managing the world of relationships and tasks (love and work). The consequences of this pattern for AvPD patients include a life that is lacking in richness, a mode of operation that is needlessly self-limiting, and a lack of emotionally meaningful relationships.

An additional way to conceptualize the dysfunctional cognitive processing of individuals with AvPD has been described by Newman (1999), who hypothesizes that such persons habitually overestimate and magnify the expected consequences of making errors of *commission*, while grossly minimizing or overlooking altogether the potential hazards of making errors of *omission*. This process is consistent with the AvPD person's typical belief that it is better not to do anything at all than to try something that might fail; 'The AvPD's credo is the antithesis of the wise saying, "Nothing ventured, nothing gained"' (Newman, 1999, p. 60). In a certain sense, this strategy is understandable. Errors of commission can be quite conspicuous, potentially leading to great embarrassment, whereas errors of omission are hidden; it is more difficult to detect the negative consequences of *not* having done something. Indeed, it is the rare patient with AvPD who presents for therapy complaining of 'avoiding too many things as a way of life.' More often, they enter treatment in an effort to reduce their symptoms of anxiety (i.e., their avoidance isn't solving their anxiety problem) and/or to address their vague sense of ennui and dissatisfaction with life. These patients begin to notice that they are 'missing out on something' compared with the people around them who seem to have fuller, richer, more active lives. They also sense that they lack the skills to achieve a more satisfying life, a belief that may in part represent a characteristic cognitive magnification of the negative, but may also be based in fact. Given that pervasive avoidance breeds ineffectiveness through sheer lack of trial-and-error practice, many persons with AvPD cannot suddenly increase their involvement in a range of life activities without committing a slew of mistakes—the very outcome they feared most of all from the very start. This can lead to a sense of being trapped, in that the patients feel unfulfilled if they do not change, but profoundly fearful if they *do* try to change.

On a broader scale, the pace of modern life in Western societies is extremely rapid. Change is ubiquitous and considered synonymous with progress. People are urged to 'keep up with the times' and 'be the first on the block . . .' Unfortunately, people with AvPD do not take kindly to change, as change threatens to make their well-worn strategies for maintaining safety, security, and familiarity obsolete. Thus the personal style of individuals with AvPD is in conflict with the environment. Therapists have to help their AvPD patients improve their confidence and abilities in being proactive, decisive, prompt, and future oriented, all the while tolerating the anxiety that is triggered along the way. The hope is that—all things considered—the patients will achieve more of a sense of accomplishment, contentment, and even excitement in life per unit of anxiety!

Research on treatment for avoidant personality disorder

In evaluating the effectiveness or efficacy of treatments for AvPD, multiple outcome criteria can be used such as: (1) degree of social interaction; (2) levels of anxiety and dysphoria; (3) changes (improvements) in beliefs specific to AvPD; and (4) degree of AvPD symptomatology as per the DSM-IV. Given the overlap between AvPD and GSP, it makes sense to measure patient progress in terms of their social skills and related cognitions and emotions. For example, short-term social skills training combined with cognitive interventions have been found to be effective in increasing the frequency of sociable behavior and decreasing social anxiety in patients with AvPD (Stravynski et al., 1982). Additional behavioral treatments (in both

individual and group modalities) that particularly focus on the AvPD patients' social anxieties and interactional difficulties have had some success as well (Alden, 1989; Stravynski et al., 1989; Renneberg et al., 1990). Interestingly, Stravynski et al. (1994) found that the addition of four *in-vivo* sessions did not enhance the outcome of an otherwise successful course of social skills training; in fact, these additional sessions were associated with a high drop-out rate.

Although the results of studies on social skills approaches (individual and group) to AvPD seem positive, the statistically significant improvements indicated by many of these studies do not necessarily translate into optimally significant clinical improvements (Alden et al., 2002). Thus, many AvPD patients made gains in treatments such as those above, but not necessarily to the point of experiencing a remission of their AvPD, or being indistinguishable from 'normals' (Alden, 1989; Renneberg et al., 1990).

A similar result can be found in the psychodynamic treatment research literature. Barber et al. (1997) found that of those patients who completed their year-long treatment of SE dynamic psychotherapy, 39% still retained their AvPD diagnosis at the end of the program. Nevertheless, the patients (as a group) demonstrated improvements on measures of depression, anxiety, general functioning, and interpersonal problems. This study was a part of a larger project at the University of Pennsylvania that also tested the efficacy of cognitive therapy with AvPD patients, as well as the efficacy of SE and cognitive therapy for obsessive-compulsive personality disorder (OCPD). Although the outcome data from the cognitive therapy modality are unpublished, the preliminary results were promising enough that the authors of the SE treatment study above were intrigued about the question of 'Which treatment suits which sort of patient best?' Thus, Barber and Muenz (1996) retrospectively examined the data from the Treatment for Depression Collaborative Research Program (TDCRP: Shea et al., 1990). The authors found that the manualized form of interpersonal psychotherapy yielded more symptomatic improvement when depressed patients were more obsessive and less avoidant, while cognitive therapy was more effective with increased levels of avoidance and decreased levels of obsessiveness. The authors hypothesize that cognitive therapists may make relatively more demands of AvPD patients to be active in the session, and between sessions (e.g., therapy homework), and that this translates in some instances into more extensive therapeutic changes with this population.

In response to the above work, Strauss (2001) examined the cognitive therapy audiotapes and data set from the aforementioned University of Pennsylvania studies on the treatment of AvPD and OCPD. She hypothesized that a uniformly smooth therapeutic alliance may *not* be the best predictor of favorable outcome, in that the therapy would be 'too easy,' with less of the changes one would expect from a therapeutic experience involving more of a struggle. Indeed, the results indicate a curvilinear relationship between variability in the therapeutic alliance and outcome, suggesting an optimal range of 'stress' between therapist and patient as being most facilitative of change. One may hypothesize that an active, directive, collaborative approach such as cognitive therapy would be most apt to induce this sort of strain in the therapeutic alliance, especially with AvPD patients who are ambivalent about change and the discomfort of actively engaging in the process.

As an illustration of the above, a single case study of cognitive-behavioral therapy for AvPD was published by Coon (1994), who found a marked decrease in Beck Depression Inventory scores from initial session to 3-month follow-up as well as modification of schemas and four of the AvPD criteria met at intake. Treatment had initially focused on goal setting, decision making, problem solving, and identification of automatic thoughts. Later (in sessions 12–22), closer attention was paid to the patient's maladaptive schemas. However, the course of treatment had its hurdles and speedbumps, with the patient missing and canceling some of the early sessions, and having some difficulties with homework and role-playing. The therapist was nonjudgmental, but stayed the course, and helped the patient address his problems in treatment within a cognitive case formulation. The patient became more engaged in treatment, and positive changes accrued and were maintained.

It is important to look at the interpatient differences *within* the diagnostic territory covered by the designation of AvPD, as such differences may account for why some of these patients improve more than others. For example, Alden and Capreol (1993) found that the AvPD subjects demonstrated differences in their interpersonal problems and that these differences influenced their response to treatments. Specifically, 'cold-avoidant' patients who had interpersonal problems related to distrustful behavior (implying a strong 'mistrust' schema) benefited from gradual exposure but not from skills training. By contrast, the 'exploitable-avoidant' patients who experienced problems being coerced and controlled by others (implying strong 'vulnerability to harm' and 'lack of individuation' schemas) benefited from both graduated exposure and skills training, particularly training focused on the development of intimate relationships.

The data seem to indicate that retention of patients with personality disorders in general (and AvPD in particular) for a complete course of treatment is difficult, yet quite important for success. For example, Greenberg and Stravynski (1985) found a link between avoidant patients' fear of ridicule and premature termination. The authors suggest that cognitive interventions should especially target this area of avoidant patients' concern in order to increase the effectiveness of treatment. In a study by Persons *et al.* (1988), more than half of the 70 patients met diagnostic criteria for a personality disorder, and—as a whole—these patients were significantly more likely to drop out of treatment early than their counterparts who did not have an Axis II diagnosis. However, those patients with concomitant personality disorders who succeeded in staying in treatment until completion showed substantial improvements that were statistically equivalent to the patients who did not have personality disorders. Similarly, Sanderson *et al.* (1994) found that those among their sample of patients with generalized anxiety disorder who also had personality disorders tended to leave therapy early. However, those who completed at least a reasonable short-term course of cognitive therapy showed a significant decrease in both anxiety and depressive symptoms. This phenomenon of early drop-out from therapy was dramatically demonstrated in the Barber *et al.* (1997) study, in which only 13 of the original 24 patients being treated for AvPD remained for the entire course of treatment (a year of weekly sessions). It makes sense that persons with avoidant habits who also fear change will have difficulties in staying in treatment. Being able to cope with the demands of therapy may be one of the most important exposures that the AvPD patient can experience on the road to recovery. Later, we will suggest some methods for engaging these patients in the process of treatment.

Therapeutic interventions for avoidant personality disorders

Psychodynamic-based models

The SE approach to AvPD puts great emphasis on giving the patients empathy for their humiliation, embarrassment, and shame surrounding interpersonal situations, and on pointing out how anxieties occurring in the transference with the therapist may provide useful information about similar anxieties in other relationships (Gabbard, 2000). Therapists help their patients explore important etiological and developmental factors pertinent to their expectations for failure, rejection, and loss of nurturance. While some focus is placed on the patient's actual past interactions with primary caregivers, additional attention is paid to the patient's unconscious impulses and fears that have led to avoidant behavior. For example, a patient may harbor an unacknowledged expectation that he will lose control in social situations, revealing primitive feelings that will lead to shame and rejection (e.g., expressing sexual interest in an inappropriate love object), and/or threat of retaliation and harm (e.g., expressing heretofore hidden anger toward a parental figure, such as an employer, mentor, or therapist).

The SE model utilizes a central concept—the Core Conflictual Relationship Theme (CCRT)—to shed light on the patients' interpersonal

style over the course of their development and life (Luborsky, 1984). The AvPD patients' penchant for wanting but fearing the seemingly risky process of getting emotionally close with others is expected to manifest itself in the therapeutic relationship. For example, the patients may respond quietly or with superficial responses (e.g., a giggle) following a heartfelt demonstration of support from the therapist, or may avoid a session out of fear that their otherwise kindhearted therapist will be harshly critical. The therapist focuses the patients' attention on these acts of avoidance in order to show them how their unconscious, automatic responses to relationship situations keep them distant and unengaged, even when the objective situation is relatively safe and secure.

Interestingly, psychodynamic approaches dovetail with cognitive-behavioral methods in emphasizing the importance of patients' gaining exposure to feared situations (Gabbard, 2000). This 'exposure' includes the *in-vivo* work involving the therapeutic relationship, where the AvPD patients may otherwise be hesitant to discuss highly emotional material, to discuss serious topics, to think about planning for the future and making personal changes, and to settle into a comfortable, open, trusting relationship with the therapist.

One of the distinguishing features of the SASB approach (Benjamin, 1993) is its emphasis on the complementary nature of social interactions, and the resultant exacerbations and polarizations in interpersonal behavior that may occur. For example, the therapist may try earnestly to encourage the AvPD person to talk about emotionally powerful material, or engage in everyday activities that involve manageable risks and potentially high rewards (e.g., going out to dinner with friends). The AvPD individual outwardly agrees with these prescriptive interventions, but then retreats and fails to follow through, owing to fears of being overwhelmed with out-of-control emotions, and of being the object of silent, social ostracism, respectively. The therapist then tries more assiduously to move the patient to make the therapeutic changes described above, which is secretly interpreted by the patient as a sign of reproach and excessive demands from the therapist. Again, the patient agrees politely in order to avoid conflict, but then does not discuss meaningful topics or follow through with the treatment plan. The therapist then becomes even more directive, and before long the two parties have unfortunately 'danced' into opposite corners where they have much less of a chance of working together. Once identified, this pattern becomes fodder for in-session discussion of the AvPD patient's typical socio-emotional interactions.

Extrapolating from the findings of Barber and Muenz (1996) and Strauss (2001) above, it may be necessary for the therapist to be moderately directive, and for AvPD patients to have the responsibility of being more goal oriented in order for the patients to move forward in therapy. If the treatment is too unstructured or exploratory without concomitant time limits, the patient's avoidant style may be given too much free reign to play itself out, session after session, thus bogging down the process of change and leading to the loss of much valuable time. It may be necessary for therapists to be more active and confrontive of the patients' avoidance (see Davanloo, 1999). The following, fictitious sample dialog serves as a brief illustration:

Therapist: What was your experience when your husband told you that he 'didn't want to hear another word' about your work stress, and that you should just 'shut up and give it a rest?'

Patient: Well, that's just my husband, you know. He doesn't like to be distracted from his reading in the evening.

Therapist: That's all well and good for him, but I asked you what *your* experience was when he made those comments to you.

Patient: He really has had to put up with my complaining about work for a long time, and he doesn't want to talk about it anymore, because he says I never do anything about it anyway.

Therapist: Do you notice that I asked you twice about *your* experience, but both of your answers focused squarely on your husband? I am interested in hearing about *you*.

Patient: (Nervously laughing) Well, you've had to hear my complaints about work too! I'll bet you're as sick of the topic as my husband is!

Therapist: So now we're talking about me? (pauses and then speaks quietly, with a friendly smile) You seem to be the missing person in all of this. It's as if you don't count. But you *do* count. Yet you're finding it very difficult to talk about *your feelings*. I have some thoughts about what you must be going through, especially because you just laughed in a tense way when you said that I must be as sick of your complaints as your husband is. I heard that. We need to talk about that. What is this whole line of questioning like for you? Can you tell me what *you're* going through, right now? I'm listening.

Cognitive-behavioral models

In some respects, the cognitive-behavioral treatment of AvPD looks very similar to the cognitive-behavioral treatment of GSP, a situation that reflects the conceptual and diagnostic overlap that has been found to exist between these two diagnostic entities (Alden *et al.*, 2002; Reich, 2000). Targets for intervention typically include the patients' inhibited social performance, their aversion to growth-related discomfort, their tendency to engage in marked procrastination, and their expectations for interpersonal censure and rejection, to name a few. Additionally, cognitive-behavioral therapists will assess, highlight, and try to facilitate the modification of the AvPD patients' specific beliefs and related schemas that maladaptively shape their perceptions of themselves and their interactions with others. For example, much attention will be paid to the patients' schemas of incompetence, social defectiveness, and vulnerability to harm (see Young, 1999), as well as such harmful beliefs as, 'If I don't think about a problem it will go away,' and 'If I never try then I can never fail' (cf. A. T. Beck *et al.*, 2001). Interestingly, cognitive therapy also focuses on the patients' avoided emotions (Newman, 1991), and thus bears some similarity to alternative models such as focused-expressive psychotherapy (Daldrup *et al.*, 1988). Imagery techniques are commonly used to heighten affect in the hope that 'hot cognitions' (see Greenberg and Safran, 1984) will be accessed that are most relevant to the patient's problems—emotion-laden thoughts that the patients usually do not notice, acknowledge, or reveal easily.

A cognitive conceptualization of a typical AvPD case often reveals that the patients demonstrate strong approach-avoidance conflicts about closeness with other people, leading to high anxiety, shying away, loneliness, and reduced opportunities to learn social skills. They have a low sense of self-efficacy—reinforced in part by their lack of practice in volunteering for challenging tasks and interpersonal engagement—along with a strong belief that others will punish them for their failures. They compensate for these problems by reducing stimulation and risk (as they see it) as much as possible. They minimize their exposure to social situations, academic/vocational tasks, interesting and novel life experiences, and even their own most important thoughts, emotions, and memories. In short, these patients fail to show up for their own lives (Newman, 1999), and become very dissatisfied with the relatively empty results.

Exposure plus rational responding

A combination of these methods is a central aspect of cognitive-behavioral intervention. Talking about the patient's difficulties is part of the process (e.g., in order to help patients address important issues), but is not considered to be a viable substitute for between-sessions interacting with others, and actively managing important but difficult tasks in everyday life. Thus, *homework* is an essential part of treatment. For example, therapists and AvPD patients can work to identify and document some of the latter's most salient examples of avoidance at home (e.g., procrastinating in writing a paper for school, in paying bills, or in washing the dishes), work (e.g., not answering e-mail memos from a supervisor, or declining a promotion with higher pay but more responsibilities), and personal relationships (e.g., not showing up for a relative's birthday party, or being 'too embarrassed' to say genuinely endearing things to a friend when the situation begged for it). Being able to face these situations and respond proactively is a vital part of the process of 'recovery' from AvPD.

At the same time, AvPD patients are hypothesized to be handicapped by negative beliefs and schemas that make it difficult for them to incorporate new

information of the sort that they would gain by engaging in the situations described above. Thus, even if they succeed in dealing actively with situations they would ordinarily avoid, individuals with AvPD may have cognitive responses that will not likely reinforce their apparent therapeutic successes. For example, they may decide that they were 'lucky' this time, but that they should not push their luck by trying again, that the other people were 'just pretending to be nice,' or that the situation was so stressful that it 'isn't worth trying to do anymore.' These sorts of cognitions need to be identified and modified in order for the AvPD patients' gains to be something more than short-lived aberrations. Thus, even when the patients complete their homework (or otherwise report therapeutic changes between sessions), therapists must ask them what they think of their new behaviors, and how much they believe they are benefiting from such changes. The goal is to help the AvPD patients 'own' the changes, to continue to engage in these new behaviors so that they learn them better, and to learn to focus on the psychological gains of such changes, rather than the concomitant anxiety.

Standard techniques such as thought-monitoring and rational responding via Dysfunctional Thought Records (DTRs: J. S. Beck, 1995) can be used to address the AvPD patients' magnified fears about errors of commission, anticipated consequences of trying to learn new things, social rejection, and the like. Similarly, DTRs and related written methods such as the Core Belief Worksheet (J. S. Beck, 1995) can be used to evaluate the patients' AvPD-related beliefs and schemas directly. In Figure 26.1, a patient uses the Core Belief Worksheet to re-examine his belief that 'It is better to ignore a problem than to dwell on it.'

CORE BELIEF WORKSHEET

Name: Anonymous

Date: Early 21st century

Old core belief: 'It is better to ignore a problem than to dwell on it.'

How much do you believe the old core belief right now? (0–100) 95

What's the most you've believed it this week? (0–100) 98

What's the least you believed it this week? (0–100) 80

New belief: 'Dealing constructively with a problem is the best way to handle it.'

How much do you believe the new belief right now? (0–100) 50

Evidence that contradicts old core beliefs and supports new belief

1) When I started therapy I wanted to quit right away, but I'm actually glad I stayed and worked on some issues.

2) By doing all that difficult work to clear up my credit card problems I'm no longer in danger of having to move to a smaller apartment.

3) The more I shy away from dealing with things, the more my self-confidence gets damaged, until the only thing I have confidence in is my 'skill' in being in denial.

Evidence that seems to support old core belief with reframe

1) I feel relieved if I stop thinking about my problems . . . but then later I feel like a coward, and I still haven't fixed anything.

2) When I dwell on a problem I get depressed . . . but I can *face* a problem without having to *dwell* on it.

3) My parents never dealt with their problems. They were the King and the Queen of Denial. So I'm just copying them. But the whole family suffered for it, and I became the Prince of Denial.

Adapted with permission from Beck, J. S. (1995). *Cognitive therapy: basics and beyond*. Guilford Press.

Fig. 26.1

Graded tasks

In order to manage the anxiety that accompanies therapeutic changes, cognitive-behavioral therapists assist their patients in structuring tasks that are graded from easiest to most challenging. In other words, patients learn that therapy generally does not involve dramatic 'breakthroughs' as much as gradual improvements. Behavioral changes and cognitive changes reinforce each other in a virtuous cycle, and the patient's emotional and interpersonal life improves in the process.

One of the overarching strategies of the cognitive-behavioral therapist is to help individuals with AvPD improve on their areas of weakness and deficit. Owing to their customary low-key behavior, aversion to change, and magnification of risk, AvPD patients often have difficulties with setting and striving toward goals, being decisive, and taking the necessary steps to grow and advance in life. Thus, therapists typically emphasize the importance of AvPD patients learning how to specify personal goals for treatment, identifying the graded steps that are required to achieve them, weighing the pros and cons for various ways of approaching these steps, cognitively and behaviorally rehearsing the enactment of these steps, and making cognitive changes so that inhibitions that might otherwise interfere with goal attainment would be minimized.

Examining the therapeutic alliance

At times, cognitive-behavioral therapists (as their psychodynamic counterparts) will examine the therapeutic alliance in the immediacy of the session. Among the goals are: (1) to access 'hot cognitions;' (2) to address the patients' sense of safety, trust, and confidence in interacting with the therapist; and (3) to highlight the process of patients' communication. For example, a patient may laugh nervously when he acknowledges that he did not follow through on his assignment. Below is a sample dialog that may follow:

Therapist: You're laughing, but I wonder what you're thinking right now.

Patient: (Keeps chuckling, but in a muted way, and looks away).

Therapist: Seriously, what are you thinking right now?

Patient: I'm kind of hopeless (keeps smiling).

Therapist: Not a pleasant thought. Not the thought I would have about you. I don't think that a homework assignment determines whether someone is hopeless or not . . . but do you? Tell me more about your thoughts about yourself.

Patient: (Long pause). This feels a little bit silly. I'm sorry I didn't do the homework. I'll try next time. What's the next agenda item (laughs)?

Therapist: This is really uncomfortable for you. You're practically leaving skid marks trying to get away from this topic . . . or these *topics*. This is not just about homework, which is important, but doesn't determine a person's worth. But this is also about how you view yourself when you have difficulties, and how you expect others—in this case, me—to view you. It's also about what to do when you feel uncomfortable. Do you get to the bottom of the discomfort and try to solve it, or do you try to get away as fast as you can? This isn't silly at all. It's real central stuff for your therapy. Can we talk about this further?

Patient: (Looking downcast). You're not going to let me get away with this, are you?

Therapist: Does it feel like a punishment, or like a criticism?

Patient: I just didn't do the homework. Can we go on to the next subject?

Therapist: (Takes some time to think). What's happening right now is so important I hope we can discuss it. I really want to know how you're feeling and what you're thinking. Even more so, I hope *you* can learn more about what you're thinking and feeling. This is not just about homework. It's about feeling badly about yourself, and expecting that others think badly about you, and then not wanting to think about it at all. If we can talk about this, I think you can get something useful out of the discussion. I'm willing to try and see. How about you?

Role-playing

Another important technique is role-playing, most often involving social situations requiring assertiveness, congeniality, or general conversational skills. Patients with AvPD often need considerable practice in acquiring or reinforcing such skills, and the therapist's office provides a unique opportunity to rehearse these behaviors without the threat of social *faux pas*. Unfortunately, AvPD patients often fear making mistakes in front of their therapists, and may even be sufficiently ashamed that they do not want to do role-plays even if nobody but themselves is around to judge. Thus, AvPD patients frequently decline to take part in role-playing, which becomes a therapeutic issue. After all, the therapy setting (arguably) is a less threatening venue than real-life situations. Thus, if the patients cannot bring themselves to engage in behavioral rehearsal exercises in session, it is unlikely that they will do so in everyday life where it is most important. Therapists cannot force their patients to take part in role-plays, but they can address the latter's fears of failure, and continue to encourage them to try the role-plays a little at a time.

Imagery

Similar to more experiential psychotherapies (e.g., Daldrup *et al.*, 1988), cognitive-behavioral therapists also recognize that persons with AvPD often demonstrate a restricted range of emotions—frequently being superficially humorous, bland, or quietly anxious (and perhaps resentful as well). In other words, the patients are avoiding their emotions as well, and would benefit from expressing them more openly, directly, and constructively in order to increase the immediacy of their interpersonal relationships as well as giving them access to greater degrees of joy and enthusiasm. In order to increase the patients' access to a broader range of meaningful emotions, cognitive-behavioral therapists sometimes employ evocative imagery exercises (Newman, 1991).

For example, a woman who presented with panic attacks and an avoidant personality style admitted that she had never properly grieved for her mother, and that she had tried 'not to think about' her guilt about how poorly she had treated her mother in her final months of life. The imagery intervention that dealt with this involved a relaxation exercise followed by the therapist guiding the patient through an imaginal trip back to her mother's hospice so she could tell her mother that she loved her and to say goodbye. During the exercise, the therapist asked the patient (whose eyes were closed) to imaginally communicate with her mother in a way that would counteract her views of herself as a 'bad daughter.' In the image, the patient was uncharacteristically emotionally demonstrative with her mother, took responsibility for having been absent during her illness, promised to treat her own kids as well as her mother had treated her, and to honor her memory in a loving way, but not with too much guilt. Postintervention debriefing suggested that the 'ocean of emotion' (as the patient described it) helped her to 'really believe' her own promises to her mother in the image. The patient reported a high degree of motivation to improve her life, and to 'be there' for others. Most important, in the coming months, this patient reported that she was not allowing her fear of panic attacks and social interactions to stop her from spending time with friends and family.

Group therapy

Group models of psychotherapy (e.g., Yalom, 1980, 1995) tend to focus more on the process of treatment in the here-and-now of the group session than on the individual etiologies of the group participants. Depending on the theoretical orientation and training of the group leader, the explanations for each group members' AvPD characteristics may focus on such factors as early-life rejection, humiliation, and shaming, schemas of incompetence and social undesirability, magnified sense of risk coupled with minimal confidence in personal resources, and the negative reinforcing value (and life inhibiting results) of avoidance. However, the purpose and function of group therapy is to use the group dynamic to test participants' expectations for negative judgment and rejection, to connect with others in a meaningful way, and to learn interactional skills that can improve interpersonal performance in everyday life. In the meantime, group members learn to tolerate the experience and expression of affect, both within themselves and in front of others.

The group therapy model arguably treats the phenomenon of AvPD as synonymous with GSP. Many groups define themselves as 'social anxiety' groups, but few ever self-label as treating AvPD (for an exception, see Renneberg *et al.*, 1990). In a group therapy model, treatment works because the opportunity for the patients to escape easily from interpersonal situations as soon as they feel anxious is greatly minimized (unless they precipitously drop out of treatment, which is a hazard in treating AvPD across all modalities, as we will touch upon below).

Group therapists (e.g., Yalom, 1995) note that as AvPD patients are fearful of socially demanding situations, they will be difficult to engage in group therapy. More specifically, they may profess to want to join such a group, but may be apt to change their minds and not show up, or drop out quickly. However, their typical problems in interacting can come to the fore quite readily in a group setting, such as when the individual thinks that everyone else in the group (including the therapist) uniformly thinks critically of them. Yalom points out that such patients fail to see others as individuals, each of whom has different preferences, opinions, and styles. Instead, the AvPD patients project their self-denigrating feelings on to all the other group members as if they were a single-minded, critical mob. One of the goals of treatment is to highlight, discredit, and change this projected 'group-think' in favor of actual interactions and authentic communication with others, each one at a time.

One of the unique challenges for the group therapy leader is to resist the temptation to 'fill in the spaces.' In other words, a group of AvPD patients may tend (collectively) to be reticent, passive, and loath to stir up an emotional or otherwise stimulating discussion. Group leaders—especially those who have been trained in a cognitive-behavioral model where being directive is often an asset—may slip into 'didactic mode' at such times, thus depriving the group of its potential to become a dynamic, interactive force among themselves. Although some groups are deliberately structured as psychoeducational in nature, this may not be the optimal approach with AvPD group members who often are all too relieved to sit back and let the therapist teach the class. On the other hand, as we have said, demanding too much role-playing and other forms of exposure to anxiety may precipitate flight from the group. Thus, finding the right balance is very important, and most likely involves building a graded-task methodology into the program.

For example, the lead author once ran an all-male GSP/AvPD group in which its participants first worked on identifying their anxiogenic thoughts in facing social and otherwise demanding situations. Next, the group members took turns practicing social interactions with each other. Finally, the group leader invited a series of female colleagues to come to successive group sessions to engage in role-play scenarios with the men, thus providing a bit of an '*in-vivo*' flavor to the social demand. Though it was sometimes difficult to get each of the patients to take part in these role-plays, not one of the group participants dropped out. However, this positive result is not always the case, as noted below.

Special difficulties in treating avoidant personality disorder

Risk of premature drop-out from therapy

Not surprisingly, persons with avoidant personality characteristics will have an increased tendency to avoid therapy itself. While it is certainly true that engaging in therapy is usually a voluntary activity, and therapists should respect their patients' autonomous choice to be in treatment or not, it is also important to be aware of the maladaptive aspects of AvPD patients' propensity for dropping out of therapy in an untimely way. The following are questions to consider:

◆ Does the patient often say, 'I almost didn't come to today's session' or otherwise express ambivalence about having shown up for the appointment?

◆ Has the patient overtly voiced concerns about the direction of treatment, and/or his or her progress in therapy, or (by contrast) have these thoughts and feelings been kept secret from the therapist?

◆ Did the patient cancel or fail to show up for an appointment directly following a therapy session that the therapist thought signified great progress?

◆ Has the patient planned for termination and/or attended an official, final session, or has he or she simply failed to show up for an appointment, and failed to return follow-up calls and letter(s) from the therapist?

In general, therapists should not blithely assume that their AvPD patients will keep their next appointment, at least not while their avoidant characteristics are still markedly active. It is wise to consider the likelihood that such patients have one foot in and one foot out of therapy at any given time during the therapeutic venture. Thus, therapists should take special care to ask their AvPD patients for feedback—about how they feel at the end of each session, how therapy is progressing in their view and how it compares with what they expected, and whether they have any doubts or misgivings about continuing. Sometimes patients are not willing to voice their complaints or problems with therapy, and thus give their therapists the superficial response, 'Everything is fine.' Still, it is worth putting out feelers of this sort, thus giving the patients overt permission to address their mixed emotions about being in treatment.

Following a particularly arduous session with an AvPD patient—the sort that might cause sufficient discomfort to dissuade him or her from returning—therapists may choose to touch base with the patient via a short phone contact. The following is a sample voicemail message that a therapist can leave so as to support the continuation of the therapeutic relationship:

> *Therapist* (phone message to patient): Hi Mr Q, this is Dr F I was thinking about our most recent meeting and how it was very stressful, but that you did some excellent work. I really look forward to continuing our discussion next Tuesday at 2:00 p.m. as we agreed. I just wanted to check in with you to let you know that I truly appreciate the effort you are making, and that I know it's going to pay off for you. Take care and I'll see you real soon.

Cognitive avoidance in session, and resultant therapist frustration

Even when AvPD patients reliably show up for their therapy sessions, it may sometimes seem that they are not really attending to what is going on. They may appear distracted or disengaged, and have relatively little to say. Therapists notice that this phenomenon is occurring when they feel as if they have to 'pull teeth' to get the patients to contribute to the therapeutic agenda and dialog, or are met with the ubiquitous answer, 'I don't know' in response to their clinical queries. Therapists can become quite frustrated with patients who respond in this way, believing that their AvPD patients are painfully lacking in insight, or are engaging in deliberate stonewalling. The hazard in such situations is that the therapists' behavior will go to one extreme or the other—either becoming too quiet and passive, allowing the sort of uncomfortable silences that the patient may interpret as rejection and punishment, or escalating the questioning to the point of sounding like an interrogator. Either way, the therapeutic alliance (such as it is) will likely be strained, thus offering 'confirmation' to the AvPD patients that they will be judged harshly if they allow themselves to be present in a conspicuous manner.

Therapists can respond to the above by being willing to say to their AvPD patients, 'I can see that this sort of discussion is not something that comes easily or naturally for you, and you may believe there are some serious drawbacks to thinking and talking about important matters in your life; I can understand that.' If empathy and a relaxed atmosphere in session are insufficient to inspire the AvPD patients to become more active, the therapist may try to offer a 'multiple choice' listing of potential topics or hypotheses to pursue. The goal is to jump-start a dialog in session, not to take sole control of the direction that therapy takes. Sometimes the patients will be responsive to such a soft sell approach, and will gradually warm to the task. However, if the AvPD patients remain excessively passive, therapists should not jump to the conclusion that therapy cannot proceed. Rather, therapists can model a comfortable reaction to silence, occasionally expressing interest in discussing any number of issues, and nicely inviting the patients to offer their ideas and feedback. If the patients often say, 'I don't know,' therapists can explain that they do not have to know for sure in order to offer some educated guesses, and that the patients' life issues are important enough to merit some thought and consideration, even if at first the patients do not know what to say. In other words, 'I don't know' should not be the end of the story; rather, it should signal the beginning of an exploration.

Homework activates the patients' incompetency schemas

One of the hypothesized active ingredients in cognitive therapy is homework (Persons et al., 1988). Thus, when patients habitually neglect to do their homework, they are likely inhibiting their potential progress in treatment, as well as their prospects for long-term maintenance of newly learned coping skills. Unfortunately, the notion of doing homework often triggers the AvPD patients' fears of failure and censure. Thus, they opt to bypass the homework (an error of omission, whose consequences they characteristically minimize), rather than take the risk of exposing their incompetence by making mistakes on between-sessions assignments (an error of commission, whose consequences they typically magnify).

When AvPD patients avoid their homework, this needs to become a therapeutic issue, as much for an exploration of their incompetency schema as the potential implications for slowed and truncated therapeutic progress. Therapists can reassure their AvPD patients that even *undone* homework can be useful, as long the patients' problems surrounding the homework are explored and discussed in an atmosphere of acceptance and hope for change. This is an argument for the continuation of the assignment of therapy homework, even when the AvPD patients rarely comply. As a caveat, therapists should temporarily back off from giving homework if the patients repeatedly fail to do it, openly state that they do not want to talk about it, and indicate (through various aspects of their demeanor) that there is a therapy-threatening rift in the therapeutic relationship.

Nevertheless, therapists can comment from time to time about the importance of patients learning to rely more upon themselves, and relatively less on the therapist. Homework is one way to facilitate this process, but therapists can also bolster their patients' self-confidence by gradually turning over control of the agenda to the patient. Further, therapists can shift from an educational style (e.g., 'Here is the method by which you can change') to a consultative style (e.g., 'Tell me how you would go about making a therapeutic change').

Conclusions

Patients who meet criteria for AvPD often evince other personality disorders such as DPD, typically look similar to patients who present with GSP or other anxiety disorders, sometimes use alcohol and other psychoactive substances in order to 'self-medicate' and otherwise avoid their experiences, and are prone to drop out of treatment as a characteristic defense. Although there is strong evidence that an avoidance-prone temperament is inherited, it has also been found that persons with AvPD experience particular difficulties during their formative years that are associated with the development of ambivalence in getting close to others. Experiences of shaming, neglect, rejection, and harsh criticism (or the chronic *perceptions* of such) can lead AvPD individuals to pursue an inconspicuous existence as a way to stay out of trouble. Although this strategy may indeed prevent overt harm, its overuse prevents the formation of self-efficacy across a wide range of life tasks, including the establishment and maintenance of open, trusting relationships. As a result, such individuals are left in a chronic state of dissatisfaction, self-reproach, and anxiety as they realize that they lack the confidence and sense of security they believe is necessary to pursue their goals.

Therapeutic modalities such as cognitive-behavioral therapies, psychodynamic therapies, and group approaches have much in common in that they recognize the importance of *exposure* to feared situations. Therapists utilize role-plays, emotionally evocative exercises (e.g., imagery), *in-vivo* interpersonal experiences, homework, and processing of the patients' hot cognitions and experiences in the therapeutic relationship in order to provide this exposure. It is also important to change the AvPD patients' maladaptive beliefs and schemas that are otherwise maintained when they fail to test them actively in session, and in everyday life.

The therapeutic relationship with AvPD patients is also very important across modalities, in that the patients often expect to be criticized, scolded, and rejected, and will typically have approach-avoidance conflicts about bonding and sharing private information with the therapist. If the therapeutic relationship is 'too easy,' it is likely that the important work is not being done. If the therapist is too directive or confrontational, the patient may abandon treatment. Finding the middle ground, in which there is a strong alliance, but also some anxiety, tumult, and exposure to high affect may be the key.

Although there have been some promising results from a limited number of outcome studies on social skills training, cognitive therapy, and short-term psychodynamic psychotherapies, it has been difficult to achieve therapeutic changes that reliably make AvPD patients indistinguishable from 'normals.' Part of the problem is the high rate of drop-out found in the literature—when AvPD patients succeed in completing their treatments they tend to do as well as patients who did not present with personality disorders. Even those who still meet criteria for AvPD at termination frequently show clinically significant reductions in anxiety and dysphoria— meaningful changes in a population that often demonstrates comorbid anxiety and mood disorders at intake.

There are indications that cognitive therapy may be particularly well-suited to treat AvPD, though more tests of this approach need to be executed and published in order to evaluate the hypothesis. In the meantime, results from trials on GSP provide some clues about what is needed to maximize positive outcomes for people whose avoidance has become an unnecessarily limiting force in their lives.

References

Alden, L. E. (1989). Short-term structured treatment for avoidant personality disorder. *Journal of Consulting and Clinical Psychology*, **57**(6), 756–64.

Alden, L. E. and Capreol, M. J. (1993). Avoidant personality disorder: interpersonal problems as predictors of treatment response. *Behavior Therapy*, **24**(3), 357–76.

Alden, L. E., Laposa, J. M., Taylor, C. T., and Ryder, A. G. (2002). Avoidant personality disorder: current status and future directions. *Journal of Personality Disorders*, **16**, 1–29.

American Psychiatric Association (1994). *Diagnostic and statistical manual of mental disorders (DSM-IV)*, 4th edn. Washington, DC: American Psychiatric Press.

Arbel, N. and Stravynski, A. (1991). A retrospective study of separation in the development of adult personality disorder. *Acta Psychiatrica Scandinavica*, **83**(3), 174–8.

Arntz, A. (1999). Do personality disorders exist? On the validity of the concept and its cognitive-behavioral formulation and treatment. *Behaviour Research and Therapy*, **37**, 97–134.

Barber, J. P. and Muenz, L. R. (1996). The role of avoidance and obsessiveness in matching patients to cognitive and interpersonal psychotherapy: empirical findings from the Treatment for Depression Collaborative Research Program. *Journal of Consulting and Clinical Psychology*, **64**(5), 951–8.

Barber, J. P., Morse, J. Q., Krakauer, I. D., Chittams, J., and Crits-Christoph, K. (1997). Change in obsessive-compulsive and avoidant personality disorders following time-limited supportive-expressive therapy. *Psychotherapy*, **34**, 133–43.

Beck, A. T., Emery, G., and Greenberg, R. L. (1985). *Anxiety disorders and phobias: a cognitive perspective*. New York: Guilford Press.

Beck, A. T., et al. (1990). *Cognitive therapy of personality disorders*. New York: Guilford Press.

Beck, A. T., et al. (2001). Dysfunctional beliefs discriminate personality disorders. *Behaviour Research and Therapy*, **39**(10), 1213–25.

Beck, J. S. (1995). *Cognitive therapy: basics and beyond*. New York: Guilford Press.

Benjamin, L. S. (1993). *Interpersonal diagnosis and treatment of personality disorders*. New York: Guilford Press.

Bowlby, J. (1973). *Attachment and loss: separation, anxiety, and anger*, Vol. 2. London: Hogarth.

Brown, E. J., Heimberg, R. G., and Juster, H. R. (1995). Social phobia subtype and avoidant personality disorder: effect on severity of social phobia, impairment, and outcome of cognitive behavioral treatment. *Behavior Therapy*, 26(3), 467–86.

Coon, D. W. (1994). Cognitive-behavioral interventions with avoidant personality: a single case study. *Journal of Cognitive Psychotherapy: An International Quarterly*, 8(3), 243–53.

Daldrup, R. J., Beutler, D. E., Engle, D., and Greenberg, L. S. (1988). *Focused-expressive psychotherapy*. New York: Guilford Press.

Davanloo, H. (1999). Intensive short-term dynamic psychotherapy—central dynamic sequence: head-on collision with resistance. *International Journal of Intensive Short-Term Dynamic Psychotherapy*, 13(4), 263–82.

Ekselius, L., Tillfors, M., Furmark, T., and Fredrikson, M. (2001). Personality disorder in the general population: DSM-IV and ICD-10 defined prevalence as related to sociodemographic profile. *Personality and Individual Differences*, 30, 311–20.

Feske, U., Perry, K. J., Chambless, D. L., Renneberg, B., and Goldstein, A. J. (1996). Avoidant personality disorder as a predictor for treatment outcome among generalized social phobics. *Journal of Personality Disorder*, 10(2), 174–84.

Gabbard, G. O. (2000). *Psychodynamic psychiatry in clinical practice*, 3rd edn. Arlington, VA: American Psychiatric Publishing, Inc.

Gilbert, P. (2002). Evolutionary approaches to psychopathology and cognitive therapy. *Journal of Cognitive Psychotherapy: An International Quarterly*, 16(3), 263–94.

Greenberg, D. and Stravynski, A. (1985). Patients who complain of social dysfunction as their main problem: I. Clinical and demographic features. *Canadian Journal of Psychiatry*, 30(3), 206–11.

Greenberg, L. S. and Safran, J. D. (1984). Integrating affect and cognition: a perspective on therapeutic change. *Cognitive Therapy and Research*, 8, 559–78.

Heimberg, R. A. (1996). Social phobia, avoidant personality disorder, and the multi-axial conceptualization of interpersonal anxiety. In: P. M. Salkovskis, ed. *Trends in cognitive and behavioral therapies*, pp. 43–61. New York: Wiley.

Luborsky, L. (1984). *Principles of psychoanalytic psychotherapy: a manual for supportive-expressive treatment*. News York: Basic Books.

Meyer, B. and Carver, C. S. (2000). Negative childhood accounts, sensitivity and pessimism: a study of avoidant personality disorder features in college students. *Journal of Personality Disorders*, 14(3), 233–48.

Millon, T. and Martinez, A. (1995). Avoidant personality disorder. In: J. W. Livesley, ed. *The DSM-IV personality disorders: diagnosis and treatment of mental disorders*, pp. 218–33. New York: Guilford Press.

Newman, C. F. (1991). Cognitive therapy and the facilitation of affect: two case illustrations. *Journal of Cognitive Psychotherapy: An International Quarterly*, 5(4), 305–16.

Newman, C. F. (1999). Showing up for your own life: cognitive therapy of avoidant personality disorder. *In-Session: Psychotherapy in Practice*, 4(4), 55–71.

Persons, J. B., Burns, B. D., and Perloff, J. M. (1988). Predictors of drop-out and outcome in cognitive therapy for depression in a private practice setting. *Cognitive Therapy and Research*, 12, 557–75.

Reich, J. (2000). The relationship of social phobia to avoidant personality disorder: a proposal to reclassify avoidant personality disorder based on clinical empirical findings. *European Psychiatry*, 15(3), 151–9.

Renneberg, B., Goldstein, A. J., Phillips, D., and Chambless, D. L. (1990). Intensive behavioral group treatment of avoidant personality disorder. *Behavior Therapy*, 21(3), 363–77.

Rettew, D. C. (2000). Avoidant personality disorder, generalized social phobia, and shyness: Putting the personality back into personality disorders. *Harvard Review of Psychiatry*, 8(6), 283–97.

Sanderson, W. C., Beck, A. T., and McGinn, L. K. (1994). Cognitive therapy for generalized anxiety disorder: significance of comorbid personality disorders. *Journal of Cognitive Psychotherapy: An International Quarterly*, 8, 13–18.

Shea, M. T., *et al.* (1990). Personality disorders and treatment outcome in the NIMH Treatment of Depression Collaborative Research Program. *American Journal of Psychiatry*, 147, 711–18.

Strauss, J. L. (2001). Patterns and impact of the alliance and affective arousal in psychotherapy: an application to cognitive therapy for avoidant and obsessive-compulsive personality disorders. *Dissertation Abstracts International: Section B: The Sciences and Engineering*, 62(5–B), 2504.

Stravynski, A., Marks, I., and Yule, W. (1982). Social skills problems in neurotic outpatients: social skills training with and without cognitive modification. *Archives of General Psychiatry*, 39, 1378–85.

Stravynski, A., Lamontagne, Y., and Lavalee, Y. J. (1986). Clinical phobias and avoidant personality disorder among alcoholics admitted to an alcoholism rehabilitation setting. *Canadian Journal of Psychiatry*, 31(8), 714–19.

Stravynski, A., Lesage, A., Marcouiller, M., and Elie, R. (1989). A test of the mechanism in social skills training with avoidant personality disorder. *Journal of Nervous and Mental Disease*, 177(12), 739–44.

Stravynski, A., Belisle, M., Marcouiller, M., Lavallee, Y., and Elie, R. (1994). The treatment of avoidant personality disorder by social skills training in the clinic or in real-life setting. *Canadian Journal of Psychiatry*, 39(8), 377–83.

Stuart, S., Pfohl, B., Battaglia, M., Bellodi, L., Grove, W., and Cadoret, R. (1998). The co-occurrence of DSM-III-R personality disorders. *Journal of Personality Disorders*, 12, 302–15.

Tillfors, M., Furmark, T., Ekselius, L., and Fredrikson, M. (2001). Social phobia and avoidant personality disorder as related to parental history of social anxiety: a general population study. *Behaviour Research and Therapy*, 39(3), 289–98.

Tran, G. and Chambless, D. (1995). Psychopathology of social phobia: effects of subtype and of avoidant personality disorder. *Journal of Anxiety Disorders*, 9(6), 489–501.

Widiger, T. A. (2001). Social anxiety, social phobia, and avoidant personality. In R. Crozier and L. Alden, ed. *International handbook of social anxiety: concepts, research, and interventions relating to the self and shyness*, pp. 335–56. London: Wiley.

Yalom, I. D. (1980). *Existential psychotherapy*. New York: Basic Books.

Yalom, I. D. (1995). *The theory and practice of group psychotherapy*, 3rd edn. New York: Basic Books.

Young, J. (1999). *Cognitive therapy of personality disorders: a schema-focused approach*, 3rd edn. Sarasota, FL: Professional Resource Exchange, Inc.

27 Dependent personality disorder

J. Christopher Perry

Introduction

Dependency includes universal personality traits, expressed in different ways to some degree over the life span. Like other mammals, humans start out being very dependent upon adults for care and protection, then evolve through maturation and learning into more self-regulating and autonomous individuals. In familial, interpersonal, and organizational settings, healthy expressions of dependency are characterized by adaptive interdependency, where individuals negotiate helping and being helped. In settings in which dependency and autonomy are either excessively encouraged, discouraged, ignored, or punished, dependency may become increasingly pronounced or pathological in its expression. When dependent behaviors are pervasive, frequent, and associated with impairment, an individual may be diagnosed with dependent personality disorder (DPD). Many individuals with DPD manage their lives by forming relationships with dominant spouses, friends, relatives, and bosses or coworkers, who in turn respond to dependency. A stable, if precarious, homeostasis in such relationships may allow the individual to function well to the outside observer. However, individuals with DPD may become symptomatic when dependent relationships are disturbed, threatened, or broken off (Perry and Vaillant, 1989), or when their own needs and feelings are increasingly ignored or punished, or failures at achievement occur (Zaretsky et al., 1997). In these instances, the individual with DPD may seek help, often precipitated by an Axis I disorder, or a painful life event. Dependency is commonly overlooked until the individual becomes symptomatic or overwhelmed with a life situation.

The psychotherapy of DPD can be quite successful, or quite lengthy and challenging depending on the patient, the therapist, their goals and alliance, as well as the technical approach employed. Although dependency issues are relevant in the treatment of many psychiatric disorders, this review is limited largely to those reports that are most relevant to the treatment of the PD.

Conceptualization

Clinical interest in dependent personality traits began with Abraham's (1924, or reprinted in Abraham, 1954) description of the oral character. The PD first appeared in a War Department Technical Bulletin in 1945 (US War Department, 1945) and later in the first edition of the *Diagnostic and statistical manual* (DSM) (1952) as a subtype of passive-aggressive PD. Since then, a large number of studies have upheld the descriptive validity of dependent personality traits, viewed as submissiveness (Presley and Walton, 1973), oral character traits (Gottheil and Stone, 1968; Kline and Storey, 1977), oral dependence (Lazare et al., 1966, 1970; van den Berg and Helstone, 1975), or passive dependence (Tyrer and Alexander, 1979), or as a constellation of both pathological and adaptive traits under the term dependency (Hirschfeld et al., 1991; Bornstein, 1992, 1998). DSM-IV (American Psychiatric Association, 1994) emphasizes two sets of traits: dependency (criteria 1–5), and insecure attachment (criteria 6–8). In a study diagnosing PDs by both DSM-IV and ICD-10 (Ottosson et al., 2002), there was moderate agreement across the two systems in diagnosing DPD

(kappa = 0.75), although ICD diagnosed almost 45% more cases, and excellent agreement between their dimensional scales (r = 0.94).

Dependent personality is common in the general population—the Midtown Manhattan Study found it in 2.5% of the entire sample (Langer and Michael, 1963), while a recent Norwegian survey found it in 1.5%, with the prevalence in women twice than in men (Torgersen et al., 2001). In clinical settings, DPD often co-occurs with other PDs, especially borderline, histrionic, and avoidant types (Hirschfeld et al., 1991; Bornstein, 1995a; Zanarini et al., 1998) and, although less frequently studied, with self-defeating, passive-aggressive, compulsive, schizotypal, and paranoid types (Bornstein, 1995a; Reich, 1996; Skodol et al., 1996), and, in the author's own research, depressive PD. Treatment should be modified accordingly. Patterns of Axis I and II comorbidity vary widely depending on sample source, reason for selection (e.g., major depression), and assessment method.

Managing the dependency that often accompanies chronic major psychiatric syndromes such as schizophrenia or unremitting depression (Bornstein, 1992; Kool et al., 2003) may have similarities with treating DPD. However, noting that Axis I disorders such as depression often increase dependency, Skodol et al. (1996) suggest that maladaptive dependency might become the focus of treatment in its own right, if it does not improve after the symptomatic disorder improves.

A factor-analytic study suggested that dependency is best characterized by three related dimensions (Hirschfeld et al., 1977). The first involves strong emotional reliance on close attachments and others. Livesley et al. (1990) labeled this dimension insecure attachment, after Bowlby's description. However, Borenstein (1997) has argued that insecure attachment is not a core aspect of DPD. Individuals with this dimension of dependency are prone to separation anxiety and will remain in relationships, even with those who mistreat them, to avoid the resurgence of feeling alone and helpless. They may act in ingratiating ways, doing whatever is asked of them in order to be liked or to secure succor. Whenever hospitalized, these individuals may transfer their attachment needs to the hospital. Prior to discharge, separation anxiety re-emerges and their presenting symptoms may recur, possibly delaying discharge (Sarwrer-Foner and Kealey, 1981). This is less likely to occur whenever the patient has an already established, good, supportive relationship outside the hospital.

A second dependent dimension is the lack of self-confidence in social situations, often accompanied by submissive behavior (Hirschfeld et al., 1977), which Livesley et al. (1990) considered the core dependency dimension. This includes having difficulty asserting oneself, agreeing with others despite believing that others are incorrect, and fearing self-expression of one's own anger, criticism, or wishes and needs. The individual may remain passive when events call for an active response. Despite this, the individual may be surprisingly able to confront anxiety-provoking situations courageously to help or protect those dependent on him or herself. In other situations, dependent individuals can be quite assertive, even aggressive, whenever striving to obtain or maintain a supportive relationship (Bornstein, 1995b).

The third dimension is the avoidance of (versus desire for) autonomy (Hirschfeld et al., 1977). Those who avoid autonomy want others to make decisions for them; otherwise, they are indecisive and have difficulty initiating or completing activities on their own. They often seek guidance and direction and thereby subordinate their freedom of choice to the will of others. The extreme opposite is often called counterdependency, in which individuals strive to be independent at all points. When ill or under extreme stress, counterdependent individuals may revert to very dependent behaviors, often accompanied by an intense sense of shame.

Dependency is moderately stable from childhood onward. Kagan and Moss (1960) found a high correlation between passive and dependent behaviors at 6–10 years of age and their continuation into young adulthood. While this was across a broader range of behaviors for women than men, cultural influences may discourage certain dependent behaviors in men. Twin studies indicate that some of the stability is due to genetic influences while others are due to specific environmental differences unique to each child (O'Neill and Kendler, 1998).

Dependent individuals experience excessive self-doubt and view themselves as incompetent and less worthy or deserving than others. They may appear overtly optimistic (Kline and Storey, 1977), but have a covert pessimistic view of their chances for self-initiated social and occupational achievement. They may be prone to ruminate on their fearful attitudes and phobic anxieties about self-assertion, social activities, independence, and abandonment (A. T. Beck et al., 1990).

A. T. Beck et al. (1990) proposed a cognitive conceptualization of DPD suggesting that the individual believes two key assumptions. First, the individual believes him or herself to be inadequate and helpless and the world to be cold, lonely, and dangerous. Second, he or she assumes that the best strategy is to find someone who is capable of dealing with the world and protecting him or her. Submissiveness and relinquishing independent decision making are considered acceptable tradeoffs for maintaining such protective relationships. Furthering this, Judith Beck (1997) suggested that the core belief in DPD about the self is that 'I am helpless' while the core belief about others is that 'others should take care of me'. Life situations that stimulate these core beliefs then trigger assumptions such as 'if I rely on myself I'll fail' and 'if I depend on others I'll survive'. These assumptions then lead to behavioral strategies of relying on others.

Some evidence supporting this was demonstrated by strong associations between DPD and specific dependent beliefs on the Personality Belief Questionnaire (A. T. Beck et al., 2001).

Whitman et al. (1954) suggested that dependent individuals may become passive whenever dependent needs are stimulated if the person finds these needs unacceptable in the situation, due either to a neurotic sense of guilt or to external frustration. As a secondary effect of frustration, the individual may become demanding in minor ways. Millon (1981) suggested that over-solicitous, controlling parents who discourage seeking rewards outside the family may discourage independence. Because dependent individuals have had a relatively good relationship with at least one parent, anxiety experienced in situations requiring independent action is counterbalanced by the expectation that someone will help. The expectation of criticism for making independent decisions, taking action, or venturing to new activities further stifles independence. Instead of channeling hostile feelings into assertive behavior, dependent individuals often smooth over troubles by acting in an especially friendly, helpful, and concerned manner. In a study of the family environment, Head et al. (1991) found some support for Millon's hypotheses in that the individuals with DPD reported that their families were low in expressiveness and high in control. Baker et al. (1996) found that DPD individuals reported early family environments that were lower in encouraging independence and higher in control over the subject than normal controls, while being lower in achievement and intellectual-cultural orientation than the environments of individuals with histrionic PD.

In a study of addicts living with their families of origin, Alexander and Dibb (1977) found that compared with control subjects, both the addicts and their parents perceived the addicts as passive, dependent, and incapable of autonomy and success. Neither the addict nor the overindulgent parent encouraged self-reliance.

Perry et al. (1989) and Waska (1997) noted that dependent individuals often act in a submissive, compliant way in order to earn others' gratitude.

This ingratiating behavior entitles them in fantasy to maintain their important attachments and protects them from abandonment and the development of separation anxiety, and entitles them to being soothed and taken care of (Waska, 1997). Despite this, they can be quite aggressive toward others when they think doing so will ingratiate themselves with authority figures or secure care or help (Bornstein, 1995b), or protect those under their care.

Epstein (1980) compared the social consequences of assertive, aggressive, passive-aggressive, and submissive behaviors. Submissive behavior (e.g., making a request accompanied by an indication that one will capitulate easily), consistently elicited high intentions to comply, low anger, and high sympathy from observers, generally equal to the levels obtained by assertive behavior. Thus, submissive behavior may meet with some success, depending on the responsiveness of others.

In a study of passive adolescents, Rosenheim and Gaoni (1977) postulated that a fear of having to mourn childhood fantasies about the future may result in a failure to make decisions, enter into personal commitments, and take independent action. Refusal to take an active stance in working toward any plan avoids having to set aside cherished, if overvalued or unrealistic, hopes for the future and avoids the sadness of mourning.

Andrews et al. (1978) suggested a biological hypothesis for dependency based on finding high levels of anxiety-proneness, emotionality, and easy fatigability in individuals with asthenic personality. This may encompass a constitutional predisposition to develop high anxiety levels under stress, often called neuroticism, which in turns disrupts learning.

Research

Efficacy and effectiveness

The treatment literature is limited largely to case descriptions, uncontrolled studies, and some controlled treatment trials with admixtures of PDs, including DPD. Across all of these, there is an apparent consensus that the treatment of DPD is often successful. This is indirectly supported by the relative lack of articles that report failures or focus on difficulties in treatment, in contrast to the plethora of such reports for other PDs.

Systematic studies including DPD indicate that treatment on average leads to improvement. Virtually all studies indicate that psychotherapy produces sizable, positive effects in PDs (Perry, 1989; Perry and Bond, 2000; Leichsenring and Leibing, 2003). This is true for both dynamic and cognitive-behavioral therapy approaches (Leichsenring and Leibing, 2003). Two related meta-analyses found a number of studies with a median of 25% (range 10–33%) of individuals with DPD, and others with large proportions of unspecified Cluster C disorders (Perry and Bond, 2000). The therapies demonstrated medium to large positive effects (generally larger than 1.0) for individual (Winston et al., 1991, 1994; Hoglend, 1993; Hardy et al., 1995; Monsen et al., 1995; Patience et al., 1995), group (Budman et al., 1996), day (Karterud et al., 1992, 2003; Piper et al., 1993; Wilberg et al., 1998), and residential treatments (Dolan et al., 1997; Krawitz, 1997). This empirically supports the earlier conclusion reached by one expert panel that the treatment of DPD is generally successful (The Quality Assurance Project, 1991).

Dependency and depression

In the Treatment of Depression Collaborative Research Program, three active treatments (imipramine, interpersonal psychotherapy, and cognitive-behavior therapy) were compared with placebo plus clinical management over 16 weeks for the treatment of acute major depressive disorder (Shea et al., 1990). Significant improvement in depressive symptoms occurred in those both with and without PDs, although there were no clear-cut differential responses to type of treatment. However, complete remission was found in fewer of the anxious cluster (33%) than of those without a PD (49%). The former also showed worse social adjustment. Thus, patients with DPD who become depressed may respond to treatment, but upon return to baseline some symptoms and social adjustment problems remain, a conclusion confirmed by other studies (Diguer et al., 1993; Hardy et al., 1995; Patience et al., 1995).

Kool *et al.* (2003) conducted a randomized trial of patients with DSM-III-R major depression, half of whom also had a PD by a self-report method. Among those scoring in the PD range, DPD was the most prevalent (38%). Patients received either antidepressive medications alone or combined with 16 sessions of Short Psychodynamic Supportive Psychotherapy (SPSS) and the percentage recovered from depression at 40 weeks was similar (44% versus 51%). In both conditions, those who recovered showed improved personality traits. However, those receiving combined treatment showed such improvement even if not recovered from their depression. In fact, dependent and several other traits (e.g., avoidant, passive-aggressive) improved more with combined treatment than pharmacotherapy alone, most evident in Cluster C disorders. This strongly supports the additive effect of psychotherapy in combined treatment on dependent traits among the depressed.

Treatment attrition

Attrition from treatment may be lower in DPD than other PDs. Shea *et al.* (1990) found that patients with anxious-cluster PDs, including DPD, had a lower attrition rate (28%) than other PD groups. Katerud *et al.* (2003) found only 16% of those with DPD dropped out of an 18-week day treatment program, lower than all PD types, except for schizoid.

Duration of treatment

There is no firm data on the optimum duration of treatment. In an examination of the natural history of open-ended dynamic psychotherapy for adults with mood and/or PDs, the author has found that DPD and significant dependent traits were associated with a median length of treatment almost twice that of those with no dependent traits of DPD (129 sessions versus 66 sessions), which was statistically significant. Karterud *et al.* (2003) examined 18 weeks of day treatment on a large sample of PDs treated at eight sites. In general PDs improved, but most did not attain healthy level scores. Among DPD specifically, Global Assessment of Functioning (GAF) improved at termination and continued to improve over 1 year follow-up (mean of 47, 52, 56). The Global Severity Index (GSI) of the Symptom Checklist-90 (revised), and a quality of life measure improved at termination and were maintained over follow-up, whereas a measure of interpersonal functioning improved but later regressed. Employment was not significantly improved over follow-up. Thus while improvement is the rule, the duration of treatment required for recovery to full, healthy functioning remains to be studied.

Key practice principles

As cultural factors influence what is considered normal dependency, the therapist should consider the cultural context of the patient. Having family members accompany the patient into a consultation might signal dependency issues in a northern American or European family, whereas the same would be absolutely the norm on the Indian subcontinent. Similarly, depending on the culture, women and men may express dependency differently, with the female stereotype showing more insecure attachment and submissiveness and the male stereotype submissiveness and especially avoidance of autonomy. This results in a tendency to overlook dependent traits in men, which may include the need to talk about every decision and seek reassurance and encouragement, or the failure to take action or move forward in a career. Failure to recognize these as dependency issues may lead to perplexing stalemates in treatment. Regardless of the treatment approach, it is important to identify the patient's specific dependent patterns.

Individual dynamic psychotherapy

In the dynamic psychotherapy literature there is apparent consensus about two central aspects in the therapy of DPD. The first is that the emergence of a dependent transference toward the therapist should be addressed in a way to promote emotional growth. The second is that therapist expectations and direct support should be used to promote self-expression, assertiveness, decision making, and independence. If both aspects are not addressed,

treatment may be incomplete (Hill, 1970; Saul and Warner, 1975; Malinow, 1981; A. T. Beck *et al.*, 1990).

At the outset of therapy, it is important to aid the development of a trusting relationship and allow the patient to begin to transfer dependent wishes on to the therapist. Hill (1970) suggested telling the patient that extra sessions may be allowed early on in therapy, especially around the patient's episodes of panic or distress. This assurance of readily available support helps the patient develop trust, and aids alliance formation. As therapy progresses, the therapist may help the patient find substitute ways of dealing with such feelings and limit extra sessions.

Alexander *et al.* (1968) found that dependency on the therapist increased from the beginning to the middle of short-term therapy and remained fairly high until termination. The high levels of dependency on the therapist necessitated working through transference issues right up until termination. In contrast, they found that the patient's dependency on outside relationships began to diminish from the middle of treatment until termination, which suggests a real effect of treatment on the resolution of dependency conflicts.

The hardest work of therapy occurs when a patient experiences increased dependency on the therapist and simultaneously has setbacks or losses in his or her outside life. Offering sympathy for the patient's distress is not helpful alone (Hill, 1970). The therapist should also encourage the patient to express real feelings and wishes and to bear the anxiety of making decisions, accepting pleasurable experiences, and dealing with episodes of anxiety. When the patient experiences frustration over his or her wish to have the therapist take a more directive role, the therapist should clarify and interpret the transference elements in addition to supporting the patient in finding more self-reliant ways to cope (Hill, 1970; Saul and Warner, 1975; Malinow, 1981; A. T. Beck *et al.*, 1990). Leeman *et al.* (1975) limit attention to transference issues in favor of focusing on relationships outside of therapy.

At this stage, the therapist should avoid taking a directive role in the patient's life; otherwise a transference–countertransference fixation might develop that simply repeats patterns from the patient's other relationships (Leeman *et al.*, 1975; Saul and Warner, 1975). This requires actively resisting the patient's repetitive requests for advice and attempts to have the therapist make decisions for the patient, something the patient expects from authority figures.

Saul and Warner (1975) described the following optimal circumstances for the therapist to give direct suggestions and encourage specific actions or solutions to problems. First, the treatment should have progressed long enough for the therapist to have a good understanding of the patient's dynamics. Second, the therapist should be aware of the state of the transference and his or her own reaction to it. Third, the patient should be at some impasse out of which a direct therapeutic intervention can mobilize the patient and prevent a repetition of feeling powerless. Given these circumstances, the therapist should help the patient conceptualize his or her own goals. If the goals are healthy, the therapist should discuss and support them. If there are conflicting goals, then it is helpful to discuss the consequences of each goal and to encourage the patient to bear the anxiety of making choices. While similar to cognitive therapy (A. T. Beck *et al.*, 1990), this approach also makes use of previous insights about the patient's motivations. The therapist may then urge the patient to commit himself or herself to actions that are within the patient's reach (e.g., taking a job) or encourage perseverance despite the urge to give up (e.g., flunking out of school). The therapist must also ensure that he or she is using his or her influence in accordance with the patient's own values, not those of the therapist.

Covert dependency on the therapist, in which the patient experiences the therapist as a benign, powerful parent figure (Goldman, 1956), can facilitate therapeutic change. The therapist's sincere interest, attention, and reliable presence may increase the patient's belief in the benevolent power of the therapist. This affects the patient's self-esteem in several ways. First, the patient may identify with the therapist and wish to be like him or her (Offenkrantz and Tobin, 1974). Idealization leads to a temporary rise in self-esteem. Second, the patient may accept and increasingly use the therapist's exploratory attitude toward his or her emotional life. Third, whenever the patient remembers or experiences hitherto unacceptable feelings for the first time, the therapist should be comprehending and accepting. This will enhance the patient's self-esteem, because the patient can identify with the more benevolent attitudes and responses of the therapist as an authority figure, rather than react according to his or her old prohibitions and ideals. This rise in self-esteem is only temporary as long as it relies largely on the reassuring presence of the therapist. However, if the patient can channel this increased self-esteem to risk trying new behaviors outside the office, he or she may experience other rewards, including approval from others. It is important for the therapist both to communicate genuine pleasure when these outside efforts succeed and to accept failures that inevitably occur. This helps the patient to shift self-perception from dependency toward social self-confidence.

Attending to the patient's defenses can inform the therapist about conflict areas requiring attention. In particular, reaction formation against feelings such as anger toward dominant others may be masked as concern. Similarly displacement may frequently divert attention away from the patient's problems to those of the people around him or her. When confronted with situations necessitating more autonomous and self-assertive functioning, the patient may lapse into help-rejecting complaining, preferring the safer experience of failure while also covertly criticizing others for their lack of care and material help. The therapist should help the patient explore the meaning of such experiences and return to the underlying feelings such as anger, disappointment, and shame. Understanding what makes such affects distressing can then lead to better tolerance of them and finally point towards more effective functioning.

During the final stage of therapy, the therapist gradually increases the level of expectations for autonomous decision making and action and for socially effective responses (Leeman and Mulvey, 1975). This includes reinforcing the individual's increasing ability to handle crises without extra sessions, to manage anxiety/panic episodes by self-soothing rather than by seeking reassurance from others (Hill, 1970). The therapist must help the patient to resolve transference wishes to be dependent and fears of aloneness, powerlessness, and others' intolerance for self-initiated expression and action, while accepting instead a more self-reliant position in relationships. Prior to termination, if the patient avoids mourning the therapeutic relationship, for instance, by fantasies that he or she was never really close to the therapist, or that the therapist will always be available, then termination will provide a crisis. The patient may feel betrayed that the therapist is after all not available, and begin to deteriorate (Werbart, 1997).

The consensus of the literature is that dynamic psychotherapy is usually helpful for the patient with DPD. Hill (1970) noted that only two of 50 cases treated showed no observable improvement. Treatment required several months to more than 2 years. Leeman and Mulvey (1975) noted that short-term (3–7 months' duration), focused psychotherapy was successful in five of six patients, although one patient required a second course of treatment. Hoglend (1993) found that more than 30 sessions were needed. Most authors used weekly sessions.

The comparative efficacy of short-term versus long-term treatment has not been adequately addressed. In general, short-term psychotherapies are most likely to succeed when a circumscribed, dynamic conflict or focus is present, the patient can form a therapeutic or working alliance rapidly, and the tendency to regress to severe dependency or acting out is limited (Malan, 1976; Davanloo, 1978; Horowitz et al., 1984; Luborsky, 1984; Strupp and Binder, 1984; Winston et al., 1991; Hoglend, 1993). Unfortunately, many patients with DPD will not meet these criteria. Short-term dynamic therapies usually require once-weekly sessions over 3–9 months.

Hoglend (1993) found that among patients with PDs, the length of treatment was more essential for long-term dynamic improvement than were patient characteristics, such as suitability, cluster category, or initial global functioning. Significant long-term dynamic changes did not appear before 30 sessions, and the amount of change correlated with the number of sessions, a finding not obtained in those without PDs. Many patients do better in longer-term, dynamic psychotherapies or psychoanalysis. These include those who have failed to improve in short-term treatments, have

multifocal conflicts or histories of significant emotional neglect or abuse. These treatments generally require two to four sessions per week over a period of several years to work through the dependent transference.

Cognitive-behavior therapy

Turkat and Carlson (1984) reported two successive behavioral treatments of a patient with DPD. The patient had initially been treated with behavioral techniques for anxiety-related complaints but had relapsed immediately after termination. The authors then reformulated the case, focusing on the dependency constructs of excessive reliance on others and deficient autonomous behavior, which they posited resulted from long-standing anxiety over independent decision making. The therapist and patient constructed a hierarchy of situations with which the patient had little experience but about which the patient was required to make independent decisions. The therapist emphasized previously taught anxiety management skills. Treatment proceeded every other week for 2 months. As therapy progressed, the patient showed decreasing levels of self-rated anxiety, and less avoidance of situations requiring independent decisions. The gains were maintained at 1-year follow-up.

A. T. Beck et al. (1990) and J. S. Beck (1997) have described cognitive-behavioral treatment for DPD. As in dynamic therapy, they view the patient–therapist relationship as a microcosm of the patient's dependent beliefs and behaviors. The therapist must foster the therapeutic alliance early and adjust the therapeutic approach somewhat to maintain it. For instance, some patients need to begin a session telling the therapist whatever is on their mind, in order to cooperate subsequently with more directed or structured tasks. The therapist formulates the case and then chooses each technique to foster accurate self-appraisal and independent decision making and behavior. The patient's dependent behavior is initially accepted, but the therapist encourages self-reflection and agenda setting for sessions.

Independence is first encouraged by helping the patient set goals for treatment. Using a Socratic method avoids directing the patient's agenda. The therapist continually challenges the patient's dichotomous thinking (e.g., 'If I am not fully successful, then I'm inadequate') to improve self-evaluation. Successful graded exposure to anxiety-provoking situations in real life challenges the patient's belief about being incompetent. Patient diaries can be used to monitor the patient's automatic thoughts, especially of inadequacy, highlighting their negative consequences. The therapist can challenge the patient to select healthier responses that aid the development of positive schemas. Relaxation training may aid in the reduction of anxiety surrounding independent reflection and decision making. Assertiveness training and role playing may help counter submissive behavior whenever real skill deficits exist.

J. S. Beck (1997) recommends a session format that includes checking the patient's mood, providing a bridge between sessions, setting an agenda for the session, reviewing any homework, discussing the items on the agenda, and then summarizing the session and giving and obtaining feedback. Patients are given work sheets that can help them combine previous work and current situations to prepare for the next session. The formulation or 'cognitive profile' plays a crucial part in helping the patient understand connections between early experiences, core beliefs, and compensatory strategies as well as reactions to current situations. Once therapist and patient have identified maladaptive core beliefs, the patient can fill out a 'core belief worksheet' each session that contrasts the old maladaptive belief with disconfirming experiences and substitutes new more flexible and adaptive beliefs. The therapist can use a variety of different techniques to help the patient discover and shape new ways of thinking and behaving, such as proposing a behavioral experiment to test a belief.

Whenever resistance to change develops, the therapist must help the patient think through ambivalence about changing, with the goal of finding constructive substitutes for the loss of old dependent habits. As treatment progresses, the dependent transference can be reduced by the addition of group therapy. Toward termination, tapering the frequency of sessions will allow the patient to feel increasingly competent without frequent visits. At termination, the fear of losing the therapist may be mitigated by offering booster sessions at infrequent intervals. Specific guidelines regarding the optimal number of sessions have not yet been developed or tested.

Marchand and Wapler (1993) conducted a retrospective study of cognitive-behavioral treatment for panic disorder with agoraphobia. A chart review diagnosis of DPD, compared with nondependent patients, was not associated with any worse response to treatment.

Overall, treatment based on a cognitive-behavioral formulation of the mechanisms for a variety of dependent features shares many features with that based on psychodynamic formulation, although the treatments differ on some specific techniques. Further case studies and treatment trials are needed to differentiate the advantages of each approach.

Group psychotherapy

Several reports suggest that group psychotherapy can be successful for the treatment of DPD. Montgomery (1971) used group therapy for dependent patients who used medications for chronic complaints such as insomnia and nervousness. All but three of 30 patients eventually discontinued medications and began to confront their anger at being dependent on the therapist. In an inpatient treatment setting for alcoholism, Poldrugo et al. (1988) found group therapy most beneficial for patients with DPD.

Sadoff and Collins (1968) employed weekly group psychotherapy for 22 patients who stuttered, most of whom had passive-dependent traits. Although the dropout rate was high, the authors found that the interpretation of passive-dependent behavior and attitudes (e.g., asking for help, believing that others are responsible for helping them) as a defense against recognizing and expressing anger proved helpful. Both stuttering and passive dependency improved in two patients who became angry and were able to confront their anger.

Torgersen (1980) studied college students who attended a weekend-long encounter group. On follow-up several weeks later, individuals who initially scored high on dependent traits had mixed responses. While the group experience left them feeling disturbed and anxious, they also reported becoming more accepting of their own feelings and opinions. No other changes were found.

Attrition may be higher in group than individual therapy for PDs (Perry and Bond, 2000), although may be less of a problem for individuals with DPD. Budman et al. (1996) demonstrated moderate improvements after an 18-month group for PDs (10% with DPD), although some changes were not evident until 6 months.

These reports suggest the usefulness of group psychotherapy in the treatment of DPD. Most clinicians employ weekly sessions of 1–11/2 hours duration. Sessions may be more frequent when group therapy is used as a major treatment modality in a day or residential treatment setting (Piper et al., 1993). Outpatient group therapy generally lasts 6 months to several years.

Day and residential therapies

Both of these modalities are useful when patients require a higher level of support and treatment intensity than is available in most outpatient therapies. Such patients often have comorbid Axis I and II disorders, and a history of refractoriness to previous treatments (Karterud et al., 1992, 2003; Piper et al., 1993; Wilberg et al., 1998). Such therapeutic approaches usually employ mixtures of individual and group therapies along with additional services, such as occupational therapy, expressive therapies, guided work experiences or counseling, and so forth. Controlled (Piper et al., 1993) and uncontrolled studies (Krawitz, 1997; Karterud et al., 1992, 2003; Wilberg et al., 1998), including Cluster C PDs, generally demonstrate large effects. Temple et al. (1997) found that interpretive group therapy was specifically helpful enabling most of a group of patients who were very dependent on day hospital improve enough for discharge to outpatient care. Day treatment duration ranges from about 18 weeks to more than a year, although a naturalistic comparison of different day treatment centers in Norway found no differences in effectiveness for PDs between longer and shorter treatment durations (Karterud et al., 2003). Residential treatment is specifically useful for those patients who have failed to improve or deteriorated with outpatient therapy, while living alone

or with family. Such patients usually require several months to a year or longer to progress to the point of living independently and benefiting from further outpatient therapy.

Family therapy

Some patients with DPD may live with family members who exert great degrees of influence over issues of support and autonomy. The family may view the patient as needing to be cared for, and the family reward and punishment contingencies maintain the patient in a dependent status. Increasing autonomy by the patient, which may include the threat of leaving home, is covertly experienced as threatening to the family. In such cases, family therapy, or periodic family meetings adjunctive to individual therapy, may help. The therapist's task is first to identify the functional relationships in the family that encourage dependency and discourage normal autonomy. The therapist must then help the family members initially develop a consensus on some modest goals for increased autonomy for the patient. As the patient begins to reach some early goals, the therapist can help the family revise the consensus. The therapist must point out discrepancies between attitudes of helping the patient and behaviors that undermine this goal. However, the alliance with the family members may become strained if the therapist takes too directive a stance. Family meetings range from once per week to once every few months, when adjunctive to individual therapy. There are no studies on the sole use of family therapy for DPD.

Challenges

Personal misfortune

One common but unpredictable occurrence in the therapy of DPD arises when the patient experiences a significant separation, loss, or diminution in personal or financial support. Such stressors often overwhelm the ability to employ newly acquired attitudes and skills, resulting in a regression in defensive functioning and an increase in dependent wishes, requests, and behaviors. This may be further exacerbated by recurrence of panic, general anxiety, somatic symptoms, or a major depressive episode. Some regression to earlier more dependent functioning is common. This may strain the therapeutic alliance if the patient perceives the therapist as insensitive to his or her emotional reactions, disappointed, impatient, or too demanding of progress. The therapist must find a balance between listening, being supportive, offering suggestions and some direction, which the patient will find helpful, while temporarily accepting this interruption in the tasks of growth. In fact, if the therapist negotiates such crises well, the alliance will be strengthened and the patient, feeling supported and understood, may return sooner than imagined to working on issues of autonomy, separation sensitivity, effective coping, and self-esteem enhancement.

Five specific challenges

The challenges in treating individuals with DPD often arise in the therapeutic relationship itself in the form of transference and countertransference problems. Five such patterns often arise in the treatment of individuals with DPD (Perry, 2001).

Repeated requests for advice and help

In the first instance, the patient entering therapy may make many demands or requests of the therapist for advice, succor, or concrete help, which the therapist is unable to meet. In one study, such patients often terminated early in therapy and were rated as having had unsuccessful outcomes (Alexander and Abeles, 1968). The therapist should give special attention to helping modulate these patients' demands early in treatment to prevent overwhelming disappointment and dropout. These patients also invite a countertransference response of emotional withdrawal and disengagement, which in turn reinforces neurotic guilt about needs.

Assumption of a directive, dominant role

A second problem may occur when the patient repeatedly attempts to put the therapist in the role of a dominant other who will both take responsibility for all decisions and tell the patient how to run his or her life (Hill, 1970; Saul and Warner, 1975). If the therapist assumes this directing countertransference role, he or she may become an external substitute for the patient's own will. Some therapists do this out of a sense of exasperation at the patient's protestations of helplessness or because of a personal wish to assume an idealized role as wise and all-knowing. This reinforces the patient's emotional reliance on the therapist without challenging him or her to learn more independent ways of coping. Directive approaches may have a useful, but limited, role during crisis interventions, but even cognitive-behavioral therapies require the therapist to foster the patient's independent decision making (A. T. Beck et al., 1990).

Compliance in order to preserve the therapeutic attachment

A third problem results when the patient avoids making real changes but stays in therapy to maintain the emotional attachment to the therapist (Leeman and Mulvey, 1975). The patient's compliant attitude toward the therapist may be mistaken for cooperation with the goals of therapy. Such individuals have tacitly refused to accept responsibility for making changes and may have their passivity reinforced if the therapist does not recognize and deal openly with this problem.

> *Case example in psychodynamic therapy*. A 47-year-old accountant presented with feelings of alienation, insecurity, and needing to please others at work and in his marriage and family of origin. Being left at a boarding school in early childhood during a prolonged period of family dislocation left him feeling alone, emotionally neglected, and needy of others help. He eagerly participated in therapy and over 5 years made several advantageous career moves—usually prompted by an external event such as a layoff—and became more assertive in his personal relationships. Nonetheless, there were crucial areas where he appeared to repeat the same well-worn themes, always bringing in a series of complaints followed by discussion, which he invariably found helpful. Yet, there was no clear progression toward an ultimate sense of autonomy, satisfaction with marriage and family, or termination of treatment.

> The therapist recognized that negative feelings expressed toward the therapist were minimal, and that the patient worked to keep the relationship comfortable, at the cost of continuing in the role of the dependent, needy one. The therapist began to interpret this pattern, that the patient reported problems followed by small successes, which he gave as gifts that served to make the therapist feel helpful, and thus maintain the relationship as it was. In fact they were all displacements and reaction formations against the harder themes of fear of abandonment, fear of hurting others and being seen as aggressive if he furthers his own wishes, envy toward those more successful, and disappointment in the therapist's limited power to change the patient's life. The therapist began to interrupt the weekly myriad of stories and point out their diversionary aim, sometimes revealing that they led him to day dream or even get sleepy, which kept them from really connecting. This mobilized the patient who responded with dysphoric feelings, but increased interest, and attention to his acceptance of the *status quo*. Focusing on these in-session phenomena led to an increase in relevant earlier memories juxtaposed with confronting changes not imagined possible. While the therapy became less comfortable for the patient, he reengaged with the more central rather than peripheral areas of conflict. The therapist also found the sessions more engaging, and progress reemerged.

Presence of a punitive relationship

A fourth problem may occur with patients who have unsatisfying, punitive relationships, commonly described as masochistic or self-defeating. The patient's repeated stories about mistreatment may evoke in the therapist a desire to control the patient's self-defeating pattern or even to punish the patient for not changing. Should the therapist challenge the patient to leave or to assert him or herself in the relationship, the patient may become extremely anxious, because of the strength of the emotional attachment or the realistic threat of a punitive response from the patient's partner, or fear of losing the therapist if he or she stays with the partner (Perry and Flannery, 1982, 1989). Such a challenge may make the patient feel trapped between pleasing the therapist and being punished by the patient's partner. It may result in panic or early termination. Instead the therapist must address the patient's fantasies that submission brings with it entitlement to

be taken care of by dominant others (Waska, 1997). The patient may resist mourning this expectation that he or she is owed the right to be taken care of, as one may have trouble giving up on a debt not repaid (Perry *et al.*, 1989).

Failure to mourn losses, especially prior to termination

A fifth problem occurs with the patient who avoids dealing with separation issues in therapy, which often involve mourning past losses or disappointments (Werbart, 1997). This may lead the patient to avoid anticipating the loss of the therapist at termination and mourning appropriately. The therapist may tacitly collude with this avoidance, because of a countertransference fantasy of always being available or fear of provoking separation panic or distress. Failure to confront the avoidance may result in a failure to make lasting dynamic changes, leaving the patient at risk for a sense of betrayal after termination, followed then by deterioration.

Conclusions

The psychotherapy of DPD is usually quite helpful. All modalities, individual, group, and residential treatment, report sizable treatment effects, as do the two major theoretical schools studied: dynamic and cognitive-behavioral. The effects on symptoms are generally large but there is less documentation in areas such as improved autonomy, healthy, nonsubmissive relationships, and successful employment. The required treatment duration leading to full recovery and healthy function still remains undetermined. This generally positive conclusion should be tempered by recognizing that there are a number of challenges in the psychotherapy of DPD that can allow improvement to plateau rather than proceed toward substantial improvement and a healthy termination. The next generation of studies, focusing on both process as well as outcome, should address these. Until then, therapists should pay particular attention to the potential for therapeutic stalemates after an initial period of improvement, and attend to particular patterns including the transference–countertransference, which may provide a key to addressing the stalemates and allow progress to resume.

References

Abraham, K. (1924). The influence of oral erotism on character formation. *International Journal of Psycho-Analysis*, **6**, 247–58.

Abraham, K. (1954). *Selected papers on psychoanalysis*, pp. 370–72. New York: Basic Books.

Alexander, J. F. and Abeles, N. (1968). Dependency changes in psychotherapy as related to interpersonal relationships. *Journal of Consulting and Clinical Psychology*, **32**, 685–9.

Alexander, B. K. and Dibb, G. S. (1977). Interpersonal perceptions in addict families. *Family Process*, **16**, 17–28.

American Psychiatric Association (1994). *Diagnostic and statistical manual for mental disorders* (*DSM-IV*), 4th edn. Washington, DC: American Psychiatric Association.

Andrews, G., Kiloh, L. G., and Kehoe, L. (1978). Asthenic personality, myth or reality? *Australian and New Zealand Journal of Psychiatry*, **12**, 95–8.

Baker, J. D., Capron, E. W., and Azorlosa, J. (1996). Family environment characteristics of persons with histrionic and dependent personality disorders. *Journal of Personality Disorders*, **10**, 82–7.

Beck, A. T., *et al.* (1990). Dependent personality disorder. In: *Cognitive therapy of personality disorders*, pp. 283–308. New York: Guilford Press.

Beck, A. T., *et al.* (2001). Dysfunctional beliefs discriminate personality disorders. *Behaviour Research and Therapy*, **39**, 1213–25.

Beck, J. S. (1997). Cognitive approaches to personality disorders. In: J. H. Wright and M. E. Thase, section ed., L. J. Dickstein, M. B. Riba, and J. Oldham, ed. *Cognitive therapy, section I of American Psychiatric Press review of psychiatry*, Vol. 16, pp. 173–1106. Washington, DC: American Psychiatric Press, Inc.

van den Berg, P. J. and Helstone, F. S. (1975). Oral, obsessive, and hysterical personality patterns: a Dutch replication. *Journal of Psychiatric Research*, **12**, 319–27.

Bornstein, R. F. (1992). The dependent personality: developmental, social, and clinic perspectives. *Psychological Bulletin*, **112**, 3–23.

Bornstein, R. F. (1995a). Comorbididty of dependent personality disorder and other psychological disorders: an integrative review. *Journal of Personality Disorders*, **9**, 286–303.

Bornstein, R. F. (1995b). Active dependency. *Journal of Nervous and Mental Disease*, **183**, 64–77.

Bornstein, R. F. (1997). Dependent personality disorder in DSM-IV and beyond. *Clinical Psychology-Science and Practice*, **4**, 175–87.

Bornstein, R. F. (1998). Depathologizing dependency. *Journal of Nervous and Mental Disease*, **186**, 67–73.

Budman, S., Demby, A., Soldz, S., and Merry, J. (1996). Time-limited group psychotherapy for patients with personality disorders: outcomes and drop-outs. *International Journal of Group Psychotherapy*, **46**, 357–77.

Davanloo, H. (1978). *Basic principles and techniques in short-term dynamic psychotherapy*. New York, Spectrum.

Diagnostic and Statistical Manual, Mental Disorders. (1952). Committee on Nomenclature and Statistics of the American Psychiatric Association. Washington, DC: APA.

Diguer, L., Barber, J., and Luborsky, L. (1993). Three concomitants: personality disorders, psychiatric severity and outcome of dynamic psychotherapy of major depression. *American Journal of Psychiatry*, **150**, 1246–8.

Dolan, B., Warren, F., and Kingsley, N. (1997). Change in borderline symptoms one year after therapeutic community treatment for severe personality disorder. *British Journal of Psychiatry*, **171**, 274–9.

Epstein, N. (1980). Social consequences of assertion, aggression, passive-aggression and submission: situational and dispositional determinants. *Behavior Therapy*, **11**, 662–9.

Goldman, A. (1956). Reparative psychotherapy. In: S. Rado and G. Daniels, ed. *Changing concepts of psychoanalytic medicine*, pp. 101–13. New York: Grune & Stratton.

Gottheil, E. and Stone, G. C. (1968). Factor analytic study of orality and anality. *Journal of Nervous and Mental Disease*, **146**, 1–17.

Hardy, G. E., *et al.* (1995). Impact of cluster C personality disorders on outcomes of contrasting brief psychotherapies for depression. *Journal of Consulting and Clinical Psychology*, **63**, 997–1004.

Head, S. B., Baker, J. D., and Williamson, D. A. (1991). Family environment characteristics and dependent personality disorder. *Journal of Personality Disorders*, **5**, 256–63.

Hill, D. E. C. (1970). Outpatient management of passive-dependent women. *Hospital and Community Psychiatry*, **21**, 402–5.

Hirschfeld, R. M. A., *et al.* (1977). A measure of interpersonal dependency. *Journal of Personality Assessment*, **41**, 610–18.

Hirschfeld, R. M. A., Shea, M. T., and Weise, R. (1991). Dependent personality disorder: perspectives for DSM-IV. *Journal of Personality Disorders*, **5**, 135–49.

Hoglend, P. (1993). Personality disorders and long-term outcome after brief dynamic psychotherapy. *Journal of Personality Disorders*, **7**, 168–81.

Horowitz, M., *et al.* (1984). *Personality styles and brief psychotherapy*. Basic Books, New York.

Kagan, J. and Moss, H. (1960). The stability of passive and dependent behavior from childhood through adulthood. *Child Development*, **31**, 577–91.

Karterud, S., *et al.* (1992). Day hospital therapeutic community treatment for patients with personality disorders. *Journal of Nervous and Mental Disease*, **180**, 238–43.

Katerud, S., *et al.* (2003). Day treatment of patients with personality disorders: experiences from a Norwegian treatment research network. *Journal of Personality Disorders*, **17**, 243–62.

Kline, P. and Storey, R. (1977). A factor analytic study of the oral character. *British Journal of the Society for Clinical Psychology*, **16**, 317–28.

Kool, S., Dekker, J., Duijsens, I. J., de Jonghe, F., and Puite, B. (2003). Changes in personality pathology after pharmacotherapy and combined therapy for depressed patients. *Journal of Personality Disorders*, **17**, 60–72.

Krawitz, R. (1997). A prospective psychotherapy outcome study. *Australian and New Zealand Journal of Psychiatry*, **31**, 465–73.

Langer, T. S. and Michael, S. T. (1963). *Life stress and mental health*. New York: The Free Press of Glencoe.

Lazare, A., Klerman, G. L., and Armor, D. (1966). Oral, obsessive, and hysterical personality patterns: an investigation of psychoanalytic concepts by means of factor analysis. *Archives of General Psychiatry*, **14**, 624–43.

Lazare, A., Klerman, G. L., and Armor, D. (1970). Oral, obsessive, and hysterical personality patterns: a replication of factor analysis in an independent sample. *Journal of Psychiatric Research*, **7**, 275–90.

Leeman, C. P. and Mulvey, C. H. (1975). Brief psychotherapy of the dependent personality. Specific techniques. *Psychotherapy and Psychosomatics*, **25**, 36–42.

Leichsenring, F. and Leibing, E. (2003). The effectiveness of psychodynamic therapy and cognitive behavior therapy in the treatment of personality disorders: a meta-analysis. *American Journal of Psychiatry*, **160**, 1223–32.

Livesley, J., Schroeder, M. L., and Jackson, D. N. (1990). Dependent personality disorder and attachment problems. *Journal of Personality Disorders*, **4**, 131–40.

Luborsky, L. (1984). *Principles of psychoanalytic psychotherapy: a manual for supportive expressive treatment*. New York: Basic Books.

Malan, D. (1976). *The frontier of brief psychotherapy: an example of the convergence of research and clinical practice*. New York: Plenum.

Malinow, K. L. (1981). Dependent personality. In: J. R. Lion, ed. *Personality disorder, diagnosis and management*, 2nd edn. Baltimore, MD: Williams & Wilkins.

Marchand, A. and Wapler, M. (1993). L'effet des troubles de la personnalite sur la reponse au traitement behavioural-cognitif du trouble panique avec agora-phobie. *Revue Canadienne de Psychiatrie*, **38**, 163–6.

Millon, T. (1981). Dependent personality disorder. In: *Disorders of personality DSM-III Axis II*. New York: John Wiley & Sons.

Monsen, J. T., Odland, T., and Eilertsen, D. E. (1995). Personality disorders: changes and stability after intensive psychotherapy focusing on affect consciousness. *Psychotherapy Research*, **5**, 33–48.

Montgomery, J. (1971). Treatment management of passive-dependent behavior. *International Journal of Social Psychiatry*, **17**, 311–17.

Offenkrantz, W. and Tobin, A. (1974). Psychoanalytic psychotherapy. *Archives of General Psychiatry*, **30**, 593–606.

O'Neill, F. A. and Kendler, K. S. (1998). Longitudinal study of interpersonal dependency in female twins. *British Journal of Psychiatry*, **172**, 154–8.

Ottosson, H., Ekselius, L., Grann, M., and Kullgren, G. (2002). Cross-system concordance of personality disorder diagnoses of DSM-IV and Diagnostic Criteria for Research of ICD-10. *Journal of Personality Disorders*, **16**, 283–92.

Patience, D. A., McGuire, R. J., Scott, A. I., and Freeman, C. P. L. (1995). The Edinburgh Primary Care Study: personality disorder and outcome. *British Journal of Psychiatry*, **167**, 324–30.

Perry, J. C. (2001). Dependent personality disorder. In: J. Gunderson and G. O. Gabbard, ed. *Treatment of psychiatric disorders*, 3rd edn, pp. 2353–68. Washington, DC: American Psychiatric Press, Inc.

Perry, J. C. and Flannery, R. B. (1982). Passive-aggressive personality disorder: treatment implications of a clinical typology. *Journal of Nervous and Mental Disease*, **170**, 164–73.

Perry, J. C. and Vaillant, G. E. (1989). Personality disorders. In: H. I. Kaplan and B. J. Sadock, ed. *Comprehensive textbook of psychiatry*, 5th edn, Vol. II, pp. 1352–87. Baltimore, MD: Williams & Wilkins Co.

Perry, J. C. and Bond, M. (2000). Empirical studies of psychotherapy for personality disorders. In: J. M. Oldham and M. B. Riba, series ed. *American Psychiatric Press review of psychiatry*, section III, Vol. 19, pp. 1–31. Washington, DC: American Psychiatric Press Inc.

Perry, J. C., Banon, E., and Ianni, F. (1999). The effectiveness of psychotherapy for personality disorders. *American Journal of Psychiatry*, **156**, 1312–21.

Piper, W. E., Rosie, J. S., Azim, H. F. A., and Joyce, A. S. (1993). A randomized trial of psychiatric day treatment for patients with affective and personality disorders. *Hospital and Community Psychiatry*, **44**, 757–63.

Presley, A. S. and Walton, H. J. (1973). Dimensions of abnormal personality. *British Journal of Psychiatry*, **122**, 269–76.

Poldrugo, F. and Forti, B. (1988). Personality disorders and alcoholism treatment outcome. *Drug and Alcohol Dependence*, **21**, 171–6.

The Quality Assurance Project. (1991). Treatment outlines for avoidant, dependent and passive-aggressive personality disorders. *Australian and New Zealand Journal of Psychiatry*, **25**, 404–11.

Reich, J. (1996). The morbidity of DSM-III-R dependent personality disorder. *Journal of Nervous and Mental Disease*, **184**, 22–6.

Rosenheim, E. and Gaoni, B. (1977). Defensive passivity in adolescence. *Adolescence*, **12**, 449–59.

Sadoff, R. L. and Collins, D. J. (1968). Passive dependency in stutterers. *American Journal of Psychiatry*, **124**, 1126–7.

Sarwer-Foner, G. J. and Kealey, L. S. (1981). Reactions to hospitalization: passive dependency factors. Recurrence of original symptoms and attempts to prolong hospitalization on the announcement of discharge. *Comprehensive Psychiatry*, **22**, 103–13.

Saul, L. J. and Warner, S. L. (1975). Mobilizing ego strengths. *International Journal of Psychoanalytic Psychotherapy*, **4**, 358–86.

Shea, M. T., *et al.* (1990). Personality disorders and treatment outcome in the NIMH Treatment of Depression Collaborative Research Program. *American Journal of Psychiatry*, **147**, 711–18.

Skodol, A. E., Gallaher, P. E., and Oldham, J. M. (1996). Excessive dependency and depression: is the relationship specific? *Journal of Nervous and Mental Disease*, **184**, 165–71.

Strupp, H. H. and Binder, J. L. (1984). *Psychotherapy in a new key: a guide to time-limited dynamic psychotherapy*. New York: Basic Books.

Temple, N., Patrick, M., Evans, M., Holloway, F., and Squire, C. (1997). Interpretive group psychotherapy and dependent day hospital patients: a preliminary investigation. *International Journal of Social Psychiatry*, **43**, 116–28.

Torgersen, S. (1980). Personality and experience in an encounter-group. *Scandinavian Journal of Psychology*, **21**, 139–41.

Torgersen, S., Kringlen, E., and Cramer, V. (2001). The prevalence of personality disorders in a community sample. *Archives of General Psychiatry*, **58**, 590–6.

Turkat, I. D. and Carlson, C. R. (1984). Data-based versus symptomatic formulation of treatment: the case of a dependent personality. *Journal of Behavior Therapy and Experimental Psychiatry*, **15**, 153–60.

Tyrer, P. and Alexander, J. (1979). Classification of personality disorder. *British Journal of Psychiatry*, **135**, 163–7.

US War Department. (1945). Nomenclature and method of recording diagnoses. *War Department Technical Bulletin*, Med, 203, **October**.

Waska, R. T. (1997). Precursors to masochistic and dependent character development. *American Journal of Psychoanalysis*, **57**, 253–67.

Werbart, A. (1997). Separation, termination process and long-term outcome in psychotherapy with severely disturbed patients. *Bulletin of the Menninger Clinic*, **61**, 16–43.

Whitman, R., Trosman, H., and Koenig, R. (1954). Clinical assessment of passive-aggressive personality. *Archives of Neurology and Psychiatry*, **72**, 540–9.

Wilberg, T., Karterud, S., Urnes, O., Pedersen, G., and Friis, S. (1998). Outcomes of poorly functioning patients with personality disorders in a day treatment program. *Psychiatric Services*, **49**, 1462–7.

Winston, A., *et al.* (1991). Brief psychotherapy of personality disorders. *Journal of Nervous and Mental Disease*, **179**, 188–93.

Winston, A., *et al.* (1994). Short-term psychotherapy of personality disorders. *American Journal of Psychiatry*, **151**, 190–4.

Zanarini, M. C., *et al.* (1998). Axis II comorbidity of borderline personality disorder. *Comprehensive Psychiatry*, **39**, 296–302.

Zaretsky, A. E., *et al.* (1997). Are dependency and self-criticism risk factors for major depressive disorder. *Canadian Journal of Psychiatry*, **42**, 291–7.

28 Psychotherapy of obsessive-compulsive personality disorder

Glen O. Gabbard and Cory F. Newman

Introduction

The symptoms of obsessive-compulsive personality disorder (OCPD) are well described in the DSM-IV (*Diagnostic and statistical manual for mental disorders*, 4th edn) classification (see Table 28.1). Most of the symptoms can be regarded as lifelong adaptations that frequently do not create a great deal of distress for the patient. Certain aspects of the condition are even adaptive, such as an emphasis on detail, work, and achievement. In some cases, family members or significant others may be instrumental in bringing the patient to the attention of a psychotherapist. Persons with OCPD are often driven workaholics who have serious problems with interpersonal intimacy. They may be conscientious to a fault, expecting others to conform to the high expectations they have of themselves. They are haunted by perfectionism and chronically feel they are not doing enough to live up to the excessive expectations they impose on themselves. They may come across as rigid, moralizing, condescending, and excessively meticulous to others. Some may be miserly, tending to hoard for future catastrophes, and lacking in generosity. Like Mr Spock of the starship *Enterprise*, people with OCPD attempt to be thoroughly logical and rational as they approach any problem. They are terrified of emotional spontaneity, and their mechanistic style can be disconcerting to others.

A long-standing historical confusion has existed between obsessive-compulsive disorder (OCD) and OCPD. Freud (1908/1959) originally regarded the constellation of symptoms typical of OCD as a neurosis connected with difficulties at the anal phase in psychosexual development. Later, when Karl Abraham (1921/1942) identified an 'anal character,' he assumed that this was simply the characterological counterpart to the obsessive-compulsive neurosis. In other words, OCD was regarded as a symptomatic neurosis, and OCPD a character neurosis. Over time, however, the relationship between the two entities has become much murkier. Whether the two have any linkage at all is quite controversial. Patients suffering from OCD are plagued with an internal drivenness to perform ritualistic behaviors and are haunted by recurring unpleasant thoughts. These symptoms are highly ego-dystonic (i.e., they are deeply distressing), and these patients wish to be relieved of the torment they cause. In stark contrast, patients with OCPD tend to have ego-*syntonic* characterological traits that they often have little interest in exploring or changing.

Recent studies suggest that a wide range of personality disorders may occur in patients with OCD. One study (Rasmussen and Tsuang, 1986) found that fewer than half of patients with OCD satisfied the criteria for OCPD. In this particular sample, mixed personality disorder with dependent, avoidant, and passive-aggressive features was the most common personality diagnosis that accompanied OCD. In another effort to determine if there was linkage between the two (Baer *et al.*, 1990), 96 patients with OCD were assessed for OCPD, and only 6% had both diagnoses. One investigation, however, suggested that OCPD is significantly more common in patients with OCD than in those with panic and major depressive disorder (Diaferia *et al.*, 1997). Another study found that obsessional symptoms were more likely to be associated with traits of OCPD than with traits of other personality disorders (Rosen and Tallis, 1995). In a Scandinavian study of comorbidity between OCD and personality disorders (Bejerot *et al.*, 1998), 36% of OCD patients were also diagnosed with OCPD.

The data accumulated to date cannot definitively determine whether or not OCD and OCPD are essentially variations of a similar fundamental pathology. Much more is known about the structural abnormalities of the brain in OCD, where there is significantly less total white matter, greater total cortex volumes, and impaired myelinization (Jenike *et al.*, 1998). In any case, the current trend within the mental health field is to approach the two disorders as though they were quite distinct, primarily because they have different treatment implications. OCD generally responds well to a combination of exposure *in vivo* and selective serotonin reuptake inhibitors. Although empirical data are lacking, OCPD generally requires psychotherapy of 40 sessions or more.

Conceptualization of the disorder

Psychodynamic/psychoanalytic

Early contributors to the psychoanalytic understanding of this character organization asserted that a constellation of character traits—parsimony, orderliness, and obstinacy—were signs of pathological regression. The castration anxiety connected with the oedipal phase of development led to a retreat to the relative safety of the anal period. These patients were regarded

Table 28.1 DSM-IV-TR criteria for obsessive-compulsive personality disorder

A pervasive pattern of preoccupation with orderliness, perfectionism, and mental and interpersonal control, at the expense of flexibility, openness, and efficiency, beginning by early adulthood and present in a variety of contexts, as indicated by four (or more) of the following:

(1) is preoccupied with details, rules, lists, order, organization, or schedules to the extent that the major point of the activity is lost

(2) shows perfectionism that interferes with task completion (e.g., is unable to complete a project because his or her own overly strict standards are not met)

(3) is excessively devoted to work and productivity to the exclusion of leisure activities and friendships (not accounted for by obvious economic necessity)

(4) is overconscientious, scrupulous, and inflexible about matters of morality, ethics, or values (not accounted for by cultural or religious identification)

(5) is unable to discard worn-out or worthless objects even when they have no sentimental value

(6) is reluctant to delegate tasks or to work with others unless they submit to exactly his or her way of doing things

(7) adopts a miserly spending style toward both self and others; money is viewed as something to be hoarded for future catastrophes

(8) shows rigidity and stubbornness

Source: Reprinted from American Psychiatric Association: *Diagnostic and Statistical Manual of Mental Disorders*, Fourth Edition, Text Revision. Arlington, VA, American Psychiatric Association, 2000. Copyright 2000, American Psychiatric Association. Used with permission.

as having had early power struggles with their mothers around toilet training that led them to have difficulty expressing aggression and stubbornness leading to an insistence on getting their own way. Orderliness was regarded as a reaction formation against an underlying wish to engage in anal messiness. The self-critical nature was related to a punitive superego resulting from the internalization of power struggles with their mothers. Other defenses linked to OCPD in this classical conceptualization were intellectualization, isolation of affect, undoing, and displacement.

As the field of psychoanalysis has evolved away from ego psychology and more in the direction of British object relations thinking and American relational theory, the emphases have changed in terms of the conceptualization of the disorder. Vicissitudes of the anal phase of psychosexual development have been superseded by a focus on problems with spontaneity and control, interpersonal difficulties, management of anger and dependency, cognitive style, self-esteem, and the problems of balancing emotional intimacy with work productivity (Shapiro, 1965; Salzman, 1968, 1980, 1983; Gabbard, 1985, 2000; Gabbard and Menninger, 1988; Horowitz, 1988; Josephs, 1992; McCullough and Maltsberger, 2001). Self-doubt is also a marker of individuals who struggle with OCPD. Their childhood experiences often have made them feel that they were not sufficiently valued or loved by their parents or caretakers. Psychoanalytic exploration may reveal that this perception is often associated with excessively high expectations of parental demonstrativeness. Hence one cannot automatically jump to the conclusion that actual coldness in the parents was pathogenic. These children may in some cases require more reassurance and affection than the ordinary child to feel loved. Psychodynamic treatment of these patients also reveals strong unfulfilled dependent yearnings and a reservoir of rage directed at parents for not being more emotionally available (Gabbard, 2000). The defense mechanism of reaction formation, associated with isolation of affect, is often employed because both anger and dependency are consciously unacceptable to the person with OCPD. In a counterdependent effort to deny the existence of dependency, they may go to great lengths to demonstrate their 'rugged individualism' and staunch independence. They may similarly attempt to master their anger completely, and their conflict over anger may lead them to appear obsequious, ingratiating, and deferential to demonstrate that they are not harboring any feelings of rage or anger.

Work has the advantage of being at least potentially under the control of the worker, so people with OCPD are much more comfortable in the work place than in human relationships. Intimacy raises the possibility that they will be overwhelmed by powerful wishes to be taken care of. Those wishes entail a risk—namely, that they will be frustrated and lead the individual to feelings of hatred and resentment. Feelings in intimate relationships, then, are threatening because they have the potential to make someone with OCPD feel 'out of control,' which is one of the worst fears that these people harbor.

People in relationships with someone who has OCPD frequently feel that they are being controlled. This tendency to control others is related, in most cases, to a fundamental concern that sources of love or support in the immediate environment are prone to disappear at the drop of a hat. The child who grows up feeling unloved evolves into an adult who feels that any love from a partner is constantly imperiled. Because of the high levels of anger and the intense destructive wishes that lurk within, an obsessive-compulsive person may worry that this anger will drive people away. This fear is coupled with a general sense of self-doubt and low self-esteem such that many people with OCPD are convinced that if a friend or lover really knew them well, he or she would be filled with contempt and loathing.

In fact, the obsessive-compulsive style of relating to others often exasperates and irritates those who have to deal with it. Josephs (1992) stresses that subordinates may be treated differently than superiors. Power differential in the relationship shapes the style of relatedness. To subordinates, people with OCPD tend to come across as hypercritical, domineering, and controlling. To superiors, they are ingratiating and obsequious in a way that is perceived as a phony effort to curry favor. Hence, the approval and love they seek is undermined, so their fear of alienating others is a self-fulfilling prophecy. They tend to feel chronically unappreciated as they strive for an approbation they never receive.

The obsessive-compulsive's quest for perfection also leads to considerable misery. Psychoanalysis or psychoanalytic therapy often reveals a barely conscious or unconscious belief that if they could only reach a transcendent stage of flawlessness, they will finally receive the esteem and approval they missed as children. They seem to have the conviction that as children they simply did not try hard enough, so as adults they then feel a chronic sense of 'not doing enough.' The parent who was perceived as never satisfied becomes introjected as a harsh superego that expects more and more from the patient. Some persons with OCPD are workaholics because they are unconsciously driven by this conviction that love and approval could finally be attained if they could reach the top of their chosen profession. Here lies part of the tragedy in persons with OCPD. Even if they do achieve extraordinary accomplishments, they are rarely satisfied with any of them. They somehow feel that success is inherently disappointing. They are driven more by a wish to gain relief from a tormenting superego than by a genuine wish for pleasure. Hence they may feel that their achievement was essentially fraudulent and that they simply deceived those around them.

Josephs (1992) has found it useful to conceptualize the complex character structure of these patients as involving a public sense of self, a private sense of self, and an unconscious sense of self. Each has one dimension that applies more to superiors and another that is linked more to relationships with subordinates. The public sense of self in relationship to superiors, for example, is that of a conscientious and responsible worker who is predictable, considerate, serious, and always socially appropriate. The public sense of self in relation to subordinates is that of a constructive mentor or thoughtful critic who provides valuable feedback for those who wish to learn. Unfortunately, the subjectively experienced sense of a public self is not what is perceived by others. The reactions of others may give rise to a private sense of self that is conscious but largely hidden from others. Persons with OCPD frequently feel that they are unappreciated and consequently are dealing with a chronic sense of narcissistic wound. The lack of approval leads them to be even more tortured by self-doubt. They must shield this insecurity from those in superior positions because they dread humiliation from bosses and supervisors. They fear that if they expose this self-doubting side, they will be seen as weak and pathetic. Existing in association with this aspect of the private sense of self is a thoroughgoing conviction of moral superiority to those who occupy subordinate positions. Because OCPD patients are so intensely defended against their aggression and sadism, they do not want to appear contemptuous. Hence, they attempt to mask this aspect of the private sense of self to avoid appearing pompous, pretentious, or hypercritical. They may even feel proud of how considerate and self-contained they are toward those who are beholden to them.

The two dimensions of the unconscious sense of self involve a controlling sadist in relation to subordinates and an obsequious masochist in relation to superiors (Josephs, 1992). The mean-spirited and sadistic wish to hurt those who do not submit to their control is entirely unacceptable to OCPD patients and therefore must be repressed. To do otherwise would be to compromise their high moral standards. When it comes to authority figures, however, these same individuals fear humiliation in the context of being submissive and longing for love. Hence, they masochistically submit to their own excessively harsh moral standards and torture themselves for not living up to these expectations. This self-torture is a way of sparing them from what they fear most, namely, control, domination, and sadistic humiliation by others. The unconscious message they give to those to whom they are subordinate is, 'You don't need to criticize me and attack me because I am already tormenting myself relentlessly.'

Cognitive/behavioral

There is some evidence that broad personality characteristics—including those that may later become dysfunctional—involve a strong hereditary component (Kagan, 1989). Nevertheless, genetics do not account for all behavioral variability, as there is an ongoing interaction with the environment and learning experiences across the lifespan. From a cognitive-behavioral standpoint, OCPD behaviors and related beliefs are learned (and/or further strengthened) over time, primarily stemming from experiences with primary caregivers during the early developmental years, and later being reinforced by broader life experiences (e.g., peers, school) and societal values.

Regarding the latter factor, it is no surprise that OCPD is fairly common in Western culture, as our society tends to reward some of the characteristics of this personality style (Simon, 1990). For example, one of the messages that children receive during their years of schooling is that if they work hard and do things extremely well, they can achieve anything and become wealthy. Later, these same children grow up to witness the extreme competitive spirit that separates the 'winners' ('the championship team,' or the best product) from the 'losers' (all the others) and learn that they must take advantage of every 'edge' they have over other students if they wish to gain entry into elite secondary schools and colleges. In other words, working hard, being busy, being in control of the situation, and avoiding mistakes at all costs are viewed as part of the recipe for success. It becomes easy to see how these behaviors and attitudes can become magnified to the point where working hard becomes working *obsessively*, with little time for rest or reflection. Competing becomes a drive for perfection, and a reluctance to cooperate and get close to others. Trying to do things well becomes a paralyzing fear of making human mistakes, and an agonizing process in making decisions. Striving to be in control of oneself and one's life situation turns into needless self-restrictions, and excessive attempts to control other people. The full clinical problem of OCPD becomes reflected by the person's rigidity in thinking style and behavioral habits, punitive perfectionism, emotional constriction, ruminative indecisiveness and doubt, and other problematic manifestations of this personality spectrum.

In general, however, relatively little has been written about OCPD in the cognitive-behavioral literature. Much more theory and research has been invested in the Axis I OCD, which typically involves more discrete, circumscribed patterns of ritualized behavior intended to reduce excessive, acute anxiety. With regard to the broader personality style of OCPD, Shapiro (1965) observed that the disorder involved a rigid, intense, focused, 'stimulus-bound' quality of thought process—a style much more amendable to technical, highly detailed tasks than to 'big picture' endeavors such as navigating a social event, or engaging in the arts. Further, those with OCPD are extremely self-conscious about what they are thinking and doing, believing that they 'should' have control over the smallest details of their functioning, and overinvesting their identity in their tasks ('I am what I do'). Shapiro also theorized that such individuals are also out of touch with their desires and wishes, and therefore experience marked subjective doubts about whether they are doing things properly, even as they steadfastly reject the well-meaning suggestions of others to 'lighten up' or do things a little differently. The result is a state of mind reflected by the apparently paradoxical thought, 'I *must* do things *this* way; but what if it's not exactly right?'

Guidano and Liotti (1983) also have written about the cognitive and emotional styles of individuals with OCPD. One of the characteristics to which they point is the individual's belief that there is an absolutely correct solution for a given problem, and that it is best to postpone acting on the problem until this clear and certain path is ascertained. Such a stance may well lead one to suffer from (in colloquial terms) 'paralysis by analysis.' Guidano and Liotti hypothesize that individuals with OCPD grew up in households in which they were given very mixed, contradictory messages from parents. When this happens, children learn that doing the 'right' thing is very elusive, and the cost for being wrong can be very high indeed. The result is a demand for certainty, and an overconcern for the smallest of details.

In general, cognitive-behavioral theorists put less emphasis on uncovering a specific etiology for OCPD symptoms, and more on a descriptive evaluation of the faulty beliefs that comprise the disorder, as well as a conceptualization of the ways in which the disorder is maintained by the current interaction of patient's beliefs with his or her environment (see J. S. Beck, 1995). For example, a number of maladaptive beliefs have been identified that are emblematic of OCPD. Clinically generated by A. T. Beck *et al.* (1990), the diagnostic specificity of these beliefs has been supported by recent empirical investigation on the discriminant validity of the Personality Beliefs Questionnaire

(PBQ: A. T. Beck *et al.*, 2001). A brief sample of these beliefs is:

- 'It is important to do a perfect job on everything.'
- 'Any flaw or defect of performance may lead to a catastrophe.'
- 'People should do things my way.'
- 'Details are extremely important.'

Similarly, Young (1999) has developed a taxonomy of schemas hypothesized to be pertinent to chronic dysfunction such as personality disorders. It may be hypothesized that the schemas common to OCPD would be *incompetence* (overconcern that mistakes or flaws will indicate an overriding lack of capability), *unrelenting standards* (such that nothing less than the highest level of performance will be allowed in oneself or in others), and *lack of individuation* (in that they fear loss of identity and control if they change any aspect of how they customarily respond).

As mentioned above, some aspects of OCPD behavior are positively reinforced by a society that values hard work and competition. However, it seems that negative reinforcement may play an even more prominent role in the maintenance of the OCPD style. Much of the extreme behavior of individuals with OCPD is driven by anxiety—about making mistakes, missing something important, and not getting it 'just right.' By focusing on details, staying true to a familiar routine, avoiding risks, and maintaining 'control,' persons with OCPD find relief when their feared outcomes do not materialize. This relief—translated as the reduction of the aversive emotion of anxiety—negatively reinforces OCPD strategies. Unfortunately, relief becomes a dominant feeling in the person's life, obscuring other important emotions such as joy and rapture. Further, the patient's ultraconservative behavioral strategies do not permit the testing of new hypotheses, thus further maintaining the *status quo*. If the OCPD patients always do the same things, they will assume that what they are doing works best—there is nothing to which to compare it. However, for the OCPD individual who is dysphoric and seeking therapy, he or she will feel 'stuck,' sometimes making statements such as, 'I know I should do things differently, but I just can't bring myself to do it.' As for the important people in their lives, they often conclude that the person with OCPD 'will never change.'

The following is a brief sample of a cognitive-behavioral conceptualization for a male, 45-year-old OCPD sufferer who is experiencing problems at work, marital difficulties, and a severe level of dysphoria that is sometimes accompanied by suicidal ideation. The therapist describes 'Ace' as a gentleman who demands perfection of himself and others, and whose emotions range from flat to dysphoric. Although his wife has complained for years that Ace is too critical and emotionally withholding, threatening to leave him on many occasions, Ace did not become depressed until he received a significant promotion at work that forced him to assume a new schedule and additional responsibilities. No longer able to do things the way he had done them for 20 years, and fearing that he was no longer capable of maintaining perfect standards, Ace lapsed into a severe depression. Ace's colleagues tried to give him some assistance, but he viewed them as patronizing and intrusive, and responded by isolating himself. He tried to compensate for his subjective sense of loss of control and competence at work by tightening the reins over his wife and kids at home, whereupon his wife informed Ace that she had contacted a divorce attorney. Ace agreed to see a therapist in order to appease his wife temporarily, but he viewed the act of consulting a therapist as an inherent failure, and his suicidal ideation worsened. Not surprisingly, his work performance suffered further, which only served to 'confirm' for Ace that he was losing control over himself and his life, and his self-reproach and hopelessness (as well as his irritability) became more pronounced. The treatment plan would focus on the suicidality first, and then the beliefs and behaviors that Ace used to punish himself and others when things would inevitably change or could not be done perfectly in life.

Outcome research

Very little research is available to guide the psychotherapist of a person with OCPD. The research that exists generally considers all Cluster C personality disorders together. For example, Svartberg et al. (2004) studied 50 patients who met criteria for one or more Cluster C personality disorders but not any of the Axis II conditions in Cluster A or B. These patients were randomly assigned to 40 sessions of short-term dynamic therapy (STDP) or cognitive therapy (CT). The therapists were full-time clinicians who were experienced at psychotherapy and who received manually guided supervision. The outcomes were evaluated in terms of interpersonal problems, core personality pathology, and symptom distress. Measures were administered repeatedly during and after treatment so that longitudinal change could be evaluated.

The whole sample of patients showed, on average, statistically significant improvements on all measures during treatment and also during the 2-year follow-up. Two years after treatment 54% of the STDP patients and 42% of the CT patients had recovered symptomatically, whereas approximately 40% in both groups had recovered in terms of interpersonal problems and personality functioning. The investigators concluded that both types of therapy have a role to play in the treatment of OCPD.

Winston et al. (1994) randomly assigned 81 patients with personality disorders to either dynamic therapy, adaptive therapy, or a wait-list control. The mean number of sessions for those treated was 40.3 sessions. Of the 81 patients, 36 were Cluster C, and 19 were diagnosed as personality disorder not otherwise specified, with Cluster C features. Some patients required longer treatment, but patients in the two therapy conditions improved significantly on all measures in comparison with wait-list controls. At follow-up (averaging 1.5 years), gains made in therapy were sustained.

In a 'follow-along' study that did not involve the use of control groups (Barber et al., 1997), 14 patients with OCPD and 24 patients with avoidant personality disorder were treated in 52 sessions of time-limited expressive-supportive dynamic psychotherapy. By the end of treatment, only 15% of the OCPD patients retained the diagnosis. OCPD patients remained in treatment significantly longer than avoidant patients and tended to improve more. The improvements that were broad based included measures of depression, anxiety, personality disorder, interpersonal problems, and general functioning.

Referring to promising data from the same series of studies conducted in the 1990s at the University of Pennsylvania noted above (that also included a cognitive therapy treatment condition), Barber and Muenz (1996) hypothesized that cognitive therapy and supportive-expressive therapy might be differentially efficacious for avoidant personality disorder and OCPD. Utilizing data published by the Treatment for Depression Collaborative Research Program (Shea et al., 1990) the authors found evidence that depressed patients with OCPD were somewhat less responsive to cognitive-behavioral therapy than to interpersonal therapy (these findings were the opposite for individuals diagnosed with avoidant personality disorder). Nevertheless, many of the OCPD patients were responsive to cognitive therapy in terms of reduced dysphoria, and the authors acknowledged that a larger 'n' would add clarity to the findings. Barber and Muenz also found that measures of the quality of the therapeutic alliance between OCPD patients and their therapists did not change significantly over the course of treatment. Perhaps this is an area for future study—how to facilitate improvements in the alliance with OCPD patients as therapy progresses.

Extrapolating from studies on cognitive therapy for Axis I mood and anxiety disorders with comorbid personality disorders, the key may be to retain the OCPD patients for a relatively longer period of treatment (e.g., 6 months to a year), as Axis II patients have been shown to benefit from a full course of cognitive therapy similarly to those without personality disorders (Dreesen et al., 1994; Sanderson et al., 1994; Hardy et al., 1995). Unfortunately, patients with comorbid personality disorders may be more apt than uncomplicated Axis I patients to drop out of cognitive therapy prematurely, before benefits can accrue (Persons et al., 1988).

These studies have some usefulness in suggesting that patients with OCPD have the potential to use psychotherapy. However, even the randomized controlled trials have relatively small samples, and in the Winston study, there was a large number of patients excluded from the trial because of rigorous inclusion criteria. Nevertheless, they point the way to further research that might shed light on what differentiates those who will respond to therapy from those who are unlikely to be helped by these psychotherapeutic interventions.

Key practice principles

Psychodynamic

A general practice principle in treating patients with OCPD is that the intrapsychic defense mechanisms will be transformed into resistances as a psychotherapy process begins. If a patient characteristically intellectualizes, for example, as a way of fending off affect, that same pattern of intellectualization will occur when the therapist attempts to explore the patient's feelings. Patients may identify facts and gather data as a way of not dealing with feelings either directly toward the therapist or outside the therapeutic situation. Because lack of control and emotional spontaneity are among the most dreaded possibilities with someone with OCPD, patients with this disorder will often attempt to maintain firm control over what transpires in the session. A typical pattern of resistance to the free flow of associations and the exploration of feelings as they spontaneously occur is to structure the session by bringing in an outline of topics the patient wishes to cover.

A useful strategy to deal with this defensive style is for the therapist to make active efforts to help the patient identify feelings. When the patient provides a long factual account of events, it is helpful for the therapist to ask, 'But what did you feel in reaction to those events?' The therapist can also be active in making observations about feelings that slip through the defensive barrier. For example, the therapist might say to a patient, 'I notice you teared up when you talked about your uncle's funeral. Could you tell me more about the feelings you had during the funeral service?' The therapist can also point out reasons that rigid defenses are necessary. In other words, the fear of spontaneity, the dread of having angry feelings that would lead to feeling out of control, and the unacceptable nature of sexual feelings may all be major contributors to the need for the defensive posture with which the patient approaches therapy.

Another key practice principle is modification of the patient's harsh superego. The patient's punitive self-critical tendencies repeatedly get in the way of open and free exploration in the treatment process. Therapists must constantly look for ways to help patients accept their humanness. Reassuring the patient of his or her essential goodness is usually not effective. A nonjudgmental stance by the therapist is essential, and from this nonjudgmental perspective, the therapist can interpret conflicts around aggression, sexuality, and dependency. While OCPD patients will repeatedly attribute punitive attitudes toward the therapist, a consistent, nonjudgmental, accepting attitude over time will help patients begin to see that they are projecting their own self-critical nature on to the therapist. There is a cumulative effect of repeated interactions in which the therapist does not behave as the patient expects, leading to a gradual internalization of the therapist associated with a corresponding modification of the patient's superego (Gabbard, 2000). A clinical example will illustrate this process:

Mr A was a 34-year-old engineer who was mechanistic in his relatedness style throughout his psychotherapy. He always made notes in the waiting room so that he would use his time fully. He was never late for his sessions and, in fact, was generally about 5 minutes early. When he came into his psychotherapy sessions, his therapist rarely had a chance to say much because Mr A followed his outline and filled up the full 50 minutes without much time to spare. Mr A would carefully watch the clock and would announce that it was about time to go when 49 minutes of the session had passed. It was clear that he needed to be in complete control over when the session ended, what transpired in the session, and the extent of the therapist's involvement.

On one particular day, Mr A encountered a minor accident en route to his therapist's office. This accident delayed him by approximately 10 minutes, so he arrived out of breath at the therapist's door, apologizing profusely for his lateness. He found his therapist reading a book at his desk while waiting for him. The therapist smiled and welcomed him into the office. The patient explained in great detail how the accident had impeded his progress toward getting to the therapist's office. Finally, the therapist interrupted his account by asking him how he felt about being late. The patient was taken off guard by the question and responded, 'How do I feel? I'm not sure I can answer that.' The therapist replied, 'Well go ahead and reflect for a moment and see if you can identify the feelings you have.' Mr A paused and finally said, 'I guess I'm feeling guilty for being late and afraid of your reaction.' His therapist asked, 'What reaction in me do you fear?' Mr A thought for a moment and replied that he assumed his therapist would be angry with him or critical of him for not being responsible enough to show up for his appointment on time. The therapist responded, 'Did I appear angry or critical when you came to my door?' The patient replied, 'No. You looked like you were enjoying reading your book.' The therapist laughed and commented that, indeed, it was a good book. He then pointed out to Mr A: 'It sounds like you attributed your own self-criticism to me. I know you are terribly harsh on yourself if you don't arrive early to everything you do. I don't happen to feel that way.'

In this vignette the therapist modifies Mr A's punitive superego by stressing the transference distortion with which he regards his therapist. He points out the origins of the criticism in the patient and how that criticism is projected on to the therapist. By clarifying that he does not actually feel that way, he makes the patient take the projection back and consider why he reacted in the way he did. The ultimate effect is to help patients acknowledge their humanness—i.e., they learn to integrate feelings, failures, and foibles into a sense of who they are without feeling that they have lost any sense of self-respect or dignity.

The patient's superego may also be modified by interpreting defensive maneuvers designed to avoid unacceptable feelings. For example, a patient who is excessively deferential to the therapist may be using reaction formation to defend against hostile feelings. At an appropriate moment the therapist may wish to interpret this defense so the patient reflects on how it serves to control unacceptable feelings. The therapist might say, 'I've noticed that when I tell you it's time to stop the session, you almost always thank me profusely for the help. I wonder if that pattern of thanking me conceals any hostility about my interrupting you and telling you it's time to go.'

The therapist also looks for opportunities to point out to OCPD patients how their defensive style interferes with pleasure outside of therapy. The tendency to overwork and to ignore intimate relationships can be an active focus of the treatment. Pointing out the patient's difficulty in prioritizing and delegating may be useful. In interpersonal relationships, the patient will describe interactions that reveal the discrepancy between how he views himself and how others view him. The therapist should systematically address the patient's behaviors, both in the transference and outside the transference, that produce certain reactions in others. For example, the therapist might say to a patient who is alienating others, 'Do you suppose that your insistence that the other employees do things exactly as you do may irritate them?' With a consistent focus of this nature, patients eventually learn that no matter how well defended they are, their controlling tendencies and hostility toward others seep out through their pores and result in problematic relationship.

Cognitive/behavioral

In cognitive therapy, patients learn to assess their own thoughts and beliefs, and to make modifications based on the evidence of their life experiences, and on the basis of an objective evaluation about what would serve to improve the quality of their lives. Some OCPD patients are adept at recognizing the demanding and punitive nature of their thoughts, while others need the therapist to offer hypotheses for their consideration. Whatever the route to better understanding, it is important for patients to come to appreciate the impact that their subjective construal of themselves and their world play on their emotions and actions. A typical intervention, therefore, is to list and examine some of the typical beliefs that OCPD patients maintain, such as 'I am a failure if I make a mistake,' and 'I must stay in complete control or else I will fall apart.' Open-ended questioning—also known as 'guided discovery' and the Socratic method—are very useful in testing such rigid, problematic beliefs. Rather than simply telling OCPD patients that their beliefs are 'maladaptive' and instructing them on what they should believe instead, cognitive therapists ask patients questions such as, 'How

else could you maintain high standards, and yet not be so punitive toward yourself or others?' or 'Under what conditions could a person such as yourself show a lot of emotions—sadness, exuberance, grief, love, and so on—and yet still feel reasonably secure, safe, and even proud of yourself?' These are important thought exercises that are intended to stretch the OCPD's conceptual comfort zone, while reducing the risk of incurring a power struggle in the therapeutic alliance.

As the patients begin to entertain new ways of thinking, therapists encourage them to test the new hypotheses in everyday life. Examples are numerous. One patient agreed that she might benefit from changing her daily routine, which led to a discussion about trying a new item on the lunch menu, driving the 'scenic' route to her mother's house on Sundays, and sometimes even calling her mother to cancel their weekly visit in favor of a recreational activity such as biking with a friend. Predictably, this patient had some misgivings, whereupon the therapist asked her to articulate her automatic thoughts. The patient stated that she might not like the new lunch item, and therefore would waste money, and that her mother might be upset with her if she took longer than usual to get to her house or postponed the visit altogether. When these sorts of thoughts are identified, the therapist's goal is not to convince the patient that she is wrong, and that being more flexible and spontaneous is right. Rather, the goal is to flesh out the patient's concerns and to evaluate them on their own merits, based on the patient's life experience. Additionally, however, the therapist tries to establish an openness to new ideas, and a willingness to explore new ways for the patient to choose to lead her life. Such new ways might very well include asserting herself with her demanding mother, learning to find diverse food choices that she might like, being less concerned about calculated gambles with small amounts of money (e.g., lunch at a cafeteria at work), and finding new activities (e.g., biking with a friend) in order to be healthier and to invest in more relationships. All of these ideas (and their implementation between sessions) will stir up more automatic thoughts and emotions, the likes of which become fodder for therapeutic discussion. The process becomes a positive feedback loop for change.

Another example is a gentleman who, after engaging in a Socratic dialog with his therapist, decided that he would try to invest more of himself in his relationships, and to write down his thoughts when he would experience time pressure to get back to his work. The therapist infused a good deal of humor into this patient's treatment, which in itself runs counter to OCPD in that it is often unexpected and off the beaten track, and involves a display of emotions. For example, when this patient said he would 'Try to have sex with [his wife] this week,' the therapist replied that the purpose was *not* so that the patient could strike the item 'Make love to wife' off his 'to do' list! The patient actually chuckled, and acknowledged that he might indeed be more concerned with getting the therapy assignment 'right' than in actually enjoying the time in bed with his spouse, assuming that she agreed to the activity! This led to a very fruitful discussion about the patient's concerns that 'the emotions were dead from both sides' in his marriage, a topic he had conspicuously avoided during 3 months of treatment. In the end, the patient scaled back his plans, and instead produced some ideas about how he would do more of 'the little things' for his wife, even if it took some time away from his work. This was viewed as a behavioral experiment that needed to be run for at least a month in order to really see what results were possible—not only in terms of the wife's responsivity, but with regard to the patient's feelings about himself as both a husband and a provider, and about his wife.

An important goal in treatment is for the OCPD patient to learn to be more tolerant of mistakes. Patients often misconstrue the intent of this goal, believing that the therapist is asking them to 'lower their standards.' Quite to the contrary, the therapist is trying to help patients to *raise* their standards in terms of risk-tolerance, willingness to do difficult tasks with uncertain outcomes, composure under duress, and benevolence toward the demonstration of human flaws in oneself and in others. The only variable the therapist is trying to attenuate is the degree of *punishment* that the patients heap on themselves as a result of their perceived miscues and shortcomings.

There is no need whatsoever to assign OCPD patients the task of doing things imperfectly on purpose. Imperfection occurs naturally in life, and its propensity for showing up at difficult moments can be used to therapeutic advantage, rather than be cursed as something terrible and devastating. The case example of Mr A is an illustration of the inevitability of imperfection. Along these lines, a useful cognitive therapy homework assignment might be for the patient to think of (and document) the things he would like to do, but usually avoids for fear of failing. Then, his task is to consider the pros and cons of trying each of these endeavors, bearing in mind his propensity for magnifying the consequences of not getting it 'right,' and underestimating the benefits of trying. Following that, the patient could then create a hierarchical list, from least threatening to most threatening, culminating in making attempts to engage in these activities, one at a time, in spite of the risk of making mistakes. As the patient proceeds through this list (which may take weeks and months to achieve), he can evaluate the process and outcome. Was it worth taking the risk? Did he learn something new and useful, even if his performance wasn't perfect? Is he better off now than he was before for having tried something new and difficult? Were the mistakes and imperfections calamitous? How did he handle the mistakes, and how is this a model for coping with mistakes in the future? As OCPD patients expand their repertoire of emotions, behaviors, and cognitions, they will experience uncertainty and missteps—experiences that can educate them further about how much is still possible in their lives, and what they're willing to go through to explore these possibilities.

Many OCPD patients are excessively indecisive as they wait for 'certainty' about the 'right' choice. This stance can lead to many missed opportunities in life that require 'taking a chance' and 'going for it.' The problematic belief underlying this problem is that there are always predetermined correct and incorrect decisions, and that it is the patient's responsibility to ascertain the difference before making the 'irreversible' choice. The following is an example of a reframe of this belief offered by a cognitive therapist for the OCPD patient's evaluation and feedback.

> When you feel paralyzed in making a decision, it is almost as if you are choosing between 'door 1' and 'door 2,' one of which is the stairway to heaven, and the other of which is the highway to hell. You believe you have to choose the right one, or forever be damned. No wonder you delay in making a decision! I would do the same thing if I had the same belief. However, perhaps the belief is faulty. Maybe there is no preordained heavenly choice or hellish path. Maybe *either* decision can work out any number of ways, for better or worse, *depending on the attitudes and behaviors you bring to the choice after having committed to it.* In other words, perhaps you have the skills and know-how to *create* the correct decision by virtue of how you deal with things after the fact. What do you think about this conceptualization? Let's think of some practical applications for your life and see how it fits, shall we?

In order to encourage patients to have greater access to—and displays of—appropriate emotionality, therapists will need to go beyond the purely semantic and action-oriented techniques of therapy at times. Merely talking abstractly about profound emotional concepts such as love and grief can take one only so far. An intellectual understanding of the role of such emotions in an OCPD patient's life is the cinematic equivalent of watching a documentary about the life and death of a beloved person. Instead, we want to metaphorically watch tearjerker movies such as *Terms of endearment* with our OCPD patients. Somehow, we have to make our interventions more emotionally evocative. In order to do this, cognitive therapists make use of imagery exercises as well as other methods sometimes associated with experiential/gestalt therapies (e.g., Daldrup *et al.*, 1988—focused-expressive psychotherapy).

For example, Newman (1991) describes the case of 'Ms B,' an emotionally constricted and overly controlled 30-year-old woman who wanted to be able to establish an intimate relationship with someone, but believed she was incapable of the necessary feelings. Discussing the issues was somewhat helpful, but Ms B still felt she could not access deeper feelings. Later in treatment, after describing the rationale for the proposed intervention in depth, the therapist walked Ms B through an evocative, combined relaxation-imagery induction, in which she was asked to remember and describe in detail (while her eyes were closed) the most significant romantic relationship she had experienced thus far in her life. As Ms B reflected on the 'one who got away' 10 years before, the therapist tried to escalate the emotionality

of the intervention by asking Ms B to imagine the boyfriend's voice, telling her how much he loved her and wanted to be with her. Then, Ms B was instructed to speak aloud to the boyfriend as if he could hear her, but to speak to him with the mature emotions and insights she had gained over the past 10 years that she did not possess at the time of the actual relationship. Finally, the therapist asked Ms B to imagine a warm embrace with the boyfriend. 'The therapist's intention was to help Ms B achieve an emotional state whereby her longing for love would be stronger than her fear of being rejected' (Newman, 1991, p. 310). Finally, Ms B (who was now weepy) was asked to state her thoughts in the moment, which included, 'This is what I want in my life . . . I don't want to be emotionally dead.' The therapist responded by playing devil's advocate, asking Ms B the question, 'Wouldn't it be [better] to go back into your nice, safe shell again?' Ms B came up with many rational responses for the therapist's implied, maladaptive entreaty. Later, she was asked to write them down in her therapy journal. This intervention took place after a number of months of therapy, when a trusting therapeutic alliance had been well established.

Reflecting on 'Ace,' the patient referred to earlier who became suicidal in response to changes in his job responsibilities and his own ineffective compensatory strategies that alienated him further from his colleagues and his family, let us summarize the interventions that were required. First, Ace's suicidality took front and center stage, as the standards of good clinical practice would dictate. However, in addition to implementing the customary, practical safeguards in case management (see Bongar, 1991), the therapist focused on Ace's perfectionism as a problem area. As a man who was very responsive to 'the facts' of a situation, Ace was attentive when the therapist educated him about the data linking perfectionism to suicide risk (Hewitt *et al.*, 1994; Blatt, 1995). Ace had always worn his perfectionism as a badge of honor. However, the therapist added, 'Your analysis is incomplete . . . you have only looked at the potential benefits of perfectionism, but not the drawbacks, nor have you tried different variations of approaches to see if there is a safer, more effective way to have high standards without the punishment.' The therapist's goal was to support Ace's goals related to accomplishment (thus counteracting his incompetency schema), while periodically monitoring the patient's reactions to the therapeutic relationship (e.g., did Ace feel that the therapist was trying to control him by suggesting therapeutic changes—a manifestation of the 'lack of individuation' schema?). Progress was evident when Ace was able to state that his perfectionism—as he practiced it—had many negative consequences. It made his family shy away from him, prevented him from ever being pleasantly surprised (because, by definition, he could never exceed his expectations), and always kept him anxious, because a single mistake could undo all the good work he had ever done. He generated two helpful flashcards as reminders to himself. They read:

> Perfectionism is the relentless, futile, lifelong pursuit of breaking even. Whoopie.

> I cannot be at my best all the time, because if I *could* be at my best all the time, it wouldn't be my best; it would be my *average*.

When Ace's acute suicidality subsided (with the help of pharmacotherapy), he and his therapist focused on gradually modifying the beliefs and behavioral habits that had so typified his 'unrelenting standards' schema. For example, Ace dwelled on the idea that he was failing at his job. As a response, Ace was given the assignment of compiling his 'collected works' (he had been a technical writer for over 20 years) and to review them as evidence of his competency and productivity. Ace kept this formidable pile of publications and departmental handbooks on his desk as a reminder that he was more than capable of being successful, and that it was unnecessary to hold himself back from learning new skills. At home, Ace had to notice when he was about to make a critical comment to his wife or kids, to resist saying anything, and instead to write these thoughts in his 'irritability journal.' Then, he had to think ahead about the pros and cons of actually making such statements to his family, and to make distinctions between helpful and unhelpful feedback. Ace then practiced (via in-session role-playing) tactful, diplomatic ways of stating his views, in advance of actually trying them at home. Ace understood that it may not be possible to reverse his wife's tentative decision to seek a marital separation, but he was going to treat her and the kids more nicely regardless.

The therapist also taught Ace how to self-induce a state of relaxation through controlled breathing and imagery of pleasant environments. Additionally, Ace generated ideas for recreational and avocational pursuits, which he pledged not to try to do perfectly! Instead, the idea to was infuse a little bit of 'down time' into his life, yet still do things that interested him and helped him to grow. Throughout this entire process, the therapist monitored Ace's thoughts about the interventions and assignments, and engaged him in empathic, collaborative dialog whenever the patient would express doubts or concerns about any of the therapeutic methods and goals. Ace understood that 'Old habits of thought and deed die hard'; thus, many repetitions of these new ways of responding in everyday life would be required.

Challenges in the treatment

Psychodynamic

One of the chief challenges therapists encounter when they treat OCPD patients is that the dutiful nature of the condition leads certain patients to try to become 'perfect' in the way they approach the therapy. They seek to produce in the therapy exactly what they think the therapist wants to hear. Their search for the therapist's approval may interfere with any authentic effort to understand themselves. McCullough and Maltsberger (2001) made the following observation: 'The patient ritualizes the therapeutic encounter and is likely to fence the therapist in by never coming late, paying the fee immediately, and becoming superficially very 'good' in the service of boxing in the treatment' (p. 2346). The therapist may have to address this style of relatedness forthrightly and even deliberately dislodge the patient from the usual rituals to try to help the patient think and speak spontaneously. For example, when a patient comes in prepared to cover several topics, the therapist might say, 'Before you get into the topics in your outline, I'd like to talk to you about something you said last time.' This type of intervention may discombobulate the patient but forces him or her to interact more authentically with the therapist.

A challenge related to the patient's efforts to be perfect is the patient's unconscious conviction that only perfection is acceptable. Therapists may need to work diligently to help such patients lower expectations of themselves and others. Patients can be helped to see that even though they may feel disappointed in themselves and others when they fall short of perfection, there is an associated relief and liberation from the fantastically high standards they have set. It may be helpful to explore with the patient whether there are any disastrous consequences for falling short of perfection and help them see that there rarely are such consequences.

Patients with OCPD may be intensely competitive with the therapist and not want to be in a position of being told things about themselves that they feel they already should know. The idea of the therapist making observations about them that were previously unknown may threaten their sense of being in control of their lives and their thoughts. The whole notion that they have an unconscious mind that may control them can be quite frightening. Patients with OCPD may discount the therapist's insights and comment that what the therapist has said is 'nothing new.' These patients may also attempt to revise what the therapist has said or pick apart the exact wording. A therapist said to a patient, 'You said yesterday that your mother was an angry woman.' The patient quickly corrected him: 'No, no, what I said was that she was a *hostile* woman.' This competitive interaction may lead to a countertransference posture in the therapist of attempting to prove that he or she is right. A kind of 'one-upmanship' may develop in the therapeutic dyad that becomes an enactment rather than a careful processing of what is going on between the two parties. Many people in the mental health professions have used obsessive-compulsive defenses in a highly adaptive way to achieve a great deal in their chosen profession. The therapists may overidentify with the patient and have a difficult time identifying the maladaptive aspects of the patient's defensive repertoire.

A major challenge involves countertransference boredom. Many therapists describe the monotonous droning of the patient with OCPD as sleep inducing. They may find their minds wandering, their eyelids getting heavy, their eyes constantly checking the clock. The absence of affect and spontaneity may give the patient's speech a mechanical feel that does not engage the therapist. The optimal approach to this common countertransference experience is to take up the patient's style of talking before sleepiness sets in. There are numerous tactful ways to bring up the patient's way of relating. One is to point out that the patient does not seem to be very interested in what he or she is talking about. Another variation is to comment that the patient does not seem to expect the therapist to be very interested in the topic. Yet a third approach is to shift gears by asking the patient directly what he or she thinks is going on in the session between the two parties.

An overall challenge and a centerpiece of dynamic therapy or analysis of patients with OCPD is helping them see how they are hiding their private sense of self behind a public presentation that is not entirely convincing to others. Therapists must 'unmask' the patient and let the patient know that the therapist can discern the struggles underneath the surface presentation. At the same time, it is critical for therapists to empathize with the shame and guilt associated with the unacceptable aspects of the private sense of self and even the unconscious sense of self. When therapists can acknowledge the underlying self-loathing of the patient, many OCPD patients feel understood and can let down their guard a bit. It may take an extended period of time in therapy, but the major challenge is to help the patients accept themselves as they are without feeling they have to be inauthentic to be acceptable.

Cognitive/behavioral

The tendency for obsessive-compulsive patients to think in all-or-none terms will likely cause them a sense of unrest with regard to ascertaining their prognosis, as well as understanding the process of therapy itself. Mental health assessment and treatment involve a certain degree of uncertainty and ambiguity. Persons who think in obsessive-compulsive terms will be very uncomfortable with this state of affairs, instead often insisting that therapists should give iron clad predictions about the time required for the patient to be 'cured.' When the therapists try to explain that this level of precision may not be possible at present, the OCPD patients may jump to the conclusion that their therapists are not knowledgeable enough, and/or that the entire field of psychotherapy is flawed beyond utility. The therapists' explanation that the patients' learning to tolerate uncertainty and ambiguity is part and parcel of the treatment may seem to them like so much double-talk.

In response, therapists may have their own dysfunctional thoughts and emotions, such as concluding prematurely that a bond cannot be formed with the patient, that the patient is so demanding as to render therapy hopelessly burdensome for the therapist, and that the therapist has only two choices: snap to attention and answer all patient's questions as if under cross-examination, or risk losing the patient in a failed attempt to engage. As one can see, the above is an example of the therapist's adopting the OCPD patient's rigid, all-or-none approach, rather than the patient modeling the therapist's openness to exploration with no guarantees. Cognitive-behavioral therapists who are aware of this potential pitfall can monitor their own thoughts so as not to abandon an approach that engages patients in collaborative empiricism and hypothesis testing. To go further, the therapists have to be aware that they may feel incompetent in the face of criticisms of OCPD patients who reject the clinician's perceived 'fuzzy' answers to their questions (e.g., 'Exactly what percentage of my depression is biological, and what percentage is psychological?'). Therapists would do well to discuss this interpersonal process with their patients, and to explore parallels with other relationships in the patient's life, rather than simply trying to tell the patients what they want to hear to reduce the criticisms.

An interesting problem involves the OCPD patient who self-selects for cognitive therapy under the assumption that it is exclusively a 'logical' therapy about thinking, but not about emotions. They may have read some of the self-help books in the field (e.g., Burns, 1980) that contain lists of types of dysfunctional thinking, and that provide methods by which to change thought patterns, and concluded erroneously that the identification and addressing of issues surrounding emotions and relationships will not be necessary. They may be very interested to utilize Automatic Thought Records (J. S. Beck, 1995; Greenberger and Padesky, 1995), but become preoccupied with relatively trivial questions of whether a particular automatic thought is an example of overgeneralization versus all-or-none thinking, rather than focus on the emotions, interpersonal context, and life issues that are reflected by their thought process. When the cognitive therapist inquires about the patients' feelings, wishes, hopes, and/or the quality of their personal relationships, the patients may feel as if they are not getting 'true' cognitive therapy and thus become dissatisfied.

Therapists can explain that the purpose of cognitive therapy is *not* to teach people to utilize logic at the *expense* of the full range of human experience. Rather, cognitive therapy chooses the patients' thinking style as a particularly useful point of entry into the entirety of their psychological system, toward the goal of helping patients live their lives more productively, functionally, and adaptively. In the case of individuals with OCPD—who may demonstrate a problematic dearth of spontaneity, flexibility, and interpersonal warmth—focusing on emotions and interpersonal relationships in therapy may in fact be the most sensible and 'logical' thing they can do.

As one of the defining characteristics of OCPD is the individual's rigid adherence to a particular set of ideas and habits, therapists will sometimes find that their OCPD patients take umbrage at the implied suggestion that 'therapists know best.' In other words, even though the patients presumably are seeking therapy in order to obtain expert professional opinions and suggestions, they may be uncomfortable with the idea that the therapist is 'right' and they are 'wrong' about how they are navigating their lives. Of course, cognitive therapists strive to work collaboratively with their patients, to validate their experiences through the expression of accurate empathy and the formulation of a solid case conceptualization, and to eschew an 'all or none' approach to problem solving and decision making in therapy. Thus, in both cognitive and dynamic therapy, the therapeutic alliance is not about 'Who is right and who is wrong?' However, as OCPD patients often see things in black and white terms, they may believe they will be unduly relinquishing control over the course of their lives if they make the kind of changes their therapists are teaching and supporting.

Therapists need to be sensitive to this possibility, lest they themselves jump to conclusions and make negative generalizations such as, 'This patient is markedly resistant to change,' or 'This patient always wants to engage in a power struggle with me, and to compete with me for control of the session.' Rather than label the patient in this way, therapists can address the patient's concerns about somehow being diminished by the process of therapy, and can work with them to generate more palatable ways to reframe their interactions. For example, one patient was able to articulate that he felt his therapist was bossing him around, and didn't respect the patient's opinions. The therapist took this as a cue to be a little less directive, and to try to conceptualize the problem with occasional reflections and thoughtful questions such as 'Do our differing views remind you of other interactions you have had in your life?' The patient noted that the therapist might try to 'take all the credit' for the patient's positive changes, just as his older brother had 'gotten all the glory' for tutoring him in math, even though it was the patient's hard work that earned him the 'A' grade. The therapist responded in such a manner as to give evidence against the patient's feared outcome—by openly reflecting on all the patient's therapeutic accomplishments to date, and showing respect and admiration to the patient for his diligence and courage in being able to make such improvements. Following this, the patient was able to add, 'You've been helpful too.' Therapist and patient then shook hands, agreeing that their teamwork was formidable.

Cognitive therapists need to observe how their OCPD patients understand and utilize their homework and other 'extra-session' tasks. The overarching purpose of homework is to provide the patients with opportunities for practicing new psychological skills without the therapist's presence. This facilitates learning in that more repetitions can be achieved than are possible solely in the therapist's office, and the patients develop a sense of self-efficacy in doing the work on their own. Patients also fill out questionnaires that can give therapists useful assessment information without taking up time in the therapy hour *per se*. However, in keeping with the OCPD

tendency to become excessively focused on the details at the expense of the bigger picture, some patients may miss the point of completing homework and mood inventories. For example, instead of using Automatic Thought Records to consider new ways to view their life situation and to solve problems, the patients get bogged down trying to determine into which precise category their dysfunctional thinking fits. Similarly, rather than using the Beck Depression Inventory (A. T. Beck *et al.*, 1961) as a quick way to assess and reveal their current mood state, they spend inordinate amounts of time splitting hairs on the items, causing more distress, and delaying the start of the therapy session. Further, OCPD patients are sometimes reluctant to do a homework assignment if they believe there is a chance of making a mistake, or if a positive outcome cannot be guaranteed. Such problematic responses go against the spirit of collaborative empiricism, and diminish the utility of these homework and assessment procedures. Nevertheless, these problems are diagnostic in and of themselves.

An interesting problem occurs when the OCPD patients try to be perfect in their treatment, such that they demonstrate they are skilled and 'good' (and therefore worthy of the therapist's high regard?), that their problems are neat and easily managed, and so that the therapist will pronounce them well (which seems more important than actually feeling well). Such patients often endorse few if any symptoms on assessment questionnaires such as the Beck Depression Inventory (A. T. Beck *et al.*, 1961) even though their life situations might suggest that more distress would be warranted and normative. They go to great lengths to be superficially agreeable, and to prepare homework that is either highly detailed, voluminous, and/or where everything has a simple, positive ending.

For example, Mr H, a high-powered businessman who met criteria both for OCPD and panic disorder (which *greatly* contradicted his sense of total control over his emotions), would repeatedly write clichés for rational responses on his Automatic Thought Records. Rather than actually generate new, original ways of thinking that might help him decatastrophize his occasional physiological spikes of arousal, or try to understand how these anxious moments were triggered, Mr H would simply write rational responses such as, 'I will not fail because failure is not an option,' and 'Whatever doesn't kill me only serves to make me stronger.' He had the most difficult time leaving the safety of these canned responses in favor of more personalized ones. In response, the therapist hypothesized that if Mr H believed he could not maintain actual control over his panic attacks, his next priority was to give the *appearance* of having such control. That Mr H might truly come to understand his feelings better, to talk to himself with more compassion, and to cope with his imperfections yet appreciate himself nonetheless was way down on his list of goals.

Conclusions

Patients with OCPD must first be carefully differentiated from patients who have OCD. Although there appears to be some degree of overlap, the conditions require different treatment approaches. OCPD is a condition that is thought to respond well to both dynamic therapy and cognitive therapy, but empirical outcome research is limited at this point. The findings of the few studies that exist are encouraging. Excessive focus on detail while missing the 'big picture,' perfectionism, and attempts to do therapy 'correctly' are challenges that both dynamic and cognitive therapists must face. Similarly, both cognitive and dynamic therapies converge around efforts to help patients see similarities between assumptions about the therapist and about others in their lives, accept the inevitability of imperfection, and eschew a 'Who's right and who's wrong' perspective on the therapeutic relationship.

References

Abraham, K. (1921/1942). Contributions to the theory of the anal character. In: *Selected papers of Karl Abraham, M.D.*, pp. 370–92. London: Hogarth Press.

Baer, J., *et al.* (1990). Standardized assessment of personality disorders in obsessive-compulsive disorder. *Archives of General Psychiatry*, **47**:826–30.

Barber, J. P. and Muenz, L. R. (1996). The role of avoidance and obsessiveness in matching patients to cognitive and interpersonal psychotherapy: Empirical findings from the treatment for depression collaborative research program. *Journal of Consulting and Clinical Psychology*, **64**(5), 951–8.

Barber, J. P., *et al.* (1997). Change in obsessive-compulsive and avoidant personality disorders following time-limited expressive-supportive therapy. *Psychotherapy*, **34**, 133–43.

Beck, A. T., Ward, C. H., Mendelson, M., Mock, J. E., and Erbaugh, J. T. (1961). An inventory for measuring depression. *Archives of General Psychiatry*, **4**, 561–71.

Beck, A. T., *et al.* (1990). *Cognitive therapy of personality disorders*. New York: Guilford Press.

Beck, A. T., *et al.* (2001). Dysfunctional beliefs discriminate personality disorders. *Behaviour Research and Therapy*, **39**(10), 1213–25.

Beck, J. S. (1995). *Cognitive therapy: basics and beyond*. New York: Guilford Press.

Bejerot, S., Ekselius, L., and von Konorring, L. (1998). Comorbidity between obsessive-compulsive disorder (OCD) and personality disorders. *Acta Psychiatrica Scandinavica*, **97**, 398–402.

Blatt, S. J. (1995). The destructiveness of perfectionism: implications for the treatment of depression. *American Psychologist*, **50**, 1003–20.

Bongar, B. (1991). *The suicidal patient: clinical and legal standards of care*. Washington, DC: American Psychiatric Association.

Burns, D. (1980). *Feeling good*. New York: William Morrow.

Daldrup, R. J., Beutler, D. E., Engle, D., and Greenberg, L. S. (1988). *Focused expressive psychotherapy*. New York: Guilford Press.

Diaferia, G., *et al.* (1997). Relationship between obsessive-compulsive personality disorder and obsessive-compulsive disorder. *Comprehensive Psychiatry*, **38**, 38–42.

Dreesen, L., Arntz, A., Luttels, C., and Sallaerts, S. (1994). Personality disorders do not influence the results of cognitive behavior therapies for anxiety disorders. *Comprehensive Psychiatry*, **35**, 265–74.

Freud, S. (1908/1959). Character and anal eroticism. In: J Strachey, trans. and ed. *The standard edition of the complete psychological works of Sigmund Freud*, Vol. 9, pp. 167–75. London: Hogarth Press.

Gabbard, G. O. (1985). The role of compulsiveness in the normal physician. *Journal of the American Medical Association*, **254**, 2926–9.

Gabbard, G. O. (2000). *Psychodynamic psychiatry in clinical practice*, 3rd edn. Washington, DC: American Psychiatric Press.

Gabbard, G. O. and Menninger, R. W. (1988). The psychology of the physician. In: G. O. Gabbard and R. W. Menninger, ed. *Medical marriages*, pp. 23–38. Washington, DC: American Psychiatric Press.

Greenberger, D. and Padesky, C. (1995). *Mind over mood*. New York: Guilford Press.

Guidano, V. F. and Liotti, G. (1983). *Cognitive processes and emotional disorders*. New York: Guilford Press.

Hardy, G. E., *et al.* (1995). Impact of Cluster C personality disorders on outcomes of contrasting brief therapies for depression. *Journal of Consulting and Clinical Psychology*, **63**, 997–1004.

Hewitt, P. L., Flett, G. L., and Weber, C. (1994). Dimensions of perfectionism and suicide ideation. *Cognitive Therapy and Research*, **18**, 439–60.

Horowitz, M. J. (1988). *Introduction to psychodynamics: a new synthesis*. New York: Basic Books.

Jenike, M. A., Baer, L., and Minichinello, W. E., ed. (1998). *Obsessive-compulsive disorders: practical management*, 3rd edn. St Louis, MO: Mosby.

Josephs, L. (1992). *Character structure and the organization of the Self*. New York: Columbia University Press.

Kagan, J. (1989). Temperamental contributions to social behavior. *American Psychologist*, **44**(4), 668–74.

McCullough, P. K. and Maltsberger, J. T. (2001). Obsessive-compulsive personality disorder. In: *Treatments of psychiatric disorders*, 3rd edn, Vol. 2, pp. 2341–52. Washington, DC: American Psychiatric Press.

Newman, C. F. (1991). Cognitive therapy and the facilitation of affect: two case illustrations. *Journal of Cognitive Psychotherapy: An International Quarterly*, **5**(4), 305–16.

Persons, J. B., Burns, D., and Perloff, J. M. (1988). Predictors of drop-out and outcome in cognitive therapy for depression in a private practice setting. *Cognitive Therapy and Research*, **12**, 557–75.

Rasmussen, S. A. and Tsuang, M. T. (1986). Clinical characteristics and family history in DSM-III obsessive-compulsive disorder. *American Journal of Psychiatry*, **143**, 317–22.

Rosen, K. V. and Tallis, F. (1995). Investigation into the relationship between personality traits and OCD. *Behaviour Research and Therapy*, **33**, 445–50.

Salzman, L. (1968). *The obsessive personality: origins, dynamics, and therapy*. New York: Science House.

Salzman, L. (1980). *Treatment of the obsessive personality*. New York: Jason Aronson.

Salzman, L. (1983). Psychoanalytic therapy of the obsessional patient. *Current Psychiatric Therapies*, **22**, 53–9.

Sanderson, W. C., Beck, A. T., and McGinn, L. K. (1994). Cognitive therapy for generalized anxiety disorder: significance of comorbid personality disorders. *Journal of Cognitive Psychotherapy: An International Quarterly*, **8**, 13–18.

Shapiro, D. (1965). *Neurotic styles*. New York: Basic Books.

Shea, M. T., *et al.* (1990). Personality disorders and treatment outcome in the NIMH Treatment of Depression Collaborative Research Program. *American Journal of Psychiatry*, **147**, 711–18.

Simon, K. (1990). Obsessive-compulsive personality disorder. In: A. T. Beck, *et al.*, ed. *Cognitive therapy of personality disorders*, pp. 309–32. New York: Guilford Press.

Svartberg, M., Stiles, T. C., and Seltzer, M. H. (2004). Effectiveness of short-term dynamic psychotherapy and cognitive therapy for Cluster C personality disorders: A randomized controlled trial. *American Journal of Psychiatry*, **161**, 810–17.

Winston, A., *et al.* (1994). Short-term psychotherapy of personality disorders. *American Journal of Psychiatry*, **151**, 190–4.

Young, J. E. (1999). *Cognitive therapy of personality disorders: a schema-focused approach*, 3rd edn. Sarasota FL: Professional Resource Exchange, Inc.

IV

Psychotherapy across the life cycle

29 Psychosocial therapies with children

Mary Target, Arietta Slade, David Cottrell,
Peter Fuggle, and Peter Fonagy

Introduction

In this chapter, we will describe and review three of the predominant approaches to working therapeutically with children: psychodynamic and play therapies, cognitive-behavioral therapy (CBT), and family therapy. Before turning to a consideration of each of these methods, however, we wish to emphasize that all psychosocial therapies with children need to be adapted to the context of maturational processes, and the social frame that supports or hinders them. Psychotherapy with children and adolescents, across orientations, aims to mobilize developmental processes appropriate to the child's age, replacing behaviors and other patterns typical of earlier development with more mature, adaptive capacities. Psychotherapy with adults also calls for an integration of constitutional, psychological, and social effects, but the developmental dimension is often seen as folded into these influences. Even though the clinician may well use a developmental model of the origins of adult difficulties (e.g., as rooted in early family experience), the difficulties themselves may not be thought about in terms of current developmental pressures, e.g., of young adulthood, mid-life, or older age. All of the interventions considered in this chapter could be thought of as ways of using the therapy situation to redirect developmental processes, and to help the child and the family create a context that facilitates these processes, which should in turn help to maintain the gains made in therapy.

Psychodynamic work with children

The origins of psychodynamic child psychotherapy

Play and playing have always been at the core of psychodynamic approaches to working with children (Klein, 1932; A. Freud, 1965; Winnicott, 1971). The reasons for this are simple: the content, structure, and function of play are viewed as providing a window to understanding the nature of the child's anxieties and conflicts, and to assessing the internal and relational capacities he has available to organize and regulate his thoughts, feelings, and intentions. Psychodynamic child psychotherapy had its earliest beginnings nearly a hundred years ago, when Sigmund Freud used the principles of psychoanalysis to understand and 'treat' (via the boy's father) the symptoms of Little Hans, a 5-year-old Viennese boy with a dread of horses (S. Freud, 1909). It was Hans's play, drawings, and fantasies that helped Freud uncover the conflicts and anxieties thought to lie beneath the child's fears, and that guided the interpretations of these fears that he passed along to the boy's father.

Freud's treatment of Little Hans was—in essence—the first psychodynamic child therapy, although his reliance upon verbal interpretation would differentiate his approach, derived directly from adult psychoanalysis, from that of psychoanalytically oriented therapy. Pioneered by his daughter, Anna, and another Viennese psychoanalyst, Melanie Klein, psychodynamic child therapy was oriented around discovering the meaning and function of the child's play. Despite enormous differences in their view of early experience and psychic organization, Freud and Klein were together to create the field of child psychoanalysis, and establish it for a time as the primary means of treating children suffering from a wide array of psychological disturbances (see Klein, 1932; A. Freud, 1966–1980). For both, play, like dreams, provided a window to the deepest parts of the child's soul, a 'royal road' to the unconscious. They and their followers were the first to fully recognize that children can express in play what they cannot express in words; indeed, until they are nearly adolescent, due to the constraints of development, and the nature of childhood defenses, play is their dominant mode of self-expression. Whereas words and insight were viewed as the primary agents of change in adult psychotherapy, the dynamic and therapeutic aspects of play were thought to be the dominant medium of change in child psychotherapy.

Dynamically oriented play therapy: aims and process

The primary aim of psychodynamic child therapy has been, from the beginning, to allow development to keep moving the child forward (A. Freud, 1965; Winnicott, 1965). Children come to therapy because— whether or not they have specific symptoms, or are more globally delayed or derailed—they are not progressing developmentally, be this manifest in their behavior, their relationships, or their capacity to learn. Most psychodynamic child therapy is aimed at freeing the child from the constraints of his conflicts, deficits, or inhibitions so that he is able to function autonomously and productively in all domains of his functioning.

In the early days of psychodynamic child therapy, verbal interpretation of the unconscious meaning of the child's play was thought crucial to symptom remission and developmental advance. The extreme of this position is best represented by Melanie Klein, who suggested that 'the child's fantasies, set forward in his play, become more and more free in response to continual interpretation' (Klein, 1932, p. 18). In this early view, resolution is only achieved via interpretation. This belief was rooted in classical psychoanalytic notions of insight and structural change, an emphasis that has diminished considerably over the course of the past 80 years, although therapists still routinely use language to make sense of children's play. Children also often talk while they play, for playing provides a safe background for talking about difficult topics. But interpretation, *per se*, is no longer emphasized as the primary agent of change in child work; rather, what is thought to be curative is enhancing the child's symbolic, imaginative, and mentalizing capacities by increasing the range, depth, and emotional richness of his play (see Rogers, 1995). This expansion of the child's capacity to acknowledge various aspects of his self-experience in the safety of play and fantasy is, many believe, what allows developmental progress. Mentalization in play leads to the development of structures for containing feelings and understanding oneself and others (Slade, 1994; Fonagy and Target, 1996b, 1998; Fonagy *et al.*, 2002a).

The capacity to play is rooted in early relationship experience (Slade, 1986, 1987, 1994). Beginning with the earliest playful exchanges with the mother, the child slowly develops the capacity to recognize that he and she have separate and unique minds, and that ideas and feelings are not concrete realities, but rather states that—in play—can be reworked and transformed (Fonagy and Target, 1996b; Target and Fonagy, 1996). The development of these capacities depends upon the establishment of intimate, secure relationships, which permit the discovery of the self and the other, and their separation. In relationships that are disturbed, however, these capacities are also disturbed; putting things into words and into play can be terrifying and disorganizing. And, lacking the presence of a comforting and organizing internalized other, symbolization becomes terrible evidence of one's separateness rather than a means to maintain contact and closeness (Winnicott, 1971; Slade, 1986).

It is for these reasons that the child's capacity to establish a relationship with the therapist (and, conversely, the therapist's capacity to establish a relationship with the child) is central to the treatment (Slade, 1994). Many children arrive knowing that their primary relationships depend upon their either *not* expressing, or disguising or distorting what they are truly thinking and feeling. The development of the capacity to play in a rich symbolic manner depends upon their experience of the therapist's willingness to both accept and contain the complexity and rawness of their actual internal world. This experience of the other as at once tolerant and regulating is what makes it possible for the child to establish the relationship that fosters the emergence of mentalization and symbolic functioning.

Play therapy is at the core two people, the child and the therapist, playing together. Children enter treatment with varying capacities to play, to talk, and to establish a relationship with the therapist. Most often these variations are linked to the nature and severity of developmental disruptions, emotional disturbance, and trauma. Sometimes the first job of the therapist is to help the child play, even a little. This may mean helping the child with the rudiments of telling a coherent story, it may mean helping him to imagine the inner life of the characters he has created, it may mean helping him find solutions in play that help to contain the intense feelings generated (Slade, 1994). But even when a child is able to play, all playing is not equal: play that is repetitive, devoid of emotion, or designed to inhibit communication (whether explicitly symbolic or not) precludes intimacy with the self or therapist, as does play that is dysregulated, fragmented, and too close to the affect it is meant to transform. In either instance, the child is unable to embrace the 'pretend mode', the space between reality and fantasy that allows for transformation, individuation, and true connection with another. Creating this 'playspace' with the therapist is the work of psychodynamic child therapy (Winnicott, 1971; Fonagy and Target, 1996b). It is important to note, in this context, that as children enter middle childhood, they may well not favor explicitly symbolic play; rather, they will choose board games or more physical forms of play, such as basketball, sewing, etc. This is not to say that such play cannot become symbolic, or at least invested with dynamic meaning and complexity that can be critical to therapeutic change (see Altman, 1997). The playspace can have all sorts of shapes, but it is the capacity to engage with the therapist in play, and in the creation of shared experience that defines real therapeutic engagement. Of course, as children age, they will begin to prefer talk over play; in fact, it is often in the context of apparently 'neutral' activities that they will begin to talk about the things that are bothering them.

Because the relationship is so central to moving development forward, regularity is thought to be an especially crucial aspect of the process of play therapy. Children are typically seen at least once a week, and many clinicians prefer to work with them twice or three times a week, because the processes inherent to the development of the capacity to pretend fully and imaginatively are complex, and require sustained periods of connection with the therapist. In many clinical settings this is simply not feasible, but there is evidence that increased frequency is critical to developmental change in seriously disturbed children (Target and Fonagy, 1994a). Equally critical to the child's progress is consistency. Children find change and disruption difficult, as their defenses are typically relatively tenuous or overly rigid (A. Freud, 1965); in either case, their capacity to engage in treatment is greatly helped by the therapist's sensitivity to the impact of changes in schedule separations and other.

Working with parents

Until relatively recently, there was little consideration in the psychodynamic child therapy literature of how to involve the parents in a child's individual treatment (this despite the fact that parents are almost always involved in children's therapy in some way). Historically, the parent and his or her actual behavior with the child were viewed as extraneous to the treatment process. This had much to do with the history of child psychoanalysis, and in particular with the emphasis within this literature upon both the privacy and exclusiveness of the of the child–therapist relationship, and upon the view that treatment was meant to affect internal processes rather than real relationships. While parents were typically seen occasionally for guidance and general 'catching up' on the child's home and school life, there was little conceptualization of how to engage dynamically the parent in the child's treatment so as to change ongoing patterns of interaction and relatedness. In the early days, this was actually frowned upon. However, as clinicians began to recognize the impact of relationships (in the extreme, trauma or abuse) upon child functioning, and as relational, attachment, and family approaches gained ascendancy, such predispositions began to change.

The first clinicians to radically confront the exclusion of parents from the child treatment process were Selma Fraiberg and her colleagues in their work on infant–parent psychotherapy (Fraiberg, 1980; Lieberman and Pawl, 1993). Called in by state welfare authorities to decide on troubled young mothers' capacities to care for their children, many of whom were showing signs of trauma and abuse at a very young age, Fraiberg and her colleagues were able to affect the parent–child relationship in direct and dramatic ways by working with parents and infants together. They believed that the baby's presence in the room galvanized maternal affects and representations in ways that were transforming and healing, and allowed mothers to separate their own projections from the babies' affiliative and attachment needs. While this approach was virtually unheard of in the late 1970s, it has now become an accepted mode of working with parents and their infants and toddlers.

Today, therapists working with pre-school and school age children continue to differ in the extent to which they involve parents in the individual psychotherapy of their children, although most believe that establishing and maintaining an alliance with parents is vital (Siskind, 1997; Slade, 1999, in press; Novick and Novick, 2002). However, therapists with differing trainings and orientations, do this differently. For some therapists, typically those who are more psychoanalytically oriented, the domain of the child's individual psychotherapy is still secluded, and parent meetings are less central to the therapy. For others, working from a more object relational and attachment framework, separate but regular (at least monthly, if not more frequently) meetings are more typical (Slade, 1999). Some therapists—following the infant–parent psychotherapy model—involve the parents in the child's actual sessions, not to talk, necessarily, but using the child's play as the means to enhancing relatedness and communication between parent and child (Slade, 1999; Oram, 2000; Chazan, 2002). (As is described in the section below, this approach has much in common with current family therapy approaches.)

The aim of most parent work is to effect change in the dynamics and functioning of the actual parent–child relationship, as such changes are believed intrinsic to development in the child. Clearly, one aspect of this work is to help parents understand critical aspects of their children's development; for example that a 4 year old's lie does not have the same significance or meaning as a 12 year old's. More important, however, successful parent work involves engaging the parent's capacity for reflective functioning (Slade, in press). Parent work helps a parent separate their own subjective experience of the child from the child's own thoughts, intentions and feelings. A parent's subjective experience of the child can be profoundly influenced by their own conflicts, or by the distorting effects of malevolent projections and representations. The work of the therapist is to help the parent hold the child and his or her subjective experience in mind, as distinct from the parent being aware only of their own perspective. This kind of work can powerfully help the parent to become better at managing the child's feelings and behaviour.

The evidence base of psychodynamic child therapy

There is rather less research available on the outcome of psychodynamic treatment than of some other approaches with children (Weisz et al., 1992). The most extensive study of intensive psychodynamic treatment was a chart review of more than 700 case records at a psychoanalytic clinic in the United Kingdom (Fonagy and Target, 1994, 1996c; Target and Fonagy, 1994a,b). The observed effects of psychodynamic treatment were impressive, particularly with younger children and those with emotional disorder or those with disruptive disorder, comorbid with anxiety. In addition, intensive treatment appeared more effective for children with emotional disorders which caused significant impairment across contexts. However, children with pervasive developmental disorders or mental retardation appeared to respond poorly to psychodynamic treatment.

Some smaller-scale studies have demonstrated that psychodynamic therapy can bring about improvement in aspects of psychological functioning beyond psychiatric symptomatology. Heinicke (1965; Heinicke and Ramsey-Klee, 1986) demonstrated that general academic performance was superior at 1-year follow-up in children who were treated more frequently in psychodynamic psychotherapy. Moran and Fonagy (Fonagy and Moran, 1990; Moran et al., 1991) demonstrated that children with poorly controlled diabetes could be significantly helped with their metabolic problems by relatively brief, intensive psychodynamic psychotherapy. In a naturalistic study, Lush et al. (1991) offered preliminary evidence that psychodynamic therapy was helpful for children with a history of severe deprivation who were fostered or adopted. Improvements were only noted in the treated group.

An important study from the University of Pisa (Muratori et al., 2003) looked at the effectiveness of an 11-session treatment program for 58 children with anxiety disorder or dysthymic disorder. The treatment was structured, focal psychodynamic psychotherapy, including both family and individual sessions. The control group were referred for community treatment. Measures were taken at baseline, 6 months (end of treatment for the experimental group), and 2 years follow-up. The two key measures were the Children's Global Assessment Scale (CGAS; completed by a blind, independent interviewer who interviewed both child and parent), and Child Behavior Check List (CBCL) completed by the parents. The results revealed a significant difference between the groups, only at follow-up, on both the CGAS and CBCL scales. In addition, the authors report a significantly lower level of service use in the experimental group during the follow-up period. This study is unique in providing a well-matched control group, to assess the effectiveness of psychodynamic psychotherapy.

Negative findings concerning the effectiveness of child psychodynamic therapy were reported by Smyrnios and Kirkby (1993). In this study no significant differences were found at follow-up between a time-limited and a time-unlimited psychodynamic therapy group and a minimal contact control group. The control group families may have had good outcomes because the minimal contact consisted of discussion of an agreed formulation and of how the family could effectively help themselves. Negative outcomes were also reported by Szapocznik et al. (1989), who compared the effectiveness of individual psychodynamic therapy or structural family therapy in treating disruptive adolescents. Both forms of treatment led to significant gains. But at 1-year follow-up, while the child functioning remained improved for both groups, family functioning had deteriorated in the individual therapy group.

Good evidence is available for the success of therapeutic approaches that can be considered indirect implementations of psychoanalytic ideas. For example, Kolvin et al. (1981) demonstrated that psychodynamic group therapy had relatively favorable effects when compared with behavior therapy and parent counseling, particularly on long-term follow-up. In a smaller-scale study of group social relations interventions, Lochman et al. (1993)

have reported similarly encouraging results. Interpersonal psychotherapy (IPT), although not a psychodynamic treatment (Klerman et al., 1984) incorporates interpersonal psychodynamic principles. Mufson et al. (1993) have manualized this therapy for depressed adolescents (IPT-A), and a clinical randomized controlled trial has been reported (Mufson et al., 1999). This included 48 referred adolescents with major depression, of whom 32 completed the protocol. The majority of drop-outs came from the control condition, which was 'clinical monitoring', effectively a waiting list. An intent-to-treat analysis showed that 75% of patients treated with IPT-A recovered, as judged by Hamilton Rating Scale scores, in comparison with 46% of those in the control group. Other studies have also found IPT to be effective for adolescents, more so on some dimensions than was CBT (Rosselló and Bernal, 1999), and sertraline (Santor and Kusumakar, 2001).

Thus, there is limited evidence on the efficacy of child psychodynamic psychotherapy. However, given the fact that each study reported has methodological shortcomings—such as small sample size, nonstandardized process and outcome assessments, nonrandom assignment, lack of adherence measures—what emerges most powerfully is the need for new outcome studies in this area, applying strict methodological criteria and samples which reflect clinical realities.

Conclusions

Psychodynamic child psychotherapy was the first psychosocial treatment specifically developed for mental disorders for children. Its ambitious aim is the developmental advancement of children whose symptoms are seen as an indication of a failure to progress socially, cognitively, or emotionally. While interpretation and insight represent an important feature of therapeutic process, more central are becoming able to play, and to establish a relationship with a therapist that is richly imbued with symbolic meaning, and aims to extend the child's capacity coherently to represent mental states. These representations allow the child to understand himself and others better, and to gain more control over what happens in his or her relationships as a result. For most child therapists, work with parents is important for both preschool and school-age children, its primary aim being to help parents understand their child's thoughts and feelings. Evidence for psychodynamic child therapy is currently limited but available studies suggest that this approach can be helpful in improving the child's development across domains of functioning, especially interpersonal understanding.

Cognitive-behavioral therapy with children

The theoretical framework of cognitive-behavioral therapy

As with other therapeutic approaches with children, CBT with children is shaped by theory, ideology, and traditions of practice. It has its theoretical underpinnings in a number of related research traditions particularly behavioral science (Herbert, 1994), social learning theory (Bandura, 1977), cognitive developmental theory (Bruner, 1990), and the cognitive theory of emotional disorders. Ideologically, CBT practice is described as following a scientific practitioner approach, which emphasizes the importance of empirical methodologies, research evidence, and formal hypothesis testing. This ideological framework has shaped specific traditions of practice such as the promotion of open collaborative practice with clients. As an example, CBT therapists encourage the development of a mutual formulation of the client's problems, professional knowledge sharing with the client, explicit explanations of the treatment model and open testing of individual focused hypotheses about what may produce change. However, compared with social constructionist approaches, CBT would be seen to adopt an expert position with its clients.

In current practice, CBT with children (and their parents) has evolved from a loosely related set of theories, research findings, beliefs, and practice traditions, resulting in a diverse set of therapeutic techniques and practice.

Some interventions emphasize the central role of children's cognitions in the etiology and maintenance of childhood disorders and thus aim to change cognitions, whereas others focus more on the behavioral mechanisms thought to be central to achieving change. Thus, Kendall (2000) has defined current practice as 'the purposeful attempt to preserve the demonstrated positive effects of behavioral therapy within a less doctrinaire context and to incorporate the cognitive activities of the client into the efforts to produce therapeutic change.'

Behavior modification and parent training

Historically, techniques of change based on behavioral theory, such as behavior modification, preceded more cognitive approaches. Behavior modification (Herbert, 1998) applies the theory of classical and operant reinforcement to a wide range of childhood clinical problems such as anxiety disorders (phobias, obsessive-compulsive disorder) conduct problems and early developmental problems (sleep disturbance, enuresis). This approach is based on the notion that problem behaviors are likely to recur if the consequences of such behaviors are rewarding to the child. Formal treatments of this kind begin with a functional analysis, in which the antecedents and consequences of problem behaviors are systematically recorded so as to determine environmental and transactional patterns and responses that support these behaviors. Interventions are planned to alter these behavioral patterns by focusing on reducing rewarding consequences, and increasing the positive consequences of pro-social behaviors. This approach is most commonly applied by working with the parent, using reported behavior of the child in the school or home environment. Improvements with respect to reduced frequency or severity of problem behaviors are explicitly celebrated or rewarded. For example, parents are encouraged not to respond to angry outbursts or tantrums in young children with 'rewarding' responses (attention, raised excitement) and to encourage more pro-social behaviors in achieving wishes or negotiating conflict.

Alternatively, treatment focuses more on the behavior and interactions taking place within the treatment session and explicitly structures sessions as opportunities to change the child's behavior. Most notable of these is the 'Parent–child Game' (Jenner, 1999) in which a therapist directly prompts parents (through a one-way screen using an earpiece) to follow behavior modification principles in changing a child's behavior.

Parent training has become one of the most widely used of the behavioral approaches. This method has been most comprehensively developed and evaluated by Webster-Stratton (Webster-Stratton et al., 1989; Webster-Stratton and Herbert, 1993). The training can be delivered to parents either individually or in a group, and is typically brief (eight to 12 sessions) with a carefully prepared curriculum for each session. Video clips are used to illustrate common parent–child conflicts, and the emphasis is on structured 'homework' exercises that facilitate the generalization of skills learned in therapy to the family environment. Initial sessions focus on positive interactions between the parent and child, particularly those that occur within the context of play. Behavioral principles of selective attention and reinforcement are illustrated and practised through homework tasks, along with more cognitive components such as problem solving, negotiating turn taking and emotional recognition.

The apparent theoretical simplicity of the original behavioral model was partly due to its nearly exclusive focus on childhood behaviors, rather than upon the relationships in which problematic behaviors occurred. This despite the fact that the intervention was almost always implemented through social interaction between the parent and child. Compared with early developments of behavior modification, current behavioral work tends to include relationship factors much more. Thus, there may be increasingly little difference between systemic interventions that encourage interactional experiments, and behavioral approaches that take account of the parent–child relationship, than may appear from theoretical descriptions of these treatment models.

Although current evidence would suggest a place for parent training in addressing the needs of children with emotional and behavioral difficulties,

the exclusive focus on the parent is clearly limiting. Greater effectiveness has been indicated for parent training programs that offer child-focused CBT alongside the parent training (Kazdin et al., 1992; Webster-Stratton and Hammond, 1997). Improved generalization and increased stability of treatment effects produced by parent work may be facilitated by greater emphasis on direct work with the child, including the child's thoughts about current difficulties, and the development of social and problem-solving skills. As will be described in the next section, these limitations have, in part, led to the development of child-based cognitive-behavioral treatments of children.

Individual cognitive-behavioral therapy with children

The CBT model is based on the proposition that childhood emotional disorders are maintained by implicit cognitive biases manifest through fixed core beliefs, dysfunctional assumptions, and automatic thoughts about the world, self, or others resulting in dysfunctional mood states, emotion or social interaction (Friedberg and McClure, 2002).

CBT with children typically has four key components, namely engagement, formulation, learning new skills, and applying change strategies (Kendall, 2000; Friedberg and McClure, 2002). The construction of a shared, comprehensible formulation is central. Problems are defined in terms of a child's thoughts, feelings, and/or behavior, usually linked to specific situations rated by frequency and severity. This enables problems to be addressed sequentially and organized in a hierarchical way that allows the child (and parent) to determine what they are able to cope with. The person (child) in a more global sense is not the problem. This definition of the problem allows for explicit understandings about the solution that is being sought and allows the possibility of the child and the parent achieving 'success' by reaching explicit targets of change. Behavioral techniques for noticing and rewarding positive change are usually integrated into this broader CBT approach.

In general, CBT sessions tend to have a more structured 'curriculum' than nondirective therapies. The therapist is active, self-disclosing where appropriate, and adopts a psychoeducational, collaborative approach in which a range of activities within the session may be suggested. Kendall (2000) uses the metaphor of the therapist as being like a sports coach in which concepts of practice, preparation, and training are often referred to. The focus is on creating change both within the session but also more crucially in generalizing change to the child's daily life. Practicing anger or anxiety management skills with the therapist in real life situations may be part of the treatment plan, as the intervention is not necessarily confined to the clinic room. In order to support the generalization of new skills to the home environment, the 'curriculum' often includes homework and record keeping tasks.

Activities initially may focus upon developing core skills such as: emotional recognition; separating thoughts, feelings, and actions; and activity monitoring and diary keeping. For example, poor discrimination between anxiety and anger feeling states may be more common in children with emotional behavioral difficulties. Similarly, improving a child's ability to regulate emotional states is likely to be dependent on their ability to monitor and notice internal states. Activities supporting strategies for change will be adopted depending on the formulation but may include a combination of behavioral and cognitive techniques such as relaxation training, problem solving, role playing, exposure, behavioral experiments, and testing the evidence for beliefs. Perhaps the most widely applied change technique is problem solving, in which children are guided to consider alternative options, to adopt a position of choice rather than powerlessness and to improve social perspective taking.

Compared with work with adults, the application of this approach to children raises a number of particular challenges. First, in contrast to adults, children are brought to therapy (Kendall, 2000). They do not make independent decisions to seek help for self-identified problems. The description of the 'problem' is constructed within a context of their families and caregivers. This is self-evident but has major implications in establishing collaborative practice with the child based on a shared formulation of a child's difficulties. Clearly, children may not 'collaborate' if they perceive the reason for therapy as being critical of them, i.e., having a 'behavior problem'. Second, compared with adults, children's ability to make changes in their lives is restricted by their dependency on parents/caregivers. Third, children's interests and styles of interaction require that therapeutic methods not rely solely only on verbal interaction (Friedberg and McClure, 2002). Some cognitive techniques for adults may be developmentally inappropriate and ineffective with children. There is a need to incorporate both the form and content of children's thinking for the cognitive components of CBT to become applicable. Thus, for younger children, their thinking and expectations of the world and others may be most readily revealed through symbolic play. Similarly, children may need narratives as a way of developing explanations about the world, rather than abstract ideas (Bruner, 1990). Thus, for example, story telling may have a greater role in cognitive restructuring than methods of Socratic questioning appropriate for adult CBT work. Finally, CBT interventions partly rely on the patient being able to report cognitive states in order that distortions can be effectively challenged. In general, children may have less practice (and less interest) in the recall of experience and monitoring internal states than adults. Clearly such therapeutic tasks need to be carefully constructed to be within their cognitive developmental abilities, although the degree to which this restricts the application of cognitive approaches even in young children is far less clear (Meadows, 1993).

Working with parents and cognitive-behavioral therapy

As already indicated, there has been a tendency in the child CBT literature to describe CBT independent of the role and relationship of parents and other family members. For example, Lochman et al. (1991) concluded that the 'most striking deficiency in CBT programs . . . has been the neglect of children's caregivers, especially parents. Intervening with these caregivers can be critical in strengthening treatment effects and in maintaining the generalization of treatment effects over time.' In addition, there is some suggestion that involvement of parents may increase treatment effectiveness (Mendlowitz et al., 1999; Barrett et al., 2001). Different CBT approaches with children have proposed different roles for parents that can be broadly identified as facilitator, co-therapist, or patient. As facilitator, the parent is predominantly involved in supporting the child's individual therapy and may meet with the therapist occasionally (Kendall, 2000). As a co-therapist the parent may be actively involved in supporting the child in learning new skills and may be central to providing behavioral feedback and rewards. In such instances, the parent is seen as closely collaborating with the therapist using agreed upon CBT techniques (March and Mulle, 1998; Mendlowitz et al., 1999). Alternatively, parents may be clients receiving treatment to cope with their own difficulties, which may be associated with the child's problem, either as part of a family approach (Barrett, 1998) or individually alongside the child's sessions (Cobham et al., 1998). Typically, parents may be offered CBT to manage their own emotional and behavioral difficulties. In practice, parents may sometimes wish to move between these different roles during a child's treatment and, although some flexibility of relationship with the family is often essential, sudden changes in parental role can be disruptive for the child. In general, much work still needs to be done in developing coherent models of CBT practice that are coherent with family roles, relationships, and individual differences.

The evidence base of behavior modification and cognitive-behavioral therapy

Overall, there is considerable evidence for the effectiveness of behavior modification, particularly with respect to conduct problems in younger children (Kazdin, 1985) and for developmental difficulties such as sleep

disturbance and enuresis (Christophersen and Mortweet, 2001). The utility of parent training has also been well supported, although the exclusive focus upon the parent clearly limits its impact. Indeed, greater effectiveness has been indicated for parent training programs that offer child-focused CBT alongside the parent training (Kazdin et al., 1992; Webster-Stratton and Hammond, 1997). Improved generalization and increased stability of treatment effects produced by parent work may be facilitated by greater emphasis on direct work with the child, directed toward the child's cognitions about current difficulties and the development of social and problem-solving skills.

There is variable empirical support for the effectiveness of CBT depending on the disorder and the developmental level of the child (Fonagy et al., 2002b). In general, as reviewed in detail in the Fonagy et al. book, the evidence for effectiveness is stronger for moderate, single problem presentations rather than complex chronic problems with high levels of comorbidity. Within these constraints, there is strong and accumulating evidence for the effectiveness of CBT (parent training) as an effective treatment for conduct problems in children under 8 years. For older children (8–12 years) the addition of problem-solving skills training for the child appears to enhance parent training approaches. Similarly, CBT is proving to be an effective treatment for general and specific anxiety disorders both delivered in individual and group settings. In addition, CBT has been shown to improve physical outcomes for children with paediatric conditions and with developmental difficulties such as sleep and toileting difficulties. Evidence for the effectiveness of CBT for depression, for conduct problems in adolescence and attentional problems is less strong. For depression, there is little evidence for pre-adolescent children. For adolescents, CBT may provide benefit for moderate levels of depression but short-term treatments need to be extended to anticipate the risk of relapse. Similarly, for conduct problems in adolescence, CBT packages such as problem-solving and social skills training are unlikely to be sufficient to address moderate to severe levels of difficulty but may contribute to the effectiveness of multimodal treatment approaches that also address family relationships and broader social environment variables such as positive leisure activities. For attentional problems, there is some evidence that CBT may enhance on-task activity and reduce disruptiveness but this is less effective than stimulant medication. However, it may contribute to an overall treatment approach and enable lower doses of medication to be effective.

Much work remains to be done to establish empirical support for many aspects of this theoretical model, as opposed to therapeutic effectiveness (Stallard, 2002). There is some evidence that children with anxiety disorders are more likely to perceive the world as threatening (Kendall and Panichelli-Mindel, 1995) and that children with conduct problems may anticipate ambiguous social situations as indicating hostility (Dodge, 1985). However, there is as of yet sufficient formal evidence either that cognitive therapy both produces cognitive change in children or that this is critical to functional improvement (Stallard, 2002). This is a crucial area for future research.

Conclusions

CBT with children currently encompasses a wide range of interventions to address childhood disorders and distress. In general, there is some evidence of the usefulness of CBT for a number of childhood disorders. More established behavioral approaches such as behavior modification and parent training increasingly include cognitive factors for both parents and children, and the child is placed in a more central position in the therapeutic endeavor. This is ideologically welcome as it conveys respect for the child's perspective and experience. However, it remains unclear whether CBT is yet addressing critical cognitive factors that lead to childhood disorders. A broader theoretical model, which includes processes of attachment, family relationships, and social developmental factors, may better capture the multiple processes that contribute to childhood distress.

Family therapy

Family and systemic therapies have, at their heart, the notion that intervention must address the interactional patterns between people as well as their intrapsychic processes. There have been many attempts at defining systemic therapies, none wholly satisfactory, but Gurman *et al.*'s (1986) definition that 'Family therapy may be defined as any psychotherapeutic endeavor that explicitly focuses on altering the interactions between or among family members and seeks to improve the functioning of the family as a unit, or its subsystems, and/or the functioning of the individual members of the family' is often quoted. This is a broad definition and one that would encompass many of the parent training programs referred to elsewhere in this chapter. As the theories and techniques underpinning therapeutic approaches to children and young people become more integrated, definitions are becoming blurred. While acknowledging that many approaches utilize systemic perspectives, this section will focus on therapies that draw on systemic, cybernetic, narrative, or constructivist/constructionist theories. As is often the case there are generally more similarities in practice than might be apparent in the theoretical descriptions.

The last 10–20 years has seen a major change from individual to family systemic therapeutic approaches to children and families in clinical practice, within both the health and social services. In the UK, there are now few child and adolescent mental health services that do not include work with families in one form or another as a major part of their approach to referred children. However, it is important to recognize that family therapy is not about the creation, or maintenance, of traditional nuclear families. Family therapists recognize the diversity of configurations that families today bring to the task of rearing children and strive to maintain a respectful and nonjudgmental approach to these differing choices.

Children and young people in family therapy

There are many excellent accounts of the history and development of systemic practice, from early more positivist roots in cybernetics, communication and systems theories, through to the so-called 'second order' therapies that incorporate constructivist and social constructionist models (Hoffman, 1981; Dallos and Draper, 2000). Although family and systemic therapies have become one of the predominant forms of working with children's emotional and behavioral problems, surprisingly little has been written about children's perceptions of family work or about ways in which children might be more fully engaged in the therapeutic process. Most therapeutic models rely heavily on verbal communication and so might be seen to exclude younger children. In the past family therapy has been criticized for ignoring children and, in effect, conducting therapy in their presence without involving them. Children's worlds are often full of play, creativity, and activity, and therapy must presumably incorporate these concepts if it is to be meaningful to children. A number of authors have written about how children might be more actively engaged in the therapeutic process: most arguing strongly for the inclusion of more play, creativity, story telling, and active involvement (O'Brien and Loudon, 1985; Zilbach, 1986; Combrinck-Graham, 1991; Gil, 1994; Wilson, 1998; Context, 2002).

Different schools of family therapy have had to address these concerns in different ways, ways that are congruent with their underlying theoretical principles. Structural family therapy (Minuchin *et al.*, 1967; Minuchin, 1974) assumes that problems in the child arise from underlying problems in the structure and organization of the family. The therapist is interested in how the family makes decisions, and how the boundaries between individuals and subsystems within the family lead to relative engagement or distancing. The therapist is often directive, attending to sequences and patterns of behavior, and seeking to bring about change using techniques such as enactment, escalation, and unbalancing.

Minuchin (1974) developed structural family therapy while working with disorganized and chaotic families in a deprived inner city (New York). Therefore, it is not surprising that he looked to provide clearer structures for families, and that therapists have found these techniques particularly helpful in working with families where children have behavioral problems. Children may not, on the surface, welcome attempts to provide clearer rules and boundaries but the active, directed approach of the therapist in structural family therapy does make it easy to engage children. Techniques such as enactment and the encouragement of family members to practice new ways of behaving and communication in the session ensure that all family members, including even quite small children are actively involved in therapy.

Brief solution-focused therapy (Berg and de Shazer, 1993) assumes that problems are maintained by the way difficulties are viewed and by the repetitive, behavioral sequences surrounding attempts to solve them. Families are seen as constantly changing and it is assumed that families will already have solutions to their own difficulties. The therapist sets clear goals with the family and focuses on solutions not problems, looking for exceptions to the 'problem-saturated' story that the child is 'always' a problem. Underlying this emphasis on competence and solutions is a focus on challenging unhelpful beliefs about the child and the problem as part of the process of generating new solutions. This focus on solutions can be helpful when working with children who are often worried that being brought for therapy is just another context in which they will be blamed for family difficulties. Solution-focused work is often active and, like structural therapies, can involve tasks and between session homework—these practical activities provide a further opportunity for children to be actively engaged.

Postmodern therapies (Andersen, 1987; Anderson and Goolishan, 1988, 1992) are informed by social constructionism and see language rather than interactional patterns as the system to focus on in therapy. Language does not just describe the family situation but can create and maintain that situation. The therapeutic style is conversational with the intention of creating change through the development of new language. The therapist takes a nonexpert role and asks questions that seek to create new possibilities or alternative understandings. 'Reflecting team' conversations are used as a means of sharing the therapy team's alternative stories and explanations with the family without imposing those ideas on the family. Such therapies are linguistically based and it can be difficult, though not impossible, to engage younger children. Reflecting teams may be confusing for younger participants, although a brief report by Marshall and Reimers (2002) suggests that teenagers, at least, find them potentially helpful, understanding, and caring.

Narrative therapy (White and Epston, 1990) draws on the way that we all make sense of our experience by creating personal accounts or narratives. Therapy is a form of conversation that encourages reflection and can transform problem-saturated narratives into more positive accounts. The emphasis on language can be off-putting for children as with other postmodern therapies but techniques such as externalization, which assist in separating the person from the problem, can help the child to feel less blamed and join the child with the family in fighting the problem. Narrative therapists also see those with problems as having expertise in solving them that may help children to feel engaged and less blamed, and the emphasis on narrative suggests the possibility of links with stories and story telling—ideas familiar to children. Narrative therapists also look for 'unique outcomes and positive exceptions' concepts similar to the search for solutions and exceptions by solution-focused therapists, and this too may help children to feel less blamed. Larner (1996) draws on child psychotherapy and narrative theory and technique to suggest ways of joining the 'child's symbolic play as narrative . . . ' to the ' . . . family story as social text in therapeutic conversation'. He quotes Anderson as describing the therapist's expertise 'being in conversation with the expertise of the client' and notes that the expertise of the child is in the ability to play.

There are a few recent studies looking at children's perspectives on therapy. Stith *et al.* (1996), for example, explored the experience of 16 children from 12 families in a qualitative study. Children, interviewed alone, wanted to be included in therapy and were keen to know more about their families, be involved in generating solutions and not feel blamed for problems. They did not want to be the sole focus of discussion. Even primary school children understood the purpose of therapy and found talking about problems helpful but their willingness to be involved increased with time and with the amount they knew about why their families were coming to therapy. Lobatto (2002) describes a thoughtful qualitative analysis of interviews of six children, aged 8–12 years, in the presence of their parents. She describes the difficulties children had in deciding how and when to participate in the therapeutic conversation, their uncertainty about the rules of therapy, and the importance of toys and play materials in maintaining a safe space for children within therapy. She echoes Wilson (1998) in suggesting the need for clearly stated ground rules about participation in therapy.

The evidence base of family therapy with young people

In general, family and systemic therapies have not been well evaluated despite their widespread use in clinical settings, and there is a need for more randomized, controlled evaluations. However, the quality of published research is similar to that concerning other psychological treatments and there are sufficient good quality studies to draw some conclusions. There is good evidence for the effectiveness of systemic therapies in the treatment of conduct disorders (particularly in older children, and in relation to offending) and substance misuse. Functional family therapy has been shown to be effective in reducing adolescent offending behavior (Alexander and Parsons, 1973; Parsons and Alexander, 1973; Barton et al., 1985; Gordon et al., 1988) in multiply offending adolescents. Follow-up into early adulthood showed improvements were maintained (Gordon et al., 1995). Multisystemic treatment (MST) comprising detailed individual assessment followed by a combination of therapeutic interventions has been demonstrated to reduce significantly recidivism when compared with treatment as usual. Improvements were maintained at 30-month follow-up and costs of MST were lower than in control groups (Borduin, 1999). MST is intensive and time consuming with sessions held in the family's home and in community locations. It is more than just family therapy, although classical family therapy interventions play a key part and is concerned, more than many interventions, with the family situated in its social context. Stanton and Shadish (1997) systematically reviewed studies of treatments for drug abuse and conclude that family–couples therapy is superior to individual counseling/therapy and peer group therapy for both adults and adolescents. Family therapy was also superior to family psychoeducation and tended to have lower drop-out rates than other treatments.

There is also good evidence for the effectiveness of systemic therapies in the treatment of anorexia nervosa in younger people. Russell et al. (1987) randomly allocated individuals with anorexia nervosa and bulimia nervosa to either family therapy or a 'nonspecific form of individual therapy' after discharge from inpatient care. At 1 year, family therapy was found to be more effective than individual therapy in patients whose illness was not chronic and had begun before the age of 19 years. Improvements were maintained at 5-year follow-up (Eisler et al., 1997). Robin et al. (1994, 1999), compared behavioral family systems therapy with a form of individual therapy for anorexia nervosa. In a random allocation study, behavioral family systems therapy produced greater weight gains and higher rates of resumption of menstruation at posttreatment and at 1-year follow-up than the comparison intervention.

In addition there is some support for the effectiveness of systemic treatments in depression, self-harm (where they may have significant cost benefits), and in chronic illness (Cottrell and Boston, 2002; Fonagy et al., 2002b). The existing research also offers some suggestions as to how systemic ideas may contribute to other therapeutic models or the development of integrated approaches. There have been reports that in controlled studies systemic therapies may reduce drop-out and increase engagement and consumer satisfaction (Szapocznik et al., 1988; Henggeler et al., 1996; Harrington et al., 1998). There is also support for the notion that parental involvement is beneficial even if parents are not in the same room as the young person as long as systemic ideas are informing therapy (Robin et al., 1994, 1999; Eisler et al., 2000). Systemic interventions may also have

positive effects that are maintained and even increase with time (Szapocznik et al., 1989). This would fit with systemic theory that addressing underlying family interactional patterns will produce lasting change and is in contrast to cognitive-behavioral treatments that require 'booster sessions' to maintain change (Fonagy et al., 2002b). These findings suggest that systemic ideas have something useful to offer other theoretical perspectives.

Conclusions

There is evidence that family and systemic therapy is an effective treatment for some young people and systemic ideas can contribute to the delivery of other treatment modalities. However, the best evaluated systemic interventions are the older 'first order' structural/strategic models, not the more recent developments using social constructionist and narrative frameworks. It is possible for systemic therapies to ignore children and young people and become marital/adult work in the presence of the child. However, the theoretical models and practical techniques of the current schools of systemic practice all acknowledge the importance of involving children and have all found creative ways of doing this. There is emerging evidence from qualitative research that even quite young children can understand, make sense of, and participate in systemic work. Careful explanation of the purpose and process of therapy, recognition of the expertise of the child and the provision of environments that are child friendly and promote play and creativity should maximize the involvement of children.

An integration: the developmental approach to psychotherapy with children

Up until now, we have considered three general approaches to working with children therapeutically. In this final section, we would like to consider a set of issues intrinsic to all psychosocial therapies for children, namely questions of development, environment, biology, and developmental psychopathology. The myriad of questions that flow from a developmental perspective are critical to any decisions regarding child treatment. For example, developmental stage (inadequately approximated by chronological age) has been found to moderate the type of psychotherapy that may suit a child with a particular problem. In a retrospective study of psychoanalytic child psychotherapy we reported larger effects for younger children than for adolescents, and a differential response to intensity of treatment (younger children responding best to more frequent sessions) (Target and Fonagy, 1994a). As another example, parenting training appears highly effective for the young child but there is far less evidence to support the use of this treatment with older children (Serketich and Dumas, 1996). By contrast, a meta-analysis of CBT interventions found significantly larger effect sizes for adolescents (aged 11–13) than younger children (7–11 years) (Durlak et al., 1991). Thus, age trends may be a critical factor in determining the most suitable and efficacious form of treatment.

Considering age trends is but one way to consider the role of developmental processes in child psychotherapy. The developmental orientation was embodied in Anna Freud's (1963, 1965) approach to psychopathology, especially her notion of developmental lines, and the idea that all symptoms must be evaluated within the context of developmental processes and their harmony or disharmony. Her descriptive approach to child disturbances created a framework for psychodynamic therapy, aimed specifically at 'scaffolding' the child's development (Kennedy and Moran, 1991; Edgcumbe, 2000). Anna Freud's formulations were criticized for being rather rigidly rooted in the classical psychoanalytic developmental theory of drives, which makes her approach seem out of place within modern child mental health services. However, there are contemporary psychoanalytic approaches that maintain this systematic, developmental perspective (Hurry, 1998). A relatively recent implementation of a general developmental focus building on Anna Freud's, but discarding the drive theory basis, is found in the work of Stanley Greenspan (2002), who identifies a number of interrelated processes contributing to the child's development, and engaged in psychological therapy, quite analogous the Anna Freud's notion of developmental lines. These include self-regulation, understanding intentions and expectations, and many other capacities.

Developmental psychopathology, the organizing discipline of child mental disorder (Cicchetti and Cohen, 1995; Toth and Cicchetti, 1999), is the inheritor of these psychoanalytic concerns. The discipline has been defined as 'the study of the origins and course of individual patterns of behavioral maladaptation' (Sroufe and Rutter, 1984). Developmental psychopathology views development as involving progressive reorganizations in response to changing environmental demands, and conceptualizes psychopathology as a breakdown of the child's and family's capacities to cope with demands for adaptation along a number of developmental pathways. Development is an active dynamic process in which meanings attributed to experiences alter their consequences, creating individual pathways that diverge in both their origins and their endings (Cicchetti and Cohen, 1995; Sameroff and Fiese, 2000), as Anna Freud tried to capture in her system of mapping developmental progress along 'developmental lines'. Developmental psychopathology aims to specify the processes underlying continuity and change; that is, its concern is with how these things happen, not simply with what happens. Thus, the focus in understanding an oppositional child is not on describing his or her behavior, but on mapping the transactional patterns between parent and child that underpin the behavior. Development is viewed as an active, dynamic process, in which the child adds meaning to experiences, and biology shapes but is also shaped by these experiences. The developmental end-point is not defined by the achievement of a stage, as in classical developmental theory (be that Freudian or Piagetian), but rather as the attainment of coherent modes of functioning within and across domains such as thinking and feeling (not on arriving at particular thoughts or feelings).

From the perspective of developmental psychopathology, then, psychological disturbance is not the result of a single cause, such as a particular type of experience. The outcomes associated with any single risk factor are extremely varied, and it is the number of serious risks rather than the nature of any one that is critical (Sameroff and Fiese, 2000). Risks are probabilistic and not causal. Male gender does not cause early childhood emotional disorder any more than female gender causes anorexia in adolescence; it is a marker for the biological, cultural, contextual processes that do cause the disorder. In addition, psychotherapy for children and adolescents, regardless of orientation, takes place in complex systems (von Bertalanffy, 1968), in which a variety of factors initiate and maintain individuals on pathways probabilistically associated with negative outcomes, and further factors differentiate those progressing to disorder A from those progressing to disorder B, and those free of disorder. A quarter of a century's research in developmental psychopathology confirms that specific problem behaviors are the result of varied pathways, including the transactional interaction of biological predisposition with lived experience (e.g., Sameroff, 1995; Cicchetti and Cohen, 1995; Alexander et al., 1996; Howard and Kendall, 1996; Henggeler et al., 1998; Mash, 1998; Sameroff, 1998). Thus, effective child therapy may not be disorder specific or risk specific.

A further complication for child psychotherapy is added by the concept of resilience. Over the past quarter of a century, substantial evidence has shown that given the same risk experience, some children succumb while others escape. Certain factors seem to produce resilience to adversity (e.g., Masten and Curtis, 2000). For example, over time most maltreated children show some self-righting tendencies in the face of extreme stresses (Cicchetti and Rogosch, 1997). Psychological therapies work by reducing risk and enhancing the developmental processes that constitute resilience. A complex interactive mix of influences is involved and there is no simple way of reducing vulnerability in a child (Rutter, 2000). Child therapies have a common assumption that the young person is proactive, construing and reconstruing their experience of the environment, within a transactional relationship whereby they affect the environment as much as the environment

affects them. The degree to which a child can engage in treatment in such an active way will, of course, depend upon their capacity for resilience.

The adoption of the developmental perspective, and particularly the notion that development is affected by a range of internal and external interacting factors, has led to substantial changes in the general approach taken by clinicians towards the psychological treatment of children. There is now room to consider the biological determinants of mental disorder, and the interaction of biological and psychosocial factors. Our developing understanding of these processes has only increased with advances in neuroscientific understanding of brain development (e.g., Schore, 1997; Siegel, 2001; Solms and Turnbull, 2002). It is now recognized that a number of disorders are at least partially irreversible because of the interaction between biological predisposition and the sensitivity of brain development to environmental influence during the first years. This suggests that psychotherapy for some childhood mental disorders may have to abandon the implicit notion of 'cure' in favor of the goal of more balanced functioning of developmental subsystems, within a systemic model.

From the framework of developmental psychopathology, the child in treatment is thus not seen as an individual. Rather, problem behaviors, either of the child or at the family level, are seen in terms of interrelated and interreacting response systems, which regulate the child's behavior and simultaneously regulate others within the system. This way of thinking is as evident in modern psychoanalytic perspectives (e.g., Hauser et al., 1984; Renik, 1993) as in cognitive-behavioral ones (Howard and Kendall, 1996). The need to take an ecological approach (Bronfenbrenner, 1979) is increasingly recognized, even when the focus is on a single aspect, such as the child's conduct problems, communication problems, or learning difficulties. There is an increased concern among clinicians even with traditional behavioral orientations with the emotional environment of the child. This includes communication patterns in the family (Gottman et al., 1997), previously of interest mainly to family therapists. A further example is the recognition of meta-cognitive controls in childhood disorders (Fonagy and Target, 1996a; Howard and Kendall, 1996). All modern therapeutic strategies aim to influence the child's functioning within his or her family or peer group through the development of capacities that might maintain improvements in relationships (Hoagwood et al., 1996).

The notion that childhood problems are best seen in terms of the interrelation of response systems implies that treatment goals must focus on the development of psychological capacities within the child and within the family system that reduce dysfunction and improve adaptation in the long term. It follows from the multifinality and equifinality of causation that the impact of child psychotherapy cannot be assessed in terms of any single variable, but a wide range of outcomes need to be considered, including the impact of changes in one relationship (subsystem) on other relationships (Emde and Robinson, 2000). Family systems are dynamic rather than stable entities. The child's dysfunction and family system interact in ways that are often difficult to predict. Family systems are also developmental entities. Their history creates predispositions in relation to, and expectations about, the future. The past does not determine the present, but rather interacts with it. The future can only be altered through addressing the interaction (Garbarino, 1995).

The developmental model also helps to focus the clinician's attention on contextual aspects of childhood disorder, and the need to consider these when planning treatment. For example, parental psychopathology (maternal depression, parental substance misuse, abnormal parental attributional styles and attitudes, etc.) constrains the effects of any treatment (e.g., Dadds et al., 1987; Frick et al., 1992; Brent et al., 1999). As nearly all interventions with children rely on the involvement of family members (whether by seeking professional help, giving medication, accepting help for themselves, or acting as agents of change in parent training programs) it is clear that the successful treatment of the parent's disorder may be necessary if the child is to benefit from treatment.

The developmental perspective on psychopathology obliges therapists to compare the posttreatment development of treated children with those developing normally, not just to generate strong prepost differences in measured behavior. For example, in one study of integrated CBT for adolescents with attention deficit hyperactive disorder, improvement following treatment was disappointing in the majority of treated cases when compared with the functioning of normal children (Barkley *et al.*, 1992). In studies of problem-solving training for children with conduct disorders, the majority of successfully treated children were still functioning outside the normal range 1 year after treatment termination (Kazdin *et al.*, 1987). These considerations echo Anna Freud's statement of aims for child psychoanalysis as returning the child to 'the path of normal development' (A. Freud, 1965). Clearly, interventions with children, wherever possible, should be judged against this developmental objective.

There are many important differences between approaches to the treatment of children. Nevertheless, there is a shared, emergent systemic perspective, which now includes the powerful biological approach, but has also produced increasing concern with the child's social and relational functioning, rather than simply with symptoms. Treatments have been extended from traditional inpatient and outpatient settings to community contexts. There is an increased tendency, across orientations, to offer treatment in context: in relation to the family and perhaps the school, rather than focusing on the child alone. We hope that the descriptions of treatment approaches within varied theoretical frameworks have highlighted both what is special about the treatment of children, and the extent to which common issues and even methods are increasingly emerging across this field of developmental psychopathology and the management of its casualties.

References

Alexander, J. F. and Parsons, B. V. (1973). Short-term behavioral intervention with delinquent families: impact on family process and recidivism. *Journal of Abnormal Psychology*, **81**, 219–25.

Alexander, J. G., Jameson, P. B., Newell, R. M., and Gunderson, D. (1996). Changing cognitive schemas: a necessary antecedent to changing behaviours in dysfunctional families? In K. S. Dobson and K. D. Craig, ed. *Advances in cognitive–behavioural therapy*, pp. 174–92. Thousand Oaks, CA: Sage.

Altman, N. (1997). The case of Ronald: Oedipal issues in the treatment of a seven-year-old boy. *Psychoanalytic Bialogues*, **7**, 725–39.

Andersen, T. (1987). The reflecting team: dialog and meta dialogue in clinical work. *Family Process*, **26**, 415–28.

Anderson, H. and Goolishan, H. (1988). Human systems as linguistic systems. *Family Process*, **27**, 371–93.

Anderson, H. and Goolishan, H. (1992). The client as the expert: a not knowing approach to therapy. In: S. McNee and K. Gergen, ed. *Therapy as a social construction*, pp. 25–39. London: Sage.

Bandura, A. (1977). *Social learning theory*. Englewood Cliffs, NJ: Prentice-Hall.

Barkley, R. A., Guevremont, D. C., Anastopoulos, A. D., and Fletcher, K. E. (1992). A comparison of three family therapy programs for treating family conflicts in adolescents with ADHD. *Journal of Consulting and Clinical Psychology*, **60**, 450–62.

Barrett, P. M. (1998). Evaluation of cognitive-behavioural group treatments for childhood anxiety disorders. *Journal of Clinical Child Psychology*, **27**, 459–68.

Barrett, P. M., Duffy, A. L., Dadds, M. R., and Rapee, R. M. (2001). Cognitive behavioural treatments of anxiety disorders in children: long term (6 year) follow-up. *Journal of Consulting and Clinical Psychology*, **69**, 135–41.

Barton, C., Alexander, J. F., Waldron, H., Turner, C. W., and Warburton, J. (1985). Generalising treatment effects of functional family therapy: three replications. *American Journal of Family Therapy*, **13**, 16–26.

Berg, I. K. and de Shazer, S. (1993). Making numbers talk: language in therapy. In: S. Friedman, ed. *The new language of change: Constructive collaboration in psychotherapy*, pp. 5–24. New York: Guilford Press.

von Bertalanffy, L. (1968). *General system theory: foundations, development, applications*. New York: George Braziller.

Borduin, C. M. (1999). Multisystemic treatment of criminality and violence in adolescents. *Journal of the American Academy for Child and Adolescent Psychiatry*, **38**, 242–9.

Brent, D. A., Kolko, D., Birmaher, B., Baugher, M., and Bridge, J. (1999). A clinical trial for adolescent depression: predictors of additional treatment in the acute and follow-up phases of the trial. *Journal of the American Academy of Child and Adolescent Psychiatry*, **38**, 263–70.

Bronfenbrenner, U. (1979). *The ecology of human development: experiments by nature and design*. Cambridge, MA: Harvard University Press.

Bruner, J. (1990). *Acts of meaning*. Cambridge, MA: Harvard University Press.

Chazan, S. (2002). *Simultaneous treatment of parent and child*, 2nd edn. London: Jessica Kingsley.

Christophersen, E. R. and Mortweet, S. L. (2001). *Treatments that work with children: empirically supported strategies for managing childhood problems*. Washington, DC: American Psychological Association.

Cicchetti, D. and Cohen, D. J. (1995). Perspectives on developmental psychopathology. In: D. Cicchetti and D. J. Cohen, ed. *Developmental psychopathology*, Vol. 1: *theory and methods*, pp. 3–23. New York: John Wiley and Sons.

Cicchetti, D. and Rogosch, F. A. (1997). The role of self-organization in the promotion of resilience in maltreated children. *Development and Psychopathology*, **9**, 797–815.

Cobham, V. E., Dadds, M. R., and Spence, S. H. (1998). The role of parental anxiety in the treatment of childhood anxiety. *Journal of Consulting and Clinical Psychology*, **66**, 893–905.

Combrinck-Graham, L. (1991). On technique with children in family therapy: how calculated should it be? *Journal of Marital and Family Therapy*, **17**, 373–7.

Context. (2002). *Context, special issue: focusing practice on children*. Kent: AFT Publishing.

Cottrell, D. and Boston, P. (2002). Practitioner review: the effectiveness of systemic family therapy for children and adolescents. *Journal of Child Psychology and Psychiatry*, **43**, 573–86.

Dadds, M. R., Schwartz, S., and Sanders, M. R. (1987). Marital discord and treatment outcome in behavioural treatment of child conduct disorders. *Journal of Consulting and Clinical Psychology*, **55**, 396–403.

Dallos, R. and Draper, R. (2000). *An introduction to family therapy*. Buckingham: Open University Press.

Dodge, K. A. (1985). Attributional bias in aggressive children. In: P. C. Kendall, ed. *Advances in cognitive-behavioural research and therapy*, Vol. 4, pp. 75–111. New York: Academic Press.

Durlak, J. A., Fuhrman, T., and Lampman, C. (1991). Effectiveness of cognitive-behavior therapy for maladapting children: a meta-analysis. *Psychological Bulletin*, **110**, 204–14.

Edgcumbe, R. (2000). *Anna Freud: a view of development, disturbance and therapeutic techniques*. London: Routledge.

Eisler, I., Dare, C., Hodes, M., Russell, G., Dodge, E., and Le Grange, D. (2000). Family therapy for adolescent anorexia nervosa: the results of a controlled comparison of two family interventions. *Journal of Child Psychology and Psychiatry*, **41**, 727–36.

Eisler, I., Dare, C., Russell, G. F. M., Szmukler, G., le Grange, D., and Dodge, E. (1997). Family and individual therapy in anorexia nervosa: a 5-year follow-up. *Archives of General Psychiatry*, **54**(11), 1025–30.

Emde, R. N. and Robinson, J. A. (2000). Guiding principles for a theory of early intervention: A developmental-psychoanalytic perspective. In: S. J. Meisels and J. P. Shonkoff, ed. *Handbook of early childhood intervention*, 2nd edn., pp. 160–78. New York: Cambridge University Press.

Fonagy, P. and Moran, G. S. (1990). Studies on the efficacy of child psychoanalysis. *Journal of Consulting and Clinical Psychology*, **58**, 684–95.

Fonagy, P. and Target, M. (1994). The efficacy of psychoanalysis for children with disruptive disorders. *Journal of the American Academy of Child and Adolescent Psychiatry*, **33**, 45–55.

Fonagy, P. and Target, M. (1996a). A contemporary psychoanalytical perspective: psychodynamic developmental therapy. In: E. Hibbs and P. Jensen, ed. *Psychosocial treatments for child and adolescent disorders: empirically based approaches*, pp. 619–38. Washington, DC: APA and NIH.

Fonagy, P. and Target, M. (1996b). Playing with reality: I. Theory of mind and the normal development of psychic reality. *International Journal of Psycho-Analysis*, **77**, 217–33.

Fonagy, P. and Target, M. (1996c). Predictors of outcome in child psychoanalysis: a retrospective study of 763 cases at the Anna Freud Centre. *Journal of the American Psychoanalytic Association*, **44**, 27–77.

Fonagy, P. and Target, M. (1998). Mentalization and the changing aims of child psychoanalysis. *Psychoanalytic Dialogues*, **8**, 87–114.

Fonagy, P., Gergely, G., Jurist, E., and Target, M. (2002a). *Affect regulation, mentalization and the development of the Self*. New York: Other Press.

Fonagy, P., Target, M., Cottrell, D., Phillips, J., and Kurtz, Z. (2002b). *What works for whom? A critical review of treatments for children and adolescents*. New York: Guilford Press.

Fraiberg, S. (1980). *Clinical studies in infant mental health*. New York: Basic Books.

Freud, A. (1963). The concept of developmental lines. *The Psychoanalytic Study of the Child*, **18**, 245–65.

Freud, A. (1965). *Normality and pathology in childhood: assessments of development*. Madison, CT: International Universities Press.

Freud, A. (1966–1980). *The writings of Anna Freud, Volumes I–VIII*. New York: International Universities Press.

Freud, S. (1909). *Analysis of a phobia in a five-year-old boy*. In: J. Strachey, trans. and ed. *The standard edition of the complete psychological works of Sigmund Freud*, Vol. 10, pp. 1–147. London: Hogarth Press.

Frick, P. J., Lahey, B. B., Loeber, R., Stouthammer–Loeber, M., Christ, M., and B. Hanson, K. (1992). Familial risk factors to oppositional defiant disorder and conduct disorder. Parental psychopathology and maternal parenting. *Journal of Consulting and Clinical Psychology*, **60**, 49–55.

Friedberg, R. D. and McClure, J. M. (2002). *Clinical practice of cognitive therapy with children and adolescents: the nuts and bolts*. New York: Guilford Press.

Garbarino, J. (1995). *Raising children in a socially toxic environment*. San Francisco: Jossey Bass.

Gil, E. (1994). *Play in family therapy*. New York: Guilford Press.

Gordon, D. A., Arbuthnot, J., Gustafson, K. E., and McGreen, P. (1988). Home-based behavioural-systems family therapy with disadvantaged juvenile delinquents. *American Journal of Family Therapy*, **16**, 243–55.

Gordon, D. A., Graves, K., and Arbuthnot, J. (1995). The effect of functional family therapy for delinquents on adult criminal behaviour. *Criminal Justice and Behaviour*, **22**, 60–73.

Gottman, J. M., Katz, L. F., and Hooven, C. (1997). *Meta-emotion: how families communicate emotionally*. Mahwah, NJ: Lawrence Erlbaum.

Greenspan, S. I. (2002). The developmental basis of psychotherapeutic processes. In: J. J. Magnavita, ed. *Comprehensive handbook of psychotherapy*: Vol. 1, *psychodynamic/object relations*, pp. 15–44. New York: John Wiley.

Gurman, A. S., Kniskern, D. P., and Pinsof, W. M. (1986). Research on the process and outcome of marital and family therapy. In: S. L. Garfield and A. E. Bergin, ed. *Handbook of psychotherapy and behavior change*, pp. 565–624. New York: John Wiley.

Harrington, R., et al. (1998). Randomized trial of a home-based family intervention for children who have deliberately poisoned themselves. *Journal of the American Academy of Child and Adolescent Psychiatry*, **37**, 512–18.

Hauser, S. T., Powers, S. I., Noan, G. G., and Jacobson, A. M. (1984). Familial contexts of adolescent ego development. *Child Development*, **55**, 195–213.

Heinicke, C. M. (1965). Frequency of psychotherapeutic session as a factor affecting the child's developmental status. *The Psychoanalytic Study of the Child*, **20**, 42–98.

Heinicke, C. M. and Ramsey-Klee, D. M. (1986). Outcome of child psychotherapy as a function of frequency of sessions. *Journal of the American Academy of Child Psychiatry*, **25**, 247–253.

Henggeler, S. W., Pickrel, S. G., Brondino, M. J., and Crouch, J. L. (1996). Eliminating (almost) treatment dropout of substance abusing or dependent delinquents through home-based multisystemic therapy. *American Journal of Psychiatry*, **153**, 427–8.

Henggeler, S. W., Schoenwald, S. K., Borduin, C. M., Rowland, M. D., and Cunningham, P. B. (1998). *Multisystemic treatment of antisocial behaviour in children and adolescents*. New York: Guilford Press.

Herbert, M. (1994). Behavioural methods. In: M. Rutter and E. Taylor and L. Hersov, ed. *Child and adolescent psychiatry: modern approaches*, pp. 858–79. Oxford: Blackwell.

Herbert, M. (1998). *Clinical child psychology: social learning, development and behaviour*, 2nd edn. New York: Wiley.

Hoagwood, K., Jensen, P. S., Petti, T., and Burns, B. J. (1996). Outcomes of mental health care for children and adolescents: I. A comprehensive conceptual model. *Journal of the American Academy of Child and Adolescent Psychiatry*, **35**, 1055–63.

Hoffman, L. (1981). *Foundations of family therapy. A conceptual framework for change*. New York: Basic Books.

Howard, B. L. and Kendall, P. C. (1996). *Cognitive-behavioral family therapy for anxious children: therapist manual*. Ardmore, PA: Workbook.

Hurry, A., ed. (1998). *Psychoanalysis and developmental therapy*. London: Karnac Books.

Jenner, S. (1999). *The parent child game: the proven key to a happy family*. London: Bloomsbury.

Kazdin, A. E. (1985). *Treatment of antisocial behavior in children and adolescents*. Homewood, IL: Dorsey Press.

Kazdin, A. E., Esveldt-Dawson, K., French, N. H., and Unis, A. S. (1987). Problem-solving skills training and relationship therapy in the treatment of antisocial child behaviour. *Journal of Consulting and Clinical Psychology*, **55**, 76–85.

Kazdin, A. E., Siegel, T. C., and Bass, D. (1992). Cognitive problem-solving skills training and parent management training in the treatment of antisocial behavior in children. *Journal of Consulting and Clinical Psychology*, **60**, 733–47.

Kendall, P. C. (2000). *Child and adolescent therapy: cognitive-behavioural procedures*. New York: Guilford Press.

Kendall, P. C. and Panichelli-Mindel, S. M. (1995). Cognitive behavioural treatments. *Journal of Abnormal Child Psychology*, **23**, 107–24.

Kennedy, H. and Moran, G. (1991). Reflections on the aims of child psychoanalysis. *The Psychoanalytic Study of the Child*, **46**, 181–98.

Klein, M. (1932). *The psycho-analysis of children*. London: Hogarth Press.

Klerman, G. L., Weissman, M. M., Rounsaville, B. J., and Chevron, E. S. (1984). *Interpersonal psychotherapy of depression*. New York: Basic Books.

Kolvin, I., et al. (1981). *Help starts here: the maladjusted child in the ordinary school*. London: Tavistock.

Larner, G. (1996). Narrative child family therapy. *Family Process*, **35**, 423–40.

Lieberman, A. F. and Pawl, J. (1993). Infant-parent psychotherapy. In: C. H. Zeanah, ed. *Handbook of infant mental health*, pp. 427–42. New York: Guilford Press.

Lobatto, W. (2002). Talking to children about family therapy: a qualitative research study. *Journal of Family Therapy*, **24**, 330–43.

Lochman, J. E., White, K. J., and Wayland, K. K. (1991). Cognitive-behavioural assessment and treatment with aggressive children. In: P. C. Kendall, ed. *Child and adolescent therapy: cognitive and behavioural procedures*, pp. 25–66. New York: Guilford Press.

Lochman, J. E., Coie, J. D., Underwood, M. K., and Terry, R. (1993). Effectiveness of a social relations intervention program for aggressive and nonaggressive, rejected children. *Journal of Consulting and Clinical Psychology*, **61**, 1053–8.

Lush, D., Boston, M., and Grainger, E. (1991). Evaluation of psychoanalytic psychotherapy with children: therapists' assessments and predictions. *Psychoanalytic Psychotherapy*, **5**, 191–234.

March, J. S. and Mulle, K. M. (1998). *OCD in children and adolescents. A cognitive-behavioural treatment manual*. New York: Guilford Press.

Marshall, R. and Reimers, S. (2002). In the centre of the looking glass: what do children think of reflecting teams. *Context*, **64**, 14–17.

Mash, E. J. (1998). Treatment of child and family disturbance: A behavioral-systems perspective. In: E. J. Mash and R. A. Barkley, ed. *Treatment of childhood disorders*, 2nd edn, pp. 3–54. New York: Guilford Press.

Masten, A. S. and Curtis, W. J. (2000). Integrating competence and psychopathology: pathways towards a comprehensive science of adaptation and development. *Development and Psychopathology*, **12**, 529–50.

Meadows, S. (1993). *The child as thinker*. London: Routledge.

Mendlowitz, S. L., *et al.* (1999). Cognitive-behavioral group treatments in childhood anxiety disorders: the role of parental involvement. *Journal of the American Academy of Child and Adolescent Psychiatry*, **38**(10), 1223–9.

Minuchin, S. (1974). *Families and family therapy*. Cambridge, MA: Harvard University Press.

Minuchin, S., Montalvo, B., Guerney, B., Rosman, B., and Schumer, F. (1967). *Families of the slums*. New York: Basic Books.

Moran, G. S. and Fonagy, P. (1987). Psychoanalysis and diabetic control: a single case study. *British Journal of Medical Psychology*, **60**, 357–72.

Moran, G., Fonagy, P., Kurtz, A., Bolton, A., and Brook, C. (1991). A controlled study of the psychoanalytic treatment of brittle diabetes. *Journal of the American Academy of Child and Adolescent Psychiatry*, **30**, 926–35.

Mufson, L., Moreau, D., Weissman, M. M., and Klerman, G. L. (1993). *Interpersonal psychotherapy for depressed adolescents*. New York: Guilford Press.

Mufson, L., Weissman, M. M., Moreau, D., and Garfinkel, R. (1999). Efficacy of interpersonal psychotherapy for depressed adolescents. *Archives of General Psychiatry*, **56**, 573–9.

Muratori, F., Picchi, L., Bruni, G., Patarnello, M., and Romagnoli, G. (2003). A two-year follow-up of psychodynamic psychotherapy for internalizing disorders in children. *J Am Acad Child Adolesc Psychiatry*, **42**(3), 331–9.

Novick, J. and Novick, K. K. (2002). Parent work in analysis: children, adolescents, and adults. Part Three: middle and pretermination stages. *Journal of Infant,Child, and Adolescent Psychotherapy*, **2**, 17–42.

O'Brien, A. and Loudon, P. (1985). Redressing the balance—involving children in family therapy. *Journal of Family Therapy*, **7**, 81–98.

Oram, K. (2000). Involving parents in the play therapy of their children. *Journal of Infant, Child, and Adolescent Psychotherapy*, **1**, 79–98.

Parsons, B. and Alexander, J. (1973). Short term family intervention: a therapy outcome study. *Journal of Consulting and Clinical Psychology*, **41**, 195–201.

Renik, O. (1993). Analytic interaction: conceptualizing technique in the light of the analyst's irreducible subjectivity. *Psychoanalytic Quarterly*, **62**, 553–71.

Robin, A. L., Siegel, P. T., Koepke, T., Moye, A., and Tice, S. (1994). Family therapy versus individual therapy for adolescent females with anorexia nervosa. *Journal of Developmental and Behavioral Pediatrics*, **15**, 111–16.

Robin, A. L., *et al.* (1999). A controlled comparison of family versus individual therapy for adolescents with anorexia nervosa. *Journal of the American Academy of Child and Adolescent Psychiatry*, **38**, 1482–9.

Rogers, A. (1995). *A shining affliction*. New York: Penguin Books.

Rosselló, J. and Bernal, G. (1999). The efficacy of cognitive-behavioral and interpersonal treatments for depression in Puerto Rican adolescents. *Journal of Consulting and Clinical Psychology*, **67**, 734–45.

Russell, G. F. M., Szmukler, G., Dare, C., and Eisler, I. (1987). An evaluation of family therapy in anorexia nervosa and bulimia nervosa. *Archives of General Psychiatry*, **44**, 1047–56.

Rutter, M. (2000). Psychosocial influences: critiques, findings and research needs. *Development and Psychopathology*, **12**, 375–405.

Sameroff, A. J. (1995). General systems theories and developmental psychopathology. In: J. Cicchetti and D. J. Cohen, ed. *Developmental psychopathology*: Vol. 1. *Theory and methods*, pp. 659–95. New York: Wiley.

Sameroff, A. J. (1998). Understanding the social context of early psychopathology. In: J. Noshpitz, ed. *Handbook of child and adolescent psychiatry*, pp. 224–35. New York: BasicBooks.

Sameroff, A. J. and Fiese, B. H. (2000). Models of development and developmental risk. In: C. H. Zeanah, ed. *Handbook of infant mental health*, pp. 3–19. New York: Guilford Press.

Santor, D. A. and Kusumakar, V. (2001). Open trial of interpersonal therapy in adolescents with moderate to severe major depression: effectiveness of

novice IPT therapists. *Journal of the American Academy of Child and Adolescent Psychiatry*, **40**(2), 236–40.

Schore, A. (1997). *Affect regulation and the origin of the self: the neurobiology of emotional development*. Hillsdale, NJ: Erlbaum.

Serketich, W. J. and Dumas, J. E. (1996). The effectiveness of behavioural parent training to modify antisocial behaviour in children: a meta–analysis. *Behaviour Therapy*, **27**, 171–86.

Siegel, D. J. (2001). Toward an interpersonal neurobiology of the developing mind: attachment relationships, 'mindsight' and neural integration. *Infant Mental Health Journal*, **22**, 67–94.

Siskind, D. (1997). *Working with parents: establishing the essential alliance in child psychotherapy and consultation*. New York: Jason Aronson.

Slade, A. (1986). Symbolic play and separation–individuation: a naturalistic study. *Bulletin of the Menninger Clinic*, **50**(6), 541–63.

Slade, A. (1987). Quality of attachment and early symbolic play. *Developmental Psychology*, **17**, 326–35.

Slade, A. (1994). Making meaning and making believe: their role in the clinical process. In: A. Slade and D. Wolf, ed. *Children at play: clinical and developmental approaches to meaning and representation*, pp. 81–110. New York: Oxford University Press.

Slade, A. (1999). Representation, symbolization and affect regulation in the concomitant treatment of a mother and child: attachment theory and child psychotherapy. *Psychoanalytic Inquiry*, **19**, 824–57.

Slade, A. (in press). *Working with parents in child psychotherapy: engaging the reflective function*. Psychoanalytic Inquiry.

Smyrnios, K. X. and Kirkby, R. J. (1993). Long-term comparison of brief versus unlimited psychodynamic treatments with children and their parents. *Journal of Consulting and Clinical Psychology*, **61**, 1020–7.

Solms, M. and Turnbull, O. (2002). *The brain and the inner world: an introduction to the neuroscience of subjective experience*. New York: Other Press.

Sroufe, L. A. and Rutter, M. (1984). The domain of developmental psychopathology. *Child Development*, **83**, 173–89.

Stallard, P. (2002). Cognitive behaviour therapy with children and young people: a selective review of key issues. *Behavioural and Cognitive Psychotherapy*, **30**(3), 297–309.

Stanton, M. D. and Shadish, W. R. (1997). Outcome, attrition and family/couples treatment for drug abuse: a meta-analysis and review of the controlled and comparative studies. *Psychological Bulletin*, **122**, 170–91.

Stith, S. M., Rosen, K. H., McCollum, E. E., Coleman, J. U., and Herman, S. A. (1996). The voices of children: pre-adolescent children's experiences in family therapy. *Journal of Marital and Family Therapy*, **22**, 69–86.

Szapocznik, J., *et al.* (1988). Engaging adolescent drug abusers and their families in treatment: a strategic structural systems approach. *Journal of Consulting and Clinical Psychology*, **56**, 552–7.

Szapocznik, J., *et al.* (1989). Structural family versus psychodynamic child therapy for problematic Hispanic boys. *Journal of Consulting and Clinical Psychology*, **57**, 571–8.

Target, M. and Fonagy, P. (1994a). The efficacy of psychoanalysis for children: developmental considerations. *Journal of the American Academy of Child and Adolescent Psychiatry*, **33**, 1134–44.

Target, M. and Fonagy, P. (1994b). The efficacy of psychoanalysis for children with emotional disorders. *Journal of the American Academy of Child and Adolescent Psychiatry*, **33**, 361–71.

Target, M. and Fonagy, P. (1996). Playing with reality II: The development of psychic reality from a theoretical perspective. *International Journal of Psycho-Analysis*, **77**, 459–79.

Toth, S. L. and Cicchetti, D. (1999). Developmental psychotherapy and child psychotherapy. In: S. W. Russ and T. H. Ollendick, ed. *Handbook of psychotherapies with children and families*, pp. 15–44. New York: Kluwer Academic/Plenum.

Webster-Stratton, C. and Hammond, M. (1997). Treating children with early-onset conduct problems: a comparison of child and parent training interventions. *Journal of Consulting and Clinical Psychology*, **65**, 93–109.

Webster-Stratton, C. and Herbert, M. (1993). What really happens in parent training? *Behaviour Modification*, **17**, 407–56.

Webster-Stratton, C., Hollinsworth, T., and Kolpacoff, M. (1989). The long-term cost effectiveness and clinical significance of three cost-effective training programs for families with conduct problem children. *Journal of Consulting and Clinical Psychology*, **57**, 550–3.

Weisz, J. R., Weiss, B., Morton, T., Granger, D., and Han, S. (1992). *Meta-analysis of psychotherapy outcome research with children and adolescents*. Los Angeles: University of California.

White, M. and Epston, D. (1990). *Narrative means to therapeutic ends*. New York: Norton.

Wilson, J. (1998). *Child-focused practice. A collaborative systemic approach*. London: Karnac Books.

Winnicott, D. W. (1965). *The maturational process and the facilitating environment*. London: Hogarth Press.

Winnicott, D. W. (1971). *Playing and reality*. London: Tavistock.

Zilbach, J. (1986). *Young children in family therapy*. Northvale NJ: Jason Aronson.

30 Psychotherapy with adolescents

Mark A. Reinecke and Stephen R. Shirk

Introduction

Psychotherapy is, in one sense, a simple endeavor. An individual and a clinician meet, and in a trusting and open manner, talk through the patient's concerns with the goal of bringing about changes in the person's thoughts, feelings, or behavior. Psychotherapy can be thought of, then, as learning and change brought about through a supportive relationship. Not all forms of psychotherapy, however, are equally effective in bringing about significant or enduring change in a person's adjustment, and the mechanisms by which psychotherapy leads to emotional, social, and behavioral improvement are not well understood. Moreover, psychotherapy with adolescents differs in a number of substantive ways from psychotherapy with adults. Adolescence is a time of transition. Processes of cognitive, social, emotional, and physical maturation can affect the nature and course of symptoms. It is necessary to adapt our psychotherapeutic approaches in order to assist adolescents in managing such changes. There is a general consensus that it is important to adopt a contextual and developmental perspective for describing, understanding, and treating adolescents.

Our understanding of the developmental psychopathology of both internalizing and externalizing disorders, for example, is rudimentary. It can be difficult, as a consequence, to use this research as a guide for clinical practice. Moreover, our understanding of processes of change in psychotherapy, predictors of response to treatment, and predictors of maintenance of gains are only beginning to emerge. From a practical perspective, it is worth acknowledging that a substantial percentage of adolescents do not benefit from psychotherapy, or do not realize a fully adequate response. Moreover, the generalizabilty of findings and approaches to community practice has not been demonstrated. What works in university research clinics may or may not be effective in community settings.

History

Although the art and science of psychotherapy with adolescents is of relatively recent origin, rapid progress has been made. Early work on psychotherapy with adolescents was based largely on psychodynamic models (Klein, 1950; Kris, 1952; S. Freud, 1953; Fraiberg, 1955; Geleerd, 1957, 1964; A. Freud, 1958; Blos, 1962, 1970; Friend, 1972; Miller, 1974). Many of the assertions of psychodynamic and psychoanalytic models have not been put to test, leading to something of a stagnation in the evolution of psychoanalytic paradigms for understanding and treating youth. With few exceptions (Moran *et al.*, 1991; Altman, 1995) theoretical and clinical development in this area has been slow during recent years.

Psychodynamic models of psychopathology tend, as a group, to be developmentally based. As Tyson and Tyson (1990) note, development occurs along a number of lines during adolescence. Psychodynamic and psychoanalytic writers traditionally view affective lability during adolescence as stemming from a developmental reorganization in the structures and functions of the ego and superego. Stage-specific defenses are needed, from this perspective, to cope with shifting moods. Changes in mood during adolescence are seen as stemming from the activation of memories of early events (Weinshel, 1970) and the recapitulation of early experiences. This notion, that adolescent development is characterized by a recapitulation, reexamination and reworking of earlier themes and conflicts, is central to many psychoanalytic models. Regression in the service of the ego (Kris, 1952), and struggles to develop a cohesive sense of self, as such, are seen as a normal part of adolescent development, and provide a way of understanding emotional and behavioral distress during this period of development. Psychodynamic theorists have proposed that the development of an adult identity stands as a central task of adolescence (Erikson, 1956).

Alternatives to psychoanalytic developmental models have emerged from several quarters over the last 30 years. Among the most prominent are models based on principles of developmental psychopathology (Cicchetti and Cohen, 1995). Rather than organizing development around phases of psychosexual maturation, these models tend to highlight age-related developmental tasks such as attachment formation, physiological and emotion regulation, mastery and cognitive competence, peer relationship formation, and identity development. From this perspective, each developmental task represents a potential challenge to be negotiated. Successful negotiation of early tasks increases the probability for better adaptation with later tasks. Secure attachment during early childhood, for example, appears to predict later peer competence. However, development is viewed as transactional and open to later influence such that early difficulties do not foreclose on the possibility of subsequent adjustment. The pivotal tasks of adolescence involve changes in physical appearance and sexuality, increased autonomy and involvement with peers, identity formation, and the development of romantic relationships.

In addition, the past few decades have witnessed the emergence of cognitive, behavioral, and family systems approaches for addressing a variety of clinically important concerns among youth (for reviews, see Hibbs and Jensen, 1996; Carr, 2000; Kazdin, 2000; Fonagy *et al.*, 2002; Reinecke *et al.*, 2003). A relatively large number of well-designed outcome studies have been completed, and an impressive body of research has been published examining both factors associated with risk for psychopathology among youth and possible mediators of therapeutic change. As research in developmental psychopathology has expanded, new and often quite specific targets for intervention have emerged. As the methodological quality of outcome and process research has improved a number of empirically supported forms of treatment have been developed. In fact, we can say with *some* confidence that *some* forms of psychotherapy may be effective for treating *some* forms of psychopathology experienced by *some* adolescents.

Developmental considerations

Early research into the efficacy of psychotherapy for treating youth borrowed heavily from research with adults. Models, methodologies, instruments, and clinical techniques that had been found useful in clinical outcome research with adults were simply applied to a new sample— children and adolescents. It quickly became apparent, however, that processes mediating the expression of behavioral and emotional difficulties among youth may differ from those of adults. Responding to this challenge, recent research has been more sensitive to developmental differences between children, adolescents, and adults.

As noted, a range of physical, social, cognitive, and emotional changes occur over the course of adolescence. These developmental changes and issues must be considered both when developing a clinical treatment plan, and when designing a clinical research project. Developmental changes include puberty, the emergence of formal operational thought, the emergence of an adult identity, increasing emphasis on relationships with peers, decreasing reliance on parents for guidance and support, the establishment of vocational goals, the emergence of sexual interests, and the consolidation of values, standards, and tacit beliefs.

Puberty

Puberty, for example, is accompanied by a range of changes, both hormonal and physical (Richards and Petersen, 1987; Richards et al., 1993). The physical transformations that accompany puberty can be confusing, exciting, and challenging. The effects of physical maturation on adjustment during adolescence, however, are complex. Significant individual differences exist in the age of onset of puberty and in the rate at which physical maturation occurs. Moreover, there can be asynchronies in development across physical, social, and emotional domains. The effects of physical maturation on psychosocial development and adaptation appear to be mediated by a number of factors including gender, age of onset of puberty, the relative maturity of peers, and cultural, familial, and community beliefs about maturation. That said, hormonal changes accompanying puberty appear to have broad effects on adolescent development. They have been associated with changes in expression of anger, oppositionality toward parents and other adults, sexual behavior, aggression, mood, self-confidence, and level of psychopathology. It is not clear, however, that relations between physical maturation and adjustment are direct. Rather, the effects of hormonal changes accompanying puberty appear to be mediated and moderated by psychological, familial, and social variables (Richards et al., 1993). The effects of puberty on adjustment are clinically important for a number of reasons. Physical maturation during adolescence has significant effects on the social status of the individual, how they view themselves, how their peers see them, and how they are viewed by their family and the larger community. Others expectations for them will change as they mature. Teenagers who appear mature may not, however, be socially, emotionally, and cognitively mature, leading to confusion and conflict. Moreover, teenagers naturally experience a range of thoughts and feelings about their physical and sexual maturation. Their thoughts, fantasies, and expectations about these changes, and their effects on their life and relationships, are worthy of discussion during psychotherapy. This is particularly important when the teen is dissatisfied with the changes in their appearance or the ways that these changes have affected their relationships with others. Physical maturation, and the social changes that accompany it have important effects on adolescent adjustment and can, as a consequence, complicate the practice of psychotherapy with adolescents.

Cognitive development

Developmental changes in reasoning also influence emotional and behavioral adaptation during adolescence. As formal operational thought emerges, for example, adolescents may be better able to reflect upon their experiences and motivations, to develop and evaluate alternative interpretations of events, and to examine critically their beliefs and attitudes. They will, as a consequence of developing hypothetico-deductive reasoning, be better able to use 'standard' insight-oriented and cognitive-behavioral interventions. As formal-operational thought emerges, however, it may be applied in an egocentric manner (Elkind, 1967). This may lead adolescents to believe that others are as concerned by their behavior and appearance as they are (an imaginary audience) or that his or her emotions are both unique and significant (the personal fable). This can be accompanied by fluctuations in affect. Egocentric thought during adolescence can be associated with a tendency to personalize events, to magnify their significance, and to misperceive their consequences. Clinically, this can contribute to emotional lability as adolescents believe their emotional experiences are 'more intense' than those of their peers. It can also contribute to difficulties trusting others (including the therapist) based on the belief that 'no one really understands me.' A central task in cognitive-behavioral psychotherapy (CBT) with adolescents, then, is to assist the individual to recognize these misperceptions and to develop more mature forms of reasoning.

Autonomy and independence

Development of autonomy, a sense of personal efficacy, and an ability to function independently of one's parents and family are central tasks of adolescence. Peer support plays a critical role in accomplishing these tasks. Adolescents' sensitivity to the norms of their peer culture, as well as a desire for acceptance by their peers, can both assist with the process of becoming independent from ones family, and can lead them to become resistant to the authority of their parents and other adults. Moreover, it can lead them to question the beliefs, attitudes, expectations, and values of their families. Clinically disturbed adolescents may, as a result, show little concern for fitting their actions to the norms of adult society. Not surprisingly, such youth can find it difficult to form a trusting relationship with a therapist. This can be exacerbated by a tendency on the part of parents and adolescents to view their problematic behavior as 'a normal part of growing up.' Adolescent oppositionality, resistance, and identification with 'negative' aspects of their peer culture may be understood, then, within a developmental context. Difficulties becoming independent from one's parents can also be problematic. Insofar as anxieties and ambivalence about autonomy from one's parents, oppositionality, fluctuating self-image, and challenging of accepted beliefs are, in many ways, normal and adaptive parts of the adolescent experience, it can be difficult for clinicians to discriminate normal, healthy adaptation and problematic behavior. The line between normative development and clinical disturbance is often a thin one. Not all adolescents experience turmoil (most, in fact, are reasonably well-adjusted socially and emotionally), and not all turmoil is maladaptive. How we conceptualize turmoil can have important effects on how we develop clinical formulations and on how we approach treatment (Elmen and Offer, 1993).

Epidemiology

Epidemiological and clinic-based studies indicate that a substantial percentage of adolescents manifest significant behavioral and emotional difficulties, and that these problems can have adverse effects on their development and adaptation. Early studies of psychiatric illness among adolescents in community samples indicated that between 10% and 20% of adolescents experience some form of psychiatric illness (Langer et al., 1974; Leslie, 1974; Gould et al., 1981; Offer et al., 1987). Unfortunately, the authors typically reported data on youth between 6 and 18 years of age, so one cannot know the rates among adolescents specifically. The Isle of Wight Study (Rutter et al., 1976), a comprehensive assessment of psychiatric symptoms in a sample of over 2000 14–15 year olds in the UK, indicated that approximately 10–15% of adolescents met criteria for a diagnosable psychiatric illness over the course of a year. More recently, a study of the prevalence of psychopathology among Canadian youth indicated that approximately 18% of 4–16-year-old children and adolescents manifest a psychiatric illness (Offord et al., 1987). Although prevalence rates vary for specific disorders, these findings are quite consistent with other studies in suggesting that, at any given time, a substantial percentage of youth manifest a significant psychiatric difficulty (Costello, 1989). Cross-cultural comparisons of rates of psychopathology among adolescents indicate that there may be differences in rates of psychopathology between countries (Bird et al., 1990; Verhulst and Achenbach, 1995; Bird, 1996).

Taken together, studies indicate that approximately 20% of children and adolescents in the USA manifest a clinically significant behavioral, emotional, or developmental difficulty at any given time. Moreover, a substantially larger percentage of youth manifest social, academic, behavioral, or emotional symptoms that, although not of sufficient duration or severity to warrant a DSM-IV diagnosis, adversely effect their adjustment and development. Many teenagers engage in behaviors (such as drug use, unprotected sex, reckless driving, smoking) that, although not diagnostic in their own right, place them at risk for a range of problems.

Many of these disorders tend to persist over time, placing adolescents at risk for adaptive difficulties during adulthood. The long-term outcomes for depression, attention deficit hyperactivity disorder (ADHD), oppositional-defiant disorder, conduct disorder, substance abuse, and many of the anxiety disorders are not positive. Although symptoms may tend to wax and wane in severity, the majority of children and adolescents do not grow out of their disorder. Depression, for example, tends to be a recurrent disorder that can persist into adulthood (Kovacs *et al.*, 1984, 1997; Harrington *et al.*, 1990; Kovacs, 1996). In a similar manner, children and adolescents with ADHD frequently develop persistent academic and social problems. Approximately 30% of adolescents with ADHD continue to meet criteria for this disorder as adults, with an additional 15–20% demonstrating subclinical symptoms that interfere with social and occupational functioning. Left untreated, the prognosis for adolescents with ADHD is poor (Gittelman *et al.*, 1985; Mannuzza *et al.*, 1993; Weiss and Hechtman, 1993). Although not all children or adolescents who develop oppositional-defiant disorder or conduct disorder follow a common developmental course, these disorders are predictive of a range of difficulties during adulthood. Adolescents with externalizing behavior disorders are at an increased risk, for example, for experiencing marital and relationship difficulties, depression, alcohol and substance abuse, poor occupational functioning, and antisocial or criminal behavior as an adult (Loeber, 1988; Quinton *et al.*, 1990; Offord and Bennett, 1994).

Anxiety disorders are common among adolescents (Kashani and Orvaschel, 1988, 1990). Community surveys indicate that between 10% and 18% of nonreferred youth manifest an anxiety disorder at any given time (Kashani and Orvaschel, 1988; McGee *et al.*, 1990). Obsessive-compulsive disorder, for example, is relatively common, occurring in approximately 1 in 200 children and adolescents in the USA (Flament *et al.*, 1988; Valleni-Basille *et al.*, 1994). Although it was once believed that these disorders were transient, it is now recognized that they can have a chronic course and that they place individuals at risk for a range of problems during adulthood (Ost, 1987; Burke *et al.*, 1990; Keller *et al.*, 1992; Orvaschel *et al.*, 1995; Last *et al.*, 1996).

Comorbidity

Comorbidity refers to the occurrence at one point in time of several psychiatric disorders. Many adolescents who meet diagnostic criteria for one psychiatric disorder simultaneously meet criteria for one or more additional disorders. Kashani *et al.* (1987), for example, reported that 100% of adolescents in their sample who met criteria for major depression also met criteria for another disorder. As a number of writers have observed, comorbidity appears to be the rule rather than the exception (Kendall and Clarkin, 1992; Reinecke, 1995).

Comorbidity is important for a number of reasons, both conceptual and practical. The co-occurrence of various clinical disorders can, for example, complicate research into the assessment, etiology, and course of individual disorders. Comorbidity also raises questions as to the validity of current taxonomic systems for classifying clinical disorders. Moreover, comorbidity can complicate the treatment process. It appears, for example, that depressed youth with a comorbid psychiatric disorder may be at increased for recurrent depression, show a poorer response to medications, be at an increased risk for social problems, and be at an increased risk for suicidal ideations and attempts. Similarly, adolescents with oppositional defiant disorder or conduct disorder often also manifest difficulties with alcohol or substance abuse, depression, or a learning disability. These conditions can impede therapeutic progress, and typically warrant additional treatment.

Depression

Studies suggest that a several forms of psychotherapy can be helpful in treating clinical depression among adolescents (for reviews see Lewinsohn and Clarke, 1999; Moore and Carr, 2000a; Curry, 2001; Fonagy *et al.*, 2002). Two approaches have received the largest amount of empirical interest and enjoy the strongest support: CBT and interpersonal psychotherapy for adolescents (also referred to as IPT-A).

Attempts have been made during recent years to develop standards for identifying treatments that are efficacious for treating clinical disorders (Task Force on Psychological Intervention Guidelines of the APA, 1995; Chambless *et al.*, 1996, 1998; Weisz *et al.*, 2000). Chambless and Hollon (1998) suggest that for a treatment to be identified as 'efficacious' it should, at a minimum, have been found to: (1) be superior to no treatment or a placebo, or equivalent or superior to an alternative treatment of documented efficacy, in a randomized controlled trial; (2) that the treatment be described in a manual; and (3) that the studies used an identified population, appropriate measures, and appropriate analyses. If these standards are met in studies completed at two or more independent sites, the treatment protocol is considered 'well established.' Attempts to identify evidence-based or empirically supported treatments has proven controversial, and have important implications for both training and clinical practice (Weisz and Hawley, 1998; Chorpita, 2003).

A substantial body of research indicates that CBT can be efficacious for treating depression among adolescents (Birmaher *et al.*, 1996; Harrington *et al.*, 1998; Lewinsohn and Clarke, 1999; Curry, 2001). Controlled outcome studies suggest that both individual and group CBT can be useful in alleviating dysphoria, and that gains may be maintained over time (Lewinsohn *et al.*, 1990; Wood *et al.*, 1996; Brent *et al.*, 1997; Birmaher *et al.*, 2000). A recent meta-analysis indicated that the effect sizes for CBT for depression among adolescents were moderate to large, and that gains were maintained for up to 2 years (Reinecke *et al.*, 1998). The efficacy of CBT for depression during adolescence appears, then, to be well-established (Curry, 2001).

Although differences exist between cognitive-behavioral protocols, they tend to emphasize the development of specific skills that can be helpful for managing depressed affect. Skills addressed include developing a goal list, monitoring one's mood, engaging in pleasant activities, development of social skills, engaging in activities that provide a sense of accomplishment or mastery, relaxation, conflict resolution and negotiation, identification of cognitive distortions or biases, identification of maladaptive thoughts, rational disputation of maladaptive thoughts, and developing realistic counterthoughts. Recently developed 'modular' approaches to CBT tailor therapeutic techniques to the specific needs of individual patients (Curry and Reinecke, 2003).

IPT, a form of psychotherapy developed by Gerald Klerman *et al.* (1984) for treating depressed adults, has been adapted for use with adolescents (Mufson *et al.*, 1993). The approach focuses on addressing common interpersonal difficulties experienced by adolescents, including challenges associated with autonomy from parents, relationships with peers, and managing the loss of significant relationships. Explicit attempts are made to identify interpersonal factors that are associated with the etiology and maintenance of the depressive episode. Information is gathered about the nature and quality of the adolescent's relationships, their expectations for the relationships, whether these expectations are being met, goals for their relationships, and how they have attempted to accomplish these goals. Particular attention is given to separations and losses, conflict, changes in roles, interpersonal deficits (including social withdrawal or isolation, social skills deficits, and social anxiety), and difficulties encountered in single family homes. Active attempts are then made to address difficulties identified in these domains.

Research on ITP-A has, to date, been positive (Mufson *et al.*, 1994, 1999; Rosselló and Bernal, 1999). Completion of a 12-week ITP-A program has been associated with a significant reduction in symptoms of depression, improved social functioning, and an increased rate of remission from the depressive episode. Moreover, gains appear to be maintained over time. Although research is limited, ITP-A is a promising approach for understanding and treating depressed youth. IPT, as such, would be identified as a 'possibly efficacious' treatment for depression among adolescents.

Psychodynamic psychotherapy has a long tradition and is widely used in clinical practice. It remains a dominant paradigm for understanding depression in many psychology, psychiatry, and social work training programs. Psychodynamic psychotherapy endeavors to treat depression by providing adolescents with insight into defenses used in coping with the expression of drives, by identifying and rectifying recurrent relationships issues, by addressing feelings of narcissistic injury, or by establishing a more coherent, integrated, and 'authentic' sense of self. Psychodynamic psychotherapy typically is nondirective, long term, and focuses upon the expression and interpretation of events within the therapeutic relationship as a means of bringing about clinical improvement.

Although it is widely used, little systematic research has been conducted examining the efficacy of psychodynamic psychotherapy with clinically depressed youth. No randomized controlled trials of these forms of psychotherapy have been published. Individual psychodynamic psychotherapy has not, then, been demonstrated to be an effective treatment for depression among adolescents. That said, preliminary evidence indicates that adolescents who receive intensive psychodynamic psychotherapy may benefit over time. Target and Fonagy (1994a,b), for example, conducted a chart review of 763 youth receiving psychoanalytic psychotherapy. Of the 65 children and adolescents who manifested a depressive disorder, over 80% demonstrated a significant reduction in symptoms at the conclusion of treatment (the average length of treatment was approximately 2 years). Given the lack of a control group and the tendency of depressive episodes to remit spontaneously within 9–12 months, however, one cannot conclude that these interventions were efficacious in alleviating the depressive symptoms. A lack of supportive evidence cannot, of course, be taken as evidence that psychodynamic psychotherapy is ineffective. Insofar as psychodynamic forms of psychotherapy are among the most widely used in clinical practice, it is unfortunate that they have not been put to empirical test. Further research on these models and approaches is urgently needed.

In conclusion, CBT and IPT appear to be effective in alleviating symptoms of depression among youth. Gains achieved appear to be reasonably stable over time. Evidence supporting the efficacy of psychodynamic and psychoanalytic psychotherapy is scant.

Case example: cognitive-behavioral therapy with a depressed adolescent

Josh Hernandez is a 15-year-old 10th grader of Hispanic-American heritage. He is enrolled in an honors program at a local magnet school. Josh is the younger of two children, and was referred for assessment and treatment by his parents due to depressed mood, a loss of interest in activities and friendships, declining academic performance, and lethargy. Josh's brother, Enrico, is a freshman at a prestigious private university. Josh's father is employed as an advertising executive and his mother is a college professor. Josh's mother noted that 'he just looks unhappy . . . and he has a great deal of difficulty getting up in the morning.' When asked to elaborate, she noted that, despite his 'enormous potential', his grades have been declining since the sixth grade. She reported that he doesn't complete his assignments, and that when he does complete his work he often forgets to turn them in. Josh's father noted that he recently failed two courses, and that he 'seems lonely and isolated.' He noted that his son has 'dropped his friendships' and that he now 'hangs with an outsider group' who are 'less ambitious.' According to his father, Josh has 'no goals' and 'doesn't seem to have future plans.' Josh's parents were also concerned by what they viewed as his 'bizarre' behavior.' They reported, for example, that he occasionally walked with a 'zombie-like' gait, that he once took a razor blade and a knife to school but 'didn't know he had them', and that he had 'lived in a computer box' in his room for several months.

Josh acknowledged his parents' concerns. He agreed that he is 'doing less of everything' and that he spends less time with his friends. He attributed this, however, to 'having less time to do stuff.' Josh's parents believe that the changes they have seen in their son's mood and behavior may have been related to the death of a maternal uncle several years before. They noted, however, that Josh and his uncle were not close, and that Josh has never spoken of his death. Josh's difficulties were subjectively severe, and were affecting his social and academic functioning. Josh's specific symptoms included:

◆ *affective:* dysphoria, anhedonia, flat affect
◆ *cognitive:* indecision, impaired concentration, forgetfulness, absence of goals, low motivation
◆ *physiological:* hypersomnia, psychomotor retardation, decreased appetite, 'zombie-like' carriage, fatigue
◆ *behavioral:* social withdrawal, poor academic performance, carrying a razor and a knife, living in a cardboard box, quiet speech, long response latencies.

Josh's medical and developmental histories were unremarkable. He was born at term after an 'easy' labor. No prenatal or perinatal complications were reported. His mother recalled that he was an 'active and cuddly' infant who 'liked audiences' and was 'warm to people.' During his preschool years he reportedly was 'very social and willing to share.' His language, motor, and self-care milestones were age appropriate. Josh's mother stated, however, that he experienced occasional nocturnal enuresis until he was 12 years of age, and that although he talked a lot at home, he 'was shy in class' and 'wouldn't talk readily to his teachers.'

Josh described his relationship with his parents as 'fine'. When asked to elaborate, he noted that they 'never argued' and that 'the only point of friction is my grades.' Josh remarked that he was 'very close' to his brother, and noted that he misses him now that he is away at college. Josh's father speculated that he may have been 'intimidated' by his older brother's academic success. Although Josh agreed that his behavior and mood had changed, and that his grades had declined dramatically during recent years, he did not feel that this represented a problem. As he stated, 'everything seems all right to me.' When asked how he felt about his failed courses, the fact that the principal now required him to take summer school, and that he would not be permitted to take driver's education until he achieved a C-average, Josh remarked, 'it's ok . . . I don't care . . . I just don't think about it much.' Josh noted that, although he was interested in dating, he did not have a girlfriend. He dismissed his classmates as 'weirdos' (who participated in school activities, focused upon maintaining their grades, and talked of applying to college). When asked about his comment that he coped with his declining grades by 'just not thinking about it', he stated 'When I'm pressured or worried by things I just ignore them, I just put it out of my mind . . . I try not to care one way or another.' Cognitive avoidance, as such, appeared to be an important coping strategy for Josh.

Assessment

Josh completed a semistructured diagnostic interview and a battery of objective self-report questionnaires as part of our initial evaluation. Reports by Josh and his parents on the K-SADS indicate that he meets DSM-IV criteria for Major Depressive Disorder, Single Episode. There was no evidence of morbid or suicidal ideations, mania, hypomania, oppositionality, conduct disorder, ADHD, alcohol or substance abuse, anxiety, or a developmental disorder. His Children's Global Assessment Scale (CGAS) score was 42.

Interestingly, no significant elevations were apparent in his responses on a battery of objective rating scales. Josh reported, for example, experiencing *no* distressing thoughts on the Hollon-Kendall Automatic Thoughts Questionnaire, other than the thought that he 'wished he was somewhere else' [than therapy]. In a similar manner, no elevations were apparent on the Young-Brown Schema Questionnaire. Josh did, however, note that he 'sometimes' worried about school, and that he felt sad, tired, and mad on the Reynolds Adolescent Depression Scale. His responses earned raw scores of 4, 5, and 6 on the Beck Depression Inventory, Anxiety Inventory, and Hopelessness Scale, respectively. These scores are within the normal range and are not consistent with reports by Josh's parents and teachers, or with observations of his behavior. They appear, as such, to underestimate Josh's current distress. This may be because of a tendency to minimize his concerns, or from a lack of reflective self-awareness.

Formulation

A number of cognitive, behavioral, and social factors appear to contribute to Josh's current difficulties. He comes from a supportive home that is characterized by high levels of motivation and accomplishment. Both of his parents are well-educated professionals, and his older brother appears to have been an academically gifted student. Josh had done quite well academically throughout elementary school, and had, following in his brother's footsteps, been enrolled in the honors program at a magnet school. Josh's difficulties first became apparent during the sixth grade, and became more prominent during his junior high school years. The timing of the changes in his mood and behavior is telling in that these years mark a transition from the relatively supportive and stable culture of elementary school to the challenging culture of junior high school. Biological and social changes during early adolescence can be difficult for many children, as can the increased demands for autonomy and self-organization.

Although Josh has a stable and supportive family, he has few friendships outside of the family. His tendency to withdraw from his childhood friends, at a time when support from peers is becoming more important, appears to have exacerbated his feelings of isolation. His tendency to denigrate them as 'weirdos' and to identify with a group of dysphoric, isolated peers who also were experiencing academic difficulties may compound his difficulties. His supports are few, and his current friends appear to model and reinforce his negative views of himself and his future.

Although Josh is a bright, capable young man, he appears to have a low sense of personal control over important outcomes in his life. As a consequence, his desire to actively address academic and social challenges is limited. He doesn't believe that his efforts will do any good. Rather than approaching problems in a thoughtful manner, he seeks to avoid them. His problem-solving motivation and perceptions of self-efficacy, as such, appear to be low.

Josh's identification with a group of peers that lack specific academic or career goals is of particular concern. He has, by spending increasing amounts of time with them, reduced his opportunities for participating in activities that would give him a sense of pleasure, enjoyment, mastery, or competence. He has, in many ways, become an outsider to the larger culture of his high school.

The development of an adult identity and vocational goals is an important task during adolescence. Josh appears to be experiencing difficulty developing goals or plans. When asked, for example, if he ever thought about his future or had fantasies about what he would like to become, remarked, 'No, never . . . I don't even think about what I'll do next weekend . . . I'll think about that when Saturday morning comes.' There may, as such, be impediments to Josh developing an adult identity. Self concept during childhood and adolescence develops, at least in part, from a conviction that one is learning tangible skills that will bring about a desired future, and that you are developing into a defined self within a broader social or community context. The adolescent must, at each step, develop a sense of competence—an awareness that his or her personal way of mastering the tasks of life are a successful and accepted variant of the larger group's identity. Adolescents are not fooled by empty praise and false encouragement. They must succeed by their own whole-hearted and tenacious efforts in mastering tasks that are important to them and that are valued by their family and culture. In this regard, Josh's parents admonishments that he has 'great potential' and that he will live up to the achievements of his parents and brother are, in the absence of actual accomplishment, hollow. By withdrawing from the social and academic challenges of adolescence, Josh has created an environment in which he feels incapable.

The process of developing an adult identity, including social and vocational goals, appears to have broken down.

Course of treatment

Josh was seen on 11 occasions over approximately $2\frac{1}{2}$ months. This was followed by four booster sessions over 2 months. His parents attended six of these therapy sessions. As in CBT with adults, sessions were problem oriented, active, and collaborative. They were strategic in that a clear and consistent focus was maintained on identifying beliefs, attitudes, attributions, and information processing deficits that may have contributed to Josh's distress, and to developing cognitive and behavioral skills.

Our first tasks were to develop a list of problems or 'targets' for therapy that Josh and his parents could agree upon, to develop a cognitive-behavioral formulation of his difficulties that could be shared with him, and to develop his motivation to participate in treatment. Insofar as Josh felt that everything was 'going all right' and that he 'didn't need treatment', these were not simple tasks. With this in mind, a patient approach, focusing upon encouraging Josh to discuss how he understood his declining grades, feelings of sadness, and social isolation, was adopted. Although he denied feeling depressed, Josh acknowledged that he often felt 'tired and bored', that he was 'upset' to have received an F in English, and that he was angry at the teacher for giving him that grade. As he stated, 'it was unjust . . . I knew the material, I just didn't turn in the work.' Whereas Josh felt that his parent's goals for treatment (i.e., develop ambition and goals; have more fun; follow-through on school assignments; be proud of his talents) were 'fine', his only goal would be to 'have more fun.' We accepted this as a reasonable goal that both Josh and his parents could support, and used it as a basis for introducing the cognitive-behavioral techniques of mood-monitoring and pleasant activities scheduling.

We began by asking Josh to make a 'daily list' of times when he felt tired, bored, or irritated. He was able to complete this and, although he was not able to identify specific thoughts or concerns at these times, readily acknowledged that his life 'pretty much is a drag.' Overcoming these feelings was, for Josh, a goal he could accept. Using this as a point of departure, we discussed at some length how his thoughts and behaviors may have contributed to his feelings of boredom and irritation, and how, if he had 'interesting, fun, or challenging things to do' his life might not be so boring. With some encouragement, Josh noted that he might be interested in trying out for a community play (he'd done well in several school productions in the past), that he was interested in designing a costume for Halloween, and that he might be interested in working to earn money to purchase video games. Using these goals as a foundation, several principles were discussed—the importance of having a clear objective, of 'persisting when the going got tough', of breaking tasks into their component parts, and of approaching problems in a flexible manner. By using goals that the teenager can accept, principles of CBT for depression among adults can be adapted for use with youth.

Although Josh did not consistently complete his cognitive homework assignments, he noted that his mood had improved when he attempted them. This was used to motivate further efforts on his part. After 4 weeks of therapy, Josh's depression scores had declined. His parents and teacher's noted the improvement in his mood, and his grade in physics had improved from an F to a C. When asked how he accomplished this, he noted that 'I worked hard, I did a lot of work . . . I got a list of the work that was missing, did it all, and turned it in.' This improvement was quite gratifying to Josh. During this time he also began participating in enjoyable activities (such as going out with friends, going to the movies with his parents, and watching boxing on cable TV) on a regular basis. Simplified forms of standard cognitive-behavioral interventions (i.e., mood monitoring, rational problem solving, and mastery-pleasure scheduling) were effective in improving his mood and in providing Josh with an enhanced sense of personal efficacy. As he noted, however, he still had 'a feeling that something's not right . . . I don't know what . . . it's a bad intuition.' This comment became a point of departure for us to introduce cognitively based techniques.

Josh's tendency to avoid thinking about distressing events in his life remained problematic. He experienced a great deal of difficulty reflecting upon his thoughts, feelings, and motivations, and so was unable to complete standard Dysfunctional Thought Records (DTRs) or 'three column' exercises. He also was unable to speculate as to what others might think when confronted with problems. Although his parents noted that he could be kind, they observed that Josh was not an empathic or sensitive young man. His rational problem-solving skills and ability to empathize with others were poorly developed, and he did not see how his thoughts might influence his emotional reactions to events. This process of cognitive avoidance was, for Josh, an active one. When asked, for example, to 'think about what went through your head the moment you learned you got the F in English', Josh turned away from the therapist and refused to respond.

We approached this difficulty obliquely, by discussing how other teenagers might solve problems in their lives. Rather than addressing his academic and social difficulties, we discussed vignettes—common problems that many teenagers might encounter. Based upon work on rational problem-solving and problem-solving motivation, we discussed how teenagers might react if they had scratched their father's car, and if they had been encouraged by friends to shoplift in a mall. A multistep problem-solving strategy was developed. Specific steps included: (1) *Relax*; (2) *Identify* the problem; (3) *Brainstorm* various solutions; (4) *Evaluate* them, look at positive and negative consequences, look at both short- and long-term effects; (5) Say '*Yes*' to one; (6) *Evaluate* whether it works. Although we intentionally had *not* discussed events in his life, Josh was open to use this RIBEYE approach, noting that it 'sounded sensible' to him.

The following week Josh remarked that he now had a goal—he wanted to look for a summer job. Given his long-standing lack of motivation and difficulty developing a vision of his future, this was a positive development. Applying the problem-solving strategies we had developed the week before, Josh developed a four-step plan for finding work. He noted that he planned to walk into neighborhood stores and talk with the managers, search for jobs on-line, check the classified ads, and talk with contacts recommended by his parents. Within a week he had found a job assembling sets for a local theatre company.

Given our success in developing Josh's rational problem-solving skills, and using them with situations that were not 'emotionally laden', we next began to explore maladaptive thoughts that may have contributed to his academic difficulties. Using a standard 'three column technique', Josh observed that he experienced a number of negative automatic thoughts when asked to complete tasks at school. These included, 'There's nothing I can do about this', 'How long do I have to endure this [work]', 'I don't know if I can do this', and 'This is going to get worse.' These thoughts were accompanied by a significant increase in feelings of anxiety. As Josh remarked, 'I start to feel really pressured and worried . . . it goes from 25% up to 100%.' He was able to recognize, as well, that his subsequent attempts to 'put it out of my mind' served to reduce his feelings of anxiety. As he stated, 'as soon as I ignore it, the feelings drop down to 0 to 10%'. Josh's cognitive avoidance, as such, appeared to serve an adaptive function.

During subsequent sessions we focused upon encouraging Josh to openly experience and express his feelings of anxiety, sadness, worry, and frustration, rather than pressing them from awareness. As he had enjoyed work in the theatre, he was encouraged to practice '*acting* happy, sad, and angry', and to note how others react. He attempted to use the rational problem-solving skills he had developed to actively cope with problems that occurred on a day-to-day basis. These interventions were accompanied by the introduction of assertiveness training activities (to reduce his passivity and social avoidance) and communications skills training (with an emphasis placed on assisting him to identify negative emotions, to describe these feelings to others, and to more clearly express his goals and desires). He and his parents were encouraged to practice the cognitive-behavioral skills he had learned, and to use contingency management techniques to motivate him to persist with tasks that were tedious or frustrating. A list of the specific cognitive-behavioral tasks we used is presented in Table 30.1.

Table 30.1 Cognitive-behavioral interventions for depression used with Josh

Development of therapeutic rapport; allow Josh and parents to feel understood
Develop shared problem list
Develop and share rationale with Josh and parents
Mood monitoring
Pleasurable events scheduling
Mastery activities scheduling
Rational problem-solving (RIBEYE)
Realistic counterthoughts (rational responding)
Social skills/address social withdrawal
Family communication (encourage expression of emotions, compromise)
Assertiveness training (to address passivity)
Review and consolidation of gains/relapse prevention
Booster/follow-up sessions

We concluded by reviewing cognitive-behavioral skills that had been the most helpful for Josh and by anticipating challenges he might face in the future. During our four booster sessions Josh noted that several techniques had been particularly useful, including goal setting, realistic thinking, rational problem-solving, and attempting to identify and develop sources of support. Josh was able to distinguishing a lapse (a 'brief problem') from a relapse ('spiraling down'), and to develop plans for coping with 'extreme problems' that might occur. As he noted, 'I've just got to not catastrophize . . . then I'll go with what works.' At the conclusion of treatment Josh was motivated to graduate from high school and stated that he hoped to attend college. He was not sure, however, where he would like to apply or what he might want to study.

At the conclusion of treatment Josh was much improved. His parents observed that he was 'very cooperative', that he 'had friends and is behaving better . . . he's polite and he's getting his work done and turning it in.' When asked about his mood they noted that he 'cheers up . . . and laughs a lot.' Josh's CGAS score at the conclusion of treatment was 72 and he no longer met diagnostic criteria for major depression.

Looking forward, several concerns remained. Specifically, his parents noted that he continued to show a 'lack of passion and direction.' This was consistent with our observation that he rarely, if ever, fantasized or thought about his future, and that he had no long-term goals or aspirations. Although his depressive episode had been successfully treated, Josh was only beginning to develop a more mature adult identity. Developing vocational goals, a capacity for more intimate personal relationships, and a sense of the possible self he would like to become were tasks that remained for him to address.

Anxiety

Several protocols have been developed for treating child and adolescent anxiety disorders. Controlled outcome studies completed over the past 15 years indicate that behavioral psychotherapy and CBT can be useful in treating generalized anxiety, school anxiety, specific phobias, panic, and obsessive-compulsive disorder among youth (for reviews see Ollendick and King, 1998; Moore and Carr, 2000b; Barrett, 2001; Piacentini *et al.*, 2003).

Based upon cognitive and behavioral models, these approaches endeavor to alleviate anxiety by teaching children and adolescents to monitor their moods, anticipate situations in which they are likely to become anxious, identify specific distressing thoughts, and respond to these cues by actively using cognitive and behavioral coping strategies. Exposure and desensitization, relaxation training, guided imagery, rehearsal of adaptive 'self-statements', and encouragement of adaptive coping attempts are frequently used. Parent and family sessions are typically included in these treatment programs, both to address parental behaviors that may be maintaining the child's anxiety and to provide them with strategies for managing their child's anxiety at home. Cognitive strategies (which focus upon reducing cognitive distortions, developing coping skills, and enhancing perceptions of control or efficacy) and behavioral approaches (which emphasize desensitization to anxiety-provoking stimuli and operant reinforcement of adaptive coping) are typically used together (Kendall et al., 1992).

Types of anxiety experienced by children and adolescents vary with age. Forms of anxiety that may be normal at one age (such as a fear of separation from parents during the toddler years) may be quite inappropriate at a later age. The most common source of anxiety during adolescence is peer rejection, and the most frequent anxiety disorders are social anxiety, panic, and agoraphobia. As adolescents develop the capacity for hypothetico-deductive reasoning, they become increasingly able to envision a range of potential threats, dangers, and sources of social embarrassment. Rates of social anxiety among adolescents are not surprising given the central importance of peer relationships for negotiating independence from one's family and for developing mature sexual relationships. Cognitive-behavioral models suggest that anxiety disorders tend, as a group, to stem from unrealistic appraisals of threats related to normative fears (Piacentini et al., 2003). It is these appraisal processes that are the focus of treatment.

CBT has been found effective for treating school phobia (Blagg and Yule, 1984; King et al., 1998), overanxious disorder (Kendall, 1994; Kendall et al., 1997), overanxious disorder and specific phobia (Barrett et al., 1996), panic disorder (Ollendick, 1995) social anxiety (Hayward et al., 2000), generalized anxiety (Cobham et al., 1998), and obsessive-compulsive disorder (March et al., 1994; Wever and Ray, 1997; deHaan et al., 1998; Franklin et al., 1998). Although few long-term follow-up studies have been completed, those that have been published are promising. Results suggest, for example, that gains achieved in CBT may be maintained for up to 3 years (Kendall and Southam-Gerow, 1996).

Whereas the large majority of these studies used individual or group therapy protocols, at least one has included a parental treatment package. Parents of anxious children and adolescents often experience high levels of anxiety themselves, and the possibility exists that this may lead parents to behave in ways that exacerbate and maintain their children's difficulties. With this in mind, Cobham et al. (1998) conducted a controlled outcome study that included a structured parental anxiety management component. As might be expected, this intervention had a significant effect, but only for those youth with highly anxious parents. The value of addressing parental anxiety when working with anxious youth is worthy of additional study. At a minimum, clinicians should attend to the moods of their patient's caregivers and the ways in which this may affect the child's adjustment. If appropriate, parents might be referred for treatment to address their feelings of anxiety.

If there is a drawback in these findings, it is that much of this work has been with prepubertal children and young adolescents (13–14 years of age). Few studies have been completed examining the treatment of anxiety among older adolescents, and samples typically include adolescents with a range of diagnoses. Moreover, psychotherapy is typically contrasted with a wait-list control, rather than another accepted form of treatment. Studies of psychotherapy for obsessive-compulsive disorder have used an open trial design, and many of the participants received concomitant medications. More formal comparisons of psychotherapy with pharmacotherapy, then, would be helpful.

Although psychodynamic psychotherapy is widely used in treating anxious youth, no controlled outcome studies have been completed examining its efficacy or effectiveness with anxious adolescents. A chart review of anxious children and adolescents completed by Target and Fonagy (1994a) indicated that a substantial percentage of youth with separation anxiety, phobias, and overanxious disorder improved over the course of treatment. Given the lack of a control group, however, it cannot be concluded that these interventions were effective in alleviating patients' anxiety.

Conduct disorder

Conduct problems, including aggressive behavior, disobedience and defiance at home and at school, and major rule violations, are among the most persistent and difficult to treat clinical problems in adolescence (Eyberg et al., 1998). They are among the most common reasons for clinical referral, reflecting their high prevalence rates (Hinshaw and Anderson, 1996) and the fact that they can be quite distressing to parents and school officials. Traditionally, serious conduct problems have been treated with long-term, dynamically informed psychotherapy aimed at offsetting major ego deficits in the form of low frustration tolerance, limited self-awareness, impaired empathy, compromised interpersonal relations, or a fragmented, noncohesive sense of self. Often psychotherapy is only one component of a broader milieu treatment, either in a residential setting, group home, or therapeutic school. Such intensive treatment is viewed as necessary because of the breadth of impairment found among conduct disordered youth. Recent evidence, however, has suggested that aggregating conduct disordered youth in residential or group treatments can have unintended, deleterious effects (Dishion et al., 1999).

Over the last two decades, substantial energy and resources have been devoted to clinical trials for conduct disordered youth (Lochman et al., 2003). A review identified 10 treatments that have been supported by controlled outcome studies (Brestan and Eyberg, 1998). However, closer inspection shows that most of these treatments were designed and implemented with children rather than adolescents, or at best, with young adolescents. For example, many of the skill training interventions such as social problem-solving training (Kazdin, 1996), parent management training (Patterson, 1976), and some forms of anger management training (Lochman et al., 1981) were designed for and principally evaluated with children ages 13 and younger. Although these treatments appear to be quite promising for altering disruptive and aggressive behavior in children, their efficacy with adolescents has not been adequately addressed. 'Upward extension' of these treatments may not be warranted given findings showing a negative association between treatment effects and age for parent management training (Strain et al., 1981).

Three treatments have been developed for and evaluated with conduct disordered adolescents. The first is *anger control training with stress inoculation* (Feindler, 1991). At the core of this intervention is the view that youth with delinquent and aggressive problems have serious difficulties with the expression and regulation of anger. The treatment, then, principally aims at teaching youth a variety of coping strategies for reducing angry arousal. Therapy focuses on helping youth to identify anger provocation cues, to suppress immediate anger responses with self-instructions, to modulate arousal with relaxation or self-instructional techniques, and to consider consequences of aggressive behavior or explosive anger. In addition, a portion of the treatment is directed toward training individuals to behave in an assertive rather than an aggressive manner. Treatment is offered in both individual and group formats, and typically is time limited (12–25 sessions). It should be noted that, although this approach emphasizes psychoeducation, the treatment is not didactic. Rather, therapists model the components of anger management, and adolescents role-play skills under varied conditions of anger arousal.

Outcome research on *anger control therapy* has produced promising but mixed results. Across three published studies (Schlichter and Horan, 1981; Feindler et al., 1984, 1986) with delinquent or seriously behaviorally disordered youth, results have shown benefits in problem-solving abilities, teacher reported self-control, and reductions in penalties for disruptive behavior in school. Not all outcome measures showed a similar pattern of benefits, and the three studies have evaluated different forms of the intervention. Thus, while promising, this cognitive-behavioral treatment is not a 'well-established' treatment. Further, given the complex nature of conduct disorder and delinquency, the relatively narrow focus of this intervention may limit its generalizability. It may lack the therapeutic scope to be a 'stand alone' treatment for these challenging clinical problems.

Among the most promising treatments for adolescent conduct disorder are family-based therapies. A growing body of research suggests that disrupted family relations, poor parental monitoring, inconsistent discipline, and cross-generational continuities may contribute to aggressive and disruptive behavior among youth (Hinshaw and Anderson, 1996). Based on these findings, family processes have been targeted for intervention. Functional family therapy draws heavily on social learning formulations of noncompliance and aggressive behavior. At the core of this intervention is the view that aggressive and disruptive behaviors are maintained through patterns of family interaction that unintentionally reinforce problem behaviors while failing to reward prosocial behaviors. One recurrent pattern involves negative reinforcement. An adolescent may, for example, respond to limits or requests with aversive behaviors such as whining, arguing, or threatening. His or her parent, in order to reduce the aversive interaction, responds by disengaging or withdrawing. The youth's aversive behavior has been reinforced by the removal of the request, and the parents' disengagement is reinforced by the reduction in aversive interactions. Not surprisingly, over time, families with conduct-disordered youth appear to be quite disengaged and lacking in cohesion. Further, youth fail to comply with parental limits and requests.

Functional family therapy (Alexander and Parsons, 1982) attempts to modify such dysfunctional family patterns by altering parental monitoring and disciplinary strategies. Similar to the approach of Patterson et al. (1992), parents are taught to use basic social learning principles for managing youth behavior. Several additional components complement the core behavioral approach including family sessions designed to improve communication and increase family reciprocity, and sessions aimed at facilitating negotiation among family members.

Several outcome studies have supported the efficacy of functional family therapy for delinquent youth. In one study (Alexander and Parson, 1973), functional family therapy was compared with client-centered family groups and psychodynamic family counseling for the treatment of juvenile offenders. Observed patterns of family interaction and youth recidivism rates were among the primary outcomes. For both sets of measures, functional family therapy outperformed the other active treatments. In fact, recidivism rates in the functional family therapy condition were approximately half the rates found in the other conditions (25% versus 47% and 50%). There have been several additional studies of functional family therapy, and the overall pattern of results has been quite promising. However, as the treatment has evolved over time, it is not clear that the required conditions for replication have been met (Chambliss and Hollon, 1998). As such, functional family therapy should be viewed as a 'probably efficacious' treatment for youth conduct problems.

Because conduct disorder is multidetermined, emerging treatments increasingly emphasize comprehensive, multicomponent interventions that address multiple pathogenic processes at multiple levels of context. Multisystemic therapy (MST; Hengeler et al., 1998) is an integrative and comprehensive approach to treating youth conduct problems and antisocial behavior. Unlike traditional, comprehensive treatments that remove the adolescent from his or her social environment through placement in residential treatment settings, MST aims at restructuring multiple levels of the youth's environment in order to promote pro-social functioning. Drawing on Bronfenbrenner's (1979) ecological model of development, individual behavior is viewed within the context of multiple, nested contexts. Relevant context is not limited to the family, as in functional family therapy, but extended to the school, neighborhood, peer group, and broader community, as well as to linkages among these systems.

MST draws upon methods from a number of empirically based treatments. For example, interventions at the family level might include communication training as well as methods from strategic or structural family therapy. Integration of specific interventions is guided by a core set of principles. MST begins with the assumption that the purpose of assessment is to understand the fit between identified problems and the functioning of multiple systems. Psychiatric diagnosis is not the primary aim, instead MST therapists attempt to identify processes at multiple levels that support or impede adaptive functioning. In turn, therapeutic interventions attempt to use systemic strengths, for example, a committed extended family, as levers for change. All interventions are present focused and action oriented. Typically, many interventions focus on specific contingencies that sustain problematic behaviors. Therapist and family agree upon specific, well-defined goals, and progress is closely monitoring, including family feedback on treatment fidelity.

A growing body of evidence supports the use of MST as a treatment for serious, conduct-disordered adolescents (Henggeler et al., 1998). Compared with treatment-as-usual, MST shows superior ability to reduce conduct problems, including the use of illicit substances. Perhaps its greatest strength resides in its power to reduce recidivism among adjudicated adolescents. It is noteworthy that long-term follow-up reveals that MST effects are sustained over time. Consequently, MST is one of the most promising treatments for conduct problems in adolescence. It is tempting to label MST as a 'well-established', empirically supported treatment. However, such a label requires replication by an independent team of investigators. Hopefully, current efforts to replicate these findings will yield comparably impressive results.

Case example: cognitive-behavioral therapy for conduct disorder

Jackie is a 14-year-old, European-American female who was referred to our clinic because of multiple school suspensions from eighth grade. According to her mother's report, Jackie was highly argumentative at home and at school, defiant in relation to teachers, and failing the majority of her courses. Her mother was also concerned about low self-esteem. An initial diagnostic assessment did not reveal a significant pattern of depressive symptoms, but did uncover long-standing difficulties with impulsivity and inattention, a common set of comorbid problems with conduct disorder. Closer evaluation also indicated a pattern of rule violation and minor acts of property destruction. Jackie acknowledged that many of her friends were using drugs and alcohol, but denied personal use. Mother and daughter agreed that they had a highly conflicted relationship, and their reports were supported by clinically elevated scores on the Issues Checklist, a measure of parent–teen conflict. Jackie's father was only peripherally involved and was reported to have substance abuse problems.

Because of her symptoms of ADHD, in addition to symptoms of conduct disorder, Jackie was referred for a medication consultation. Second, in order to address Jackie's problematic interactions with teachers, her social problem-solving skills were targeted for intervention in individual therapy. Third, her mother was involved in parent management training to deal with Jackie's disruptive behavior at home and at school. In order to manage school behavior, a collaborative program was developed between Jackie's mother and school personnel involving the use of a weekly report card for assignments and behavioral outbursts. In brief, school personnel systematically monitored her behavior while her mother delivered consequences (largely positive) for gradual improvement in homework and self-regulation.

In individual sessions, the therapist attempted to engage Jackie in social problem-solving training. Like many young teens with conduct problems, Jackie was a reluctant participant in therapy. As a result, her therapist worked very slowly to build rapport by closely listening to Jackie's 'weekly tales' of her adventures with peers, and with substantial talk about music and fashion. With the gradual development of rapport, her therapist attempted to identify what Jackie might want from their meetings. Jackie acknowledged that she didn't want to 'flunk' for a second time, and her therapist amplified what it would mean to be 15 and still in middle school. Together they decided to spend a portion of each session on developing new strategies for coping with the demands of school.

Initially her therapist had Jackie identify problematic situations at school. Again, her problems with attention made self-monitoring difficult, but with medication, her ability to examine situations improved. Most of the difficult situations involved perceptions that she was being treated unfairly by a teacher. Her typical solution was to vent her anger by cursing or walking out of class. Integrating methods from cognitive therapy, her therapist introduced the concept of negative automatic thoughts and assigned Jackie the task of catching these rapid cognitions when she felt anger. Although Jackie was disinclined to complete homework, she readily reviewed situations in session. The primary goal at this point was to encourage Jackie to consider alternative interpretations of evocative situations in order to reduce immediate responding. Next her therapist introduced basic problem-solving steps including; breaking down the problem, defining the desired outcome, brainstorming alternative solutions, evaluating the solutions in terms of consequences, and implementing a plan. Problem-solving training began with hypothetical situations then proceeded to situations Jackie encountered at school or at home. With each plan, Jackie and her therapist role-played variations on different situations with the therapist providing feedback, or modeling alternative strategies.

After about 4 months (15 sessions) of working individually with Jackie and her mother, dyadic sessions were started in an effort to reduce mother–daughter conflict. Early sessions revealed problematic communication behaviors, including rampant use of sarcasm, verbal attacks, and put-downs by both mother and daughter. Drawing on the marital communication literature, the therapist modeled active listening skills and practiced these skills with the dyad over a series of sessions. After Jackie and her mother rated the intensity of various conflicts, the therapist began with a low intensity issue (washing the dishes), and introduced problem-solving communication (similar to what Jackie had been working on individually). The therapist closely monitored problematic communication, e.g., verbal put-downs, and stopped their interaction when breaks in problem solving occurred. It should be noted that the therapist was lavish in her praise for the dyad when they successfully negotiated low intensity conflicts. In addition, she assigned positive joint activities for mother and daughter each week. Gradually, the dyad worked on increasingly intense conflicts as they acquired more of the basic skills, and could monitor their own breaches in problem solving.

After 6 months of treatment, scores on the Issues Checklist showed a substantial reduction in problem intensity, although problem frequency remained elevated compared with adolescent norms. Jackie had been suspended from school only one time during the 6-month course of treatment, in contrast to three suspensions during the month proceeding treatment. Both mother and daughter reported an improved relationship, and Jackie was promoted to high school at the end of the school year.

Limitations of the literature

Over the last two decades, there has been substantial progress in the field of psychotherapeutic treatments for adolescent disorders. A major trend has been the development of specific treatments for specific diagnostic groups. The assumption that a single form of therapy—be it psychodynamic, behavioral, or family therapy—can be generically applied to a broad range of adolescent problems has been laid to rest. Similarly, the assumption that all forms of therapy are equally effective has not been supported. This is not surprising given recent research in developmental psychopathology. Evidence indicates that psychopathology among youth is multiply determined, that there are a range of developmental pathways or trajectories for each disorder, and that different combinations of factors are implicated in the development and maintenance of different conditions. There is simply too much diversity in pathogenic processes that contribute to and maintain different disorders to allow us to maintain that all forms of psychotherapy are equally effective. Our understanding of developmental psychopathology, however, is far from complete. Research into factors that place individuals at risk for developing specific conditions and that exacerbate or maintain their difficulties will serve as a sound foundation for developing more effective treatments. Much work, however, remains to be done.

A major limitation of the current literature stems from the design and goals of efficacy trials. Randomized controlled trials are designed to demonstrate that specific interventions can be effective for treating specific

clinical problems in specific populations. In an effort to demonstrate the effects of specific treatments, the requirements of experimental control can result in clinical trials that are less than 'clinically representative'. Findings from randomized controlled trials completed in research clinics may or may not, as a consequence, be generalizable to community clinics or private practice settings. The inclusion and exclusion criteria for patients with particular disorders, for example, can result in samples that differ in important ways from typical clinical referrals where high levels of comorbidity and low levels of family functioning are common. Similarly, therapists with limited caseloads are trained to deliver a specific, well-defined intervention, are closely monitored, and are carefully supervised. Unfortunately, such a high commitment to treatment integrity is not possible in many clinical practice settings. Thus, a major limitation of, and a major question for, psychotherapy researchers involves the transportability of these promising approaches to 'clinically representative' practice. That said, several points are worth noting. First, many efficacy trials do include patients that are seriously impaired and highly symptomatic. The promising results of MST trials cannot be discounted, for example, because the participants did not manifest serious conduct problems. In fact, most youth in these studies were court involved. Second, it is worth acknowledging that the generalizability of treatment effects is a scientific and technical question. It is one that will be resolved through systematic research rather than partisan debate. Finally, research in cardiology, oncology, and more recently, psychiatry indicates that treatment integrity and clinician expertise may be associated with improved outcomes, at least when working with more severely ill patients. It is not enough, as such, to demonstrate that empirically supported therapies can be effective in community settings; it will also be necessary to train clinicians in their use and to encourage them to use these approaches appropriately.

A second limitation involves the assessment of outcomes. Although clinical trials are more systematic in gathering objective outcome data than typical clinical practice, several shortcomings are worthy of note. First, the field has been far too concerned with symptom reduction. Most studies include multiple measures of specific symptoms associated with particular disorders (e.g., self-report and interview measures of depressive symptoms) without adequate attention to functional outcomes that are related to long-term adaptation. For example, research on outcomes for youth with major depression would be well advised to include measures of peer relationships, family functioning, and academic performance as indicators of change. Second, few studies have provided evidence of long-term stability of gains. Outcomes typically are assessed at posttreatment and 6–12 months later. For many disorders, especially those with a remitting/recurring pattern, long-term follow-up assessments are needed. Admittedly this is a costly enterprise, but evidence that emerging treatments divert youth from deviant developmental pathways over the long haul would be a powerful incentive for their dissemination and implementation.

A range of adolescent disorders and a number of widely practiced forms of therapy have not been adequately evaluated. Although anxiety, depressive, and conduct disorders make up the bulk of adolescent referrals, there are a number of clinical problems that deserve increased attention. One set of problems that often emerge during adolescence are the eating disorders, bulimia and anorexia nervosa. Research on treatments for these problems in adolescence lags behind research with adults (LeGrange, 2003). Again, given important developmental differences between adolescents and adults, it is not clear that treatments developed with adults can be readily extended to adolescents. The fact that most adolescents live with their family and interact with them on a daily basis is no small consideration.

Similarly, research on treatments for adolescents with posttraumatic stress disorder is virtually nonexistent. As many adolescent females have a history of sexual abuse or assault, work in this area is sorely needed. Moreover, a history of trauma can complicate the treatment of other clinical conditions. A significant percentage of youth with depression, anxiety, or substance abuse problems, for example, have experienced abuse or neglect, or come from environments characterized by violence. These experiences can contribute to the development of maladaptive coping strategies and can interfere with the treatment process. Finally, research on treatments for adolescents with varying combinations of comorbid disorders is needed. Research in community clinic settings indicates that most referred youth present with three or more diagnosable disorders (Weisz et al., 1998). Relatively little is known about the treatment of such multiproblem youth. Questions about the ordering, integration, and decision rules for applying multiple interventions are clearly underdeveloped.

As noted, a number of widely used treatments have received little attention in the research literature. Most prominently, psychodynamic psychotherapy with adolescents has received scant attention in clinical trials. Given the large adult literature on psychodynamic and psychoanalytic psychotherapies, and the development of psychodynamic psychotherapy protocols (Luborsky, 1984) it is evident that these approaches can be systematically evaluated in clinical trials (Barber and Crits-Christoph, 1993; Crits-Christoph and Connolly, 1998). However, because of the therapeutic allegiances of most investigators, dynamic treatments are rarely studied. When they are, they are often addressed in poorly designed trials or case reports. A new generation of psychodynamic investigators is needed to address this substantial gap in the literature. Similarly, many forms of family therapy have received little systematic evaluation. Although there is a growing body of research on structural and behavioral family therapies, systemic, strategic, and narrative therapies have been understudied. Although case studies represent a reasonable starting point for treatment development, evidence-based practice requires a higher standard of evaluation.

Future directions

Clearly, the most pressing question for psychotherapy research with adolescents involves the evaluation of promising, efficacious treatments under clinically representative conditions. Can treatments that have been shown to be efficacious in research clinics provide the same benefits to clinically referred youth in community settings? If not, what types of modifications need to be made to produce positive outcomes? Can community practitioners deliver efficacious treatments with sufficient fidelity such that beneficial outcomes will be realized? How much training and supervision is needed to produce positive outcomes in clinical practice? In brief, how flexible are these promising treatments? Will the demanding conditions of everyday practice undercut their integrity and dilute their effectiveness? These are some of the questions to be addressed by the next generation of clinical trials.

One major issue that is likely to emerge in the effort to evaluate treatments under clinically representative conditions involves treatment engagement and attrition. It is a sad fact that most youth referred for treatment receive no more than one session of psychotherapy (Gould et al., 1985). Research on attrition from community clinics reveals high levels of early attrition, estimated between 40 and 70% (Armbruster and Kazdin, 1994). Obviously, treatments cannot be expected to produce significant effects when minimally or partially completed. Thus, a critical question involves identifying processes that enable patients to receive an adequate dose of treatment.

Emerging research shows that the development of a positive, working alliance between youth, parents, and their therapist may hold the key to treatment engagement and completion (Kazdin et al., 1997; Garcia and Weisz, 2002). Further, a recent meta-analysis of relationship predictors of treatment outcomes (Shirk and Karver, 2003), shows that relationship variables are modest, but consistent, predictors of treatment outcomes across a range of treatments for youth. An important question, then, naturally arises—which therapist actions and strategies promote a positive, working alliance, and with which patients? Although a growing number of studies have examined alliance-outcome relations in youth treatment, virtually no research on alliance development and therapist facilitating behaviors has been published (Shirk and Russell, 1998). Psychodynamic theorists (e.g., Meeks, 1971) have long emphasized the fragile nature of the therapeutic alliance with adolescents, yet emerging treatment models rarely address this

issue in any detail. In part, this reflects the absence of evidence, beyond single case narratives, to support specific recommendations. Thus, research is needed to examine sequences of early therapeutic interactions to identify specific therapist behaviors and styles that promote alliance formation with adolescents.

Such studies could be part of a new research agenda focused on linking specific therapeutic processes with treatment outcomes.

Conclusions

We can be optimistic about the benefits of psychotherapy for treating anxiety and depressive disorders experienced by adolescents. The treatment of conduct disorder remains a vexing problem, but the emergence of comprehensive and systematic interventions, such as MST, hold significant promise.

The number and quality of psychotherapy outcome studies has increased dramatically over the past 10 years. Unfortunately, this growth has largely been limited to behavioral, cognitive-behavioral, and interpersonal approaches. Well-designed studies of psychodynamic, psychoanalytic, and systemic therapies are lacking, as is research into processes mediating therapeutic change among youth. Case reports and open trials can be useful in the initial stages of developing a treatment approach. They are entirely inadequate, however, as a basis for developing evidence based treatment guidelines or for refining existing treatment programs. The efficacy and effectiveness of psychotherapeutic interventions with adolescents can only be demonstrated though randomized controlled outcome studies that use a range of sensitive outcome measures. To be sure, recent attempts to develop guidelines for evidence-based clinical practice have proven controversial. Conducting clinical research can be daunting, and the generalizability of findings from university clinics to community settings has not been demonstrated. Moreover, it is quite clear that even the best empirically supported treatment programs are less than fully adequate. All are in need of refinement. That said, our treatment practices can only develop if they are subjected to careful, objective scrutiny.

As we have seen, a substantial body of evidence now exists indicating that psychotherapy can be beneficial for adolescents with behavioral and emotional difficulties. More important questions, however, remain—Are some forms of treatment more effective than others? Are some interventions more effective than others for specific problems? Are there developmental, cultural, or gender differences in response to treatment? How can we understand the relative equivalence of different forms of psychotherapy? Are variations in therapeutic technique needed as a result of developmental changes in cognitive, social, and emotional functioning over the course of adolescence? What are the moderators and mediators of therapeutic change? Although we do not have clear answers to many of these questions, the findings we have reviewed allow us to draw a number of tentative conclusions.

1. Therapy works.

2. Not all forms of treatment are created equal—some appear to be more effective than others.

3. Although preliminary findings are promising, controlled comparative outcome studies and process research are needed.

4. Strategic, problem-focused forms of therapy are more effective than nondirective, long-term treatments.

5. The successful treatment of adolescent conduct disorder requires attention to the broad contexts that maintain problematic behavior.

6. There appears to be a dose–response relationship—regular, active participation in therapy is associated with better outcomes.

7. An active, collaborative therapeutic relationship may facilitate clinical improvement.

8. Patients perceptions of efficacy, competence, and optimism may mediate outcome.

9. The social environment (both family and peers) is important. It is important to attend to both stressors and social supports.

Behavioral, emotional, and social difficulties experienced by adolescents can have pernicious effects that persist into adulthood. It is important, then, to include long-term assessments as a part of both clinical practice and research. We should, at the same time, attempt to insure that our interventions have broad, positive effects on adolescents' development.

We should, in short, adopt the broad view. We should keep both the forest and the trees in view. Our treatments may be narrow in the sense that they are designed to reduce immediate distress, to alleviate specific symptoms, and to prevent negative outcomes over a short period of time. These are not unimportant goals. At the same time, adolescents behave in ways that shape their environment and their experiences. We all do. As a consequence, specific interventions may have a larger effect on the adolescent's social, educational, and emotional adjustment. Psychotherapy, then, may serve as a transition or inflection point in the adolescent's life. It may place them on a more positive or adaptive developmental trajectory. Our challenge, then, is to develop interventions that both alleviate immediate distress and that support the long-term development of our patients.

We return, then, to the question with which we began—What constitutes an effective treatment? The answer depends, of course, on how one defines 'effective.' This, in turn, depends on our goals for treatment, what we view as acceptable evidence, our definition of 'objectivity', and what we consider to be an acceptable design or methodology for accumulating evidence. To say that a treatment is not 'empirically supported' or 'evidence based' is not to say that it is without support. Many forms of evidence—including open trials, case series, clinical observations, and professional consensus—are accepted as reasonable by many individuals.

To be sure, reduction of symptomatology is an important goal. As important, however, are the effects of our interventions on the social, academic, and emotional development. In reviewing the results of psychotherapy outcome research approximately 10 years ago Reinecke (1993, p. 397) noted that 'Our goal, in the larger sense, is not simply to assist the adolescent in resolving immediate concerns, but also to support ongoing development—to assist him or her in developing the capacity to form mature, trusting relationships and to function effectively as an adult—in short, to love and to work.' These sentiments remain true today. The effects of an intervention can be assessed in a number of ways, and broader effects may not be apparent for some time after the treatment has been completed. Moreover, interventions can be useful even if they do not alleviate the individual's presenting problems. Consider, for example, the suicidal adolescent. An intervention that reduces the risk of further suicide attempts may be quite beneficial, even if feelings of sadness or anxiety persist. An intervention that prevents an ominous outcome, or which places an adolescent on a more adaptive developmental path, may be quite beneficial. Documenting these effects, however, can be challenging.

A number of innovative and efficacious interventions have been developed during recent years. Our goal, as clinicians and scholars, is to refine, develop, evaluate, and disseminate them such that they can be used to alleviate distress and enrich the lives of adolescents.

References

Alexander, J. and Parsons, B. (1973). Short-term behavioral intervention with delinquent families: impact on family process and recidivism. *Journal of Abnormal Psychology*, **51**, 219–25.

Alexander, J. and Parsons, B. (1982). *Functional family therapy: principles and procedures*. Monterey, CA: Brooks Cole.

Altman, N. (1995). *The analyst in the inner city: race, class, and culture through a psychoanalytical lens*. Hillsdale, NJ: Analytic Press.

Armbruster, P. and Kazdin, A. (1994). Attrition in child psychotherapy. In: T. Ollendick and R. Prinz, ed. *Advances in clinical child psychology*, pp. 81–108. New York: Plenum.

Barber, J. and Crits-Christoph, P. (1993). Advances in measures of psychodynamic formulations. *Journal of Consulting and Clinical Psychology*, **61**, 574–85.

Barrett, P. (2001). Current issues in the treatment of childhood anxiety. In: M. Vasey and M. Dadds, ed. *The developmental psychopathology of anxiety*, pp. 304–24. New York: Oxford University Press.

Barrett, P., Dadds, M., and Rapee, R. (1996). Family treatment of childhood anxiety: a controlled trial. *Journal of Consulting and Clinical Psychology*, **64**, 333–42.

Bird, H. (1996). Epidemiology of childhood disorders in cross-cultural context. *Journal of Child Psychology and Psychiatry*, **37**, 35–49.

Bird, H., *et al.* (1990). Impairment in the epidemiological measurement of childhood psychopathology in the community. *Journal of the American Academy of Child and Adolescent Psychiatry*, **29**, 796–803.

Birmaher, B., Ryan, N., Williamson, D., Brent, D., and Kaufman, J. (1996). Childhood and adolescent depression: a review of the past 10 years. Part II. *Journal of the American Academy of Child and Adolescent Psychiatry*, **35**, 1575–83.

Birmaher, B., *et al.* (2000). Clinical outcome after short-term psychotherapy for adolescents with major depressive disorder. *Archives of General Psychiatry*, **57**, 29–36.

Blagg, N. and Yule, W. (1984). The behavioral treatment of school refusal: a comparative study. *Behavior Research and Therapy*, **22**, 119–27.

Blos, P. (1962). *On adolescence: a psychoanalytic interpretation*. New York: Free Press.

Blos, P. (1970). *The young adolescent: clinical studies*. New York: Free Press.

Brent, D., *et al.* (1997). A clinical psychotherapy trial for adolescent depression comparing cognitive, family and supportive therapy. *Archives of General Psychiatry*, **54**, 877–85.

Brestan, E. and Eyberg, S. (1998). Effective psychosocial treatments of conduct disordered children and adolescents: 29 years, 82 studies, and 5272 kids. *Journal of Clinical Child Psychology*, **27**, 180–9.

Bronfenbrenner, U. (1979). *The ecology of human development*. Cambridge, MA: Harvard University Press.

Burke, C., Burke, J., Regier, D., and Rae, D. (1990). Age at onset of selected mental disorders in five community populations. *Archives of General Psychiatry*, **47**, 511–18.

Carr, A., ed. (2000). *What works with children and adolescents? A critical review of psychological interventions with children, adolescents, and their families*. London: Routledge.

Chambless, D. and Hollon, S. (1998). Defining empirically supported therapies. *Journal of Consulting and Clinical Psychology*, **66**, 7–18.

Chambless, D., *et al.* (1996). An update on empirically validated therapies. *The Clinical Psychologist*, **49**, 5–18.

Chambless, D., *et al.* (1998). Update on empirically validated therapies II. *The Clinical Psychologist*, **51**, 3–16.

Chorpita, B. (2003). The frontier of evidence-based practice. In: A. Kazdin and J. Weisz, ed. *Evidence-based psychotherapies for children and adolescents*, pp. 42–59. New York: Guilford Press.

Cicchetti, D. and Cohen, D. (1995). Perspectives on developmental psychopathology. In: D. Cicchetti and D. Cohen, ed. *Developmental psychopathology: theory and methods*, Vol. 1, pp. 3–20. New York: Wiley.

Cobham, V., Dadds, M., and Spence, S. (1998). The role of parental anxiety in the treatment of child anxiety. *Journal of Consulting and Clinical Psychology*, **66**, 893–905.

Costello, E. (1989). Developments in child psychiatric epidemiology. *Journal of the American Academy of Child and Adolescent Psychiatry*, **28**, 836–41.

Crits-Christoph, P. and Connolly, M. (1998). Empirical basis of supportive-expressive psychodynamic psychotherapy. In: R. Bornstein and J. Masling, ed. *Empirical studies of the therapeutic hour*. Washington, DC: American Psychiatric Association Press.

Curry, J. (2001). Specific psychotherapies for childhood and adolescent depression. *Biological Psychiatry*, **49**, 1091–100.

Curry, J. and Reinecke, M. (2003). Modular therapy for adolescents with major depression. In: M. Reinecke, F. Dattilio, and A. Freeman, ed. *Cognitive therapy with children and adolescents*, 2nd edn, pp. 95–127. New York: Guilford Press.

Dishion, T., McCord, J., and Poulin, F. (1999). When interventions harm: peer groups and problem behaviors. *American Psychologist*, **54**, 755–64.

Elkind, D. (1967). Egocentrism in adolescence. *Child Development*, **38**, 1025–34.

Elmen, J. and Offer, D. (1993). Normality, turmoil, and adolescence. In: P. Tolan and B. Cohler, ed. *Handbook of clinical research and practice with adolescents*, pp. 5–19. New York: Wiley-Interscience.

Erikson, E. (1956). The concept of ego identity. *Journal of the American Psychoanalytic Association*, **4**, 56–121.

Eyberg, S., Edwards, D., Boggs, S., and Foote, R. (1998). Maintaining the treatment effects of parent training: the role of booster sessions and other maintenance strategies. *Clinical Psychology: Science and Practice*, **5**, 544–54.

Feindler, E. (1991). Cognitive strategies in anger control: interventions for children and adolescents. In: P. Kendall, ed. *Child and adolescent therapy: cognitive behavioral procedures*, pp. 66–87. New York: Guilford Press.

Feindler, E., Marriot, S., and Iwata, M. (1984). Group anger control training for junior high school delinquents. *Cognitive therapy and research*, **8**, 299–311.

Feindler, E., Ecton, R., Kingsley, D., and Dubey, D. (1986). Group anger control training for institutionalized psychiatric male adolescents. *Behavior Therapy*, **17**, 109–23.

Flament, M., *et al.* (1988). Obsessive-compulsive disorder in adolescence: an epidemiological study. *Journal of the American Academy of Child and Adolescent Psychiatry*, **27**, 764–71.

Fonagy, P., Target, M., Cottrell, D., Phillips, J., and Kurtz, Z. (2002). *What works for whom? A critical review of treatments for children and adolescents*. New York: Guilford Press.

Fraiberg, S. (1955). Some considerations in the introduction to therapy in puberty. *Psychoanalytic Study of the Child*, **10**, 264–86.

Franklin, M., *et al.* (1998). Cognitive-behavioral treatment of pediatric obsessive-compulsive disorder: an open clinical trial. *Journal of the American Academy of Child and Adolescent Psychiatry*, **37**, 412–19.

Freud, A. (1958). Adolescence. *Psychoanalytic Study of the Child*, **13**, 255–78.

Freud, S. (1953). *A case of hysteria*. In: J. Strachey, ed. and trans. *The standard edition of the complete psychological works of Sigmund Freud*, Vol. 7, pp. 1–122. London: Hogarth Press.

Friend, M. (1972). Psychoanalysis of adolescents. In: B. Wolman, ed. *Handbook of child psychoanalysis: research, theory, and practice*, pp. 297–363. New York: Van Nordstrand Reinhold.

Garcia, J. and Weisz, J. (2002). When youth mental health care stops: relationship problems and other reasons for ending outpatient treatment. *Journal of Consulting and Clinical Psychology*, **70**, 439–43.

Geleerd, E. (1957). Some aspects of psychoanalytic technique in adolescence. *Psychoanalytic Study of the Child*, **12**, 263–83.

Geleerd, E. (1964). Adolescence and adaptive regression. *Bulletin of the Menninger Clinic*, **28**, 302–8.

Gittelman, R., Mannuzza, S., Shenker, R., and Bonagura, N. (1985). Hyperactive boys almost grown up: I. Psychiatric status. *Archives of General Psychiatry*, **42**, 937–47.

Gould, M., Wunsch-Hitzig, R., and Dohrenwend, B. (1981). Estimating the prevalence of childhood psychopathology: a critical review. *Journal of the American Academy of Child and Adolescent Psychiatry*, **20**, 462–76.

Gould, M., Shaffer, D., and Kaplan, D. (1985). The characteristics of dropouts from a child psychiatry clinic. *Journal of the American Academy of Child and Adolescent Psychiatry*, **24**, 316–28.

deHaan, E., Hoogduin, K., Buitelaar, J., and Keijsers, G. (1998). Behavior therapy versus clomipramine for the treatment of obsessive-compulsive disorder in children and adolescents. *Journal of the American Academy of Child and Adolescent Psychiatry*, **37**, 1022–9.

Harrington, M., Fudge, H., Rutter, M., Pickles, A., and Hill, J. (1990). Adult outcomes of childhood and adolescent depression. *Archives of General Psychiatry*, **47**, 465–73.

Harrington, R., Whittaker, J., and Shoebridge, P. (1998). Psychological treatment of depression in children and adolescents: a review of treatment research. *British Journal of Psychiatry*, **173**, 291–8.

Hayword, C., Varady, S., Albano, A., Thieneman, M., Henderson, L., and Schatzberg, A. (2000). Cognitive behavioral group therapy for female socially phobic adolescents: results of a pilot study. *Journal of the American Academy of Child and Adolescent Psychiatry*, **39**, 721–6.

Henggeler, S., Schoenwald, S., Borduin, C. Rowland, M., and Cunningham, P. (1998). *Multisystemic treatment of antisocial behavior in children and adolescents*. New York: Guilford Press.

Hibbs, E. and Jensen, P., ed. (1996). *Psychosocial treatments for child and adolescent disorders: empirically based strategies for clinical practice*. Washington, DC: American Psychological Association.

Hinshaw, S. and Anderson, C. (1996). Conduct and oppositional defiant disorders. In: E. Mash and R. Barkeley, ed. *Child psychopathology*. New York: Guilford Press.

Kashani, J. and Orvaschel, H. (1988). Anxiety disorders in mid-adolescence: a community sample. *American Journal of Psychiatry*, **145**, 960–4.

Kashani, J. and Orvaschel, H. (1990). A community study of anxiety in children and adolescents. *American Journal of Psychiatry*, **147**, 313–18.

Kashani, J., *et al.* (1987). Depression, depressive symptoms, and depressed mood among a community sample of adolescents. *American Journal of Psychiatry*, **144**(7), 931–4.

Kazdin, A. (1996). Problem-solving and parent management training in treating aggressive and antisocial behavior. In: E. Hibbs and P. Jensen, ed. *Psychosocial treatments for child and adolescent disorders: empirically based strategies for clinical practice*, pp. 377–408. Washington, DC: American Psychological Association.

Kazdin, A. (2000). *Psychotherapy for children and adolescents: directions for research and practice*. New York: Oxford University Press.

Kazdin, A., Holland, L., and Crowley, M. (1997). Family experience of barriers to treatment and premature termination from child therapy. *Journal of Consulting and Clinical Psychology*, **65**, 453–63.

Keller, M., Lavori, P., Wunder, J., Beardslee, W., and Schwarts, C. (1992). Chronic course of anxiety disorders in children and adolescents. *Journal of the American Academy of Child and Adolescent Psychiatry*, **31**, 595–9.

Kendall, P. (1994). Treating anxiety disorders in children: results of a randomized clinical trial. *Journal of Consulting and Clinical Psychology*, **62**, 100–10.

Kendall, P. and Clarkin, J. (1992). Introduction to special section: comorbidity and treatment implications. *Journal of Consulting and Clinical Psychology*, **60**, 833–4.

Kendall, P. and Southam-Gerow, M. (1996). Long-term follow-up of a cognitive-behavioral therapy for anxiety-disordered youths. *Journal of Consulting and Clinical Psychology*, **64**, 724–30.

Kendall, P., *et al.* (1992). *Anxiety disorders in youth: cognitive-behavioral interventions*. Needham Heights, MA: Allyn and Bacon.

Kendall, P., *et al.* (1997). Treating anxiety disorders in youth: a second randomized clinical trial. *Journal of Consulting and Clinical Psychology*, **65**, 366–80.

King, N., *et al.* (1998). Cognitive-behavioral treatment of school-refusing children: a controlled evaluation. *Journal of the American Academy of Child and Adolescent Psychiatry*, **37**, 395–403.

Klein, M. (1950). *The psychoanalysis of children*. London: Hogarth Press.

Klerman, G., Weissman, M., Rounsaville, B., and Chevron, E. (1984). *Interpersonal psychotherapy of depression*. New York: Basic Books.

Kovacs, M. (1996). The course of childhood-onset depressive disorders. *Psychiatric Annals*, **26**, 326–30.

Kovacs, M., Feinberg, T., Crouse-Novak, M., Paulauskas, S., and Finkelstein, R. (1984). Depressive disorders in childhood: I. A longitudinal prospective study of characteristics and recovery. *Archives of General Psychiatry*, **41**, 229–37.

Kovacs, M., Devlin, B., Pollock, M., Richards, C., and Mukerji, P. (1997). A controlled family history study of childhood-onset depressive disorder. *Archives of General Psychiatry*, **54**, 613–23.

Kris, E. (1952). *Psychoanalytic explorations in art*. New York: International Universities Press.

Langer, T., Gersten, J., and Eisenberg, J. (1974). Approaches to measurement and definition in epidemiology of behavior disorders: ethnic background and child behavior. *International Journal of Health Services*, **4**, 483–501.

Last, C., Perrin, S., Hersen, M., and Kazdin, A. (1996). A prospective study of childhood anxiety disorders. *Journal of the American Academy of Child and Adolescent Psychiatry*, **35**, 1502–10.

LeGrange, D. (2003). The cognitive model of bulimia nervosa. In: M. Reinecke and D. Clark, ed. *Cognitive therapy across the lifespan: evidence and practice*. Cambridge: Cambridge University Press.

Leslie, S. (1974). Psychiatric disorder in young adolescents of an industrial town. *British Journal of Psychiatry*, **125**, 113–24.

Lewinsohn, P. and Clarke, G. (1999). Psychosocial treatments for adolescent depression. *Clinical Psychology Review*, **19**, 329–42.

Lewinsohn, P., Clarke, G., Hops, H., and Andrews, J. (1990). Cognitive-behavioral treatment for depressed adolescents. *Behavior Therapy*, **21**, 385–401.

Lochman, J., Nelson, W., and Sims, J. (1981). A cognitive-behavioral program for use with aggressive children. *Journal of Clinical Child Psychology*, **10**, 146–8.

Lochman, J., Magee, T., and Pardini, D. (2003). Cognitive-behavioral interventions for children with conduct problems. In: M. Reinecke and D. Clark, ed. *Cognitive therapy across the lifespan: evidence and practice.* Cambridge: Cambridge University Press.

Loeber, R. (1988). Natural histories of conduct problems, delinquency, and associated substance abuse: evidence for developmental progressions. In: B. Lahey and A. Kazdin, ed. *Advances in clinical child psychology*, Vol. 11. New York: Plenum Press.

Luborsky, L. (1984). *Principles of psychoanalytic psychotherapy: a manual for supportive–expressive treatment.* New York: Basic Books.

Mannuzza, S., *et al.* (1991). Hyperactive boys almost grown up: V. Replication of psychiatric status. *Archives of General Psychiatry*, **48**, 77–83.

March, J., Mulle, K., and Herbel, B. (1994). Behavioral psychotherapy for children and adolescents with obsessive-compulsive disorder: an open trial of a new protocol-driven treatment package. *Journal of the American Academy of Child and Adolescent Psychiatry*, **33**, 333–41.

McGee, R., *et al.* (1990). DSM-III disorders in a large sample of adolescents. *Journal of the American Academy of Child and Adolescent Psychiatry*, **29**(4), 611–19.

Meeks, J. (1971). *The fragile alliance.* New York: Krieger.

Miller, D. (1974). *Adolescence: psychology, psychopathology, and psychotherapy.* New York: Aronson.

Moore, M. and Carr, A. (2000a). Depression and grief. In: A. Carr, ed. *What works with children and adolescents? A critical review of psychological interventions with children, adolescents, and their families*, pp. 203–32. London: Routledge.

Moore, M. and Carr, A. (2000b). Anxiety disorders. In: A. Carr, ed. *What works with children and adolescents? A critical review of psychological interventions with children, adolescents, and their families*, pp. 178–202. London: Routledge.

Moran, G., Fonagy, P., Kurtz, A., Bolton, A., and Brook, C. (1991). A controlled study of the psychoanalytic treatment of brittle diabetes. *Journal of the American Academy of Child and Adolescent Psychiatry*, **30**, 926–35.

Mufson, L., Moreau, D., Weissman, M., and Klerman, G. (1993). *Interpersonal psychotherapy for depressed adolescents.* New York: Guilford Press.

Mufson, L., Moreau, D., and Weissman, M. (1994). Modification of interpersonal psychotherapy with depressed adolescents (IPT-A): phase I and II studies. *Journal of the American Academy of Child and Adolescent Psychiatry*, **33**, 695–705.

Mufson, L., Weissman, M., Moreau, D., and Garfinkel, R. (1999). Efficacy of interpersonal psychotherapy for depressed adolescents. *Archives of General Psychiatry*, **56**, 573–9.

Offer, D., Ostrov, E., and Howard, K. (1987). Epidemiology of mental health and mental illness among adolescents. In: J. Noshpitz, ed. *Basic handbook of child psychiatry*, Vol. 5, pp. 82–8. New York: Basic Books.

Offord, D. and Bennett, K. (1994). Conduct disorder: long-term outcomes and intervention effectiveness. *Journal of the American Academy of Child and Adolescent Psychiatry*, **33**, 1069–78.

Offord, D., *et al.* (1987). Ontario Child Health Study: II. Six month prevalence of disorder and rates of service utilization. *Archives of General Psychiatry*, **44**, 832–6.

Ollendick, T. (1995). Cognitive-behavioral treatment of panic disorder with agoraphobia in adolescents: a multiple baseline analysis. *Behavior Therapy*, **26**, 517–31.

Ollendick, T. and King, N. (1998). Empirically supported treatments for children with phobic and anxiety disorders. *Journal of Clinical Child Psychology*, **27**, 156–67.

Orvaschel, H., Lewinsohn, P., and Seeley, J. (1995). Continuity of psychopathology in a community sample of adolescents. *Journal of the American Academy of Child and Adolescent Psychiatry*, **34**, 1525–35.

Ost, L. (1987). Age of onset in different phobias. *Journal of Abnormal Psychology*, **96**, 223–9.

Patterson, G. (1976). *Living with children: new methods for parents and teachers.* Champaign, IL: Research Press.

Patterson, G., Reid, J., and Dishion, T. (1992). *A social learning approach: anti-social boys.* Eugene, OR: Castalia.

Piacentini, J., Bergman, R., and Aikins, J. (2003). Cognitive-behavioral interventions in childhood anxiety disorders. In: M. Reinecke and D. Clark, ed. *Cognitive therapy across the lifespan: evidence and practice.* Cambridge: Cambridge University Press.

Quinton, D., Rutter, M., and Gulliver, L. (1990). Continuities in psychiatric disorders from childhood to adulthood in children of psychiatric patients. In: L. Robins and M. Rutter, ed. *Straight and devious pathways from childhood to adulthood.* Cambridge: Cambridge University Press.

Reinecke, M. (1993). Outpatient treatment of mild psychopathology. In: P. Tolan and B. Cohler, ed. *Handbook of clinical research and practice with adolescents*, pp. 387–410. New York: Wiley-Interscience.

Reinecke, M. (1995). Comorbidity of conduct disorder and depression among adolescents: Implications for assessment and treatment. *Cognitive and Behavioral Practice*, **2**, 299–326.

Reinecke, M., Ryan, N., and DuBois, D. (1998). Cognitive-behavioral therapy of depression and depressive symptoms during adolescence: a review and meta-analysis. *Journal of the American Academy of Child and Adolescent Psychiatry*, **37**, 26–34.

Reinecke, M., Dattilio, F., and Freeman, A. (2003). *Cognitive therapy with children and adolescents: a casebook for clinical practice*, 2nd edn. New York: Guilford Press.

Richards, M. and Petersen, A. (1987). Biological theoretical models of adolescent development. In: V. Van Hasselt and M. Hersen, ed. *Handbook of adolescent psychology*, pp. 34–52. Trowbridge: Pergamon Press.

Richards, M., Abell, S., and Petersen, A. (1993). Biological development. In: P. Tolan and B. Cohler, ed. *Handbook of clinical research and practice with adolescents*, pp. 21–44. New York: Wiley-Interscience.

Rosselló, J. and Bernal, G. (1999). The efficacy of cognitive-behavioral and interpersonal treatments for depression in Puerto Rican adolescents. *Journal of Consulting and Clinical Psychology*, **67**, 734–45.

Rutter, M., Tizard, J., Yule, W., Graham, P., and Whitmore, K. (1976). Research report: Isle of Wight studies, 1964–1974. *Psychological Medicine*, **6**, 313–32.

Schlichter, K. and Horan, J. (1981). Effects of stress inoculation on the anger and aggression management skills of institutionalized juvenile delinquents. *Cognitive Therapy and Research*, **5**, 359–65.

Shirk, S. and Karver, M. (2003). Prediction of treatment outcome from relationship variables in child and adolescent therapy: a meta-analytic review. *Journal of Consulting and Clinical Psychology*, **71**, 452–64.

Shirk, S. and Russell, R. (1998). Process issues in child psychotherapy. In: A. Bellack and M. Hersen, ed. *Comprehensive clinical psychology*, Vol. 5, pp. 57–82. Oxford: Pergamon.

Strain, P., Young, C., and Horowitz, J. (1981). Generalized behavior change during oppositional child training: an examination of child and demographic variables. *Behavior Modification*, **5**, 15–26.

Target, M. and Fonagy, P. (1994a). The efficacy of psychoanalysis for children with emotional disorders. *Journal of the American Academy of Child and Adolescent Psychiatry*, **33**, 361–71.

Target, M. and Fonagy, P. (1994b). The efficacy of psychoanalysis for children: developmental considerations. *Journal of the American Academy of Child and Adolescent Psychiatry*, **33**, 1134–44.

Task Force on Psychological Intervention Guidelines of the American Psychological Association. (1995). *Template for developing guidelines: interventions for mental disorders and psychosocial aspects of physical disorders.* Washington, DC: American Psychological Association.

Tyson, P. and Tyson, R. (1990). *Psychoanalytic theories of development: an integration.* New Haven: Yale University Press.

Valleni-Basille, L., Garrison, C., Jackson, K., Waller, J., McKeown, R., Addy, C., and Cuffe, S. (1994). Frequency of obsessive-compulsive disorder in a community sample of young adolescents. *Journal of the American Academy of Child and Adolescent Psychiatry*, **33**, 782–91.

Verhulst, F. and Achenbach, T. (1995). Empirically based assessment and taxonomy of psychopathology: *European Child and Adolescent Psychiatry*, **4**, 61–76.

Weinshel, E. (1970). Some psychoanalytic considerations on moods. *International Journal of Psychoanalysis*, **51**, 313–20.

Weiss, G. and Hechtman, L. (1993). *Hyperactive children grown up*. New York: Guilford Press.

Weisz, J. and Hawley, K. (1998). Finding, evaluating, refining, and applying empirically supported treatments for children and adolescents. *Journal of Clinical Child Psychology*, **27**, 206–16.

Weisz, J., Huey, S., and Weersing, R. (1998). Psychotherapy outcome research with children and adolescents: the state of the art. In: T. Ollendick and R. Prinz, ed. *Advances in clinical child psychology*, pp. 49–91. New York: Plenum.

Weisz, J., Hawley, K., Pilkonis, P., Woody, S., and Follette, W. (2000). Stressing the (other) three Rs in the search for empirically supported treatments: review procedures, research quality, relevance to practice and the public interest. *Clinical Psychology: Science and Practice*, **7**, 243–58.

Wever, C. and Rey, J. (1997). Juvenile obsessive-compulsive disorder. *Australian and New Zealand Journal of Psychiatry*, **31**, 105–13.

Wood, A., Harrington, R., and Moore, A. (1996). Controlled trial of a brief cognitive-behavioral intervention in adolescent patients with depressive disorders. *Journal of Child Psychology and Psychiatry*, **37**, 737–46.

31 Psychotherapy during the reproductive years

Joan Raphael-Leff

> The communal life of human beings had, therefore, a two-fold foundation:
> the compulsion to work . . . and the power of love
>
> Freud, *Civilisation and its discontents* (1930, p. 101)

Introduction: 'love, work, and play'

In recent times, 'reproductive years' are elongated at both ends—from premature puberty to well past middle-age. Hopefully, throughout this extended period we continue to grow—strive to learn, develop, change—and ultimately (albeit, intermittently) achieve a form of wisdom unavailable in youth. For some, creativity invested in love, work, and play extends to procreation, offering evocative opportunities to reprocess past experiences. Nonparents express their 'generative identity' and nurturing capacities in other ways. The love–work–play trajectory spans goal-oriented achievements, reliant in early adulthood on external affirmation, to progressively more personalized values in later life. Frequently, growth is spurred by critical life experiences of shake-up and self-doubt, especially during transitional phases and mid-life. Development is consolidated by 'stocktaking' after each transition, acknowledging one's capacities, limitations, and inevitable demise. *Maturation is defined as increased integration of personal incongruities and acceptance of the irreversibility of time.*

This chapter addresses the use of psychotherapy to foster development in people whose childhood traumatic experiences and/or disordered transitions across the adult life course have distorted or inhibited their growth process. Disorders occur within the contemporary psychosocial context of diverse, rapidly changing life-styles and unequal access to both external and internal resources. Disturbances range from posttraumatic stress, anxiety, phobic disorders, psychosomatic, addictive, narcissistic, and borderline states to psychotic manifestations. *In common most therapies focus on releasing a sense of agency by altering pathogenic mental connections.*

Presuppositions of psychotherapy

Some basic assumptions, albeit held to varying extent by different schools of thought, underpin therapeutic treatments:

◆ Motivated to seek meaning, healing, and reciprocity, most human beings share a propensity to love, desire, and suffer.

◆ As adults we constantly renegotiate boundaries in social contacts, using self-other regulatory mechanisms to demarcate degrees of intensity and safe distance with our lovers, family, friends, carers, community, society, and internalized memorabilia.

◆ Proficiency in adult relationships rests on a sense of inner security, which in turn is rooted in the quality of early care and later formative experiences and the way these continue to be processed in adulthood.

◆ Conversely, unprocessed issues from the past are repeatedly and blindly played out as we engage others to enact scenes from our internal worlds, seeking to provoke similar affective responses.

◆ Imagined and actual traumatic impingements intensify mental distress. Emotional disorders severely affect more than a quarter of all adults at some point during their lifetime. Periods of heightened vulnerability—*transitions* (for instance, our children's adolescence, our own midlife), or *life events* (such as marriage, retirement, births, and deaths) inevitably involve disruption, necessitating reappraisal for the individual and often, renegotiations for the whole family.

◆ A person's self-esteem, internal resources, fantasies, and type of defensive strategies, as well as the quality of his/her emotional relationships at any one time will determine the significance of both phase-specific predicaments (such as promotion at work, or grandparenthood) and responses to unforeseen painful crises (of health, loss, economic, or psychosocial traumata).

◆ While elaborating new levels of comprehension we revisit old conflicts and anxieties, and in addition to experience-evoked strategies, persistent unconscious issues resurface at each new phase, as a trait or defensive tendency.

◆ In general, the *meaning* ascribed to each life event determines its impact. Responses may range from confusion, inertia, regression or defensive retrenchment and compulsive repetition, to posttraumatic growth and healthy recovery after the initial shock.

◆ The degree of disturbance and capacity for reorganization fluctuate across the life cycle in accordance with concurrent circumstances and age-related comorbidity risks; the nature of personal aspirations and flexibility of one's own approach to attaining these.

Psychotherapy, which provides emotional support and fosters understanding, can boost resilience in people susceptible to retraumatization.

Disturbances of adult relating

For each of us, childhood attachments provide an enduring template of the constitutive process of give and take within which representations of self and others are formed. If original carers were overtaxed, depressed, and unresponsive, or deficient, persecutory, and abusive due to their own psychohistories or troubled by life events or disasters—childhood maturational processes are interrupted, resulting not only in stunted growth but in *internalization of the faulty relationship as a distorted expectation*. Unless this is addressed, adult intimacy continues to be modeled on the original experience (and its denial), with enactment of both the desired compensatory (idealized) relationship and its cruel, perverse, or deficient counterpart.

Love and intimacy

While many people achieve a flexible spectrum of relating, for most patients intimacy is a prime area of concern. Working therapeutically with these individuals or couples, we realize that love is fundamental, and like all primary affects including anger, fear, and surprise, it has both universal physiological components and diverse individual and cultural manifestations.

Many people come into therapy having discovered the pernicious nature of the compulsion to repeat the past, which threatens to destroy new relationships.

In the West, personal expectations of intimacy are also influenced by bombardments of flamboyant erotic imagery, larger-than-life passions, and a cacophony of lyrical narratives that provide the cultural backdrop of symbolic representations of 'love'. Indeed, there is some concern about the 'tyranny' of a milieu that so invades and controls the most private recesses of the human mind through its proliferate media, commercial and service instruments, displacing the authority of religion and elders with transmission of 'manufactured fantasies of total gratification' (Lasch, 1978). *Some contemporary discontent and difficulty in finding satisfaction in love, work, and play stems from persuasive media communications—articulating primitive illusions of unconditional love and everlasting sexual excitement, which resonate with our own cherished infantile fantasies.*

Today's message of 'Love as a crucible for identity' is ambiguous—juxtaposing 1960s images of hedonistic free choice and sexual exploration with nineteenth century romantic ideas of mature conformity, duty, and loyalty. The composite mythology poses a dilemma, endorsing adulthood as both 'a prolonged adolescent-like period of continuing crisis, challenge and change' (Swidler, 1980, p. 130), and a search for sexual perfection. This blend of individualistic exploratory 'self-actualization' and self-centered indulgent materialism contrasts with social obligation, ethical responsibility, and a sense of global accountability. Precariously poised in the twenty-first century, we occupy a world of contradictions, uncertainty, and cynical leadership, with disturbing antidotes of fundamentalist terrorism or arrogant military triumphalism. Poignantly, faced with mortal danger, victims distil their emotions sending messages saying simply: 'I love you'.

Unconscious contracts

> . . . I can give you no idea of the important bearing of this first object [the mother] upon the choice of every later object, of the profoundest effects it has in its transformations and substitutions in even the remotest regions of our sexual life.
>
> Freud (1917, p. 314)

On an individual level falling in love in adulthood is a form of *re-cognition*, investing a 'familiar' stranger with heightened emotions transferred from internal figures and unconscious projections that attempt to probe and occupy the other, hoping to activate the desired archaic response. Sexual partners are often unconsciously selected not only for their resemblance to early 'objects' of desire but for their 'transformational' capacity to re-evoke early solicitations. The search is a 'memorial' one of surrendering to the other as a 'medium' to alter the self (Bollas, 1979). (This is also the evocative basis of transference in psychotherapy.) Each partner brings to intimate sexual encounters their cumulative past including emotional relationships, unresolved conflicts, and unfulfilled cravings that they wish to satisfy alongside hopes of adult development. Healthy unions that respect difference and allow each partner to flourish, facilitate further growth despite the pull to repeat and gratify unprocessed archaic desires.

Every couple acquires an identity of its own in addition to the distinctiveness of each of the mates. The twosome becomes the repository of both partners' conscious and unconscious sexual fantasies and desires, wishes, and wants. This potential joint system undergoes vicissitudes 'of gratitude and guilt, of stereotyping and conventionality, of deceptiveness and long-range destructive and self-destructive scenarios' (Kernberg, 1993, p. 653). One source of tension in adult relationships that persist over time, is a potential mismatch between needs of the couple and each partner's personal transformational hopes—both to play out childhood myths and to relinquish these and expand their own self-definition. The latter may clash with the *dyad*'s requirement to preserve equilibrium in the face of growing family and occupational responsibilities (see Gould, 1993).

In addition to explicit social expectations and each partner's implicit personal aspirations—love relationships in early adulthood include persistent *collusive unconscious 'contracts'*. When contested by one partner, these are transferred to new relationships by the other. The significant other may personify 'lost', repudiated, or dangerous parts of the self. Their 'pact' may provide breakaway from negative aspects of their respective archaic parents, may mutually confirm each other's shaky sense of identity by boosting defiance, or promote reciprocal idealization, fostering an illusion of dyadic fusion or a means of denying separateness (see Dicks, 1963; Clulow *et al.*, 1986; Raphael-Leff, 2005)—a spectrum reflecting the severity of joint pathology. Erotic desire and sexual activity further shifts the boundaries, temporarily blurring psychosomatic, gendered, and transpersonal distinctions.

Unconscious contracts are very difficult to disentangle especially when the partners' respective underpinning configurations dovetail. If these persist into parenthood, to avoid recognizing the pathological nature of their interaction the couple may enlist the new baby in fantasy enactments. Assessment for *couple therapy* must therefore evaluate the nature of their 'shared internal world' and their capacity to confront pain rather than evade it (Lanman, 2003).

Breakdown of intimate relationships

In recent years there has been a dramatic shift to *cohabitation* as the first mode of union in Britain, and although three in five permanent relationships do result in marriage, 35% of couples living together dissolve within 10 years, followed by an average of 3 years alone before starting a new relationship (ISER Report, 2000/1). Ironically, the high level of failed marriages is ascribed to more negative behavior following premarital cohabitation with its greater autonomy (Coghan and Kleinbaum, 2002). Failure is also attributed to factors such as premarital sex, racial, and religious heterogamy. However, the picture is complex. The US National Survey of Family Growth indicates that marriages contracted after 1980 are becoming more stable, possibly due to rising age at marriage and increased cohabitation (Heaton, 2002). But, according to the US Census, almost half of all couples in first marriages divorce and a further fifth separate. American second marriages have a 10% higher rate of divorce (and one in three children come from 'broken' homes). The British Office for National Statistics indicates that about 70% of subsequent UK marriages end in divorce, and 50% of these occur between ages 35 and 55.

Numerous studies find women more disappointed in marriage, which does not match the nurturing and relational intimacy of their unconscious expectations. Seemingly, men are less aware of the build up of problems and less accepting of the end of a relationship, continuing to sustain unrealistic expectations of reconciliation and suffering increased health and psychological problems following the break up (Gorell Barnes, 1998). Nonetheless, with therapy and/or delineation of their emotional priorities, many (childless) individuals eventually go on to happier relationships. When offspring are involved, a common pattern in separation among both married and unwed couples is that children mostly reside with their mothers, with decreasing contact with noncustodial fathers (despite governmental decrees on shared parental responsibility even in failed adult partnerships). In almost half the cases, separation may lead to paternal withdrawal or lack of access (Cockett and Tripp, 1994), estrangement and loss of contact within two years (Simpson *et al.*, 1995), and even denial of paternity. In fact USA and UK surveys find that one-third to one-half of men's children from previous relationships go unmentioned by nonresident fathers compared with custodial mothers' reports.

Parting may come as a welcome end to quarrelling, but often involves reduced economic security, geographical relocation and for a child, a disrupted family, change of school, friends, neighborhood, loss of relatives, and restructured network. Faced with a preoccupied, sad or angry resident parent with no other emotional support, a child may resort to role reversal to comforting the jilted adult (see Gorell Barnes *et al.*, 1998). Separation anxiety, depression, and psychosomatic symptoms are not uncommon following a divorce, as are less visible symptoms of low self-esteem and often irrational self-blame for the break up. Pre- or postseparation *family therapy or conciliation counseling* may be indicated. However, during the conflictual process of separation, therapists may be drawn into unconscious identifications (Wallerstein, 1990) and countertransferential roles (judge, magician, or servant), which render them ineffectual (Vincent, 1995).

Abusive relationships

Recent widespread disclosure of *domestic violence* and *sexual abuse* demonstrate the potential dangers of asymmetrical intimate relationships with devastating consequences for defenseless victims—long-lasting impairments in their emotional, physical, psychosexual, and interpersonal functioning. Violence and victimization are implicated as both cause and consequence of family breakdown, community disintegration, isolation, and alcoholism or substance abuse. Child-bearing raises the risk, with increased vulnerability, dependence, and raised tensions. Given ubiquitous antenatal health provision pregnancy is also a prime time for detection and intervention (Reading, 2003). Abused mothers of young babies require therapeutic intervention. Special *group sessions* in aggression-control benefit motivated perpetrators. Victims in refuge accommodation are usually offered *brief* and *time-limited counseling* or *outpatient group psychotherapy*. Those who have been exposed to extreme and repeated exploitation by intimates require *longer-term clinical care* to overcome distrust and achieve internal reparative work. In cases of chronic violation and extreme emotional harm, extended *psychodynamic treatment* is justified by elevated risk of repeated victimization and transgenerational transmission (Dutton and Holzworth-Munroe, 1997). Inconsistent government and nongovernmental organization responses to domestic violence and child protection concerns indicate a need for more comprehensive interagency guidelines (Waugh and Bonner, 2002) to both alleviate long-lasting psychological distress and prevent recurrent crises and medical interventions.

As in perversions and prejudicial attacks, a central essential aspect of most deviant practices is *dehumanization*. In a world where women feel powerless as agents in an adult world, they may employ their power as mothers to inflict emotional and bodily harm on their children. *Perverse mothering* often follows on intergenerational propagation of sadomasochistic pathology where the mother who treats her child as part of herself also maltreats her child as an expression of her own self-hatred (Welldon, 2002). Sexual abuse, prostitution, eating disorders, self-mutilation, and compulsive exercising similarly reflect attempts to both self control and to attack the body-self. *Munchausen by proxy*, another a perverse use of a child as an extension, is fatal in about 10% of cases. *Psychotherapeutic treatment* is fraught with issues of control, deception, and corruption which pressurises the therapist to act abusively rather than think (Lloyd-Owen, 2003). Male offenders usually lack the maternal masochistic identification with the victim. The victims of pedophiles' sexual and violent abuse are usually genetically unrelated; in extreme cases a sadistic component leads to homicide. Invariably, adult abusers were maltreated children, and retrospective studies reveal that childhood sexual exploitation rarely occurs as an isolated feature but is associated with physical and emotional abuse, neglect, and household dysfunction (Dong *et al.*, 2003).

Preventative measures are as necessary as corrective ones to break the transgenerational cycle.

'Lifespan' psychology

In complex societies, sociocultural fragmentation and rapid changes necessitate constant emotional reworking. As adults we each belong to numerous reference groups. Mental health is affected by extent of clash or compartmentalization among these, as well as our intrapsychic unconscious affiliations and social status within them. Psychosexual mores determine compatibility or conflict in work/parenting demands and personal issues of domestic/public gender politics. Social prominence or marginalization are affected by personality, mobility, and/or discriminatory minority status within ethnic, class, sex, and age stratified hierarchies. However, we are never passive recipients nor does psychic development occur solipsistically. Growth is instigated by internalizing losses (Freud, 1917) and by identifying

constraints and assimilating tensions within the psychosocial matrix in which we are both embedded and emanate our own emotional forces.

Life-course challenges

Psychodynamic theories of adult maturation stress both cognitive development towards wisdom and affective growth towards mature love (Erikson, 1980; Emde, 1985; Stevens-Long, 1990; Kernberg, 1993). Some themes are applicable across the reproductive years, although a medley of challenges now replace previous phase-specific 'psychological tasks' (e.g., Erikson, 1950; Jaques, 1965) and some growth issues are suspended or defy the expected sequence:

◆ *Adolescence:* a prolonged search for identity is stirred up by puberty, role confusion, and multiple choices, exemplified by idealization of mentors and use of peer group both to escape a sense of inadequacy, and as an experimental arena to explore self-definition and sexual identity.

◆ *Early adulthood:* given today's (ostensible) equal opportunity, many women as well as men prioritize education and career ambitions over intimacy. A healthy search for love is instigated by greater stability and tolerance of loss (versus feared isolation).

◆ *Maturing adulthood:* desire to reproduce reflects readiness to nurture (versus stagnation anxieties or desires for generational lineage). Postponed reproduction or waived parenthood suggests expanding 'generative identity' and/or increasingly antithetic conditions of domesticity and work attainments.

◆ With rising longevity and postmenopausal reproduction, *midlife crisis* may equally accompany retirement, belated parenthood, discovery of irreversible infertility, or empty nest syndrome.

◆ A *late adult crisis* usually follows challenges to bodily integrity, with death's ultimate inescapability forcing reappraisal of one's accrued sense of order, ethics, and personalized meaning to counter despair.

Emotional upheavals stimulate psychic reorganization and formative reconfigurations of identity. Maturation builds on reworked concerns, self-reflection, and integration of change. Lifelong confrontation with 'developmental challenges' (Settlage *et al.*, 1988) and resolution of conflicts bring a series of commensurate changes in *self-representation*. Although shifting, fragmented, and elusive, identity nevertheless has a subjective continuity. We bring old emotions into new situations, investing them with unresolved issues transferred from the past and recreate archaic scenarios in the present. Insight is enhanced by withdrawing projections and confronting human frailty and complexity. The hallmark of maturity is one of diminishing omnipotence and increasing agency. *Accepting one's own contradictions, failures, and destructiveness increases the desire to contribute and conversely, acknowledging one's own input to difficulties fosters meaningful new choices.*

Psychosocial backdrop to disturbance

Social forces structure our lives, with influences beyond our ken forming us and shaping our decisions. This 'social unconscious' (Hopper, 2003) remains unexplored due to personal resistances, 'normative reticence', and ideological constraints. Over the last few decades, breakdown of traditional structures in postindustrialized societies has resulted in disordered life-course sequences. Britain is a prime example: improved nutrition has lowered the age of menarche, and despite Western demarcation of adolescence as a prolonged transitional period of maturation, earlier sexual activity, relaxed social mores, and diminished restrictions means Britain now has the highest rate in Europe of *very young teenage mothers* [triple that of France and Sweden, quadruple that of Italy, six times that of the Netherlands, and 10 times that of Switzerland! (Kiernan, 1997)] with associated emotional and socioeconomic hardships. Conversely, with access to further education and career promises, many women postpone child-bearing until their mid-thirties or beyond and a whole industry of fertility treatments has arisen to assist waning fecundity. These technological innovations in turn pose false hopes adding tension to the anguish of infertility. Successful interventions create further unprecedented doubts and emotional distress, as new kinship categories and ethical dilemmas arise.

Modern-day maternal career expectations often vie with the infant's needs, which have changed little over the millennia. Serial cohabitation replaces marriage, with a rise in unwed and same-sexed parents. Social stratification leaves new parents unprepared for the impact of a baby on their lives. More importantly, *smaller families deny people opportunities to rework and resolve their own infantile issues in the presence of babies before having their own.*

'Life-style' decisions

Worldwide, changing demographic and socioeconomic parameters of the reproductive years include urbanization, which alters family patterns, dispersing extended families and forming viable, yet often isolated, small and emotionally intense nuclear units. Even in developing countries birth rates have declined substantially, largely due to changing attitudes, abortion, and efficient contraception. Safer childbirth and decreased infant mortality diminish the need to have many children to ensure some will survive. Earlier puberty and longer life expectancy shift commencement of adulthood and extend its upper range and versatility well beyond menopause. However, adulthood is no longer synonymous with childbearing and the rate of *childlessness-by-choice* is estimated at 12–20% across Europe.

Psychologically, 'life-style' decisions are never straightforward, and inflated expectations influenced by media depictions and sociopolitical changes often contribute to frustration, disillusionment, and depression. Rising unemployment, housing shortages, deteriorating transport, poor education, and health service facilities have become a feature of what I call 'de-developing' as well as developing countries. And data from cross-national surveys in 'restructuring societies' such as Brazil, Chile, India, and Zimbabwe show that common mental disorders are about twice as frequent among the poor (Patel *et al.*, 1999). Women in all societies are 1.5–3 times more likely than men to develop depressive and anxiety disorders (Ustun, 2000) peaking during the reproductive years, with postpartum and other psychiatric disturbances across the lifespan (Swartz, 2003)—explained not by biological factors but childhood adversity and/or psychosocial entrapment in marriage and motherhood (Brown *et al.*, 1995; Craig and Pathare, 2000). Sex discrimination is rife—there are still disproportionately few female tertiary students even in the West, and worldwide the market reveals earning differentials, segregated work conditions, and postmaternal downward occupational mobility, for professional women too. Even in privileged Europe, gender equity for parents remains a myth, with women struggling to fulfill often conflicting domestic and work roles, both in traditional (largely Catholic) southeastern European countries (where the fertility rate has now dropped below 1.7 births per woman), and in the more generously state-endowed northwestern European countries (see Hobcraft and Kiernan, 1995). On the other hand, the Western trend towards postponed, concentrated parenthood, thrusts young children into their parents' midlife crises and juxtaposes adolescent offspring's turmoil with parental elderliness. Coupled with social mobility and geographical migration resulting in dispersal and loss of extended families and support systems it fosters *an intensely interdependent and overburdened couple relationship and/or parent–child bond.*

Conversely, in many third world and particularly sub-Saharan African countries, the life span of adults is now *declining* to four decades (!) due to famine, violence, and disease, especially AIDS, in addition to dietary deficiencies and maternal mortality. Healthy life expectancy at birth varies both within social groups and between societies [29.5 years in Sierra Leone, 33.8 years in Afghanistan to 69.9 in the UK and 73.8 in Japan (WHO, 2003)]. With 29.4 million HIV/AIDS sufferers worldwide (10 million of whom are between ages 10 and 24!), increasingly, grandparents care for orphaned toddlers and, as the mid-generation die off, numerous child-headed households are left to cope with emotionally devastating aftermaths of adult wars and sexually transmitted diseases.

Finally, disturbances of the reproductive years relate to changing attitudes about the quality and duration of intimate relationships and a contemporary, often colliding quest for self-actualization, contributing to the complexity of (post)modern life. Given all these factors it is no longer meaningful to think in terms of normative 'life cycle' frameworks. Therapists working with adult patients across the reproductive years, from adolescent sexuality to postmenopausal childbearing, must identify ongoing developmental challenges. *Emotional disturbances occur within this matrix of rapidly changing psychosocial demands, cultural and ethnic resource variations, and gender/cross-generational differences in overstrained nuclear families.*

Procreation

Pregnancy, whether planned or not, immediately throws sexual difference into relief, in even the most egalitarian of couples. It is in her swelling body that their joint baby is growing, she who feels nauseous and mediates contact. An expectant father may be absent or ignorant of his status. If present he too undergoes emotional processes related to the gestation, including salient preconscious self/baby representations shaped by his own fantasy baby and internal model of parenting. This may or may not coincide with hers, leading to synchronous or diverging parental practices within the couple. On her own or in a couple, every pregnant woman engages with, or disengages herself from, age-old female mysteries and anxieties of formation, transformation, separation, and birth (Raphael-Leff, 1993/2001). Unlike her counterpart in previous generations or in traditional societies, a Western woman is often unprepared for pregnancy, having had little exposure to female lore, labor, and birth stories nor even watched a baby suckling. In her steep learning curve, clinic appointments replace rituals and protective ceremonies, and midwives—wise women guides.

Instigated by antenatal investigations such as ultrasound screening (which reveals the baby's movements before she experiences these), amniocentesis (disclosing the baby's sex), HIV testing and/or tests diagnosing complications, emotions tend to run high at various points during the pregnancy. Some negative information prompts immediate decisions about discontinuing the pregnancy and whatever option is chosen leads to long-lasting emotions, self-doubts, recriminations, and guilt. Other fraught issues stem from reawakened torments, or a couple's discrepant representations of the baby (idealized to maligned), or overidentification with an envied or feared, vulnerable, 'starving', or 'claustrophobic' fetus. Psychosexual anxieties about the internal 'parasite', apprehension about the inexorable birth, extreme jealousy, and rage may indicate concerns about *redistribution of love*—being displaced by the baby. Very young or vulnerable women may be overwhelmed by the emotional strain. Anxieties accompany delivery and choice of options often reflect semiconscious concerns. A woman may elect Cesarean section to protect herself and/or baby from inflicting damage; survivors of sexual abuse may fear that pain and intimate physicality of labor will retrigger dormant 'body memory' reactions; a water-birth may symbolize maternal rebirth.

Finally, disagreement between expectant partners over their respective parenting orientations or divergent responses to unexpected events such as emergency surgery or prematurity, may reflect deeper discord, which untreated results in couple conflict or resentment of parenting. *Perinatal couple counseling* is indicated.

Antenatal disturbances

The higher incidence of antenatal depressive symptoms in inner cities are also associated with socioeconomic disadvantage—no educational qualifications, unemployment and poor support or no partner in second or subsequent pregnancy (Bolton *et al.*, 1998). For the woman who actually has another inside her, distinctions between self and other, outer, and inner may blur. While most expectant mothers experience a variety of mixed feelings fluctuating over the course of a day if not an hour, some pregnant women take a *fixed* stance. This may center around *depressive issues* of feeling insufficiently nurturing; or *persecutory anxieties* about being depleted and exploited by the baby (if intolerable these lead to fetal abuse or an abortion to expel the tyrant). *Obsessional defenses* geared to regulating closeness become jeopardized by the ultra-intimacy of having two people in one body. *Compulsive actions* fail to ward off danger, and the struggle to keep good and bad apart is imperiled by the uncontrollable 'invader' who threatens to reveal her hidden badness. *Intrusive thoughts* break through, with a risk of enacting these antenatally in physical attacks on the fetus, or in postnatal violence or sexual abuse (Raphael-Leff, 1997). Expectant fathers, too, are prone to emotional disturbances (Lovestone and Kumar, 1993), in addition to experiencing envy of the woman or fetus. 'Talking cures' are a treatment option for psychiatric disorders in pregnancy as both medication and maternal illness may have an adverse effects on the fetus (Cott and Wisner, 2003).

There is a substantial overlap between depression and anxiety in the pre- and postpartum periods (Da Costa *et al.*, 2000) but antenatal depression possibly has a *higher* prevalence than postnatal depression, which it frequently precedes (Evans *et al.*, 2001). Although no causal connection can be sustained by available evidence (Oates, 2002) in addition to direct effects on the fetus of alcohol and substance abuse in pregnancy (Siney, 1999) there is a growing body of work linking maternal antenatal emotional disturbance and later behavioral problems in the offspring. Prenatal depression has even been claimed to produce differing effects on fetus and newborn according to ethnicity and socioeconomic status. In a longitudinal study of over 10 000 women that examined antenatal disturbance separately from postnatal depression, anxiety in late pregnancy was found to pose an independent risk associated with behavioral/emotional problems in the child at 4 years of age (O'Connor *et al.*, 2002). *Preventive interventions* in pregnancy and *perinatal therapy* consisting of individual or joint sessions that continue after the birth, benefit expectant mothers or parents experiencing emotional overload, irresolvable antagonism or revival of previous troubling experiences.

High-risk categories are *conflicted pregnancies*, including unplanned, untimely, or highly ambivalent. *Emotional sensitization*, including conception by donor gametes or following on prolonged infertility; family history of obstetric complications, or psychiatric treatment. *Complicated pregnancies*, including eating disorders or substance abuse, multiple fetuses, concurrent life events such as bereavement or eviction, socioeconomic problems, and lack of emotional support (Raphael-Leff, 1993/2001, p. 193). Similarly, people encountering *perinatal losses*, whether abortion, miscarriage, stillbirth, neonatal death, and abnormalities often feel the need for *grief counseling*. A therapeutic atmosphere in which to examine and express their feelings of shock, sorrow, guilt, shame, and/or desperation is essential as these are often negated in a conspiracy of silence or placation ('you can always have another baby') by well-meaning friends and professionals alike (Raphael-Leff, 1993).

Perinatal disturbances

In the West of every 1000 women having a baby it is estimated that two develop puerperal psychosis, 17 will already be psychiatric patients, 100–150 experience postnatal depression or persecution, 300–400 suffer mood disturbance and temporary emotional distress. While some female postnatal disturbance is attributed to hormonal fluctuations, *birth of a baby is in itself a highly arousing experience for carers of either sex*. Exposure to the infant's urgent crying and nonverbally expressed needs often touches a raw nerve in the adult, conflating demands and their evocation. Direct contact with the smells and feel of primary substances may reactivate in the adult implicit 'procedural' memories in feeling. Paradoxically, to function sensitively, the parent must remain receptive to these and draw on them to empathically understand the baby's needs. However, if the adult is overwhelmed by his/her own infantile feelings or too susceptible to the baby's, parenting becomes problematical (Raphael-Leff, 2000a).

With a first baby, a couple's sudden shift from intimate dyad to triad retriggers old mother/father/child issues of *inclusion/exclusion*, and now

that the new parents are in the powerful position on the triangle, they may inflict ancient jealousies and unresolved sibling rivalries on their dependent baby and each other. The ever-present third, both stranger and part of themselves, enriches yet disrupts the intimate sexual partnership. For women, a new baby 'ruins' postindustrial life-styles and careers. The cost is high: by keeping the child, a mother loses half her expected lifetime's income and not surprisingly, compensates by unrealistically high expectations of motherhood (Leach, 1996). A women who has cared for her own narcissistic mother since childhood, may feel unwilling to mother the baby and/or envious of the care she herself provides. Feeling endangered by the infant's fragility or neediness a father or mother may withdraw emotionally or physically. These problems are well served by *parent–infant therapy*, *couple* or *individual psychodynamic therapy*. Conversely, when issues of *dominance/submission* are enacted in violent or sexual maltreatment of the baby, *crisis intervention* is crucial, at times necessitating removal of the offender or the baby from the family.

As in all disturbances, *when resources are scarce, mental health priorities must focus on prevention, identification of high-risk cases, and early referral for treatment*. In many societies, well-baby clinics exist and primary health carers are in a prime position to identify infant disorders such as disturbances of sleep, feeding disorders, traumatic stress, failure to thrive, persistent crying, and behavioral complaints, which both contribute to, but are also symptomatic of family dysfunction. In these cases *developmental guidance* may be the first call of action, especially with very anxious inexperienced parents. This involves *supportive counseling* by community nurse, health visitor, or therapist whose observation of the parent–child involves spontaneous 'advocacy' (speaking on behalf of the nonverbal baby), and commentary about ongoing interaction fostering freedom to experiment with new ways of relating, affirmed by the infant's responses. More contemplative carers can use *brief parent–infant therapy*. The nonjudgmental 'holding' of a therapeutic relationship can help them reflect on painful issues in their own infancy and ways these may be impinging emotionally on their current interaction with the baby. Such external support and insight can eliminate 'ghosts' that have come to occupy the nursery (Fraiberg *et al.*, 1975). All communication involves mismatches and the mother–infant capacity for co-creative processes and 'interactive repair' (Tronick, 2003) is enhanced when negative internal representations alter in the adult. (Interestingly, 'distorted' representations have a better outcome than 'detached' ones.)

In cases where the family disturbance stems from a carer's deep-seated unconscious representations of the baby as a *defective baby-self*, long-term *psychodynamic individual therapy* offers a safe haven to work through infantile experiences associated with these attributions and to regain ownership of them. In families where the disturbance is clearly related to the partners' interactive dovetailing, *conjoint couple* or *family therapy* will enable them to identify their patterns.

Special cases

About 2% of childbearing couples suffer loss of a baby through *miscarriage, stillbirth, or SIDS* (sudden infant death syndrome). *The process of mourning perinatal losses is hampered by the unknowable and the inexplicable*. Death in the midst of procreation seems an obscene 'nonevent' and unmanageable feelings include love–hate conflicts, grievances, and excessive or inhibited grief (Bourne and Lewis, 2003). *Crisis support, grief counseling*, and information about diverse reactions and gender differences in mourning help parents feel less guilty, ashamed and stupefied, and less likely to rush into a replacement pregnancy. The need for *individualized, compassionate midwifery care* in the pregnancy following neonatal loss is also stressed by a joint Australian-Canadian study of a Special Delivery Service program and supportive healthcare services (Caelli *et al.*, 2002).

Birth of a *special needs baby* constitutes a potential trauma for the parents whose guilt, grief, and anger reactions will be influenced by a complex interplay of intrapsychic and external factors (such as severity and correctability of the defect, how they discovered it, and the nature of the medical procedures required). As with all trauma, parents tend to experience an initial sense of shock, disappointment, anger, and injury to self-esteem followed by a period of painful intrapsychic dis-equilibrium. After mourning both the wished-for-child and their own losses there is a gradual restoration of intrapsychic equilibrium and capacity to value the child as separate rather than a negative extension of the parent (Mintzer *et al.*, 1984). According to need, *antenatal preparatory counseling, early postnatal support, grief work,* or *longer-term therapeutic contact* may be indicated and/or access to a *support-network* of like-minded parents may be helpful, at different points over the years.

Increasingly *AIDS* is becoming an issue when linked to maternity in one of three ways:

1. An HIV positive woman chooses to conceive—to 'fulfill' her 'feminine destiny', compensate her for the illness, create an illusion of immortality or leave a living legacy behind her when she dies.

2. A woman discovers through antenatal screening that she is HIV positive following rape or voluntary sexual contact (one in three in Southern Africa).

3. A woman whose partner is HIV positive chooses to conceive or finds herself pregnant with anxieties that she and/or the baby may develop the virus.

From supervision of midwives, therapists, and counselors on different continents, in all three situations *the juxtaposition of a life threatening illness with life-giving pregnancy is an impossible aporia.* Disclosure of HIV in the context of pregnancy is accompanied by stages akin to mourning—shock, confusion, denial, abandonment, anger, and mixed feelings about her own survival. Annihilation anxiety mingles with guilt about bringing an orphan into the world, remorse at possibly infecting her baby, shame about having to break the news to her family (with the social stigma of AIDS still rife), and anxieties about the uncertain course ahead, including treatment (or its unavailability). Fear that pregnancy will exacerbate the illness, ambivalence about the need for a C-section, fantasies cum reality of her body and milk being poisonous and experience of unknown side effects, often lead to inconsistent treatment of the baby who is both overinvested and envied yet repudiated. Clearly the need for *supportive counseling* is great but not often acknowledged as an ongoing perinatal need by overstretched service providers. (Work in Soweto demonstrates the effectiveness of trained lay befrienders and leaderless *support groups.*) The bereavement process in children of parents with AIDS is complicated by secrecy, shame, ostracism, and neglect. Behavioral symptoms such as stealing, self-harm, truancy, and drug taking may be relieved by *grief work* that offers the child stability and possibilities for open communication (Aronson, 1996).

Postpartum mood disorders

There is a threefold increased rate of depression within 5 weeks of delivery (Cox *et al.*, 1993) with prevalence rates of 10–22% for severe depression. Symptomatology (unrelated to age, marital status or education, although increased by lack of confidante) includes diminished pleasure, depressed mood, energy loss, guilt, and sense of worthlessness. Depression also has a high comorbidity with anxiety disorders, substance abuse, and eating disorders. However, wide community studies of new mothers indicate that about half of those who meet operational clinical criteria for psychiatric 'caseness' remain undetected by family doctors and other professionals.

Apart from the sufferer's distress, psychological effects on the partner and parenting is of ongoing concern. High rates of couple disharmony, conflict, and separation are associated with assortative mating, and contemporaneous psychiatric morbidity in partners (Burke, 2003). Serious mental illness in primary caregivers has long-term repercussions. *Assessment of parenting capacity* must focus on the level of disturbance, instability, paranoia and impulse control, responsibility and the degree to which a child is involved in the parental psychopathological system (Gopfert *et al.*, 1996), or deprived by the quality of their emotional functioning. *Results show disturbed parents are less responsive, less attuned, at times rejecting or hostile, inconsistent, or ineffectual* (Mowbry and Lennon,

1998). Specific studies of adverse effects of *postnatal depression* find that the child's cognitive development and sociability are impaired long after resolution of the maternal illness (Murray and Cooper, 1997). When associated with vulnerability factors such as psychosocial adversity and marital discord, the risk increases (Brown *et al.*, 1995) and untreated parental illnesses persist with 30% still suffering at 1-year postpartum (Pitt, 1968) with chronic depression or recurrent relapses.

Health visitors and other primary carers find that not surprisingly, mothers who are worn down by persistent socioeconomic deprivation and chronic depression are often apathetic, demoralized and powerless, displaying emotional numbness, low self-confidence, depression and insensitivity to, and/or overreliance on, their children for support. Conversely, perfectionistic mothers with good social skills often go undetected by professionals as they hide their severe depression under a façade of bright coping mechanisms. When these fail, reluctance to admit defeat or ask for help carries a high risk of *suicide.* Finally, in cases of persecutory driven illness, where the baby becomes incorporated in the paranoid or depressive system, *infanticide* is a danger.

Given that early infancy is deemed a critical period for emotional development, and that neuropsychological evidence reveals that the developing brain itself is affected by maltreatment, over- or understimulation (Schore, 1999) early detection and speedy treatment are imperative. In most Western countries, the regular high scrutiny of antenatal care offers an opportunity to identify women at risk for both puerperal psychosis (with 50% chance of recurrence) and other forms of postnatal disturbance, if midwives and traditional birth attendants are trained. *Couple therapy during pregnancy* as well as *postnatal parent–infant or family therapy* help prevent family dysfunction hardening into an established and intractable interactional pattern. *Family intervention programs* aim to improve parental functioning ante- or postnatally. Some attempt to 'optimize' the relationship and to address the child's emotional, cognitive, linguistic, and social needs, through home visits, *mother–infant group intervention* and a variety of toddler's stimulation groups and community-liaison supervised work rehabilitation (Heinicke *et al.*, 2001). Disturbed parents may benefit from specialized *group therapy* (Puckering *et al.*, 1994).

Psychiatrically disturbed parents of older children

Research has confirmed the raised risk of emotional and behavioral disturbance in children of a mentally ill parent (Marks *et al.*, 2002). The association is strongest in cases of *personality disorder* and chronic or recurring depression in the parent. Although some depressed mothers manage to sustain warm, even excessively affectionate relationships with their 'savior' child (Radke-Yarrow *et al.*, 1988) *affective disorders* restrict the capacity to engage sensitively. Children suffer from the depressed parent's persistent unhappiness, emotional preoccupation and self-blame, or the overactivity, grandiosity, denial, and contempt of mania (Pound, 1996). The inconsistencies of *bipolar illness* are thus particularly confusing. Owing to domestic disruptions the admission rate of children to care is high, with a 44% chance of psychiatric disorder in adulthood versus 2% noncare controls (Rutter and Quinton, 1984). *A high genetic loading is responsible for some morbidity in adulthood but the deficits in care, the tense, unhappy, or unpredictable domestic atmosphere, and the anxieties about the parent's welfare result in defensive organization in the offspring.*

Two main patterns of dysfunction in children of chronically depressed parents are overidentification and depression (1.6 times that of matched controls) with poor self-esteem or an 'oppositional syndrome' (Pound, 1996) of detachment, substance abuse, and/or antisocial behaviors (more common in boys). Protective factors enable some children to develop well despite the presence of psychotic manifestations within their families. Of central importance are dispositional attributes, family cohesion, and the relationship to the non ill parent and other warm supportive figures and an intimate confiding friendship with a peer. The child's personal resources of resilience, compassion, high self-esteem and self-reflectiveness are both protective assets and outgrowths of coping with psychopathology.

In the UK, 28% of (urban) family-practice attenders and 50% of psychiatric outpatient populations have a *personality disorder*, presenting with a variety of symptoms such as violence, anxiety and depression, self-mutilation, sexual disinhibition, substance abuse, and eating disorders. This narrow repertoire of habitual coping strategies adversely affects flexibility of response in relating. Conduct disorders and a high risk of chronic delinquency are more common in children of personality disordered parents, who often themselves suffered from ineffective parenting, harsh discipline, and childhood sexual abuse and/or violence. *Across studies, a triad of demoralizing factors recurs in association with psychiatric disorders: environmental hardships, poor or deteriorating relationships of cohabitation and early trauma or cumulative adversity* (see Cox et al., 1987; Brown et al., 1995).

When one member of a family has *schizophrenia* the effect of an atmosphere of negative 'expressed emotions' on maintaining illness and exacerbating psychotic relapses has been demonstrated, as has *family intervention* to improve communication patterns and to foster recognition of each family member's differing needs (Kuipers et al., 2002). When hostility and criticism are predominant features of interaction *family therapy* is indicated.

Perils of parenting

Parent to child transmission clearly operates over several generations. Less clear is the *effect of the child on the parent*, and the two-way impact of their exchange. At the best of times the arduous nature of parenting can feel persecuting when resources are depleted. When an unsupported parent is also highly sensitive and confused or delusional, the child's ordinary neediness may seem like a criticism of his/her poor parenting, which is then projected back into the child as hostile condemnation. Internalized, this in turn reinforces the child's sense of unentitlement and low self-esteem.

On the positive side, although it poses emotional challenges and unmanageable risks for both vulnerable parents and susceptible infants, caregiving, especially of very young children, also offers *new opportunities for reworking rather than enacting old grievances*. Through parenting collusive partners may differentiate from each other and acknowledge their own parents as both a reproductive couple and idiosyncratic individuals in their own right.

Parents' unresolved developmental issues are often reactivated as the child reaches an equivalent phase (Benedek, 1959). These weak links constitute the parental flash point, sometimes necessitating *therapy*. But, often, within the safety of a secure couple relationship, mothers and fathers can utilize the upsurge of revitalized emotions to liberate themselves from past restrictions, deprivations, and irrational prohibitions. In the absence of a loving extended family, parents benefit from creating one, by establishing a community of like-minded friends, joining an existing *self-support group* or participating in *groups exploring parenthood*, which offer encouragement pre- and postnatally, and at different stages of the child's development. Once again, presence of *a confidante* for a single mother, or resilience of the relationship for a couple, and their capacity to *share* both perils and pleasures of parenting will determine their mental health and emotional climate in the home.

Fathers

Dads are often relegated to a secondary position, treated as supporter or breadwinner, or in psychoanalytic parlance seen as the 'third' element, necessary to break the 'symbiosis' of the pre-oedipal mother–child dyad. Nonetheless, from the mid-seventies the literature reveals burgeoning awareness the father's affiliation in his own right, effects of his absence, and 'hunger' for the reality of this relationship (Gurwitt, 1976; Layland, 1981; Herzog, 1982; Lewis, 1986; Glasser, 1985; Cath et al., 1989). The relatively few longitudinal infant observations within families that do include the father, note both paternal input and parental rivalry over the baby (Yogman, 1982; Boston and Carter, 2002; Cardenal et al., 2002).

Researchers' sexual bias is reflected in studies. By contrast to 72 types of child psychopathology attributed directly to maternal care (Caplan and McCorquodale, 1985) only 1% of empirical clinical investigation is dedicated to fathers (Phares and Compas, 1992). These few studies indicate that paternal alcoholism, detachment, absence, panic disorders, and/or depression (Field et al., 1999) have deleterious effects, particularly on 'externalizing' behavioral problems in older children (Connell and Goodman, 2002). On the other hand, children of highly motivated involved fathers show increased cognitive competence, empathy, less sex stereotyped beliefs, and more internal control (see Pruett, 1992; Lamb, 1997). Effects of involuntary male primary care due to high unemployment is yet to be studied.

Parental orientations

Unlike tightly orchestrated traditional patterns, contemporary parenting allows for choice among a variety of ideologies and differing conceptions of caregiving. First time parents are often unprepared for the demands of parenthood—lacking babycare skills possessed by a 4 year old in developing societies. Furthermore, with smaller nuclear families and social mobility, many Westerners lack not only the supportive network, but the emotional experience of exposure to babies while growing up. As a result, most arrive at the point of parenthood with few realistic guidelines and many archaic grievances and irrational expectations intact, having failed to process their own infantile feelings in the evocative presence of an infant before the birth of their own.

In nondirective societies, such as our own at the moment, *the choice of goals and priorities informing a new parent's mode of parenting will be determined by their own unconscious internal model and current beliefs* (in addition to socioeconomic constraints). Like developmental theories, these internal paradigms vary from belief in the newborn as benign and vulnerable, to assumptions about innate aggression and need for socialization. Maternal orientations (predictable from pregnancy) include facilitation, regulation, and reciprocation (Raphael-Leff, 1986, 2005). A woman of the *Facilitator* orientation treats motherhood as a vocation and herself as uniquely able to fathom her infant's needs because of their close communion during pregnancy and breastfeeding. Therefore, keeping her baby in close proximity at all times, she devotes herself to adapting, spontaneously gratifying needs as they arise. Conversely, a *Regulator* mother tends to regard mothering as one role among many she performs. As she believes the newborn is undiscriminating and treats mothering as a learned skill, shared care is possible. Unlike the Facilitator who locates security in providing exclusive care, a Regulator establishes security in predictability. She introduces a routine that allows for consistent transferability between co-carers to regulate the adaptable baby and train him/her to fit in with social demands. Paternal orientations, too, include *Participators* who relish providing primary baby care and *Renouncers* who see it as 'women's work' until the child is older, when his paternal influence will be required. *Reciprocators* of either sex do not adapt (like the Facilitator) nor expect the baby to adapt (like the Regulator), but treat each incident as requiring thoughtful negotiation and responsive compromise.

Sympathetic partners (whatever their personal orientation) serve a protective function for each other. Conversely, when partners' ideas about caregiving clash, postnatal distress is often related to disjunctive dynamics between them or to obstacles preventing expression of their own optimal parenting style. Thus *enforced separation* from her baby (due to economic necessity or a medical problem) may precipitate depression in a Facilitator, while *enforced togetherness* (such as unemployment) triggers it in a Regulator (Raphael-Leff, 2005). A Participator partner relished by the Regulator, may feel persecutory to the Facilitator if he undermines the exclusivity of her care. Conversely, a traditional husband who forbids her to work, or the absence of help with child care and consequent lost sense of 'personhood', evokes postnatal distress in a would-be Regulator. A Renouncer may jealously guard his rights, feeling that his wife's excessive devotion to their baby detracts from his portion. An envious Participator father may unconsciously sabotage his wife's capacity to breastfeed. Fathers are not exempt from postnatal disturbance, which is often externalized in acting out and high alcohol consumption, and as noted by GP's and researchers alike, an increased incidence of psychosomatic symptoms and psychiatric morbidity (Lovestone and Kumar, 1993). Therapists and health professionals too, tend to be adherents of one particular orientation and puzzled by, or disapproving of parents who hold a different stance.

Lone parents and reconstituted families

Almost a quarter of American and British families are mother-headed. This may be due to death, desertion, separation, or choice. Interviews with over 5000 British women found a threefold risk of depression among single mothers (Targosz *et al.*, 2003). Four nationally representative studies of lone motherhood cite reduced income as the single most important disadvantage and cause of negative outcome.

Widowhood means children are affected by maternal bereavement as well as paternal loss and may feel excluded, especially where the topic of death is deliberately avoided. Secrecy, evasion, and lack of communication compound bewilderment leading to guilt, inability to mourn, and a pervasive sense of incompleteness. *Family grief counseling* may be indicated. Shared grief reduces adverse effects but offspring and surviving parent are often at different stages in their mourning (Robinson, 1996) and introduction of a step-parent may result in polarization, and unconscious splitting of the dead ideal and live substitute (Gorell Barnes *et al.*, 1998).

Desertion has long-term traumatic effects on the remaining partner's self-esteem especially when the disappearance is unanticipated and involves mystery. In addition to a sense of puzzlement, like the jilted parent, the abandoned children may feel guilt, rage, disillusionment, loss of an ideal, hopes, and expectations. In addition, she may experience intense feelings of jealousy and loneliness, with possible depression. *Individual or family therapy* may be necessary to prevent creeping role-reversal of the child caring for the distressed parent.

The quality of lone parenting as a result of *parental separation* is determined by both partners' capacity to resolve their own conflicts and the degree of preparation, explanation, and subsequent discussion with the child(ren). The latter's ability to sustain a mental relationship is crucial, at times in the face of the remaining parent's erasure of traces of the absent one and/or severing of contact. For both resident parent and child, psychological processes may involve a range of feelings from relief through shame, envy, rage, and grief affected very much by their resilience, the circumstances of separation, and degree of emotional support available. Open communication rather than denial of loss helps adjustment. Similarly, much is determined by the lone parent's inner state—psychosexual contentment with the separation, capacity to reflect, and curiosity, liveliness, and enjoyment of the parenting relationship.

When family disintegration coincides with crucial developmental transitions such as pregnancy in the woman or a child's entry to puberty, adaptive challenges and stresses are compounded, and in the latter case, associated with problems such as truancy, uncontrolled aggression, school drop out, teenage pregnancy, and minor delinquency. The lone parent may feel overburdened by these. However, although severe psychological and behavioral problems are two to three times more prevalent in children from divorcing families, 70–80% do not manifest severe or enduring problems (Hetherington and Stanley-Hagan, 1999). Nonetheless, multiply disadvantaged children are at high risk of developing conduct disorders, especially in adolescence. *Most studies attribute better adjustment to parents capable of providing a relatively conflict-free emotional climate of separation with cooperative shared supportive and consistent care.* Given strong evidence that during the painful conflictual process of separation itself many children experience difficulties with peers and schoolwork, *mediation or 'conciliation' counseling* to help incompatible partners cum parents to separate appropriately seems to be as important as *couple therapy* to help others to stay together.

Men are likely to 're-partner' more quickly. However, as 90% (!) of children live with their mothers they are most affected by *her* choices such as introduction of a stepfather and/or *'reconstituted' step family*. Women are

deemed 'less inept' at introducing a new partner and outcome studies indicate relative ease of accepting step-fathers compared with step-mothers, especially before age 7 and if the household routine is maintained in the previous style. Stepmothers generally fare worse, are often demonized with mythical 'wicked' malevolence, and doomed to fail, due to higher expectations that women act as emotional carers for traumatized kids (Robinson, 1996). Jealousy over lost intimacy with the lone biological parent and rivalry with new children raises emotional issues that may require *therapeutic help* (see Gorell Barnes *et al.*, 1998).

In all these situations there is no single pathway of adaptation, no set sequences of stresses, or timescale for resolution. Much is dependent on connection to an extended family and particularly the role of grandparents in mitigating the disintegration of an old way of life, maintaining links, and establishing order and closeness in the new one. In families with very young children, secrecy may prevail with fictions regarding true paternity engineering a break with the past. Conversely, when the separation coincides with a child's entry to adolescence, the double emotional adaptation may result in withdrawal and avoidance or increased turbulence, including arguments, hostility about displacement and possible violence. When *family therapy* is not an option, young people's *walk-in counseling clinics* may provide a neutral place for airing grievances and discussion.

In addition to these disrupted families, another group of fatherless children are those raised from the outset by a single mother. Longitudinal studies comparing one and two parent families find that *single mothers by choice* express greater warmth towards their child(ren) who, unsurprisingly are also found to be more secure and unlikely to develop emotional or behavioral problems (although they perceived themselves to be *less* cognitively and physically competent than peers living with two parents). Similarly, lone lesbian mothers, who in addition, engage in more interaction with the child compared with heterosexual single mothers (Golombok *et al.*, 1997). Findings suggest that children of lone mothers are not disadvantaged in relation to their mothers, but express lower self-esteem related to absence of a second adult.

Infertility

The contemporary increase in fertility problems is almost equally distributed between men and women. Subfertility is partly a natural function of aging due to postponement of childbearing, and partly attributable to environmental toxins, increased intake of medications, and after-effects of a rising incidence of sexually transmitted diseases. Only a very small proportion of cases of 'unexplained' infertility may be attributable to psychological causes, and this is decreasing with refined diagnostic techniques. However, when people *are* referred for psychotherapy for *psychogenic inhibition of fertility*, *psychodynamic treatment* can be effective in addressing the underlying unconscious prohibitions and associations (Christie and Morgan, 2003).

The majority of people suffer from the *psychological impact* of any/all of four aspects of infertility itself:

◆ the prolonged period of trying to conceive

◆ the blow of infertility assessment and diagnosis

◆ the unremitting demands and increasingly bizarre nature of treatment procedures

◆ and the outcome—whether accommodating to enforced childlessness, or to birth of a child after so much hope and anxiety (Raphael-Leff, 1992, 2001).

Contraception has fostered an illusion of control over fertility. Discovering that conception does not necessarily follow emotional readiness for a baby can feel devastating. Dawning realization that something is wrong often leads to mortification, and disagreement within the couple as to whether to seek help or give up on the idea of having children. One partner may feel satisfied with the richness of their life or resigned to fate. Or anxious about shameful exposure and/or fearful of bodily incursion during investigations. The other may ache for a child or feel desperately hurt and cheated. *Counseling or couple therapy* can explore these differences enabling some resolution—whether rewarding 'child-free' lives, or a decision to pursue treatment.

Investigations can be prolonged and involve physically invasive, painful, and humiliating procedures, including postcoital tests and reports to a third party about their private lovemaking. Scrutiny activates sexual problems and impotence. *Psychosexual counseling* addresses tensions exacerbated by routine hospital procedures (Pengelly *et al.*, 1995). Old feelings of disgrace and incapability come flooding back, as attitudes towards the omnipotent parents of childhood are transferred on to the fertile experts. *Diagnosis* produces a further self-deprecating sense of feminine insufficiency or, conflating virility and potency, masculine embarrassment about quality of sperm. Partners experience shame at needing help 'to do what any animal can'. Feeling singled out a couple may isolate themselves in secrecy, deeming themselves outcasts from the human race, overwhelmed by powerful emotions of envy, rage, sadness, and despair. Seeking meaning, the past is scanned for punishment-deserving misdemeanors, and animosity festers in self-recriminations or accusations. *An existential crisis occurs at being last of a genealogical line.* When only one partner is infertile and resents the asymmetry of their positions, this leads to further acrimony, self-sacrificial separation demands/declarations and even threatened suicide. *Individual* or *couple therapy* becomes imperative to restore equilibrium and reappraise their resources in the light of the new situation. Evaluation after 6 months of *cognitive-behavior therapy* found an improvement in sperm concentration, a reduction in thoughts of helplessness and a decrease in marital distress (Tuschen-Caffier, 1999). At this junction too, some will opt for medical treatment, others will accept childlessness together, or negotiate the fostering/adoption route or indeed, decide to separate.

Treatment brings yet another host of emotional roller-coasters, with recurrent cycles of hope and despair, elation and deflation. Beguiled by promise of increasingly fantastic solutions, the momentum often prevents the couple's pause to reconsider personal needs. Nonetheless, they periodically reassess their desire for parenthood, weighing up the emotional, physical, and financial toll of their predicament against the intensity of their wish for a child. Lucky ones conceive; others continue to pursue conception, often well into menopause. Some desist from IVF treatment, allowing fate to take its course. Resigning themselves to childlessness, some grieve their losses, take up contraception again, finding emotionally rewarding avenues apart from parenting. Yet others now invest their energies in pursuing increasingly unattainable adoption of a baby. A proportion go on to seek solutions that may involve receiving donated gametes/fertilized embryo, or surrogate gestation. In these cases reproduction becomes a medically orchestrated production, with long-term emotional repercussions for offspring and parents.

Because assisted reproductive 'success' is often measured by conception, *parenthood* following prolonged infertility may come as a surprise, fraught with the sudden switch of self-image and extensive demands, often involving treatment-induced twins or triplets and complications due to prematurity. Nevertheless, a study of IVF mothers rate them as highly attentive and the infants more playful (Papaligoura and Trevarthen, 2001), perhaps because of the emotional investment of producing them. In all cases, provision of a *therapeutic space* for individuals/couples/families to think about the ramifications of their ordeals benefits all involved.

Finally, to the question of why some people are so devastated by the inability to conceive while others adjust, albeit with sadness. This seems related to 'generative identity'. I propose that childhood recognition of the limitations of *sex* (being male or female), *genesis* (not self-made), *generation* (only adults procreate), and *generativity* (it takes two) can take three courses, either: (1) acquiescence and promise of future reproduction; (2) denial, leading to gender dysfunctions; or (3) a poetic leap into creativity as a means of imaginatively overcoming restrictions and deferment. In adulthood, infertility hits hardest those who have unconsciously invested all their potential creativity in deferred procreativity (Raphael-Leff, 1997, 2001).

The 'third individuation'

Mid-life crisis

The mid-life paradox is that of 'entering the prime of life, the stage of fulfillment, but at the same time the prime and fulfillment are dated. Death lies beyond' (Jaques, 1965, p. 504). Somewhere between 35 and 45 most of us begin to realize that half of life is over. Points of reference change with the individual's realization that s/he 'has stopped growing up, and has begun to grow old' (Jaques, 1965, p. 505). Taking stock we register unachieved youthful dreams and the unlikelihood of our anticipated outstanding contribution.

Mid-life reevaluation is precipitated by changing relationships to elderly or dead parents, to childlessness or self-reliant children. Shocked by illness or unexpected deaths we register signs of the biological clock's slowing down in our own bodies. Crisis may take the form of self-doubts, uncontrolled weeping, panic attacks, fear of loss or accidents, nonspecific anxieties, and resistance to change. *Pertinent catalysts are failure of personal ideals and collapse of defensive illusions of reversibility, correctability and invincibility.* Memory loss, discovery of one's ineffectuality at work or elsewhere, lack of influence over colleagues, politicians, or family members accompany growing awareness of one's own mortality. The quandary begins with a sense of irritation, confusion, and futility, which is then suppressed, or denied by manic counteractivity, but nevertheless returns with increasing insistence and urgency. Although dissatisfaction or meaninglessness is often pinned on environmental factors, ultimately we come to identify interior origins of our own state of mind. In health the process forms a cyclical sense of defendedness against 'alienation'. As conflicts we try to resolve prematurely gradually build up, this leads either to inauthentic solutions and 'stagnation', or to a courageous self-examination promoting 'regeneration' and a gradual shift from reliance on external to internal referents (Polden, 2002).

Elaboration and enrichment

Freud's is one of the earliest depictions of a mid-life crisis. His self-analysis began aged 40 after the emotional upheaval instigated by his father's death. Delineating shared origins of dreams and symptoms, he combined his ambition to be a scientist and theoretician with his youthful dream of becoming a great healer (Lohser and Newton, 1996). Some years later, the 37-year-old Jung described both the pain of his split from Freud, and the fruitfulness of his psychological turmoil eventually leading to individuation (Jung, 1930). Like Freud's generalization from recognizing oedipal residues and intimations of mortality in himself, Jung also emphasized applicability of his theories to others. Erikson (1980) indicates that vicissitudes of growth following crises are determined by the subject's capacity to be identified with others. *The ability to feel that one belongs to a whole—a family, a society, the human race—makes the idea of one's individual finitude tolerable.*

The psychological scene of the reality and inevitability of one's own eventual personal demise is defined by Jaques (the psychoanalyst who invented the phrase 'mid-life crisis'), as its central and crucial feature. Death—at the conscious level—instead of being a general conception, or an event experienced in terms of the loss of someone else, becomes 'a personal matter, one's own death, one's own real and actual mortality' (Jaques, 1965).

Self-transformation induced by the changing sense of time includes reappraising the past and questioning future actions. By liberating ourselves in middle adulthood from the codes and regulations of those who formed us, we gain freedom but have to relinquish illusions of absolute safety and familiar assumptions that guided us (Gould, 1993). Reexamination of values and expectations occurs with a gradual acceptance of becoming an 'elder' (Settlage *et al.*, 1988). Preoccupation with time restrictions and aging instigate a powerful *intrapsychic shift from being left to leaving*, culminating in late adulthood coming to grips with illness/death of contemporaries and oneself (Colarusso, 2000). Grandparenthood may form a narcissistic buffer against old age, providing emotional refueling and a sense of genetic continuity as well as a screen against separation anxiety regarding the shrinking self and world. It offers a benign means of denying imperfections in oneself by selective identification with desirable qualities of the grandchild (Cath *et al.*, 1989). Likewise, the mature individual may achieve a form of wisdom that enables him or her to become a 'keeper of meaning', guiding others in the preservation of past cultural achievements (Vaillant and Koury, 1993).

Part of mid-life development takes place within intimate relationships wherein unconscious heritage and irrational forces from the past are recognized as obsolete 'scripts'. *Healthy relationships are predicated on respect for separateness and ability to tolerate difference and integrate contradictions.* In couples, this depends on *synchronous* rather than asymmetrical personal growth of both partners, who also simultaneously work at deepening the relationship itself. However, separations after collapse of long-term commitment or a partner's death may prompt growth. In the absence of the Other (unconsciously relied on to process or 'hold' one's feelings) inhibited people may experience an upsurge of autonomy or recognize their emotional vulnerabilities (see Polden, 2002).

Similarly, a time comes in middle age when we begin to question the unrewarding achievement-oriented busyness of our pressured lives. Typically, resistance to insight in middle age externalizes internal conflicts on to relationships or work situations. Initially, the solution seems to lie in life-style modifications—drastic changes of environment, job, and/or partner. Excitement of an illicit sexual passion, romantic escape to sea or countryside, compulsive activity or conversely, withdrawal from work in absenteeism or stress-related illness. However, when the erotic affair becomes domesticated or the new place overfamiliar, mid-life discontent returns with a vengeance as the external solution fails and internal patterns reassert their defensive hold. The definition of mid-life depression as *'inhibition of feared aggression in the face of loss of status'* (Polden, 2002, p. 226) links the destructive grip of depressive guilt, self-doubt, and helplessness to breakdown of defensive coping mechanisms. *Psychotherapy* explores how avoidant or ambivalent defenses were originally developed to combat early insecurity.

Late onset disorders

Although men continue to be fertile until their 80s, a common feature of later years noted by a variety of practitioners and researchers is *a decrease in gender dimorphism*. The phantasmic integration (possibly eased in both sexes by biochemical changes and hormonal reductions) of feminine and masculine aspects of the self, which might have been suppressed earlier in adulthood. Jung (1930) described 'psychic androgeny' after a 6-year period of numerous dreams and intrapsychic struggles, during which he coined the term *'anima'* to describe his own feminine muse.

This shift towards 'psychic bisexuality' (as Freud called it) is not without its stresses, particularly in macho men, who passionately pursue overt masculinity. An Older Adult Program at Northwestern Medical School found that first hospital admissions for acute psychiatric illness in men aged 55–65 revealed similar early histories underpinning a variety of presenting symptoms, ranging from severe alcoholism, diffuse anxiety states, to significant and often suicidal depression or paranoid psychosis in a wide socioeconomic and ethnic spectrum of patients. Hemmingway is cited as an example of this syndrome. The common denominator of breakdown is a sense of 'manhood at risk'. Case histories reveal repudiated early identification with a 'destructively dominating' gender-defying mother while at the same time unconsciously retaining her 'driving ego ideal' for him to resemble the maternal grandfather. Simultaneously, denied affection for, yet identification with, the defeated fathers (Gutmann, 1990). Male late onset disturbance begins with threatened reemergence of early feminine traits, usually connected to increasing mid-life independence of a previously submissive, needy wife for whom he served as Protector. As cultural acceptance of female assertiveness increases, the equivalent crisis in women is recognizable as a feature of hysteria, obsessionality, or manic disinhibition.

The major form of psychic disability in older people worldwide is *depression*, peaking around mid-life and again in old age. Many times more prevalent in women, depression is consistently linked to stressful life events entailing losses: breakdown of marriage or bereavement; menopause, loss of sexual attractiveness and fertility; failed hope of having a child or loss of identity related to 'empty nest' sense of worthlessness, and/or declining professional recognition with belated motherhood or retirement. In women late onset psychoses too, tends to be depressive.

Loss and individuation

A *'third individuation'* (Oldham, 1988) occurs when, caring for aging parents, middle-aged 'children' are suffused with revived recollections of the invincible parents of childhood. Watching them falter brings home human frailty and the inevitability of pain and eventual death. Illness, separation, and loss inevitably arouse intimations of mortality and lack of a parental buffer between self and grave shifts one generation. *Loss of living repositories of early experience leads to poignant awareness of one's own faulty archival memory and potentialities that are no longer possible.* Regression and turmoil, resurfaced unresolved parent–child conflicts sometimes results in prolonged 'melancholia' rather than mourning. Bereavement, with adult reworking of the integrative 'depressive position' (Klein, 1940), leads to relinquishing omnipotent forms of mental functioning, allowing appreciation of long denied losses. This new crisis often brings mature people to *analysis or therapy* with great benefit. Accepting loss brings liberation and the further stage of autonomy achieved by confronting one's own mortality and limitations.

Interestingly, studies of *spousal loss* in mid- and later-life find that bereaved partners who showed little grief after their spouses died were the best adapted over a 7-year follow-up, apparently related to realistic adult expectations. Although grief reactions are varied and not highly predictable from the dynamics of mourning, they are intrinsically self-limiting. The less stunting the marital relationship prior to the death, the more limited the grieving, and the greater the probability of personal growth (Lieberman, 1993). Prolonged grief responses involve the highest dependency, guilt, and anger toward the deceased and benefit from *bereavement counseling/therapy*.

Sex differences are striking with 25–30% of successful suicides following spousal death occurring in men over 65; far fewer occur in older women seemingly due to their anticipation of widowhood and preparation for loss. Women tend to place more emphasis on relatedness than men, engaging others in emotionally satisfying ways that bring about a 'postspousal individuation' (Colorusso, 2000)—flowering follows mourning, learning to be alone as opposed to lonely. Others dedicate themselves to grandmotherhood, travel, or study, or find new creative resources within themselves and a sense of liberation.

Relationship to time and memory

Time is relative. If in healthy adulthood the 20s are a transition period in which attitudes toward time are still strongly influenced by childhood experience and physical growth, the 30s constitute an adult watershed. Now too old to die young (Dorfman, M., 1994, personal communication), time sense is dominated by mid-life themes, as signs of physical aging shatter childhood and adolescent notions of time in unlimited supply, which is gradually replaced by 'the shift from time left to live to time lived' (Neugarten, 1979, p. 890). As puberty forces psychic reorganization, so dwindling fertility changes the sense of self. Approaching 40 the shift from 'physical progression in childhood to physical retrogression in adulthood' is integrated. A poignant emotional sophistication experienced by a healthy individual as 'an exquisite mental state which, perhaps more than any other, defines what it means to be human' (Boschan, 1990).

Time operates on memories, bringing trauma within the purview of the self. Freud's theory of *'nachträglichkeit'* locates psychic-metabolization of experience in 'retranscription'—stratified reframing or recontextualization of memory at each new developmental phase ('successive registrations represent the psychic achievement of successive epochs of life' (Freud, Dec. 6, 1896). A central feature of the emotional upheaval of later life is reformulation of past experience within a different sense of human temporality; and acceptance of irreversibility and finitude.

The intensity of a mid-life crisis clearly relates to disturbances in defenses that have served to deny death. Patients with predominantly narcissistic pathology often stop and 'freeze' time both to negate their own finitude and to protect themselves from contact with emotions, their own and others'. As omnipotent control of time fails, they are confronted with ticking of the biological clock and inevitability of death. In therapy they reveal the threat of destruction posed by others and a narcissistic difficulty in subject/object discrimination (Boschan, 1990). Similarly, confrontation with the fact that time is running out for the achievement of grandiose dreams, may result in despair. Finally, Time stretches ahead to be filled. In women, relative longevity raises the odds they may live as long after menopause as before it (Greer, 1991), and those who have lived in the shadow of others may feel invisible or suicidal in their absence.

Psychoanalytic or psychodynamic therapy fosters the central task of accepting reality limitations and overcoming the fear of death (presented symbolically as fear of psychic death), which may release creativity, depending on the quality of internal relationships. Integration of essentially realistic positive internalizations in the course of therapy creates a benign psychological context that enables the individual to cope more effectively with subsequent vicissitudes of the life cycle that begin with a mid-life crisis and continue throughout aging and senescence (Blatt and Blass, 1990).

Psychotherapy in mid- and later-life

Both the old idea of phase-specific maturational tasks and contemporary emphasis on a potential for continuous (albeit nonlinear) growth have fostered growing acceptance of *older adult therapy* (contrary to Freud's pessimism about nonamenable rigidity). Indeed, therapy is sought for specifically age-related issues—such as diminution of potency, changing marital relations and/or empty nest syndrome; retirement or loss of effectiveness at work; aging, the race against time and the inevitability of death. *'Developmental tasks' achieved by mid-life relate to 'love, work, and play': ability to enjoy one's sexuality; capacity to relate to people in depth; awareness of one's ambivalence and concern about aggression towards one's loved ones; satisfaction in hard work, leisure and meaningfulness of life.* Failure in any of these indicate pathological defenses (Jaques, 1965; King, 1980; Hildebrand, 1982; Kernberg, 1993; Limentani, 1995).

In conclusion, exceedingly rapid contemporary sociocultural changes, complex postmodern admixtures, and fragmentation create disordered life cycle sequences and disrupted intrapsychic and psychosocial adaptive systems. Seen in this context, disturbances often form a defensive reorganization, breakdown, or arrest with a potential for reformulation and change. *Therapy in later life* offers space for contemplation for those who cannot find it in solitude. When the capacity to enjoy being alone has not been acquired in the childhood presence of a loving nonimpinging carer, it may have to be learned (and fear of solitude unlearned) in the presence of a therapist (Winnicott, 1958). *The invariable ingredients in all types of therapy are provision of a safe confidential space and reliable, neutral but caring therapist.* Growth of the therapist by confronting suppressed aspects of his/her self stirred up while sitting with the patient, will reflect both intrapsychic and interpersonal pressures.

While *cognitively oriented therapies* rely on guided reformulations of maladaptive patterns to install more rational ones, *psychodynamic treatments* encourage emotional reexperiencing of past configurations within the therapeutic sanctuary, and freedom to explore anything that arises in the mind, however irrational. Words (and silence) within the 'playground' of therapy often disclose unprocessed archaic forces coexisting alongside increasing sophistication. Older adults who can relinquish certitude and overcome resistance to ambiguity, gradually form newly discovered unconscious linkages thereby enriching a well worn narrative of love, work, and play.

References

Aronson, S. (1996). The bereavement process in children of parents with AIDS. *Psychoanalytic Study of the Child*, **51**, 422–35.

Benedek, T. (1959). Parenthood as a developmental phase: a contribution to libido theory. *Journal American Psychoanalytic Association*, **7**, 389–417.

Blatt, S. J. and Blass, R. B. (1990). Attachment and separateness: a dialectical model of the products and processes of development throughout the lifecycle *Psychoanalytic Study of the Child*, **45**, 107–27.

Bollas, C. (1979). The transformational object, *International Journal of Psycho-Analysis*, **60**, 97–107. (Also in *The Shadow of the Object* 1987, London: Free Association.)

Bolton, H. L., Hughes, P. M., Turton, P., and Sedgwick, P. (1998). Incidence and demographic correlates of depressive symptoms during pregnancy in an inner London population, *Abstracts*, **19**, Dec. 4.

Boschan, P. (1990). Temporality and narcissism. *International Review of Psycho-Analysis*, **17**, 337–49.

Boston, M. and Carter, U. (2002). 'Daddy and me'—observing a young couple and their baby, from birth to two years. *Infant Observation—The International Journal of Infant Observation and its Applications*, **5**, 16–38.

Bourne, S. and Lewis, E. (2003). Pregnancy after stillbirth or neonatal death: psychological risks. In: J. Raphael-Leff, ed. *Parent-infant psychodynamics—wild things, mirrors and ghosts*, Ch. 22, pp. 275–83. London: Whurr, 2003. (Originally in *Lancet* 1984, 31–3.)

Brown, G. W., Harris, T. O., and Hepworth, C. (1995). Loss, humiliation and entrapment among women developing depression: a patient and non-patient comparison, *Psychological Medicine*, **25**, 7–21.

Burke, L. (2003). The impact of maternal depression on familial relationships. *International Review of Psychiatry*, **15**, 243–55.

Caelli, K., Downie, J., and Letendre, A. (2002). Parent's experience of midwife-managed care following the loss of a baby in a previous pregnancy. *Journal of Advanced Nursing*, **39**, 127–36.

Caplan, P. and McCorquodale, I. (1985). Mother blaming in major clinical journals. *American Journal of Orthopsychiatry*, **55**, 345–53.

Cardenal, M., Di Carlo, C., and Ganara, C. (2002). Play and the function of the father *Infant Observation, The International Journal of Infant Observation and its Applications*, **5**, 556–69.

Cath, S. H., Gurwitt, A., and Gunsberg, L. (1989). *Fathers and their families*. Hillsdale, NJ: The Analytic Press.

Christie, G. and Morgan, A. (2003). Love, hate and the generative couple. In: J. Haynes and J. Miller, ed. *Inconceivable conceptions—psychological aspects of infertility and reproductive technology*, Ch. 9, pp. 86–103. London: Bruner-Routledge.

Clulow, C., Dearnley, B., and Balfour, F. (1986). Shared fantasy and therapeutic structure in a brief marital therapy. *British Journal of Psychotherapy*, **3**, 124–43.

Cockett, M. and Tripp, J. (1994). Children living in re-ordered families (review). *Social Policy Research Findings*, No. 45, February: The Exeter Study, London: Joseph Rowntree Foundation.

Coghan, C. L. and Kleinbaum, S. (2002). Toward a greater understanding of the cohabitation effect. *Journal Marriage and Family*, **64**, 180–92.

Colarusso, C. A. (2000). Separation-individuation phenomena in adulthood: general concepts and the fifth individuation. *Journal American Psychoanalytic Association*, **48**, 1467–89.

Connell, A. and Goodman, S. (2002). The association between psychopathology in fathers versus mother and children's internalising and externalising behaviour problems: a meta analysis. *Psychological Bulletin*, **128**, 746–73.

Cott, A. D. and Wisner, K. L. (2003). Psychiatric disorders during pregnancy. *International Review of Psychiatry*, **15**, 217–30.

Cox, A. D., Puckering, C., Pound, A., and Mills, M. (1987). The impact of maternal depression in young children. *Journal of Child Psychology and Psychiatry*, **28**, 917–28.

Cox, J. L., Murray, D., and Chapman, G. (1993). A controlled study of onset, duration and prevalence of postnatal depression. *British Journal of Psychiatry*, **163**, 27–31.

Craig, T. and Pathare, S. (2000). Gender differences in the experience and response to adversity. In: T. Harris, ed. *Where inner and outer worlds meet—psychosocial research in the tradition of George W Brown*, pp. 211–26. London: Routledge.

Dicks, H. V. (1963). Object relations theory and marital studies. *British Journal of Medical Psychology*, 36, 125–9.

Da Costa, D., Larouche, J., Drista, M., and Brender, W. (2000). Psychosocial correlates of prepartum and postpartum depressed mood. *Journal of Affective Disorders*, 59, 31–40.

Dong, M., Anda, R. F., Dube, S. R., Giles, W. H., and Felitti, V. J. (2003). The relationship of exposure to childhood sexual abuse to other forms of abuse, neglect and household dysfunction during childhood. *Child Abuse and Neglect*, 27, 625–39.

Dutton, D. G. and Holzworth-Munroe, A. (1997). The role of early trauma in males who assault their wives. In: D. Cicchetti and S. L. Toth, ed. *Developmental perspectives on trauma: theory, research and intervention*. Rochester Symposium on Developmental Psychology, 8, pp. 370–401.

Emde, R. N. (1985). From adolescence to midlife: remodeling the structure of adult development. *Journal American Psychoanalytic Association*, 33(Suppl.), 59–112.

Erikson, E. H. (1950). *Childhood and society*. New York: W. W. Norton.

Erikson, E. H. (1980). On the generational cycle an address. *International Journal of Psycho-Analysis*, 61, 213–23.

Evans, J., Heron, J., Francomb, H., Oke, S., and Golding, J. (2001). Cohort study of depressed mood during and after childbirth. *British Medical Journal*, 323, 257–60.

Field, T., Hussain, Z., and Malphurs, J. (1999). *Infant Mental Health Journal*, 20, 322–32.

Fraiberg, S., Adelson, E., and Shapiro, U. (1975). Ghosts in the nursery: a psychoanalytic approach to the problems of impaired mother-infant relationships. *Journal of the American Academy of Child Psychiatry*, 14, 387–421.

Freud, S. (1896/1985). J. M. Masson, ed. *The complete letters of Sigmund Freud to Wilhelm Fliess 1887–1904*. Cambridge, MA: Belknap, Harvard.

Freud, S. (1917). Mourning and melancholia. In: J. Strachey, trans. and ed. *The Standard Edition of the complete psychological works of Sigmund Freud*, Vol. 14. London: Hogarth Press, 1955.

Freud, S. (1930). Civilisation and its discontents. In: J. Strachey, trans. and ed. *The Standard Edition of the complete psychological works of Sigmund Freud*, Vol. 21. London: Hogarth Press, 1955.

Glasser, M. (1985). The 'weak spot'—some observations on male sexuality. *International Journal of Psycho-Analysis*, 66, 405–14.

Golombok, S., Tasker, F., and Murray, C. (1997). Children raised in fatherless families from infancy: family relationships and socioemotional development of children of lesbian and single heterosexual mothers. *Journal of Child Psychology and Psychiatry*, 38, 783–92.

Gopfert, M., Webster, J., and Seeman, M., ed. (1996). *Parental psychiatric disorder—distressed parents and their families*. Cambridge: Cambridge University Press.

Gorell Barnes, J. (1998). *Family therapy in changing times*. Basic Texts in Counselling and Psychotherapy. London: MacMillan.

Gorell Barnes, J., Thompson, P., Daniel, G., and Burchardt, N. (1998). *Growing up in step-families*. Oxford: Clarendon Press.

Gould, R. (1993). Transformational tasks in adulthood. In: G. H. Pollock and S. I. Greenspan, ed. *The course of life. Vol. VI. Late adulthood*. Madison, CT: International Universities Press.

Greer, G. (1991). *The change*. London: Hamish Hamilton.

Gurwitt, A. (1976). Aspects of prospective fatherhood—a case report. *Psychoanalytic Study of the Child*, 31, 237–71.

Gutmann, D. (1990). Psychological development and pathology in later life. In: R. A. Nemiroff and C. A. Colarusso, ed. *New dimensions in adult development*, pp. 170–85. New York: Basic Books.

Healy, K. and Kennedy, R. (1993). Which families benefit from inpatient psychotherapeutic work at the Cassel Hospital? *British Journal of Psychotherapy*, 9, 394–404.

Heaton, T. B. (2002). Factors contributing to increasing marital stability in the US. *Journal of Family Issues*, 23, 392.

Heinicke, C. M., Finemean, N. R., Ponce, V. A., and Guthrie, D. (2001). Relation-based intervention with at-risk mothers: outcome in the second year of life. *Infant Mental Health Journal*, 22, 431–9.

Herzog, J. (1982). Patterns of expectant fatherhood: a study of the fathers of a group of premature infants. In: S. Cath, A. Gurwitt, and J. M. Ross, ed. *Father and child—developmental and clinical perspectives*, pp. 301–14. Boston: Little, Brown and Co.

Hetherington, E. M. and Stanley-Hagan, M. (1999). The adjustment of children with divorced parents: a risk and resiliency perspective. *Journal of Child Psychology and Psychiatry and Allied Disciplines*, 40, 129–40.

Hildebrand, P. (1982). Psychotherapy with older patients. *British Journal of Medical Psychology*, 55, 19–25.

Hobcraft, J. and Kiernan, K. (1995). *Becoming a parent in Europe*. Discussion paper WSP 116, Welfare State Programme. London: LSE.

Hopper, E. (2003). *The social unconscious: selected papers*. London: Jessica Kingsley Publishers.

ISER Report. (2000/1). Colchester, UK: University of Essex.

Jaques, E. (1965). Death and the mid-life crisis. *International Journal of Psychoanalysis*, 46, 502–14.

Jung, C. G. (1930). The stages of life. In: *Modern man in search of a soul*. London: Routledge, 1984.

Kernberg, O. (1993). The couple's constructive and destructive superego functions. *Journal of the American Psychoanalytic Association*, 41, 653–77.

Kiernan, K. (1997). Becoming a young parent: a longitudinal study of associated factors. *British Journal of Sociology*, 48, 406–28.

King, P. (1980). The life cycle as indicated by the nature of the transference in the psychoanalysis of the middle-aged and elderly. *International Journal of Psycho-Analysis*, 61, 153–60.

Klein, M. (1940/1988). Mourning and its relation to manic-depressive states. In: *Love, Guilt and Reparation*. London: Virago.

Kuipers, E., Leff, J., and Lam, D. (2002). *Family work for schizophrenia—a practical guide*. London: Gaskell Press (Royal College of Psychiatrists).

Lamb, M. E. (1997). The development of father-infant relationships. In: *The role of the father in child development*, 3rd edn. New York: Wiley and Sons.

Lanman, M. (2003). Assessment for couple psychoanalytic psychotherapy. *British Journal of Psychotherapy*, 19, 309–24.

Lasch, C. (1978). *The culture of narcissism*. New York: Norton and Co.

Layland, W. R. (1981). In search of a loving father. *International Journal of Psycho-Analysis*, 62, 215–24.

Leach, P. (1996). Who comes first—partner or child? In: C. Clulow, ed. *Partners becoming parents—talks from the Tavistock Marital Studies Institute*, pp. 32–43. London: Sheldon Press.

Lewis, C. (1986). *Becoming a father*. Milton Keynes: Open University Press.

Lieberman, M. A. (1993). A reexamination of adult life crises: spousal loss in mid- and late life. In: G. H. Pollock and S. I. Greenspan, ed. *The course of life*, Vol. 6: *late adulthood*, pp. 69–110. Madison, CT: International Universities Press.

Limentani, A. (1995). Creativity and the Third Age. *International Journal of Psycho-Analysis*, 76, 825–33.

Lloyd-Owen, D. (2003). Perverse females: their unique psychopathology. *British Journal of Psychotherapy*, 19, 285–97.

Lohser, B. and Newton, P. M. (1996). *The unorthodox Freud: the view from the couch*. New York: Guilford Press.

Lovestone, S. and Kumar, R. (1993). Postnatal psychiatric illness: the impact on partners. *The British Journal of Psychiatry*, 163, 210–16.

Marks, M. N., Hipwell, A., and Kumar, R. (2002). Implications for the infant of maternal puerperal psychiatric disorders. In: M. Rutter and E. Taylor, ed. *Child and adolescent psychiatry*, 4th edn, pp. 858–77. Oxford: Blackwell Science.

Mintzer, D., Als, H., Tronick, E. Z., and Brazelton, T. B. (1984). Parenting an infant with a birth defect—the regulation of self-esteem. *Psychoanalytic Study of the Child*, 39, 561–89. (Also in J. Raphael-Leff, ed. *Parent-infant psychodynamics—wild things, mirrors and ghosts*. London: Whurr, 2003.)

Mowbry, B. J. and Lennon, D. P. (1998). Puerperal psychosis: associated clinical features in psychiatric hospital mother-baby unit. *Australian and New Zealand Journal of Psychiatry*, 32, 287–90.

Murray, L. and Cooper, P., ed. (1997). *Post partum depression and child development*, London: Guilford Press.

Neugarten, B. (1979). Time, age and the life cycle. *American Journal of Psychiatry*, 136, 887–94.

Oates, M. (2002). Adverse effects of maternal antenatal anxiety on children: causal effect or Developmental continuum? *British Journal of Psychiatry*, **180**, 478–9.

O'Connor, T. G., Heron, J., Glover, V., and the Alspac Study Team (2002). Antenatal anxiety predicts child behavioral emotional problems independently of postnatal depression. *Journal of American Academy of Child and Adolescent Psychiatry*, **41**, 1470–7.

Oldham, J. M. (1988). The middle years. Panel, G. Ahem and W. Jacobson, reporters. *Bulletin Association of Psychoanalytic Medicine*, **27**, 77–80.

Papaligoura, Z. and Trevarthen, C. (2001). Mother-infant communication can be enhanced after conception by in-vitro fertilisation. *Infant Mental Health Journal*, **22**, 591–604.

Patel, V., Araya, R., de Lima, M., Ludermir, A., and Todd, C. (1999). Women, poverty and common mental disorders in four restructuring societies. *Social Science and Medicine*, **49**, 1461–71.

Pengelly, P., Inglis, M., and Cudmore, L. (1995). Infertility: couples' experiences and the use of counselling in treatment centres. *Psychodynamic Counselling*, **1**, 4.

Phares, V. and Compas, B. E. (1992). The role of fathers in child and adolescent psychopathology: make room for daddy. *Psychological Bulletin*, **111**, 387–412.

Pitt, B. (1968). 'Atypical' depression following childbirth. *British Journal of Psychiatry*, **114**, 1325–35.

Polden, J. (2002). *Regeneration—journey through the mid-life crisis*. London: Continuum.

Pound, A. (1996). Parental affective disorder and childhood disturbance. In: M. Gopfert, J. Webster, and M. V. Seeman, ed. *Parental psychiatric disorder—distressed parents and their families*, pp. 201–18. Cambridge: Cambridge University Press.

Pruett, K. (1992). Latency development in children of primary nurturing fathers—eight-year follow-up. *Psychoanalytic Study of the Child*, **47**, 85–101.

Puckering, C., *et al.* (1994). Process and evaluation of a group intervention for mothers with parenting difficulties. *Child Abuse Review*, **3**, 299–310.

Raphael-Leff, J. (1986). Facilitators and Regulators: conscious and unconscious processes in pregnancy and early motherhood. *British Journal of Medical Psychology*, **59**, 43–55.

Raphael-Leff, J. (1992). The baby-makers: an in-depth single-case study of conscious and unconscious psychological reactions to infertility and 'baby-making'. *British Journal of Psychotherapy*, **8**, 266–77.

Raphael-Leff, J. (1993). *Pregnancy—the inside story*. London: Karnac, 2001.

Raphael-Leff, J. (1997). Procreative process, placental paradigm and perinatal psychotherapy, *Journal of the American Psychoanalytic Association* (Female Psychology Supplement), **44**, 373–99.

Raphael-Leff, J. (2000a). 'Climbing the walls': puerperal disturbance and perinatal therapy. In: J. Raphael-Leff, ed. *Spilt milk—perinatal loss and breakdown*, pp. 60–81. London: Institute of Psychoanalysis, London: Routledge.

Raphael-Leff, J. (2000b). 'Behind the shut door'—a psychoanalytical approach to premature menopause. In: D. Singer and M. Hunter, ed. *Premature menopause—a multidisciplinary approach*. London: Whurr publishers.

Raphael-Leff, J. (2001). 'Gift of gametes'—intrapsychic, interpersonal and ethical implications of donated gametes. In: K. W. M. Fulford, D. Dickenson, and T. M. Murray, ed. *Healthcare ethics and human values*, pp. 79–96. Oxford: Blackwell.

Raphael-Leff, J. (2002). Egg donation. In: M. A. Alizade, ed. *The embodied female*, pp. 53–65. London: Karnac Press.

Raphael-Leff, J. (2003). Parent-infant psychodynamics—wild things, mirrors and ghosts. London: Whurr.

Raphael-Leff, J. (2005). *Psychological Processes of Childbearing*, 4th edn. London: Emma Freud Centre.

Radke-Yarrow, M., Richters, J., and Wilson, W. E. (1988). Child development in a network of relationships. In: R. A. Hinde and J. Stevenson-Hinde, ed. *Relationships within families: mutual influences*, pp. 48–67. Oxford: Oxford University Press.

Reading, R. (2003). The prevalence of domestic violence in pregnant women. *Child Care, Health and Development*, **29**, 314–15.

Robinson, M. (1996). Parents becoming partners. In: C. Clulow, ed. *Partners becoming parents—talks from the Tavistock Marital Studies Institute*, pp. 159–68. London: Sheldon Press.

Rutter, M. and Quinton, D. (1984). Parental psychiatric disorder: effects on children. *Psychological Medicine*, **14**, 853–80.

Settlage, C., *et al.* (1988). Conceptualizing adult development. *Journal of the American Psychoanalytic Association*, **36**, 347–69.

Schore, A. (1999). *Affect regulation and the origin of the self: the neurobiological aspects of emotional development*. Hillsdale, NJ: Lawrence Erlbaum.

Simpson, B., McArthy, P., and Walker, J. (1995). *Being there: fathers after divorce*. Newcastle: Relate Centre for Family Studies, University of Newcastle.

Siney, C., ed. (1999). *Pregnancy and drug misuse*, 2nd edn. London: Hale Books for Midwives.

Stevens-Long, J. (1990). Adult development: theories past and future. In: R. A. Nemiroff and C. A. Colarusso, ed. *New dimensions in adult development*, pp. 125–69. New York: Basic Books.

Swartz, K. L. (2003). Psychiatric disorders through a woman's lifespan. *International Review of Psychiatry*, **15**, 203–4.

Swidler, A. (1980). Love and adulthood in American culture. In: N. Smelser and E. Erikson, ed. *Themes of work and love in adulthood*, pp. 120–47. Cambridge, MA: Harvard University Press.

Targosz, S., *et al.* (2003). Lone mothers, social exclusion and depression. *Psychological Medicine*, **33**, 715–22.

Tronick, E. Z. (2003). 'Of course all relationships are unique': how co-creative processes generate unique mother-infant and patient-therapist relationships and change other relationships. *Psychoanalytic Inquiry*, **23**, 475–91.

Tuschen-Caffier, B., Florin, I., Krause, W., and Pook, M. (1999). Cognitive-behavioral therapy for idiopathic infertile couples. *Psychotherapy and Psychosomatics*, **68**, 15–21.

Ustun, T. B. (2000). Cross-national epidemiology of depression and gender. *The Journal of Gender-Specific Medicine*, **3**, 54–8.

Valliant, G. E. and Koury, J. (1993). Late mid-life development. In: G. H. Pollock and S. I. Greenspan, ed. *The Course of life*. Vol. VI. *Late Adulthood*. Madison, CT: International Universities Press.

Vincent, C. (1995). Consulting to divorcing couples. *Family Law*, **25**, 678–81.

Wallerstein, J. S. (1990). Transference and countertransference in clinical intervention with divorcing families. *American Journal of Orthopsychiatry*, **60**, 337–45.

Waugh, F. and Bonner, M. (2002). Domestic violence and child protection: issues in safety planning. *Child Abuse Review*, **11**, 282.

Welldon, E. (2002). *Sadomasochism*. Ideas in Psychoanalysis. Cambridge, UK: Icon Books.

WHO Report. (2003). *Healthy life expectancy for 191 nations*. Geneva: WHO/OMS.

Winnicott, D. W. (1958). The capacity to be alone. *International Journal of Psycho-Analysis*, **39**, 416–20. (Also in *The Maturational Processes and the Facilitating Environment*, pp. 29–36. London: Hogarth Press.)

Yogman, M. Y. (1982). Observations on the father-infant relationship. In: S. Cath, A. Gurwitt, and J. M. Ross, ed. *Father And child: developmental and clinical perspectives*, pp. 101–22. Boston: Little and Brown.

32 Psychotherapy with older adults

Joan M. Cook, Dolores Gallagher-Thompson, and Jason Hepple

Historical overview

The application of psychotherapy to older adults began with much skepticism. Sigmund Freud believed that psychological treatment of individuals over the age of 50 was ineffective (Freud, 1904/1959). To substantiate this view he put forth claims that older adults have limitations in ego or cognitive functioning; analysis would have to deal with a relatively longer lifetime and thus would go on indefinitely; and analysis would occur at a time when it was no longer essential to be psychologically healthy. Although Abraham (1919/1927) was the first psychoanalyst to acknowledge and convey optimism about the psychological treatment of older adults, the views of Freud dominated clinical thinking at that time. However, in 1929 Lillien Martin pioneered the provision of psychotherapy to older adults at the San Francisco Old Age Counseling Center (Martin, 1944). This was the first psychotherapy program for older individuals in the USA. Martin's directive and inspirational techniques centered on overcoming pessimism by adopting the 'will-to-do' attitude.

In 1959, Rechtschaffen provided a landmark review of psychotherapy with older adults. In addition to providing a thoughtful summary of anecdotal and case report data, he argued that older adults are heterogeneous in terms of both their internal and external strengths and resources, as are young adults, and challenged the widely held notion that older adults could not benefit from psychological intervention. Since Rechtschaffen's review, this line of work has continued to grow with a number of key summaries of the then current state of the psychotherapy field (Brink, 1986; Knight, 1986; Gallagher-Thompson and Thompson, 1995). Two reviews stand out for their comprehensiveness (Teri and McCurry, 1994; Gatz *et al.*, 1998). In particular, Gatz *et al.* (1998) categorized psychological treatments for older adults in terms of empirically validated criteria developed by the American Psychological Association's (APA) Division of Clinical Psychology and offered important guidance for empirically-based practice.

In addition to the accumulation of general scientific knowledge of the psychology of older adults (i.e., cognitive functioning, stress, and coping, etc.; for a historical review of the growth and development of the psychological study of older adults, see Cook *et al.*, 1998), the field of geriatric mental health intervention research has blossomed, particularly in the area of depression. The completion of randomized and quasi-randomized controlled trials of psychotherapy with older adults represents an excellent step forward in the direction of more effectively serving the elderly population. Furthermore, there is a strong federal push in the USA for the geriatric mental health intervention field to move away from the traditional clinical trials model towards a more public health model of treatment (Lebowitz and Harris, 2000), and to place greater emphasis on treatments that are more broadly accessible and acceptable, rather than confined to the select samples of older adults that have been studied in clinical trials in specialty settings.

Changing demographics

Demographic projections estimate that the number and proportion of older adults in the population is increasing in industrialized countries. In North America, the proportion of the population over 65 years of age is predicted to grow from 12.3% in 2000 to 20.2% in 2035 with the population over 80 years of age rising from 3.2% in 2000 to 6.0% by 2035. (All demographic data provided by United Nations, 2003). Among those over 65 years of age in 2035, women will out number men in an approximate ratio of 1.7:1. The elderly dependency ratio, the number of older adults to working adults, was 19 to 100 in 2000, and is predicted to grow to 33 to 100 by 2035. By 2035 there will be an estimated 261 000 people over 100 years in North America.

Europe has more of a demographic crisis than North America. In the UK in 2035, for example, the elderly dependency ratio will be 37 to 100 adults of working age. In all industrialized countries, however, the trend towards an increasing elderly dependency ratio fizzles out in 2035 with the proportion of over 65 years old stabilizing by 2050. Over the next 30 years, the aging population will create a significant rise in the number of dependent older people. By 2035 in North America there will be 85 million older people. Approximately 10% are expected to need institutional care. The 30–40% living alone are expected to have an increased need for social and medical services (Grundy, 1989). This translates to an extra 4 million nursing or residential homes and approximately 15 million additional older people living alone. It is essential to plan ahead for these changing demographics, whose greatest acceleration towards an aging population will be between 2015 and 2025 before gradually reaching a static position in 2050.

Myths and actualities of aging

Western societies have only recently begun to identify ageism as a source of prejudice and discriminatory practice. On the surface this is surprising given that aging is universal, although demographically, older people have traditionally been a minority group. Denial-based psychological defenses may serve the purpose of separating the self from an unrealistically idealized concept of older people in an attempt to avoid the realities of one's own aging (Hepple, 2003a). There are numerous stereotypes about older adults, which can adversely affect a psychotherapist's attitude and behavior. Namely, that older adults are: (1) a homogeneous group; (2) generally alone and lonely; (3) sick, frail, and dependent on others; (4) living in segregated housing for the elderly or nursing homes; (5) often cognitively impaired; (6) often depressed; (7) difficult and rigid; and (8) not coping well with the physical and intellectual decline associated with aging (APA Working Group on the Older Adult, 1998). Overidealized stereotypes of older adults can similarly be unhelpful by minimizing the challenges of aging ('You are only as young as you feel,' for example). On the contrary, older adults are a heterogeneous group who, in general, maintain close contact with family, live independently, and adjust well to the challenges of aging (APA Working Group on the Older Adult, 1998). Usually, older adults' personalities stay consistent throughout the life span, with proportionally few suffering from major mental health problems (APA Working Group on the Older Adult, 1998). Although there may be some decline in intellectual abilities, debility is typically not severe enough to cause problems in daily living.

Major psychotherapeutic orientations and their efficacy with the elderly

In this section, theoretical perspectives and relevant empirical evidence are briefly summarized. For those general therapeutic orientations that are well known, the actual description of the therapy is limited. For those treatments that are primarily or only used in older adults, a more detailed account is provided.

Cognitive-behavioral therapy

Cognitive-behavioral therapy (CBT) has been one of the most widely studied and efficacious treatments for older adults. Though it includes a variety of interventions ranging from the cognitive work of Beck et al. (1979) to the behavioral work of Lewinsohn et al. (1976), its most common application is a blend of both cognitive and behavioral techniques. The conceptualization underlying CBT is that much of psychopathology is learned and maintained by a combination of distorted, dysfunctional thinking about oneself and the world and reduced behavioral or environmental reinforcement. Thus, therapeutic intervention seeks to change unhelpful thinking, increase positive behaviors, and reduce negative actions. CBT is typically highly structured, directive, time-limited, and focused on current problems.

The CBT model has been widely used for many disorders in older adults and reported in case reports and empirical investigations. A series of studies by Gallagher-Thompson et al. have shown that CBT is highly efficacious for depression (Thompson et al., 1987; Gallagher-Thompson and Steffen, 1994; Thompson et al., 2001; for a more thorough summary see Teri et al., 1994). In particular, there is evidence for its efficacy with depressed outpatients and inpatients, the medically ill as well as healthy, in individual or group format, and when delivered by a trained therapist or self-taught through bibliotherapy (Scogin et al., 1987, 1989, 1990). Relative to the stringent criteria of the APA Task Force on empirically supported treatments, CBT was identified as 'probably efficacious' for treatment of depression in community residing older adults who are cognitively intact, have minimal comorbidities, and are not suicidal (Gatz et al., 1998). In addition, cognitive-behavioral forms of therapy have demonstrated efficacy for alleviating sleep disturbances (for review see Morin et al., 1994 and Gatz et al., 1998), generalized anxiety (Wetherell et al., 2003), and behavioral problems associated with dementia (Teri et al., 1998; Allen-Burge et al., 1999). A case example illustrating the use of CBT with a depressed elder is presented later in this chapter.

Psychodynamic and interpersonal therapies

A wide variety of treatments are offered under the rubric of psychoanalytic/dynamic therapy, including insight-oriented and supportive approaches. Many of them concern the historical causes and larger patterns of current behavior, restoration of healthy defenses and positive self-perception, and examination of the client–therapist relationship. This treatment is typically less directive, and often seeks to help identify and resolve unsettled issues from earlier in development and explore their impact on current functioning.

From a psychodynamic perspective there are some unique developmental tasks and transferences to be addressed in therapy with older adults. These age-appropriate themes include grieving for losses, fear of physical illness, disability and death, and guilt and despair over past failures (Pfeiffer and Busse, 1973; Hildebrand, 1995). One specific developmental tension that is beautifully illustrated in Shakespeare's *King Lear* and *The Tempest*, is the dialectic between the decline and sense of impending death that is associated with aging versus growth and liberation (Deats, 1996; Hildebrand, 2000). Transference issues are atypical, but may reflect concerns related to one's family of procreation (i.e., spouse and children) rather than one's family of origin; while countertransference may be influenced by unresolved issues with parents, one's own fears of aging and/or negative cultural stereotypes regarding aging (Gallagher-Thompson and Thompson, 1996).

Unfortunately few empirical investigations have examined the efficacy of psychodynamic therapy for use in older adults. A study by Thompson et al. (1987) demonstrates that brief psychodynamic psychotherapy is equally efficacious in the treatment of major depressive disorder in older people as behavioral and cognitive interventions. Seventy percent of subjects showed remission or significant improvement after 16–20 treatment sessions compared with minimal spontaneous improvement in a delayed-treatment control group. Although it has an extremely small sample size and no control group, the work of Lazarus et al. (1984, 1987) provides some promise that psychodynamic therapy is useful for older adults (for an excellent though less current review, see Newton et al., 1986).

One time-limited integrative therapy with a heavy influence on psychodynamic conceptualization and technique is cognitive analytic therapy (CAT; Ryle, 1990). This structured therapy has two primary influences, as its name implies, cognitive-behavioral and psychoanalytic. CAT is gaining popularity in the UK and Europe, and its application with older adults has recently been discussed (Hepple, 2002). Its premise is that experience about oneself in relation to others becomes internalized in early development as a repertoire of reciprocal roles that act as templates for subsequent interactions. Insight and change are promoted through the exploration of these experiences in the here and now, particularly the therapeutic relationship, using a variety of cognitive, behavioral, interpretative and creative tools and techniques. CAT has not yet been formally evaluated, but has been suggested as potentially beneficial for treatment-resistant depression or dysthymia, stable personality difficulties with traumatic or abusive antecedents, and somatization disorders (Hepple, 2002).

Interpersonal psychotherapy (IPT) has multiple theoretical underpinnings, including psychodynamic, and has received empirical support with older adults (Klerman et al., 1984). This treatment is manual-based, highly structured, and short term. Its underlying premise is that regardless of the etiology of psychopathology, understanding and renegotiating relationships plays a key role in reducing symptoms, restoring function and possibly preventing future disturbance. IPT focuses on current relationships in four general problem areas: role transition, role dispute, abnormal grief, and interpersonal deficit.

Monthly IPT sessions demonstrated efficacy as a monotherapy and in combination with antidepressant pharmacotherapy as a maintenance treatment strategy to prolong recovery and prevent recurrence of major depression (Reynolds et al., 1999). The older patients in this randomized clinical trial had had current major depression and at least one prior episode during the past 3 years. Combination of IPT and antidepressant medication not only improved duration of recovery but social adjustment as well (Lenze et al., 2002).

In addition to a review of IPT as applied to late-life depression, Miller et al. (2001) have reported preliminary findings on IPT combined with antidepressants in cognitively impaired depressed elders. Uncomplicated bereavement-related depression also responds well to IPT (Miller et al., 1994). Additionally, this type of counseling has been shown effective in the treatment of subsyndromal depression in postsurgical patients following hospital discharge (Mossey et al., 1996).

Reminiscence/life review therapy

Reminiscence therapy (RT) involves recalling the past as a way to increase self-esteem and social connection. RT typically occurs in a group format in which individuals are encouraged to remember and share memories of the past, with personal artifacts, newspapers, and/or music often used to stimulate memories. These sessions are frequently structured with the therapist picking the topic. This very popular counseling tool is regularly used with well elderly to gain perspective on their lives and thus is popular in senior centers, residential settings, and retirement communities rather than as clinical intervention for those older adults with major mental health or personality disorders (Thorton and Brotchie, 1987; Gatz et al., 1998).

Life review therapy (LRT: Butler, 1963), a more intense type of RT, involves the reworking of past conflicts in order to gain a better understanding and acceptance of the past. These types of therapies are based on the work of Erik Erikson (1959, 1982) and his eight-stage model of psychosocial development. The underlying premise is that an older adult can be helped through the last stage of Erikson's model, ego integrity versus despair. It is thought that if older adults can satisfactorily formulate and accept personalized answers to existential questions such as, 'Who am I?' and 'How did I live my life?', they will achieve integrity. As this treatment is so individualized, it is difficult to manualize; however, Haight and Webster (1995; Webster and Haight, 2002) have done so. Although LRT involves various therapeutic approaches, not all of which are clearly defined (Haight et al., 1997), effect sizes of 1.05 have been reported for LRT versus no treatment in controlled therapy studies of geriatric depression. However, superiority over a no treatment comparison condition does not demonstrate specific efficacy for the particular brand of therapy. A case series of older trauma survivors with posttraumatic stress disorder successfully treated with LRT was recently reported (Maercker, 2002); thus, this may be a good therapy for clients that need to focus on/confront past trauma issues.

Other psychosocial interventions

Unfortunately, the application of family therapy with older individuals remains underdeveloped, and research investigating its efficacy is virtually nonexistent (Qualls, 1995; Knight and McCallum, 1998). One area in which there may be an increased demand and relevance is therapy with families caring for a cognitively impaired elderly member (Bonjean, 1988; Qualls, 2000). Individual and family therapy for spouse-caregivers and families of Alzheimer disease patients was efficacious in postponing nursing home placement. Family therapy may be used as a separate modality or to elicit family members' involvement as facilitators of individual therapy for older individuals.

Another area in need of further investigation is the application and provision of psychotherapeutic services to those with cognitive impairment. A significant minority of the elderly population experience limitations in their cognitive abilities due to progressive dementia, and many of these individuals also experience comorbid emotional distress. Owing to their cognitive deficits, such as memory loss or decreased capacity for judgment and problem solving, persons with dementia are usually not considered to be good candidates for traditional psychotherapy. However, the symptoms and behaviors of persons with dementia should not be viewed solely as manifestations of biology, but rather, as being affected by social, psychological, and environmental contexts as well (Kasl-Godley and Gatz, 2000). Thus, patients with dementia are able to derive some benefit from psychological interventions. Various CBT, environmental, and supportive interventions may help cognitively impaired older adults reduce disruptive behaviors and excess disabilities, increase or maintain positive behaviors, improve memory or learn coping skills to manage loss of cognitive skills, increase quality of life, reduce excessive burden on health-care delivery systems, alleviate symptoms of depression or anxiety, or help adjustment to multiple losses (Gatz et al., 1998; Kasl-Godley and Gatz, 2000). Research on the degree to which cognitive deficits operate as moderators to limit their use (e.g., within what ranges of cognitive dysfunction traditional talk therapies can be used effectively, and with what modifications) is needed.

Many psychosocial interventions currently in use with older adults with dementia are based on uncontrolled case studies and anecdotal reports. However, there are some studies examining the feasibility of conducting therapy or the effectiveness of therapy for particular purposes with older adults (for reviews, see Cheston, 1998; Gatz et al., 1998). Use of behavioral and environmental treatments for behavior problems and memory and cognitive retraining for some forms of late-life cognitive impairment may be effective. However, there is much dispute about cognitive training, in particular. Support groups and CBT can assist those with early-stage dementia to foster coping strategies and reduce distress. RT may provide mild to moderate stage individuals with interpersonal connections. Behavioral approaches and memory training target specific cognitive and behavioral impairments and help to optimize remaining abilities.

One intervention that is often used with memory-impaired older adults is reality orientation (RO), which involves exposing cognitively impaired patients to stimuli that facilitate orientation to time or place (for a manual, see American Hospital Association, 1976). The most widely used type of

RO takes place anywhere from once a week to several times a day and involves the rehearsal of basic orientation facts such as the day, date, time, and the weather. In 24-hour RO, patients are reoriented on the nursing home units throughout the day, either by staff or environmental cues such as big clocks and calendars.

Other types of therapies such as problem-solving therapy and eclectic approaches are also being applied to older individuals. For more information, the interested reader might seek Duffy (1999) or Frazer and Jongsma (1999).

Updates and recent areas of inquiry and application

Depression and suicide

As previously noted, the most widely researched disorder in the geriatric mental health field is depression. In 1991, the US National Institute of Health convened a panel of experts from the biomedical and behavioral sciences to address the diagnosis and treatment of depression in late life (National Institutes of Health Consensus Development Panel on Depression in Late Life, 1992). Since then, an update from the consensus conference has been published (Lebowitz et al., 1997) as have numerous reviews, including Areán and Cook (2002). Despite widespread knowledge of the efficacy of major treatment modalities for some disorders or problems occurring in old age, there are still numerous areas in the field in need of further investigation. A brief review of the noteworthy areas follows.

Most industrialized countries report that suicide rates rise increasingly with age, with the highest rates occurring for men age 75 and older (Pearson and Conwell, 1995). In a comparison of age differences in suicidal intent in psychological autopsy studies, older adults were more likely to have avoided intervention and taken precautions against discovery and were less likely to communicate their intent to others, as well as less likely to have a history of previous attempts (Conwell et al., 1998). These distinctive features present a challenge to detecting and treating high-risk elderly. Although suicide in older adults is a major public health problem, there are as yet no effective interventions for reducing suicidal behaviors in this population (Pearson and Brown, 2000). However, given the strong relationship of depression as a risk factor for suicide, improving the detection and treatment of late life depression in primary care settings, where older adults often seek treatment for emotional difficulties, seems to be a promising approach (Brown et al., 2001).

Grief

Studies of bereavement-related distress, now referred to as complicated or traumatic grief reactions, have begun (Frank et al., 1997). Clinical researchers at the University of Pittsburgh's Western Psychiatric Institute and Clinic have completed an open treatment trial of traumatic grief therapy conceptualized and treated similar to exposure therapy for posttraumatic stress disorder (e.g., reliving the moment of death, saying goodbye to the deceased, and in vivo exposure to situations that clients have been avoiding since the death) (Shear et al., 2001). This protocol appears to be a promising intervention for debilitating grief in older adults.

Alcohol abuse and dependence

Alcohol abuse is common among older adults, with roughly 12% of older women and 15% of older men regularly drinking in excess of limits recommended by the National Institute of Alcoholism and Alcohol Abuse (i.e., no more than one drink per day; Adams et al., 1996). Hazards of drinking among older adults may include increased risk for falls, accidents, and interference with medications. Alcohol abuse may also present differently in the elderly, as the level of drinking necessary to be considered hazardous is lower than the level for younger people, and many late-onset alcoholics do not develop dependence (Levin et al., 2000). However, there is reason to hope that elder-specific interventions can lead to reductions in alcohol consumption (Blow and Barry, 2000). Several large-scale projects have shown promising outcomes with interventions of varying length, most notably Project GOAL—Guiding Older Adult Lifestyles (Fleming *et al.*, 1999), the Gerontology Alcohol Project (Dupree *et al.*, 1984), and the Michigan Outcomes Study (Barry *et al.*, 2001). Project GOAL demonstrated that 15–20 minutes of physician provided advice and education about the negative consequences of excessive drinking can significantly reduce frequency of excessive drinking. More lengthy interventions utilize motivational interviewing techniques (Miller and Rollnick, 1991) and/or skills training (Dupree and Schonfield, 1999). Structured nonconfrontational techniques that reinforce values incompatible with drinking (e.g., maintaining good health) and teach coping skills for avoiding alcohol in high-risk situations (e.g. bereavement) have shown comparable outcomes among older and younger adults (Blow and Barry, 2000). More effort is needed to bring these interventions into primary care and community settings.

Other disorders

Techniques for treating certain mental health problems, such as anxiety disorders, prescription medicine misuse (i.e., benzodiazepine), personality disorders, and psychoses, have been sorely lacking (Gallo and Lebowitz, 1999). Epidemiological evidence indicates that anxiety disorders are more prevalent than either depression or severe cognitive impairment among older adults (Regier *et al.*, 1988). However, despite its prevalence, very little psychotherapy intervention research has been conducted on anxiety (for reviews, see Niederehe and Schnieder, 1998; Wetherell, 1998).

One noteworthy investigation was the randomization of older adults with generalized anxiety disorder (GAD) to the CBT group, a discussion group organized around worry-provoking topics, or a waiting period (Wetherell *et al.*, 2003). Older adults in both active conditions improved relative to the waiting-list; however, CBT showed large effects while the discussion group showed medium-sized effects. These results provide limited support for the superiority of CBT to a comparison intervention.

Additionally, a version of CBT that targets the needs of older adults with GAD in the primary care setting was preliminary tested against usual care (Stanley *et al.*, 2003). Outcome data suggested significant improvements in worry and depression after CBT relative to usual care.

Mohlman *et al.* (2003) are the first to test the efficacy of CBT as compared with an enhanced version (ECBT) that included learning and memory aids such as homework reminders and troubleshooting calls, and a weekly review of all concepts and techniques for treatment of late-life GAD. ECBT resulted in improvement on more measures and yielded larger effect sizes than standard CBT, when each was compared against a wait-list control group. These findings provide evidence that content and procedural modifications may be necessary to maximize the effectiveness of CBT therapy with older people with mild cognitive impairments.

Prescription medication misuse may be a particular problem for older adults, in particular the use of benzodiazepines (Gallo and Lebowitz, 1999). Anxiolytic medications are the most common treatment for anxiety in older adults and benzodiazepines figure prominently (Blazer *et al.*, 1991). In addition, benzodiazepines are commonly prescribed and used for depression, insomnia, and other sleep disturbances in older individuals. Despite the expressed concern of the American Psychiatric Association (1990) Task Force Report on Benzodiazepine Dependency regarding the 'appropriate therapeutic use, toxicity, abuse and risk of inducing a drug-dependent state' in older adults, there are reasons to believe that use is high and often inappropriate (Hanlon *et al.*, 2002). The serious negative side-effect profile, including associations with significant morbidities such as sleep disturbance, cognitive difficulty, impairment in activities of daily living, motor vehicle crashes, and problems with gait (e.g., accidental falls and fall-related fractures) has been well-established (Bertz *et al.*, 1997; Hemmelgarn *et al.*, 1997; Hanlon *et al.*, 1998; Ray *et al.*, 2000). Though pharmacotherapy has been successful in reducing or eliminating benzodiazepine misuse, CBT has also been shown effective in helping older individuals successfully discontinue or reduce inappropriate use (Gorenstein *et al.*, in press; Morin *et al.*, 1995).

As in younger populations, older adults with personality disorders may be less willing to engage, adhere, and benefit from traditional mental health interventions (Lynch *et al.*, 2003). Although to date no outcome study has specifically focused on treating personality disorders in older adults, evidence from case reports and data on effects of personality pathology on treatment of depression suggests that this is a worthy area of future investment (for a recent review, see DeLeo *et al.*, 1999). Pilot data provides preliminary evidence for the feasibility of applying dialectical behavior therapy (Linehan, 1993) to depressed older adults, a significant minority of whom meet criteria for a personality disorder (Lynch *et al.*, 2003). It has been suggested that the increase in life events and disability found in later life may 'unmask' maladaptive personality traits that have been dormant in mid-life; the concept of reemergent borderline personality traits (Hepple 2003b for a review of this area). Distress and behaviors arising from this can often be misconstrued as resulting from organic pathology. A clinical case example is presented later to help illustrate this point.

Although there is a large scientific knowledge base on schizophrenia among younger adults, much less is known about late-life schizophrenia and its treatment (Palmer *et al.*, 1999). What is known about its treatment is mainly pharmacological, the use of conventional neuroleptics and the newer serotonin–dopamine antagonists (Jeste and McClure, 1997). However, recently Patterson *et al.* (2003) developed and evaluated a psychosocial intervention to improve everyday living skills of older patients with schizophrenia and other chronic psychoses. Preliminary findings suggest that older patients with longstanding psychotic disorders may benefit from participation in this skills-training program.

Long-term care

There are a growing number of older individuals who reside in long-term care settings. A US network termed Psychologists in Long-Term Care has developed standards for psychological practice in long-term care facilities (Lichtenberg *et al.*, 1998). Other guidelines and resources for professionals exist, such as information on competency determinations, work within the structure of an interdisciplinary team, and staff development (US Department of Veterans Affairs, 1997; Gallagher-Thompson *et al.*, 2000b; Zeiss and Gallagher-Thompson, 2003).

Recommended modifications or adaptations of treatment

There are numerous physical, psychological, cognitive, social, developmental, and environmental factors that can impact the choice and delivery of psychotherapy to older adults. Most older adults have at least one chronic medical illness, some degree of functional impairment/disability, an increasing frequency of loss events, and a decrease in controllability of these losses (e.g., financial limitations, diminished sensory capacities, decreased mobility, retirement, widowhood, and change in residence). The complexity of these intermingling influences often merit special therapeutic consideration.

Although some mental health interventions are comparable with those used with younger individuals, it is often necessary to adapt therapies to address special considerations unique to older adults. For example, psychotherapy with older adults often occurs at a slower pace due to possible sensory problems and slower learning rates (Gallagher-Thompson and Thompson, 1996). This means that repetition is very important in the learning process, and information should be presented in both verbal and visual modalities (i.e., on chalk boards and hand-outs) in order to help older patients encode and retain information. Older clients should also be encouraged to take notes to help aid memory retention and thus increase efficacy of therapy (Knight and Satre, 1999). Assignments may need to be in bold print or sessions tape-recorded for review. Additionally, psychotherapy with older adults often requires a collaborative style with few clearly outlined goals and a more active or task-focused approach (Gallagher-Thompson and Thompson, 1996).

The goals of psychotherapy with older adults should be continually highlighted to reinforce the purpose and facilitate the direction of treatment. It may also be necessary to facilitate therapy for those with sensory problems, particularly hearing and vision impairments. Thus, adaptations such as pocket talkers to assist in hearing or eliminating glare for the sight impaired should be made available. Rather than giving suggestions or expecting the client to infer answers, Knight and Satre (1999) suggest that as there is a normal age decline in fluid intelligence, therapists may need to lead the older adult to conclusions.

When determining if and which modifications are needed, it is important to separate the effects of maturation from the effects of cohort (Knight and Satre, 1999). Maturational effects include similarities that are developmentally common or specific to older adulthood, such as adjusting to chronic illness and disability, or loss of friends and family due to death. Cohort effects are specific to a certain birth-year-defined group. For example, in the USA, early-born cohorts have lower educational levels and less exposure to psychological concepts (Knight and Satre, 1999). Psychotherapists working with older people need to be aware of maturational and cohort differences in the expression and treatment of psychological problems. Additionally, therapists working with older adults should learn about chronic illness and its psychosocial impact, management of chronic pain, factors influencing adherence to medical treatment, rehabilitation methods, and assessment of behavioral signs of negative medication effects (Knight and Satre, 1999).

Assessment should always include current mental and cognitive status (for further information on modifications of assessment techniques for use with older adults, see Zarit and Zarit, 1998). A brief screen of cognitive functioning, such as the Mini-Mental State Exam (MMSE; Folstein et al., 1975), can measure suitability for treatment, as well as identify patients in need of more extensive neuropsychological testing. It is also imperative to consider the medical status of and social support available to older adults, as these may affect presentation and treatment of pathology (APA Working Group, 1998). Formal testing, such as the MMSE, requires normative data specific to older adults in the reference group of the person being tested (e.g., education, race, gender). Without such normative data, 'normal' aging processes are impossible to distinguish from pathology or impairment (Dougherty and Chamblin, 1999).

Providing psychological services to older adults often requires flexibility in scheduling, location and collaboration. Older adults often have a greater chance of hospitalization or reduced mobility, responsibility to care for infirm relatives, or a reluctance to travel in bad weather conditions, all of which may necessitate missed therapy sessions (APA Working Group on the Older Adult, 1998). Thus, brief, occasional hospital visits, telephone sessions, or letters may need to be made at times to maintain contact. Access to building and acceptable transportation services should be made available (Hepple, 2002). Additionally, because older adults often have concurrent physical and social problems, consultation and coordination with other health service providers is often necessary (APA Working Group on the Older Adult, 1998).

At times, when an older adult becomes temporarily dependent upon a caregiver for assistance, it may be crucial to engage the caregiver in aspects of the treatment. An example of this is the pivotal work by Teri et al. (1997) of treating depression in older dementia patients via training caregivers in behavioral interventions. An excellent case example, which describes in detail a systematic course of CBT for a depressed female caregiver of an Alzheimer's disease patient, is described elsewhere (Dick and Gallagher-Thompson, 1995). Goals of that treatment, not uncommon to other caregiver stress experiences, included setting limits and making time for personal needs. Treating the caregiver in individual or group, dyadic or brief educational sessions can be directly beneficial to the caregiver and indirectly helpful to the care recipient. If a caregiver is taught to understand and more effectively cope with emotions such as frustration and anger, they may be less distressed and better able to provide effective care (Gallagher-Thompson et al., 1992).

Because many older adults have experienced increased loss of family members or friends compared with younger individuals, clinical lore suggests that the therapeutic relationship becomes a vital source of support as well as information. For this reason, it has been suggested that rather than traditional termination, ending sessions be spread out and booster sessions be offered (Gallagher-Thompson and Thompson, 1996). A suggested acronym to help therapists working with older adults provide respectful and appropriate therapy is MICKS: 'a) use Multimodal teaching, b) maintain Interdisciplinary awareness, c) present information more Clearly, d) develop Knowledge of aging challenges and strengths, and e) present therapy material more Slowly' (Crowther and Zeiss, 1999).

Clinical lore also suggests that many older adults hold negative stereotypes about mental health and psychotherapy, which may result in reluctance to accept or engage in therapy, limitations in self-disclosure and endorsement of symptoms. Some of these myths follow: only crazy people seek mental health treatment; psychological problems indicate moral weakness; therapy constitutes an invasion of privacy; adults, especially men do not share their feelings or show weakness to strangers; adults do not need to ask for help; and therapy has no relevance (Glantz, 1989). Thus, one additional adaptation for therapy with older adults may be to have an introductory orientation/socialization into psychotherapy. Here incorrect assumptions or fallacies can be corrected, and roles and expectations established. It is important to remember that there is much more commonality between the young and the old than there are differences, and that older people have a huge diversity of life experience having matured in a world of unprecedented change, where wars, mass migration, and rapid technological development changed many aspects of life beyond recognition for many individuals. Psychotherapists, although benefiting from the specialized skills and approaches utilized in work with older people, need to bear in mind that what is shared with their older clients is humanity and that what is different may take some understanding.

Case illustrations

How best to choose an optimal form of psychotherapy for an older adult patient is influenced by a number factors, including diagnosis, cognitive functioning, and psychological-mindedness. Choice of therapy is often based on therapist awareness of and training in available therapies. However, considerations impacting the choice and delivery of intervention include knowledge of efficacy of intervention with older adults, likelihood of effectiveness for the particular patient (e.g., skills), severity and timing of problem (e.g., acute versus chronic), timing of intervention, patient preference and motivation, and ethnic and cultural considerations (Hepple et al., 2002). Other factors to consider are previous treatment history and response. Two case illustrations are presented here from two different theoretical orientations, CBT and CAT.

Cognitive-behavioral therapy

Although several excellent examples of CBT and its application to older adults have been presented elsewhere in case report form (Dick and Gallagher-Thompson, 1995; Crowther and Zeiss, 1999; Karel et al., 2002), a brief highlighted review of a treatment case is described here to help illustrate the applicability of CBT conceptualization and practice with older individuals. A manual that describes this approach is available for both therapist and client (Dick et al., 1995; Thompson et al., 1995). Additionally, Coon and Gallagher-Thompson (2002) utilize case vignettes to illustrate CBT homework challenges and successful approaches to address adherence barriers.

Mrs W was a 79-year-old, widowed, retired, Caucasian woman who sought treatment for depression at the Older Adult and Family Center at the VA Palo Alto Health Care System. Her symptoms at this time warranted a diagnosis of major depressive disorder and dependent personality features. Mrs W's husband had passed away about 2 years prior and her two sons had moved to a different state. She reported intense feelings of loneliness, disappointment, and frustration that her physical ailments (i.e., congestive heart failure with edema and shortness of breath) had made her less mobile and more dependent on others.

A program of individual weekly CBT was initiated beginning with an introduction to the CBT model and Mrs W was encouraged to apply the skills learned in session outside of therapy (i.e., via homework assignments). In order to help reduce depressive thoughts about herself, she was taught to use a daily thought record, and trained in challenging negative beliefs. In order to increase engagement and enjoyment in pleasant events, the client was taught to the use mood monitoring and activity tracking.

The first session, included thorough history taking, a description of current problems, and completion of assessment measures, such as the MMSE (Folstein *et al.*, 1975), and the Beck Depression Inventory (BDI; Beck and Steer, 1987). At the end of the first session, the therapist presented an introduction to the cognitive-behavioral model of depression (e.g., how thoughts and behaviors affect functioning, see Figure 32.1) and using materials the client had talked about gave examples of the antecedent, belief, and emotional consequences. The client was easily able to summarize the model and was asked to read material on CBT.

At the beginning of every session, Mrs W completed the BDI to monitor depressive symptomatology. In the second session, the collaborative nature of the relationship between the therapist and client and the importance of practicing new skills learned in session (e.g., homework) were discussed, specific goals of therapy were outlined, and the CBT model was revisited. Mrs W was reminded that CBT was a short-term treatment and that goals must be manageable within the time allowed. Her target complaints were she would like to be cured of her depression and would like to find more satisfying things to do with her life. In session 3, Mrs W was taught how to notice and monitor 'unhelpful thoughts' following stressful events. This involved introducing her to an unhelpful thought diary (three columns: antecedent, belief, and emotional consequences). In order to help Mrs W understand the impact and strength of her thoughts on her mood, she was taught to assign a belief rating from 0 (not strong at all) to 100 (completely true) to each thought. A useful analogy was used to help her understand the effects of unhelpful thoughts on mood: listening to a radio station with a headset. It was explained that if the headset is clear, if it is correctly connected to the radio receiver and positioned securely on one's head, then the station will come in clearly (Thompson *et al.*, 1995). It was further explained that if the headset is not on properly, there may be misinterpretation of the signal or information from the radio. A list of unhelpful thoughts entitled 'Signals from your negative headset' was given to Mrs W and the therapist explained negative distortions such as attaching negative labels of oneself, having unrealistic expectations for oneself, viewing a situation in terms of extreme outcomes, and tendency to blow events out of proportion. The therapist and Mrs W worked together to identify examples from the patient's current life. Over the next several sessions, Mrs W was taught how to challenge her unhelpful thoughts (e.g., challenging their validity). She was given a list of techniques entitled 'Fine tuning your signal' that included challenges such as engaging in specific behaviors to obtain additional information in challenging unhelpful assumptions, considering alternatives, and weighing the advantages and disadvantages of maintaining a current thought, emotion, or behavior.

Through individual sessions and homework assignments, Mrs W was able to challenge her own thinking as well as allow the therapist to provide her with new information that challenged her unhelpful thoughts. Mrs W was able to recognize that she was recognizing only negative aspects of her current situation and discounting positive accomplishments (see Box 32.1 for partial completion of homework assignment). She was attaching

a negative label to herself and sending herself negative messages, such as 'I'm dumb,' because of age-associated impairments. Attributing these limitations to aging and not to self was a step toward recovery for Mrs W.

Mrs W did not drive and since her husband's death had abandoned pleasant activities due, in part, to transportation problems. It was important to get her reactivated behaviorally. Mrs W completed the Older Person's Pleasant Events Schedule (OPPES; Hedlund and Gilewski, 1980; Gallagher and Thompson, 1981) a self-report measure designed to measure frequency of engagement in pleasant activities and perceived enjoyment of the activities regardless of whether or not they had been undertaken. She was encouraged to take part in events that once gave her pleasure in which she was no longer engaging (i.e., take an art and computer class) and to increase socialization by broadening her opportunities for social contact. The therapist helped Mrs W arrange transportation to a local senior center to better occupy her daytime hours, a time during which she was home alone. She reported that doing so lessened her feelings of loneliness and her dependency on other care providers. Additionally, Mrs W was encouraged to reconnect with friends from her childhood via telephone and postal

Box 32.1 An excerpt from cognitive-behavioral therapy homework with depressed older woman

'I'm dumb.'

A. Where's the evidence?

B. What are alternative explanations?

1A. I have trouble opening bottle caps, fastening doors, putting cartons together, folding maps. Things just about anyone can do.

1B. I am not mechanically inclined. My hands are also stiff, sore, and fingers are bent and misshapen. It is hard for me to get a good grip on jar and bottle caps. Also reduced strength. Also the anemia makes me weak.

2A. I don't have a VCR because I have no idea how to hook one up or even play it. I'd like to have one too! I had to have my son hook up my TV and hi fi because I couldn't understand the instructions. The same with telephones, clocks, etc. When my husband was alive, he always did it.

2B. Again, I am and never have been mechanically inclined. I've always depended on my sons and husband to do things. I think I will have to be more patient and take more time reading and following the instructions.

3A. I had a beautiful brand new sewing machine that I couldn't use because I couldn't understand the directions for doing all the stitches, or for putting the various attachments on. I could do straight stitching but that's all.

3B. Much the same as the above. I went to the store for lessons on how to do these things. However, the instructor did the exercises and just let me watch. I do better with hands on experience and I should have told them to let me do it while they watched and guided me. I have to do the maneuvers as well as the instructions.

4A. I never was able to knit or crochet or do any kind of fancy work. I can't even get the 'hang' of sewing any more.

4B. Knitting, crocheting, or fancy work were just not too interesting. I just couldn't get the feel for them. I do or did a lot of other kinds of artwork. Flower arranging, beautifully decorated gift packages, Resin art. I could sew pretty well. I was an excellent cook, not good at baking, but I could do many other kinds of cooking. I kept my family well fed, and they always enjoyed my cooking. So did my friends. I gave beautiful dinner parties, holiday parties, etc.

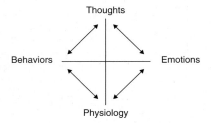

Fig. 32.1 Cognitive-behavioral model.

mail. Mrs W completed a 15-session course of CBT for depression. At the end of treatment she noted that she had made significant gains in reducing her depression and had regained previously forgotten hobbies.

Cognitive analytic therapy

Mrs S was a woman in her late seventies who presented to mental health services in the UK for the first time following the death of her husband. She complained of feelings of depression, panic, 'nameless dread,' and a variety of unexplained physical symptoms. She felt suicidal at times and had taken an overdose of sleeping tablets on two occasions. She found it very difficult to be alone at home and her nocturnal calls to neighbors, her daughter, and emergency services had become problematic. After two admissions to an older persons' psychiatric inpatient unit the team felt at a loss as to how to help Mrs S. She did not show signs of pervasive depression and often acted as the 'life and soul' of the unit, entertaining other patients with her dramatic and musical skills. Her mobility deteriorated, however, although staff felt this was under 'voluntary control' and she needed a great deal of staff time and attention for physical care.

As discharge approached, her physical abilities seemed to deteriorate and she became more anxious, depressed, and in need of reassurance. Attempts at discharge to her home resulted in a rapid escalation of suicide threats and emergency phone calls, resulting in readmission.

Following a series of individual sessions with a psychologist using a CAT approach, it became clear that Mrs S had a borderline personality constellation that had reemerged following the death of her husband whom she had nursed for many years. She was the oldest of five siblings and had to become a 'parental child' towards her siblings to avoid her mother's criticism and physical abuse. In session 3 she disclosed sexual abuse occurring over many years by her father (which she had not disclosed to anyone before). Disclosing this material was very upsetting for Mrs S but staff noticed that her physical problems and dependency improved and she was more likely to talk about real feelings rather than physical symptoms or 'nameless dread'. By processing the core pain of the abuse, even at this stage of her life, Mrs S was able to gain insight into her patterns of somatization and becoming 'the manipulator' to escape from the distress of helplessness, anger, and guilt. Figure 32.2 highlights this pattern.

The emotional pain had been uncovered in late life due to her husband's death and the breakdown of Mrs S's defensive procedure in which she behaved 'as if' she were an ideal care provider to her husband (and deny her own needs). After the sessions ended Mrs S was able to choose to move into a residential home setting and did not re-present to services in the following 5 years.

Needs for investigation and future direction

There are numerous areas in need of further investigation in the treatment and provision of services for older adults with mental disorders, including issues of ethnicity and cultural diversity and how and where psychotherapeutic services can best be provided to older adults.

Relatively little is known about ethnic and cultural diversity in older individuals and how these factors may influence psychotherapy engagement, adherence, and outcome. This is particularly important as the number of ethnically and culturally diverse elders is projected to increase (US Department of Health and Human Services, 2001), and the significant minority in need of mental health services have not been well represented in mental health clinics or in psychosocial research (Areán and Gallagher-Thompson, 1996). Several authors have discussed psychotherapists' need for cultural competence in the provision of clinical services to these elders and the barriers to recruiting and retaining them in treatment (Areán and Gallagher-Thompson, 1996; Lau and Gallagher-Thompson, 2002). One innovative culturally-competent intervention for older adults is a program for caregivers of culturally diverse backgrounds (e.g., African American,

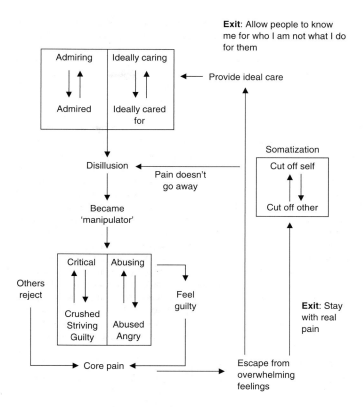

Fig. 32.2 Mrs S's diagram.

Hispanic American, Asian American, and Native American/Alaska Native) who are caring for a relative with Alzheimer's disease or another form of dementing illness (Gallagher-Thompson et al., 2000a).

Certainly there may be modifications or adaptations of treatment based on ethnic and cultural considerations, but specific changes leading to increased effectiveness have not been determined. Improved treatment for these individuals undoubtedly requires an understanding of the context of their lives, including historical events that have impacted them. Baker (1994) reminds the geriatric mental health field that within ethnicities, there is diversity and that it is important to seek specific information about life circumstances rather than make assumptions based on group stereotypes.

Preliminary research suggests that ethnic elders are much less likely than Caucasians to seek or participate in psychotherapy (Yeo and Hikoyeda, 1993). Despite limited knowledge, there is a great need for more information. One area that may affect mental health practice in need of further investigation is assessing and improving social supports, usually through extended family and organized religion communities. Though not typical terrain for psychotherapists, these areas are often important to ethnically and culturally diverse elders.

Epidemiological studies indicate that older individuals in need of psychiatric services are often underserved. In the UK and the USA, referral to and delivery of psychotherapeutic services to the elderly is low (George et al., 1988; Murphy, 2000). Older adults are less likely to seek mental health services than younger adults, and they typically present symptoms of emotional distress in their physicians' office (Goldstrom et al., 1987). This may be due to a host of influences, including accessibility and reimbursement patterns. One opportunity and challenge to the field is how and where psychotherapeutic services can best be provided to this population. Innovative ways of improving the availability of mental health services for older adults, such as telehealth or telephonic use of therapies, mental health treatment in managed primary care (Gallo and Lebowitz, 1999), home and community-based interventions (Rabins et al., 2000), and the inclusion of psychotherapists on integrated teams (Zeiss and Gallagher-Thompson, 2003) are vast. Hopefully, the geriatric mental health intervention field will continue to flourish in their provision of services to older individuals, and will be joined by more colleagues in the future.

Conclusions

The older adult segment of the populations in industrialized countries is becoming larger and more diverse. This may translate to increased need for services for this age group. Psychotherapy, once thought fruitless for older adults, has been shown effective for an array of mental health disorders and problems in this population. The majority of therapists lack formal training in geropsychology and perceive themselves as needing additional training (Qualls *et al.*, 2002). Although there are many commonalities in working with younger and older adults, there are also certain distinctive factors about older individuals that affect prevalence of mental health conditions, risk factors, assessment, and treatment. Psychotherapists who are interested in working with older individuals should familiarize themselves with the myths and actualities of aging, including understanding maturational and cohort differences, understand which therapies are empirically supported, and become familiar with and attentive to the potential modifications of assessment and treatment.

References

Abraham, K. (1919/1927). The applicability of psycho-analytic treatment to patients at an advanced age. In: D. Bryan and A. Strachey, trans. *Selected papers on psychoanalysis*, pp. 312–17. New York: Brunner/Mazel.

Adams, W., Barry, K., and Fleming, M. (1996). Screening for problem drinking in older primary care patients. *Journal of the American Medical Association*, **276**, 1964–7.

Allen-Burge, R., Stevens, A. B., and Burgio, L. D. (1999). Effective behavioral interventions for decreasing dementia-related challenging behavior in nursing homes. *International Journal of Geriatric Psychiatry*, **14**, 213–32.

American Hospital Association. (1976). *The way to reality: guide for developing a reality orientation programme*. Chicago, IL: American Hospital Association.

American Psychiatric Association Task Force on Benzodiazepine Dependency. (1990). *Benzodiazepine dependence, toxicity, and abuse*. Washington, DC: Author.

American Psychological Association Working Group on the Older Adult. (1998). What practitioners should know about working with older adults. *Professional Psychology: Research and Practice*, **29**, 413–27.

Areán, P. A. and Cook, B. L. (2002). Psychotherapy and combined psychotherapy/ pharmacotherapy for late life depression. *Biological Psychiatry*, **52**, 293–303.

Areán, P. A. and Gallagher-Thompson, D. (1996). Issues and recommendations for the recruitment and retention of older ethnic minority adults into clinical research. *Journal of Consulting and Clinical Psychology*, **64**, 875–80.

Baker, F. M. (1994). Psychiatric treatment of older African-Americans. *Hospital and Community Psychiatry*, **45**, 32–7.

Barry, K., Oslin, D., and Blow, F. (2001). Alcohol problems in older adults. *Prevention and management*. New York: Springer.

Beck, A. T. and Steer, R. A. (1987). *Manual for the revised Beck Depression Inventory*. San Antonio, TX: Psychological Corporation.

Beck, A. T., Rush, J., Shaw, B., and Emery, G. (1979). *Cognitive therapy of depression*. New York: Guilford Press.

Bertz, R. J., *et al.* (1997). Alprazolam in young and elderly men: sensitivity and tolerance to psychomotor sedative, and memory effects. *Journal of Pharmacology and Experimental Therapeutics*, **281**, 1317–29.

Blazer, D., George, L. K., and Hughes, D. (1991). The epidemiology of anxiety disorders: an age comparison. In: C. Salzman and B. D. Lebowitz, ed. *Anxiety in the elderly: treatment and research*, pp. 17–30. New York: Springer Publishing.

Blow, F. and Barry, K. (2000). Older patients with at-risk and problem drinking patterns: new developments in brief interventions. *Journal of Geriatric Psychiatry and Neurology*, **13**, 115–23.

Brink, T. L. (1986). *Clinical gerontology: a guide to assessment and intervention*. New York: Haworth Press.

Bonjean, M. J. (1988). Psychotherapy with families caring for a mentally impaired elderly member. In: C. S. Chilman and E. W. Nunnally, ed. *Chronic illness and disability. Families in trouble series*, Vol. 2, pp. 141–55. New York: Sage.

Brown, G. K., Bruce, M. L., Pearson, J. L., and the PROSPECT Study Group (2001). High-risk management guidelines for elderly suicidal patients in primary care settings. *International Journal of Geriatric Psychiatry*, **16**, 593–601.

Butler, R. N. (1963). The life review. An interpretation of reminiscence in the aged. *Psychiatry*, **26**, 65–76.

Cheston, R. (1998). Psychotherapeutic work with people with dementia: a review of the literature. *British Journal of Medical Psychology*, **71**, 211–31.

Conwell, Y., *et al.* (1998). Age differences in behaviors leading to completed suicide. *American Journal of Geriatric Psychiatry*, **6**, 122–6.

Cook, J. M., Hersen, M., and Van Hasselt, V. B. (1998). Historical perspectives. In: M. Hersen and V. Van Hasselt, ed. *Handbook of clinical geropsychology*, pp. 3–17. New York: Plenum Press.

Coon, D. W. and Gallagher-Thompson, D. (2002). Encouraging homework completion among older adults in therapy. *Journal of Clinical Psychology*, **58**, 549–63.

Crowther, M. R. and Zeiss, A. M. (1999). Cognitive-behavior therapy in older adults: a case involving sexual functioning. *Journal of Clinical Psychology*, **55**, 961–75.

Deats, S. M. (1996). The problem of aging in *King Lear* and *The Tempest*. *Journal of Aging and Identity*, **1**, 87–98.

DeLeo, D., Scocco, P., and Meneghel, G. (1999). Pharmacological and psychotherapeutic treatment of personality disorders in the elderly. *International Psychogeriatrics*, **11**, 191–206.

Dick, L. P. and Gallagher-Thompson, D. (1995). Cognitive therapy with the core beliefs of a distressed, lonely caregiver. *Journal of Cognitive Psychotherapy: An International Quarterly*, **9**, 215–27.

Dick, L. P., Gallagher-Thompson, D., Coon, D. W., Powers, D. V., and Thompson, L. W. (1995). *Cognitive-behavioral therapy for late life depression: a client manual*. Palo Alto, CA: Older Adult and Family Center, Veterans Affairs Palo Alto Health Care System.

Dougherty, L. and Chamblin, B. (1999). Assessment as an adjunct to psychotherapy. In: P. Lichtenberg, ed. *Handbook of assessment in clinical gerontology*, pp. 91–110. New York: John Wiley and Sons.

Duffy, M., ed. (1999). *Handbook of counseling and psychotherapy with older adults*. New York: Wiley.

Dupree, L. and Schonfeld, L. (1999). Management of alcohol abuse in older adults. In: M. Duffy, ed. *Handbook of counseling and psychotherapy with older adults*, pp. 632–49. New York: John Wiley and Sons, Inc.

Dupree, L., Broskowski, H., and Schonfeld, L. (1984). The gerontology alcoholism project: a behavioral treatment program for elderly alcohol abusers. *The Gerontologist*, **24**, 510–16.

Erikson, E. H. (1959). *Identity and the life cycle*. New York: Norton.

Erikson, E. (1982). *The life cycle completed*. New York: Norton.

Fleming, M., Baxter-Maxwell, L., Barry, K., Adams, W., and Stauffacher, E. (1999). Brief physician advice for alcohol problems in older adults. A randomized community-based trial. *The Journal of Family Practice*, **48**, 378–84.

Folstein, M. F., Folstein, S. E., and McHugh, P. R. (1975). Mini-Mental State: a practical method for grading the cognitive state of patients for the clinician. *Journal of Psychiatric Research*, **12**, 189–98.

Frank, E., Prigerson, H. G., Shear, M. K., and Reynolds, C. F. (1997). Phenomenology and treatment of bereavement-related distress in the elderly. *International Clinical Psychopharmacology*, **12**, S25–9.

Frazer, D. W. and Jongsma, A. E. (1999). *The older adult psychotherapy treatment planner*. New York: Wiley.

Freud, S. (1904/1959). On psychotherapy. In: J. Riviere, trans. *Collected papers*: Vol. 1. *Early papers on the history of the psycho-analytic movement*, pp. 249–63. New York: Basic Books.

Gallagher-Thompson, D. and Steffen, A. M. (1994). Comparative effects of cognitive-behavioral and brief psychodynamic psychotherapies for depressed family caregivers. *Journal of Consulting and Clinical Psychology*, **62**, 543–9.

Gallagher, D. and Thompson, L. W. (1981). *Depression in the elderly: a behavioral treatment manual*. Los Angeles, CA: University of Southern California Press.

Gallagher-Thompson, D. and Thompson, L. W. (1995). Psychotherapy with older adults in theory and practice. In: B. Bongar and L. E. Beutler, ed. *Comprehensive textbook of psychotherapy: theory and practice*, pp. 359–79. New York: Oxford University Press.

Gallagher-Thompson, D. and Thompson, L. W. (1996). Applying cognitive-behavioral therapy to the psychological problems of later life. In: S. H. Zarit and B. G. Knight, ed. *A guide to psychotherapy and aging: effective clinical interventions in a life-stage context*, pp. 61–82. Washington, DC: American Psychological Association.

Gallagher-Thompson, D., et al. (1992). *Controlling your frustration: a class for caregivers*. Palo Alto, CA: Department of Veterans Affairs Medical Center.

Gallagher-Thompson, D., et al. (2000a). Development and implementation of intervention strategies for culturally diverse caregiving populations. In: R. Schulz, ed. *Handbook on dementia caregiving: evidence–based interventions for family caregivers*, pp. 151–85. New York: Springer Publishing.

Gallagher-Thompson, D., Cassidy, E. L., and Lovett, S. (2000b). Training psychologists for service delivery in long-term care settings. *Clinical Psychology: Science and Practice*, 7, 329–36.

Gallo, J. J. and Lebowitz, B. D. (1999). The epidemiology of common late-life mental disorders in the community: themes for the new century. *Psychiatric Services*, 50, 1158–66.

Gatz, M., et al. (1998). Empirically validated psychological treatments for older adults. *Journal of Mental Health and Aging*, 4, 9–46.

George, L. K., Blazer, D. G., Winfield–Laird, I., Leaf, P. J., and Fischbach, R. L. (1988). Psychiatric disorders and mental health service use in later life: Evidence from the epidemiologic catchment area program. In: J. A. Brody and G. L. Maddox, ed. *Epidemiology and aging*, pp. 189–219. New York: Springer.

Glantz, M. D. (1989). Cognitive therapy with the elderly. In: A. Freeman, K. Simon, K. Simon, L. Beutler, and H. Arkowitz, ed. *A comprehensive handbook of cognitive therapy*, pp. 467–89. New York: Plenum Press.

Goldstrom, I. D., et al. (1987). Mental health services use by elderly adults in a primary care setting. *Journal of Gerontology*, 42, 147–53.

Gorenstein, E. E., et al. (in press). Cognitive-behavioral therapy for management of anxiety and medication in older adults. *American Journal of Geriatric Psychiatry*.

Grundy, E. (1989). Longitudinal perspectives on the living arrangements of the elderly. In: M. Jefferys, ed. *Growing old in the twentieth century*, pp. 128–47. Routledge, London.

Haight, B. K. and Webster, J. D., ed. (1995). *The art and science of reminiscence: theory, research, methods, and applications*. Washington, DC: Taylor and Francis.

Haight, B. K., Coleman, P., and Lord, K. (1997). The linchpins of a successful life review: structure, evaluation, and individuality. In: B. K. Haight and J. D. Webster, ed. *The art and science of reminiscing. Theory, research, methods, and applications*, pp. 179–92. Washington, DC: Taylor and Francis.

Hanlon, J. T., et al. (1998). Benzodiazepine use and cognitive function among community-dwelling elderly. *Clinical Pharmacology and Therapeutics*, 64, 684–92.

Hanlon, J. T., et al. (2002). Use of inappropriate prescription drugs by older people. *Journal of the American Geriatrics Society*, 50, 26–34.

Hedlund, B. and Gilewski, M.(1980). *Development of pleasant and unpleasant events schedule for older adults: a validation study of short forms for use with elderly individuals*. University of Southern California. Unpublished Manuscript.

Hemmelgarn, B., Suissa, S., Huang, A., Boivin, J. F., and Pinard, G. (1997). Benzodiazepine use and the risk of motor vehicle crash in the elderly. *Journal of the American Medical Association*, 278, 27–31.

Hepple, J. (2002). Cognitive analytic therapy. In: J. Hepple, J. Pearce, and P. Wilkinson, ed. *Psychological therapies with older people: developing treatments for effective practice*, pp. 128–59. Hove, East Sussex: Brunner-Routledge.

Hepple, J. (2003a). Ageism in therapy and beyond. In: J. Hepple and L. Sutton, ed. *Cognitive analytic therapy and later life: a new perspective on old age*, pp. 45–66. Hove, East Sussex, England: Brunner-Routledge.

Hepple, J. (2003b). Borderline traits and dissociated states in later life. In: J. Hepple and L. Sutton, ed. *Cognitive analytic therapy and later life: a new perspective on old age*, pp. 177–200. Hove, East Sussex, England: Brunner-Routledge.

Hepple, J., Wilkinson, P., and Pearce, J. (2002). Psychological therapies with older people: An overview. In: J. Hepple, J. Pearce, and P. Wilkinson, ed. *Psychological therapies with older people: developing treatments for effective practice*, pp. 161–76. Hove, East Sussex, England: Brunner-Routledge.

Hildebrand, P. E. (1995). *Beyond mid-life crisis: a psychodynamic approach to aging*. London: Sheldon Press.

Hildebrand, P. E. (2000). Shakespeare at the Sorbonne. *Journal of European Psychoanalysis*, 10–11, 59–67.

Jeste, D. V. and McClure, F. S. (1997). Psychoses: diagnosis and treatment in the elderly. In: L. S. Schneider, ed. *Developments in geriatric psychiatry. New directions for mental health services*, No. 76, pp. 53–70. San Francisco, CA: Jossey-Bass.

Karel, M. J., Ogland–Hand, S., Gatz, M., and Unützer, J. (2002). *Assessing and treating late-life depression: a casebook and resource guide*. New York: Basic Books, Inc.

Kasl-Godley, J. and Gatz, M. (2000). Psychosocial intervention for individuals with dementia: an integration of theory, therapy, and a clinical understanding of dementia. *Clinical Psychology Review*, 20, 755–82.

Klerman, G. L., Weissman, M. M., Rounsaville, B. J., and Chevron, E. (1984). *Interpersonal psychotherapy of depression*. New York: Academic Press, Basic Books.

Knight, B. (1986). *Psychotherapy with older adults*. Newbury Park, CA: Sage.

Knight, B. G. and McCallum, T. J. (1998). Psychotherapy with older adult families: the contextual, cohort-based/specific challenge model. In: I. H. Nordhus, G. R. VandenBos, S. Berg, and P. Fromholt, ed. *Clinical geropsychology*, pp. 313–28. Washington, DC: American Psychological Association.

Knight, B. G. and Satre, D. D. (1999). Cognitive behavioral psychotherapy with older adults. *Clinical Psychology: Science and Practice*, 6, 188–203.

Lau, A. W. and Gallagher-Thompson, D. (2002). Ethnic minority older adults in clinical and research programs: Issues and recommendations. *Behavior Therapist*, 25, 10–11, 16.

Lazarus, L. W., et al. (1984). Brief psychotherapy with the elderly: a review and preliminary study of process and outcome. In: L. W. Lazarus, ed. *Clinical approaches to psychotherapy with the elderly*, pp. 15–35. Washington, DC: American Psychiatric Press.

Lazarus, L. W., et al. (1987). Brief psychotherapy with the elderly: a study of process and outcome. In: J. Sadavoy and M. Leszcz, ed. *Treating the elderly with psychotherapy*, pp. 265–93. Madison, CT: International Universities Press.

Lebowitz, B. D. and Harris, H. W. (2000). Efficacy and effectiveness: From regulatory to public health models. In: I. Katz and D. Oslin, ed. *Annual review of gerontology and geriatrics: focus on psychopharmacologic interventions in late life*, 19, 3–12.

Lebowitz, B. D., et al. (1997). Diagnosis and treatment of depression in late life: consensus statement update. *Journal of the American Medical Association*, 278, 1186–90.

Lenze, E. J., et al. (2002). Combined pharmacotherapy and psychotherapy as maintenance treatment for late-life depression: effects on social adjustment. *American Journal of Psychiatry*, 159, 466–8.

Levin, S., Kruger, J., and Blow, F. (2000). Substance abuse among older adults: a guide for social service providers. *Treatment Improvement Protocol (TIP) Series*, Vol. 26. US Department of Health and Human Services (SAMHSA): Rockville, MD.

Lewinsohn, P. M., Biglan, T., and Zeiss, A. (1976). Behavioral treatment of depression. In: P. Davidson, ed. *Behavioral management of anxiety, depression and pain*, pp. 91–146. New York: Brunner/Mazel.

Lichtenberg, P.A., et al. (1998). Standards for psychological services in long-term care facilities. *The Gerontologist*, 38, 122–7.

Linehan, M. M. (1993). *Cognitive-behavioral treatment of borderline personality disorder*. New York: Guilford Press.

Lynch, T. R., Morse, J. Q., Mendelson, T., and Robins, C. J. (2003). Dialectical behavior therapy for depressed older adults: a randomized pilot study. *American Journal of Geriatric Psychiatry*, 11, 33–45.

Maercker, A. (2002). Life-review technique in the treatment of PTSD in elderly patients: Rationale and three single case studies. *Journal of Clinical Geropsychology*, 8, 239–49.

Martin, L. J. (1944). *A handbook for old age counselors*. San Francisco: Geertz.

Miller, M. D., *et al.* (1994). Applying interpersonal psychotherapy to bereavement-related depression following loss of a spouse in late life. *Journal of Psychotherapy Practice and Research*, 3, 149–62.

Miller, M. D., *et al.* (2001). Interpersonal psychotherapy for late-life depression: past, present, and future. *Journal of Psychotherapy Practice and Research*, 10, 231–8.

Miller, W. and Rollnick, S. (1991). *Motivational interviewing*. Guilford Press: New York.

Mohlman, J., *et al.* (2003). Standard and enhanced cognitive-behavior therapy for late-life generalized anxiety disorder: two pilot investigations. *American Journal of Geriatric Psychiatry*, 11, 24–32.

Morin, C. M., Culbert, J. P., and Schwartz, S. M. (1994). Nonpharmacological interventions for insomnia: a meta-analysis of treatment efficacy. *American Journal of Psychiatry*, 151, 1172–80.

Morin, C. M., Colecchi, C. A., Ling, W. D., and Sood, R. K. (1995). Cognitive behavior therapy to facilitate benzodiazepine discontinuation among hypnotic-dependent patients with insomnia. *Behavior Therapy*, 26, 733–45.

Mossey, J. M., Knott, K. A., Higgins, M., and Talerico, K. (1996). Effectiveness of a psychosocial intervention, interpersonal counseling, for subdysthymic depression in medically ill elderly. *Journal of Gerontology*, 51A, M172–8.

Murphy, S. (2000). Provision of psychotherapy services for older people. *Psychiatric Bulletin*, 24, 184–7.

National Institutes of Health Consensus Development Panel on Depression in Late Life. (1992). Diagnosis and treatment of depression in late life. *Journal of the American Medical Association*, 268, 1018–24.

Newton, N. A., Brauer, D., Gutmann, D. L., and Grunes, J. (1986). Psychodynamic therapy with the aged: a review. *Clinical Gerontologist*, 5, 205–29.

Niederehe, G. and Schneider, L. S. (1998). Treatments for depression and anxiety in the aged. In: P. E. Nathan and J. M. Gorman, ed. *A guide to treatments that work*, pp. 270–87. New York: Oxford University Press.

Palmer, B. W., Heaton, S. C., and Jeste, D. V. (1999). Older patients with schizophrenia: challenges in the coming decades. *Psychiatric Services*, 50, 1178–83.

Patterson, T. L., McKibbin, C., Taylor, M., Goldman, S., Davila–Fraga, W., Bucardo, J., *et al.* (2003). Functional Adaptation Skills Training (FAST): a pilot psychosocial intervention study in middle-aged and older patients with chronic psychotic disorders. *American Journal of Geriatric Psychiatry*, 11, 17–23.

Pearson, J. L. and Brown, G. K. (2000). Suicide prevention in late life: Directions for science and practice. *Clinical Psychology Review*, 20, 685–705.

Pearson, J. L. and Conwell, Y. (1995). Suicide in late-life: challenges and opportunities for research. *International Psychogeriatrics*, 7, 131–6.

Pfeiffer, E. and Busse, E. (1973). Mental disorders in late life—affective disorders: paranoid, neurotic, and substantial reactions. In: E. Busse and E. Pfeiffer, ed. *Mental illness in later life*, pp. 107–44. Washington, DC: American Psychiatric Press.

Qualls, S. H. (1995). Clinical interventions with later-life families. In: R. Blieszner, and V. H. Bedford, ed. *Handbook of aging and the family*, pp. 474–87. Westport, CT: Greenwood Press.

Qualls, S. H. (2000). Therapy with aging families: Rationale, opportunities and challenges. *Aging and Mental Health*, 4, 191–9.

Qualls, S. H., Segal, D. L., Norman, S., Niederehe, G., and Gallagher-Thompson, D. (2002). Psychologists in practice with older adults: current patterns, sources of training, and need for continuing education. *Professional Psychology: Research and Practice*, 33, 435–42.

Rabins, P. V., *et al.* (2000). Effectiveness of a nurse–based outreach program for identifying and treating psychiatric illness in the elderly. *Journal of the American Medical Association*, 283, 2802–9.

Ray, W. A., Thapa, P. B., and Gideon, P. (2000). Benzodiazepines and the risk of falls in nursing home residents. *Journal of the American Geriatrics Society*, 48, 682–5.

Rechtschaffen, A. (1959). Psychotherapy with geriatric patients: a review of the literature. *Journal of Gerontology*, 14, 73–84.

Regier, D. A., *et al.* (1988). One-month prevalence of mental disorders in the United States: based on five Epidemiologic Catchment Area sites. *Archives of General Psychiatry*, 45, 977–86.

Reynolds, C. F., *et al.* (1999). Nortriptyline and interpersonal psychotherapy as maintenance therapies for recurrent major depression: a randomized controlled trial in patients older than 59 years. *Journal of the American Medical Association*, 281, 39–45.

Ryle, A. (1990). *Cognitive analytic therapy: active participation in change. A new integration in brief psychotherapy*. Chichester: Wiley.

Scogin, F., Hamblin, D., and Beutler, L. (1987). Bibliotherapy for depressed older adults: a self help alternative. *The Gerontologist*, 27, 383–7.

Scogin, F., Jamison, C., and Gochneaur, K. (1989). Comparative efficacy of cognitive and behavioral bibliotherapy for mildly and moderately depressed older adults. *Journal of Consulting and Clinical Psychology*, 57, 403–7.

Scogin, F., Jamison, C., and Davis, N. (1990). Two-year follow-up of bibliotherapy for depression in older adults. *Journal of Consulting and Clinical Psychology*, 58, 665–7.

Shear, M. K., *et al.* (2001). Traumatic grief treatment: a pilot study. *American Journal of Psychiatry*, 158, 1506–8.

Stanley, M. A., *et al.* (2003). Cognitive-behavior therapy for late-life generalized anxiety disorder in primary care—preliminary findings. *American Journal of Geriatric Psychiatry*, 11, 92–6.

Teri, L. and McCurry, S. M. (1994). Psychosocial therapies. In: C. E. Coffey and J. L. Cummings, ed. *The American Psychiatric Press Textbook of Geriatric Neuropsychiatry*, pp. 662–82. Washington, DC: American Psychiatric Press.

Teri, L., Curtis, J., Gallagher-Thompson, D., and Thompson, L. W. (1994). Cognitive/behavior therapy with depressed older adults. In: L. S. Schneider, C. F. Reynolds, B. Lebowitz, and A. Friedhoff, ed. *Diagnosis and treatment of depression in the elderly: proceedings of the NIH consensus development conference*, pp. 279–91. Washington, DC: American Psychiatric Press.

Teri, L., Logsdon, R. G., Uomoto, J., and McCurry, S. M. (1997). Behavioral treatment of depression in dementia patients: a controlled clinical trial. *Journals of Gerontology Series B—Psychological Sciences and Social Sciences*, 52, P159–66.

Teri, L., *et al.* (1998). Treatment for agitation in dementia patients: a behavior management approach. *Psychotherapy*, 35, 436–43.

Thompson, L., Gallagher, D., and Breckenridge, J. S. (1987). Comparative effectiveness of psychotherapies for depressed elders. *Journal of Consulting and Clinical Psychology*, 55, 385–90.

Thompson, L. W., Gallagher-Thompson, D., and Dick, L. P. (1995). *Cognitive-behavioral therapy for late life depression: a therapist manual*. Palo Alto, CA: Older Adult and Family Center, Veterans Affairs Palo Alto Health Care System.

Thompson, L. W., Coon, D. W., Gallagher-Thompson, D., Sommer, B. R., and Koin, D. (2001). Comparison of desipramine and cognitive/behavioral therapy in the treatment of elderly outpatients with mild-to-moderate depression. *American Journal of Geriatric Psychiatry*, 9, 225–40.

Thorton, S. and Brotchie, J. (1987). Reminiscence: a critical review of the literature. *British Journal of Clinical Psychology*, 26, 93–111.

United Nations. (2003). *Population division of the Department of Economic and Social Affairs of the United Nations Secretariat, World Population Prospects: the 2002 Revision and World Urbanization Prospects*. http://esa.un.org/unpp, 11 March 2003.

US Department of Health and Human Services Mental Health: Culture, Race, and Ethnicity. (2001). *A supplement to mental health: report of the Surgeon General*. Rockville, MD: US Department of Health and Human Services, Substance Abuse and Mental Health Services Administration, Center for Mental Health Services.

US Department of Veterans Affairs. (1997). *Assessment of competency and capacity of the older adult: a practice guideline for psychologists*. National Center for Cost Containment (NTIS no. PB-97-147904). Milwaukee, WI: US Department of Veterans Affairs.

Webster, J. D. and Haight, B. K. (2002). *Critical advances in reminiscence work from theory to application*. New York: Springer Publishing.

Wetherell, J. L. (1998). Treatment of anxiety in older adults. *Psychotherapy: Theory, Research, Practice, Training*, 35, 444–58.

Wetherell, J. L., Gatz, M., and Craske, M. G. (2003). Treatment of generalized anxiety disorder in older adults. *Journal of Consulting and Clinical Psychology*, 71, 31–40.

Yeo, G. and Hikoyeda, N. (1993). *Differential assessment and treatment of mental health problems: African American, Latino, Filipino, and Chinese American elders*. Stanford, CA: Stanford Geriatric Education Center Working Paper Series No. 13.

Zarit, S. H. and Zarit, J. M. (1998). *Mental disorders in older adults: fundamentals of assessment and treatment*. New York: Guilford Press.

Zeiss, A. M. and Gallagher-Thompson, D. (2003). Providing interdisciplinary geriatric team care: what does it really take? *Clinical Psychology: Science and Practice*, 10, 115–19.

V

Issues in specific populations

33 Psychotherapy for medical patients

C. A. White and P. M. Trief

Introduction

Physical illnesses are associated with an increased risk of experiencing psychological problems and disorders. People who are medically ill often have to endure debilitating treatments that can further contribute to this increased risk. Deterioration in quality of life and family functioning can also occur. The practice of psychotherapy for psychological and psychiatric problems that are secondary to physical illness is, in many cases, relatively straightforward and mirrors the principles and procedural elements of the application of such therapies in people without comorbid physical illness. In some instances, though, clinicians need to be aware of known certain issues in the application of a particular psychotherapeutic model to patients with psychological and psychiatric comorbidities and when applied to physical syndromes such as chronic pain or irritable bowel syndrome (IBS). This chapter will outline the issues relating to the application of psychotherapy for people with concurrent medical disorders, first from the perspective of the more common psychotherapy modalities and then within the context of the medical problems and disorders that therapists are most likely to encounter in their clinical work.

The field of clinical health psychology has been rapidly expanding in recent years. Important extensions have included the refinement of psychotherapies targeted at problems of treatment adherence (Horne and Weinman, 1999) and also the application of psychotherapeutic strategies to modify physical risk factors such as smoking and diet (Miller *et al.*, 1997). Indeed, some psychotherapeutic interventions have developed as a result of work that has associated the etiology, genesis, and/or course of physical health problems with psychological processes (Wiklund and Butler-Wheelhouse, 1996). It has also been suggested that psychological factors may influence the extent to which physical illnesses result in mortality (Katon, 1996; Ormel *et al.*, 1999; Wulsin *et al.*, 1999). Although this chapter will refer to such work when it is relevant, the consideration of psychotherapies to modify health behaviors is outside the scope of this chapter and interested readers are referred elsewhere (Ogden, 2000).

Core psychopathology among physically ill

The prevalence of psychological disorders among people with physical illnesses is higher than that seen within the general population (Martin, 2001; Chew-Graham and Hogg, 2002). In some cases, these disorders account for the psychological disorders that patients experience (e.g., an affective disorder due to a general medical condition) but by far the most common psychological disorders are those that present comorbidly with medical problems. These are adjustment disorders, anxiety disorders, and affective disorders. Adjustment disorders occur in approximately one-fourth of general medical patients and a further 12% of people experience symptoms of anxiety and depressive disorders. It is commonly accepted that prevalence estimates vary enormously (by as much as 40%) depending upon the strategies that are used to estimate the presence and severity of psychopathology. Studies that use self-report measures of anxiety and depressive symptomatology tend to produce higher estimates than studies that use standardized diagnostic classification systems such as the International Classification of Diseases (World Health Organization, 1992) and Diagnostic and Statistical Manual (American Psychiatric Association, 1994). Researchers have sometimes failed to address the potential confounding nature of somatic symptoms, which has resulted in a similar tendency to overestimate the prevalence of problems. The capacity of physical ill health and associated treatment to precipitate posttraumatic stress reactions is being increasingly recognized and the prevalence of PTSD among those with medical illness might be as high as 10%. Depressive disorders occur in approximately one-third of people with physical health problems and are more likely to occur in the presence of a life-threatening illness or when the problems are part of a chronic course. People who are exposed to treatment that is associated with unpleasant side-effects (e.g., prolonged pain or changed appearance) and people whose physical illnesses occur in the context of social adversity or low social support are at particular risk of comorbid psychosocial morbidity with a predominant depressive component (Smith, 2003). These reactions may also occur as a direct result of biological influences: the physical disorders themselves (e.g., a depressive episode mediated by thyroid dysfunction) or a medication-induced phenomenon (e.g., an anxiety reaction related to corticosteroids).

Psychopathology among the physically ill is often not detected (van Hemert *et al.*, 1993), especially because clinicians have difficulty in distinguishing psychopathological symptoms from normal reactions, for various reasons. For one, patients may withhold information about their psychiatric symptoms. Also, some health professionals in highly medicalized settings are not sensitive enough toward the psychosocial dimensions of patient care and fail to recognize the necessity of identifying comorbid conditions. When managing psychological disorders among the medically ill, psychotherapy is one of a range of therapeutic strategies than can be implemented. Psychotropic medication can be prescribed alone or as an adjunct to psychotherapy. In considering which psychotherapy to apply to those who are both medically and psychologically unwell, it is important to take into account both the key features of the therapy being considered and of the medical illness that has been diagnosed. The next section of this chapter will describe major psychotherapeutic modalities in working with the medically ill.

Psychotherapies with physically ill patients

Overview

This section will outline, in basic terms, the defining features of four modalities of psychotherapy that are most commonly applied to the psychosocial morbidity associated with a primary medical illness. The aims of assessment, the particular issues relating to the conceptualization of problems of the medically ill and key factors in psychotherapy implementation will be addressed within each section.

Cognitive-behavioral psychotherapy

There are a number of factors that make cognitive-behavioral psychotherapy (CBT) particularly suited to addressing the problems associated with comorbid physical and psychosocial morbidity. CBT has demonstrated efficacy, is the treatment of choice, and/or has an established role in the management of the most common psychopathologies outlined above (DeRubeis and Crits-Cristoph, 1998). Healthcare providers are increasingly advocating that patients adopt an active self-management approach (Tattersall, 2002). This is in keeping with the CBT emphasis on skill acquisition. Individual response to illness is closely linked with cognitive factors such as symptom perception (Lacroix et al., 1991). Disease-specific illness representations often account for variability in emotional reactions (Prohaska et al., 1987) and self-care behaviors (Petrie et al., 1996). Patient beliefs are often related to behavioral aspects of interaction with the healthcare system (Ridsdale et al., 1999). A patient that has been experiencing fatigue, shortness of breath, a skin rash, and a headache may believe that these symptoms are all the result of different medical conditions, when this may not be the case. This perception of symptoms will have an influence on behavior. If someone believes that their shortness of breath and fatigue might be related to a viral illness then they will have a different behavioral response than someone who believed themselves to have an anxiety disorder.

Although there is a significant amount of evidence on the efficacy of CBT as an intervention for anxiety and depressive disorders, many of these studies have been conducted with patients without significant medical problems. There is no reason to expect CBT to be any less effective in treating psychological morbidity when it coexists with medical problems. However, it is only in the areas of functional syndromes, cancer, and chronic pain that research has specifically established CBTs effectiveness. Cognitive-behaviorally based therapies have been shown to improve anxiety and depressive symptoms experienced by cancer patients (Greer et al., 1992; Moorey et al., 1998), to reduce pain and additional use of psychological services among those with noncardiac chest pain (NCCP) (van Peski-Oosterbaan et al., 1999), and to have a positive impact on the full range of biopsychosocial variables associated with chronic pain (Morley et al., 1999). It has also been applied to the management of symptoms of asthma (Grover et al., 2002) and in a group based format for older adults with chronic obstructive pulmonary disease (Kunik et al., 2001). Enright (1997) has suggested that there is almost no medical or disorder that cannot be understood and treated using CBT. This is particularly reflected in the assessment phase of therapy where adjustment to illness and secondary psychological morbidities are assessed according to the contributory feelings, thoughts, and behavior.

Assessing thoughts and behavior

The primary purpose of assessment within CBT is to elicit information for later synthesis within the case formulation (or conceptualization). Assessment should utilize a mix of observation, data from self-report questionnaire, semistructured interview, clinical interview, and the completion of diaries (White, 2001). Questionnaires are a particularly useful way of identifying information. An individual's behavior provides a number of clues to cognitive and emotional dimensions and can inform other elements of the process. Diaries can often be individually constructed for patients based on their symptoms and individual problem profiles. They also help patients appreciate the importance of beginning to work on their problems outside treatment sessions (and enable therapists to identify potential obstacles to the later implementation of therapy homework). The problem list is a very useful way of structuring the assessment session and assessment process (Persons, 1989). The act of exploring cognitive and behavioral dimensions of a problem is illustrated in the following session extract:

Therapist: So you have found that you cannot do the things that you used to do any more—this is one of the ways in which it has been difficult to get used to life after the operation

Patient: Yes, it is really dreadful

Therapist: How have you been feeling when you cannot do the things you used to? (elicit emotions)

Patient: Oh, very tired . . . exhausted (patient gives physical sensations which can be noted, but not emotions)

Therapist: So physically you have been tired and exhausted . . . is that all the time or just when it is difficult to do things?

Patient: Just when I need to do certain things about the house

Therapist: How does it make you feel emotionally, in your mood when you can't do the things that you used to do?

Patient: Oh fed up, down . . . really sad

Therapist: And when you are feeling this way—down and sad . . . What sorts of things do you think about—what passes through your mind? (elicit thoughts)

Patient: Mm . . . (sighs) . . . that I will never get over this, things will never get better

Therapist: When you think this way . . . what do you do, what is your reaction?

Patient: I just sit and do nothing . . . it all seems so pointless

The clinician can help the patient respond to the thought, 'It's all so pointless' and modify his behavior (of sitting and doing nothing).

Problem list assessment can then be complemented by the administration of a self-report measure, observational data, or a self-completed diary. Enquiry about childhood illnesses, parental health and parental responses to illness is often helpful when working with the medically ill as it provides information on early influences on representations of illness and medical treatments. Medical history is very important and including this as part of the assessment is a very helpful way of gaining information on the potential for interaction between medical historical events, patients' thoughts, feelings, and behavior. This information may also relate to other significant life events, thoughts and feelings about medical and nursing staff, satisfaction with treatment, communication skills of staff, understanding of relevant medical information, and current medical management. People who are not willing to consider any potential relationship between psychological variables and their medical problems (even at the level of coping) are likely to find engagement in CBT difficult. When there is doubt about the suitability of CBT, therapists may wish to offer a finite number of sessions to such patients, toward the end of which they can collaboratively decide whether or not to continue treatment.

Conceptualization

White (2001) has distinguished problem level and case level within the process of case formulation. Problem level formulation involves the application of cognitive-behavioral theory and principles to account for the main factors contributing to the occurrence, severity, and nature of problems at the situation-specific level. A case level formulation aims to synthesize the information contained in multiple problem level formulations and seeks to integrate this with historical information on the problems, details on core cognitive structures, the patient's life history and their current living situation. Critical incidents are essential components of a case level formulation and provide a rich source of information regarding the ways in which hypothesized cognitive mechanisms can manifest particular psychosocial problems as a result of the interface between belief and life event. They are usually easy to identify in that they are associated with the onset, exacerbation or recurrence of physical and/or psychosocial problems. There are a number of cognitive-behavioral theories and models that therapists can choose from to assist with the conceptualization and formulation of the psychological problems associated with chronic medical problems. The framework proposed by Padesky and Greenberger (1995) is particularly helpful for the construction of problem level formulations in CBT. The inclusion of a component consisting of physical variables makes it particularly useful in that it acknowledges the importance of taking physical symptoms into account.

There are obviously many strategies that are utilized within CBT. For the purpose of illustrating elements of therapy the focus of this section will be on generic themes that are often implicated in psychosocial adjustment to physical illness. These themes will be highlighted within the following case example regarding the application of CBT with symptoms of an affective disorder presenting in a patient with severe cardiac disease.

Case example

Assessment

Mr R was a 55-year-old man who was referred to the first author with symptoms of a major depressive disorder that had responded only partially to antidepressant medication. He had had four previous myocardial infarctions and had undergone coronary artery bypass graft (CABG) surgery on three occasions. He had experienced repeated admissions to medical wards from the Accident and Emergency Department (Emergency Room) where he had presented with chest pain. He believed that something had gone wrong with his surgery. He reported a 'constant pain' in his chest and lumbar regions, unremitting and unreactive to external circumstances. He described times when his chest pain became more severe, starting with feelings of fatigue and exhaustion. These sensations were followed by shivering, shaking, and hot/cold sensations. He talked of this 'coming out of the blue' and occurring approximately twice per day. He said that he could not get a 'good full day' and that his pain would occasionally wake him from sleep. He said that the episodes had been occurring approximately seven times per day for a period of 2 months prior to assessment. He described the pain as 'sharp', 'cramping', 'crushing', 'squeezing', and 'nauseating'. He presented as being extremely preoccupied with his cardiac disease, chest pain, and the degree to which this was interfering with his life.

The following assessment measures were administered during the initial assessment phase: Beck Depression Inventory (BDI); Beck Anxiety Inventory (BAI); Beck Hopelessness Scale (BHS); Ways of Coping Checklist (WCC); and the McGill–Melzack Pain Questionnaire (MMPQ). Mr R was unable to walk without tiring easily and he was unable to complete jobs he wished to begin around his house. He also reported being unable to plan ahead for the future due to a belief that he would become ill and that he would be a burden to other people. Mr R described the consequences of his continued experience of symptoms to be frustration. He was finding it increasingly difficult to trust medical staff involved with his care. His main coping strategies at the time of assessment were using medication and sitting or lying down in a quiet area.

Conceptualization

Mr R's depressive symptoms were hypothesized to have begun when his expectations of his CABG surgery differed from the actual outcome. This discrepancy seemed to have activated a belief that he was likely to die—imminently—due to cardiac disease. Earlier experiences where family members had died seemed to contribute to the development of this belief which became reinforced when a medical practitioner told him that it was not possible to survive a fifth myocardial infarction (he had had four already). The hopelessness that he experienced following belief activation resulted in a reluctance to engage in any activity and an attentional bias toward pain. His depressive symptoms were hypothesized as being maintained by inactivity and cognitive distortions.

Therapy

At the end of first meeting the interactive nature of chest pain and arousal was discussed. Mr R believed that his pain was present all of the time, a probable overgeneralization. Therefore, prospective monitoring was indicated as a way of providing further information on the pattern of pain symptoms, which would allow him to test accurately the validity of his belief (testing beliefs was an important part of therapy). The patient was instructed to monitor his pain hourly for 7 days using a scale from 0 to 10 where 0 indicated 'no pain at all' and 10 indicated 'worst pain ever'. At the next session Mr R was surprised to learn that there were times when he experienced no pain and, indeed, that all his ratings were 5 or less and 85% of them were 0 or 1. Mr R's BDI scores reduced from 30 (severe) to 17 (mild) which he attributed to the pain monitoring exercise. This exercise also provided powerful evidence of the unhelpful nature of some of his depressed thinking Mr R also believed that he was unable to do anything and that he was unable to cope effectively with his chest pain. His clinician

decided to intervene with these cognitions in the same way: by monitoring his episodes of pain, recording chest pain severity before and after his attempts to cope with it. Once again Mr R disconfirmed his dysfunctional ideas and recognized the importance of testing the validity of his automatic thoughts regarding the consequences of his cardiac disease instead of unequivocally accepting them as true.

Mr R was particularly concerned about his tendency to procrastinate, especially about tasks that he wanted to do around the house. He was able to identify the following cognitions: 'It should be done in 2 days'; 'I'll never do it in the time I've got', 'I cannot do anything in the time available'. When asked what he thought might have to change for him to be able to increase his activity levels and complete tasks, he responded 'certain aspects of the tasks, the time I set aside to do them or the way I look at them'. Therapy focused on dividing an activity into smaller steps and testing negative automatic thoughts using an 'antiprocrastination' sheet. Given sustained symptomatic improvement, it was decided to begin to focus on the successful components of the intervention and how he might use these if there were similar difficulties in the future. In doing this Mr R identified the following to be of therapeutic value: reminding himself of how pain improves with rest, breaking activities down into smaller tasks, being flexible about how much and when to do things, and monitoring to determine the validity of thoughts.

Group psychotherapy

The belief that people can learn from, and feel most supported by, others who share their illness-related problems led to the emergence of group psychotherapies for medical patients. Groups became popular in the early 1970s, promoted as unique and cost-effective treatments. Most early reports described loosely structured educational groups (Parsell and Tagliareni, 1974; Wood et al., 1978). However, education only appeared to increase anxiety for some groups (Wallace and Wallace, 1977) and knowledge was often forgotten (Rahe and Ward, 1985). Other groups were modeled on those for psychiatric patients and aimed at breaking through defensive denial; however, these were often problematic and uncomfortable for medical patients (Ibrahim et al., 1974). Improved mood and mutual support resulted when group discussion focused on coping with the illness, and when the goals were increased knowledge (Rahe et al., 1979; Bucher et al., 1984; Stern et al., 1984; Blumenthal, 1985; Crawford and McIver, 1985; Gamsa et al., 1985). More structured interventions soon followed, such as Spiegel's supportive-expressive therapy for cancer patients (Spiegel et al., 1981) and Sobel and Worden's Omega Project (Sobel and Worden, 1982). The group content expanded to include relaxation (Heinrich and Schlag, 1982), coping skills (Telch and Telch, 1986; Edgar et al., 2001), and stress management (Fawzy et al., 1990a) training. Overall, studies showed that group participants, as compared with no-group controls, demonstrated better knowledge of, and emotional adjustment to, their illness, with some evidence of reduced morbidity and mortality (Spiegel et al., 1981; Fawzy et al., 1993; Linden et al., 1996; Fawzy and Fawzy, 1998).

Suitability for groups

As many studies use convenience samples of patients the issue of suitability for group has not received sufficient attention. One must first understand the goals of group involvement. Cassileth (1995) describes two classes of goals for psychotherapeutic interventions for cancer patients that apply to the varied group models. The first are 'process goals', i.e., to provide skills and tools to help patients deal with their illness. Examples include: providing disease-related information, and teaching skills and providing opportunities for patients to experience/express emotions, to address the 'meaning' of the illness, to establish a sense of coherence and control, and to promote improved family communication. The second class are 'primary goals', that include decreasing physical and emotional sequelae of disease, and treatment (e.g., pain, nausea, depression, anxiety), and thus enhance adjustment, acceptance and quality-of-life. Skills to manage pain and mood, such as relaxation, activity pacing, distraction, and pleasant event scheduling, address these goals.

Given these broad goals, it may seem that most people might benefit from groups. In a study of 400 cancer patients in a coping skills group, it was found that coping skills training improved quality of life and mood and subgroup analysis found that gender, education, religion, marital status and prior self-help experience did not affect outcome (Cunningham et al., 1993). A few studies have suggested that patients with low internal locus of control (Zakus et al., 1979) or high hypochondriasis (Moore et al., 1984) may not benefit from a group. It has also been suggested that such patients may have a negative impact on the effectiveness of the group for other members, suggesting that they should be excluded.

The question of homogeneity of groups has also been raised, i.e., should groups be disease, or even stage-of-disease, specific? The vast majority of studied groups address one specific disease, e.g., cancer or heart disease. A report of a group of heterogeneous cancer patients notes that greater satisfaction was found with diagnosis-specific meetings (Petersson et al., 2000). As most groups include a strong didactic component, and much of the benefit derives from contact with others with similar experiences, combining patients with varied diseases in one group is counter-intuitive. However, Jon Kabat-Zinn (1990) has adopted this approach to teach mindfulness meditation to patients in large heterogeneous groups and reports notable success. A related question is when should group be chosen over individual treatment? In a nonrandomized study of melanoma patients, those in a group showed greater improvement than those seen individually (Fawzy et al., 1996). In contrast, a study of breast and colon cancer patients showed significantly greater benefit for individual versus group treatment. In this study, patients were randomly assigned to Nucare (a short-term psychoeducational coping skills training intervention) presented either individually or in a group format, or to a support group or no intervention control. Individual Nucare patients showed significantly greater improvements in well-being; however, type of cancer, gender, and patient choice of format were all factors that affected the results, and authors noted significant difficulties in establishing functioning groups (Edgar et al., 2001). In two other studies (one a meta-analysis), no differences in emotional distress between group and individually treated patients were found (Cain et al., 1986; Sheard and Maguire, 1999). These conflicting findings fail to clarify the issue. Clinical expertise suggests that the decision to recommend group versus individual treatment should be made within the therapist's conceptualization of the patient—considering the degree to which the patient is likely to be able to engage in, and benefit from, group involvement. In addition, one must take into account the patient's preference, which is affected by personality, openness, and need for social support, and such logistical considerations as time, cost, and access.

There is also the question of what type of group to develop. Few studies have actively compared different types of groups. One study compared group coping skills instruction to a support group and to no treatment. They found coping skills training (CST) patients improved, support group patients remained the same and no treatment controls deteriorated (Telch and Telch, 1986). CST included instruction in relaxation, stress management, assertive communication, problem solving, pleasant activity planning, and affect regulation. Further research is needed to determine which types or lengths of groups, or types of leaders, benefit which patients, or in what ways these benefits may manifest.

Given limited mental health resources, should groups be offered to all patients (the standard in most studies) or only to those individuals who show evidence of significant distress or difficulty coping? A meta-analysis of cancer trials noted that only four of 25 trials specifically recruited subjects suffering, or at risk of, high distress (Sheard and Maguire, 1999). Simonton and Sherman (2000) propose a group model for cancer patients that tailors the intervention to the patient's stage of illness and medical treatment. They recommend brief, educational groups for newly diagnosed patients, time-limited skills training groups for those in, or recently discharged from, active medical treatment, and longer-term, less-structured groups that emphasize support and emotional expression for patients later in the process. Similarly, Harper et al. (1999) propose providing an open attendance, ongoing support group for cardiac patients that welcomes family members. They recommend focused discussion of themes that consistently emerge such as: frustration at life-style limitations, anger at overprotectiveness of family members, anger at self for lack of adherence, and sadness about losses that accompany medical illness.

Finally, the issue of appropriate outcome remains unresolved. Most reports assess psychosocial outcomes, such as changes in anxiety, depression, coping skills, knowledge, and adherence. However, Spiegel's well-known follow-up of metastatic breast cancer group members that found significantly longer survival time (36.3 months for group members versus 18.9 months for no treatment controls) led to a great deal of interest in the effect of group social support on morbidity and mortality, described by Andersen as the Biobehavioral Model of cancer stress and disease course (Andersen, 2002). Andersen's model explores how disease endpoints, (e.g., recurrence, disease-free interval, mortality) can be affected by psychological (e.g., stress), behavioral (e.g., adherence), and biologic (e.g., immune response activity) factors. Studies of the effect of group interventions on these variables are inconsistent, with some showing improved survival time and immunologic response for cancer group members (Spiegel et al., 1989; Fawzy et al., 1990b, 1993), but others failing to demonstrate such a connection (Ilnyckyj et al., 1994; Cunningham et al., 1998; Edelman et al., 1999; Schrock et al., 1999; Goodwin et al., 2001).

Using group process therapeutically

In addition to education and skills training, group therapy can foster interactions and opportunities that are highly meaningful for medical patients (Blake-Mortimer et al., 1999). Group process refers to this ebb and flow of relationships and discussions. The process occurs around common patient themes that, when attended to by the group leader, can foster growth and opportunities for change.

The most important process is enhanced social support through group cohesion. Illness often fosters social withdrawal and isolation, yet evidence is strong that social connections are important to health (Mulder et al., 1992; Smith and Ruiz, 2002). The unique caring bonds that are forged with similarly ill individuals who can form a close-knit unit are consistently reported by patients as being highlights of the group experience (Spiegel, 1993; Harper et al., 1999). A second process fostered in group is the expression of emotions. Emotional expression has been associated with better coping and adjustment, and even with improved medical outcomes (Pennebaker and Beall, 1986; Smyth, 1998; Smyth et al., 1999). The group leader's words, and behaviors modeled by emotionally expressive group members, can allow the experience and expression of deepest feelings within a safe environment.

Group patients can also learn to adopt active coping styles. They may discuss ways to improve communication with family members, which has been shown to reduce distress in cancer patients (Spiegel et al., 1983). Or, stress reduction skills (Gier et al., 1988; Bennett et al., 1996) can be modeled, practiced, and reinforced, as members encourage and guide each other. This process leads to enhanced feelings of control and optimism. Similarly, discussion about life-style changes due to illness, disability and even the possibility of their own death will help some members grieve their losses and face their fears, while others may find a sense of meaning and purpose by helping others (Yalom, 1985; Greenstein and Breitbart, 2000; Wiens and Kellogg, 2000).

Case example

Anne was a 69-year-old woman who had ovarian cancer. She had attended three 8-member support group sessions and had been quiet. When encouraged to speak, she said that she just wanted to listen, that she was 'dealing with my cancer quite well' and didn't need to talk. At one particular session, another member, Barbara, was absent. The therapist informed the group that Barbara was in the hospital, that her cancer had recurred and she was not doing well. The group was quiet. The therapist asked how they were feeling. At that point, Anne burst into tears. The following is an extract from the group therapy session:

Anne: I thought I was doing okay but this really sets me back. I knew I shouldn't come to a group like this, that it would be depressing and people would die. I don't think I can handle that.

Therapist: How do others feel about Barbara's recurrence and illness?

Cathy: It's hard to hear about. Barbara seems like such a nice person. It isn't fair! And, it makes me scared. I knew before that my odds weren't good, but knowing someone who is having a recurrence is really terrifying! It could be me next.

Anne: That's just how I feel. I try to be positive and optimistic, but it's hard to do that when this happens.

Therapist: Are others trying to feel positive all the time? Is that hard? Does it work?

Donna: I think it's good to try to be positive, but we have to be realistic too. And, it definitely isn't good to hide your bad feelings and fears. That just adds more stress.

Anne: But what do you do when your family tells you to think positive thoughts, they don't want to hear any negative thinking?

Donna: I just tell them that I'm trying to be optimistic, but they have to realize that I'm scared, and sad, and that those feelings are important too. I think they don't want to hear that I'm scared because they're scared too. The closest times have been when we all say what we're really feeling, even if we cry together. That seems to help us be able to laugh together, too. I know that sounds weird . . .

Anne: No, it doesn't. I know just what you mean. I think I have to sit down and really talk to my family and let them know where I'm at. It will be hard, but I think we'll all be better off than pretending. Thanks. That's what I'll do.

This is an example of using the group to help patients vent their feelings and learn from each other how to handle them, even when the feelings are negative and difficult to experience. Note that the therapist's role is to foster discussion between group members, by looking for common experiences and encouraging members to talk. In a well-functioning group, the therapist often has little to say, as the members talk to each other, raise issues openly, share positive coping efforts, and support each other's growth. The group went on to discuss other communication issues, as well as their fears about death, pain and loss of function. At the end of the session, they decided to make a card for Barbara to let her know they were thinking about her and missed her.

Psychodynamic therapies

Psychoanalytic concepts can be utilized successfully to formulate the clinical problems of the medically ill and to inform practice when applied as a therapy (Grossman, 1984/5).

Conceptualization

The threat of pain, disfigurement, limitations, and death associated with medical illness can result in anxiety, depression, and problems with adaptation and coping, even for psychologically healthy individuals. A psychodynamic perspective contributes two major areas of focus (Postone, 1998; Straker, 1998). Illness is, above all, a challenge to one's sense of self, a threat to the ego (Backman, 1989a). A psychodynamic approach focuses on understanding the unique psychological issues that an individual brings to the illness experience. Early childhood experiences that define one's self can yield core conflicts that may be triggered by serious illness. Thus, patients may be especially distressed in dependent situations, or vulnerable to conflict with authority figures. The patient role can exacerbate these dependency/authority conflicts. Other common intrapsychic conflicts that can be rekindled by a medical illness involve separation/abandonment and trust.

Also, a psychodynamic perspective includes awareness of each individual's unique defensive structure (Viederman, 1974; Straker and Wyszynski, 1986). Defenses are ways, often unconscious, that we routinely try to manage distressing emotions, block conflicts from awareness and thus maintain our sense of self. Examples include denial, regression, repression of affect, and intellectualization, as well as humor and spiritual seeking. When defenses break down patients become emotionally overwhelmed and unable to cope proactively (Backman, 1989b). The psychodynamic therapist typically meets individually with the patient, although many group therapists also work from a psychodynamic perspective. A major goal is to enable the patient to experience distressing emotions, and express them within

a nonjudgmental, supportive relationship. The therapist also helps him/her explore underlying conflicts, and understand their expression within current relationships. This process moves patients from rigid, limiting defenses to proactive, positive coping efforts.

Common transference and countertransference issues

The therapeutic relationship is key to the process. Patients experience deep trust within the relationship, can let defenses down and open up to emotional exploration. Patients may transfer old feelings and ways of relating established with parents on to the therapist, causing distortions and conflict. Illness often fosters dependency on the therapist, who can become idealized as the 'only one who understands'. Patients can become extremely angry when the nurturance they seek is not provided by their therapist. Patients who have unresolved authority issues will often resist therapists' efforts to guide or explore. The opportunity to work through these issues, to accept mature relationship boundaries, to face dependency needs or work with, not against, an authority figure can provide significant opportunities for emotional growth (Stoute *et al.*, 1996). Therapists also develop countertransference feelings, i.e., emotional responses to patients that may be rooted in therapists' own needs and conflicts. The therapist may feel out of control and helpless to impact the illness. They may be uncomfortable with medical changes, e.g., scars, blood, amputations. They may fear loss and sadness if the patient dies. They may struggle with a need to nurture the patient and foster an unhealthy dependency. And, therapists will use their own defenses to cope with these feelings, which may help or hinder the therapeutic relationship.

What is different about the intervention?

Psychodynamic psychotherapy is often referred to as 'the talking cure'. Yet, all therapeutic approaches involve talking, so what's the difference? Psychodynamic psychotherapy emphasizes the uniqueness of the individual, especially in two domains. The therapist pays attention to the patient's deepest unexpressed feelings, to help him/her understand and process those feelings. It is theorized that when the patient does not need to expend emotional energy defending against feelings he/she is better able to cope with illness-related distress. Also, psychodynamic psychotherapy highlights unresolved childhood conflicts. By helping patients understand the role that these conflicts play in current relationships, the patient can gather and experience appropriate support and reestablish a sense of personal control.

Case example

PM was a 45-year-old single white female who had been diagnosed with type 1 diabetes at age 11. Type 1 diabetes is a metabolic disease, patients must inject insulin regularly throughout the day and closely monitor their blood sugar levels, diet, and activity. Diabetes frequently leads to various medical complications including eye, heart, and kidney disease. At the time of psychotherapy assessment PM's complications included uncontrolled high blood pressure, digestive problems, eye disease (retinopathy), and end-stage renal (kidney) disease (ESRD). Patients with ESRD must undergo hemodialysis, a process in which they are connected to a machine for several hours that cleanses their blood of impurities. She had commenced hemodialysis three times weekly 1 year prior to attendance for assessment. She presented with symptoms of major depressive disorder, including depressed mood, anhedonia, decreased appetite (10 pound weight loss), terminal insomnia, guilt, memory and concentration problems, and passive suicidal thoughts (i.e., 'Sometimes, I wish I wouldn't wake up') but no intent or plan. She had been in poor control of her diabetes since diagnosis, with poor adherence to recommended diet, exercise, and BG testing. Evidence of significant weight gain indicated that she was not consistently restricting fluid intake as is required. She was on Prozac, and other medications for her medical problems.

The patient had been chronically dysthymic since her early adulthood, intermittently treated with psychotherapy and antidepressants. She became more seriously depressed when she began dialysis and was seeking therapy for 'emotional support'. She had been school-phobic as a child and highly anxious when separated from her mother. Academically, she was an excellent student; in high school she was valedictorian. However, when she left home for college, she became depressed and anxious, returned home, and took 8 years to complete her 4-year degree. Her mother died suddenly (unknown cause) when she was aged 21. She described that relationship as 'extremely close, she was the only person who really loved me'. Her relationship with her father was described as 'distant, I don't bother him and he doesn't bother me'. She had two older siblings, lived with her father, and worked as a waitress. She had no close friends. Her history suggested that she had difficulty separating from her mother, and that attachment and loss themes were central to her intrapsychic experience. Her mother's sudden and unexplained death contributed to these conflicts, as she was unable to work successfully through the individuation process to develop her intellectual potential and establish herself as an independent adult. Her unmet dependency needs and grief over her mother's death caused significant emotional distress, but she had low tolerance for negative affect. She defended against these feelings by acting-out. For example, when she watched a TV show about a mother–daughter relationship and became sad, she binged on sweet foods. The core conflict was around dependency issues, and the process focused on the transference, as PM tried to draw the therapist into the maternal role. Hemodialysis also rekindled dependency and attachment issues. The therapist maintained a supportive and caring stance within a well-defined relationship, interpreted her acting-out behaviors, and attempted to help her develop other ways of coping with distress. The limits of the relationship engendered anger at the therapist. As she was encouraged to express these angry feelings, the therapist interpreted the anger as being rooted in unresolved anger towards her mother, whom she felt had 'abandoned' her. She was then able to experience those feelings, and the sadness she also felt. The patient's opportunity to work through these unresolved feelings without fear of loss of the relationship was a major focus of treatment.

Family therapy

Having someone who is physically ill within the family can have a significant impact on one or more members of the immediate and extended family (McCorkle et al., 1993; Kissane et al., 1994). It can be as psychologically demanding to be a family member as a patient—and sometimes more so (Soskolne and Kaplan De-Nour, 1989; Astudills et al., 1996). In most cases family members act as a helpful resource to support and assist the patient (Xiaolian et al., 2002). Indeed, families are often very involved with decision-making about treatment and tend to provide one another with emotional support throughout the duration of the physical illness. There are, however, some circumstances where illness results in problems within the family (Lyons et al., 1995). In some instances it will be necessary to consider family therapy targeted at the family system. Family therapy has traditionally been applied to the psychosocial needs of families with a physically ill child (Finney and Bonner, 1993; Wood, 1994), to children and adolescents (Cottrell and Boston, 2002) and with mental health problems (Barrett et al., 1996), though this has been changing over the past two decades with 'medical family therapy' developing the focus on families who have a member with a chronic illness or disability (Doherty et al., 1994).

Assessment

Basic information on family composition is essential for any assessment that might result in family therapy for families with a medically ill member. This is a core competency within the prequalification training of most mental health professionals. This information can then be used to explore important dimensions of family response to illness. There are usually some members of the family who have more frequent contact with the person being assessed, who demonstrate greater empathy and understanding, who offer more practical support and in whom the patient will find it easier to confide. Each family member has his or her own understanding of the index patient's experience of illness and, while it will not always be possible to speak with each member of the family at the same time, it is important to gather as much information as possible about different perspectives.

Clinicians should consider the impact of the illness on each family member. The assessment process will need to take account of the age and developmental stages of the constituent family members.

Family 'myths' are also important. These may relate to beliefs that are held about the disposition of a family member ('She has always been vulnerable and unable to deal with stress') or processes within the family ('We function best when we avoid talking about disagreements'). These often influence and may mirror beliefs shared by the medically ill patient. This is sometimes referred to as the 'family world view' or the 'family paradigm'. Clinicians may not come into contact with all members of the family at the one time (as might traditionally be the case in an outpatient family therapy clinic) and it might take some weeks to build up a picture of how a particular family has responded to illness. Therapists should determine the ways in which families have addressed problems in the past as this may lead to the identification of successful strategies or assist the therapist in recognizing characteristic problems and/or responses to problems within the family system.

In general, families (as do individuals) tend to cope with conflict or problem situations in similar ways throughout life. This is usually by directly confronting the situation in some way or by avoiding the situation. Family members can be asked 'Which of these styles would have best characterized your way of resolving problems when you were growing up?' and asked to provide examples of the ways in which other people might perceive their family to have reacted to other significant events. Clinical staff who work within inpatient settings are in the unique position of being able to meet many family members in the course of their involvement with inpatient care. They often make observations that can be useful in conceptualizing family response to illness. Therapists need to appreciate the way in which individuals within the family are reacting to the index patient and they need to take time to explore each of these individually. This will assist with the formulation of a shared understanding of the family's way of responding to illness and the difficulties that the family unit is facing.

Conceptualization

It is important to think of family case conceptualization both in terms of family factors and illness specific factors. There may also be issues that are specific to the psychosocial presentation. For example, a 41-year-old male developed multiple sclerosis and major depressive disorder. The conceptualization needed to take account of the course, severity, and symptoms of his illness, family factors and reactions, and psychosocial issues contributing the overall presentation. It was important to identify the patient's neurological symptoms, the distress of his children who believed he was going to die, and the impact on the family of the patient's inactivity, complicated by his depressive belief that he would fail at any task he tried.

Complex consequences can develop when family members have differing illness representations. Misunderstandings that are the product of such differing views of physical illness can contribute to distress or, in some cases, to major family conflict. Family members may also have different feelings about the way in which the index patient responds to his or her illness. Most families will gain mastery of the situation in the initial phases. Some families have difficulty modifying their initial response to the illness when the acute phase has passed (Kreutzer et al., 2002). It is important to track responses within the family, with particular emphasis on the extent to which these responses seem to take account of changes in illness course, treatment or prognosis.

Using the family system therapeutically

Most family oriented interventions seek to enhance communication and facilitate relationships that are sensitive to the emotional and psychological dimensions of being physically ill. Therapeutic work often focuses upon enabling families to ensure that physical illness does not become a dominant feature in influencing all relationships and responses to everyday events. Families can find it useful to focus on the identification of shared assets and to engage in a process whereby they begin to prioritize the problems that face them. The majority of families are able to maintain a degree of stability, ensuring that the nonmedical needs of the family are addressed. Therapeutic time may need to be devoted to reinforcing the nonmedical needs of the patient (and possibly those of key family members). This is particularly the case when a conceptualization reveals that families have been neglecting well-being as individuals and within a family.

Contrasts and conclusions

The first section of this chapter has considered two important dimensions relating to the provision of psychotherapies with those who are medically ill. The first relates to the predominant therapeutic modality. The next is related to the focus of the therapeutic relationship and whether it will be individually based or encompasses more than one person. The process of assessment, case conceptualization, and therapeutic work will not only differ according to these dimensions but will also be influenced by the nature of the medical illness that patients are experiencing. The next section of the chapter outlines the issues relating to the provision of psychotherapy with common presenting physical disorders.

Specific disorders

Cancer

Cancer-related psychosocial morbidity

Faulkner and Maguire (1994) have suggested that psychosocial adjustment to cancer is associated with six hurdles: (1) managing uncertainty about the future; (2) searching for meaning; (3) dealing with a loss of control; (4) having a need for openness; (5) needs for emotional support; and (6) needs for medical support. They suggest that a failure to deal with these results in psychosocial problems. Increasing medical advances have meant that people with cancer are now tending to live longer than used to the case, a factor that means that cancer is increasingly being conceptualized as a chronic illness. Patients who are told that they have cancer experience distress, but some have a normal adjustment reaction with limited distress that does not cause lasting psychological problems. Others experience psychological problems that significantly interfere with their quality of life; some of these will develop symptoms of an adjustment disorder, major depressive disorder, or an anxiety disorder (Derogatis et al., 1983).

Cancer treatment is also associated with a number of psychosocial concerns, some of which comprise quality of life and contribute to anxiety or depression. Nonphysical treatment side-effects such as anger, anxiety, or apprehension are often rated by patients as being more severe than physical side-effects such as nausea or hair loss (Coates et al., 1983). Indeed, some patients drop out of chemotherapy because of psychological problems (Gilbar and Kaplan de Nour, 1989). Some treatment procedures (e.g., bone marrow transplantation) result in psychological problems because of the particular demands that accompany them (Andyknowski et al., 1995). Many patients have to face treatment regimens that are difficult to tolerate, may involve behavioral demands such as frequent hospital visits and levels of motivation that may be difficult to generate or sustain. Advances in drug therapies have resulted in a reduction in the incidence of nausea and vomiting associated with chemotherapy. However, conditioned nausea and vomiting do still occur and aversions to food can also develop. Even after the end of treatment, patients' lives may be affected throughout the follow-up period, as they attend appointments to determine whether the cancer has returned.

Some psychological problems are more commonly experienced at particular times during the patient's 'cancer journey': at diagnosis, during the early months of treatment, at the end of treatment, at the discovery that the cancer has spread, or at recurrence. Some patients find that they notice persistent negative psychological consequences only at the end of treatment (Ell et al., 1989; Arai et al., 1996). Most, however, do not experience any lasting negative psychological consequences. Others develop an increased vulnerability to future psychosocial problems as a result of the impact of an episode of cancer and cancer treatments. Some become more avoidant in their thinking about illness, having greater illness concerns and diminished capacity to work. Cella and Tross (1986) provide a useful framework for understanding the stages that someone with cancer may pass through.

Problem-focused psychotherapies

Psychoeducational and cognitive-behavioral interventions are the most commonly 'problem-focused' therapies for cancer patients. Most of the empirically validated psychological interventions for cancer-related morbidity have been short term, structured, and problem focused (Devine and Westlake, 2003; Meyer and Mark, 1995). Psychoeducational interventions are typically of short duration and concentrate on didactic teaching of skills and strategies. This is in contrast to cognitive-behaviorally based therapies that include instruction in specific skills and strategies but that are based on a cognitive and behavioral conceptualization of the individual patient. These therapies typically seek to help patients reduce their emotional distress by fostering control and regulating affective responses via the application of behavioral strategies (e.g., activity scheduling) or cognitive strategies that address distortion in thinking and/or enable people to test and develop more helpful alternatives to their dysfunctional ideas (Antoni et al., 2001; Moorey and Greer, 2002; Nezu et al., 2003).

Supportive-expressive psychotherapies

Supportive-expressive therapy has been traditionally delivered in a group and in the context of research activity that has sought to evaluate the impact of participation in such groups on survival (Classen et al., 2001). One of the major goals of this modality is to enable individuals to express all emotions (negative and positive) (Giese-Davis et al., 2002). Based on the premise that most people tend to avoid the fear and anxiety associated with the possibility of death, supportive-expressive therapy enables someone to express and tolerate the affect associated with thoughts of death and dying. This has been referred to as 'detoxifying death' (Spiegel and Classen, 2000). It has been suggested that therapy with this focus may be more appropriate for patients with advanced cancer.

Integrative approaches to psychotherapy in cancer

Kissane et al. (1997) have integrated elements of cognitive, supportive, and existential therapies in group therapy, including elements of Spiegel's work (i.e., the development of a supportive network and addressing issues of death) with an existential focus on the management of uncertainty and awareness of one's own mortality. Supportive-expressive work shares some similarities with other modalities. The 'detoxification' of death, for example, enables patients to express their feelings about death. It can also, from a cognitive perspective, provide patients with evidence about the impact and consequences of the expression of emotion. In practice, most clinicians tailor therapy to the individual, taking account of the presenting problems, and emphasize particular educational, supportive, expressive, or existential elements. Watson and Burton (1998) and Barrowclough (1999) provide helpful overviews of how psychological interventions can be applied in cancer settings.

Psychotherapy and survival

Over the past two decades, various researchers have examined the influence of psychosocial factors on mortality and the potential benefits of psychological intervention on survival. Spiegel's well-known follow-up of metastatic breast cancer led to a great deal of interest in the effect of group social support on morbidity and mortality (Spiegel and Classen, 2000). Other studies of group interventions have been inconsistent, with some showing improved survival time and immunologic response for cancer group members (Spiegel et al., 1989; Fawzy et al., 1993; Fawzy et al., 1995), but others failing to demonstrate such a connection (Ilnyckyj et al., 1994; Cunningham et al., 1998; Edelman et al., 1999; Schrock et al., 1999; Goodwin et al., 2001). The debate continues (Yalom, 1985; Spiegel, 2001; Sampson, 2002) and further research to address these issues is being carried out (Kissane et al., 2001; Cunningham and Edmonds, 2002). Walker et al. (2000) has reported that a relaxation-based intervention prolonged survival. Patients may request psychotherapy to prolong their survival but clinicians cannot ethically claim to prolong survival by directly influencing disease-specific biological processes. On the other hand, psychotherapy might have a positive impact on treatment adherence or mood and might influence host defenses or ameliorate chemotherapy induced immunosuppression. Walker *et al.* (1999) have shown that greater mood disturbance is associated with poorer response to chemotherapy. Watson *et al.* (1999) have demonstrated that high helpless/hopelessness scores on the Mental Adjustment to Cancer Scale are associated with a moderately detrimental effect on survival. It is therefore possible that psychotherapy targeted at helplessness and/or hopelessness might produce moderate survival benefits.

Psychotherapy with dying patients

The establishment of a psychotherapeutic relationship with someone who has an incurable disease can be overwhelming to the clinician (Anderson and Barrett, 2001). There are also some circumstances when the procedural elements of psychotherapy may seem irrelevant in the face of the uncontrollable nature of impending death. However, experienced therapists can significantly enhance the quality of life of someone with an incurable disease, if they vary therapy appropriately. It is often insensitive to focus upon the customary therapeutic elements such as defense mechanisms, conflicts, or automatic thoughts when someone is dying. Instead 'being with' a dying patient, listening to his/her thoughts and feelings, may be most helpful. Facilitating emotional expression is important, therapists should not underestimate the value of sensitively combining listening and emotional expression with more structured and problem-oriented therapy tasks (such as addressing dysfunctional thinking about cancer or death). Therapists sometimes avoid the latter on the basis of a belief that to use problem-focused therapeutic strategies is to dismiss the distressing reality of incurable disease.

Future practice and research issues

Newell *et al.* (2002) have stated that the results of their systematic review of psychological therapies for cancer patients 'lead them to be considerably less enthusiastic, . . . , than do the results of other recent reviews' (p. 581) and that these other reviews have included trials with many methodological shortcomings. They have suggested that future studies on psychotherapy with cancer patients should strive to meet a series of 10 indicators to reflect good practice in the conduct of randomized controlled trials (see Table 33.1).

Diabetes

Diabetes is a serious chronic illness that can result in blindness, amputations, heart disease, and stroke. Individuals with diabetes must control blood glucose (BG) through vigilant self-care, including frequent blood tests, dietary control, exercise, foot care, and medications. Results from two ground-breaking studies convincingly demonstrated that intensive efforts to change behavior to maintain tight BG control can delay or prevent

Table 33.1 Newell *et al.* (2002) suggested quality indicators for conducting randomized controlled trials of psychological therapies in cancer

Ensure adequate concealment of allocation

Ensure patients are randomly selected

Ensure patients are blinded to their experimental group

Ensure care providers are blinded to patients' experimental group

Ensure all other treatments, expect the trial intervention, are equivalent

Ensure care providers' adherence to the study protocol

Provide detailed loss to follow-up information

Minimize the percentage of patients excluded from analyses

Conduct intention-to-treat analyses

Ensure study outcomes are measured in a manner blinded to patients' experimental groups

complications (The Diabetes Control and Complications Trial Research Group, 1993; United Kingdom Prospective Diabetes Study Group, 1998). Another landmark study showed that intensive behavior change to promote weight loss and increase activity can even prevent diabetes onset of those at risk (Knowler *et al.*, 2002).

Diabetes-related psychosocial morbidity

More than most diseases, patient self-management behaviors strongly affect the outcome and course of diabetes and it is important to recognize the psychological disorders that are frequently comorbid with diabetes. Major depressive disorder is diagnosed twice as often in people with diabetes as in healthy people (Popkin *et al.*, 1988; Wells *et al.*, 1989; Weyer *et al.*, 1989; Gavard *et al.*, 1993). Research has demonstrated a clear link between depression and high BG (hyperglycemia) (Lustman *et al.*, 2000b), and that depression may not improve without treatment, often persists and, once treated, is likely to recur (Kovacs *et al.*, 1997; Lustman *et al.*, 1997; Peyrot and Rubin, 1999). It is unclear if the link involves hormonal changes common to both diabetes and depression, the effect of chronic high BG levels, and/or the psychological burdens of the disease, including loss of autonomy, shame, fear, and anxiety about future complications. However, it is clear that the hopelessness of depression can negatively impact self-care. Studies suggest that psychopharmacological and psychotherapeutic treatment improves depression and may also improve BG control (Lustman *et al.*, 1998, 2000).

Anxiety disorders are also more common in individuals with diabetes and associated with high BG levels, although this area warrants further research attention (Peyrot and Rubin, 1997). This may reflect endocrine changes related to the activation of the sympathetic nervous system common to both diabetes and anxiety disorders. A study that demonstrated antianxiety medications improved BG control, even for individuals without a diagnosed anxiety disorder, supports this hypothesis (Lustman *et al.*, 1995). Alternatively, anxiety may be the psychological response to a disease with debilitating and frightening complications. Daily and major life stresses have also been implicated in poor self-care and hyperglycemia (Gonder-Frederick *et al.*, 1990; Aikens *et al.*, 1992; Viner *et al.*, 1996; Lloyd *et al.*, 1999). In a recent study it was shown that stress management training can improve BG control (Surwit *et al.*, 2002), but results in this area are less consistent.

Eating disorders

Young women with diabetes (usually type 1) are particularly vulnerable to comorbid eating disorders, which are associated with a high likelihood of poor BG control and complications (Rodin *et al.*, 1986; Rydall *et al.*, 1997; Daneman *et al.*, 1998). Insulin use is associated with weight gain, which may enhance sensitivity to body image in our weight-conscious society. As diabetes requires constant attention to diet, one can hide an eating disorder that is caused by other factors. Also, women can 'purge' by manipulating insulin. If a young woman binge eats, she can deliberately take a smaller dose or skip insulin, so the body is purged of excess calories without inducing vomiting. Thus, one cost of comorbid eating disorder may be hyperglycemia.

Quality of life

In addition to assessing these major mental illnesses, researchers have demonstrated that diabetes and its consequences place significant emotional and cognitive burdens on patients, leading to impaired quality of life for many who may not have a diagnosable mental illness (Polonsky *et al.*, 1995; Rubin, 2000). Health-related quality of life is defined as how one's life is affected by disease and health. It includes factors such as how much a disease impacts how well an individual functions physically, emotionally, and socially. Psychotherapy is often recommended to help patients accept and proactively manage these issues to improve their overall quality of life (Delamater, 2000).

Cognitive-behavioral approaches to self-management

As managing diabetes involves making major behavioral changes, the psychological intervention research has grown. One controlled study of psychoanalytic treatment of children with type 1 diabetes demonstrated improved BG control following intensive inpatient treatment that included three to four times per week psychoanalytic treatment for an average of 15 weeks (Moran *et al.*, 1991). However, most of the intervention studies have focused on cognitive-behavioral training programs that target these behaviors, commonly referred to as diabetes self-management education. These interventions have been shown to result in reduced healthcare costs and hospitalizations, improved knowledge, self-care, quality of life, and BG control (Rubin *et al.*, 1989, 1993; Clement, 1995). A large body of research specifically focuses on changes in eating and exercise to promote weight loss (Jeffery *et al.*, 2000). In individual or group sessions, strategies that promote life-style change are taught, behavior change is reinforced, and obstacles to change are addressed. These strategies include: focusing on a specific self-care behavior (e.g., BG testing); setting clear and reasonable goals; stimulus control strategies (e.g., not stocking high fat foods); behavioral contracting; and enhancing social support and reinforcement. More broadly defined 'coping skills training' identifies specific cognitive strategies to deal with situations that make adherence difficult, e.g., teaching assertiveness to deal with peer pressure to eat inappropriate foods. These interventions can result in behavior change and improve BG control, diabetes self-care, and quality of life in the short term, but concerns exist about lasting benefits.

CBT has also been used as an intervention for depressed individuals with diabetes, much as for other groups (Lustman *et al.*, 1997, 1998). By challenging and correcting irrational beliefs, and teaching positive coping skills, such as relaxation, cognitive reappraisal and realistic self-talk, therapists help depressed diabetes patients resolve their depression, which can also result in improved BG control.

Family therapy

Family environment factors, such as high cohesion, low conflict, and good communication skills, relate to BG control, adherence, and other clinical outcomes (Herskowitz *et al.*, 1995). Most research has been with children and adolescents with type 1 diabetes (Hauser *et al.*, 1990; Jacobson *et al.*, 1994). The role of the family for adults, and children with type 2, is only beginning to be studied (Trief *et al.*, 1998), but early data support the importance of family support for coping with diabetes (Trief *et al.*, 2001, 2002).

Family therapy interventions are generally aimed at improving family communication and decreasing family conflict. Studies with type 1 adolescents and parents has aimed to encourage parents to share responsibility for diabetes self-care (Anderson *et al.*, 1999), enhancing problem-solving abilities, communication and conflict resolution skills (Wysocki *et al.*, 2000). While family therapy interventions are often evaluated by measuring their impact on BG control, the importance of psychosocial outcomes, such as decreased parent–child conflict and increased parental involvement, are also emphasized.

Group therapy

Meeting with others to share feelings and thoughts about coping with the burdens of diabetes, and to discuss problem-solving techniques, can reduce anxiety and isolation, enhance adjustment and promote self-management skill building. Studies with adolescents have found that BG control improves and diabetes-related distress decreases when adolescents are involved in a peer group support program (Anderson *et al.*, 1989; Grey *et al.*, 1998).

Group therapy is also valued as a practical, cost- and time-efficient way of reaching patients with diabetes. Therefore, most of the adult research examines interventions that are delivered in a group format, such as coping skills training (Rubin *et al.*, 1993), behavioral weight loss programs (Jeffrey *et al.*, 2000), stress management training (Surwit *et al.*, 2002) and BG awareness training (Cox *et al.*, 1989). However, these studies have not compared group with individual therapy, and one cannot conclude group therapy is more effective than individual.

Future directions

While evidence supports the value of psychotherapeutic interventions for patients with diabetes, many research and clinical issues need to be addressed and are outlined in two systematic reviews (Delamater *et al.*, 2001; Gonder-Frederick *et al.*, 2002). The psychotherapy literature is sorely lacking in two areas. Given the evidence of high psychosocial morbidity, research should explore interventions for individuals with diabetes and comorbid psychiatric diagnoses, e.g., depression, anxiety, and eating disorders. These patients are often excluded from intervention studies, when they need more, not less, help. Other populations that are often ignored include minorities and the elderly. The incidence of diabetes is high in minority groups, for example, the prevalence of diabetes among African-Americans is almost twice that of non-Hispanic white people (Diabetes Quick Stats—website of the American Diabetes Association— http://www.diabetes.org). Minority patients often have poorer BG control and a higher rate of complications and it is predicted that, for American Indians and Hispanics, diabetes may soon become the leading cause of death (Gilliland *et al.*, 1997). Therefore, culturally sensitive and effective psychotherapies should be developed to address their needs (Brown, 1998). Similarly, psychotherapy with elderly patients is rarely reported, yet we know that they have unique needs and experience significant barriers to care (Moritz *et al.*, 1994; Wandell and Tovi, 2000).

Chronic pain

Pain is the most common reason that patients seek medical intervention, estimated to be the primary complaint for 80% of US medical visits (National Center for Health Statistics and Koch, 1986). Pain that is benign (i.e., not cancer related) and has persisted longer than 6 months was routinely labeled 'chronic' (Sternbach, 1974), but recent evidence that a 3-month cut-off predicts functional outcome has changed the definition (Turczyn, 1992). Chronic pain is associated with diseases of every organ system, traumatic injuries, and medical procedures, and has significant medical, emotional, and financial consequences. Chronic pain research focuses on back and neck pain, osteoarthritis, rheumatoid arthritis, headache, temporomandibular joint pain, fibromyalgia, and NCCP. However, most research studies focus on chronic back pain and arthritis due to the number of sufferers and high financial costs. For example, chronic back pain is estimated to cost $85 billion per year in the US (Cats-Baril and Frymoyer, 1991), while the direct and indirect costs of arthritis are estimated at $64.8 billion (Yelin and Callahan, 1995).

Psychosocial morbidity in chronic pain

Psychological problems associated with chronic pain include depression, anxiety, anger, and social isolation (Gamsa, 1990; Polatin *et al.*, 1993). In turn, psychosocial factors have been shown to affect pain perception, level of disability, emotional adaptation, and response to treatment (Himmelstein, 1995). Many individual and environmental factors have been found to affect outcome, e.g., family pain history (Gamsa and Vikis-Freibergs, 1991), childhood trauma history (Schofferman *et al.*, 1993), litigation/compensation status (Tait *et al.*, 1990), and work stress/satisfaction (Truchon and Fillion, 2000). The role of depression and anxiety has received the most attention.

Depression

Chronic pain and depression have been linked in numerous studies (Romano and Turner, 1985; Magni *et al.*, 1990). Early work defined chronic pain as a 'depressive equivalent', i.e., an acceptable way for the individual to express emotional distress (Blumer and Heilbronn, 1982). However, research has not supported this idea. In one study of 200 chronic back pain patients screened for psychiatric disorder, researchers found that depression may have preceded the chronic back pain in 54% of depressed patients, but it was a consequence of pain in 46% of the sample (Polatin *et al.*, 1993). In studies with arthritis patients, the rate of depression has also been found to be high (23% of rheumatoid arthritis patients, 10% of osteoarthritis patients) (Abdel-Nasser, 1998). Evidence is growing that depression relates to both disease activity and level of physical disability (Beckham *et al.*, 1992; Parker *et al.*, 1992), and is a significant risk for younger rheumatoid arthritis patients (Wright *et al.*, 1998) and those who have lost their ability to engage in important activities (Katz and Yelin, 1995). Similarly, studies show that 30–50% of patients with fibromyalgia suffer from clinical depression (Hudson et al., 1985).

Anxiety

There are two major ways to understand the role that anxiety may play in pain perception and disability. The first, proposed by Turk (2002), extends the work on 'anxiety-sensitivity' (AS) to chronic pain patients. AS is defined as an individual's predisposition to fear the symptoms of anxiety, based on the belief that these symptoms will be harmful (Reiss and McNally, 1985). Turk proposes that patients with high anxiety sensitivity are especially vigilant to pain, and that this leads to higher levels of emotional arousal when even minor pain is perceived. Those with a heightened fear of pain interpret their pain symptoms as signs of serious underlying pathology, which contributes to greater fear. They then avoid activities that increase pain and its associated anxiety. This pain avoidance can, in turn, lead to greater fear, physical limitations, deconditioning, and impaired quality of life. This theory is supported by research that has shown that fear-avoidance beliefs are significant, and sometimes the best, predictors of higher pain level, greater functional limitation, poorer physical performance, and lower likelihood of return to work (Reiss and McNally, 1985; Waddell et al., 1993; Crombez et al., 1999a,b; Alobaidi, 2000).

Others have explored the role that nonspecific stress may play in chronic pain, especially for arthritis patients. Longitudinal studies have lent support to earlier cross-sectional research that suggested that stress and arthritis symptoms co-vary. In two longitudinal studies of arthritis patients, Zautra and colleagues found that symptomatic changes in pain and joint tenderness were predicted by level of interpersonal stress, although level of depression and marital support were also important (Zautra et al., 1999; Zautra and Smith, 2001). Some studies have suggested that stress plays a more significant role for those with rheumatoid arthritis than with osteoarthritis, but more work needs to be done (Zautra et al., 1994; Hirano et al., 2001).

This literature, coupled with evidence that different subgroups of pain patients vary on psychosocial factors (Turk and Rudy, 1990; Johansson and Lindberg, 2000) and demonstrate different behavioral responses to treatments (Rudy et al., 1995; Epker and Gatchel, 2000), has led to the recommendation that, in addition to a biomedical diagnosis, pain patients be assigned a psychosocial diagnosis (Turk and Rudy, 1990; Jamison et al., 1994).

Focus on pain

Turk and Okifuji (2002) point to a growing emphasis on the cognitive processes that affect pain and disability, processes that focus on the pain. They highlight three areas that have received the greatest research support; patient appraisals, fears and pain self-management skills, all closely linked to the AS literature cited earlier.

Appraisal refers to the meaning and beliefs that the patient holds about the pain. If a patient believes that pain is a sign of serious pathology, he may avoid physical activities, including those necessary for adequate rehabilitation (Turk and Okifuji, 1996). Similarly, patients who have fears and anxieties about their pain are likely to avoid health-promoting behaviors (e.g., exercise, pleasurable activities), so that these fear avoidance beliefs promote worry (McCrackern and Gross, 1993), avoidance (Crombez et al., 1999a,b), and disability (Waddell et al., 1993). In addition, pain-related fear appears to enhance physiological arousal (Vlaeyen et al., 1995), including the reactivity of spinal musculature (Burns et al., 1997), and may thus directly contribute to increased pain severity.

A complementary construct is pain management self-efficacy, a term to describe the conviction that one can successfully perform skills that have been shown to decrease and control pain (Dolce et al., 1986b; Turk and Okifuji, 2002). Self-efficacy ratings have been associated with exercise and activity levels (Dolce et al., 1986a; Council et al., 1988), disability ratings (Lorig et al., 1989), pain perception (Keefe et al., 1997), and depression (Schiaffino and Revenson, 1995). Work that has shown that treatment outcomes can be predicted by changes in self-efficacy (Lorig et al., 1993;

Keefe et al., 1999) has drawn increased attention to this construct that focuses on pain.

Common processes in pain psychotherapy

The processes involved in pain psychotherapy evolve from the understanding of pain-related psychopathology outlined above. Patients come into therapy looking for pain relief. They learn that other important outcomes of pain psychotherapy are improvements in function, mood, self-esteem, interpersonal relationships, and quality of life. The overall focus is to improve the individual's ability to cope with the pain and its consequences. This is accomplished by addressing the skills deficits and pain-related cognitions that interfere with positive coping.

Therapists attempt to intervene in several ways. They may try to change the individual's appraisal of the pain. This can be accomplished by encouraging active exercise despite moderate pain increases. Patients are also taught the principles of 'pacing' their activity level. Many try to 'push through the pain' by persisting in a strenuous, pain-aggravating task. This results in a cycle of pain–activity–increased pain–inactivity, and fosters frustration and fear. When patients pace their activities, i.e., do something for a shorter period, then rest, then return to the task, they learn that they can do more without 'paying for it later'. They also learn that pain is not always a signal of serious pathology and increases in pain need not cause increased anxiety. This process helps patients become less fearful of the pain and of future reinjury, and enhances feelings of self-efficacy and control.

Pain management skills are also emphasized. This commonly involves relaxation training, possibly with EMG biofeedback. Most patients recognize that tension makes their pain worse, and that pain and its consequences increases tension. By learning to deeply relax they can resolve the tension-related component of their pain, and establish a sense of control over their pain. Additional stress management skills include identification of stressors and ways to manage life stress.

Other cognitive coping skills taught include attention-diversion, i.e., teaching patients to manage pain by distracting themselves from it, and assertiveness, i.e., teaching patients to assert their needs with family and friends. There is ample evidence that pain coping skills training leads to improved outcomes. For example, Lorig et al. (1993) and Keefe et al. (1999) have completed several studies of self-help interventions with arthritis patients and found that changes in self-efficacy relate to improved pain management outcomes. Parker et al. (1995) also found that stress management training with rheumatoid arthritis patients resulted in long-term improvements in pain, health, coping, and self-efficacy. Similar results have been obtained in coping skills training with patients who suffer from chronic low back pain (e.g., Flor et al., 1992; Hildebrant et al., 1997), headaches (Holroyd and Lipchik, 1999), temporomandibular joint pain (Dworkin et al., 1994), and with other pain groups.

A caveat: Although people in pain typically seek psychotherapy for pain management, one must remember that they, like other psychotherapy candidates, are dealing with other issues that may cause, or contribute to, their distress. They may be depressed because of marital conflict, or experiencing posttraumatic stress symptoms related to early childhood abuse. As a psychotherapist, one must attend to the unique issues that a patient presents and not limit the focus to only the most obvious one.

Future psychotherapy and research issues

The US Congress has designated the period 2001–11 as 'The Decade of Pain Control and Research', attesting to the importance now placed on helping patients cope with pain and its consequences. Two reviews note many future research and practice directions (Keefe et al., 2002; Turk and Okifuji, 2002). One important area, among many others, involves establishing whether the early identification of depression and intensive depression treatment, will affect pain-related outcomes, including the pain itself, disability, or medical utilization. A second area would involve having researchers identify subgroups of patients based on their psychosocial and behavioral profiles and then develop specific, targeted psychosocial interventions for each subgroup CBT that would be more effective in reducing pain than a general approach (Turk and Okifuji, 2001).

Functional syndromes

This section will outline the main issues pertaining to psychotherapy with patients who have symptoms of IBS, chronic fatigue syndrome (CFS), and symptoms of NCCP.

Irritable bowel syndrome

There are numerous syndromal descriptions of what have become known as functional gastrointestinal disorders. The most commonly known is IBS that presents with persistent abdominal pain, altered bowel habits, and abdominal distension. It is believed to have point prevalence of 20% (Camilleri and Choi, 1997). It is believed that a general medical practitioner in the UK sees, on average, eight patients presenting with IBS each week. A proportion of female patients with these symptoms have experienced childhood sexual abuse. The evidence for the effectiveness of psychotherapies in treating the functional bowel disorders is equivocal. Talley *et al.* (1996) have highlighted various methodological weaknesses of work to evaluate psychotherapy in this area.

However, most guidance documents on the management of IBS recommend psychotherapy. Short-term dynamic therapy has been shown to be effective in reducing IBS symptoms and associated psychopathology (Svedlund *et al.*, 1983; Guthrie *et al.*, 1991). These therapies focus upon enabling patients to make links between physical symptom experiences and intrapsychic factors. Relaxation (Whorwell *et al.*, 1984; Blanchard *et al.*, 1993), cognitive therapy (Greene and Blanchard, 1994; Payne and Blanchard, 1995), have all demonstrated positive impacts on IBS symptoms, though there are some negative studies for CBT (Blanchard *et al.*, 1992a,b). Cognitive therapeutic approaches to functional bowel disorders involve engagement of the patient in monitoring their gastrointestinal symptoms and, in doing so, considering both the potential links between physical and psychosocial factors and idiosyncratic beliefs about symptom presence and course. Case conceptualizations often make links between primary anxiogenic thoughts and beliefs (e.g., 'I am going to collapse') and secondary IBS-specific appraisals (e.g., 'I am losing control of my bowels') that further contribute to the process of anxiogenesis and the generation of symptom episodes. CBT is more likely to be successful when patients are able to make links between elements of their bowel symptom experiences and related thoughts, emotions, or behavioral responses. Psychotherapy has been shown to improve health-related quality of life at no additional cost (Creed *et al.*, 2003). Svedlund (2002) suggests that given dynamic psychotherapy, hypnosis, CBT, and relaxation, have each resulted in successful outcomes, psychotherapists should use the technique with which they are most experienced.

Chronic fatigue syndrome

CFS is a descriptive term for the experience of physical and mental fatigue that persists for at least 6 months and is associated with reductions in activity. Acceptance of the relevance of psychotherapeutic work is a particular challenge with CFS patients (Bentall *et al.*, 2002). CFS patients may exhibit resistance to suggestions that consideration be given to psychosocial experiences, believing that this questions the legitimacy of their symptoms. The provision of an underlying rationale for psychotherapeutic work is particularly important. Prevailing opinion is that this should be based on a biopsychosocial formulation that acknowledges all of these influences on the experience of symptoms (Johnson, 1998).

Behavioral interventions focus upon enabling patients to sustain graded increases in their activity levels, including exercise, once some stability has been observed in daytime activity level. Cognitive interventions target beliefs that are related to symptom experiences (e.g., 'I need to rest to conserve my energy before activity'). Cognitive-behavioral therapies incorporating these interventions have been demonstrated to be the most effective (Allen *et al.*, 2002; Whiting *et al.*, 2001).

Noncardiac chest pain

Patients with NCCP constitute almost half of the new referrals to cardiology clinics (Bass and Mayou, 1995). CBT has been shown to be effective for this group of patients when implemented in both research and general hospital outpatient settings (Mayou and Sharpe, 1997). Almost all psychotherapy literature for NCCP is cognitive-behavioral in focus. Patients and therapist work to discover how patients' life experiences, beliefs, thoughts, emotions, and behavior might be relevant to the understanding of why they experience cardiac symptoms in the absence of cardiac pathology (or in addition to or in excess of objective cardiac disease). This information is ultimately linked with the modification of cognitive-behavioral mediating factors. Patients with NCCP often report anxiogenic misinterpretations of physical sensations such as 'I am having a heart attack' or 'I am going to collapse'. These cognitions may also be experienced in the form of images. Patients also report behaviors that they have developed in an attempt to manage their symptoms, including regular use of heart or blood pressure monitoring equipment, palpation of their chest wall, taking aspirin or limiting activity when they experience discomfort. These behaviors actually serve to exacerbate the problem as they reinforce the idea that the sensations are dangerous.

The most common strategies used in demonstrating cognitive-behavioral mediation of cardiac symptoms are those that help the patient develop a benign explanation for their chest pain: that rather being due to a potentially fatal cardiac problem, it may be due to hyperventilation, muscle tension, and catastrophic thinking. First the clinician introduces the idea of collaboratively working together to explore experiences within the session. The role of catastrophic thinking can be demonstrated by using flashcards containing words pertaining to their unique anxiogenic thoughts (collapse, heart attack, pain, crushing). Patients are encouraged to read these words and notice any physical sensations that they experience. Patients that experience symptoms of anxious arousal can reflect upon the way in which focusing upon salient words has resulted in their experiencing autonomic symptoms. Patients are then encouraged to list the sensations that they attribute to cardiac symptoms. This is then used to compare the sensations that they experience during the session as a result of behavioral or cognitive manipulation (though patients are not told that this is going to happen). Situations that have been avoided because of previously held beliefs can be confronted using the techniques of graded exposure and/or within the framework of a behavioral experiment. Behaviors that have become habitual because of beliefs about increased risk of heart problems are then more easily extinguished. Anxiogenic thoughts can be evaluated as patients become increasingly aware that their problems are best construed as anxiety symptoms and not cardiac symptoms.

Future practice and research issues

The emergence of data to support psychotherapy for common functional disorders results in a challenge and service planners and for clinicians who need to help patients to accept psychotherapy as a legitimate treatment and as one that does not minimize their suffering. It has been suggested that new conceptual frameworks and greater integration of psychotherapeutic treatments within medicine might facilitate greater integration with medical practice and acceptability to people who experience these symptoms (Salmon, 2000; Sharpe and Carson, 2001; De Gucht and Fischler, 2002).

Neurological disorders

Patients who have experienced symptoms of a neurological disorder often encounter problems with anxiety and fears that can be traced to the sudden onset of the condition and related concerns of experiencing a similar future episode (Newson-Davis *et al.*, 1998). Patients may also become preoccupied that they will die and/or suffer further brain damage. This is most clearly appreciated in considering the clinical presentation of epilepsy or a cerebrovascular accident. There are also neurological disorders that have a more insidious onset (such as multiple sclerosis and motor neuron disease) and are more gradually progressive. These present with a different range of concerns, relating more to incapacity and eventual slow death. There are few clinical practice guidelines on psychotherapy with this group of patients. Most interventions focus on psychoeducation (Korner-Bitensky et al., 1998).

Clinicians treating patients who experience such disorders need to take account of the direct influence of neurological dysfunction on psychological functioning, such as in the case of emotional disinhibition or impaired intellectual functioning that can occur following a cerebrovascular event. Although there have been attempts to influence the nature and severity of neurological events such as seizures, research to examine this has been of poor quality and has generally concluded that there is no effect of psychotherapeutic techniques on symptom occurrence (Ramaratnam et al., 2003). There is some evidence to suggest that positive benefits are more likely to be found, as would be expected, on mood and quality of life.

Although there is a paucity of research on psychotherapy and neurological disorders there has been some recent work to examine psychotherapeutic work with families. Glass et al. (2000) have been developing a therapeutic protocol for families one of whose members has suffered a stroke. Their intervention is based on a family systems perspective with a specific emphasis on addressing the needs within the family to accommodate care giving and support for the neurologically impaired family member. They make specific attempts to encompass professional carers within an expanded systemic conceptualization that they refer to as the 'problem defined system'. This intervention aims to increase patient efficacy and control; promote social support; reduce stress and maximize system cohesion; and enhance problem-solving effectiveness. The implementation of psychotherapeutic modalities covered in this chapter may be difficult with a stroke patient if the neurological disorder has resulted in neuropsychological problems such as aphasia. Therapists may have to adapt standard components of therapy and enable people to express themselves using other means (e.g., writing). Laatsch (1999) has developed this approach in her work to integrate cognitive rehabilitation therapy techniques in psychotherapy with patients experiencing neuropsychological impairment. This approach aims to blend psychotherapy and cognitive retraining in patients who have experienced a stroke or sustained a head injury.

Conclusions

The recognition that physical illness can result in the development of psychological disorder has led to developments in the application and study of psychotherapy for the medically ill. Although most therapeutic modalities have been developed for application with one form of medical illness or another, the predominant focus within the literature has been on cognitive-behaviorally based therapies with the most common presenting physical disorders such as cancer, chronic pain, and diabetes. Group-based supportive therapy and group psychotherapies have been studied mostly within oncology settings and found to be particularly suited to the needs of people facing feelings and issues associated with death and dying. Work in this area has also been applied to functional somatic syndromes such as IBS and although most evidence comes from cognitive-behavioral approaches, psychodynamic therapy demonstrates considerable promise in the management of functional gastrointestinal disorders. Many therapists working with the medically ill elect to adopt a multimodal approach to psychotherapy—choosing to tailor their interventions to the particular physical disorder, psychosocial morbidity, and presenting psychological problems that are presented. Further research in this area is now required to determine the active ingredients of effective psychotherapy for the medically ill and to refine the evidence base for psychodynamic and family systems therapies in physically ill adults.

Acknowledgments

This chapter is dedicated to Andrew John McPhail (1967–2003). The authors wish to thank Audrey McDonald for her assistance with preparation and to Angela Hissett, Medical Library, Ailsa Hospital for her assistance in identifying literature referenced in the chapter.

References

Abdel-Nasser, A. M., et al. (1998). Depression and depressive symptoms in rheumatoid arthritis patients: an analysis of their occurrence and determinants. British Journal of Rheumatology, 37, 391–7.

Aikens, J. E., Wallander, J. L., Bell, D. S., and Cole, J. A. (1992). Daily stress variability, learned resourcefulness, regimen adherence, and metabolic control in type 1 diabetes mellitus: evaluation of a path model. Journal of Consulting and Clinical Psychology, 60, 113–18.

Allen, L. A., Escobar, J. I., Gara, M. A., and Woolfolk, R. L. (2002). Psychosocial treatments for multiple unexplained physical symptoms: a review of the literature. Psychosomatic Medicine, 64(6), 939–50.

Alobaidi, S. M., Nelson, R. M., Al-awadhi, S., and Al-Shuwaie, N. (2000). The role of anticipation and fear of pain in the persistence of avoidance behaviour in patients with chronic low back pain. Spine, 25, 1126–31.

American Psychiatric Association (1994). Diagnostic and statistical manual of mental disorders, 4th edn (revised). Washington DC: American Psychiatric Press.

Andersen, B. L. (2002). Biobehavioural outcomes following psychological interventions for cancer patients. Journal of Consulting and Clinical Psychology, 70, 590–610.

Andersen, B. L., Kiecolt-Glaser, J. K., and Glaser, R. (1994). A biobehavioural model of cancer stress and disease course. American Psychologist, 49, 89–404.

Anderson, B. J., Wolf, F., Burkhart, M., Cornell, R., and Bacon, G. (1989). Effects of peer-group intervention on metabolic control of adolescents with IDDM: randomized outpatient study. Diabetes Care, 12, 179–183.

Anderson, B. J., Brackett, J., Ho, J., and Laffel, L. M. (1999). An office-based intervention to maintain parent-adolescent teamwork in diabetes management: Impact on parent involvement, family conflict, and subsequent glycemic control. Diabetes Care, 22, 713–21.

Andrykowski, M. A., et al. (1995). Returning to normal following bone marrow transplantation: outcomes, expectations and informed consent. Bone Marrow Transplantation, 15, 573–81.

Antoni, M. H., et al. (2001). Cognitive-behavioural stress management intervention decreases the prevalence of depression and enhances benefit finding among women under treatment for early-stage breast cancer. Health Psychology, 20, 20–32.

Arai, Y. M., et al. (1996). Psychological aspects in long term survivors of testicular cancer. Journal of Urology, 155, 574–8.

Backman, M. E. (1989a). Challenges to the Self. In: M. E. Backman, ed. The psychology of the physically ill patient: a clinician's guide, pp. 15–22. New York: Plenum Press.

Backman, M. E. (1989b). Psychosocial issues and medical illness. In: M. E. Backman, The psychology of the physically ill patient: a clinician's guide, pp. 7–14. New York: Plenum Press.

Barrett, P. M., Dadds, M. R., and Rapee, R. M. (1996). Family treatment of childhood anxiety: a controlled trial. Journal of Consulting and Clinical Psychology, 64(2), 333–42.

Barrowclough, J. (1999) Cancer and emotion. An introduction to psycho-oncology. Chichester: John Wiley and Sons.

Bass, C. and Mayou, R. A. (1995). Chest pain and palpitations. In: R. A. Mayou, C. Bass, and M. Sharpe, ed. Treatment of functional somatic symptoms, pp. 328–52. Oxford: Oxford University Press.

Beckham, J. C., et al. (1992). Depression and level of functioning in patients with rheumatoid arthritis. Canadian Journal of Psychiatry, 37, 539–43.

Bennett, R. M., *et al.* (1996). Group treatment of fibromyalgia: a 6 month outpatient program. *Journal of Rheumatology*, **23**, 521–8.

Bentall, R. P., Powell, P., Nye, F. J., and Edwards, R. H. (2002). Predictors of response to treatment for chronic fatigue syndrome. *British Journal of Psychiatry*, **181**, 248–52.

Blake-Mortimer, J., Gore-Felton, C., Kimerling, R., Turner-Cobb, J. M., and Spiegel, D. (1999). Improving the quality and quantity of life among patients with cancer: a review of the effectiveness of group psychotherapy. *European Journal of Cancer*, **35**, 1581–6.

Blanchard, E. B., *et al.* (1992a). Prediction of outcome from cognitive-behavioural treatment of irritable bowel syndrome. *Behaviour Research and Therapy*, **30**(6), 647–50.

Blanchard, E. B., *et al.* (1992b). Two controlled evaluations of multicomponent psychological treatment of irritable bowel syndrome. *Behaviour Research and Therapy*, **30**(2), 175–89.

Blanchard, E. B., Greene, B., Scharff, L., and Schwaz-McMorris, S. P. (1993). Relaxation training as treatment for irritable bowel syndrome. *Biofeedback and Self Regulation*, **18**(3), 125–32.

Blumenthal, J. A. (1985). Psychologic assessment in cardiac rehabilitation. *Journal of Cardiopulmonary Rehabilitation*, **5**, 208–15.

Blumer, D. and Heilbronn, M. (1982). Chronic pain as a variant of depressive disease: the pain-prone patient. *Journal of Nervous and Mental Disease*, **170**, 381–406.

Bucher, J., Smith, E., and Gillespie, C. (1984). Short-term group therapy for stroke patients in a rehabilitation center. *British Journal of Medical Psychology*, **57**, 283–90.

Burns, J. W., Wiegner, S., Derleth, M., Kiselica, K., and Pawl, R. (1997). Linking symptom-specific physiological reactivity to pain severity in chronic low back pain patients: a test of mediation and moderation models. *Health Psychology*, **16**, 319–26.

Cain, E. N., Kohorn, E. I., Quinlan, D. M., Latimer, K., and Schwartz, P. E. (1986). Psychosocial benefits of a cancer support group. *Cancer*, **57**, 183–9.

Camilleri, M. and Choi, M. G. (1997). Review article: irritable bowel syndrome. *Alimentary Pharmacology and Therapeutics*, **11**, 3–15.

Cassileth, B. R. (1995). The aim of psychotherapeutic intervention in cancer patients. *Supportive Care*, **3**, 267–9.

Cats-Baril, W. L. and Frymoyer, J. W. (1991). The economics of spinal disorders. In: J. W. Frymoyer, ed. *The adult spine: principles and practice*, pp. 85–105. New York: Raven Press.

Cella, D. F. and Tross, S. (1986). Psychological adjustment to survival from Hodgkin's disease. *Journal of Consulting and Clinical Psychology*, **54**, 616–22.

Chew-Graham, C. A. and Hogg, T. (2002). Patients with chronic physical illness and co-existing psychological morbidity: GPs' views on their role in detection and management. *Primary Care Psychiatry*, **8**(2), 35–9.

Classen, C., *et al.* (2001). Supportive-expressive group therapy and distress in patients with metastatic breast cancer: a randomized clinical intervention trial. *Archives of General Psychiatry*, **58**, 494–501.

Clement, S. (1995). Diabetes self-management education. *Diabetes Care*, **18**, 1204–14.

Coates, A., *et al.* (1983). On the receiving end—patient perception of the side effects of cancer chemotherapy. *European Journal of Cancer and Clinical Oncology*, **19**, 203–8.

Cottrell, D. and Boston, P. (2002). Practitioner review: the effectiveness of systemic family therapy for children and adolescents. *Journal of Child Psychology and Psychiatry and Allied Disciplines*, **43**(5), 573–86.

Council, J. R., Ahern, D. K., Follick, M. J., and Kline, C. L. (1988). Expectancies and functional impairment in chronic low back pain. *Pain*, **33**, 323–331.

Cox, D. J., *et al.* (1989). Effects and correlates of blood glucose awareness training among patients with IDDM. *Diabetes Care*, **12**, 313–18.

Crawford, J. D. and McIver, G. P. (1985). Group psychotherapy: benefits in multiple sclerosis. *Archives of Physical and Medical Rehabilitation*, **66**, 810–13.

Creed, F., *et al.* (2003). The cost-effectiveness of psychotherapy and paroxetine for severe irritable bowel syndrome. *Gastroenterology*, **124**(2), 303–17.

Crombez, G., Vlaeyen, J. W., and Heuts, P. H. (1999). Pain-related fear is more disabling than pain itself: evidence on the role of pain-related fear in chronic back pain disability. *Pain*, **80**, 329–39.

Crombez, G., Vlaeyen, J. W. S., Heuts, P. H. T. G., and Lysens, R. (1999). Fear of pain is more disabling than the pain itself: further evidence on the role of pain-related fear in chronic back pain disability. *Pain*, **80**, 529–39.

Cunningham, A. J. and Edmonds, C. (2002). Group psychosocial support in metastatic breast cancer (letter). *New England Journal of Medicine*, **346**(16), 1247–8.

Cunningham, A. J., Lockwood, G. A., and Edmonds, C. V. I. (1993). Which cancer patients benefit most from a brief, group, coping skills program? *International Journal of Psychiatry in Medicine*, **23**, 383–98.

Cunningham, A. J., *et al.* (1998). A randomized controlled trial of the effects of group psychological therapy on survival in women with metastatic breast cancer. *Psycho-Oncology*, **7**, 508–17.

Daneman, D., Olmsted, M., Rydall, A., Maharaj, S., and Rodin, G. (1998). Eating disorders in young women with type 1 diabetes: prevalence, problems and prevention. *Hormone Research*, **50** (Suppl.), 79–86.

De Gucht, V. and Fischler, B. (2002). Somatization: a critical review of conceptual and methodological issues. *Psychosomatics*, **43**, 1–9.

Delamater, A. M. (2000). Quality of life in youths with diabetes. *Diabetes Spectrum*, **13**, 42–7.

Delamater, A. M., *et al.* (2001). Psychosocial therapies in diabetes: report of the Psychosocial Therapies Working Group. *Diabetes Care*, **24**, 1286–92.

Derogatis, L. R., *et al.* (1983). The prevalence of psychiatric disorders among cancer patients. *Journal of the American Medical Association*, **249**, 751–7.

DeRubeis, R. J. and Crits-Christoph, P. (1998). Empirically supported individual and group psychological treatments for adult mental disorders. *Journal of Consulting and Clinical Psychology*, **66**, 37–52.

Devine, E. C. and Westlake, S. K. (2003). Meta-analysis of the effect of psycho-educational interventions of pain in adults with cancer. *Oncology Nursing Forum*, **30**, 75–89.

Diabetes Control and Complications Trial Research Group (1993). The effect of intensive treatment of diabetes on the development and progression of long-term complications in insulin-dependent diabetes mellitus. *New England Journal of Medicine*, **329**, 927–86.

Doherty, W. J., McDaniel, S. H., and Hepworth, J. (1994). Medical family therapy: an emerging arena for family therapy. *Journal of Family Therapy*, **16**, 31–46.

Dolce, J. J., Crocker, M. F., Moletteire, C., and Doleys, D. M. (1986a). Exercise quotas, anticipatory concern and self-efficacy expectancies in chronic pain: a preliminary report. *Pain*, **24**, 365–75.

Dolce, J. J., *et al.* (1986b). The role of self-efficacy expectancies in the prediction of pain tolerance. *Pain*, **27**, 261–72.

Dworkin, S. F., *et al.* (1994). Brief group cognitive-behavioural intervention for temporomandibular disorders. *Pain*, **59**, 175–87.

Edelman, S., Lemon, J., Bell, D. R., and Kidman, A. D. (1999). Effects of group CBT on the survival time of patients with metastatic breast cancer. *Psycho-Oncology*, **8**, 474–81.

Edgar, L., Rosberger, Z., and Collet, J.-P. (2001). Lessons learned: outcomes and methodology of a coping skills intervention trial comparing individual and group formats for patients with cancer. *Inernational Journal of Psychiatry in Medicine*, **31**, 289–304.

Ell, K., *et al.* (1989). A longitudinal analysis of psychological adaptation among survivors of cancer. *Cancer*, **63**, 406–13.

Enright, S. J. (1997). Cognitive behavior therapy—clinical applications. *British Medical Journal*, **314**, 1811–16.

Epker, J. and Gatchel, R. J. (2000). Coping profile differences in the biopsychosocial functioning of patients with temporomandibular disoders. *Psychosomatic Medicine*, **62**, 69–75.

Faulkner, A. and Maguire, P. (1994). *Talking to cancer patients and their relatives.* New York: Oxford University Press.

Fawzy, F. I. and Fawzy, N. W. (1998). Group therapy in the cancer setting. *Journal of Psychosomatic Research*, **45**, 191–200.

Fawzy, F. I., *et al.* (1990a). A structured psychiatric intervention for cancer patients. I. Changes over times in methods of coping and affective disturbance. *Archives of General Psychiatry*, **47**, 720–5.

Fawzy, F. I., *et al.* (1990b). A structured psychiatric intervention for cancer patients. II Changes over time in immunological measures. *Archives of General Psychiatry*, **54**, 489–517.

Fawzy, F. I., *et al.* (1993). Malignant melanoma. Effects of an early structured psychiatric intervention, coping, and affective state on recurrence and survival 6 years later. *Archives of General Psychiatry*, **50**(9), 681–9.

Fawzy, F. I., *et al.* (1995). Critical review of psychosocial interventions in cancer care. *Archives of General Psychiatry*, **52**, 100–13.

Fawzy, F. I., Fawzy, N. W., and Wheler, J. G. (1996). A post-hoc comparison of the efficiency of a psychoeducational intervention for melanoma patients delivered in a group versus individual formats: an analysis of data from two studies. *Psycho-Oncology*, **5**, 81–9.

Finney, J. W. and Bonner, M. J. (1993). The influence of behavioural family intervention on the health of chronically ill children. *Behaviour Change*, **9**, 157–70.

Flor, H., Fydrich, T., and Turk, D. C. (1992). Efficacy of multidisciplinary pain treatment centers: a meta-analytic review. *Pain*, **49**, 221–30.

Gamsa, A. (1990). Is emotional disturbance a precipitator or a consequence of chronic pain? *Pain*, **42**, 183–95.

Gamsa, A. and Vikis-Freibergs, V. (1991). Psychological events are both risk factors in, and consequences of, chronic pain. *Pain*, **44**, 271–7.

Gamsa, A., Braha, R. E., and Catchlove, R. F. (1985). The use of structured group therapy sessions in the treatment of chronic pain patients. *Pain*, **22**, 91–6.

Gavard, J. A., Lustman, P. J., and Clouse, R. E. (1993). Prevalence of depression in adults with diabetes: an epidemiological evaluation. *Diabetes Care*, **16**, 1167–78.

Gier, M. D., Levick, M. D., and Blazina, P. J. (1988). Stress reduction with heart transplant patients and their families: a multidisciplinary approach. *Journal of Heart Transplantation*, **7**, 342–7.

Giese-Davis, J., *et al.* (2002). Change in emotion-regulation strategy for women with metastatic breast cancer following supportive-expressive group therapy. *Journal of Consulting and Clinical Psychology*, **70**(4), 916–25.

Gilbar, O. and De-Nour, K. (1989). Adjustment to illness and dropout of chemotherapy. *Journal of Psychosomatic Research*, **33**, 1–5.

Gilliland, F. D., Owen, C., Gilliland, S. S., and Carter, J. S. (1997). Temporal trends in diabetes mortality among American Indians and Hispanics in New Mexico: birth cohort and period effects. *American Journal of Epidemiology*, **145**, 422–31.

Glass, T. A., *et al.* (2000). Psychosocial intervention in stroke: families in recovery from stroke trial (FIRST). *American Journal of Orthopsychiatry*, **70**(2), 169–81.

Gonder-Frederick, L. A., Carter, W. R., Cox, D. J., and Clarke, W. L. (1990). Environmental stress and blood glucose change in insulin-dependent diabetes mellitus. *Health Psychology*, **9**, 503–15.

Gonder-Frederick, L. A., Cox, D. J., and Ritterband, L. M. (2002). Diabetes and behavioural medicine: the second decade. *Journal of Consulting and Clinical Psychology*, **70**, 611–25.

Goodwin, P. J., *et al.* (2001). The effect of group psychosocial support on survival in metastatic breast cancer. *New England Journal of Medicine*, **345**(24), 1719–26.

Greene, B. and Blanchard, E. B. (1994). Cognitive therapy for irritable bowel syndrome. *Journal of Consulting and Clinical Psychology*, **62**, 576–82.

Greenstein, M. and Breitbart, W. (2000). Cancer and the experience of meaning: a group psychotherapy program for people with cancer. *American Journal of Psychotherapy*, **54**, 487–99.

Greer, S., *et al.* (1992). Adjuvant psychological therapy for patients with cancer: a prospective randomised trial. *British Medical Journal*, **304**, 675–80.

Grey, M., *et al.* (1998). Short-term effects of coping skills training as adjunct to intensive therapy in adolescents. *Diabetes Care*, **21**, 902–8.

Grossman, S. (1984/5). The use of psychoanalytic theory and technique on the medical ward. *International Journal of Psychoanalytic Psychotherapy*, **10**, 533–48.

Grover, N., *et al.* (2002). Cognitive behavioural intervention in bronchial asthma. *Journal of the Association of Physicians of India*, **50**, 896–900.

Guthrie, E. A., *et al.* (1991). A controlled trial of psychological treatment for the irritable bowel syndrome. *Gastroenterology*, **100**, 450–7.

Harper, W., Groves, J., Gilliam, J., and Armstrong, C. (1999). Rethinking the place of psychological support groups in cardiopulmonary rehabilitation. *Journal of Cardiopulmonary Rehabilitation*, **19**, 18–21.

Hauser, S. T., *et al.* (1990). Adherence among children and adolescents with insulin-dependent diabetes over a four-year longitudinal follow-up: II Immediate and long-term linkages with the family milieu. *Journal of Pediatric Psychology*, **15**, 527–42.

Heinrich, R. L. and Schlag, C. C. (1982). Stress and activity management: group treatment for cancer patients and spouses. *Journal of Consulting and Clinical Psychology*, **33**, 439–46.

van Hemert, A. M., Hengeveld, M. W., Bolk, J. H., Rooijmans, H. G., and Vandenbroucke, J. P. (1993). Psychiatric disorders in relation to medical illness among patients of a general medical out-patient clinic. *Psychological Medicine*, **23**, 167–73.

Herskowitz, D. R., *et al.* (1995). Psychosocial predictors of acute complications of diabetes in youth. *Diabetic Medicine*, **12**, 612–18.

Hildebrant, J., *et al.* (1997). Prediction of success from a multidisciplinary program for chronic low back pain. *Spine*, **22**, 990–1001.

Himmelstein, J. S., *et al.* (1995). Work-related upper extremity disorders and work disability: clinical and psychosocial presentation. *Journal of Occupational and Environmental Medicine*, **37**, 1278–86.

Hirano, D., Nagashima, M., Ogawa, R., and Yoshino, S. (2001). Serum levels of IL-6 and stress related substances indicate mental stress condition in patients with RA. *Journal of Rheumatology*, **12**, 35–43.

Holroyd, K. and Lipchik, G. (1999). Psychological management of recurrent headache disorders: Progress and prospects. In: R. J. Gatchel and D. C. Turk, ed. *Psychosocial factors in pain: critical perspectives*, pp. 193–212. New York: Guliford Press.

Horne, R. and Weinman, J. (1999). Patients' beliefs about prescribed medicines and their role in adherence to treatment in chronic physical illness. *Journal of Psychosomatic Research*, **47**(6), 555–67.

Hudson, J. I., *et al.* (1985). Fibromyalgia and major affective disorder: a controlled phenomenology and family history study. *American Journal of Psychiatry*, **142**, 441–6.

Ibrahim, M. A., *et al.* (1974). Management after myocardial infarction: a controlled trial of the effect of group psychotherapy. *International Journal of Psychiatry in Medicine*, **5**, 253–68.

Ilnyckyj, A., Farber, J., Cheang, J., and Weinerman, B. H. (1994). A randomized controlled trial of psychotherapeutic intervention in cancer patients. *Annals of the Royal College of Physicians and Surgeons of Canada*, **27**, 93–6.

Jacobson, A. M., *et al.* (1994). Family environment and glycemic control: a four-year prospective study of children and adolescents with insulin-dependent diabetes mellitus. *Psychosomatic Medicine*, **56**, 401–9.

Jamison, R. N., Rudy, T. E., Pentzen, D. B., and Mosley, T. H. Jr. (1994). Cognitive-behavioural classifications of chronic pain: replication and extension of empirically derived patient profiles. *Pain*, **57**, 277–92.

Jeffery, R. W., *et al.* (2000). Long-term maintenance of weight loss: current status. *Health Psychology*, **19**, 5–16.

Johansson, E. and Lindberg, P. (2000). Low back pain patients in primary care: subgroups based on the Multidimensional Pain Inventory. *International Journal of Behavioural Medicine*, **7**, 340–52.

Johnson, S. K. (1998). The biopsychosocial model and chronic fatigue syndrome. *American Psychologist*, **53**(9), 1080–2.

Kabat-Zinn, J. (1990). *Full catastrophe living: using the wisdom of your body and mind to face stress, pain, and illness*, p. 453. New York: Delacorte Press.

Katon, W. (1996). The impact of major depression on chronic medical illness. *General Hospital Psychiatry*, **18**, 215–19.

Katz, P. and Yelin, E. H. (1995). The development of depressive symptoms among women with rheumatoid arthritis: the role of function. *Arthritis and Rheumatism*, **38**, 49–56.

Keefe, F. J., Lefebvre, J. C., Maixner, W., Salley, A. N., and Caldwell, D. S. (1997). Self-efficacy for arthritis pain: relationship to perception of thermal laboratory pain stimuli. *Arthritis Care and Research*, **10**, 177–84.

Keefe, F. J., *et al.* (1999). Spouse-assisted coping training in the management of knee pain in osteoarthritis: long-term follow-up results. *Arthritis Care and Research*, **12**, 101–11.

Keefe, F. J., *et al.* (2002). Recent advances and future directions in the biopsychosocial assessment and treatment of arthritis. *Journal of Consulting and Clinical Psychology*, **70**, 640–55.

Kissane, D. W., Bloch, S., Clarke, D. M., and Smith, G. C. (2001). *Australian RCT of group therapy for breast cancer.* Presented at the American Psychiatric Association Annual Meeting, New Orleans.

Kissane, D. W., *et al.* (1994). Psychological morbidity in the families of patients with cancer. *Psycho-Oncology*, **3**, 47–56.

Kissane, D. W., *et al.* (1997). Cognitive-existential group therapy for patients with primary breast cancer-techniques and themes. *Psycho-Oncology*, **6**, 25–33.

Knowler, W. C., Barrett-Connor, E., Fowler, S. E., *et al.* (2002). Reduction in the incidence of type 2 diabetes with lifestyle intervention or metformin. *New England Journal of Medicine*, **346**, 393–403.

Korner-Bitensky, N., Tarasuk, J., Nelles, J., and Bouchard, J. M. (1998). The impact of interventions with families poststroke: a review. *Topics in Stroke Rehabilitation*, **5**(3), 69–85.

Kovacs, M., Obrosky, D. S., Goldston, D., and Drash, A. (1997). Major depressive disorder in youths with IDDM: a controlled prospective study of course and outcome. *Diabetes Care*, **20**, 45–51.

Kreutzer, J. S., Kolakowsky-Hayner, S. A., Demm, S. R., and Meade, M. A. (2002). A structured approach to family intervention after brain injury. *Journal of Head Trauma Rehabilitation*, **17**(4), 349–67.

Kunik, M. E., Braun, U., Stanley, M. A., Wristers, K., Molinari, V., Stoebner, D., and Orengo, C. A. (2001). One session cognitive behavioral therapy for elderly patients with chronic obstructive pulmonary disease. *Psychological Medicine*, **31**(4), 717–23.

Laatsch, L. (1999). Application of cognitive rehabilitation techniques in psychotherapy. In: K. G. Langer, *et al.*, ed. *Psychotherapeutic interventions for adults with brain injury or stroke: a clinician's treatment resource*, pp. 131–48. Madison, CT: Psychosocial Press/International Universities Press.

Lacroix, J. M., *et al.* (1991). Symptom schemata in chronic respiratory patients. *Health Psychology*, **10**, 268–73.

Linden, W., Stossel, C., and Maurice, J. (1996). Psychosocial interventions for patients with coronary artery disease. *Archives of Internal Medicine*, **156**, 745–52.

Lloyd, C. E., *et al.* (1999). Association between stress and glycemic control in adults with type 1 (insulin-dependent) diabetes. *Diabetes Care*, **22**, 1278–83.

Lorig, K., Chastain, R. L., Ung, E., Shoor, S., and Holman, H. R. (1989). Development and evaluation of a scale to measure perceived self-efficacy in people with arthritis. *Arthritis and Rheumatism*, **36**, 439–46.

Lorig, K. R., Mazonson, P. D., and Holman, H. R. (1993). Evidence suggesting that health education for self-management in patients with chronic arthritis has sustained health benefits while reducing health care costs. *Arthritis and Rheumatism*, **32**, 37–44.

Lustman, P. J., *et al.* (1995). Effects of alprazolam on glucose regulation in diabetes: results of a double-blind, placebo-controlled trial. *Diabetes Care*, **18**, 1133–9.

Lustman, P. J., Griffiths, L. S., and Clouse, R. E. (1997). Depression in adults with diabetes. *Seminars in Clinical Neuropsychiatry*, **2**, 15–23.

Lustman, P. J., Griffith, L. S., Freedland, K. E., Kissel, S. S., and Clouse, R. E. (1998). Cognitive behaviour therapy for depression in type 2 diabetes mellitus. A randomized, controlled trial. *Annals of Internal Medicine*, **129**, 613–21.

Lustman, P. H., Freedland, K. E., Griffith, L. S., and Clouse, R. E. (2000a). Fluoxetine for depression in diabetes: a randomized double-blind placebo-controlled trial. *Diabetes Care*, **23**, 618–23.

Lustman, P. J., *et al.* (2000b). Depression and poor glycemic control: a meta-analytic review of the literature. *Diabetes Care*, **23**, 934–42.

Lyons, R. F., Sullivan, M. J. L., and Ritvo, P. G. (1995). *Relationships in chronic illness and disability.* Thousand Oaks, CA: Sage Publications.

Magni, G., Caldieron, C., Rigatti-Luchini, S., and Merskey, H. (1990). Chronic musculoskeletal pain and depressive symptoms in the general population. An analysis of the 1st National Health and Nutrition Examination Survey data. *Pain*, **43**, 299–307.

Martin, F. (2001). Co-morbidity of depression with physical illnesses: a review of the literature. *Mental Health Care*, **4**(12), 405–8.

Mayou, R. and Sharpe, M. (1997). Treating medically unexplained physical symptoms. *British Medical Journal*, **315**, 561–2.

McCrackern, L. M. and Gross, R. T. (1993). Does anxiety affect coping with chronic pain? *Clinical Journal of Pain*, **9**, 253–9.

Meyer, T. J. and Mark, M. M. (1995). Effects of Psychosocial interventions with adult cancer patients: A meta-analysis of randomized experiments. *Health Psychology*, **14**, 101–8.

Miller, N. H., Smith, P. M., DeBusk, R. F., Sobel, D. S., and Taylor, C. B. (1997). Smoking cessation in hospitalised patients. Results of a randomised trial. *Archives of Internal Medicine*, **157**(4), 409–15.

Moore, M. E., Berk, S. N., and Nyparer, A. (1984). Chronic pain: inpatient treatment with small group effects. *Archives of Physical and Medical Rehabilitation*, **6**, 356–61.

Moorey, S. and Greer, S. (2002). *Cognitive behaviour therapy for people with cancer.* New York: Oxford University Press.

Moorey, S., *et al.* (1998). A comparison of adjuvant psychological therapy and supportive counselling in patients with cancer. *Psycho-Oncology*, **7**, 218–28.

Moran, G., Fonagy, P., Kurtz, A., Bolton, A., and Brook, C. (1991). A controlled study of psychoanalytic treatment of brittle diabetes. *Journal of the American Academy of Child and Adolescent Psychiatry*, **30**, 926–35.

Moritz, D. J., *et al.* (1994). The health burden of diabetes for the elderly in four communities. *Public Health Reports*, **109**, 782–90.

Morley, S., *et al.* (1999). Systematic review and meta-analysis of randomised controlled trials of cognitive behaviour therapy and behaviour therapy for chronic pain in adults, excluding headache. *Pain*, **80**, 1–13.

Mulder, C. L., Pompe, G. van der Spiegel, D., Antoni, M. H., and DeVries, M. J. (1992). Do psychosocial factors influence the course of breast cancer? A review of recent literature, methodological problems and future directions. *Psycho-Oncology*, **1**, 155–67.

National Center for Health Statistics and Koch, H. (1986). *The management of chronic pain in office-based ambulatory care: National Ambulatory Medical Care Survey.* Advance data from Vital and Health Statistics, No. 123 (DHHS Publication No. PHS 86-1250). Hyattsville, MD: Public Health Service.

Newell, S. A., Sanson-Fisher, R. W., and Savolainen, N. J. (2002). Systematic review of psychological therapies for cancer patients: overview and recommendations for future research. *Journal of the National Cancer Institute*, **94**(8), 558–84.

Newson-Davis, I., Goldstein, L. H., and Fitzpatrick, D. (1998). Fear of seizures: an investigation and treatment. *Seizure*, **7**(2), 101–6.

Nezu, A. M., *et al.* (2003). Project genesis: assessing the efficacy of problem solving therapy for distressed cancer patients. *Journal of Consulting and Clinical Psychology*, **71**(6), 1036–48.

Ogden, J. (2000). *Health psychology: a textbook.* Buckingham: Open University Press.

Ormel, J., *et al.* (1999). Onset of disability in depressed and non-depressed primary care patients. *Psychological Medicine*, **29**, 847–53.

Padesky, C. and Greenberger, D. (1995). *Mind over mood. A cognitive therapy manual for clients.* New York: Guildford Press.

Parker, J. C., *et al.* (1992). Psychological factors, immunologic activation, and disease activity in rheumatoid arthritis. *Arthritis Care and Research*, **5**, 196–201.

Parker, J. C., *et al.* (1995). Effects of stress management on clinical outcomes in rheumatoid arthritis. *Arthritis and Rheumatism*, **38**, 1807–18.

Parsell, S. and Tagliareni, E. M. (1974). Cancer patients help each other. *American Journal of Nursing*, **74**, 650–1.

Payne, A. and Blanchard, E. B. (1995). A controlled comparison of cognitive therapy and self help support groups in the treatment of irritable bowel syndrome. *Journal of Consulting and Clinical Psychology*, **63**(5), 779–86.

Pennebaker, J. W. and Beall, S. K. (1986). Confronting a traumatic event: toward an understanding of inhibition and disease. *Journal of Abnormal Psychology*, **95**, 274–81.

Persons, J. (1989). *Cognitive therapy in practice. a case formulation approach.* Norton.

van Peski-Oosterbann, A. S., *et al.* (2000). Cognitive behavioural therapy reduced noncardiac chest pain and use of psychological services. *ACP Journal Club*, **132**, 8.

Petersson, L. M., Berglund, G., Brodin, O., Glimelius, B., and Sjoden, P. O. (2000). Group rehabilitation for cancer patients: satisfaction and perceived benefits. *Patient Education and Counselling*, **3**, 219–29.

Petrie, K. J., *et al.* (1996). Roles of patients' view of their illness in predicting return to work and functioning after myocardial infarction: longitudinal study. *British Medical Journal*, 312, 1191–4.

Peyrot, M. and Rubin, R. R. (1997). Levels and risk of depression and anxiety symptomatology among diabetic adults. *Diabetes Care*, 20, 585–90.

Peyrot, M. K. and Rubin, R. R. (1999). Persistence of depressive symptoms in diabetic adults. *Diabetes Care*, 22(3), 448–52.

Polatin, P. B., Kinney, R. K., Gatchel, R. J., Lillo, E., and Mayer, T. G. (1993). Psychiatric illness and chronic low-back pain. *Spine*, 18, 66–71.

Polonsky, W. H., *et al.* (1995). Assessment of diabetes-related distress. *Diabetes Care*, 18, 754–60.

Popkin, M. K., Callies, A. L., Lentz, R. D., Colon, E. A., and Sutherland, D. E. (1988). Prevalence of major depression, simple phobia, and other psychiatric disorders in patients with long-standing type I diabetes mellitus. *Archives of General Psychiatry*, 45, 64–8.

Postone, N. (1998). Psychotherapy with cancer patients. *American Journal of Psychotherapy*, 52(4), 412–24.

Prohaska, T. R., Keller, M. L., Leventhal, E. A., and Leventhal, H. (1987). Impact of symptoms and aging attribution on emotions and coping. *Health Psychology*, 6(6), 495–514.

Rahe, R. H. and Ward, H. W. (1985). Brief group therapy in myocardial infarction rehabilitation. *Journal of Cardiopulmomary Rehabilitation*, 5, 208–15.

Rahe, R. H., Ward, H. W., and Hayes, V. (1979). Brief group therapy in myocardial infarction rehabilitation; three to four year follow-up of a controlled trial. *Psychosomatic Medicine*, 41, 229–42.

Ramaratnam, S., Baker, G. A., and Goldstein, L. (2003). Psychological treatments for epilepsy. *Cochrane Database of Systematic Reviews*, 1, 2003.

Reiss, S. and McNally, R. J. (1985). The expectancy model of fear. In: S. Reiss and R. R. Bootzin, ed. *Theoretical issues in behaviour therapy*. New York: Academic Press.

Ridsdale, L., Mandalia, S., Evans, A., Jerrett, W., and Osler, K. (1999). Tiredness as a ticket of entry: the role of patients' beliefs and psychological symptoms in explaining frequent attendance. *Scandinavian Journal of Primary Health Care*, 17(2), 72–4.

Rodin, G. M., Johnson, L. E., Garfinkel, P. E., Daneman, D., and Kenshole, A. B. (1986). Eating disorders in female adolescents with insulin-dependent diabetes mellitus. *International Journal of Psychiatry and Medicine*, 16, 49–57.

Romano, J. M. and Turner, J. A. (1985). Chronic pain and depression: Does the evidence support a relationship. *Psychological Bulletin*, 97, 18–34.

Rubin, R. R. (2000). Diabetes and quality of life. *Diabetes Spectrum*, 13, 21–3.

Rubin, R. R., Peyrot, M., and Saudek, C. (1989). Effect of diabetes education on self-care, metabolic control, and emotional well-being. *Diabetes Care*, 12, 673–9.

Rubin, R. R., Peyrot, M., and Saudek, C. (1993). The effect of a diabetes education program incorporating coping skills training on emotional well-being and diabetes self-efficacy. *Diabetes Educator*, 19, 210–14.

Rudy, T. E., Turk, D. C., Kubinski, J. A., and Zaki, H. S. (1995). Differential treatment responses of TMD patients as a function of psychological characteristics. *Pain*, 61, 103–12.

Rydall, A. C., Rodin, G. M., Olmsted, M. P., Devenyi, R. G., and Daneman, D. (1997). Disordered eating behaviour and microvascular complications in young women with insulin-dependent diabetes mellitus. *New England Journal of Medicine*, 336, 1849–54.

Salmon, P. (2000). Patients who present physical symptoms in the absence of physical pathology: a challenge to existing models of doctor-patient interaction. *Patient Education and Counselling*, 39, 105–13.

Sampson, W. (2002). Controversies in cancer and the mind: effects of psychosocial support. *Seminars in Oncology*, 29(6), 595–600.

Schiaffino, K. M. and Revenson, T. A. (1995). Relative contributions of spousal support and illness appraisals to depressed mood in arthritis patients. *Arthritis Care and Research*, 8, 80–7.

Schofferman, J., Anderson, D., Hines, R., Smith, G., and Keane, G. (1993). Childhood psychological trauma and chronic refractory low-back pain. *Clinical Journal of Pain*, 9, 260–5.

Schrock, D., Palmer, R. F., and Taylor, B. (1999). Effects of a psychosocial intervention on survival among patients with stage I breast and prostate cancer: a matched case-control study. *Alternative Therapies and Health Medicine*, 5, 49–55.

Sharpe, M. and Carson, A. (2001). 'Unexplained' somatic symptoms, functional syndromes, and somatization: do we need a paradigm shift? *Annals of Internal Medicine*, 134(9 Pt 2), 926–30.

Sheard, T. and Maguire, P. (1999). The effect of psychological interventions on anxiety and depression in cancer patients: results of two meta–analyses. *British Journal of Cancer*, 80, 1770–80.

Simonton, S. and Sherman, A. (2000). An integrated model of group treatment for cancer patients. *International Journal of Group Psychotherapy*, 50, 487–506.

Smith, G. C. (2003). The future of consultation-liaison psychiatry. *Australian and New Zealand Journal of Psychiatry*, 37(2), 150–9.

Smith, T. W. and Ruiz, J. M. (2002). Psychosocial influences on the development and course of coronary heart disease: current status and implications for research and practice. *Journal of Consulting and Clinical Psychology*, 70, 548–68.

Smyth, J. M. (1998). Written emotional expression: effect sizes, outcome types, and moderating variables. *Journal of Consulting and Clinical Psychology*, 66, 174–84.

Smyth, J. M., Stone, A. A., Hurewitz, A., and Kaell, A. (1999). Effects of writing about stressful experiences on symptom reduction in patients with asthma or rheumatoid arthritis: a randomized trial. *Journal of the American Medical Association*, 281, 1304–9.

Sobel, H. J. and Worden, J. W. (1982). *Practitioner's manual: helping cancer patients cope*, pp. 1–32. New York: Guilford Press.

Spiegel, D. (1993). Psychosocial intervention in cancer. *Journal of the National Cancer Institute*, 85, 1198–205.

Spiegel, D. (2001). Mind matters: Group therapy and survival in breast cancer (Editorial). *New England Journal of Medicine*, 345, 1767–8.

Spiegel, D. and Classen, C. (2000). *Group therapy for cancer patients: a research-based handbook of psychosocial care*. p. 303. New York: Basic Books.

Spiegel, D., Bloom, J. R., and Yalom, I. (1981). Group support for patients with metastatic cancer. *Archives of General Psychiatry*, 38, 527–533.

Spiegel, D., Bloom, J. R., and Gottheil, E. (1983). Family environment of patients with metastatic carcinoma. *Journal of Psychosocial Oncology*, 1, 33–44.

Spiegel, D., *et al.* (1989). Effect of psychosocial treatment on survival of patients with metastatic breast cancer. *Lancet*, 14, 888–91.

Stern, M. J., Plionis, E., and Kaslow, L. (1984). Group process expectations and outcome with post-myocardial infarction patients. *General Hospital Psychiatry*, 6, 101–8.

Sternbach, R. A. (1974). *Pain patients: Traits and treatments*. New York: Academic Press.

Stoute, B., Shapiro, T., and Viederman, M. (1996). Developmental arrest and maternal loss in an adolescent girl with lupus erythematosus and terminal renal failure. *American Journal of Psychiatry*, 153, 1476–82.

Straker, N. (1998). Psychodynamic psychotherapy for cancer patients. *Journal of Psychotherapy Practice and Research*, 7, 1–9.

Straker, N. and Wyszynski, A. (1986). Denial in the cancer patient: a common sense approach. *Internal Medicine for the Specialist*, 7(3), 150–5.

Surwit, R. S., *et al.* (2002). Stress management improves long-term glycemic control in type 2 diabetes. *Diabetes Care*, 25, 30–4.

Svedlund, J. (2002). Functional gastrointestinal diseases. Psychotherapy is an efficient complement to drug therapy. (Swedish). *Lakartidningen*, 99(3), 172–4.

Svedlund, J., Sjodin, I., Ottosson, J. O., and Dotevall, G. (1983). Controlled study of psychotherapy in irritable bowel syndrome. *Lancet*, ii, 589–92.

Tait, R. C., Chibnall, J. T., and Richardson, W. D. (1990). Litigation and employment status: effects on patients with chronic pain. *Pain*, 43, 37–46.

Talley, N. J., Owen, B. K., Boyce, P., and Paterson, K. (1996). Psychological treatments for irritable bowel syndrome: a critique of controlled treatment trials. *American Journal of Gastroenterology*, 91(2), 277–83.

Tattersall, R. L. (2002). The expert patient: a new approach to chronic disease management for the twenty-first century. *Clinical Medicine*, 2(3), 227–9.

Telch, C. F. and Telch, M. J. (1986). Group coping skills instruction and supportive group therapy for cancer patients: a comparison of strategies. *Journal of Consulting and Clinical Psychology*, 54, 802–8.

Trief, P. M., Grant, W., Elbert, K., and Weinstock, R. S. (1998). Family environment, glycemic control, and the psychosocial adaptation of adults with diabetes. *Diabetes Care*, 21, 241–5.

Trief, P. M., Himes, C. L., Orendorff, R., and Weinstock, R. S. (2001). The marital relationship and psychosocial adaptation and glycemic control of individuals with diabetes. *Diabetes Care*, **24**, 1384–9.

Trief, P. M., Wade, M. J., Britton, K. D., and Weinstock, R. S. (2002). A prospective analysis of marital relationship factors and quality of life in diabetes. *Diabetes Care*, **25**, 1154–8.

Truchon, M. and Fillion, L. (2000). Biopsychosocial determinants of chronic disability and low-back pain; a review. *Journal of Occupational Rehabilitation*, **10**, 117–42.

Turczyn, K. M. and Drury, T. F. (1992). Inventory of pain data from the National Center for Health Statistics. Vital and Health Statistics-Series 1: Programs and collection procedures, **26**, 1–66.

Turk, D. C. (2002). A diathesis-stress model of chronic pain and disability following traumatic injury. *Pain Research and Management*, **7**, 9–19.

Turk, D. C. and Okifuji, A. (1996). Perception of traumatic events, compensation status, and physical findings: impact on pain severity, emotional distress, and disability in chronic pain patients. *Journal of Behavioural Medicine*, **19**, 435–453.

Turk, D. C. and Okifuji, A. (2002). Psychological factors in chronic pain: evolution and revolution. *Journal of Consulting and Clinical Psychology*, **70**, 678–90.

Turk, D. C. and Rudy, T. E. (1990). Toward an empirically derived taxonomy of chronic pain patients: integration of psychological assessment data. *Journal of Consulting and Clinical Psychology*, **56**, 233–8.

United Kingdom Prospective Diabetes Study Group (1998). Intensive blood-glucose control with sulphonylureas or insulin compared with conventional treatment and risk of complications in patients with type 2 diabetes. *Lancet*, **352**, 837–53.

Viederman, M. (1974). Adaptive and maladaptive regression in hemodialysis. *Psychiatry*, **37**, 68–77.

Viner, R., McGrath, M., and Trudinger, P. (1996). Family stress and metabolic control in diabetes. *Archives of Disease in Childhood*, **74**, 418–21.

Vlaeyen, J. W., Haazen, I. W., Schuerman, J. A., Kole-Snijders, A. M. J., and vanEck, H. (1995). Behavioural rehabilitation of chronic low back pain: comparison of an operant treatment, an operant-cognitive treatment and an operant-respondent treatment. *British Journal of Clinical Psychology*, **34**, 95–118.

Waddell, G., Newton, M., Henderson, I., Somerville, D., and Main, C. J. (1993). A Fear Avoidance Beliefs Questionnaire (FABQ) and the role of fear-avoidance beliefs in chronic low back pain and disability. *Pain*, **52**, 157–68.

Walker, L. G., *et al.* (1999). Psychological, clinical and pathological effects of relaxation training and guided imagery during primary chemotherapy. *British Journal of Cancer*, **80**, 262–8.

Walker, L. G., Ratcliffe, M. A., and Dawson, A. A. (2000) Relaxation and hypnotherapy: long term effects on the survival of patients with lymphoma. *Psycho-Oncology*, **9**, 355–6.

Wallace, N. and Wallace, D. C. (1977). Group education after myocardial infarction: Is it effective? *Medical Journal of Australia*, **2**, 245–7.

Wandell, P. E. and Tovi, J. (2000). The quality of life of elderly diabetic patients. *Journal of Diabetes and its Complications*, **14**, 25–30.

Watson, M. and Burton, M. (1998). *Counselling patients with cancer*. Chichester: John Wiley and Sons.

Watson, M., *et al.* (1999). Influence of psychological response on survival in breast cancer: a population-based cohort study. *Lancet*, **354**, 1331–6.

Wells, K. B., *et al.* (1989). The functioning and well-being of depressed patients: results from the medical outcomes study. *Journal of the American Medical Association*, **262**, 914–19.

Weyer, S., Hewer, W., Pfeifer-Kurda, M., and Dilling, H. (1989). Psychiatric disorders and diabetes: results from a community study. *Journal of Psychosomatic Research*, **33**, 633–40.

White, C. A. (2001). *Cognitive behaviour therapy for chronic medical problems: a guide to assessment and treatment in practice*. New York: John Wiley and Sons Ltd.

Whiting, P., Bagnall, A. M., Sowden, A. K., Multrow, C. D., and Ramirez, G. (2001). Interventions in the treatment and management of chronic fatigue syndrome: a systematic review. *Journal of the American Medical Association*, **286**(11), 1360–8.

Whorwell, P. J., Prior, A., and Faragher, E. B. (1984). Controlled trial of hypnotherapy in the treatment of severe refractory irritable bowel syndrome. *Lancet*, **ii**, 1232–4.

Wiens, B. A. and Kellogg, J. S. (2000). Implementation of a therapy group at a camp in southern Illinois for children with burn injuries. *Journal of Burn Care and Rehabilitation*, **21**, 281–7.

Wiklund, I. and Butler-Wheelhouse, P. (1996). Psychosocial factors and their role in symptomatic gastroesophageal reflux disease and functional dyspepsia. *Scandinavian Journal of Gastroenterology–Supplement*, **31**(220), 94–100.

Wood, B. L. (1994). One articulation of the structural family therapy model: a biobehavioural family model of chronic illness in children. *Journal of Family Therapy*, **16**, 53–72.

Wood, P. E., Milligan, M., Christ, D., and Liff, D. (1978). Group counselling for cancer patients in a community hospital. *Psychosomatics*, **19**, 555–61.

World Health Organization (1992). *The ICD-10 Classification of Mental and Behavioural Disorders. Clinical descriptions and diagnostic guidelines*. Geneva: World Health Organisation.

Wulsin, L. R., Vaillant, G. E., and Wells, V. E. (1999). A systematic review of the mortality of depression. *Psychosomatic Medicine*, **51**, 6–17.

Wysocki, T., *et al.* (2000). Randomized, controlled trial of behaviour therapy for families of adolescents with insulin-dependent diabetes mellitus. *Journal of Pediatric Psychology*, **25**, 23–33.

Xiaolian, J. Chaiwan, S., Panuthai, S., Yijuan, C., Lei, Y., and Jiping, L. (2002). Family support and self-care behaviour of Chinese chronic obstructive pulmonary disease patients. *Nursing and Health Sciences*, **4**(1–2), 41–9.

Yalom, I. (1985). *The theory and practice of group psychotherapy*, 3rd edn. New York: Basic Books.

Yelin, E. and Callahan, L. (1995). The economic cost and social and psychological impact of musculoskeletal conditions. *Arthritis and Rheumatism*, **38**, 1351–62.

Zakus, G., *et al.* (1979). A group behaviour modification approach to adolescent obesity. *Adolescence*, **14**, 481–9.

Zautra, A. J. and Smith, B. W. (2001). Depression and reactivity to stress in older women with rheumatoid arthritis and osteoarthritis. *Psychosomatic Medicine*, **63**, 687–96.

Zautra, A. J., Burleson, M. H., Matt, K. S., Roth, S., and Burrows, L. (1994). Interpersonal stress, depression, and disease activity in rheumatoid arthritis and osteoarthritis patients. *Health Psychology*, **13**, 139–48.

Zautra, A. J., Hamilton, N. A., Potter, P., and Smith, B. (1999). Field research on the relationship between stress and disease activity in rheumatoid arthritis. *Annals of the New York Academy of Sciences*, **876**, 397–412.

34 Gender issues in psychotherapy

Carol C. Nadelson, Malkah T. Notman, and Mary K. McCarthy

As in all areas of health care, gender is an important variable in the treatment of a variety of psychiatric symptoms and disorders. Gender is mediated by psychosocial factors and the physiological and metabolic differences between men and women. Gender can influence the patient's choice of caregiver, the 'fit' between caregiver and patient and the sequence and content of the clinical material presented. It may also affect the diagnosis, treatment selection, length of treatment, and even the outcome of treatment.

In this chapter we will focus first on normal development and the interaction of gender and the environment, then on how the sexes experience the life cycle in different ways, and finally explore how one's values and gender influence psychotherapeutic treatment in many ways, closing with a review of the psychotherapy literature on gender and treatment variables.

Introduction

Despite heroic efforts to reconceptualize existing paradigms, the dichotomy between 'brain disease' and 'mind disease' continues to be prevalent. There is growing support, however, for an interactional construct that unifies brain and mind, biologic and psychosocial, based on increasingly sophisticated and complex scientific data and conceptualization. As Eisenberg (1995) has stated, 'Nature and nurture stand in reciprocity, not opposition. All children inherit, along with their parents' genes, their parents, their peers, and the places they inhabit'. This idea about reciprocity and interaction of nature and nurture applies to gender differences.

Evidence of gender differences in the nervous system, beginning in fetal life, suggests that from birth boys and girls may not perceive and experience the world in the same way. For example, females are better at language skills such as verbal fluency and grammar, classically left-hemisphere functions, while males, on average, are more facile at spatially related tasks such as picture assembly and block design, typically right-hemisphere processes (Siegel, 1999). Gender differences in neural maturity and organization influence behavior and reactions in infants. These, in turn, can affect caretakers responses, further reinforcing differences. Because experience can modify the structure and function of neurons and neuronal networks, and can even change gene expression, these differences in caretaker responses serve to further alter the growth and development of neuronal pathways (Kandel, 1999).

Another area in which the integration of biological and psychosocial phenomena has relevance has been shown in the data accumulating on the consequences of early abuse. Early childhood physical and sexual abuse is associated with brain dysfunction, primarily of the limbic system (Hull, 2002). Teicher *et al.* (1993) concluded that their 'findings are consistent with a complex biopsychosocial hypothesis: namely, that sociological factors leading to early abuse may result in biological alterations in the development of the central nervous system, with these alterations manifesting as persistent behavioral disturbances that are in turn associated with long-term psychiatric sequelae and a proclivity for the intergenerational transfer of abusive and aggressive behavior'. Moreover, some data on the experience of childhood trauma suggest that each sex is affected differently.

Women report more problems with self-esteem, relationships, and work, and men are at higher risk to act out the abuse by becoming perpetrators themselves (Glasser *et al.*, 2001).

Studies also demonstrate that brain metabolism and function are affected by psychotherapy. These findings reinforce our understanding of the plasticity of the brain: that it can functionally organize and reorganize, and that it is affected by behavior and experience (Baxter *et al.*, 1992; Schwartz *et al.*, 1996; Thase *et al.*, 1996; Brody *et al.*, 2001; Martin *et al.*, 2001).

These data further underscore that the distinction between the biological and the psychosocial is both artificial and misleading.

Gender and early development

Early influences and endowments, both biological and psychosocial, are important in the shaping of personality. In childhood, the presence or absence of continued stable care, styles of child rearing, the responsiveness and nurturance of people in the environment, physical health and illness, loss, and trauma, as well as biological endowment, are all determinants of the ultimate configuration of personality.

The effects of particular cultural practices, including gender differences in child rearing, are also manifested very early in life and affect development. Gender differences in parental behavior, especially related to male and female roles, are powerful developmental forces (Rogers *et al.*, 2002). Ideas about the determinants of gender identity have changed from the early views that the major determinants of gender development were anatomic genital differences, to a view that there are differing developmental experiences and paths. Complex processes take place beginning in the prenatal period, including the hormonal environment, the structure of the family, the presence and roles of other siblings, the mother's past pregnancies, and many aspects of the child's relationship with others.

Gender identity development starts early, with prenatal expectations of parents and others about the child's gender and its meaning. By the second and third year of life, a child's developmental goals include a sense of independence to explore the world and the formation of a stable self-image in the setting of a consistent, predictable, and close relationship with parents and others. Important aspects of this developmental phase are the formation of an internalized image of the parent that remains even when the parent is physically absent, and the ability to sustain a sense of closeness in the face of other conflicting feelings.

Gender identity and gender role

The concepts of gender identity and gender role have become important in treatment (Stoller, 1976; Person and Ovesey, 1983). Gender identity is the internalized sense of maleness or femaleness, and the knowledge of one's biological sex, including the associated psychological attributes. It begins to evolve in early childhood and appears to be firmly established by the age of about 18 months. It derives from many influences, including identifications with parents and their attitudes, expectations, and behaviors, as well as biological and cultural factors (Money and Ehrhardt, 1972; Kleeman, 1976; Hines and Green, 1991).

Gender role is a cultural construct referring to the expectations, attitudes, and behaviors that are considered to be appropriate for each gender in that particular culture. There are enormous differences in the roles and expectations of men and women in different societies. Some societies dictate more rigid and fixed roles than others and not all value the same traits or see traits as gender specific in the same ways. For example, despite their smaller size and lesser physical strength, women in some cultures are assigned the heavy work. The role consistently assumed by women across cultures is child-rearing (LeVine, 1991). During early development, in all cultures, the mother remains the primary caregiver of young children. Thus, the earliest bond is more likely to be made with her. She becomes the primary identification figure in early childhood, for both boys and girls. Thus, for girls, the first identification is with the parent of the same sex. For boys, the first identification is with the parent of the opposite sex.

As girls grow up, this same-sex identification does not have to change in order for a feminine gender identity to consolidate. That is, girls learn a maternal identification. In order for a boy to consolidate his masculine identity, however, he must shift his primary identification away from his mother and develop identification with a male figure. In this process he moves away from his early attachment. The complex process of establishing a male identity, and the separation from early attachments that seems necessary to the process of the development of a masculine identity, may be factors accounting for the higher incidence of gender identity disorders in males (American Psychiatric Association, 1987).

Many of these developmental differences have been thought to be important determinants of the personality differences that have been observed between men and women (Chodorow, 1978). For men, the pull toward an early attachment to their mother can feel regressive and create a wish for distance and separation from these early ties. Closeness and intimacy can seem threatening, as if leading inevitably to regression (Chodorow, 1978). Clinically, we often see qualitative differences in intimacy, dependency, and attachment between men and women. Although girls usually function better as students in the primary grades than do boys, and they present fewer behavior problems and less overt psychopathology, these characteristics also represent conformity to social stereotypes. Girls are often expected to be more compliant and conforming, and the later repercussions appear to be that the activity and ambition that lead to a sense of competence and self-esteem can be inhibited (Wellesley College Center for Research on Women, 1992).

For girls, the continuity of attachment to their mothers, or primary caregivers, and the fear of loss of love by manifesting open aggression may make it more difficult to establish autonomy and independence while holding on to important relationships. Aggression, competitiveness, and anger may be difficult to manage because relationships can be threatened (Chodorow, 1978; Miller et al., 1981; Gilligan, 1982). It can be difficult for women to express themselves freely, especially when they experience anger and aggression, and, at the same time, to preserve relationships. This may be seen later in life in a woman's conflict about aggression, manifested in her difficulty in being appropriately assertive and in her inhibited risk-taking behavior (Nadelson et al., 1982).

At times, women may also fail to act in their own best interests because of their desire to preserve relationships, even if these are abusive. For some women this can result in behavior that may continue to put them at risk for victimization (Carmen et al., 1984; Jaffe et al., 1986; van der Kolk, 1989). The threat of loss, then, may motivate behavior that can be interpreted as masochistic. For women, the conflict experienced around aggression can result in turning aggression on themselves, such as occurs in the form of excessive self-criticism, with diminished self-esteem. Culturally supported passivity, with consequent feelings of helplessness can be risk factors for depression.

For girls, problems in the development of self-esteem appear to be intensified in adolescence. Gilligan (1987) found that there are gender differences in self-concept and identity in adolescence. Males generally define themselves in terms of individual achievement and work and females more often in relational terms.

Gilligan found that in mid-adolescence girls experienced a crisis of connection, with conflicts between selfish or individual solutions to relational problems and selflessness or self-sacrifice. This period is also one in which girls become more vulnerable to depression than do boys: by age 15, females are about twice as likely as males to have an episode of depression. It is a time when they begin to assume adult feminine identities and roles. Cyranowski et al. (2000) proposed an explanatory model that links adolescent girls' changing hormonal milieu, which may biochemically stimulate affiliative needs, with the dramatic role transitions of adolescence and the 'sensitization' of some girls to the depressogenic effects of negative life events. In any case, the coalescence of biological and psychosocial factors makes it necessary to integrate and not polarize our conceptualization of development.

Body image and reproduction

As puberty approaches, girls and boys experience their reproductive identities in different ways. For girls, menarche signals a capacity for pregnancy. This change also brings a potential vulnerability for the girl that is not in the boy's experience. It is both a positive experience and a source of risk and anxiety. A girl also develops a new 'organ', breasts, transforming her body. This has no parallel in the boy (Notman et al., 1991). Menarche, for a girl, is an organizer of her sense of sexual identity. It is also an undeniable physical experience, and it can be a source of pleasure and conflict about growing up and being feminine. The adolescent girl in Western cultures is bombarded with media images of woman who are loved because of their physical appearance. A specific model of physical attractiveness continues to be more important for women than for men, for whom strength and performance are more valued. For both, however, self-esteem and self-confidence rest heavily on physical attributes and body image, especially during adolescence.

Conflicts around self-image and body image become more prominent during adolescence and can be expressed differently for boys and girls. Discomfort with body image, and fear and ambivalence about mastery, independence, separation from family, and adulthood, including sexuality, are difficult issues that are thought to contribute to the dramatic incidence of eating disorders in adolescent girls, who may literally attempt to starve themselves back into childhood.

Gender differences in life cycle events

Women's life cycles are closely connected to their reproductive potential in a way that differs from most men's life cycles. The acknowledgment of a woman's reproductive capacity is usually an important component of her sense of identity and femininity, regardless of whether or not she actually bears children. The knowledge that there is a finite time period for reproduction also influences her concept of time and her life cycle. She must make decisions about career and family in a way that men do not (Nadelson and Notman, 1982a,b; Notman and Lester, 1988; Notman et al., 1991). This difference can obviously affect her emotional state and her decision to seek treatment, as well as the issues that will be raised in the course of treatment (Nadelson, 1989a). It is rare, for example, for a man in his 30s to seek treatment to resolve a decision about having children; this is not uncommon for women.

Pregnancy as a life event marks a transition to motherhood and raises many issues for a woman, including her relationship and identification with her own mother. This transition may parallel a man's experience of fatherhood, but the life event is not the same. For example, the ante- and postpartum period increases the woman's vulnerability to specific psychiatric disorders, particularly depression (O'Hara, 1995; Janowsky et al., 1996).

Infertility is also a different experience for men and women, and there are different issues to consider in treatment. Historically, and in some cultures today, women have been 'blamed' for infertility. A woman's pregnancy has also been viewed as a confirmation of a man's masculinity and potency. Infertility can be as threatening and distressing a problem for a man as for a woman, but in different ways. Social norms have also supported men's resistance to involvement in infertility workups and treatment. Thus, failures occur when couples attempt to conceive and there has been inadequate evaluation or treatment.

Menopause is a marker of the life cycle that does not occur in the same way for men. Stereotyped expectations about women's life cycle and the attribution of midlife symptoms to menopause have resulted in the confusion of the experiences of this time of life, such as concerns about aging, family changes, shifts in expectations, and retirement, with the effects of physiological event of cessation of menses. Menopause has been linked with depression and loss, but there is no evidence supporting that this is an inevitable connection. Those women who become depressed in midlife are generally those who have had depressions at other times in their lives.

The peak incidence of depression in women, in fact, is in early adulthood (Weissman, 1991). Estrogen replacement therapy does not address psychiatric problems, and many women have been referred to menopause clinics for treatment of depression or other symptoms whose problems are not related to the menopause itself. Responses to menopause are also strongly influenced by cultural expectations, and in many cultures, women regard the cessation of menses and childbearing with relief.

Hysterectomy has also been considered a procedure that produces a high risk for depression. Here, too, depression is not linked to the procedure. Most of the data supporting the link have not attended to the woman's age, diagnosis (e.g., cancer), the type of procedure performed (e.g., whether it is accompanied by oophorectomy and thus precipitates an abrupt menopause), or other circumstances, such as other events in a woman's life (McKinlay and McKinlay, 1989).

Values and treatment

Personal and societal values affect standards of normality and influence the perception, diagnosis, and treatment of mental disorders and emotional problems (Nadelson and Notman, 1977, 1982b; Person, 1983a). Labeling a behavior as deviant or psychopathological reflects a judgment about normality and affects the way a symptom is understood and whether and how it is treated.

Although there have been changes in how normality, mental illness, and deviancy are conceptualized, evidence suggests that there continue to be differences in what is considered normal for men and women. Broverman et al. (1970) in their classic study, found that when male and female psychotherapists were asked to describe a mentally healthy person, psychological health was more closely associated with descriptions of 'healthy, mature, socially competent' men than with concepts of maturity or mental health in women. In both male and female therapists, standards of what was mentally healthy more closely approximated stereotypical description of the normal male than those of the normal female ('normal' was thus equated with 'like a man').

Although concepts and standards of what is considered 'normal' masculine and feminine behavior have shifted somewhat, these changes in expressed values and attitudes are not necessarily integrated into a cohesive view of normality for either men or women. Even if treaters consciously adopt gender-neutral attitudes, their unconscious views about what is 'normal' may remain unchanged. Those behaviors and attitudes of the patient that are markedly different from the therapist's may be judged as pathological, and this can affect treatment (Nadelson and Notman, 1977).

In all areas of health, values are communicated to patients in both overt and subtle ways in the process of evaluation and referral as well as during treatment (Nadelson and Notman, 1977; Person, 1983a,b). In psychotherapy, therapists communicate values by their selection of material to question or to comment on, by the timing of their interpretations, and by their affective reaction to the content of what is said by the patient. A patient's

life experiences can be viewed differently by male and female therapists, particularly if these experiences are gender specific (Shapiro, 1993). For example, the therapist may emphasize or ignore the patient's references to menstruation, taking drugs, or engaging in risky sexual behavior. On the basis of values a therapist may respond more to the relationship-related problems of women patients and to the work-related concerns of men. By responding this way, the therapist in effect expresses a judgment of what is important and to whom, and consequently may misinterpret the importance of these issues for the patient.

Person (1983a,b) suggested that certain kinds of material are not consciously withheld, but 'overlooked'. Supervisors report that trainees may ignore certain material or interpret behavior as 'regressed' or 'primitive' because the trainees fail to understand the critical importance of a particular life event that may have to do with gender. For example, one senior resident, in presenting couples therapy case to a supervisor, discussed the difficulty the husband was having with his wife's 'regressive' behavior. The resident described the wife as 'borderline'. It was only at the end of the supervisory session that the resident casually reported that the wife was scheduled for a hysterectomy the next day. This particular example raises many questions, such as the following: Would the anxious male patient have communicated his anxiety in a way that is more likely to be recognized by a male therapist? If a male patient were to have a similar response to a prostatectomy, would it have been judged to be 'regressed'? Would a male resident have failed to mention a male patient's surgery in a similar supervisory circumstance?

Gender also affects treatment priorities and approaches. It has been suggested, for example, that concern about some more characteristically male behavior, such as violence related to alcohol abuse, may lead to the development of treatment methods that are more suitable for men. These methods may also be used for women, although there is evidence that they are less effective for women (Reed, 1991; Weisner, 1991). More attention may be paid to treating the adolescent schizophrenic or substance-abusing male, because of the threat of violence, than to treating the seriously handicapped but less-threatening female with posttraumatic stress disorder, depression, or substance abuse.

Women with alcoholism tend to seek specific alcohol-related treatment less often than men, are less likely to seek help from specialized alcohol treatment resources (Greenfield, 2002), and when they do, most treatment approaches are male oriented and do not account for psychological and behavioral factors affecting women that can be barriers to seeking care (Kauffman et al., 1995). For example, treatment programs attempt to dissociate abusers from their drug-using peers, placing women abusers at a disadvantage as they are more likely to live with substance-abusing partners who discourage or prevent them from seeking help, with threats or actual physical and/or sexual abuse. The female partners of male abusers are less likely to be abusers. Most treatment programs also expect total abstinence as part of the treatment plan. This is impossible for most female abusers who continue to live in drug- and alcohol-abusing situations. In addition, treatment approaches use confrontation to get complete disclosure in 12-step programs, a style that is often not comfortable for women. Many groups use aggressive and punitive methods including shouting and verbal assault, which are not as accepted by women who respond better to relational involvement in treatment programs (Comtois and Ries, 1995). Women find women's groups more helpful, and they frequently don't attend mixed sex groups, or they don't participate. As women's substance use occurs more frequently at home and is less public than it is for men, their abuse is often not known by family and friends so they are not encouraged to seek treatment. The fact that women are more likely to be primary caregivers for dependent children and others also makes it less likely that they will come to treatment if they lack childcare or fear losing custody of their children.

Gender also affects diagnosis. If there is a disruption in early life such as a serious illness, a major loss, trauma, or family dysfunction, both sexes may have a greater vulnerability to psychopathology, particularly depression and personality disorders (Adler, 1985; Zanarini et al., 1989). In women, one of the syndromes that has been seen as related to the conflict about autonomy and independence, and the sense of vulnerability to loss, is agoraphobia, which is more commonly diagnosed in women than in men (Symonds, 1971; Bourdon et al., 1988). Although this syndrome may have biological determinants as well, it may represent anxiety about moving out into the world and feeling alone. Depression is more frequently diagnosed in women than in men (Weissman, 1991). In contrast, disturbances involving violent, aggressive behavior, and problems with impulsiveness are more often diagnosed in men (Weissman, 1991), perhaps because of conflicts around intimacy and their socialization toward aggression. These findings raise questions about the factors affecting the process of diagnosis itself, particularly, although not exclusively, with Axis II disorders. Because these disorders more generally reflect clusters of observed personality characteristics rather than specific symptoms, the incidence figures may reflect biases and sex-role stereotypes (Adler et al., 1990; Sprock et al., 1990). It is interesting to note, in this regard, that approximately 75% of those diagnosed with borderline personality disorder are women (Gunderson et al., 1991). Male patients who have the characteristics of borderline personality disorder are often diagnosed as having narcissistic or antisocial personality disorder.

Gender and choice of therapist

Patients give many reasons for their choice of therapist. These reasons are often based on stereotyped views such as that men tend to perpetuate patriarchal values, or that women are more nurturant. It is also true that some patients have no particular preference regarding the therapist's gender and could work equally well with either gender in therapy.

However, if the patient has a preference, for a woman, the choice to be treated by a woman can represent a wish to restore the relationship with her mother or to have a better mother. A desire to see only a male can be based on the desire to avoid this maternal kind of relationship or the anxiety that these feelings arouse, or may reflect anxiety about the intense attachment that may be evoked by a woman (Nadelson and Notman, 1991).

The search for a role model has also been an important determinant of choice of therapist (Person and Ovesey, 1983). Women frequently feel that a woman therapist would be more responsive to their wishes for achievement, success, and self-actualization or that, because she has faced similar conflicts, she could empathize with them more easily. Women may also request to see a woman because they want permission to succeed in certain goals, particularly those involving their work. Permission, explicit or implicit, can result in improvement and can enable the patient to compete and succeed, even if the issues are not taken up specifically and explicitly (Person and Ovesey, 1983). Although this idea may facilitate the development of an alliance it does not, by itself, resolve the patient's difficulties (Notman et al., 1978). Men may search for a role model in a therapist for different reasons, such as a wish to learn how to be a good father, because for many men there have been more role models for achievement and success outside of the family rather than inside (Pollack et al., 1998).

Identification with a therapist is also important. Although the reasons for the choice may be based on stereotypes, without regard for the characteristics of the specific therapist, the patient's feeling of greater comfort or empathy can facilitate the initial development of a positive therapeutic alliance.

More recently, concerns about sexualization and sexual relationships in treatment have become important factors in requests based on gender. For those patients who have actually been abused in a previous treatment, trust can be severely damaged. It may be particularly difficult for such patients to see anyone who serves as a reminder of the previous experience. Women therapists are often asked to see women patients who have had sexual involvements with male therapists (Person and Ovesey, 1983). Although it does occur, women are less likely to become sexually involved with their patients, either male or female, than are men (Holroyd and Brodsky, 1977; Gartrell et al., 1986; Gabbard, 1989).

Sexual orientation has also become a consideration. Many gay individuals request treatment from gays, who they feel will not only better understand and empathize with them, but be less likely to judge their sexual object choice as pathological (Krajeski, 1984). Although there has been controversy about the appropriateness of this disclosure, some therapists have indicated that disclosure of their sexual orientation to patients may be beneficial in therapy (Gartrell, 1984; Isay, 1989).

Choosing a therapist of a particular gender with the expectation that this will resolve the patient's problems can also be a resistance to therapy. A woman may want to see a woman for treatment because she feels unlovable and unattractive to men and can, in this way, avoid the experience of confronting her feelings (Thompson, 1938). A woman may seek a woman therapist initially because she wants support, and later devalue the therapist or find herself in an angry, competitive interaction, which can be a repetition of her relationship with her mother (Notman et al., 1978). She may be unaware of the origins of her feelings or the reasons for her choice of therapist. Although there are conscious reasons for choices, unconscious factors or needs such as fear of anger or a search for mothering may be important and should be considered in the initial encounter with a patient.

Not only do some patients make gender a priority in choosing a therapist, but some therapists also make gender-based recommendations regarding the choice of a therapist. For example, because some women victims of sexual abuse find it difficult to work with men, some clinicians suggest that they should be treated by women. Others believe that adolescents should be treated by someone of the same sex because sexual issues are so pressing, embarrassing, and intrusive at this life stage that they can interfere with therapeutic progress. Many support the view that women should be treated by women in order to avoid being misunderstood or treated from a male-oriented perspective. This may oversimplify the effects of gender and minimize the necessary working through of ambivalence and conflict in the therapeutic relationship.

Stereotypes and expectations about women affect male patients as well. A man may seek treatment from a woman in order to avoid a competitive or authoritarian relationship with a man, to avoid homosexual feelings, or because he has had poor relationships with women in the past and wants to work these out with a woman. His expectations may be that a woman will provide the cure for his problems with intimacy.

Some women may choose a male therapist who may not focus on or confront certain problems in an effort to avoid being labeled as sexist. These therapists have described feeling intimidated by the successful women who are their patients. They may not feel free to raise questions about the motivation or specific behavior of such a patient, fearing accusations about being sexist or unsympathetic. Some women avoid female therapists who they fear might confront them more directly about this behavior.

The therapeutic process

Understanding the concept of transference can clarify aspects of the therapist–patient relationship that may otherwise be difficult to comprehend. A patient brings attitudes and feelings to the relationship from past experiences with important figures, such as parents, which may be problematic and need to be addressed in therapy. For example, the patient may bring the need to please or to gain love by acquiescence or seductive behavior into the therapist–patient relationship. If not recognized as transference, the clinician may see this as a genuine reaction to the therapist rather than a pattern of response to someone in authority carried over from past relationships.

The classical conceptualization of transference assumed that both maternal or paternal transference could be developed toward both male and female therapists. Thus, the therapist's gender was not a particularly salient consideration. Freud came to believe that transference responses to a male analyst differed from those to a female analyst (Freud, 1931/1961). Subsequently, Horney emphasized the importance of the competitive transference with the same-sex analyst, and Greenacre stated that strong wishes regarding the choice of analyst with regard to gender should be respected, but also carefully analyzed because prior wishes, expectations, and fantasies could affect not only the choice but the course of the analytic process (Greenacre, 1959; Horney, 1967). Zetzel (1970) indicated that transference repeats the patient's actual identification with the parent of his or her own sex, and the wish for love from the parent of the other sex. Kernberg (1998) indicated that the therapist can 'collude' with the culture to reinforce gender stereotypes. For example, a narcissistic male patient with a female analyst may develop an intense erotization of the relationship to avoid feeling dependent and to destroy the analyst's authority, thereby preserving for the patient the conventional relationship of dominant male and subservient female.

One study evaluated the development of transference in 47 cases of same-gender and cross-gender therapist/patient dyads in psychoanalytic psychotherapy. Each therapist was interviewed about two of their cases at 4- and 6-month intervals over a 2-year period. Two judges, a male and a female, rated each of the interviews on the emergence of transference paradigms, such as maternal/paternal relationship themes. The authors found that patients have a strong inclination to develop an initial transference consistent with the therapist's gender, and in opposite-gender dyads, therapists, especially female therapists, have a strong bias against perceiving themselves in the opposite-gender role. In addition, the more experienced therapists were more likely to report opposite-gender transference. The current psychoanalytic view is that the person of the therapist is important and that therapy is affected by real characteristics of the therapist, the patient, and the transference (Gruenthal, 1993).

Therapists often do not attend sufficiently to the transference issues that encourage or inhibit discussion of particular material. This insufficient attention may be based on a number of factors, including gender. It can be seen at any phase in a therapeutic interaction and can occur with any patient or in any treatment modality. Many women feel that it is more difficult for a man to empathize with some issues that are gender specific; this may also be true for women who must empathize with male issues (Horner, 1992).

Women report that they do not tell male therapists details of menstrual-related symptoms or even discuss concerns about hysterectomy or past histories of abortion or miscarriage. These 'censorships' create the potential for inappropriate treatment.

The persistence of conventional sex-stereotyped attitudes and behaviors can be seen clinically. A male therapist who accepts the traditional male gender role may experience strong negative countertransference to a male patient who freely expresses emotion (Wisch and Mahlik, 1999). The concerns of a woman who decides to have children late in life or is ambivalent about childbearing, or those of the man, who wants custody of his young children, are still often not appreciated. Therapists treating women may see themselves as advocates for a woman's right to have both family and career and may not fully acknowledge their patients' conflicts about balancing the two. The woman executive who wants to have a baby but has recently undertaken a very demanding job may need to explore why she chose to make that commitment at the time she did, just as a woman of 40 with an established career who suddenly decides to have a baby and feels she must give up her career would do well to understand this behavior. Both women may be acting defensively as well as making positive choices.

MB was 40. Her two children were in high school. She had worked as a librarian before they were born and recently had taken some computer courses to update her library skills. She was hoping to get a job as a librarian for a high-level medical department but was worried that the responsibility of the role would be beyond her recently acquired skills. Her male therapist enthusiastically supported her return to work and the career opportunities it offered. This seemed both unusual and helpful to MB. It had seemed not politically correct to talk about her ambivalence. As she was preparing to start her new job she discovered she was pregnant. Although this did not mean she could not work, it represented an unconscious return to a safer role.

Changing therapists

Change or reassignment of a therapist on the basis of gender has been widely discussed and is often recommended. Some have suggested that a change of therapist might mobilize a stalemated situation. Transfers on the basis of the therapist's gender have also been made when there is a therapeutic impasse or failure.

A hospital nurse had become depressed after her supervisor left the hospital. She had had unacknowledged but intense feelings of affection and dependency about this supervisor. She went into therapy with a woman psychiatrist who was supportive. A gesture of handing the nurse a Kleenex was perceived as reaching out to her and evoked strong feelings and a maternal transference. Her depression lifted, and she began to make career plans for further schooling elsewhere. However, she found it difficult to leave, in particular to end the therapy, because of her dependence and anxiety at separation. It seemed like an impasse. The therapist referred the patient to a supportive male therapist. That relationship was less intense, and stirred up a less dependent transference. She was able to negotiate the termination and went on to school.

This is an example of a situation where the gender of the therapist made a difference.

Unless there has been a sexual interaction, however, it is rare that gender itself is the significant variable in the majority of cases that are not successful. A transfer based on gender may be a way of avoiding responsibility for failure or dealing with the embarrassment of negative outcome. Because gender affects trust, and even compliance, in other modes of treatment, as well as in psychotherapy, change in the treater based on gender might be helpful in some situations.

Gender choice in couples and family therapy

As with other forms of therapy, gender may be a consideration in the choice of a therapist for couples or families. This issue is frequently dealt with by having couples and family therapy performed by male–female therapist dyads. In general, as with individual therapy, issues related to gender choice should be clarified and addressed. A couple with marital difficulties may request a female therapist because it is the wife who has made the call and it is her preference, perhaps because she feels intimidated by men or because she fears that she could be left out of the male dyad if the therapist were male. On the other hand, the husband may choose a woman or comply with his wife's choice of a female therapist because he is more comfortable and less threatened by women, because he does not take the therapy seriously, or because he has negative feelings about women. The choice of a male therapist for some couples may re-create, in the transference, a paternal or authoritarian relationship or even the fantasy of possible sexual abuse. This can be a special problem if abuse has actually occurred.

During the course of therapy, attention must be paid to bias regardless of whether the therapist is male or female. Transference issues in couples and family therapy are multiple and more complex because there are more people directly involved in the therapy. For example, each partner, and the couple as a unit, will have different transference reactions to the therapist and to each other. If there are additional family members involved, they, too, will add to the transference complexity.

Changes in family patterns have also presented an increasing array of challenging issues for therapy. For example, the stress and demands of dual-career or commuting families, especially those with two achievement-oriented partners, can create enormous tension. This may be a greater source of conflict if the wife is earning more money, or if there is a job offer for either partner in another city. Because the husband's work has traditionally been the motivating factor in a relocation, a wife's job offer can create tensions, especially involving competition. A wife who achieves success later in life can be on a different timetable than her husband, who may wish to retire earlier.

The therapist can be influenced by his or her attitudes and values about divorce, marriage, and custody. The increasing divorce and remarriage rates have brought a larger number of so-called reconstituted or recombined families. The members of these families often experience divided and conflicted loyalties between their family of origin and their new family. There are also unexpected pressures related to childbearing at different phases of the life cycle with many of these relationships. For example, a woman in her late 30s without children may marry a man in his 50s with grown children, and the couple may be in conflict about having additional children. Although they may have previously agreed that this was not an option, the wife, who is younger, may change her mind, and marital problems ensue.

As men gain permission for expression of their dependent needs and wishes for nurturance, they experience conflicts that are not dissimilar from those that women have traditionally encountered. For instance, a few men now take paternity leave, but risk their careers as most employers see such men as less committed to their careers and therefore less worthy of promotion. The man caught in an unsatisfying and even destructive marriage may find himself torn between a new and gratifying relationship and the potential loss of the intimacy and experience of his children's growth if he leaves his family. The alternatives are to remain in the marriage, leave and attempt to gain custody, or work out joint arrangements.

Feminist critiques of family therapy express concerns about the structural/hierarchical dominant role of males in the family, mother blaming, assumptions about sharing power and responsibility embedded in systemic concepts, and assumptions about therapist neutrality (Nutt, 1992; Stabb *et al.*, 1997). Family therapy has recently been criticized for biased treatment of men—for example, for reinforcing the socialized limitations of male roles (Stabb *et al.*, 1997).

Group therapy

As with couples and family therapy, there are gender issues in group therapy. When group therapy is sought or recommended, the gender of the group therapist is not frequently considered, although the gender composition of the group often becomes an important factor. There are some data suggesting that group behavior both between group members and with the leader is affected by gender (Mayes, 1979; Bass, 1990; Forsyth *et al.*, 1997). McNab (1990) reported that men set themselves apart to a greater extent than women at the start of group therapy and become integrated into the group later.

Women often seek women's groups because in groups of men or even in mixed groups they feel powerless, intimidated, and uncomfortable about speaking up. One need only look at classrooms, professional meetings, and business groups to recognize that women speak less often than men, and when they do speak, their comments are more often ignored or attributed to others. Women report the same experiences, regardless of professional status or income (Nadelson, 1987). They may feel supported and less anxious in same-sex groups, although mixed groups may be helpful in confronting these problems of professional development. Most often single-sex groups have been used for support and consciousness-raising. Both male and female self-help groups often form around a specific focus (e.g., substance abuse, divorce, family violence) and use problem-solving approaches.

Therapy groups with both male and female leaders permit men and women to deal with transference issues, both as peers and as leaders. It is important, however, that the leaders' relationship with each other, just as with male and female therapists in family therapy, be a facilitating rather than inhibitory factor. Mistrust, competition, and anger that are not addressed in either leader or group members can be unproductive and inhibitory to group process.

Psychotherapy treatments and outcome

There are abundant data indicating that women have a greater incidence of some mental disorders and men of others. A 1991 report from the US Institute of Medicine cited gender differences that have been replicated (Weissmann, 1991; Kessler *et al.*, 1994). A summary of current epidemiology on gender differences can be seen in Table 34.1.

Table 34.1 Gender differences in lifetime prevalence of psychiatric disorders (Burt and Hendrick, 2001)

Disorder	Prevalence in %		Reference
	Women	Men	
Depression	21.3	12.7	Kessler *et al.* (1994)
Dysthmia	8.0	4.8	Kessler *et al.* (1994)
Bipolar disorder			
bipolar 1	0.9	0.7	Weissman *et al.* (1991)
bipolar 2	0.5	0.4	
Seasonal affective disorder	6.3	1.0	Rosenthal *et al.* (1984)
Panic disorder	5.0	2.0	Kessler *et al.* (1994)
Social phobia	15.5	11.1	Kessler *et al.* (1994)
Generalized anxiety disorder	6.6	3.6	Kessler *et al.* (1994)
Schizophrenia	1.7	1.2	Weissman *et al.* (1991)
Anorexia nervosa	0.5	0.05	Walter and Kendler (1995) Garfinkel (1995)
Bulimia	1.1	0.1	Garfinkel *et al.* (1995)
Alcohol dependence	8.2	20.1	Kessler *et al.* (1994)
Alcohol abuse without dependence	6.4	12.5	Kessler *et al.* (1994)
Drug dependence	5.9	9.2	Weissman *et al.* (1991)
Drug abuse without dependence	3.5	5.4	Weissman *et al.* (1991)
Antisocial personality	1.2	5.8	Kessler *et al.* (1994)

In terms of treatment, most of the early research on treatment outcome did not consider gender as a salient variable. This is beginning to change, particularly in the biological areas of psychiatry.

In the psychotherapy literature, while there is increasing emphasis on outcome, gender has not been well studied. The analysis and interpretation of outcome data considering gender and psychotherapy, as with any outcome data, require consideration of a number of variables, including therapist/patient selection mechanisms and match, type of treatment, treatment goals, therapeutic process, length of treatment, measured and perceived therapeutic outcome, and patient satisfaction.

Most of the data on gender and therapeutic outcome have come from short-term types of treatment. Investigators in these studies have attempted to use easily controllable treatment techniques and protocols and to include patients with specific diagnoses, and they have assessed specific outcomes that are often behavioral, such as a decrease in alcohol intake or impulsive behavior, or measurable with specific objective criteria, such as depression or anxiety scales. Because affective and intrapsychic processes have been less amenable to the kinds of measures traditionally employed, there are many fewer studies of long-term psychotherapy and psychoanalysis.

Cavenar and Werman (1983) in their early critique of studies of psychotherapy outcome emphasized the importance of specifying the treatment approach. They indicated that the gender of the therapist may be more relevant in modalities such as supportive psychotherapy, in which identification with the therapist and restoration of defenses are more critical. With insight-oriented psychotherapy, the goal of self-understanding and the difference in process may change the way interpretations are made and perceptions evolve.

Mogul (1982) suggested that therapist sex matters least in traditional psychoanalysis. The issue, however, may have more to do with the alliance and the transference than the modality or the diagnosis (Gruenthal, 1993; Kernberg, 1993; Shapiro, 1993). Person (1983a) suggested that gender effects are more subtle in psychoanalysis than in psychotherapy but may be just as pervasive.

The popular belief is that women patients do better in therapy with women therapists because women therapists are more relational, empathic, and less likely to disempower women patients. There is empirical evidence on both sides of the efficacy argument for a gender effect in treatment, with most studies concluding that there is none (Zlotnick et al., 1998; Huppert et al., 2001). There are, however, no data from naturalistic studies.

One controlled study (Zlotnick et al., 1996) on the effect of gender on short-term treatment of depressed patients found no effect on level of depression at termination, attrition rates, or patient's perception of the therapists' degree of empathy early in treatment and at termination. Likewise, patients' beliefs that a male or female therapist would be more helpful, and their match or mismatch in the study protocol, were not significantly associated with the measures of treatment process or outcome employed. Gender did not interact with therapist level of experience. It is possible that a patient's perception of a specific therapist is influenced not by gender stereotypes but rather by the patient's experience with the specific person.

Studies conducted two decades ago reported little outcome difference by gender of patient or therapist for short-term psychotherapy (Abramowitz et al., 1976; Orlinsky and Howard, 1976; Gurri, 1977; Blasé, 1979; Goldenholz, 1979; Malloy, 1979). Kirshner et al. (1978) studied a large number of therapist–patient matches in short-term individual psychotherapy and found that female patients showed greater responsiveness to psychotherapy and that greater patient satisfaction and self-rated improvement occurred with female therapists. More improvement was seen in attitudes toward careers, academic motivation, academic performance, and family relations. At the same time, however, these researchers also reported that the female patients of female therapists were less likely to describe their therapists as competent than were the patients of other gender dyads. When therapist experience and gender were considered, more experienced therapists seemed to have had better therapeutic results and showed fewer gender effects than did less experienced therapists, regardless of sex.

Other controlled studies of short-term psychotherapy have reported that female therapists formed a more effective therapeutic alliance than did male therapists (Jones and Zoppel, 1982) and that patients treated by female therapists reported more symptomatic improvement (Jones et al., 1987). However, these differences may be attributable to methodologic differences and outcome measures. In the study reporting a gender difference in symptoms (Jones et al., 1987), male therapists saw recently bereaved women who had lost a husband or father. Thus, the reported effects may have been related to the specific circumstances in which the symptoms originated or to the effect of seeing a male therapist as a possible replacement for the lost husband or father. Some studies used self-reports; others manualized treatment (Zlotnick et al., 1998). Given the rigid training and protocols used in these studies, naturalistic responses or differences in attitudes and behaviors might not emerge.

Gender also may affect treatment selection. Women, because of life cycle events such as pregnancy, may want to avoid psychopharmacological treatments altogether and yet be in need of acute effective treatment for depression and anxiety. Cognitive-behavioral psychotherapy and interpersonal psychotherapy are both short-term, focused psychotherapies found to be effective in controlled, clinical trials for the treatment of depressive and anxiety disorders and are useful modalities for the pregnant or postpartum patient who wishes to breastfeed (Beck et al., 1979; Klerman et al., 1984; Frank et al., 1993; Stuart and O'Hara, 1995; Spinelli, 2001). A recent study suggests that men and women may benefit from different modalities (Ogrodniczuk et al., 2001). Men responded more to interpretive therapy while women's symptoms responded to supportive psychotherapy. The authors suggest that the two different psychotherapies facilitated trust and a willingness to work: for men, on introspection and the examination of uncomfortable emotions, and for women, on problem solving within a more collaborative and personal relationship.

With regard to referral trends, much of the literature derives from methodologically problematic studies that are now dated. More current work continues to suggest, however, that males are more likely to be referred to a male therapist and that female therapists get fewer referrals of male patients (Mayer and deMarneffe, 1992). This finding implies that gender stereotypes continue to operate.

Other studies of gender differences focus on additional variables. For example, one study (Thase et al., 1994) reported that patients with higher pretreatment levels of depressive symptoms, especially women, had poorer outcomes. Another investigation (Frank et al., 1993) reported that among patients with recurrent depression, men demonstrated a more rapid response to treatment than did women. Still other research indicates that posttreatment outcomes are similar for men and women, that male and female patients suffering from major depression had generally similar outcomes over time-limited courses of cognitive-behavioral therapy (Sotsky et al., 1991; Thase et al., 1996), and that men and women have similar responses to different treatment modalities (Ogrodniczuk et al., 2001). Samstag et al. (1998) reported that the women in their sample were more likely to have either good overall outcome or to drop out of therapy, whereas the men were more likely to remain regardless of outcome. They suggest that this is consistent with reports in the literature indicating that women attend more to relational cues (Gilligan, 1982; Gilligan et al., 1991). A further analysis of their data suggested that the subjective meaning of the alliance seemed to be the most critical factor. These data certainly suggest that more study is needed on gender effects.

Psychotherapy research has more often used female patients, and as noted above, frequently does not consider other salient variables (e.g. age, race). There are also differences of opinion about the importance of therapist experience, with some studies showing that experience is an important variable and that it interacts with gender. Thus, the gender of a less experienced therapist may have a more negative impact on outcome than the gender of a more experienced therapist. There are data suggesting that less experienced female therapists do better with women than less experienced male therapists. The theoretical orientation of a therapist may also be important. For example, some data indicate that therapists who are most effective tend to embrace a psychological orientation and eschew biological treatments but that therapy (especially for depression) is longer with these psychologically oriented therapists (Blatt et al., 1996). Some studies reveal that both men and women prefer therapists of their own gender (Simons and Helms, 1976).

Conclusions

It is apparent that gender is an important treatment variable and that attention to gender effects together with better understanding of the complex interaction of gender and other variables will shed light on the therapeutic process and contribute to greater therapeutic effectiveness.

References

Abramowitz, S., et al. (1976). Sex bias in psychotherapy: a failure to confirm. American Journal of Psychiatry, 133, 706–9.

Adler, D. A., Drake, R. E., and Teague, G. B. (1990). Clinician's practices in personality assessment: does gender influence the use of DSM-III axis II? Comprehensive Psychiatry, 31(2), 125–33.

Adler, G. (1985). Borderline psychopathology and its treatment. New York: Jason Aronson.

American Psychiatric Association. (1987). Diagnostic and mental disorder, 3rd edn (revised). Washington, DC: American Psychiatric Association.

Bass, A. (1990). Studies find workplace still a man's world. Boston Globe, March 12, 39.

Baxter, L. R. Jr, et al. (1992). Caudate glucose metabolic rate changes with both drug and behavior therapy for obsessive-compulsive disorder. Archives of General Psychiatry, 49, 681–9.

Beck, A. T., Rush, A. J., Shaw, B. F., and Emery, G. (1979). Cognitive therapy of depression. New York: Guilford Press.

Blasé, J. (1979). A study on the effects of sex of the client and sex of the therapist on client's satisfaction with psychotherapy. Dissertation Abstracts International, 49, 6107-B.

Blatt, S. J., *et al.* (1996). Characteristics of effective therapists: further analyses of data from the National Institute of Mental Health Treatment of Depression Collaborative Research Program. *Journal of Consulting and Clinical Psychology*, **64**, 1276–84.

Bourdon, K., Bloyd, J., Rae, D., Burns, B., Thompson, J., and Locker, B. (1988). Gender differences in phobias: results of the ECA community survey. *Journal of Anxiety Disorders*, **2**, 227–41.

Brody, A. L., *et al.* (2001). Regional brain metabolic changes in-patients with major depression treated with either paroxetine or interpersonal therapy. *Archives of General Psychiatry*, **58**, 631–40.

Broverman, I., *et al.* (1970). Sex role stereotypes and clinical judgments of mental health. *Journal of Consulting and Clinical Psychology*, **34**, 1–7.

Burt, V. K. and Hendrick, V. C. (2001). *Concise guide to women's mental health*, 2nd edn. Washington, DC: American Psychiatric Publishing.

Carmen, E., Reiker, P., and Mills, T. (1984). Victims of violence and psychiatric illness. *American Journal of Psychiatry*, **141**, 378–9.

Cavenar, J. J. and Werman, D. (1983). The sex of the psychotherapist. *American Journal of Psychiatry*, **140**, 85–7.

Chodorow, N. (1978). *The reproduction of mothering: psychoanalysis and the sociology of gender*. Berkeley, CA: University of California Press.

Comtois, K. A. and Ries, R. K. (1995). Sex differences in dually diagnosed severely mentally ill clients in dual diagnosis outpatient treatment. *American Journal of Addiction*, **4**, 425–53.

Cyranowski, J. M., *et al.* (2000). Adolescent onset of the gender differences in lifetime rates of major depression: a theoretical model. *Archives of General Psychiatry*, **57**, 21–7.

Eisenberg, L. (1995). The social construction of the human brain. *American Journal of Psychiatry*, **152**, 1563–75.

Forsyth, D. R., Heiney, M. M., and Wright, S. S. (1997). Biases in appraisals of women leaders. *Group Dynamics: Theory, Research, & Practice*, **1**, 98–103.

Frank, E., Kupfer, D. J., Cornes, C., and Morris, S. M. (1993). Maintenance interpersonal psychotherapy for recurrent depression. In: G. L. Klerman and M. M. Weissman, ed. *New applications of interpersonal psychotherapy*, pp. 97–9. Washington, DC: American Psychiatric Press.

Freud, S. (1931/1961). Female sexuality. In: J. Strachey, trans. and ed. *The standard edition of the complete psychological works of Sigmund Freud*, Vol. 21, pp. 221–43. London: Hogarth Press.

Gabbard, G. O. (1989). *Sexual exploitation in professional relationships*. Washington, DC: American Psychiatric Press.

Garfinkel, P. E. (1995). Eating disorders. In: H. I. Kaplan and B. J. Saddock, ed. *Comprehensive textbook of psychiatry*, 6th edn, p. 1364. Baltimore, MD: Williams & Wilkins.

Garfinkel, P. E., *et al.* (1995). Bulimia nervosa in a Canadian community sample: prevalence and comparisons of subgroups. *American Journal of Psychiatry*, **152**, 1052–8.

Gartrell, N. (1984). Issues in psychotherapy with lesbian women. In: *Work in progress*, 83–04. Wellesley, MA: Stone Center for Developmental Services and Studies, Wellesley College.

Gartrell, H., *et al.* (1986). Psychiatrist-patient sexual contact: results of a national survey, I: revalence. *American Journal of Psychiatry*, **143**, 1126–31.

Gilligan, C. (1987). Adolescent development reconsidered. In: C. Irwin, ed. *New directions for child development: Adolescent social behavior and health*, pp. 63–92. San Francisco: Jossey-Bass.

Glasser, M., *et al.* (2001). Cycle of child sexual abuse: links between being a victim and becoming a perpetrator. *British Journal of Psychiatry*, **179**, 482–94.

Goldenholz, N. (1979). The effect of the sex of therapist-client dyad upon outcome of psychotherapy (Abstract). *Dissertation Abstracts International*, **40**, 492B.

Greenacre, P. (1959). Certain technical problems in the transference relationship. *Journal of the American Psychoanalysis Association*, **7**, 484–502.

Greenfield, S. (2002). Women and alcohol use disorders. *Harvard Review of Psychiatry*, **10**, 76–85.

Gruenthal, R. (1993). The patient's transference of the analyst's gender: projection, factuality, interpretation, or construction. *Psychoanalytic Dialogues*, **3**, 323–41.

Gunderson, J., Zanarini, M., and Kisiel, C. (1991). Borderline personality disorder: a review of data on DSM-III-R descriptions. *Journal of Personality Disorders*, **5**, 340–52.

Gurri, I. (1977). The influence of therapist sex, client sex, and client sex bias on therapy outcome (abstract). *Dissertation Abstracts International*, **38**, 898–9B.

Hines, M. and Green, R. (1991). Human hormonal and neural correlates of sex-typed behaviors. In: *Review of Psychiatry*, pp. 536–55. Washington, DC: American Psychiatric Press Inc.

Holroyd, J. and Brodsky, A. (1977). Psychologist's attitudes and practices regarding erotic and nonerotic physical contact with patients. *American Journal of Psychology*, **32**, 843–9.

Horner, A. (1992). The role of the female therapist in the affirmation of gender in male patients. *Journal of the American Academy of Psychoanalysis*, **20**, 599–610.

Horney, K. (1967). *Feminine psychology*. H. Kelman, ed. New York: Norton.

Hull, A. M. (2002). Neuroimaging findings in post-traumatic stress disorder: systematic review. *British Journal of Psychiatry*, **181**, 102–10.

Huppert, J. D., *et al.* (2001). Therapists, therapist variables, and cognitive-behavioral therapy outcome in a multi-center trial for panic disorder. *Journal of Consulting and Clinical Psychology*, **69**, 747–55.

Isay, R. A. (1989). *Being homosexual: gay men and their development*. New York: Farrar, Straus, Giroux.

Jaffe, P., *et al.* (1986). Family violence and child adjustment: a comparative analysis of girls' and boys' behavioral symptoms. *American Journal of Psychiatry*, **143**, 74–7.

Janowsky, D. S., Halbreich, U., and Rausch, J. (1996). Association among ovarian hormones, other hormones, emotional disorders, and neurotransmitters. In: M. F. Jensvold, U. Halbreich, and J. A. Hamilton, ed. *Psychopharmacology and Women: Sex, Gender and Hormones*, pp. 85–106. Washington, DC, American Psychiatric Press, Inc.

Jones, E. E. and Zoppel, C. (1982). Impact of client and therapist gender on psychotherapy process and outcome. *Journal of Consulting and Clinical Psychology*, **50**, 259–72.

Jones, E. E., *et al.* (1987). Some gender effects in a brief psychotherapy. *Psychotherapy*, **24**, 336–52.

Kandel, E. R. (1999). Biology and the future of psychoanalysis: a new intellectual framework for psychiatry revisited. *American Journal of Psychiatry*, **156**, 505–24.

Kauffman, E., Dore, M. M., and Nelson-Zlupko, L. (1995). The role of women's therapy groups in the treatment of chemical dependence. *American Journal of Orthopsychiatry*, **65**, 335–63.

Kernberg, O. (1998). The influence of the gender of patient and analyst in the psychoanalytic relationship. *Journal of the American Psychoanalytic Association*, **48**, 859–83.

Kessler, R. C., *et al.* (1994). Lifetime and 12-month prevalence of DSM-III-R psychiatric disorders in the United States: results from the National Comorbidity Survey. *Archives of General Psychiatry*, **51**, 8–19.

Kirshner, L., Genack, A., and Hauser, S. (1978). Effects of gender on short-term psychotherapy. *Psychotherapy Theory, Research and Practice*, **15**, 158–67.

Kleeman, J. (1976). Freud's views on early female sexuality in the light of direct child observation. *Journal of the American Psychoanalytic Association*, **24**, 3–27.

Klerman, G. L., Weissman, M. M., Rounsaville, B. J., and Chevron, E. (1984). *Interpersonal psychotherapy for depression*. New York: Basic Books.

van der Kolk, B. A. (1989). The compulsion to repeat the trauma: re-enactment, revictimization, and masochism. *Psychiatric Clinics of North America*, **12**(2), 389–411.

Krajeski, J. (1984). Psychotherapy with gay and lesbian patients. In: E. Hetrick and T. Stein, ed. *Innovations in psychotherapy with homosexuals*, pp. 75–88. Washington, DC: American Psychiatric Press.

LeVine, R. A. (1991). Gender differences: interpreting anthropological data. In: M. T. Notman and C. C. Nadelson, ed. *Women and men: new perspectives on gender difference*, pp. 1–8. Washington, DC: American Psychiatric Press Inc.

Malloy, T. (1979). The relationship between therapist-client interpersonal compatibility, sex of therapist, and psychotherapeutic outcome (Abstract). *Dissertation Abstracts International*, **40**, 456B.

Martin, S. D., *et al.* (2001). Brain blood flow changes in depressed patients treated with interpersonal psychotherapy or venlafaxine hydrochloride. *Archives of General Psychiatry*, **58**, 641–48.

Mayer, E. L. and deMarneffe, D. (1992). When theory and practice diverge: gender-related patterns of referral to psychoanalysts. *Journal of the American Psychoanalytic Association*, **40**(2), 531–85.

Mayes, S. (1979). Women in positions of authority: a case study of changing sex roles. *Signs*, **4**, 556–68.

McKinley, S. M. and McKinlay, J. B. (1989). The impact of menopause and social factors on health. In: B. Hammond, F. Hazeltine, and I. Schiff, ed. *Menopause: evaluation, treatment and health concerns*. New York: A. R. Liss.

McNab, T. (1990). What do men want? Male rituals of initiation in group psychotherapy. *International Journal of Group Psychotherapy*, **40**, 139–54.

Miller, J. B., Nadelson, C. C., Notman, M. T., and Zilbach, J. (1981). Aggression in women: a reexamination. In: S. Klebanow, ed. *Changing concepts in psychoanalysis*, pp. 157–67. New York: Gardner Press.

Mogul, K. (1982). Overview the sex of the therapist. *American Journal of Psychiatry*, **139**, 1–11.

Money, J. and Ehrhardt, A. A. (1972). *Man and woman, boy and girl: the differentiation and dimorphism of gender identity from concept to maturity*. Baltimore, MD: Johns Hopkins University Press.

Nadelson, C. C. (1989a). Issues in the analysis of single women in their thirties and forties. In: R. Liebert and J. Oldham, ed. *The middle years*, pp. 105–221. New Haven, CT: Yale University Press.

Nadelson, C. C. (1989b). Women in leadership roles: development and challenges. In: S. Feinstein, ed. *Adolescent psychiatry*, Vol. 14, pp. 28–41. Chicago, IL: The University of Chicago Press.

Nadelson, C. C. and Notman, M. T. (1977). Psychotherapy supervision: the problem of conflicting values. *American Journal of Psychotherapy*, **31**, 275–83.

Nadelson, C. C. and Notman, M. T. (1982a). To marry or not to marry. In: C. Nadelson and M. Notman, ed. *The woman patient*, Vol. 2, pp. 111–20. New York: Plenum Press.

Nadelson, C. C. and Notman, M. T. (1982b). Social change and psychotherapeutic implications. In: C. Nadelson and M. Notman, ed. *The woman patient*, Vol. 3, pp. 3–16. New York: Plenum Press.

Nadelson, C. C. and Notman, M. T. (1991). The impact on psychotherapy of the new psychology of men and women. In: A. Tasman, ed. *The American Psychiatric Press review of psychiatry*, Vol. 10, pp. 608–26. Washington, DC: American Psychiatric Press.

Nadelson, C. C., Notman, M. T., Baker-Miller, J., and Zilbach, J. (1982). Aggression in women: conceptual issues and clinical impressions. In: M. T. Notman and C. C. Nadelson, ed. *The woman patient*, Vol. 3, pp. 17–28. New York: Plenum Press.

Notman, M. T. and Lester, E. P. (1988). Pregnancy theoretical considerations. *Psychoanalytic Inquiry*, **8**(2), 139–59.

Notman, M. T., Nadelson, C. C., and Bennett, M. (1978). Achievement conflict in women: psychotherapeutic considerations. *Psychotherapy and Psychosomatic*, **29**, 203–13.

Notman, M. T., Klein, R., Jordan, J. V., and Zilbach, J. J. (1991). Women's unique developmental issues across the life cycle. In: A. Tasman and S. M. Goldfinger, ed. *American Psychiatric Press review of psychiatry*, pp. 556–77. Washington, DC: American Psychiatric Press Inc.

Nutt, R. L. (1992). Feminist family therapy: a review of the literature. *Topics in Family Psychological Counseling*, **1**, 13–23.

Ogrodniczuk, J. S., Piper, W. E., Joyce, A. S., and McCallum, M. (2001). Effect of patient gender on outcome in two forms of short-term individual psychotherapy. *Journal of Psychotherapy Practice and Research*, **10**, 69–78.

O'Hara, M. W. (1995). *Postpartum depression: causes and consequences*, pp. 1–13. New York: Springer-Verlag, Inc.

Orlinsky, D. and Howard, K. (1976). The effects of sex of therapist on the therapeutic experiences of women. *Psychotherapy: Theory, Research and Practice*, **13**, 82–8.

Perry, J. C. and Herman, J. L. (1993). Trauma and defense in the etiology of borderline personality disorder. In: J. Paris, ed. *Borderline personality disorder: etiology and treatment*, pp. 123–40. Washington, DC: American Psychiatric Press Inc.

Person, E. (1983a). Women in therapy: therapist's gender as a variable. *International Review of Psycho-Analysis*, **10**, 193–204.

Person, E. (1983b). The influence of values in psychoanalysis: the case of female psychology. In: L. Grinspoon, ed. *Psychiatry update: the American Psychiatric Association annual review*, Vol. 2, pp. 36–49. Washington, DC: American Psychiatric Press.

Person, E. and Ovesey, L. (1983). Psychoanalytic theories of gender and identity. *Journal of the American Academy of Psychoanalysis*, **22**(2), 103–226.

Pollack, W. S. and Levant, R. F. (1998). *New Psychotherapy for Men*. New York: John Wiley & Sons.

Raine, R., Goldfrad, C., Rowan, K., and Black, N. (2002). Influence of patient gender on admission to intensive care. *Journal of Epidemiology and Community Health*, **56**, 418–23.

Reed, B. G. (1991). Services research and drug-involved women: concepts, questions, and options. In: *Assessing future research needs mental and addictive disorders in women*, pp. 91–7. Washington, DC: Institute of Medicine.

Rogers, C. M. and Ritter, J. M. (2002). The power of perception: children's appearance as a factor in adults' predictions of gender-typical behavior. *Social Development*, **11**, 409–26.

Rosenthal, N. E., *et al.* (1984). Seasonal affective disorder: a description of the syndrome and preliminary findings with light therapy. *Archives of General Psychiatry*, **41**, 72–80.

Samstag, L. W., *et al.* (1998). Early identification of treatment failures in short-term psychotherapy: an assessment of therapeutic alliance and interpersonal behavior. *Journal of Psychotherapy Practice and Research*, **7**, 126–39.

Schwartz, J. M., *et al.* (1996). Systematic changes in cerebral glucose metabolic rate after successful behavior modification treatment of obsessive-compulsive disorder. *Archives of General Psychiatry*, **53**, 109–13.

Shapiro, S. (1993). Gender-role stereotypes and clinical process: commentary on papers by Gruenthal and Hirsch. *Psychoanalytic Dialogues*, **3**, 371–87.

Siegel, D. J. (1999). *The developing mind*, pp. 190–2. New York: Guilford Press.

Simons, J. A. and Helms, J. E. (1976). Influence of counselor's marital status, sex and age on college and non-college women's preference. *Journal of Counseling Psychology*, **23**, 380–6.

Sotsky, S. M., *et al.* (1991). Patient predictors of response to psychotherapy and pharmacotherapy: findings in the NIHM Treatment of Depression Collaborative Research Program. *American Journal of Psychiatry*, **148**, 997–1008.

Spinelli, M. (2001). Interpersonal psychotherapy for antepartum depressed women. In: K. Yonkers and B. Little, ed. *Management of psychiatric disorders in pregnancy*, pp. 105–21. London: Arnold Press.

Sprock, J., *et al.* (1990). Gender weighting of DSM-III-R personality disorder criteria. *American Journal of Psychiatry*, **147**(5), 586–90.

Stabb, S. D., Cox, D. L., and Harber, J. L. (1997). Gender-related therapist attributions in couples' therapy: a preliminary multiple case study investigation. *Journal of Marital Family Therapy*, **23**, 335–46.

Stoller, R. J. (1976). Primary femininity. *Journal of the American Psychoanalysis Association*, **24**(5, Suppl.), 59–78.

Stuart, S. and O'Hara, M. W. (1995). Interpersonal psychotherapy for postpartum depression. *Journal of Psychotherapy Practice and Research*, **4**, 18–29.

Symonds, A. (1971). Phobias after marriage—women's declaration of dependence. *American Journal of Psychoanalysis*, **31**, 144–52.

Teicher, M. D., *et al.* (1993). Early childhood abuse and limbic system ratings in adult psychiatric outpatients. *Journal of Neuropsychiatry and Clinical Neuroscience*, **5**, 301–6.

Thase, M. E., *et al.* (1994). Do depressed men and women respond similarly to cognitive behavior therapy? *American Journal of Psychiatry*, **151**, 500–5.

Thase, M. E., *et al.* (1996). Abnormal electroencepoalographic sleep profiles in major depression: association response to cognitive behavior therapy. *Archives of General Psychiatry*, **53**, 99–108.

Thompson, C. (1938). Notes on the psychoanalytic significance of the choice of the analyst. *Psychiatry*, **1**, 205–16.

Walter, E. E. and Kendler, K. S. (1995). Anorexia nervosa and anorexia-like syndromes in a population-based female twin sample. *American Journal of Psychiatry*, **152**, 64–71.

Weisner, C. (1989). Treatment services research and alcohol problems: treatment entry, access, and effectiveness. In: *Assessing future research needs: mental and addictive disorders in women*, pp. 85–90. Washington, DC: Institute of Medicine.

Weissman, M. M. (1991). Gender differences in the rates of mental disorders. In: *Assessing future research needs: mental and addictive disorders in women*, pp. 8–13. Washington, DC: Institute of Medicine.

Weissman, M. M., *et al.* (1991). Affective disorders. In: *Psychiatric disorders in America: the Epidemiologic Catchment Area Study*, pp. 53–80. New York: Free Press.

Wellesley College Center for Research on Women. (1992). *How schools short-change girls.* Washington, DC: American Association of University Women.

Wenger, N. K. and Speroff, L. P. B. (1993). Cardiovascular health and disease in women. *New England Journal of Medicine*, **329**(4), 247–56.

Wisch, A. F. and Mahalik, J. R. (1999). Male therapists' clinical bias: influence of client gender roles and therapist gender role conflict. *Journal of Counseling Psychology*, **46**, 51–60.

Zanarini, M., *et al.* (1989). Childhood experiences of borderline patients. *Comprehensive Psychiatry*, **30**, 18–25.

Zetzel, E. R. (1970). The doctor-patient relationship in psychiatry. In: *The capacity for emotional growth*, pp. 139–55. New York: International Universities Press.

Zlotnick, C., *et al.* (1996). Gender, type of treatment, dysfunctional attitudes, social support, life events, and depressive symptoms over naturalistic follow-up. *American Journal of Psychiatry*, **153**, 10–17.

Zlotnick, C., *et al.* (1998). Does the gender of a patient or the gender of a therapist affect the treatment of patients with major depression? *Journal of Consulting and Clinical Psychology*, **66**, 655–9.

35 Sexual orientation and psychotherapy

Sidney H. Phillips, Justin Richardson, and Susan C. Vaughan

Introduction

Setting aside a chapter to explore the implications of our patient's sexual orientation on their psychotherapy suggests that the treatment of gay, lesbian, and bisexual patients differs from the work we do with our heterosexual patients. In many ways, of course, it doesn't. Much of our daily work focuses on the mitigation of mental disorders and of life challenges that transcend the categories of sexual orientation. Nevertheless, gay, lesbian, and bisexual individuals do bring to their treatments particular life experiences that are less common in the lives of heterosexual patients and that can profoundly shape the goals and the techniques of their psychotherapies.

The mental health profession has its own developmental history that also contributes to the challenges clinicians face in treating these patients. Although attitudes regarding homosexuality have changed rapidly in the last few decades, we have behind us a long history of considering homosexuality a sin, a crime, a form of degeneracy, and—our own contribution to this list—a psychiatric disorder. Despite the removal of homosexuality from the American Psychiatric Association's nosology in 1973, this legacy still casts a shadow over our efforts to understand our gay patients as clinicians and as a profession.

Perhaps what is unique about homosexual and bisexual people would disappear in an unbiased society. But in our current world, conventional judgments about gender, the necessity for hiding and secrecy, and the presumption that all children will turn out to be heterosexual make for common developmental challenges in the lives of gay and lesbian patients, which, in turn, lead to particular clinical presentations and unique technical challenges for the therapist. In this chapter we examine each of these areas to define a psychotherapeutic approach to gay, lesbian, and bisexual patients that has, at its core, the goal of promoting the healthy integration of our patients' sexual orientation into their personality as a whole.

Developmental perspectives relevant to treating adults

Conducting therapy commonly stimulates, in the mind of clinicians and patients alike, a wish for answers to questions such as, 'How did this happen?' or 'Where does this come from?' The pursuit of answers to such questions has a rich history with at least two complementary trends: one plumbing the clinical situation for information about psychological development, the other drawing on empirically derived developmental data to inform clinical work. Both practices have been roundly criticized: the former as an unreliable and unverifiable method of inquiry, the latter as incapable of capturing the most essential aspect of observable developmental events—their meaning (Auchincloss and Vaughan, 2001; Tyson, 2002).

With these cautions in mind, some authors who treat gay and lesbian adults have drawn upon commonalities in their patients' life histories to construct developmental lines or nodes that they consider common to the experience of homosexual individuals. Others have looked to allied fields for empirically validated developmental data and have attempted to integrate those data with their clinical experience.

The result is a rich collection of observations and hypotheses, which, though they lack a common epistemological foundation, can be helpful to the clinician in a few important ways. First, as predictors of themes that may be important in the lives of gay and lesbian patients, these theories can guide the therapist's listening, helping her look for salient experiences her patients may not yet be able to articulate. And second, a familiarity with common developmental events in gay and lesbian lives can help the clinician predict the sorts of transferences that may develop over the course of a treatment and understand those that do.

Gender role

The development of many gay and lesbian individuals may diverge from that of their heterosexual peers in the earliest years of life. Gay and lesbian adults in various cultures are more likely to recall gender nonconformity in childhood than heterosexual adults (Whitam and Zent, 1984; Whitam and Mathy, 1991). One notable aspect of their atypicality that has received particular attention is the common aversion to rough and tumble play among prehomosexual boys and the interest in such play among prehomosexual girls.

The gender role nonconformity of many prehomosexual boys has been found to include preference for social interactions with girls and women over boys and men, interest in doll play, cross-dressing, adornment, an aptitude for color and texture, and emotionality (Corbett, 1996; Isay, 1999). Similarly, many prehomosexual girls have been described as showing little interest in girls' toys and clothes, a preference for boys' company, and for typically boyish styles of dress (Whitam and Mathy, 1991).

This nonconformity has been considered to derive in part from biological influences, such as the prenatal organizing effects of sex steroids (although there is more direct evidence of steroids influencing play preference in girls than in boys) acting in concert with early experiences and identifications in childhood (Ehrhardt, 1985; Isay, 1999; Friedman, 2001).

Gender identity

The prehomosexual child's sense of his or her own gender identity is shaped by the unfolding of his or her temperament, play preferences, and identifications throughout the course of childhood. Unlike children with gender identity disorder, the majority of prehomosexual children do not appear to doubt that they are male or female. However, in the context of the rigid and highly conventional notions of how boys and girls should behave typical among early school-age children their nonconformity can create in prehomosexual children a troubling sense of gender defectiveness (Richardson, 1999).

For example, while a boy who feels more comfortable playing with girls and dolls and fears getting hit with the ball on the playground may not doubt that he is a boy, he may feel that he is behaving in a girlish way. Friedman (1988) has described this common experience as a sense of 'unmasculinity' while Corbett (1996) has referred to it as an 'experience of gender otherness.'

Early relationships with parents

The clash of prehomosexual children's gender role nonconformity with their parents' expectations for their behavior and the mismatch between their temperament and that of their same sex parent can lead to tension and conflict in those early relationships. For example, an early school-age boy who is afraid of loud noises or being flipped upside down may find an afternoon in the backyard with his father an uncomfortable, even frightening, experience. His father, who discovers that he just can't get his son to enjoy playing with him, who sees his son hurry up back into his mother's arms when given the chance, may start to feel rejected by his boy. Father and son may withdraw from each other, each with feelings of failure, isolation, and anger (Friedman and Downey, 2002). Similarly, some gender nonconforming girls may have difficulty in their relationships with mothers who are persistently critical of or uncomfortable around their daughter's boisterous play (Vaughan, 1998).

Whether the same-sexed parent is thought of as a prehomosexual child's primary erotic object, as Isay (1987) has suggested, or as a figure whose attention and affection, while not erotic, is yearned for by the child, as Friedman and Downey (2002) believe, most authors have described the disruptions that arise in these relationships as having potentially serious negative consequences for the developing prehomosexual child (see, for example, Goldsmith, 1995, 2001). Among those commonly described are lingering damage to the individual's self esteem and a difficulty establishing love relationships in adulthood (Isay, 1999; Friedman and Downey, 2002).

Peer experiences in childhood

Childhood experiences in the world of peers often compound these difficulties, particularly for gender nonconforming prehomosexual boys. Boys' society has been described as a hierarchical one, with athletic prowess and boldness one of the major determinants of a boy's place in the social order. Gender nonconforming boys are typically relegated to the lowest strata of this society where they are vulnerable to being shamed and scapegoated routinely by their peers. For many adult homosexual patients, these negative experiences are crucial to their self concept and their anticipations of experiences with other men, including gay men, and persist as traumatic memories they may never have disclosed to anyone.

Gender nonconforming prehomosexual girls seem to suffer less from teasing or exclusion by their peers during middle and late childhood perhaps in part because girls' society during these ages appears to be more tolerant of gender role differences (Friedman and Downey, 2002). Unlike the almost always negatively viewed 'sissy-boys,' the bold behavior of tomboys can be seen as a desirable trait, occasionally giving these girls the status of peer leaders and making these prepubertal years a time tomboys can safely pursue and profit from close relationships with peers (Zevy, 1999).

Early and middle adolescence

As with all children, gay and lesbian children entering early adolescence experience the physical changes associated with puberty coupled with growing awareness of their own sexuality. Gay and lesbian adolescents may be troubled to find that they are attracted to same sex peers or that they have homosexual masturbatory fantasies. Budding sexuality may allow them for the first time to comprehend what is actually behind the life-long sense of being different than others (Floyd et al., 1999).

Parental responses to the physical changes of puberty may be especially important for homosexual youth. For example, many lesbians describe strong bonds with their fathers in childhood and time spent pursuing common interests such as sports or working on cars, but as these girls enter puberty, many find that their fathers retreat, no longer finding it acceptable to play in the same manner with a 'young lady' that they did with their younger daughters. Many lesbians describe a sense of loss of this important relationship and of feeling betrayed by their bodies as a consequence (Vaughan, 1998).

Typical situations of this developmental period such as sleepovers and experiences in physical education and locker rooms may prove both intensely erotic as well as disturbing as to gay and lesbian youths as these adolescents strive to prevent others from discovering the nature of their secret differences. The fact that society is organized around the presumption of heterosexuality creates a unique and distressing situation for gay and lesbian youths, who are sexually overstimulated while simultaneously feeling a strong sense of shame (that frequently accompanies self-recognition of homosexuality) and a concomitant need to hide.

Gay and lesbian adolescents are often in the awkward position of being attracted to same-gender peers without initially knowing whether their peers are attracted to them. Partly because of this uncertainty, homosexual adolescents may find themselves secretly falling in love with their same-gender, heterosexual friends. These 'love affairs from afar' are usually unconsummated exercises in frustration and can have a substantive developmental impact on an individual's later capacity to form and sustain loving, intimate relationships in adulthood as demonstrated in the following vignette.

Ms A, a woman in her late thirties, presented with anxiety and confusion over her relationship with K, her female partner of 8 years. Several months prior to Ms A's entering psychotherapy, K had suffered a depressive episode after being tapered off an antidepressant medication that she had taken for several years. In her irritable, depressive state, K had been withdrawn and harshly critical of Ms A and their relationship, leaving Ms A feeling emotionally battered. Eventually K recognized that she was in the midst of a depressive relapse, resumed her medication, and recovered. K was then eager to 'forget about' her criticisms of and withdrawal from her partner, but Ms A had been so shaken by K's attacks that she found herself unable to let go so easily of the hurt she felt. Ms A noticed at that time that she was intensely attracted to men and had masturbatory fantasies of heterosexual intercourse. Prior to this, Ms A had been monogamous and had had only fleeting thoughts about men. These secret feelings persisted and troubled Ms A and prompted her presenting for psychotherapy.

Following Ms A's first therapy session, she precipitously and tearfully 'confessed' to K about her recent interest in men and wondered if they should break up. During the opening phase of treatment, the therapist linked Ms A's sexual desires for men with her feeling both abandoned by and resentful of K during her irritable bout of depression. Ms A revealed that the secretive nature of her masturbatory fantasies had made her feel extremely guilty, which seemed to confirm the therapist's formulation that these fantasies were partly Ms A's retaliation against K for her critical attacks.

Ms A then revealed a similar experience had occurred during adolescence. She had developed a crush on L, her best friend in high school. At sleepovers, the two girls cuddled in physically intimate though not overtly sexual ways. Even though she realized L was interested in boys, Ms A could not stop herself from impulsively blurting out her desire to have sex with her. The friendship dissolved practically overnight and left Ms A heartbroken. The therapist was then able to show Ms A how her 'confession' of her heterosexual fantasies to K, which threatened shattering their long-term relationship, had recapitulated the earlier adolescent experience where the sudden revelation of sexual feelings with L had led to the loss of her first love relationship. These insights helped Ms A understand at a deeper emotional level what was at stake in her relationship with K. The heterosexual fantasies faded from importance as Ms A and K gradually rekindled their love and passion for one another.

As the homosexual youth begins high school and enters mid-adolescence, other distinctive problems arise. Social context clearly proves a powerful determinant of how gay and lesbian youths will weather these years. In those few social milieus in which being gay or lesbian tends to be seen as an alternative but equally valid developmental pathway as heterosexuality, gay and lesbian adolescents will tend to have adequate adult support and role models for how to achieve a healthy gay identity. For example, the presence of gay–straight alliances in schools that are progressive about homosexuality often helps to foster acceptance of the full range of sexual self-expression. Such programs are generally only possible in areas where adults appreciate and understand that such an approach will not result in greater numbers of homosexual children but rather better self-esteem and an earlier capacity for an integrated sense of self in those who are gay or lesbian.

Late adolescence and young adulthood

As homosexual adolescents complete their high school years and leave home for work or for college, they may experience a sense of freedom to define who they are and to surround themselves with people who may be more capable of supporting their growing sense of gay identity. When they are able to enter a milieu where same-sex attraction, dating, and partnering are more acceptable, they may be able to accomplish two key developmental tasks: coming out with the sense of identity integration that it both reflects and provides and falling in love/beginning the search for a life partner.

Beginning the process of coming out is a necessary precursor to beginning the process of finding a mate, and how well the coming out process goes may determine how the gay or lesbian youth feels about himself as a potential life and sexual partner for another. The search for intimacy characteristic of young adulthood may be postponed in homosexuals. Delays in the coming out process itself or the fact that the gay or lesbian adolescent has been denied the opportunities to date those he wants to date prior to leaving home may create such developmental delays. Ready access to drugs and alcohol for late adolescents and young adults can be problematic as gay men and lesbians in their late teens and early twenties may use such substances to override their sense of discomfort with themselves, sometimes putting themselves at risk for HIV and other STDs.

Coming out later in life

While most gay men and lesbians will come out during their teens, twenties, and early thirties, a subset do not come out until later in life. Those who come out later in life seem to belong to two distinctive subgroups. Members of the first group are well aware of long-standing, if not lifelong homosexual feelings and may have grappled with internalized homophobia and feelings of shame and self-loathing that prevented the evolution and consolidation of a healthy gay identity earlier in life. Alternatively, they may have long been aware of homosexual longings but hoped that heterosexual marriage or having children would lessen the importance of these feelings or may have decided that they wanted the social acceptance and protection of a heterosexual life-style (Isay, 1996).

The second group seems to be a distinctive set of women in their forties and beyond who are often completely unaware of homosexual feelings earlier in life and do not feel that they have struggled with their identities but who suddenly, in midlife and perhaps in the context of a heterosexual marriage that lacks intimacy, find themselves in love with a woman with whom they have developed a close relationship (Notman, 2002). They are often startled to find that there is an erotic component to such a relationship but often describe themselves as curious to explore this added dimension of what originally began as a friendship with a confidante.

Middle age and beyond

Many gay men and lesbians find that having accomplished important developmental tasks such as coming out, forming bonds and relationships within the gay and lesbian community, forging a positive gay identity and finding a partner, their concerns—and their developmental pathways—once again converge with those of their heterosexual cohorts (Kertzner, 2001). Their strong homosexual identity is gradually subsumed into a wider set of identities (and to an overall sense of being human) as they become increasingly integrated into the larger community. Having children may speed this process as many gay men and lesbians find that this gives strong common ties to other parents regardless of their sexual orientation of those parents. Concerns about caring for aging parents, maintaining a strong primary relationship over time, and aging itself are examples of mid and late life issues that are universal.

Clinical presentations

In the 30 years since American psychiatry accepted homosexuality as a potentially healthy form of loving and sexuality, clinicians—freed from seeing their patients' orientation as their pathology—have identified a wide range of needs in their gay, lesbian, and bisexual patients. Accordingly, a literature has grown up in which psychotherapists have described the most common clinical presentations they've faced with their homosexual patients and shared the results of their innovative efforts to respond to them.

In the following pages we summarize some of the most useful of these insights to have emerged. Most of these contributions come from the consulting rooms of psychodynamic psychotherapists and psychoanalysts, and as with other similarly derived theories of technique, the question of their validity remains empirically unanswered. Instead, we consider the following to be provisional yet, nevertheless, well supported findings in so far as they capture a clinical consensus among those most experienced in treating homosexual patients. Where outcome data are available, as is the case with some cognitive-behavioral interventions, we report it.

Internalized homophobia

Many gay and lesbian patients bring to their psychotherapy a persistent pattern of conscious and unconscious shame and self-hate organized around the knowledge that they are gay. Some will arrive describing their struggle with internalized homophobia as the reason they have sought out treatment. Others may only discover their difficulties with it as a result of years of treatment. For most, however, the mitigation of sexual orientation-associated shame will be an important therapeutic goal.

Adolescents and adults vary widely in the complexity of the underpinnings of their homophobia. Some patients may come to the recognition that they are gay after a healthy childhood in which they received the necessary support to achieve a solid foundation of self-worth. Having absorbed their culture's prevailing negative views towards gay people, the discovery of same-sex attractions in adolescence may activate anxiety, depression, and a subsequent struggle to revise their notions of themselves or of gay and lesbian people. But they will be bolstered in this process by a basic conviction in their own goodness and lovability.

Cognitive-behavioral approaches may be well suited for these patients as their internalized homophobia can be framed as a pervasive negative schema toward homosexuality. Some cognitive-behavioral therapists consider such homophobia to be a conditioned emotional response that can be treated with cognitive restructuring (Spencer and Hemmer, 1993; Purcell et al., 1996, pp. 401–2). Various cognitive-behavioral approaches such as identifying thinking errors, cognitive restructuring, and behavioral experiments can help patients confront their self-blaming cognitions and pathological core beliefs while relaxation techniques and stress reduction may decrease distress and increase their quality of life (Safren et al., 2001a).

For other patients, internalized homophobia will be a more layered phenomenon, built up over the course of childhood and adolescent development. Their feeling that being gay renders them defective typically condenses early experiences of gender difference, rejection by the same sex parent, harassment by peers in grade school, and shame over homosexual attractions in early and middle adolescence. In some cases, other experiences of trauma and neglect originally unrelated to the patient's sexual orientation may retrospectively become organized into this constellation of self-hate for being gay.

Among the commonest ramifications of internalized homophobia are difficulty maintaining a love relationship; difficulty integrating sexual pleasure with love; and self-consciousness about the masculinity or femininity of one's speech, behavior, and body. In those with more severe developmental traumas and unconscious guilt, internalized homophobia may manifest itself through self-destructive behavior, including drug and alcohol abuse and unsafe sex. Healthier patients may, by contrast, be well adjusted to the demands of work and successful in love, but may harbor unconscious negative self-evaluations that result in a gnawing sense of inadequacy.

The treatment of internalized homophobia combines supportive and insight-oriented interventions in a balance titrated to the immediate needs of the particular patient. Supportive maneuvers include the facilitation of the coming out process (described below), the therapist's expression of an accepting view of the patient's past and present gender nonconformity (Isay, 1999) and homosexuality (Frommer, 1994), psychoeducation about sexual orientation and its development, and empathic support as the patient describes possibly for the first time to anyone some of the shaming and frightening experiences of her development. These techniques will play a relatively greater role in work with patients whose treatment is less complicated by early and marked developmental injuries.

Insight-oriented approaches (whether psychodynamic or cognitive) focus on helping the patient unravel the various strands of shame and guilt that have come together to form his homophobia (Downey and Friedman, 1995; Friedman and Downey, 1995). In this process, the unconscious beliefs that may underlie the patient's shame ('My father withdrew from me, because I was overly emotional. Being overly emotional is gay and wrong.') can be made conscious, challenged, and gradually modified by the patient and therapist. This treatment approach, also conducted in the context of the therapist's affirming stance, will constitute the greater portion of the work with patients whose homophobia condenses earlier traumatic experiences.

The following vignette demonstrates the mitigation of shame related to homosexuality in a psychoanalytic treatment:

> When Mr B first presented for analysis at 24 years of age, he described conscious, romantic, and erotic attraction to and arousal for male peers since early adolescence. He deeply desired a loving, intimate relationship with a man, yet he reported having fled good prospects for reasons he did not fully understand. He felt chronically unhappy about this. In the sixth year of an 8-year analysis the patient described his childhood 'obsession' with seeing his handsome father's muscular body. He reported numerous episodes of trying to catch glimpses of his father's getting in or out of the shower. Over the ensuing weeks, he told his analyst in detail—alternating with protests of intense shame—of a conscious, erotic fantasy he recalled from childhood and adolescence. His fantasy was that he would be in the shower with his father who would lift him face-to-face and press him up against his soapy, hairy, muscular chest, gradually sliding him down to enter him anally with his erect penis.

> In the session, the patient yelled out in angry distress how humiliated he felt to admit that he liked anal sex: 'I like to get fucked—okay?! Are you happy now, you fucker?' It was rare for him speak so frankly. The therapist replied within the transference: 'You experience me as the humiliating fucker, penetrating you with my interpretations.' 'Yes,' he said, though calmer now, 'maybe you really get off on being top dog here.' It took many more months of analysis of his shame—touching on themes such as top/bottom, big/little, adult/child, 'dirty' anal sex/'clean' vaginal sex—for this analysand to acknowledge to himself and to his analyst with some semblance of acceptance how passionately aroused in so many variations he was by other men's bodies.

Facilitation of the coming out process

Many patients who seek therapy in pain over their sexual orientation have (consciously or not) chosen to come to treatment as a part of the larger process of coming out. For them, therapy can play an important part by helping them move through this crucial developmental process.

The phrase 'coming out' has come to mean the social and psychological process of acquiring a gay identity. Often conceptualized as a developmental line or a sequence of stages, coming out is generally considered to include realizing that one is gay, disclosing that fact to others, establishing social relationships with other gay people, coming to value positively one's homosexuality, subsuming that identity to a wider set of identities (and to an overall sense of being human), and integrating oneself into the larger community (Coleman, 1982; Cass, 1989).

For many gay and lesbian individuals who do not seek out treatment for their fear or shame about being gay, coming out will be psychotherapy enough. Dramatic and lasting improvement in their self-esteem and self-expression as well as their ability to love and work often result. For those individuals who encounter obstacles along the way to self-disclosure and creating a community of gay friends and supports, psychotherapy can be helpful by identifying and removing those barriers.

The individual therapist can explore with the patient the possible implications of talking openly with parents, siblings, children, friends, and coworkers about the patient's orientation. Where such disclosures would not endanger the patient, they can be gently encouraged and the resistances to making them explored. The therapist can also help the patient find a way into friendships with gay peers. A gay or lesbian group psychotherapy may be especially helpful for those who have difficulty creating their own peer group.

The gender nonconforming child

Occasionally, a parent will seek treatment for a child—most commonly a boy—whose gender nonconformity has become a focus of worry in the family. Some of these parents ask that their child's behavior be rendered more typical; some, considering it an indication of future homosexuality, will want the therapist to prevent that outcome; and others seek therapy as a way to protect their child from harassment. In all cases the first task of the clinician is to assess the child's behavior and the nature of the family system of which it is a part.

A small group of gender nonconforming children will meet the diagnostic criteria for gender identity disorder (GID). Their nonconformity, which may consist of inflexible, repetitive, and insistent cross-gendered behavior suffused with anxiety or aggression, has been understood as an effort to defend against extreme anxiety in the face of a felt separation from the opposite sex parent and merits clinical attention in the form of individual and family therapy (Coates and Woolfe, 1995). Most gender nonconformity in childhood, however, is not pathological and presents, instead, as pleasurable self-expression and flexible play. This distinction, which can be difficult to make, has been the subject of some controversy (Richardson, 1999; Zucker, 1999).

In cases of healthy gender nonconformity, many parents will benefit from expressing their fears and learning from a sympathetic expert about the development of sexual orientation. Other parents will require more extended therapeutic interventions exploring the meaning to them of their child's atypicality (Friedman and Downey, 2002).

Therapists can also help nonconforming children resist the damaging effects of peer harassment. The clinician can help counter the attitudes of peers with open support of the child's interests and help the child develop new ways of responding to peers. Gender nonconforming children face a difficult choice between proudly pursuing their interests and changing their behavior to decrease negative attention. The sensitive clinician can help a child craft a well-considered response to this dilemma. In the case of severe harassment, the clinician may advocate for a change in the child's social milieu (Friedman, 1997).

The family of the homosexual adolescent

The parent or parents of a homosexual adolescent who has just come out or whose homosexuality has just been discovered by his family may also seek treatment. As with gender nonconformity, it is essential to delineate the reason for seeking treatment, to educate the parents, and to focus the treatment appropriately. For example, the family of the homosexual adolescent may be seeking treatment for the adolescent with the goal of making sure he or she turns out to be heterosexual. In this case, it is the clinician's job to educate the family, pointing out that most professional associations condemn such attempts as unethical because of the lack of evidence that such change from homosexual to heterosexual is actually possible and the risk that such attempts at change will increase depression and anxiety while decreasing self-esteem (Bernstein and Miller, 1995; Shidlo et al., 2001). Allowing the parents to mourn their lost image of who their child is and will become can be crucially important in helping them to begin to accept and support their homosexual adolescent. Support groups such as Parents, Families, and Friends of Lesbians and Gays (PFLAG) can provide a helpful forum for families struggling to accept homosexuality in a loved one and can encourage them to begin to fight the homophobia and heterosexism in society that adversely affects their child.

One essential principle to keep in mind when a child has just come out to his or her parents is the inherent mismatch in phase of development that is likely to result in hurt and frustration on both sides. The adolescent telling his parents he is homosexual has most likely known and dealt with this aspect of himself for some time and is disclosing it at a point where he feels it is more important to be authentic, whatever the interpersonal risks, than to continue to hide such a key aspect of his identity. In other words, the telling itself is the end result of an internal process that represents a step toward psychological integrity and wholeness. Parents, in contrast, may have little or no inkling of their child's homosexuality and may be caught off guard as they quickly try to formulate a response to a disclosure that shatters their image of who the child is. Many parents recall reacting with dismay, disappointment, and despair, reactions that they later wish they could undo as they see their hurtful impact on their child. Highlighting this disparity between coming out and finding out may help to mitigate this situation and improve relations between parent and child.

It is possible that parents, upon hearing of their child's homosexuality for the first time, may become abusive and punitive or may withdraw support from the adolescent, sometimes kicking them out of the house or refusing to pay for schooling. As shifts in society's acceptance of homosexuality have helped to move the average age of coming out in a younger and younger direction, more adolescents are at risk as they may come out before they are actually psychologically or fiscally capable of living independently. In situations of such extreme parental reactions, clinicians must be prepared to involve social services to ensure that the adolescent is safe and living in an abuse-free environment. In this case, the clinician's perspective that the parents' reaction is homophobic in nature and that one can live an equally fulfilling, valid, and valuable life as a gay man or lesbian will be key in psychologically protecting the adolescent. Cognitive-behavioral interventions that target coping with chronic stress such as problem-solving techniques can also be helpful in these situations (Safren et al., 2001a, p. 220).

The heterosexually married homosexual adult

The heterosexually married homosexual adult may seek treatment at a point of crisis in the marriage, perhaps after a homosexual affair or encounter has come to light, or may seek treatment as the result of an ongoing inner psychological process when the conflict between inner desires and the reality of the heterosexual relationship become too much to bear. The question of 'why now?' is especially important in understanding the factors that lead a homosexual adult in a long-standing marriage to seek treatment at a given time. When a third, same-sex sexual partner of the heterosexual married individual is also involved, evaluating the qualities of this tie and attempting to understand the pressures being exerted by the same-sex partner may also be clinically relevant.

It is important in the initial evaluation of such a patient to decide whether a couples-oriented focus or an individual approach is more appropriate and for the clinician to resist the patient's (or spouse's) sense of urgency that the situation be quickly resolved but to press for adequate time for psychological exploration before taking definitive action. One important factor in the evaluation process is whether the spouse of the heterosexually married homosexual has known or suspected his or her partner's homosexuality and whether there is any potential for compromise within the partnership regarding the issue of the homosexuality. For many, such a revelation triggers a desire for an immediate divorce while others may be willing or able to tolerate a transition period while the issues are sorted out or even a restructuring of the marital agreement, which allows for the expression of same-sex sexual relationships alongside the preservation of the marital bond. The decision to divorce generally involves moving from many years of denial of one's sexuality and requires giving up the social respectability provided by marriage and eventually coming out to those—often including children—who know the homosexual individual as heterosexual and who are likely to feel unsettled or betrayed by the revelation.

If divorce seems likely, it is important for the clinician to help the patient limit the extent to which the patient's guilt and the spouse's anger lead to legal and financial concessions that are not in the patient's best long-term interests.

The adult homosexual seeking to start a family

Although many gay men and lesbians will form partnerships and start families without seeking clinical assistance, occasionally a couple or individual will come to treatment to explore concerns about having children. A couple seeking to start a family often present with concerns about the state of their current relationship and the potential emotional, sexual, and financial impact of children on their union. In these cases, work with the couple will be similar to that of a heterosexual couple seeking assistance at such a transition point, with the caveat that a gay or lesbian couple may lack the societal approbations, ranging from familial encouragement to legal protections, that a heterosexual couple takes for granted.

Gay and lesbian couples may also present with issues specific to their homosexuality. The de facto infertility of a homosexual couple—their inability to conceive and bear a child together as a couple—is often a hidden reason for mourning and may be helpful to elucidate in treatment. Decisions such as who will carry a child in the case of a lesbian couple or who will father a child in the case of a gay male couple as well as struggles over whether to involve a known sperm or egg donor or whether to adopt. Modern reproductive technologies allow potential creative answers to these issues once the couple has dealt with the underlying psychological issues (such as mixing the sperm of two gay men during artificial insemination or in vitro fertilization with a surrogate or having a lesbian serve as an egg donor for her partner), but dealing with the underlying issues may also make such questions recede in importance in the minds of the couple. Seemingly practical questions about how to conceive or what a child will call each partner frequently hide deeper concerns about competition within the pair or unresolved tensions about gender.

Having children demands of gay men and lesbians that they achieve an even greater level of resolution of their own internalized homophobia than coming out and forming a partnership did earlier in life. For example, wondering whether having gay or lesbian parents is fair to the child or attempting to create parenting scenarios that involve a third, opposite-sex parental figure on the grounds that two same-sex parents are inadequate to the task of raising a child are common lingering expressions of internalized homophobia that can be usefully explored in couples or individual psychotherapy. Having children also often precipitates another round of coming out and working through within the families of gay men and lesbians as, for example, the parents and siblings of the couple decide whom to tell about their new grandchild or nephew. Addressing these vestiges of homophobia within the couple and the family system may allow the couple to deal more effectively with the very real issues of gay and lesbian parenting, including the antihomosexual bias that parents and children can be faced with in the school or community.

The HIV-positive patient

While the patient with HIV may or may not come to treatment to focus on issues specifically related to his HIV-positive status, living with HIV/AIDS creates the stress typical of living with any chronic life-threatening illness as well as the stigma associated with homosexuality and sexually transmitted disease. Fear of suffering and death, the diminution of expectations of longevity and accomplishment in life, the fear of rejection by family and friends, and dealing with the loathing and prejudice of society are common themes in the HIV-positive patient in treatment (Blechner, 1997).

Being HIV positive can also create a sense of being damaged, bad, or sick that resonates powerfully with the patient's original responses to his own homosexuality. Gay men who are HIV positive and seeking a partner frequently view themselves as 'damaged goods' when it comes to forming an intimate long-term relationship, assuming no partner would want to contend with their HIV disease and the specter of AIDS. Becoming involved with an HIV-positive partner may ameliorate fears of infecting—and thereby potentially killing—the loved other but creates different concerns such as facing illness and mortality and threat of loss of the partner.

Negative core beliefs about the self—such as an HIV-positive patient's conception of himself as defective and unlovable—can usefully be targets of cognitive approaches to case conceptualization and treatment. The labeling of inaccurate inferences or distortions may help the patient become aware of the unreasonableness of such automatic patterns of thought (Beck and Freeman, 1990, p. 80). Cognitive probes and questioning may be used to elicit such automatic thoughts (p. 81). As an example, when John expresses reluctance to invite a man out on a date, the cognitive therapist might ask the patient to imagine out loud here and now in the session how his prospective date would react. 'Oh, I know what he would say'. He'd say 'I don't want to be involved with someone who is going to die. I'm out of here.' Here the therapist has identified an automatic thought: 'HIV-infected people will all die.' Such automatic thoughts can then be tested with the therapist who carefully attends to the possibility of exaggeration and catastrophizing. Relaxation techniques can also be useful with patients who are anxiously worried about the impact of their diagnosis on various aspects of their lives (Beck and Freeman, 1990, pp. 79–94). Outcome studies demonstrate the efficacy of cognitive therapy for depressed patients with HIV (Lee *et al.*, 1999; Safren *et al.*, 2001b; Blanch *et al.*, 2002; Molassiotis *et al.*, 2002).

Interpersonal psychotherapy has been shown to have particular advantages for HIV patients (Markowitz *et al.*, 1998). Interpersonal therapy relates mood changes to environmental events and resultant changes in social roles. For example, the interpersonal therapist defines depression as a medical illness and then assigns the patient both the diagnosis and the sick role. She then 'engages the patient on affectively laden current life issues, and frames the patient's difficulties within an interpersonal problem area: grief, role dispute, role transition, or interpersonal deficits. Strategies then address these problem areas, focusing in the present on what the patients want and what options exist to achieve this' (Markowitz *et al.*, 1998).

Exploratory psychodynamic treatments, including psychoanalysis may be usefully employed with the HIV-positive patient grappling with these issues. In patients with frank AIDS, evaluation and treatment should focus on helping patients receive life-enhancing medical care, resolving troubling psychological issues and making the best use of whatever time is left.

A clinical vignette illustrates the psychodynamic approach with a patient with end-stage AIDS:

A 33-year-old successful business executive with a year-long history of Kaposi's sarcoma, Mr C presented with complaints of anxiety a few weeks after being discharged from the hospital after his first bout of pneumocystis pneumonia. The bout had been serious, requiring endotracheal intubation and forced ventilation of his lungs while he recovered. There was much material, seemingly as scattered and diffuse as his anxiety: not feeling close to his lover since the hospitalization; the lover's positive HIV antibody test; his law suit against his company, which had fired him while he was in the intensive care unit; and so on. There were questions about which 'new age crystal' to use today, which relaxation tape to listen to, and how many times to visit his acupuncturist. All of this was spoken of in a chatty way and was woven in and out of discussion of his traditional medical treatment. Two dynamic themes permeated his speech, though neither was directly mentioned: (1) intense guilt and shame about his homosexuality for which AIDS seemed (to the patient) to be the punishment, and (2) enormous anxiety about death. Both were taken up and explored psychotherapeutically in some depth. This vignette focuses on the latter theme.

The prognosis at the time of Mr C's treatment was gloomy for patients with Kaposi's sarcoma and pneumocystis pneumonia and he was well aware of this. Natural enough, one might think, to be anxious about death while living with a potentially fatal illness. The therapist asked him to describe his fears in as great detail as he could. Mr C began, somewhat to the therapist's surprise, to depict his inner landscape. There was a figure—not human, maybe animal—hooded in formless darkness except for glowing eyes. This is what came to mind when he became anxious about his own death.

The material wandered to his sixth year. He had pet hamsters that he kept in a cage on the back porch. He returned home one day to find no hamsters present in the screened-in porch where he had let them roam. There was a hole in the screen leading into the backyard. He followed the trail to the bloody remnant of one furry, dismembered limb. He ran back into the house screaming in terror and sobbing inconsolably. 'Why terror?' the therapist inquired. He did not know.

Then yet another story from the patient's childhood emerged. At age 2 years, he went to a store with his parents. A colorful neon light in the front window attracted his attention. He grabbed on to the nearby electrical cord that had exposed wires and received a massive electrical shock for several seconds until he was forcibly knocked away from the cord. Consciously he remembered nothing of this incident, though he had been told about the time he 'almost died' and had seen photographs of himself with bandaged, badly burned hand. The therapist and Mr C then spoke in detail of the connections between these three experiences.

They began to consider that, though amnesic for the electrocution, Mr C seemed to carry forward some mental representation of this near-death trauma, which may then have informed his terrified reaction to his hamsters' death (perhaps via the homology from burned hand to dismembered limb). The childhood terror carried forward yet again and infiltrated his natural concerns and fear of dying from his present illness. The therapist and patient together reconstructed the dark, formless animal with glowing eyes (of neon?) as the unseen, fantasied predator who ate his hamsters, a childhood embodiment of death that haunted him still, invoking fears of a violent, abrupt, and painful death. Having analyzed the unconscious roots of his fears about death in this way, Mr C was able to think and speak more freely about his own death with his therapist, his lover, and his family. This led to his experiencing much greater self-control over the way he lived his life and to a marked reduction in his anxiety.

The patient seeking sexual orientation change

Given the prevalence of antihomosexual bias in society at large and of internalized homophobia among gay men and lesbians, it should not be surprising that some homosexual adults seek out therapy with a wish to become heterosexual. The treatment of choice in these cases takes the patient's wish to change rather than his homosexuality as the target of therapeutic attention. Patients seeking to change the direction of their sexual attractions should be informed that attempting to do so is unlikely to be successful (particularly in males) and may further compound the patient's distress. Instead, the clinician can explain, psychotherapy may offer the patient help in the form of a deeper understanding of his sexual feelings, his attitudes towards them, and the choices before him about disclosing or acting on his attractions.

The therapy may then proceed as a treatment of internalized homophobia and a facilitation of the coming out process as described above. Not all patients will choose to pursue these goals or be able to achieve them. Particularly among patients whose acceptance of their homosexuality implies a departure from deeply held religious beliefs or the loss of a crucial relationship (as may be the case with some heterosexually married patients), the open acceptance of one's orientation may entail such sacrifice that a patient will choose to continue efforts to suppress his desires. Even in these cases, however, a supportive therapist empathic to the patient's conflicts may help ease the pain inherent in what will inevitably be experienced as a compromised life.

Technical considerations

The psychotherapist's attitude: neutral, affirmative, and 'reparative' psychotherapies

The psychodynamic psychotherapist's attitude toward homosexuality in general and homosexual individuals in particular may well be determinative in whether an insight-oriented psychotherapy can be effective. While blatant prejudice against gay and lesbian people would certainly be an obvious contraindication for a therapist to work with this population, subtler forms of conscious and unconscious homophobia are often present within a therapist regardless of his or her sexual orientation. Mitchell (1996) observes that a therapist's pursuit of being bias-free is a futile and disingenuous ideal. He suggests that we serve our patients better by remaining open to discovering and rediscovering our prejudices and affinities as inevitable aspects of the therapeutic inquiry (p. 71). Neutrality is a fundamental principle of psychoanalytic treatment that asserts that the therapist should resist imposing his or her own values on the patient. This principle is meant to protect patients from therapists' using their authority and influence deliberately to shape or guide patients' beliefs, choices, or actions.

In reaction to decades of biased treatment approaches for homosexual individuals, a group of therapists—influenced culturally both by the gay liberation movement and the antihomosexual bias within psychoanalysis—decided that dynamic psychotherapy had never been conducted under the principle of neutrality with regard to sexual orientation. They proposed an alternative principle—gay affirmative psychotherapy. Gay affirmative psychotherapy categorically rejected any effort to change a person's sexual orientation from heterosexual to homosexual and established an affirmative psychotherapeutic stance that emotionally communicates to the patient the therapist's belief that homosexuality is a natural developmental end point for some individuals (Frommer, 1994, p. 215).

In reaction to gay affirmative psychotherapy, a contemporary version of the earlier directive-suggestive approach (also known as 'conversion therapy') has emerged. This approach is known as reparative therapy (see Nicolosi, 1991, 1993) and is based on the assumption that homosexuality is a mental disorder that can be changed through treatment. These approaches are controversial because they require the patient to regard core aspects of the self—i.e., homosexual desires—as pathological. For a detailed account of the extremely problematic nature of sexual conversion therapy, see Bernstein and Miller (1995), Roughton (1999), and Shidlo *et al.* (2001).

Roughton (1999) has made a strong case for reclaiming the value of neutrality in psychodynamic psychotherapy for gay and lesbian individuals. He emphasizes the need for searching self-reflection by all psychotherapists who work with homosexual individuals to recognize currents of antihomosexual bias, cultural heterosexism, and ignorance of the norms of gay life within themselves. Thus, neutrally conducted psychoanalytic psychotherapy allows for the possibility that a patient might begin treatment thinking that he or she is homosexual (or conflicted about sexual orientation) and eventually realize heterosexuality is the orientation of his or her sexual desire (Roughton, 2001).

The patient's request for a gay or lesbian therapist and the therapist's self-disclosure

Given the many decades of discrimination against homosexual individuals within mainstream psychotherapy—both cognitive and psychodynamic—it is not surprising that the gay and lesbian communities are wary of insight-oriented psychotherapies. While some prospective patients have consequently avoided dynamic therapy altogether, others have tried to protect themselves from biased treatment by seeking out openly gay or lesbian therapists.

Ironically, such patients are attempting to insure that they receive the type of therapy that is authentically neutral with regard to issues of sexual orientation. It does not necessarily follow that homosexual patients could only receive competent and compassionate treatment from openly homosexual therapists, but the history of prejudice within psychoanalysis (e.g., the so-called 'reparative therapies') is well known in the gay and lesbian community and serves as a cautionary tale.

The patient's learning of the therapist's homosexuality seems to have a magnetizing effect on conflicts from virtually all developmental periods and thus may act as an organizing principle of transference wishes and defenses. As these conflicts realign in reaction to this discovery, some things become easier to talk about; some things harder, pointing the way to exploration of resistance. Exploration of the patient's conscious resistance to speak about the therapist's homosexuality often reveals the patient's fear of divulging old prejudices against homosexuality that he worries will offend the therapist. Such material may also lead to discovery of a wellspring of unconscious internalized homophobia that presents an opportunity for superego exploration that can yield far-reaching therapeutic effect.

For example, a 26-year-old gay man was told by a referring therapist that the psychotherapist to whom he was referred was openly gay. The patient did not mention he knew about his therapist's homosexuality until several months later in treatment. The patient acknowledged that he thought this might 'embarrass' the therapist as such information was 'private and personal and none of my business.' The therapist helped the patient to consider that what ostensibly was protecting the therapist's 'privacy' was actually a way to protect the patient's 'private and personal' fantasies about the therapist. This intervention helped to bring under psychotherapeutic scrutiny new material concerning the patient's internalized homophobia and how it restrained currents of curiosity and fantasy about the therapist.

Transference and countertransference

The heart of psychodynamic or psychoanalytic psychotherapy is the psychotherapist's attention to and understanding of both the patient's transference and the therapist's inevitable reaction to it, which is known as the countertransference. By transference, we refer to the conscious and unconscious attitudes, feelings, and fantasies that the patient has about the therapist. These attitudes, feelings, and fantasies (such as sexual, affectionate, aggressive, competitive ones) about the therapist carry the pathogenic core—the conflicted wishes and fears and pathological object relations—from the patient's childhood and adolescence. In the context of a trusting and safe relationship with a judiciously frustrating, supportive psychotherapist, the ghosts of childhood conflicts, traumas, and relationships reawaken and come back to life as though they were occurring in the present in relation to the therapist. Reciprocally, the countertransference entails the therapist's conscious and unconscious attitudes, feelings, and fantasies towards the patient in reaction to the patient's transference. The transference and countertransference often bear a close relation to one another—knowledge of the countertransference, for example, often yields important and illuminating information about the patient's transference.

Patients often struggle against recognizing and admitting these intimate reactions towards their therapist. They often try to conceal these feelings and thoughts from themselves as well as their therapists. This reluctance to admit and discuss such reactions is known as the resistance to the transference. Resistance is often first detected by a shift in the free flowing associations the patient has during a session. Instead of speaking easily, the patient becomes halting about a particular subject or abruptly changes the subject altogether. Technically, the psychotherapist then focuses on precisely those feelings and thoughts that make the patient reluctant to speak what has come to mind. Such nodes of resistance are diffused throughout the material and are especially present in symptoms. Thus, psychotherapeutic exploration of these resistance nodes is often informative about the types of problems that brought the patient for treatment in the first place.

The transference and the resistance against it, then, become central to the therapeutic endeavor in psychoanalytic psychotherapy. Isay (1989), for example, has shown persuasively how resolution of diverse symptomatology during the therapy of gay men depends on their becoming conscious of, and accepting emotionally, their homoerotic, incestuous fantasies and desires for their fathers (p. 46). These homoerotic, incestuous feelings and fantasies may first come to light through discovery of erotic feelings for the therapist. Isay (1989) notes how 'defenses against these erotic feelings may lead to a distortion of the gay man's perception of other men and to a fear of intimacy and may be the most important cause of inhibited and impoverished relations in adulthood' (p. 39).

The reenactment in the transference of this type of overstimulation and the defensive struggles against it give rise to characteristic countertransference reactions in the therapist. The therapist may unwittingly collude with patients in their dissociative defenses against overstimulation by becoming distracted, bored, or sleepy. Or the therapist may experience a version of the sexual overstimulation itself by feeling mild sexual arousal accompanied by explicit erotic fantasies about the patient or a displacement figure. Therapists may react with shame and/or guilt to such fantasies. As the following vignette illustrates, when recognized and brought under self-analytic scrutiny by the therapist, these reactions—both the arousal and the shame and/or guilt—can prove extremely illuminating with regard to the patient's early, warded-off experiences of everyday overstimulation (see Phillips, 2001, 2002).

Mr D was a handsome, muscular, 20-year-old college student who presented for psychotherapy because of depression about his homosexuality. He felt unmanly and embarrassed that he was drawn to and aroused by other men. He thought coming out to his family would 'cure' him of his conflicts about his sexual orientation but paradoxically found that his family's loving and accepting reaction only worsened his dilemma. Now he had to acknowledge his conflicts about being gay were within him, and he wanted help in feeling better about himself so that he could enjoy a mutual, romantic, sexual relationship with another man.

From the beginning, the therapist noticed he was attracted to the patient's boyish good looks and diffidence. The patient usually wore a sleeveless T-shirt and short pants to therapy sessions and spoke graphically—alternating with intense expressions of shame—about his surreptitious, sexual exploits with other male college students. The therapist found himself feeling both attracted to the patient as well as uncharacteristically ashamed of such feelings. The shame was puzzling as the therapist felt in no danger of acting on any of his fantasies. The therapist silently thought this might relate to important experiences in the patient's past and resolved to see what developed.

As the patient spoke more about his past, he described a long-standing sexual attraction to his brother with whom he had shared a bedroom growing up. The patient described repeated experiences in childhood of feeling 'spurned' when his brother preferred playing with his own friends rather than with the patient. Here was one component of what was being reenacted in the transference and countertransference. In the psychotherapy, Mr D was taking the role of the athletic, attractive brother and unconsciously assigning his own childhood role to the therapist. In this way, the patient was conveying to the therapist—by inducing him actually to feel it in sessions—the past attraction, arousal, excitement towards the brother as well as the frustration, shame, disappointment, and feeling 'spurned.' This same interaction was being repeated in the present in Mr D's symptomatic difficulty in allowing himself a mutually enjoyable sexual and romantic relationship with a peer.

The therapist used these clues in the transference–countertransference reenactment to show the patient how he was repeating in his present love life these old conflicts from his past frustrated 'love affair' with his brother. As the patient became aware of this pattern, he felt freed up to permit himself openly to date and fall in love with an available, caring man.

Management of dangerous behaviors

Tactful, direct confrontation of patients who openly acknowledge unsafe sexual practices is crucial to helping some patients—heterosexual or homosexual—confront their denial of their own destructiveness through exposure to HIV or other sexually transmitted diseases. Thorough clinical evaluation of such a patient is essential so as not to miss the diagnosis of a major psychiatric illness (such as bipolar disorder or addictions). Complex characterological pathology may be present, in which case psychodynamic or cognitive psychotherapeutic exploration of symptomatic destructive behaviors may be the preferred treatment over direct confrontation and psychoeducation.

The following vignette illustrates the psychodynamic approach to a patient engaging in unprotected sex:

A 47-year-old man presented with hypochondriacal anxiety and the fear that he had contracted HIV. Concerned about his 25-year history of frequenting homosexual hustler bars and aware of the recent death of a distant acquaintance, Mr E

worried that symptoms of an upper respiratory viral syndrome represented pneumocystis pneumonia or that seemingly innocuous bumps on the skin were Kaposi's sarcoma. Complete evaluations by an experienced internist and an immunologist turned up no sign of disease but were only mildly and transiently reassuring to the patient. He, thus, was referred for psychotherapeutic evaluation.

Mr E's mental status examination revealed no evidence of psychotic process, bipolar disorder, or addiction. Though he recognized there was no 'logical' basis for his fears, he remained anxious. Remarkably soon after the therapy began, the panic about contracting HIV began to fade and was replaced with anxiously reported material about his sexual life. Mr E reluctantly mentioned his predilection for sadomasochistic sexual activity with hustlers. When asked about those practices by his therapist, Mr E protested that it would be far too embarrassing to ever discuss such a thing with his therapist.

Mr E's practice of unprotected sex with hustlers was a secret that he controlled, usually divulging only to those who would participate fully and share in the enactment of the secret, thereby avoiding the shame and humiliation of revealing it as well as protecting him from losing control over the use of this powerful and important part of his mental life. Shame and humiliation and the need to control the secret entered the transference as forceful resistances. It became clear that he was inviting his therapist to extract the secret from him for what the patient imagined was the therapist's own voyeuristic excitement, re-creating in the transference the sadomasochistic couple of his sexual enactments, with the therapist experienced as the hustler. Over time, the therapist was able to interpret the patient's enactment as an important defense of his, to turn what made him anxious into a harmless game.

Trying to approach patients such as Mr E merely by re-educating them about safer sexual practices and reinforcing the risks of their behavior can paradoxically worsen the risk of infection rather than lowering it. The clinician's well-intentioned 're-education' about his risky sexual behavior fits too seamlessly into the defensive structure of the patient's personality, a game-like inner world that seeks to turn real danger into harmless play. The unsuspecting clinician may counsel such a patient to 'play it safe', emphasizing 'safe,' and yet this type of patient hears 'play it safe,' emphasizing 'play,' as in 'it's just a game' or 'nothing serious' or 'no real danger.'

As with Mr E. the transference–countertransference in such cases is likely to be a sadomasochistic one, including pressure to violate the psychotherapeutic frame. Consultation and/or ongoing supervision from an experienced psychotherapist will assist the therapist from foundering on the dangerous shoals of boundary violations or patient exploitation (Gabbard and Lester, 1995, p. 193). Careful attention to maintenance of boundaries and countertransference scrutiny and regulation can result in a workable therapeutic alliance that allows the patient safely to explore likely childhood traumas and deprivations that have chronically been reenacted in current symptomatology. As these patients often do not present for psychotherapeutic treatment openly reporting their sexual risk taking, they underscore the importance of tactfully eliciting a careful sexual history in all patients.

In order to deaden painful internalized homophobia, self-loathing, and shame related to homosexuality, some patients turn to illicit drugs and/or alcohol. The therapist must explicitly ask the patient about a history of drug and alcohol use and abuse both in the past and present. If a drug or alcohol problem is present and of sufficient severity that it impairs social, occupational, or interpersonal functioning, medically supervised detoxification, drug/alcohol rehabilitation, and/or relapse prevention and recovery programs (such as Alcoholics Anonymous or Narcotics Anonymous) may be necessary in the context of ongoing supportive psychotherapy.

Compulsive sexuality can put the individual at risk for contracting HIV and presents the therapist with a serious management problem. Compulsive sexuality can be used to anesthetize psychic pain, stave off emotional conflict, or stabilize a fragmenting sense of self. Formulating such behaviors as compulsions offers psychodynamic psychotherapists powerful therapeutic leverage (Dodes, 1996). The therapist helps the patient to understand that the internal moment of crisis that triggers the desperate, compulsive search for sexual partners is a sense of traumatic helplessness reawakened from the past by a similar, resonant experience in the present. Behavioral therapy has also been shown to be a helpful treatment strategy with compulsive sexuality (McConaghy *et al.*, 1985; Konopacki and Oei, 1988). For a detailed discussion of the nature and management of sexual disorders, the reader is referred to Chapter 17 (this volume).

Conclusions

Perhaps more than any other encounter in clinical practice, the meeting of a therapist with a gay patient has long been configured by social forces. Those forces have shifted over the past few decades, both mercifully—as with the increased acceptance of gay people into social institutions—and disastrously, with the emergence of HIV.

As the realities that impinge on our patients continue to change, so will their needs for us evolve. Clinicians who work with homosexual patients must surely be humbled by the powerful effect of cultural factors far beyond their control on their daily work with patients. But they may also enjoy the hope that the biases that lie at the root of so many of the problems they struggle to repair may diminish, even perhaps one day, vanish.

Loewald (1960) wrote memorably of the benefit to the patient of the therapist's holding in mind a view of him as one day becoming healthier, more capable. Those who devote hours treating patients who have suffered from bigotry and rejection may find it similarly helpful to keep in mind that some day, at least in this one small area, society itself may improve.

References

Auchincloss, E. and Vaughan, S. (2001). Psychoanalysis and homosexuality: do we need a new theory. *Journal of the American Psychoanalytic Association*, **49**(4), 1157–86.

Beck, A. T. and Freeman, A. (1990). *Cognitive therapy of personality disorders*. New York: Guilford Press.

Bernstein, G. S. and Miller, M. E. (1995). Behavior therapy with lesbian and gay individuals. In: M. Hersen, R. M. Eisler, and P. M. Miller, ed. *Progress in behavior modification*, Vol. 30, pp. 19–45. Newbury Park, CA: Sage.

Blanch, J., *et al.* (2002). Assessment of the efficacy of a cognitive-behavioural liaison psychiatry department. *Psychotherapy and Psychosomatics*, **71**(2), 77–84.

Blechner, M. (1997). Psychodynamic approaches to AIDS and HIV. In: M. Blechner, ed. *Hope and mortality: psychodynamic approaches to AIDS and HIV*, pp. 3–62. Hillsdale, NJ: Analytic Press, Inc.

Cass, V. C. (1989). Homosexual identity formation: a theoretical model. *Journal of Homosexuality*, **4**, 219–35.

Coates, S. W. and Wolfe, S. M. (1995). Gender identity disorder in boys: the interface of constitution and early experience. *Psychoanalytic Inquiry*, **15**, 6–38.

Coleman, E. (1982). Developmental stages of the coming out process. *Journal of Homosexuality*, **7**, 2–3.

Corbett, K. (1996). Homosexual boyhood: notes on girlyboys. *Gender and Psychoanalysis*, **1**, 429–61.

Dodes, L. M. (1996). Compulsion and addiction. *Journal of the American Psychoanalytic Association*, **44**, 815–35.

Downey, J. I. and Friedman, R. C. (1995). Internalized homophobia in lesbian relationships. *Journal of the American Academy of Psychoanalysis*, **23**, 435–47.

Ehrhardt, A. A. (1985). Gender differences: a biosocial perspective. *Psychology and Gender*, **32**, 37–57.

Floyd, F., Stein, T., Harter, K., Allison, A., and Nye, C. (1999). Gay, lesbian, and bisexual youths: Separation-individuation, parental attitudes, identity consolidation, and well-being. *Journal of Youth and Adolescence*, **28**, 719–39.

Friedman, R. C. (1997). Response to Ken Corbett's 'Homosexual boyhood': notes on girlyboys. *Gender and Psychoanalysis*, **2**, 487–94.

Friedman, R. C. (2001). Psychoanalysis and human sexuality. *Journal of the American Psychoanalytic Association*, **49**(4), 1115–32.

Friedman, R. C. and Downey, J. I. (1995). Internalized homophobia and the negative therapeutic reaction in homosexual men. *Journal of the American Academy of Psychoanalysis*, **23**, 99–113.

Friedman, R. C. and Downey, J. I. (2002). *Sexual orientation and psychoanalysis: sexual science and clinical practice*. New York: Columbia University Press.

Frommer, M. (1994). Homosexuality and psychoanalysis: technical considerations revisited (with commentaries by O. Renik and C. Spezzano). *Psychoanalytic Dialogues*, **4**, 215–51.

Gabbard, G. O. and Lester, E. P. (1995). *Boundaries and boundary violations in psychoanalysis*. New York: Basic Books.

Goldsmith, S. J. (1995). Oedipus or Orestes? Aspects of gender identity development in homosexual men. *Psychoanalytic Inquiry*, **15**, 112–24.

Goldsmith, S. J. (2001). Oedipus or Orestes? Homosexual men, their mothers, and other women revisited. *Journal of the American Psychoanalytic Association*, **49**, 1269–87.

Isay, R. A. (1987). Fathers and their homosexually inclined sons in childhood. *Psychoanalytic Study of the Child*, **42**, 275–94.

Isay, R. A. (1989). *Being homosexual: gay men and their development*. New York: Farrar Strauss Giroux.

Isay, R. A. (1996). *Becoming gay: the journey to self-acceptance*. New York: Pantheon.

Isay, R. A. (1999). Gender in homosexual boys: some developmental and clinical considerations. *Psychiatry: Interpersonal and Biological Processes*, **62**(2), 187–94.

Kertzner, R. (2001). The adult life course and homosexual identity in midlife gay men. *Annual Review of Sex Research*, **12**: 75–92.

Konopacki, W. P. and Oei, T. P. (1988). Interruption in the maintenance of compulsive sexual disorder. *Archives of Sexual Behavior*, **17**(5), 411–19.

Lee, M. R., Cohen, L., Hadley, S. W., and Goodwin, F. K. (1999). Cognitive-behavioral group therapy with medication for depressed gay men with AIDS or symptomatic HIV infection. *Psychiatric Services*, **50**(7), 948–52.

Loewald, H. (1960). On the therapeutic action of psychoanalysis. *International Journal of Psychoanalysis*, **41**, 16–33.

Markowitz, J. C., *et al.* (1998). Treatment of depressive symptoms in human immunodeficiency virus-positive patients. *Archives of General Psychiatry*, **55**(5), 452–7.

McConaghy, N., Armstrong, M. S., and Blaszczynski, A. (1985). Expectancy, covert sensitization and imaginal desensitization in compulsive sexuality. *Acta Psychiatrica Scandinavica*, **72**(2), 176–87.

Mitchell, S. (1996). Gender and sexual orientation in the age of postmodernism: the plight of the perplexed clinician. *Gender and Psychoanalysis*, **1**, 45–74.

Molassiotis, A., Callaghan, P., Twinn, S. F., Chung, W. Y., and Li, C. K. (2002). A pilot study of the effects of cognitive–behavioral group therapy and peer support/counseling in decreasing psychologic distress and improving quality of life in Chinese patients with symptomatic HIV disease. *AIDS Patient Care and STDS*, **16**(2), 83–96.

Nicolosi, J. (1991). *Reparative therapy of male homosexuality: a new clinical approach*. Northvale, NJ: Jason Aronson.

Nicolosi, J. (1993). *Healing homosexuality: case stories of reparative therapy*. Northvale, NJ: Jason Aronson.

Notman, M. (2002). Changes in sexual orientation and object choice in midlife women. *Psychoanalytic Inquiry*, **22**, 182–95.

Phillips, S. H. (2001). The overstimulation of everyday life: I. New aspects of male homosexuality. *Journal of the American Psychoanalytic Association*, **49**(4), 1235–67.

Phillips, S. H. (2002). The overstimulation of everyday life: II. Male homosexuality, countertransference, and psychoanalytic treatment. *The Annual of Psychoanalysis*, **30**, 131–45.

Purcell, D. W., Campos, P. E., and Perilla, J. L. (1996). Therapy with lesbians and gay men: a cognitive behavioral perspective. *Cognitive and Behavioral Practice*, **3**, 391–415.

Richardson, J. (1999). Finding the disorder in gender identity disorder. *Harvard Review of Psychiatry*, **7**, 43–50.

Roughton, R. (1999). Repair, analyze, or affirm? Reflections on treatment for gay men. Presented at the meeting of the American Psychoanalytic Association, New York City, December 17, 1999.

Roughton, R. (2001). Four men in treatment: an evolving perspective on homosexuality and bisexuality, 1965 to 2000. *Journal of the American Psychoanalytic Association*, **49**, 1187–217.

Safren, S. A., Hollander, G., Hart, T. A., and Heimberg, R. G. (2001a). Cognitive-behavioral therapy with lesbian, gay, and bisexual youth. *Cognitive and Behavioral Practice*, **8**, 215–23.

Safren, S. A., *et al.* (2001b). Two strategies to increase adherence to HIV antiretroviral medication: life-steps and medication monitoring. *Behaviour Research and Therapy*, **39**(10), 1151–62.

Shidlo, A., Schroeder, M., and Drescher, J., ed. (2001). *Sexual conversion therapy: ethical, clinical, and research perspectives*. New York: The Haworth Medical Press.

Spencer, S. B. and Hemmer, R. C. (1993). Therapeutic bias with gay and lesbian clients: a functional analysis. *The Behavior Therapist*, **16**, 93–97.

Tyson, P. (2002). The challenges of psychoanalytic developmental theory. *Journal of the American Psychoanalytic Association*, **50**, 19–52.

Vaughan, S. (1998). Psychoanalytic and biological perspectives on lesbian patients: why developmental themes are more important in psychotherapy. *Harvard Review of Psychiatry*, **6**(3), 160–4.

Whitam, F. L. and Mathy, R. M. (1991). Childhood cross-gender behavior of homosexual females in Brazil, Peru, the Philippines, and the United States. *Archives of Sexual Behavior*, **20**, 151–70.

Whitam, F. L. and Zent, M. (1984). A cross-cultural assessment of early cross-gender behavior and familial factors in male homosexuality. *Archives of Sexual Behavior*, **13**, 427–39.

Zevy, L. (1999). Sexing the tomboy. In: M. Rottnek, ed. *Sissies and tomboys: Gender nonconformity and homosexual childhood*. pp. 80–195. New York: New York University Press.

Zucker, K. J. (1999). Commentary of Richardson's 1996 setting limits on gender health. *Harvard Review of Psychiatry*, **7**, 34–42.

36 Cross-Cultural psychotherapy

Pedro Ruiz, Irma J. Bland, Edmond H. Pi, and Felicity de Zulueta

Introduction

During the last 10–15 years, there has been an extensive globalization process that has affected most areas of the world, and has also impacted on all aspects of society, including health care. Concomitantly, there has additionally been a strong migration process from developing countries and regions toward industrialized nations. This migratory process began after World War II, and has intensified during the last two to three decades (Ruiz, 1995a). In the USA this process has led to a multiethnic and multicultural growth as never seen before in this country. This pluralistic transformation of the American society has been manifested in all aspects of life, including the healthcare system.

This situation is not unique of the USA. In Europe, something very similar is currently happening. An estimated 500 000 illegal immigrants enter the European Union annually (Walt, 2002). During the year 2000, 680 300 legal immigrants entered the European countries. In 2002, the legal migration to Europe has been as follows: Italy: 181 300; Great Britain: 140 000; Germany: 105 300; France: 55 000; the Netherlands: 53 100; Sweden: 24 400; Greece: 23 900; Spain: 20 800; Ireland: 20 000; Austria: 17 300; Belgium: 12 100; Portugal: 11 000; Denmark: 10 100; Luxembourg: 3600; and Finland: 2400. The easy mobility between the countries of the European Union makes this situation more complex and relevant.

On a parallel basis, and in many ways as a result of this globalization and migratory process, cross-cultural psychiatry has also grown extensively during the last two to three decades. In this context, World War II helped to realize the complexity and magnitude of psychiatric disorders and conditions. It also helped to focus on the specific characteristics of psychiatric disorders, as they were manifested among soldiers from different ethnic and cultural backgrounds (Ruiz, 1995a). Several books and journals focusing on cross-cultural psychiatry were published following the termination of World War II (Opler, 1959; Ruiz, 1995b), as well as the creation of the Joint Commission on Mental Illness and Health in 1955 and the Action for Mental Health Proposal in 1961 (Ruiz, 1995b). Additionally, the American Psychiatric Association, via its Board of Trustees, approved in 1969 a position statement officially delineating 'transcultural psychiatry' as a specialized field of study (American Psychiatric Association, 1969). The Canadian Psychiatric Association concomitantly approved this position statement. Along these lines, during the last two to three decades the world medical literature has clearly witnessed an extensive scientific growth in the field of cross-cultural psychiatry. In this respect, it is important to define for the benefit of our readers the terms ethnicity, race, and culture.

- *Ethnicity* refers to a subjective sense of belonging to a group of persons who share a common origin. Thus, ethnicity becomes a component of one's sense of identity, and, therefore reflects a series of clinical and social manifestations pertaining to a person's self-image and intrapsychic life (Ruiz, 1998a).

- *Race* is defined as the conceptual process in which human beings chose to group themselves based primarily on their common physiognomy. Physical, biological, and genetic connotations are part of this concept (Ruiz, 1998a).

- *Culture* is defined as a set of meanings, behavioral norms, values, everyday practices, and beliefs used by members of a given group in society as a way of conceptualizing their view of the world and their interactions with the environment. In this respect, language, religion, and social relationships are manifestations of one's own culture (Alarcon and Ruiz, 1995; Ruiz, 1998a, b; Gonzalez *et al.*, 2001).

Based on this premise, in this chapter we address psychotherapy within the boundaries of cross-cultural psychiatry. We focus on the most relevant psychotherapeutic issues pertaining to the major cultural and ethnic groups in America, including African-American patients, Hispanic patients, and Asian-American patients. Finally, we discuss psychotherapeutic issues with respect to the ethnic migrant patients from western Europe, especially England.

We should underline once more that the psychotherapeutic issues discussed in these cultural and ethnic groups are generic and relevant to other ethnic and cultural groups as well. Although specific manifestations might be different in each ethnic and cultural subgroup the understanding from a theoretical and clinical perspective is universal. In other words, it has theoretical and clinical applicability to all ethnic and cultural groups around the world. We also hope that this chapter will stimulate further interest in this very relevant subspecialty field within psychiatry, and that further investigational efforts will result from these renewed interests.

Psychotherapy with African-American patients

African-Americans are a heterogeneous group of individuals of multiple skin hues, hair textures, cultural backgrounds, ideologies, levels of education, and economic status. As a collective however, they share the history of the enslavement of their ancestors, and its legacy of segregation, oppression, and racial discrimination. African-Americans differ in the degree to which they claim their history, the sense of continuity with their historical past, resolution of conflicts about their past and present, the level of integration of racial identity, and the healthy adaptation regarding their race. While the history of slavery and the struggles of racism are unique, as experienced in the lives of African-Americans, the psychological impact of traumatic and demoralizing experiences is not. Unresolved issues in this area create conflict, as well as emotional and narcissistic vulnerability for which compensatory defenses are erected. This siphons off creative energy interferes with the consolidation of a positive sense of self, and limits a full affective participation and healthy adaptation in life. We must give legitimacy to the uniqueness of these experiences, expand our therapeutic inquiry, and gain further insight into their impact on the psychological lives of our individual patients. Only then can we assure the effective application of psychotherapy with African-American patients, with adequate working through of areas of conflict, affirmation of racial identity, and the restoration of the sense of self and human dignity.

Stress, coping, and adaptation

In doing psychotherapy with African-Americans, one must understand well the stress they face and their coping and adaptation styles. While sociological changes have gradually begun to shift the balance in some ways, the residuals of segregation and racism create, in the psychotherapeutic setting, a chronically stressful environment for African-Americans. It remains a social milieu in which they must continually demand equal status, equal resources, and equal opportunity, and then prove their worthiness. African-Americans must work harder to find ways to affirm and validate the self, struggle constantly against negative stereotypes, and must continue to function despite a sense of emotional vulnerability. Many succumb to despair and all of its self-destructive influences (substance abuse, violence, crime, etc.) in a desperate search for self, while simultaneously externalizing the internally felt defective sense of self. Others have found creative ways to cope and to adapt.

Greene (1994) describes the multiple social stressors, cultural imperatives, and psychological realities faced by the African-American woman as she attempts to fulfill her role as provider, protector, caretaker, and nurturer, with little external validation, personal nurturing, comfort, or support. African-American women have attempted to cope with these stresses through a sense of connectedness with family and community, through hope in a better life for their children, and through their spirituality. A major form of adaptation for many African-American women has been stoicism, the internalized ego ideal of the 'strong black woman'.

The struggle for African-American men is even more tortuous. Grier and Cobbs (1980) describe the conundrum that the African-American man faces from early childhood at the hands of his own mother. The African-American mother must rear her son in such a way that inevitably crushes his natural ambition, defiant spirit, and aggressiveness, and discourages his maturity and independence in order to assure his physical survival. Subsequently, from birth to death the African-American man must fight for his physical and psychological survival, while on a journey of self-discovery, personal empowerment, and reconciliation with his past and the realities of his existence. White and Cones (1999) define this task as consisting of: (1) a search for self and masculine identity; (2) the challenge of sustaining intimacy and involvement in relationships; (3) coping with the realities of racism; (4) maintaining black consciousness; and (5) finding adaptive possibilities within the African-American way of being, while integrating African-American and European American life-styles. Many African-American men have made this journey channeling their passion and anger into intellectual and creative contributions, sociopolitical activities or Afrocentric community involvement. Many others continue to search for self and to define their masculinity through gang activities, an endless cycle of projected self-hatred, or 'go for bad' masculinity (White and Cones, 1999). Still others succumb in despair, immobilized, having given up, subsumed in drugs and alcohol.

Although influenced by a particular culture, the basic role of the family is universal. The role of the family is to provide basic physical resources for its members; loving affection; a sense of safety and security; to define values, roles, responsibilities, and competencies; and to serve as positive mirrors and models of idealization to facilitate consolidation of self-esteem in their children. The balance of stresses are different for poor and middle class African-American families, but both must cope with societal barriers that limit access to needed resources and the struggles and burdens of its individual members to maintain some sense of self and human dignity, which in combination undermine the family's ability to develop fully the system functions that it must serve.

The ascension into the middle class has created a different challenge and burden, and with it the fantasy that having arrived with education and financial resources, that race would not matter. A new challenge of adaptation has been necessary for the black middle class. Coner-Edwards and Spurlock (1988) examine the stress and crisis that this ascension has created for African-American families, and the multiple ways in which they have attempted to cope and adapt to their new found status, particularly their 'survivors guilt', and issues regarding identity and class affiliation.

Access to psychotherapeutic treatment

For some time African-Americans were systematically excluded from psychotherapeutic interventions solely based on race and social class (Yamamoto and Steinberg, 1981). Therapists low expectations, interactive factors with patients, e.g., problems developing the therapeutic alliance, or difficulties for majority therapists in working through troubled transactions with African-American patients led to early dropouts (Mohl et al., 1991). Still today, access to psychotherapeutic treatments are restricted by patient mistrust, lack of awareness and education about the effectiveness of these interventions, limited financial resources, and by the therapist bias and selection factors. Additionally, a large percentage of African-Americans are uninsured and dependent on public mental health services in which access to psychotherapeutic treatments are limited or nonexistent.

Jackson and Greene (2000) consider psychodynamic theories to be ethnocentric, based on white, upper middle class, European standards, which perpetuate sex-role stereotypes, pathologize difference, and fail to provide a depth understanding of the 'experience of the other'. They attempt to analyze and reformulate traditional psychodynamic theories regarding African-American women, to explicate the complexities, and to dispel myths. They agree, however, that African-Americans function no differently on an unconscious level, psychologically, than others. Also, that the real task is to expand our theoretical paradigms and therapeutic inquiry to take into account the impact of historical, social, political, and real life experiences of African-Americans, to understand better the psychodynamic underpinnings of their psychological experiences, and to more accurately guide the education and training of future clinicians. Foulks et al. (1995) develop the argument that a supportive-expressive psychotherapy that conforms to standardized guidelines is more effective and discuss factors that can lead to optimal outcomes in a cross-cultural context. Although they do not negate the usefulness of 'ethnic specific' therapies where feasible, they do caution against the proliferation of an array of 'ethnic-specific' therapies that avoid the task of the effective application of psychotherapy across cultures.

Engagement and development of the therapeutic alliance

Regardless of the specific type of psychotherapeutic treatment, no effective process can occur without engagement and the establishment of a therapeutic alliance with the patient. Bland and Kraft (1998) examine the therapeutic alliance from a psychoanalytic perspective, and demonstrate common problems in its development across cultures. They illustrate how clearly perceived differences (such as race with a black patient and a white therapist) create an experience of social distance for both patient and therapist. This mobilizes mistrust and anxiety in the patient thus decreasing self-disclosure, and causing anxiety in the therapist that leads to potential countertransference enactments. Only by openly acknowledging this potential impediment is the therapist able to gain credibility with the patient, which can facilitate empathic bonding, development of the therapeutic alliance and ultimately leads to a successful treatment outcome (Bland and Kraft, 1998).

Racially matched versus cross-matched therapeutic dyads

The therapist's empathy, ability to listen, experience, and skill are the best determinants of the effective application of psychotherapy, including with African-American patients. While no empirical comparative studies have demonstrated the differential superiority of racially matched versus cross-matched therapeutic dyads of patient and therapist, some articles have suggested certain advantages in the conduct of psychotherapy when the patient and therapist are alike, and there is the perception of commonality (whether real or imagined) on the part of the patient. Foulks et al. (1995) in a study of more than 120 African-American, cocaine-dependent men treated with supportive-expressive psychotherapy in a racially matched therapeutic dyad, observed ease of engagement, more natural establishment of empathy, and lessen negative countertransference. Patients also appeared to experience affirmation of self and racial identity, which facilitated the therapeutic process. Jones (1982) found no differences in psychotherapy outcome as a function of client–therapist racial match, although there were differences in therapy process. Comas Diaz and Jacobsen (1991) caution against potential over-resonance, overidentification, and countertransference collusion in racially matched therapeutic dyads. Racial match may be more critical under specific circumstances, e.g., when there are high levels of mistrust, narcissistic issues, identity conflicts or extreme tentativeness in the commitment to therapy (Bland and Kraft, 1998).

Transference and countertransference: working through troubled transactions

Because of their history, experiences, and struggles with prejudice and discrimination, African-Americans may enter psychotherapy with white therapists with several plaguing questions (at times conscious, at times unconscious): (1) Can I trust this person? (2) Can I reveal my true self? (3) Will I be understood? (4) Will I be judged negatively? (5) Will I be exploited? While these may be similar to questions of any patient, African-Americans' real and pervasive experiences with racism give these questions unique meaning and intensity. This, in conjunction with the individual's specific intrapsychic conflicts, may lead to transference and early phase resistance manifested as anger and failure to self disclose. This creates anxiety in the therapist, whose need to be helpful is thwarted and if not correctly understood can result in countertransference enactments. The therapist may prematurely judge the patient as unmotivated, unpsychologically minded, and unsuitable for treatment (Bland and Kraft, 1998). By rejecting the patient before being rejected, the therapist contains his own anxiety, avoids acknowledging his anger, and wards off rejection and the associated narcissistic injury. Evans (1985) cautions against premature interpretation of race focused content in treatment as defense and resistance, and encourages deeper exploration of these issues. Grier and Cobbs (1980) suggest that, although for different reasons, both white and black therapists may unconsciously avoid exploration of these issues because it is too painful. Black therapists may fear overidentification and resonation with their patients' vulnerability, despair, and anger, while white therapists may fear mobilization of feelings of guilt and an assault from the patient's angry feelings. Whether white or black, the therapist must be aware of and able to manage his own countertransference reactions. Only then is he/she able to be available to the patient and to provide a secure container for expression of the patient's affective experiences (including race focused issues), to help the patient work through conflicts, to develop more effective coping mechanisms, to work through negative internalizations, and to develop a more positive, confident, and competent sense of self.

Integration of the sense of self and racial identity in psychotherapy

Most scholars are beginning to agree that race is a cultural invention that serves to stratify the social system and has no intrinsic relationship to actual human physical characteristics (Smedley, 1999). Negative stereotypes have been attached to the physical, mental, and moral characteristics of African-Americans based on race. Despite its negative effect, racial identity for African-Americans is an important part of their sense of self and identity. The sense of connectedness as members of a group with a shared history, experiences, and world view has helped them to bear the common struggles of their black reality. At the same time, it has created psychological distress and conflict, which has interfered with the internalization and consolidation of a positive sense of self and racial identity. Thus, in psychotherapy, the formation of a positive sense of self and racial identity for African-Americans is a dynamic process over time involving a transformation of an internalized negative sense of self and various levels of conflict about 'blackness', to a more positive integrated sense of self and racial identity.

Cross (1991) has described four stages in this process of racial identity formation, each corresponding to a set of feelings, beliefs, and attitudes of the individual regarding being black. Stage 1 (preencounter): there is a sense of neutrality or the denial of blackness, 'human beings who just happen to be black'; stage 2 (encounter): a series of positive or negative, but decisively felt experiences compel the individual to turn to his racial group membership and identification with his blackness; stage 3 (immersion): there is a vortex of change with idealization and immersion in black interests, involvements, activities, in search of self and black group membership; and stage 4 (internalization): there is a resolution of conflicts and transformation of negative self feelings, firmly grounded in a sense of pride, self-acceptance, and deep sense of connection to the black community with a tolerance of diversity and acceptance of others and their views. Wherever the individual African-American is or settles along this continuum has a decisive influence on his sense of self, group membership, and resolution of conflicts about his blackness. This issue thus needs to be understood and addressed when doing psychotherapy with African-American patients.

African-Americans cannot be divorced from their history or their real life experiences with racism. Our knowledge base and the literature continue to expand regarding the interface of black reality and the psychology of African-Americans. We need to utilize this knowledge to expand our theoretical paradigms, and to guide psychotherapeutic inquiry in order to provide more effective applications of psychotherapy with African-Americans. Clinical reports suggest that African-Americans respond favorably to psychotherapy treatments. More research is needed to demonstrate clinical effectiveness, as well as how treatments may need to be modified (US Department of Health and Human Services, 2001a).

Psychotherapy with Hispanic patients

In accordance to the Census of 2000 (US Bureau of the Census, 2000a), there are about 32.2 million of Hispanics living in the USA. This number represents 12.5% of the total US population, which is 281.4 million. Hispanics, however, are not a monolithic group; about 58.5% are of Mexican origin, 9.6% are Puerto Ricans, 4.8% are Central Americans, 3.8% are South Americans, 3.5% are Cubans, 2.2% are Dominicans, 0.3% are Spaniards, and 17.3% are from other Hispanic origins. In some cities of the USA, Hispanics represent the majority of the population. For instance, Hispanics represent 77% of the population in El Paso, 66% in Miami, and 59% in San Antonio.

A sociodemographic factor of concern for Hispanics is the number of female-headed households; 39.4% of the Puerto Rican families and 26.8% of the Central and South American families are headed by females, as compared only with 14.2% of Caucasian families. Additionally, Hispanic families have an average annual income of $30 735 in comparison with $44 366 for the Caucasian families. Also, only 10.3% of Hispanics reach an educational level of college/university in comparison with 24.6% for Caucasians. Finally, 21.7% of Hispanic families live under the poverty level, in comparison with only 5.7% of Caucasian families. These sociodemographic characteristics certainly have much relevance in diagnosing and treating Hispanic populations, particularly in a psychotherapeutic setting.

The meaning of symptoms

In psychotherapy, the concept of symptom formation has a very important meaning and significance. In this respect, it is important to understand the meaning of symptoms for a large number of Hispanics. For many Hispanics, some psychiatric symptoms are perceived as manifestations of strength, and thus to be cherished and retained (Ruiz, 1982). For instance, hallucinatory experiences could be perceived as a manifestation of 'mediunity', and therefore as a religious gift with potential healing powers. Attempts to eradicate this type of symptomatology in a psychotherapeutic setting might lead to resistances and challenges to the appropriate development and maintenance of the therapeutic alliance. From a different perspective, certain other symptoms can manifest themselves differently among some Hispanic patients. For instance, depressive symptomatology may be manifested by Hispanics as fatigue, headaches, body aches, and feelings of weakness and exhaustion; that is, primarily about somatic lines. Likewise, anxiety, in and of it self, may not be recognized well by some Hispanic patients. In these cases, anxiety could be manifested as dizziness, heart palpitations, and feelings of fainting (Abad and Boyce, 1979). Similarly, anger may be manifested among Hispanics as nervousness or malaise. Also, manifestations of aggression are not well tolerated or socially acceptable. In all of these situations, the meaning of symptoms needs to be well understood, and thus managed accordingly in the psychotherapeutic setting.

Conceptualization of mental illness

For many Hispanics, the conceptualization of mental illness is different than for other ethnic groups, especially Anglo-Saxons. Etiologically, Hispanics might perceive mental illness either as a supernatural phenomenon or associated to certain religious beliefs. For instance, psychosis may be explained by Hispanics as a manifestation of being possessed by spirits (Ruiz, 1977). This belief tends to be quite common among Hispanics from the Caribbean basin who believe in Spiritism (Ruiz, 1985). Likewise, some Hispanics might perceive mental illnesses as a result of God's punishment (Ruiz, 1998a). In these cases, the appropriate management of 'guilt' within the psychotherapeutic relationship is of paramount importance. In certain religions, as in the Pentecostal Church, psychiatric symptoms such as hallucinations might be perceived and conceptualized as 'miracles'. For many Pentecostals, 'miracles' are a welcomed expectation rather than a manifestation of psychiatric illnesses. The appropriate understanding and management of these situations will certainly lead to a good outcome when doing psychotherapeutic interventions with Hispanic patients.

Understanding family dynamics

As in any other ethnic group, family dynamics are very unique, and require appropriate understanding and management when doing psychotherapy with Hispanic patients. Hispanics place high value on the family as a central point of their lives (Ruiz, 1982). Contrary to the American culture where the nuclear family represents the core element of the family structure, the extended family network tends to predominate among Hispanics and, thus, given high priority and relevance by them (Ruiz, 1982). Among Hispanics, the extended family includes not only all relatives, but friends, neighbors, and coworkers as well. This extended family network system can be very beneficial among families from low socioeconomic levels.

For Hispanic children who reside and grow up in the USA, this type of extended family network system offers them the opportunity to bond at an early age not only with his/her parents but with grandfathers, cousins, aunts and uncles, and even godparents and friends as well (Pumariega and Ruiz, 1997). Contrary to the American culture, which is individualistic and gives a high priority in achieving independence, the Hispanic culture is oriented towards a strong family and an extended family unity and gives a high priority to the achievement of interdependence. These cultural differences need to be taken in full consideration when offering psychotherapy to members of a Hispanic family; particularly, among first and second generations of Hispanic families. However, as members of Hispanic families achieve high levels of acculturation in the USA, a different psychotherapeutic perspective should also be entertained.

A dynamic factor that must also be taken into consideration when doing psychotherapy with Hispanic patients is that of 'machismo' (Ruiz, 1995a). Among traditional Hispanic families, it is common to observe a male-oriented hierarchical system. In these families, the father is sought when discipline of the children is needed; the mother is always a source of support and nurture; boys and girls are raised with different behavioral and occupational expectations; also, the expectation of 'male responsibility' is an issue of honor. While acculturation and generations tend to change Hispanic families substantially, the impact of traditional values needs to be given full consideration when psychotherapeutically treating Hispanic patients.

Language considerations

When doing psychotherapy with patients with a native language different than the language of the therapist certain factors need to be considered. It is known that Hispanic patients who speak in a language different than their native language are likely to be perceived as more depressed, more psychotic and with more cognitive impairment than patients who speak the same language of their therapists (Marcos et al., 1973). Language barriers can also lead to underutilization of mental health services, diagnostic errors, and poor mental health care (Gomez et al., 1985). However, it has additionally been reported that psychotherapeutic success can also be achieved when treating patients in their own language or using an acquired language (Gomez et al., 1982). It must be acknowledged, however, that patients could switch from the native language into the acquired language when dealing with emotionally charged psychotherapeutic issues. This is a way of avoiding affectively charged discussions; that is, as a manifestation of resistance (Marcos and Albert, 1976). It must also be noted that the use of interpreters do not offer a good solution to the problem of language barriers as interpreters tend to bring distortions into the translation process; this is primarily based on their own emotional needs and conflicts (Marcos, 1979; Laval et al., 1983).

Finally, the pattern of 'small talk' (la platica) observed among the Hispanic population at large must also be acknowledged. Among Hispanics, it is common to observe them speak for a while about irrelevant topics before they proceed to discuss serious and important matters (Ruiz, 1998b). The knowledge of this communication pattern is of great importance in the psychotherapeutic setting; otherwise, therapists might blame 'resistance' as the cause of this phenomenon or as a lack of interest in the psychotherapeutic treatment.

Nonverbal communication pattern

Hispanics tend to use a lot of nonverbal means of communication when trying to speak with other persons (Ruiz, 1998b). Unfortunately, this pattern of communication often leads to recommendations for somatic therapies rather than psychotherapy. This pattern is, however, culturally related. Thus, once understood it does not represent a deterrent for psychotherapeutic intervention. In many ways, this phenomenon could also be related to another phenomenon that is commonly observed among Hispanics; that is, an increased manifestation of functional somatization. This somatization phenomenon has been well studied among Hispanics and reported in the medical literature (Escobar, 1987; Canino et al., 1992). This cultural characteristic among Hispanics certainly has a major impact on the manifestation of symptoms among Hispanics. For instance, during the manifestations of depressive and anxiety symptomatology as previously discussed. Once understood, it should not represent a barrier to psychotherapy interventions among Hispanic patients.

Culture and the therapeutic alliance

Culture can play a beneficial as well as nonbeneficial role vis-à-vis the development and maintenance of a strong therapeutic alliance. For therapists who have little expertise about the cultural heritage of his/her patients, the development of a strong therapeutic alliance will be a major challenge, and most probably will lead to noncompliance with the recommended psychotherapeutic interventions. Actually, it has been demonstrated that among patients in psychotherapy who have rooted nonmedical beliefs about the causes of their illnesses, the rates of noncompliance and psychotherapy termination is much higher than among those who do not have it (Foulks et al., 1986). Kernberg (1968) understood quite well these problems when he underlined the importance of understanding both the latent and the manifested transference within a cultural matrix.

Hispanic populations, like any other ethnic groups, have their unique cultural characteristics. Thus, when psychiatrically treating Hispanics, particularly along the lines of psychotherapy interventions, it is imperative that psychotherapists be vested in these culturally related characteristics. This cultural understanding and sensitivity on the part of psychotherapists is essential to achieve a beneficial psychotherapeutic outcome.

Psychotherapy with Asian-American patients

It is estimated that more than half of the world's 6.17 billion population is Asian. In the USA, the Asian population is increasing rapidly. Between 1970 and 1990 it nearly quadrupled to 7 million, and from 1990 to 2000 it grew to 10 million; that is, about 3.5% of the US population. Immigration accounts for three-fourths of the rapid growth of the US Asian population; currently, six of 10 US Asians are foreign-born (US Bureau of the Census, 2000b). The overwhelming majority of Asians reside in metropolitan areas (inside or outside central cities) in two western states (California and Hawaii) and three nonwestern states (New York, Texas, and Illinois).

Asians, however, are a very heterogeneous group with different ethnicities, languages, dialects, cultures, religious beliefs, levels of education, and socioeconomic classes. Owing to their migratory experience and history, Asians, including both new immigrants and persons whose families have been here for generations, also vary in terms of acculturation and assimilation. The major Asian groups in the USA are Chinese, Filipino, Asian Indian, Vietnamese, Korean, Japanese, Burmese, Cambodian, Hmong, Laotian, Thai, and Tongan (US Bureau of the Census, 2000b).

Asians speak over 100 languages and dialects. Sixty-seven percent of Asians residing in the USA speak a language other than English at home. Given the high proportion of recent immigrants, more than 35% of Asian households are linguistically isolated (US DHHS, 2001a). Asians also have a bimodal distribution of socioeconomic resources such as income and education. Some Asians clustered in the high income and education categories while others are in the low income and education categories (US Bureau of the Census, 2000b).

Utilization of psychiatric treatment for Asian patients

Asian-Americans have the lowest rates of mental health utilization among US ethnic populations. This underrepresentation in mental health care is characteristic of most Asian groups, regardless of gender, age, and geographic location (US DHHS, 2001b). As Asians tend to underutilize or even avoid mental health care, they have been perceived as a well adjusted 'model minority' and with little or no need for mental health services. However, so far, there is a lack of data specifically addressing the utilization of psychotherapeutic intervention among Asians.

While the majority of people with mental health problems, regardless of race or ethnicity, demonstrate a reluctance to receive treatment, the stigma and shame surrounding mental illness are particularly powerful barriers for Asians to utilize mental health services. As mental disorders are considered taboo, it is stigmatizing to admit psychopathology and to utilize mental health services, even among third and fourth generations of US Asian families (Yamamoto and Acosta, 1982). Additional barriers and deterrents include the Asian tradition of caring for ill members within the family, protecting the family's name and honor, delayed confrontation, racism, fear of discrimination, and differences in language and communication. Some Asian cultures even view suffering as inevitable, and hence may lack an understanding of the need for early intervention and preventive measures. Among those who use mental health services, their conditions often have become severe and chronic by the time they seek treatment, and thus are more often diagnosed as psychotic disorders than among other ethnic groups. Thus they are more likely to require psychopharmacotherapy (Lin et al., 1982; Sue et al., 1991; Kitano et al., 1997; Pi and Gray, 2000). This suggests that Asians delay seeking mental health services until problems become very serious, and those with less severe symptoms may not seek mental health treatment such as psychotherapy.

Cultural context of Asian patients

Recognizing the heterogeneity and diversity of the Asian population in the USA, caution must be exercised in making generalizations about them. Factors such as demographic variables, cultural backgrounds, generational issues, unique life-styles, and assimilation and acculturation levels must be taken into consideration when doing psychotherapy with Asian patients.

Culturally determined health beliefs and practices can profoundly influence psychiatric treatment. A critical issue is whether or not Asians manifest symptoms similar to those found in Western societies. Cultural influences on symptom manifestation are often observed among Asians, which may mislead clinicians who are not familiar with such a phenomenon (Lin, 1996). For example, Asians with a strong somatizing tendency are likely to express their problems in somatic or behavioral terms rather than in emotional ones (Lin, 1996). Thus, they may receive a physical health diagnosis and fail to receive appropriate psychotherapeutic treatment.

The Asian population in the USA is diverse. Some Asian families have remained strongly traditional, while others have assimilated to a considerable extent into 'mainstream' American culture. Significant differences exist between Asian and Western cultures. Asian cultures emphasize the value of responsibility, moderation, restraint, attending to others, fitting in, and harmonious interdependence with others (Markus and Kitayama, 1991). On the other hand, Western culture values independence, individualism, and spontaneity (Sue and Zane, 1987). Asians under the influence of their traditional cultures and philosophies encourage self/inner control to maintain social and familial harmony rather than openly expressing emotions.

An individual's view of psychopathology influences the seeking of particular treatment modalities. Asians tend to have a multifaceted view of the causation of mental illness. For instance, views such as: hereditary, physiological, biochemical, psychological, social, nutritional, infectious, religious, moralistic, and imbalance of energy (Yin and Yang or cold and hot) explanations. Asians believe that mental illness is associated with organic or somatic factors and that mental health involves the avoidance of morbid thoughts (Sue et al., 1976). Asians are also more likely to express somatic symptoms when seeking treatment, sometimes referred to as 'somatization overpsychologization' (Sue and Sue, 1974; White, 1982). Somatization is a 'face-saving' mechanism used to gain assistance for emotional problems they dare not openly express (Mattson, 1993). Often what is verbalized is different from the underlying problem. Many Asians also view Western psychotherapies as attributing psychopathology to intrapsychic or interpersonal conflicts, a concept that is incongruent to the Asian emphasis on somatic factors. Asians may prefer to seek biological therapies over psychotherapies (Sue and Sue, 1987). Even in the presence of Western mental health services, Asian cultures are more holistically oriented. Asians frequently use complementary methods of indigenous or alternative remedies, such as herbal medicine and 'hot' and 'cold' foods. Traditional or folk healing practices such as meditation and religious healing may be relied on as the primary treatment and tried first for psychiatric symptoms. Also, religious values and spirituality are sources of comfort for Asians. Asians who seek Western mental health treatment may still maintain many of their healing traditions, including the notion of brief intervention, magical cures, and concurrent consultation with many other healers. Thus, long-term recovery strategies and persistence with a given treatment modality may not be well understood by them.

One of the most important characteristics of Asian cultures is their family values, such as family cohesiveness and stability. In relation to empathy and transference in the treatment of the family, especially in those who are not acculturated to the mainstream culture, empathy needs to be applied to both the individual and his or her family. A family-oriented approach that recognizes the family unit and getting family members involved in psychotherapeutic interventions is an essential element of a successful healing process; particularly in working with issues involving two or more family generations.

Language plays a very important role in psychotherapy. How to communicate in a culturally palatable, sensitive, or competent way is always a challenging clinical issue when working with culturally and linguistically diverse Asian patients; especially with less acculturated Asian patients who also have limited English proficiency. Bilingual interpreters are often involved in the evaluation and treatment process, but not without difficulties and problems. The best solution may be to match bilingual psychotherapists with Asian patients. Transference and countertransference (both positive and negative) reactions must, however, be carefully addressed (Yamamoto et al., 1993).

Regarding the issue of therapist–patient match or 'fit' in the process of psychotherapy, one should not automatically assume that the patient prefers an Asian therapist. For Asians who are already acculturated into the mainstream US majority culture, Western psychotherapeutic modalities can be readily applied with little modification; although the traditional cultural values still need to be considered during the course of psychotherapy.

Integration of multiethnic and multicultural modalities of treatment with Asian patients

The issue of which type of psychotherapy should be applied to patients from different ethnic or cultural groups, as well as their appropriateness, has been raised. Psychodynamic psychotherapy has sometimes been criticized as inappropriate and ineffective with nonwhites, and empirically high dropout rates and less than optimal outcomes have been reported (Trujillo, 2000). Many Asians believe that therapists from the traditional US mental health system cannot help them (Root, 1985), and thus are skeptical toward Western forms of psychotherapy. There are, additionally, many common myths regarding the provision of psychotherapy to Asian patients. These include the myth that psychodynamic psychotherapy is inappropriate for patients belonging to different cultural traditions and that long-term psychotherapy is ineffective. Studies have reported that compliance with psychotherapy may, however, be more problematic among non-Western than Western populations. For example, some Asians believe that the Western therapies are too confrontational (Sue and Sue, 1987), and Asians tend to prefer psychotherapists who provide structure, guidance, and direction rather than nondirective advice and interactions (Atkinson et al., 1978).

Sue and Zane (1987) have pointed out that the role of culture and cultural techniques in psychotherapy is perhaps the most difficult issue facing the mental health field. Cultural knowledge and techniques are frequently applied in inappropriate ways, with psychotherapists acting on insufficient knowledge or overgeneralizations. They suggest that cultural knowledge and culture-consistent strategies should be linked to two basic processes: credibility and giving. Credibility refers to an Asian patient's perception that the therapist is both effective and trustworthy. Giving refers to the Asian patient's perception that something of significant value was received from the psychotherapeutic encounter. Asians need to feel a direct benefit or 'gift' from the treatment and a direct relationship between work in psychotherapy and the alleviation of problems. Some of the 'gifts' (immediate benefits) may include anxiety reduction, depression relief, cognitive clarity, reassurance, hope and faith, skills acquisition, developing a coping perspective, and goals setting (Sue and Zane, 1987). Also of normalization; that is, a process to realize that thoughts, feelings, or experiences are common, and that many individuals encounter similar experiences (Sue and Morishima, 1982). A balance between cultural knowledge and these two therapeutic processes is necessary in order to achieve positive psychotherapy outcomes and to prevent Asian patients from dropping out of treatment.

It is not possible to pick one 'right' or 'specific' form of psychotherapy for all Asians; although there are culture-specific psychotherapies in Asia, such as Morita therapy. Morita therapy is a very unique form of psychotherapy used primarily in Japan. Morita therapy does not address psychological conflicts or use psychotherapy techniques such as transference or dream analysis; its main objective is to free the patient from excessive self-preoccupation and intellectualizations as well as help the patient accept things as they are (Fujii et al., 1993). Also, cognitive-behavioral psychotherapy was found to be effective and accepted by Asians (O'Hare and Tran, 1998; Dai et al., 1999). It should be acknowledged that each psychotherapeutic strategy has its applicability and strengths. Within Asian patients, some will respond and some will not. It is also important to recognize that the inclusion of concepts, values, beliefs, and problem-solving procedures that are congruent with an individual's culture make psychotherapy more effective (Fisher and Jome, 1998).

There is limited evidence regarding psychotherapy outcomes for Asians. It appears that Asians who attend ethnic-specific services and receive culturally-sensitive psychotherapeutic modalities stay in treatment longer than Asians who attend mainstream psychotherapy services. The ethnic matching of therapists with Asian patients has also been associated with an increased use of mental health services and with favorable treatment outcomes (Sue et al., 1991; US DHHS, 2001b). There is increased awareness of the need to provide culturally-competent, relevant, responsive, and meaningful psychotherapy. Cultural sensitivity/competency must avoid stereotyping diverse Asian groups and must also allow therapists to have the ability to empathically connect with people who are different from them. Thus, an exact ethnic or cultural match or fit between Asian patients and therapists may not be necessary except for those patients who are less acculturated. Also, it is not necessary to eliminate any differences that do exist. We should not make groups indistinguishable one from the other, but should make a concerted effort to understand and respect differences. Forcing or imposing assimilation is ineffective in the healing process of psychotherapy.

Certainly there is no single or special psychotherapeutic modality or style for all Asians, for a subgroup of Asians, or for Asians only. Mental health professionals who provide psychotherapy to Asians must not automatically assume that their distinct cultural characteristics require different treatment approaches, to be reinvented for each group and totally different from traditional Western psychotherapeutic modalities. Some psychotherapeutic principles and issues, such as empathy, transference, and countertransference are universal and applicable to all cultural groups. Until we have better research data examining the effectiveness of each psychotherapeutic modality in treating Asians, the standard of practice should go beyond cultural differences and be applied to all ethnic groups.

At present, the field of psychotherapy for Asians, as for other cultural groups, ranges from the conventional to the mystical. There is a paucity of empirical information on the effectiveness of therapeutic modalities targeting Asian patients. We must let scientific evaluation make determinations about which psychotherapies and provided by whom are best applied to what types of problems (Kendall, 1998). Given the significant growth in the Asian population in the USA, continuous efforts must be made to expand the science base, including research that confirms the efficacy of evidence-based psychotherapies for Asian patients.

Psychotherapy with European migrant patients

A few years ago, only a small proportion of the patients referred to the outpatient psychiatric service at Maudsley Hospital in London, UK, were from ethnic minority groups. In the last 2 years, however, an increasing numbers of asylum seekers and refugees have been referred to Maudsley Hospital, thus the therapeutic approaches had to be changed to suit their needs. The clinical problems are compounded by the fact that the migrants who are currently referred to Maudsley Hospital come from a host of different countries and cultures in the Middle East, eastern Europe, Africa and South America. In this regard, traumatic events will affect different responses in individuals depending on the cultures in which they live and the use of posttraumatic stress disorder (PTSD) as a diagnostic label can be criticized for medicalizing emotional experiences and life events. However, this diagnosis continues to be used for two reasons: (1) it provides a professional explanation for these individuals' sometimes incoherent statements to the authorities and useful evidence for their asylum request, and (2) PTSD is an attachment disorder that attends to both the physical, mental, and cultural components of the asylum seeker's presentation. In this context, one can conclude that PTSD is essentially a dissociative disorder that results from the failure to integrate trauma into the declarative memory system. As a result, trauma can become organized at a sensory and somatic level and the traumatic response can be unconsciously triggered off and physically re-experienced without the conscious memories to accompany it.

Judith Herman (1992) defined the victims of the chronic form of PTSD as those who had survived 'A history of subjection to totalitarian control over a prolonged period'. Examples include prisoners of war, concentration camp survivors, and 'those subjected to totalitarian systems in their domestic life'. Their symptoms involve changes in affect regulation, changes in consciousness such as amnesia for traumatic events, transient dissociate episodes, experiences of depersonalization or derealization, and reliving experiences through flashbacks or intrusive thoughts. Accompanying these thoughts are changes in self-perception, a sense of having been defiled or stigmatized, and of being different from what the person was and from other people.

Shame may play a much more important role in the suffering of many of the asylum seekers and refugees; particularly if they come from families and communities that endorse shaming as a way of punishing children and ostracizing adults. For instance, Kosovan and other east European women who were raped during the Balkans war are customarily abandoned by their humiliated husbands and their communities.

Special treatment issues

The core of the therapeutic approach at Maudsley Hospital is to ensure that the patient is given a sense of control and responsibility throughout the treatment program. This is to counteract the sense of helplessness induced by traumatic experiences. With ethnic minorities, this means making the individual feel as secure as possible within a foreign context. To achieve this, it is essential to bear in mind the fact that these people may have a constellation of psychological problems that generally fall into three groups: (1) problems arising from displacement, such as cultural bereavement, isolation, unmet expectations of life in the UK, changing roles in the family leading to a clash of values, the stress of the asylum-seeking process, and racism in their new community; (2) major mental health problems; that is, patients may have had mental health problems before their move to the UK or they may have been precipitated by the move such as a psychotic illness (they will often hide such a history as it often means social ostracization in their home communities); and (3) mental health problems stemming from traumatization (in this context, the asylum seekers or refugees may have witnessed or been the victims of torture, rape, or other atrocities in their home country; they may have lost family members or friends through traumatic bereavements or they may have taken part in atrocities with resulting emotional problems). A history of past political oppression will mean that patients will be very worried about issues of confidentiality. These fears must be attended to. Those who have been tortured may feel very anxious in the presence of doctors as the latter are often involved in the torture of political prisoners.

Some of these manifestations reflect a Western categorization of mental health problems and may not reflect the refugees' perception of their problems and distress. For this reason it is so important to listen and to take note of the patients' accounts and explanations of their problems, and not to impose the psychotherapists views and beliefs upon them. Similarly, our labeling of an experience as a pathological symptom may not reflect what patients think and feel. For example, a Somalian woman described night visits by her dead family with whom she would communicate; she saw these visions as comforting.

If the patient is known not to speak the language of the therapist, an interpreter is booked in for the session. Family members and especially children should not be used as interpreters as the patients may not want members of the family to know the cause of their distress. For example, many women who have been raped do not want their husbands or members of their communities to know as this would mean being thrown out of their community and thereby add to their sense of isolation and fear. This will have implications in terms of the choice of interpreter as well.

The first obstacle to the doctor–patient attachment relationship with asylum seekers, can be the linguistic divide. If a patient cannot speak good English, they will feel quite helpless and even paranoid in the interview. An interpreter who both speaks the patient's language and who is of the right social group is essential. In some cases, bilingual patients who are proficient in English may choose to use their second language which can act as a 'linguistic defense' protecting people from disturbing associations and emotions linked to their mother tongue (Zulueta, 1995).

To counteract the overwhelming sense of helplessness experienced by many patients, they are taught relaxation techniques using tapes, guided imagery, and the establishment of a safe place. These experiences can be comforting and facilitate the attachment process between therapist and patient as well as providing some symptomatic relief. Asylum seekers also need to be given information about their rights, services that are available, and community support groups.

Patients with complex PTSD often resort to destructive patterns of behavior in order to cope with their symptoms. A thorough assessment needs to be done in relation to their capacity for self-harm or the dangers that they might bring upon themselves by engaging in treatment. Sorting this out may require quite a long period of stabilization. For example, with asylum seekers, the need for a home, community services, legal support, and attention to substance abuse and physical health issues is essential before any trauma work can be contemplated. This used to be done by the staff but is now carried out by other services.

Standard trauma work usually requires a patient to confront their traumatic experience as well as the feelings and cognitive distortions that accompany it. To do this asylum seekers are offered a choice of therapies: narrative reprocessing, psychodynamic psychotherapy with a marked cognitive input, focused group therapy, and family therapy. The latter is particularly important for some patients whose irritability and potential for violence can be very frightening for their partner and children. Medication is offered as a 'life jacket' to cope with the difficulties of the therapeutic journey.

The treatment of asylum seekers, refugees, and migrant ethnic minorities is one of the most interesting and challenging areas of work in the field of psychiatry. However, techniques and approaches need to be adapted to people from other cultures and languages.

Conclusions

In this chapter, we have described the impact of globalization in the migration process that began after World War II. Likewise, we have underlined the growth of the field of cultural psychiatry in the last two to three decades, as well as its association with the migration and the globalization process. We have also focused on the psychotherapeutic process with emphasis on multiethnic and multicultural factors. In this context, we have used the examples of the African-American, the Hispanic, and the Asian patients who reside in the USA. It is, however, obvious that these examples also have much validity in other parts of the world; particularly, in western Europe.

Obviously, it should be understood that no one fixed set or school of psychotherapy can be simply and effectively applied to patients from all of the many diverse cultures (i.e., no one size fits all). Thus, the thing to remember about the content of this chapter is that culturally speaking we are not one world. Thus, in understanding how to successfully diagnose and treat persons from a cultural dimension different from one's own, theoretical concepts and clinical experiences must be supplemented by the awareness and appreciation of the patients' cultural condition. This is certainly not easy to do; however, if psychotherapists do not understand and show respect and sensitivity for the deeply held values and normative perceptions of the patients they treat, they are stretching the patients' cultural world view upon the mental health criteria of the psychotherapists' cultures. If this happens, even though with the best of the psychotherapists intentions, the result can be treatment failure and frustration for both patients and psychotherapists; worse, it can also, at times, do harm.

References

Abed, V. and Boyce, E. (1979). Issues in psychiatric evaluations of Puerto Ricans: a socio-cultural perspective. *Journal of Operational Psychiatry*, **10**, 28–39.

Alarcon, R. D. and Ruiz, P. (1995). Theory and practice of cultural psychiatry in the United States and abroad. In: J. M. Oldham and M. B. Riba, ed. *Review of Psychiatry*, Vol. 14, pp. 599–626. Washington, DC: American Psychiatric Press, Inc.

American Psychiatric Association (1969). Position statement on the delineation of transcultural psychiatry as a specialized field of study. *American Journal of Psychiatry*, **126**, 453–5.

Atkinson, D. R., Maruyama, M., and Matsui, S. (1978). The effects of counselor race and counseling approach on Asian Americans' perceptions of counselor credibility and utility. *Journal of Counseling Psychology*, **25**, 76–83.

Bland, I. J. and Kraft, I. (1998). The therapeutic alliance across cultures. In: S. O. Opaku, ed. *Clinical methods in transcultural psychiatry*, pp. 266–78. Washington, DC: American Psychiatric Press Inc.

Canino, I. A., Rubio-Stipec, M., Canino, G., and Escobar, J. I. (1992). Functional somatic symptoms: a cross-ethnic comparison. *American Journal of Psychiatry*, **62**, 605–12.

Comas Diaz, L. and Jacobsen, F. F. L. (1991). Ethnocultural transference and countertransference in the therapeutic dyad. *American Journal of Orthopsychiatry*, **61**, 392–402.

Coner-Edwards, A. F. and Spurlock, J. (1988). *Black families in crisis: The middle class*. New York: Brunner/Mazel.

Cross, W. E. (1991). *Shades of black diversity in African-American identity*. Philadelphia, PA: Temple University Press.

Dai, Y., *et al.* (1999). Cognitive behavioral therapy of depressive symptoms in early Chinese Americans: a pilot study. *Community Mental Health Journal*, **35**, 537–42.

Escobar, J. I. (1987). Cross-cultural aspects of the somatization trait. *Hospital and Community Psychiatry*, **38**, 174–80.

Evans, D. A. (1985). Psychotherapy and black patients: problems of training, trainees and trainers. *Psychotherapy*, **22**, 457–60.

Fisher, A. R. and Jome, L. M. (1998). Reconceptualing multicultural counseling: universal healing conditions in a culturally specific context. *Counseling Psychologist*, **26**, 525–88.

Foulks, E. F., Persons, J. B., and Merkel, R. L. (1986). The effect of patients' beliefs about their illnesses on compliance in psychotherapy. *American Journal of Psychiatry*, **193**, 340–4.

Foulks, E. F., Bland, I. J., and Shervington, D. (1995). Psychotherapy across cultures. In: J. M. Oldham and M. B. Riba, ed. *Annual Review of Psychiatry*, Vol. 14, pp. 511–28. Washington, DC: American Psychiatric Press Inc.

Fujii, J. S., Fukushima, S. N., and Yamamoto, J. (1993). Psychiatric care of Japanese Americans. In: A. C. Gaw, ed. *Culture, ethnicity and mental illness*, pp. 305–45. Washington, DC: American Psychiatric Press Inc.

Gomez, E. A., Ruiz, P., and Laval, R. (1982). Psychotherapy and bilingualism: is acculturation important? *Journal of Operational Psychiatry*, **13**, 13–16.

Gomez, R., Ruiz, P., and Rumbaut, R. D. (1985). Hispanic patients: a linguo-cultural minority. *Hispanic Journal of Behavioral Sciences*, **7**, 177–86.

Gonzalez, C. A., Griffith, E. E. H., and Ruiz, P. (2001). Cross-cultural issues in psychiatric treatment. In: G. O. Gabbard, ed. *Treatment of psychiatric disorders*, 3rd edn, Vol. I, pp. 47–67. Washington, DC: American Psychiatric Press Inc.

Greene, B. (1994). African American women. In: L. Comas Diaz and B. Greene, ed. *Women of color: integrating ethnic and gender identities in psychotherapy*, pp. 10–29. New York: Guilford Press.

Grier, W. H. and Cobbs, P. M. (1980). Black rage. New York: Basic Books.

Herman, J. (1992). *Trauma and recovery: the aftermath of violence from domestic abuse to political terror*. New York: Basic Books.

Jackson, L. C. and Greene, B. (2000). *Psychotherapy with African American women: innovation in psychodynamic perspectives and practice*. New York: Guilford Press.

Jones, E. E. (1982). Psychotherapists' impressions of treatment outcome as a function of race. *Journal of Clinical Psychology*, **38**, 722–31.

Kendall, P. C. (1998). Empirically supported psychological therapies. *Journal of Consulting and Clinical Psychology*, **66**, 3–6.

Kernberg, O. (1968). The treatment of patients with borderline personality organization. *International Journal of Psychoanalysis*, **49**, 600–19.

Kitano, H. H. L., Shibusawa, T., and Kitano, K. J. (1997). Asian American elderly mental health. In: K. S. Markides and M. R. Miranda, ed. *Minorities, aging, and health*, pp. 300–7. Thousand Oaks, CA: Sage.

Laval, R. A., Gomez, E. A., and Ruiz, P. (1983). A language minority: Hispanic American mental health care. *American Journal of Social Psychiatry*, **3**, 42–9.

Lin, K. M. (1996). Cultural influences on the diagnosis of psychotic and organic disorders. In: J. E. Mezzich, A. Kleinman, H. Fabrega, and D. L. Parron, ed. *Culture and psychiatric diagnosis: a DSM-IV perspective*, pp. 35–8. Washington, DC: American Psychiatric Press Inc.

Lin, K. M., Innui, T. S., and Kleinman, A. (1982). Sociocultural determinants of the help-seeking behavior of patients with mental illness. *Journal of Nervous and Mental Disease*, **170**, 78–85.

Marcos, L. R. (1979). Effect of interpreters on the evaluation of psychotherapy in non-English-speaking patients. *American Journal of Psychiatry*, **136**, 171–4.

Marcos, L. R. and Alpert, M. (1976). Strategies and risks in psychotherapy with bilingual patients: the phenomenon of language independence. *American Journal of Psychiatry*, **133**, 1275–8.

Marcos, L. R., Urcuyo, L., Kesselman, M., and Alpert, M. (1973). The language barrier in evaluating Spanish-American patients. *Archives of General Psychiatry*, **29**, 655–9.

Markus, H. R. and Kitayama, S. (1991). Culture and the self: implications for cognition, emotion, and motivation. *Psychological Review*, **98**, 224–53.

Mattson, S. (1993). Mental health of Southeast Asian refugee women: an overview. *Health Care Women International*, **14**, 155–65.

Mohl, P. C., *et al.* (1991). Early dropouts from psychotherapy. *Journal of Nervous and Mental Disease*, **179**, 478–81.

O'Hare, T. and Tran, T. V. (1998). Substance abuse among Southeast Asians in the US: implications for practice and research. *Social Work in Health Care*, **26**, 69–80.

Opler, M. K. (1959). *Culture and mental health: cross-cultural studies*. New York: Macmillan.

Pi, E. H. and Gray, G. E. (2000). Ethnopsychopharmacology for Asians. In: J. M. Oldham and M. B. Riba, ed. *Ethnicity and psychopharmacology*, Review of Psychiatry Series, Vol. 19, pp. 91–112. Washington DC: American Psychiatric Press Inc.

Pumariega, A. J. and Ruiz, P. (1997). The Cuban American child. In: J. D. Noshpitz, ed. *Handbook of child and adolescent psychiatry*, Vol. IV, pp. 515–22. New York: John Wiley & Sons, Inc.

Root, M. P. (1985). Guidelines for facilitating therapy with Asian American clients. *Psychotherapy*, **22**, 349–56.

Ruiz, P. (1977). Culture and mental health: a Hispanic perspective. *Journal of Contemporary Psychotherapy*, **9**, 24–7.

Ruiz, P. (1982). The Hispanic patient: sociocultural perspectives. In: R. M. Becerra, M. Darno, and J. I. Escobar, ed. *Mental Health and Hispanic Americans*, pp. 17–27. New York: Grune & Stratton, Inc.

Ruiz, P. (1985). Cultural barriers to effective medical care among Hispanic–American patients. *Annual Review of Medicine*, **36**, 63–71.

Ruiz, P. (1995a). Assessing, diagnosing and treating culturally diverse individuals: a Hispanic perspective. *Psychiatric Quarterly*, **66**, 329–41.

Ruiz, P. (1995b). Cross-cultural psychiatry: foreword. In: J. M. Oldham and M. B. Riba, ed. *Review of Psychiatry*, Vol. 14, pp. 467–76. Washington, DC: American Psychiatric Press Inc.

Ruiz, P. (1998a). New clinical perspectives in cultural psychiatry. *Journal of Practical Psychiatry and Behavioral Health*, **4**, 150–6.

Ruiz, P. (1998b). The role of culture in psychiatric care. *American Journal of Psychiatry*, **155**, 1763–5.

Smedley, A. (1999). 'Race' and the construction of human identity. *American Anthropologist*, **100**, 690–702.

Sue, S. and Morishima, J. K. (1982). *The mental health of Asian Americans*. San Francisco, CA: Jossey-Bass.

Sue, S. and Sue, D. (1974). MMPI comparisons between Asian-American and non-Asian students utilizing a student health psychiatric clinic. *Journal of Counseling Psychology*, **21**, 423–7.

Sue, D. and Sue, S. (1987). Cultural factors in the clinical assessment of Asian Americans. *Journal of Consulting and Clinical Psychology*, **55**, 479–87.

Sue, S. and Zane, N. (1987). The role of culture and cultural techniques in psychotherapy: a critique and reformation. *American Psychologist*, **42**, 37–45.

Sue, S., Wagner, N., Ja, D., Margullis, C., and Lew, L. (1976). Conceptions of mental illness among Asian and Caucasian-American students. *Psychological Reports*, **38**, 703–8.

Trujillo, M. (2000). Cultural psychiatry. In: B. J. Sadock and V. A. Sadock, ed. *Comprehensive textbook of psychiatry*, 7th edn, pp. 492–9. Baltimore, MD: Lippincott Williams and Wilkins.

US Bureau of the Census (2000a).

US Bureau of the Census (2000b). The Asian and Pacific Islander population in the United States: March 2000 (Update) (PPL-146).

US DHHS (2001a). *Mental health: culture, race, and ethnicity. a supplement to mental health: a report of the Surgeon General*, pp. 105–6. Washington, DC: US DHHS.

US DHHS (2001b). *Mental health: culture, race, and ethnicity. Executive summary. A supplement to mental health: A report of the Surgeon General*, pp. 5–12. Washington, DC: US DHHS.

Walt, V. (2002). Europe fights tide of immigrants. *USA Today*, p. 24, **June 24**.

White, G. M. (1982). The role of cultural explanations in 'somatization' and 'psychologization.' *Social Science Medicine*, **16**, 1519–30.

White, J. L. and Cones, J. H. (1999). *Black man emerging. facing the past and seizing a future in America*. New York: W. H. Freeman and Co.

Yamamoto, J. and Acosta, F. X. (1982). Treatment of Asian Americans and Hispanic Americans: similarities and differences. *American Academy of Psychoanalysis*, **10**, 585–607.

Yamamoto, J. and Steinberg, A. L. (1981). Ethnic, racial, and social class factors in mental health. *Journal of the National Medical Association*, **73**, 231–40.

Yamamoto, J., Silva, J. A., Justice, L. R., Chang, C. Y., and Leong, G. B. (1993). Cross-cultural psychotherapy. In: A. C. Gaw, ed. *Cultural ethnicity, and mental illness*, pp. 101–24. Washington, DC: American Psychiatric Press Inc.

Zulueta de, F (1995). Bilingualism, culture and identity. *Group Analysis*, **28**, 179–90.

VI

Special topics

37 Implications of research in cognitive neuroscience for psychodynamic psychotherapy

Drew Westen

Virtually all psychotherapies rely on some mixture of the following:

- exposure to new or anxiety-provoking stimuli, ideas, feelings, or behaviors;
- efforts at understanding and reworking problematic ways of thinking, feeling, and behaving;
- efforts at behavior change that may in turn catalyze cognitive and emotional change (as well changes in the behavior of others);
- interaction with another person (or group of people) who may provide a supportive environment, act in ways that disconfirm past expectations about relationships, or offer new ways of interacting.

All of these processes rely on learning, memory, and cognitive change, which suggests that relevant developments in the basic sciences should be useful in conceptualizing, reformulating, and adding to our repertoire of psychotherapeutic interventions. The extraordinary progress in cognitive neuroscience (and the related, emerging field of affective neuroscience) in the last decade has as yet led to only a handful of studies directly relevant to psychotherapy (e.g., research linking changes in brain to changes in depression or anxiety responses; e.g., Brody *et al.*, 2001; Goldapple *et al.*, 2004). However, *basic* science data generated thus far may have substantial implications for the therapeutic practice, both by supporting long-held clinical hypotheses about the way neural networks function and by challenging exclusive use of therapeutic practices that focus primarily on only a handful of systems that regulate thought, emotion, and behavior.

This chapter begins with a brief description of how psychologists, cognitive scientists, and cognitive neuroscientists have come to understand learning, memory, and cognition. (Although one could profitably focus on the cellular level, given that all learning ultimately involves changes in synaptic connections, gene expression, etc., the focus here is primarily on molar processes likely to translate more directly into implications for psychotherapeutic interventions.) It then briefly describes potential implications for psychodynamic psychotherapy. (For an expanded presentation of some of these ideas, see Westen, 2000a,b, 2002; Westen and Gabbard, 2002a,b; Gabbard and Westen, 2003.)

Learning, memory, and the evolution of cognitive neuroscience

This section briefly describes the evolution of conceptions of learning, memory, and cognition of relevance to contemporary theory and research in cognitive neuroscience. It focuses on how earlier research inspired contemporary approaches to treatment. The chapter then examines implications of more recent developments for all forms of psychotherapy.

Classical and operant conditioning

The first systematic approach to learning emerged from the laboratories of Pavlov, Skinner, and hundreds of other researchers who studied what came to be known as classical and operant conditioning. For much of the first half of the twentieth century, researchers from a behavioral tradition argued that the most complex behaviors reflect a handful of learning mechanisms shared by humans and other animals that could be understood without reference to internal mental processes. The animal learns in *classical conditioning* to produce a relatively automatic response when a previously neutral stimulus (the conditioned stimulus) is repeatedly paired with a stimulus that innately (prior to learning) produces a similar response (a conditioned response). The best known example occurred in Pavlov's experiments, in which dogs learned to salivate at the sound of a tone that tended to precede presentation of meat. The animal learns in *operant conditioning* to associate certain behaviors with *consequences*—reinforcers and punishers—that increase or decrease the likelihood of the behavior recurring. In general, classical conditioning tends to involve involuntary reactions, whereas operant conditioning involves voluntary behaviors that a person or animal performs or inhibits to obtain or avoid rewarding or aversive consequences.

The understanding of classical and operant conditioning led, in the 1950s and 1960s, to the development of behavior therapies aimed at altering conditioned emotional responses and maladaptive behaviors. Classically conditioned emotional responses are involved in many forms of psychopathology, particularly in anxiety disorders (e.g., in the startle responses and intense anxiety and autonomic reactivity that occur when patients with posttraumatic stress disorder encounter 'triggers' that resemble in some way those present during a traumatic event). Some of the earliest behavioral treatments emerged directly from research on classical conditioning processes, as researchers and clinicians developed *exposure* techniques to try to break associative links between stimuli (or imagined stimuli, as in flashbacks of traumatic events) and intense negative feelings, particularly fear and anxiety (Wolpe, 1958). Exposure means presenting the person with the feared stimulus and preventing him or her from escaping the initial feelings of anxiety or panic. Over time, if the person cannot escape exposure, the intense emotional reaction irrationally associated with an objectively nonthreatening stimulus will generally wane if not extinguish entirely. Using exposure to treat conditioned emotional responses in anxiety disorders has been demonstrated to be quite efficacious (Barlow, 2002).

Behavior therapists similarly learned to use principles of operant conditioning to treat a range of problems, such as maladaptive parenting strategies that fostered rather than curtailed aggression. Most behavioral treatments use both classical and operant principles to promote behavior change. For example, effective treatments of anxiety disorders tend to address not only classically conditioned emotional responses but also the avoidance mechanisms patients develop through operant conditioning to escape frightening experiences (e.g., agoraphobic avoidance of situations associated with panic attacks). Thus, behavior therapists typically combine exposure to threatening stimuli (aimed at extinguishing a classically conditioned response) with response prevention (preventing the patient from escaping the feared stimulus and hence extinguishing a response learned via operant conditioning).

Serial (conscious) processing of information: the cognitive revolution

Although highly productive, the behaviorist enterprise ultimately ran aground as the dominant perspective in experimental psychology as researchers increasingly recognized anomalies that could not be understood without reference to mental processes. Buoyed by developments in artificial intelligence (and the development of high-speed computers), cognitive science began to displace behaviorism in a scientific revolution that began in the late 1950s (see Robins *et al.*, 1999). Based on the metaphor of the mind as a computer, researchers developed a serial processing model of cognition—that is, a model in which information passes sequentially (serially) through a series of three memory stores (Atkinson and Shiffrin, 1968). This three-stage model, now sometimes called the 'modal model' (Healy and McNamara, 1996), provided the theoretical basis for cognitive research for 30 years.

According to this model, following a brief initial stage of sensory registration that retains information for a fraction of a second, information is held in short-term memory, which can maintain roughly seven pieces of information in consciousness for about 30 seconds (Miller, 1956). (The move to 10-digit local phone numbers in the US in the 1990s, necessitated by the proliferation of fax and computer lines, has posed a challenge to the limits of human short-term memory.) The next stage is long-term memory, from which information, if properly processed (e.g., memorized in a way that is meaningful), is retrieved as needed into short-term memory. Although information may remain in long-term memory indefinitely, in general, the more frequently and recently information has been used, the easier it is to retrieve.

Researchers offered a number of theories and metaphors to describe the way information is stored in long-term memory. One emphasizes *associative networks*: pieces of information are associatively connected with one another, so that activating one node (unit of information) on a network spreads activation to related nodes. Suppose a participant in an experiment is presented ('primed') with the word *bird* and subsequently asked to press a button as soon as she recognizes each of a series of words. With priming, she will respond more quickly to the word 'robin' than to the word 'butter.' The reason is that bird and robin are located along the same network of associations, so that activating one spreads activation to the other. Another way researchers have described the organization of memory is in terms of *schemas*, patterns of thought that guide perception and memory. Thus, if an eye witness to an accident is asked how quickly a car *smashed* into another car, she is likely to estimate a higher speed than if asked how quickly the car was going when it *hit* the other car, because 'smash' activates a schema that implies high impact (Loftus *et al.*, 1975).

This information-processing model offers a general view not only of memory but of thinking—that is, of the processes by which people manipulate remembered information to solve problems. According to the model that dominated the field for 30 years (and remains the foundation of many cognitive models of thought and decision making, with some caveats; see Markman and Gentner, 2000), when people want to make a decision, they use short-term memory to maintain current information, retrieve relevant information from long-term memory, and perform various operations on the information held there (Newell and Simon, 1972; Klahr and Simon, 2001). Thus, problem solving involves parsing a problem into an initial state (how things currently are), a goal state, and potential operators that might transform the initial state into the goal state.

This way of thinking about cognition provided the zeitgeist within which cognitive approaches to psychotherapy developed in the 1960s (e.g., Ellis, 1962; A. T. Beck, 1967, 1995). Early cognitive models of therapy tended to presume a serial model of cognition, in which people feel and act based on the thoughts that come into consciousness (or on 'automatic thoughts' that lie just outside the periphery of awareness but can be readily retrieved with proper cueing). An important goal of these therapies is to change dysfunctional attitudes, views of the self, and things people say to themselves that are associated empirically with negative mood states such as depression and dysfunctional behaviors such as bulimic binge–purge cycles. Although the information processing models of the 1960s and 1970s were relatively silent

about the kinds of classical and operant learning processes studied by behaviorists, in clinical practice by the late 1970s cognitive-behavioral approaches began to emerge that integrated behavioral techniques with cognitive strategies designed to change dysfunctional thinking patterns.

The second cognitive revolution

In the last decade the modal model has undergone considerable evolution in four interrelated respects, which probably constitute more of a revolution than an evolution in thinking. The first change is a shift away from a serial processing model. In the modal model, stages of memory storage and retrieval occur sequentially, one at a time, with most of the 'real' work of cognition done by bringing information into short-term memory. Contemporary researchers, however, recognize that most processing occurs outside of awareness, as the brain processes multiple pieces of information in parallel. Serial processing, in this view, is the task of a specialized memory system, *working memory* (a construct that evolved from the construct of short-term memory, referring to a 'work space' in which the individual can consciously manipulate information; see Baddeley, 1995; Richardson, 1996).

A second and related shift is from conceiving of memory as involving 'stores' (places where memories are 'kept') to a view of memory and cognition as involving multiple *circuits or systems*. For example, when a person sees an object, cortical circuits involving the occipital and lower (inferior) temporal lobes are involved in breaking it into component parts and comparing it with familiar objects, and a second circuit running from the occipital lobes through the upper (superior) temporal and parietal lobes attempts to pinpoint its location in space. The person is never aware of using different circuits to identify an image and locate it in space, because both circuits are part of a broader neural circuit that integrates the information—and does this so quickly that the person has no phenomenological experience of anything other than the immediate recognition of having seen a squirrel running across the road. This conception of memory systems is bolstered by research showing that memory for episodes (e.g., remembering what happened yesterday), memory about the emotional meaning of stimuli (e.g., whether something has consistently been associated with pain), memory for procedures (e.g., playing a piece on the piano), and working memory constitute neurologically distinct memory systems. For example, memory for episodes requires an intact hippocampus, but a person with hippocampal damage can still associate a stimulus with an emotional response, even though he may have no memory for having ever encountered it (e.g., Bechara *et al.*, 1994). Working memory, in contrast, is readily disrupted by lesions to the dorsolateral prefrontal cortex, which is involved in deliberate conscious thinking and decision making.

A third major shift has occurred with the recognition of the existence of two ways that memory can be expressed, either explicitly (via conscious recall or recognition) or implicitly (in behavior, independent of conscious control). *Explicit memory* refers to conscious memory for ideas, facts, and episodes. *Implicit memory* refers to memory that is observable in behavior but is not consciously brought to mind (Roediger, 1990; Schacter, 1992, 1998). One kind of implicit memory is *procedural memory*, which refers to 'how to' knowledge of procedures or skills, such as how close to stand to another person or how to respond when someone reaches out his or her hand for a handshake. Another kind of implicit memory involves *associative memory*. For example, priming subjects with an infrequently used word such as *syncopate* among a long list of words renders them more likely a week later to respond with the correct word when asked to fill in the missing letters of the word fragment, S-----ATE. This occurs even though they may lack any conscious recollection of whether *syncopate* was on the list a week earlier (Tulving *et al.*, 1982). Essentially, the network of associations still has some residual activation, leading to memory expressed in behavior but not in conscious recollection.

A fourth shift involves a change in metaphor. Cognitive psychologists in the late 1950s and early 1960s saw in the computer a powerful metaphor for the human mind. Today, cognitive scientists are turning to a different metaphor: *mind as brain*. In this view, memory is not so much a matter of 'storing' something somewhere in the brain and later retrieving it (as in a computer file) than a process by which an experience activates a set of neurons distributed throughout the brain that can in turn be reactivated by similar experiences or efforts at recollection. In this view, memory is simply a *potential* for reactivation of a set of neurons that together constitute a representation. The notion of using the brain as a metaphor for the mind may seem today obvious if not tautological; however, metaphors of mind have tended to follow understanding in other domains, particularly in the physical sciences. Freud, for example, certainly knew that what he referred to as mental processes occur through the actions of brain processes, and he developed some complex models of neural excitation that appear today to be remarkably prescient in multiple respects (Freud, 1966; Pribram and Gill, 1976; Westen, 1998). However, because knowledge of the brain was so primitive, he turned to metaphors from physics to explain how mental 'dynamics' function. Similarly, the information processing theorists of the 1960s through 1980s tended to draw their inspiration from computer technology. Not until knowledge of the brain expanded exponentially in the last two decades did brain processes become potential metaphors for mental processes.

The notion of mind as brain is central to *connectionist*, or *parallel distributed processing*, models of perception, memory, and thinking (Rumelhart *et al.*, 1986; Kunda and Thagard, 1996; Smith, 1998). Connectionist models suggest that most information processing occurs in parallel, outside of awareness, as multiple components of a thought, memory, or perception are processed simultaneously. Representations are *distributed* throughout the brain over many sets of neurons processing different aspects of a thought, perception, or memory, rather than 'located' in any particular part of the brain. Knowledge lies in the connections among these neural units or nodes, which, like neurons, can either inhibit or activate each other. Cognitive activity involves a process of *constraint satisfaction*, in which the brain simultaneously and unconsciously processes multiple features of a stimulus, attended to by different nodes or sets of nodes in a network that provides *constraints* on the conclusions that can be drawn. The brain then draws the best tentative conclusion it can based on the available data. In other words, it equilibrates to the solution that provides the best 'fit' to the data. Thus, if a patient is crying, the clinician's interpretation of that crying as tears of pain or joy will depend on auditory and semantic cues processed simultaneously (in parallel).

Connectionist models have the advantage of building in a way of modeling both the chronic ways people tend to process information and moment to moment changes in the way they view important people and experiences in their lives (see Barsalou, 1999). One of the virtues of connectionist models is their suggestion that representations, such as a person's representations of significant others, are not static. Rather, the representation of a significant other activated at any given point depends on the context. Thus, the same person can represent his wife as impossible to deal with at one time but a source of loving support at another, depending on aspects of his 'wife network' activated by the current situation, his feeling state, and so forth. At the same time, the chronic activation of a way of seeing something or someone—that is, the frequent activation of a set of neurons representing some aspect of that person—will create an *attractor state*, a pattern of neural firing that is readily activated under particular circumstances. Thus, a patient with a critical parent may be 'primed' to hear his therapist's comments as criticisms because a network representing self-being-criticized-by-parental-figure is an attractor state that 'attracts' the brain to this interpretation. In this view, then, a representation is not something 'stored' in the brain. It is a *potential for reactivation* of a set of neural units that have been activated together in the past. Activating part of that network may reproduce much of the original experience (as in an episodic memory, e.g., of a time the parent was critical, or more directly in a flashback in posttraumatic stress disorder) or may influence the way the person interprets current experiences.

Implications for psychodynamic psychotherapy

Although psychoanalytic practice has largely evolved from the consulting room independent of experimental research, in many respects, recent developments in the cognitive neurosciences have breathed new empirical life into psychodynamic forms of psychotherapy, bolstering the basic science behind them even if the applied science (treatment research) lags far behind. The second cognitive revolution documented perhaps the most central psychoanalytic hypothesis, and the one that distinguished it from other approaches to the mind and treatment for a century: that unconscious associative networks and unconscious procedures (e.g., defenses, motives) influence thought, feeling, and behavior outside of awareness. The research evidence is now clear that much of the way people view themselves and others is implicit or unconscious; that their brains are frequently 'triggered' or 'primed' to behave or interpret events in certain ways based on the implicit activation of networks of which they have no awareness; that they can have emotional reactions of which they are unaware; that they can regulate emotions outside of awareness to avoid painful feelings (what psychoanalysts call defense); and that the same event can trigger contradictory thoughts, feelings, or actions consciously and unconsciously (such as negative racial attitudes in people who consider themselves free of racism, or devalued views of self in patients who present with grandiosity) (Westen, 1998).

Mapping and changing implicit networks

Fundamental to all psychoanalytic forms of treatment is the effort to map the idiosyncratic associative networks that may be relevant to the patient's sources of distress. The goal, as first enunciated by Freud, was to give the patient more freedom to make conscious, explicit choices. Indeed, in describing the process of open-ended, long-term therapy to patients, it can be very useful to offer a simple explanation such as the following:

> Much of what we do reflects the way thoughts and feelings have gotten connected in our minds. But we have no direct access to those connections. So you find yourself bingeing and then vomiting but don't really know why you're doing it and can't find a way to stop. In many ways, our task together is to map those connections in your head, so we can figure out what's leading you to do things you'd rather not do and to begin developing new connections.

The existence of unconscious or implicit networks—which tend to be resistant to change because they reflect longstanding regularities in the person's experience and allow him or her to navigate the world in ways that feel predictable (even if sometimes rigid, inaccurate, or otherwise maladaptive)—provides perhaps the best empirical justification for long-term therapies. Deeply engrained views of the self, others—called 'internal working models of relationships' in research on attachment (see, e.g., Bowlby, 1973; Main *et al.*, 1985; Fonagy *et al.*, 2002) and object representations in theory and research on interpersonal functioning more broadly in psychoanalysis (see, e.g., Greenberg and Mitchell, 1983; Westen, 1990, 1991; Blatt *et al.*, 1997)—may take months or years to identify in their various manifestations. The same is true of problematic ways of regulating emotions (defenses) that are triggered automatically and may lead to a cascade of internal and interpersonal events.

For example, patients with prominent passive–aggressive features are often unaware of both their anger and the ways they put other people in uncomfortable positions—which in turn lead others to become angry at or avoid them. This, in turn, makes the patient more angry and passive–aggressive. Consciously, these patients view themselves as helpless victims of indifferent or mean-spirited others; unconsciously, they provoke precisely the behavior that makes them feel mistreated. Breaking into these kinds of self-sustaining spirals—into what Wachtel (1997) calls *cyclical psychodynamics*—can take a long time, because the patient cannot report them. Such dynamics may become most apparent—and most workable as a treatment issue—when they show up in the therapeutic relationship (Luborsky and Crits-Christoph, 1998).

Techniques for exploring associative networks: free and directed association

Thus, contemporary research in cognitive neuroscience corroborates some central psychoanalytic assumptions that have been the source of tremendous controversy for a century. At the same time, this research also poses some important challenges for psychodynamic psychotherapy and suggests potential refinements in theory and technique (see Westen, 2002; Westen and Gabbard, 2002a; Westen and Gabbard, 2002b; Gabbard and Westen, 2003). For example, research in cognitive neuroscience suggests precisely why the psychoanalytic practice of exploring patients' associations to symptoms, feelings, or events—asking them what comes to mind—can often be very useful: people cannot report on their implicit networks, and they typically invent plausible but often inaccurate explanations if called upon to do so (e.g., when asked, 'Why do you think you felt that way?'; Nisbett and Wilson, 1977). On the other hand, this same body of research suggests limits to free association as a therapeutic technique, on two grounds.

First, although free association can be essential in exploring implicit networks, it may do very little to illuminate or alter explicit (conscious) beliefs, procedures, or ways of behaving that operate through the action of different neural networks. As argued below, with limited therapeutic time (even for patients treated more than once a week), attention to implicit processes inherently comes at the expense of attention to explicit processes, which can also wreak havoc on a person's quality of life, and nothing guarantees that even emotionally important change in implicit expectations, motives, feelings, or conflicts will alter conscious habits of thought or behavior that have attained functional autonomy over years or decades of use. This recognition is precisely what led Aaron Beck (1976) to develop cognitive therapy for depression.

Second, research in cognitive science suggests that what is on a person's (unconscious) mind at any time is a join function of what is *chronically* on his mind (much of which is likely, in fact, to reflect concerns forged in childhood) and what is *recently* on his mind, which may or may not be related to the concerns that brought the patient to treatment. In other words, the particular associations that emerge in any analytic hour if the patient follows what Freud called the 'fundamental rule' of psychoanalysis (namely, to say whatever comes to mind) may or may not prove useful to explore, depending on what has been activated recently in and out of the consulting room. Any given set of associations reflects some combination of clinically meaningful signal and clinically less meaningful noise, and one cannot always distinguish the two. *Over time* one would expect important material to be reflected repeatedly in the patient's associations, as chronically activated networks influence the patient's thought, feeling, and behavior in the treatment. However, waiting for important material to emerge, particularly in the context of therapeutic interventions (particularly interpretations) that shape subsequent associations, is likely to be an inefficient process.

Patients can also avoid doing things associated with anxiety, such as allowing themselves to fall in love because doing so is associated with anxiety or fear of rejection. As a result, some of the most important networks may never be activated to the extent necessary for useful exploratory work until the patient actually exposes herself to the feared situation. Under such circumstances, the therapist may do well to encourage the patient to approach what she fears, to alter the patient's associative networks and/or to bring material to the fore in the patient's associations that are most important in maintaining maladaptive patterns. Freud himself noted that people do not get free of their fears unless they confront them, and he practiced a much more active mode of therapy than practiced by subsequent generations of analysts for many years. As many psychoanalytically oriented clinicians now recognize, good treatment probably requires a balance of exploration and exhortation at the service of further exploration and behavioral change (see Wachtel, 1997; Gabbard and Westen, 2003).

One useful way to employ associative techniques in once- or twice-weekly psychotherapy, where one does not have the luxury to explore whatever associations come to mind at any given time, is what might be called *directed free association*, in which the therapist targets particular thoughts, feelings, or memories for further associative work (see Westen, 2000b).

For example, one patient had a pattern of becoming excited about some plan (e.g., spending the evening out with friends) but then finding himself depressed and unable to imagine that he would really enjoy doing it. (For a

sophisticated cognitive-dynamic explanation of the way patients shift between such 'states of mind,' see Horowitz, 1979.) As a result, the patient experienced few pleasures in life. After the pattern became clear, I routinely asked him to imagine as vividly as possible what he initially thought and felt when he was excited about the plan or to picture the moment he found himself feeling depressed and uninterested in pursuing it. I would ask him to walk me through the episode or image moment by moment or scene by scene, taking associations along the way, much as Freud would have explored a dream, encouraging him to report whatever he felt at the time and whatever thoughts, feelings, images, or memories emerged as he pictured the experience. Doing so led to a series of associations and memories in which he wished for something that subsequently fell through and his corresponding fear of hoping for enjoyment, as well as survivor guilt around a mentally retarded sister who could never have such pleasures and toward whom he felt a mixture of love and (largely unacknowledged) resentment.

Understanding transference processes

Data from the cognitive neurosciences may also help shed new light on psychoanalytic constructs such as transference. The connectionist notion of representations as potentials for reactivation—as sets of neurons that have been activated in the past and are hence more readily activated as a unit in the future—offers a mechanism to explain the long-held psychoanalytic position that patients are likely to express important conflicts, defenses, motives, and interpersonal patterns in their relationship with the therapist (Westen and Gabbard, 2002b). To the extent that the therapeutic situation or relationship matches prototypes from the past, it is likely to activate similar responses (for empirical evidence, see Andersen and Baum, 1994; Luborsky and Crits-Christoph, 1998). It should therefore not be surprising if important relational patterns emerge in a relationship in which the patient self-discloses and becomes attached in an intimate but asymmetrical relationship with another who is trying to be helpful, nurturant, and attentive primarily to his or her needs. Inherent in the *cognitive situation* of the therapeutic relationship is the likelihood that the therapist will be experienced as an authority figure, an attachment figure, or an object of love or affection, which renders exploration of the therapeutic relationship of particular use if the patient is presenting with problems that include interpersonal components (which is nearly always the case).

Important dynamics are likely to emerge relatively quickly and persistently in patients with rigid maladaptive patterns of interpersonal functioning, cognition, and emotion regulation. For example, narcissistic patients tend to manifest particular patterns when interacting with their therapists regardless of the therapist's theoretical understanding or technical approach. Empirically, clinicians of all therapeutic orientations report that narcissistic patients need excessive admiration from them, vacillate between idealizing and devaluing them, and need to be special to the therapist at the same time as being sadistic and hostile and feeling criticized by the therapist (Bradley *et al.*, in press). Correspondingly, therapists of all theoretical orientations report similar countertransference reactions to their narcissistic patients: They tend to feel annoyed, manipulated, used, criticized, and as if they are 'walking on eggshells' with the patient, and correspondingly frequently fight their impulses to be sadistic themselves or to drift off during sessions (Betan *et al.*, in press).

Conclusions

Perhaps the most important lesson to be learned from developments in the cognitive neurosciences is that clinicians need to attend in psychotherapy to both implicit processes (emphasized by psychoanalysis and to some extent by both cognitive and behavior therapy) and explicit processes (emphasized by cognitive therapy). One cannot assume that the same techniques likely to change explicit thought processes will change implicit networks and vice versa (Westen, 2000b; Gabbard and Westen, 2003). Indeed, data from the cognitive neurosciences suggest that implicit and explicit processes often reflect neuroanatomically distinct brain systems, and that what registers implicitly and explicitly can be very different.

Psychotherapists and treatment researchers need to think more carefully about, and study empirically, the tradeoffs inherent in attention to implicit and explicit processes in psychotherapy. Every time clinicians explore the meaning of a self-critical statement, they are choosing not to try to alter an explicit process directly. Every time they explore the meaning of an anxiety symptom, they are only indirectly, if at all, using exposure techniques that might be applied therapeutically in much more direct ways to alter the feeling state. Conversely, every time clinicians draw a patient's attention to a self-critical statement as a way of trying to alter current mood or address an explicit way the patient talks to herself, and every time they use exposure techniques to try to change an affective association, they are altering the conditions that would allow optimal exploration of its implicit meanings. What is exciting about developments in cognitive neuroscience is that they may help clinicians, theorists, and researchers begin to address crucial issues such as this by calling attention to multiple systems that will likely require multiple types of therapeutic intervention.

Preparation of this chapter was supported in part by NIMH grants MH62377 and MH062378 to the author.

References

Andersen, S. M. and Baum, A. (1994). Transference in interpersonal relations: inferences and affect based on significant-other representations. *Journal of Personality*, **62**, 459–97.

Atkinson, R. and Shiffrin, R. (1968). Human memory: a proposed system and its control processes. In: K. W. Spence and J. T. Spence, ed. *The psychology of learning and motivation*, Vol. 2, pp. 89–195. New York: Academic Press.

Baddeley, A. D. (1995). Working memory. In: M. S. Gazzaniga, ed. *The cognitive neurosciences*, pp. 755–64. Cambridge, MA: MIT Press.

Barlow, D. (2002). *Anxiety and its disorders*, 2nd edn. New York: Guilford Press.

Barsalou, L. W. (1999). Perceptual symbol systems. *Behavioral and Brain Sciences*, **22**, 577–660.

Bechara, A., Damasio, A. R., Damasio, H., and Anderson, S. W. (1994). Insensitivity to future consequences following damage to human prefrontal cortex. *Cognition*, **50**, 7–15.

Beck, A. T. (1967). *Depression: clinical, experimental, and theoretical aspects*. New York: Harper and Row.

Beck, A. T. (1976). *Cognitive therapy and the emotional disorders*. New York: International Universities Press.

Beck, A. T. (1995). Cognitive therapy: past, present, and future. In: M. J. Mahoney, ed. *Cognitive and constructive psychotherapies: theory, research, and practice*, pp. 29–40. New York: Springer.

Betan, E., Zittel, C., Heim, A., and Westen, D. (in press). The structure of countertransference phenomena in psychotherapy: an empirical investigation. Unpublished manuscript, Emory University.

Blatt, S. J., Auerbach, J. S., and Levy, K. N. (1997). Mental representations in personality development, psychopathology, and the therapeutic process. *Review of General Psychology*, **1**, 351–74.

Bowlby, J. (1973). *Separation*, Vol. 2. London: Hogarth Press.

Bradley, R., Heim, A., and Westen, D. (in press). Transference phenomena in the psychotherapy of personality disorders: an empirical investigation. Unpublished manuscript, Emory University.

Brody, A., *et al.* (2001). Regional brain metabolic changes in patients with major depression treated with either paroxetine or interpersonal therapy: preliminary findings. *Archives of General Psychiatry*, **58**(7), 631–40.

Ellis, A. (1962). *Reason and emotion in psychotherapy*. New York: Lyle Stuart.

Fonagy, P., Gergely, G., Jurist, E. L., and Target, M. (2002). *Affect regulation, mentalization, and the development of the self*. New York, NY: Other Press.

Freud, S. (1966). Project for a scientific psychology. In: J. Strachey, ed. *The standard edition of the complete psychological works of Sigmund Freud*, Vol. 1, pp. 281–397. London: Hogarth Press.

Gabbard, G. and Westen, D. (2003). On therapeutic action. *International Journal of Psycho-Analysis*, **84**, 823–41.

Goldapple, K., *et al.* (2004). Modulation of cortical-limbic pathways in major depression. *Archives of General Psychiatry*, **61**, 34–41.

Greenberg, J. R. and Mitchell, S. (1983). *Object relations in psychoanalytic theory*. Cambridge, MA: Harvard University Press.

Healy, A. F. and McNamara, D. S. (1996). Verbal learning and memory: does the modal model still work? *Annual Review*, **47**, 143–72.

Horowitz, M. (1979). *States of mind: analysis of change in psychotherapy*. New York: Plenum.

Klahr, D. and Simon, H. A. (2001). What have psychologists (and others) discovered about the process of scientific discovery? *Current Directions in Psychological Science*, **10**, 75–9.

Kunda, Z. and Thagard, P. (1996). Forming impressions from stereotypes, traits, and behaviors: a parallel-constraint-satisfaction theory. *Psychological Review*, **103**, 284–308.

Loftus, E. F., Altman, D., and Geballe, R. (1975). Effects of questioning upon a witness' later recollections. *Journal of Police Science and Administration*, **3**, 162–5.

Luborsky, L. and Crits-Christoph, P. (1998). *Understanding transference—The core conflictual relationship theme method*, 2nd edn. Washington, DC: American Psychological Association.

Main, M., Kaplan, N., and Cassidy, J. (1985). Security in infancy, childhood, and adulthood: a move to the level of representation. *Monographs of the Society for Research in Child Development*, **50**(1/2), 66–104.

Markman, A. B. and Gentner, D. (2000). Thinking. *Annual Review of Psychology*, **52**, 223–47.

Miller, G. (1956). The magical number seven, plus or minus two: some limits on our capacity for processing information. *Psychological Review*, **63**, 81–97.

Newell, A. and Simon, H. A. (1972). *Human problem solving*. Englewood Cliffs, NJ: Prentice-Hall.

Nisbett, R. E. and Wilson, T. D. (1977). Telling more than we can know: verbal reports on mental processes. *Psychological Review*, **84**, 231–59.

Pribram, K. and Gill, M. (1976). *Freud's project reassessed*. New York: Basic Books.

Richardson, J. T. E. (1996). Evolving concepts of working memory. In: J. T. E. Richardson, R. W. *et al.*, ed. *Working memory and human cognition*. New York: Oxford University Press.

Robins, R. W., Gosling, S. D., and Craik, K. H. (1999). An empirical analysis of trends in psychology. *American Psychologist*, **54**, 117–28.

Roediger, H. L. (1990). Implicit memory: retention without remembering. *American Psychologist*, **45**, 1043–56.

Rumelhart, D. E., McClelland, J. L., and PDP Research Group. (1986). *Parallel distributed processing: explorations in the microstructure of cognition*: Vol. 1. *Foundations*. Cambridge, MA: MIT Press.

Schacter, D. L. (1992). Understanding implicit memory: a cognitive neuroscience approach. *American Psychologist*, **47**, 559–69.

Schacter, D. L. (1998). Memory and awareness. *Science*, **280**, 59–60.

Smith, E. R. (1998). Mental representation and memory. In: D. T. Gilbert, S. T. Fiske, and G. Lindzey, ed. *Handbook of social psychology*, Vol. 1, pp. 391–445. New York: McGraw-Hill.

Tulving, E., Schacter, D. L., and Stark, H. A. (1982). Priming effects in word-fragment completion are independent of recognition memory. *Journal of Experimental Psychology: Learning, Memory, and Cognition*, **8**, 336–42.

Wachtel, P. (1997). *Psychoanalysis, behavior therapy, and the relational world*. Washington, DC: American Psychological Association Press.

Westen, D. (1990). Towards a revised theory of borderline object relations: contributions of empirical research. *International Journal of Psycho-analysis*, **71**, 661–93.

Westen, D. (1991). Social cognition and object relations. *Psychological Bulletin*, **109**, 429–55.

Westen, D. (1998). The scientific legacy of Sigmund Freud: toward a psychodynamically informed psychological science. *Psychological Bulletin*, **124**, 333–71.

Westen, D. (2000a). Commentary: Implicit and emotional processes in cognitive-behavioral therapy. *Clinical Psychology—Science and Practice*, **7**, 386–90.

Westen, D. (2000b). Integrative psychotherapy: integrating psychodynamic and cognitive-behavioral theory and technique. In: C. R. Snyder and R. Ingram, ed. *Handbook of psychological change: psychotherapy processes and practices for the 21st century*, pp. 217–42. New York: Wiley.

Westen, D. (2002). Implications of developments in cognitive neuroscience for psychoanalytic psychotherapy. *Harvard Review of Psychiatry*, **10**, 369–73.

Westen, D. and Gabbard, G. O. (2002a). Developments in cognitive neuroscience: I. Conflict, compromise, and connectionism. *Journal of the American Psychoanalytic Association*, **50**, 53–98.

Westen, D. and Gabbard, G. O. (2002b). Developments in cognitive neuroscience: II. Implications for theories of transference. *Journal of the American Psychoanalytic Association*, **50**, 99–134.

Wolpe, J. (1958). *Psychotherapy by reciprocal inhibition*. Palo Alto, CA: Stanford University Press.

38 Psychotherapy research

Mark Aveline, Bernhard Strauss, and William B. Stiles

Introduction

In principle, clinicians and researchers have a common purpose; they want practice to be as effective, relevant, and safe as possible. One of the most important contributions that research can make to this end is to minimize bias. Clinicians, however experienced, have a relatively small pool of experience from which to draw conclusions that they hope will improve their practice. The range of patients (clients) is limited in variety and severity of problem, stage and life situation; their ideas on what therapy can achieve is narrowed by restrictions in type or types of therapy practiced and the constraining imperatives of the clinical settings in which they work. Any judgment is likely to be based on partial evidence and heavily influenced by recent selective experience. Research can help individual clinicians, researchers, and other stakeholders stand to one side of their inevitable bias and take a fresh look at what is revealed. Research can also enhance the validity of impression, elucidate processes, and provide evidence to confirm and disconfirm received clinical wisdom.

Research can help one think again about what actually happens in therapy—the outcomes and processes—and how and why they happen. All psychotherapy is an experiment. Interactions occur; clinicians make their best judgment on what to do next; what happens is reviewed in the light of experience and new judgments are made, the effects of what is done or not done is reviewed in turn. On a pragmatic level, it is an experiment, influenced by feedback and judged against the markers of progress, e.g., enhanced alliance, deepened empathy, fuller understanding, problem resolution, and patient satisfaction. Research is a systematic form of experiment in which the significance of elements in the clinical story is tested by being held constant or varied or brought into prominence for detailed scrutiny. Finally, research is an essential element in reliable communication between colleagues; it brings to the table the discipline of clear definition, the benefit of transparent methodology, the value of access to the experience of others through shared results, and the potential for replication and further testing of conclusions.

Of course, this 'best of all possible worlds' ideal is difficult to achieve. Most times the answers provided by research are small, sometimes contradictory, increments in knowledge, a few of which add to our understanding of complex issues. Rarely are results definitive; studies generally breed more questions than answers. Grand epiphanous ideas have to be scaled down to what can be achieved in the available time and resource. For good methodological reasons, what is studied may not be representative of everyday clinical practice. Results may take years to arrive and have limited generalizability: they have to be interpreted in light of clinical and social context, researcher bias and allegiance. Sometimes however, research can meet the seven desiderata of being representative, relevant, rigorous, refined, realizable, resourced and revelatory (Aveline *et al.*, 1995). Then the rewards can be great for the labor of doing research.

For the practitioner, research begins with pressing clinical questions whose answers may improve practice. Research may focus on *qualitative* questions, e.g.:

- What is the effect of making this or that intervention in a session?
- Does the effect persist from one session to the next?

- What is the relationship between sessions that go well or badly to outcome at termination?
- What are the contributory factors and how do they interact?
- In what way do patients, therapists, and significant others perceive sessions or the therapy differently?
- How may a patient's intrapsychic or interpersonal conflicts be formulated? Can this be done reliably? Can such formulations benefit clinical practice?
- How do patients' narratives alter over time and what relationship does this have to psychotherapy theory.
  Or on *quantitative* questions, e.g.
- Is this treatment more effective than other treatments?
- How does the efficacy of new therapies conducted under experimental conditions translate into clinical effectiveness in everyday work?
- What extra gain can a patient expect to derive from a therapy that lasts for 50 as opposed to 25 sessions?
- Does the gain justify the cost of the larger investment in time and duration?
- Do different forms of gain accrue with different durations of therapy?
- Do different therapies have different effects?
- Which patients with what conditions do best with what therapy?
- What training is necessary to maximize gain or minimize harm from therapy?

Studying process is the subject of qualitative research. In focus, it is in the same domain as that considered by a clinician in internal or external supervision; the difference is in the degree of systematization. Quantitative research provides an empirical, often controlled, means of validating and refining psychotherapy theory and practice.

Having set out a rationale for doing research, we consider basic principles of methodology and give a brief history of the field before summarizing what we know about outcomes and process. Then we discuss how to implement evidence into clinical practice. Finally, we anticipate future directions. An appendix contains guidance on how to read a research paper.

Methodology of psychotherapy research

In researching clinical problems in psychotherapy, investigators can call upon a wide range of methodologies, some well established in classical empirical research in medicine and psychology and some breaking new ground in their exploration of subjectivity and individual meaning. Each has potentials and limitations in providing significant answers.

The method chosen depends on where one is in the cycle of developing or refining a therapy. New ideas for practice begin with clinical observation or theoretical inference. The hypothesized therapeutic effect might be evaluated through observational single case studies. Should these generate large *effect sizes* (see Roth and Fonagy, 1996, pp. 379–8), this would indicate that there could be something worthwhile in the innovation. The next step would be small-scale single group designs, i.e., uncontrolled naturalistic studies. A major step up in rigor would be to move to a randomized controlled trial (RCT); this is an acid test of *efficacy* (see below). Results under controlled conditions, however, do not necessarily generalize to everyday clinical practice. *Effectiveness* has to be established through field trials; these establish *generalizability* (see implementing evidence into clinical practice). Finally, *dismantling* studies tease out what are the effective ingredients in the practice being studied. Qualitative studies at each stage can be a rich source of ideas about the process of change.

Going through the sequence once is not enough. New perspectives arising from the findings at various stages prompt new paths through the cycle; studies need to be repeated to test the robustness of the findings. All this has to be evaluated against a standard of *clinically significant change* (see Outcome section), a more stringent and relevant standard than simple statistical significance (Jacobson and Truax, 1991; Ogles *et al.*, 2001).

The difference between efficacy and effectiveness is crucial in understanding the divergence between research and service planning.

Efficacy versus effectiveness

Outcome studies are commonly divided into studies determining the *efficacy* of a treatment versus studies focusing on a treatment's *effectiveness* (Seligman, 1995; Strauss and Kächele, 1998; Lambert and Ogles, 2004).

Efficacy is determined by (randomized) clinical trials in which as many variables as possible are controlled in order to demonstrate unambiguously the relationship between treatment and outcome, and potentially infer causal relationships from the findings (Strauss and Wittmann, 1999).

Efficacy studies emphasize the *internal validity* of the experimental design through random assignments to treatments, controlling the types of patients included with respect to their diagnosis (commonly excluding patients with comorbid disorders), through using manualized treatments, pretraining the therapists in the study clinical practice, and monitoring adherence to the treatment manual. These parameters ensure uniformity of therapy and enable other researchers to replicate the investigation. The price of high *internal validity* is usually poor *external validity*; the nature of the intervention is clear and consistent but unrepresentative of everyday practice and, thus, the findings of the study may not generalize. An example of an important efficacy study is the NIMH Collaborative Depression Study (Elkin, 1994; Krupnick *et al.*, 1996; Ogles *et al.*, 2001) in which patients with major depressive disorder were randomly assigned to four treatments: imipramine + clinical management, placebo + clinical management, cognitive-behavior therapy (CBT), interpersonal psychotherapy (IPT). One surprising result was that there was little evidence for the superiority of one treatment in contrast to the placebo condition. At least two explanations have been put forward to account for this 'negative result'. One is that 'placebo' was not inert—it involved frequent contact with therapists, albeit of a supportive nature. It is possible that 'nonspecific' therapy effects may have been making a contribution to good outcomes even in this arm. Second, as many other studies have shown that CBT *is* superior to placebo, it has been suggested that this result may have been a fault of the 'quality control' in this study, and that CBT was poorly delivered in one center. All of which goes to show how complex a business it is to mount a large-scale psychotherapy evaluation study of this sort.

Effectiveness studies, on the other hand, focus on clinical situations and the implementation of a treatment in clinical settings. Such studies emphasize the external validity of the experimental design: patients usually are not preselected, treatments commonly are not manualized, the duration of the treatment and other setting-related characteristics are not controlled. These *clinically representative* studies show how interventions perform in routine clinical practice (Shadish *et al.*, 1997). Their weakness is the converse of the strength of efficacy studies; it is difficult to know what was done, when, and how. The variability inherent in effectiveness studies makes it much harder to disentangle what were the therapeutic elements

and replicate the work in other settings. An example of an effectiveness study is the German multisite study on inpatient psychotherapy for patients with eating disorders (Kächele *et al.*, 2001). Questions examined in this prospective, naturalistic design included: What is the effectiveness of inpatient psychodynamic therapy for eating disorders? What factors determine the length of treatment? How do treatment duration and intensity contribute to effectiveness? Can such effects be attributed to specific patient characteristics?

Naturalistic or effectiveness studies are the principal research approach for the assessment of outcome in treatments that are hard to assess within a controlled clinical trial, either because of formal characteristics (e.g., treatment length) or because of ethical reasons (e.g., impracticalities in randomizing subjects to treatments) such as inpatient treatments or long-term psychoanalysis. Examples of representative effectiveness studies from the psychoanalytical field are as the Menninger Psychotherapy Research Project (Wallerstein, 1986), the Heidelberg Psychosomatic Clinic Study (Fonagy, 2001), or the Berlin Multicenter Study on psychoanalytic oriented treatments (Rudolf, 1991) (see the 'open door review of outcome studies in psychoanalysis', Fonagy, 2001).

Study design concepts

Randomized controlled trials

The first question usually asked about any psychotherapy is: 'does it work?' The most widely respected way to answer this question is by a *randomized controlled trial* (RCT).

RCTs are an adaptation of the experimental method, which is the closest science has come to a means for demonstrating causality. The logic of the experimental method is that if all prior conditions except one (the *independent variable*) are held constant (controlled), then any differences in the outcome (the *dependent variable*) must have been caused by the one condition that varied. For example, if one patient is given psychotherapy and another identical patient is not, but is treated identically in all other respects, then any differences in their outcomes must have been caused by the therapy. Difficulties arise in applying the experimental method to study psychotherapy because no two people are identical and because it is impossible to treat two people identically in all respects except for the theoretically specified treatment (Haaga and Stiles, 2000).

RCTs address the differences among patients statistically. Rather than comparing single patients, investigators randomly assign patients to groups that are to receive the different treatments, on the assumption that any prior differences that might affect the outcomes will be more-or-less evenly distributed across the groups. Even though individuals' outcomes might vary within groups (because patients are not identical), any mean differences between groups beyond those due to chance should be attributable to the different treatments.

Researchers have attempted to standardize psychotherapeutic treatments by constructing treatment manuals (e.g., Beck *et al.*, 1979; Elliott *et al.*, 2004) and by assessing treatment delivery via studies of adherence and competence (e.g., Shapiro and Startup, 1992; Startup and Shapiro, 1993; Waltz *et al.*, 1993).

Some investigators speak of *quasi-experimental* designs (T. D. Cook and Campbell, 1979), which refer to comparisons between groups of patients who were not randomly assigned—for example, groups of patients who seem generally comparable but were assigned to different treatments on some other basis, perhaps because they appeared before or after the introduction of a new program or because of scheduling constraints or because they were treated at different sites. Such designs are often more feasible than strict RCTs; indeed they may appear as *natural experiments,* in which apparently similar groups happen to receive contrasting treatments. In such cases, however, there are always variables that were confounded with the variable of interest, so the evidence of causality is, to some degree, ambiguous.

Correlational process-outcome studies

Another major genre in psychotherapy research is the process-outcome study, which uses a correlational approach. Correlational studies are those in which two (or more) variables are observed, and the degree to which they covary is assessed.

In a widely cited article, Yeaton and Sechrest (1981) argued that effective psychotherapeutic treatments should contain large amounts of helpful change ingredients (*strength*) and should be delivered in a pure manner (*integrity*). If the theory underlying the treatment is correct, then delivering interventions with strength and integrity should be effective in producing client change. This view of process-outcome relations has been called the *drug metaphor* (Stiles and Shapiro, 1989; Stiles and Shapiro, 1994). This logic suggests that clients who receive a larger quantity or greater intensity of the helpful ingredients (process variables) should show greater improvement (outcome variables), so that process and outcome should be positively correlated across patients. Much process-outcome research has adopted this drug metaphor and sought to assess the relationship of process ingredients with outcome by correlating the process and outcome measures. It has been assumed that this method would allow researchers to determine which process components are the active ingredients, which should be positively correlated with outcome, and are merely inert flavors and fillers, uncorrelated with outcome (Orlinsky *et al.*, 1994). Some, however, including ourselves, suggest that this reasoning may be misleading (e.g., Stiles, 1988; Stiles *et al.*, 1998).

Case study

Since long before Freud, case studies have been a standard tool for investigating the theory and practice of psychotherapy. Although they are vulnerable to significant bias and distortion, as investigators unintentionally (or intentionally) perceive and report data selectively, case studies have always been a principal source of ideas and theories about psychotherapy (Aveline, in press).

Theoretically, based case studies can be confirmatory as well as exploratory. Interpretive and hypothesis-testing research are alternative strategies for scientific quality control on theory (Stiles, 1993, 2003). In hypothesis-testing research, scientists extract or derive one statement (or a few statements) from a theory and compare this statement with observations. If the observations match the statement (that is, if the scientists' experience of the observed events resembles their experience of the statement), then people's confidence in the statement is substantially increased, and this, in turn, yields a small increment of confidence in the theory as a whole. In case studies, however, investigators compare a large number of observations based on a particular individual with a correspondingly large number of theoretical statements. Such studies ask, in effect, how well the theory describes the details of a particular case. The increment or decrement in confidence in any one statement may be very small. Nevertheless, because many statements are examined, the increment (or decrement) in people's confidence in the whole theory may be comparable with that stemming from a statistical hypothesis-testing study. A few systematically analyzed therapy cases that match a clinical theory in precise or unexpected detail may strongly support a theory, even though each component assertion may remain tentative when considered separately.

Quantitative versus qualitative

Qualitative research differs from traditional quantitative research on human experience in several ways. Results are typically reported in words rather than primarily in numbers. This may take the form of narratives (e.g., case studies) and typically includes a rich array of descriptive terms, rather than focusing on a few common dimensions or scales. Investigators use their (imperfect) empathic understanding of participants' inner experiences as data. Events are understood and reported in their unique context; theory is generated from data. Materials may be chosen for study because they are good examples rather than because they are representative of some larger population. Sample size and composition may be informed by emerging results (e.g., cases chosen to fill gaps; data gathering continued until new cases seem redundant). One well-known form of qualitative research is *grounded theory* (Glaser and Strauss, 1967).

Grounded theory starts not from a pre-existing theory or hypothesis, but 'bottom up' from experience-near observations. It tries to derive theoretical categories from the commonalities that are generated from a multitude of such observations. These categories are then 'back-tested' against the raw experiential data, and if they stand up, gives confidence that the theoretical principles that emerge are based in reality, not prior preconceptions of the researcher or clinician. The whole thrust therefore is an attempt to circumvent the inherent observer bias found in psychotherapy, in which, Kleinian therapists see 'Kleinian' material in their clients, Jungians find 'Jungian' themes, and so on.

Emancipation or enhancement of the lives of participants may be considered as a legitimate purpose of the research. As a consequence of these characteristics, interpretations are always tentative and bound by context (Stiles, 2003).

Scientific versus hermeneutic

A scientific theory can be understood not as an organized edifice of facts but as an understanding that is shared to varying degrees by those who have propounded it or been exposed to it. In this view, research is cumulative not because each new observation adds a fact to an edifice but because each new observation that enters a theory changes it in some way. The change may be manifested, for example, as a greater or lesser confidence in theoretical assertions, as the introduction or revised meanings of terms, or as differences in the way particular ideas are phrased or introduced. In this view, theory can be considered as the principal product of science and the work of scientists as quality control—insuring that the theories are good ones by comparing them with observations (Stiles, 2003). If science is understood in this way, theory is just as central in interpretative (qualitative) research as it is in hypothesis-testing research.

Not all qualitative investigators of psychotherapy see quality control on scientific theory as their main activity. Some instead use alternative forms of discourse that can be described as *hermeneutic*, after Hermes, the messenger (e.g., Rennie, 1994a,b; Rhodes *et al.*, 1994; McLeod and Lynch, 2000). This alternative discourse form represents a distinct sort of intellectual activity, entails different goals and procedures, and yield distinct products. The goal of hermeneutic discourse can be described as *deepening*. The activity consists in understanding what the target material, such as some text or concept, has meant or could mean to other people. Put another way, it is unpacking the experiences that have been or could be embodied in the words and other signs of the target material. Insofar as most words have very long histories, this process is potentially endless. Packer and Addison (1989) and Rhodes *et al.* (1994) described this process of unpacking as the hermeneutic circle-observing, interpreting, reviewing through the new interpretation, revising, and so forth. The product is thus a series of reinterpretations, leading to ever-deeper understandings but not necessarily to a unified synthesis (Hillman, 1983; Woolfolk *et al.*, 1988). The exploration of alternatives is itself the product of the activity rather than a means of developing a particular theory. The understanding achieved is valued for its depth—the richer appreciation—not necessarily because it is more simple or unified.

Cautionary points

- *Reductionism*. The trade-off between the grand idea and a do-able study is simplification. Problems arise when the essence of the natural complexity of human problems is fractured by the pragmatics of doing research. The large picture is lost sight of in attending to the micro-focus; the fascinating minute process may be irrelevant to the overall outcome.

- *Nonrepresentativeness*. In order to control variables or simply live within the constraint of the available resource, selective choices are made of type and intensity of disorder, duration of therapy and experience and competence of therapists, which simplify the clinical field, and result in nonrepresentative findings with limited generalizability.

- *Context*. RCTs are snapshots in time, capturing the performance of sets of patients and therapists. Generalizing conclusions from one set to another needs to be done cautiously as much of the variance lies with the particularity of each set. Even within a service that evaluates its performance over time periods that are appropriate for the practiced therapy and demonstrates effectiveness, the healing therapists who contributed to the success may long since have gone.

◆ *Mistaking what is studied for what is important.* It is easy to assume that what is positively correlated is causally related. Unappreciated important intervening (*confounding*) variables may lurk out of sight, yet to be discovered.

◆ *False positivism.* By virtue of objectified methodology, there is a risk of giving false certainty to the external world when the inner world is essentially subjective and idiosyncratic.

◆ *Emphasis on mental disorders.* Categorical diagnosis implies that disorders are discrete entities with possibly different etiologies and treatments. The categorical view, which is an import from medicine, does not necessarily fit the 'problems in living' presentations that are the province of psychotherapy and a major part of the work of psychiatry. It overemphasizes difference between conditions and underplays the alternative view that the great range of nonpsychotic symptomatology is better seen a single manifestation of disturbance whose origins need to be understood and formulated (Aveline, 1999).

◆ *Comorbidity.* On grounds of practicality or an intention to concentrate on 'pure' disorders, many studies specifically exclude comorbidity and, in particular, Axis II disorders. This is not representative of the real world. Also, from a psychodynamic perspective, how a person reacts to the world is a function of their personality; Axis II depicts exaggerated forms of personality dimensions.

◆ *Therapeutic change is not linear.* Early in the development of physics, sequential rules were thought to govern processes; outcomes were the predictable consequence of interactions; cause and effect were linked in a *pas de deux*. Just as Heisenberg's uncertainty principle guides—if that is the right word—modern physics, so does uncertainty rule in psychotherapeutic interactions. Progress may be followed by regression, the gain of symptom reduction blunts the spur of discomfort, life choices are perceived in new light as fresh insights are gained, intentionality alters, and significant others in the subject's life have their own influential agendas. Similarly, therapy interventions are not linear but hermeneutic.

◆ *Manualization* prioritizes internal validity over external validity. It increases reliability and replicability, but may decease reflexivity. If the manual is highly prescriptive, therapist responsiveness may be limited, thereby restricting a key factor in successful therapy. Except in training, clinicians rarely follow manuals to the letter in everyday clinical practice.

◆ *Randomization* may conflict with subject preference for therapy. It is also difficult to provide comparable control interventions.

◆ *Measures.* Symptoms are easier to measure than problems in relationship and, in their generic form, are a good marker of distress. They need to be supplemented by domain-specific measures including that of interpersonal functioning.

◆ *Statistical problems.* In order to have the possibility of significant results, trials must have sufficient *power* (Cohen, 1977). For example, a comparison of two treatments with a 50% chance of detecting a true difference between groups (a 'median effect' in Cohen's terms) would require 64 subjects in each group (Shapiro *et al.*, 1995). All studies have subject attrition but often the attrition is selective and, if not allowed for, biases the results. Studies should report results based on *intention to treat*, i.e., include all potential clients, encompassing those that fail to start, or drop out at an early stage, as well as 'finishers'. In addition simple prepost testing does not give robust results. What is needed is *clinically significant change*. Significance results are poor guides for clinical practice. Better statistics are *relative risk, confidence intervals* and *numbers needed to treat* (NNT, R. J. Cook and Sackett, 1995; Altman, 1998; Jacobson *et al.*, 1999). The latter refers to the number of patients who would need to have been effectively treated in order to produce benefit compared with an untreated (i.e., spontaneously recovering) group—the smaller the NNT the more useful a therapy is considered to be.

◆ *Allegiance effects.* Clinicians and researchers often have loyalties to the therapy being studied. This introduces significant, systemic bias in favor of the preferred approach. Allegiance should be declared in write-ups.

◆ *Group results do not predict individual reaction.* Research findings can inform practice but cannot be an absolute guide to what therapy to recommend at assessment or, in clinical practice, what to do for the best in a therapy session. This is an important caveat to set against the enthusiasm of health purchasers and planners for what they may see as the hard facts of empirical research.

◆ *Therapy is not the only change factor in patients' lives.* Unpredictable negative or positive events in someone's life may lead to change unrelated to therapy.

Ethical considerations

Research has to be ethical. Subjects should be seen as equals with a vital interest in process and outcome. Their interest is considered explicitly when approval is sought from the relevant Ethical Committee. If subjects are to be randomized to treatments, the clinicians have to be confident that the alternatives are of equal value, i.e., there is equipoise (Lilford and Jackson, 1995); they, also, need to consider how the patient might differentially value what is on offer (Lilford, 2003). The possibility of doing harm must be minimized. This does not mean that interventions have to be risk-free; this would be impossible with an active intervention such as psychotherapy but the risks need to be anticipated and the subject given sufficient information to make an informed choice. Some research designs specifically allow for subject preference.

Traditionally, detailed case accounts have been the source of theory and the way for clinicians to illustrate their work. However regulatory bodies in medicine, psychology, psychotherapy, and counseling are increasingly restrictive in allowing case-material to be published without the written consent of the subject. One can imagine that consent might not be given in the very cases that would be the most valuable for learning but which were problematic in some way for the original therapy dyad. A solution needs to be found that balances privacy and the legitimate needs of the field. Fortunately, for the most part, subjects give consent when the purpose is explained or they see a draft of what is to be written and have opportunity to comment.

The British Association for Counselling and Psychotherapy has adopted as policy an excellent framework for ethical practice in general (Bond *et al.*, 2002) which has now been supplemented by specific research guidance (Bond, 2004).

A brief history of the field

Orlinsky and Russell (1994) divided the history of psychotherapy research into four phases, marked by the publication of distinct sets of synthetic reviews of the field and distinct types of major research projects.

◆ Phase I (c. 1927–54) was a pioneering period, characterized as *establishing a role for scientific research*, in which investigators began tabulating therapeutic outcomes and (in the 1940s) recording psychotherapy sessions for process research.

◆ Phase II (c. 1955–69), characterized as *searching for scientific rigor*, was marked by investigators 'developing objective methods for measuring the events of recorded therapy sessions' and 'demonstrating effectiveness in controlled experiments' (p. 193).

◆ Phase III (c. 1970–83), characterized as *expansion, differentiation, and organization*, was marked by the growth of scientific organizations devoted to psychotherapy research and by increasing conceptual and methodological sophistication, as well as innovation, illustrated in comparative outcome studies, phenomenological and task-analytic approaches to process, and the use of meta-analytic reviewing techniques.

◆ Phase IV (c. 1984–94 and beyond), characterized as *consolidation, dissatisfaction, and reformulation*, has been a period in which continuing growth in the sophistication of methods that now seem traditional has been accompanied by fundamental doubts about their appropriate application to the human enterprise of psychotherapy, and the proposal of alternatives. Some of these issues are touched upon in our section on Methodology.

Barkham (2002) sees the progression moving from *justification* (is psychotherapy effective?) to *specificity* (which psychotherapy is effective) to *efficacy* and *cost-effectiveness* (how can therapies be made more effective?) to *effectiveness* and *clinical significance* (how can the quality/delivery of therapy be improved?).

What we know about outcomes

The term *outcome* describes all aspects of changes that patients can make during psychotherapy. The specific definition of outcome depends on the perspective of the stakeholder assessing the outcome (i.e., the patient, his or her social group, the therapist, representatives of the healthcare system, such as insurance companies, or the society as a whole). It also depends on the specific goals of a treatment or a treatment model (Ambühl and Strauss, 1999).

Ideally, outcome should be measured using multiple criteria, dimensions, measures, and modes, all on multiple occasions. Outcome should be related to the circumstances of a problem, the specific symptoms associated with the problem, and long-term consequences of a treatment. Schulte (1995) has proposed a classification system for the assessment of treatment success that differentiates content and methodological dimensions (see Table 38.1).

Measures related to the causes of a problem (the 'defect' such as impaired ego-functions, a discrepancy between perceived and ideal self, or specific cognitive strategies) mostly reflect the theoretical basis of the treatment model and are therefore school specific. On the level of symptoms, a wide variety of disorder-specific measures, independent of the theoretical model, are available. Finally, on the level of consequences, Schulte (1995) proposes outcome measures that are related to the 'sick role' (i.e., the utilization of healthcare services, or the subjective experience of the sick role) and to the impairment of normal roles (i.e., related to work, social activities, social relationships).

Methodological design structures the investigation and determines the generalizations that can be made across time, settings, behaviors, and subjects. An essential component is operationalization, i.e., decisions that have to be made about the specific methods or instruments used to measure change and the definition of outcome criteria, e.g., the amount of change that has to be reached or degree of goal attainment in order for it to be significant.

Table 38.1 Conceptual and methodological aspects of outcome measurement (according to Schulte, 1995)

Dimension	Content	Method
Level	Causes and defect —school-specific measures	Operationalization —data source —measures
	Symptoms —disorder-specific measures —general symptom measures	Outcome criteria —criteria for significant change —goal attainment Efficiency Change over time
	Consequences —sick role —impairment of normal roles	Design of data collection —time and setting of measurement

General outcomes of psychotherapy

Historically, outcome research dates back to the 1930s when clinicians started to tabulate systematically the benefits achieved by their patients, e.g., Fenichel at the Berlin Psychoanalytical Institute (Fenichel, 1930). Many outcome studies were stimulated by a provocative article that Eysenck published in 1952 in which he drew the conclusion that psychotherapy was no more effective than spontaneous remission (Eysenck, 1952). It took considerable time and numerous research efforts until McNeilly and Howard (1991) using Eysenck's original data set were able to show that psychotherapy produced the same recovery rate after 15 sessions as spontaneous remission after 2 years!

Our knowledge about the outcomes of psychotherapy is based on numerous comparative treatment efficacy as well as effectiveness studies. After several decades of research, the controversy about the general outcome of psychotherapy has largely been ended through the use of meta-analyses. Meta-analyses provide a tool for summarizing single studies on the efficacy and effectiveness of psychotherapeutic treatment by the application of methods and principles of empirical research to the process of reviewing literature. This procedure usually results in a summary statistic, the *effect size*, which quantifies the cumulative effects demonstrated within the single studies included in the review.

In a recent summary of the outcome literature, Lambert and Ogles (2004) concluded: 'While the methods of primary research studies and meta-analytic reviews can be improved, the pervasive theme of this large body of psychotherapy research must remain the same—psychotherapy is beneficial. This consistent finding across thousands of studies and hundreds of meta-analyses is seemingly undebatable.' (p. 148).

One milestone in the development of the meta-analytic methodology was the publication of M. L. Smith *et al.*'s (1980) article summarizing 475 single studies on the outcome of psychotherapy. The authors reported an average effect size of 0.85 for the comparison of treated and untreated groups. The statistic indicates that the average person treated in psychotherapy is better off than 80% of untreated people.

Following M. L. Smith *et al.*'s report, a large number of meta-analyses have been conducted that summarize the general effects of psychotherapy as well as the effects of treatments for specific disorders (e.g., anxiety disorders or depression) and of specific treatment models (e.g., CBT or psychodynamic therapy). In a review of a total of 302 meta-analyses of different treatments, Lipsey and Wilson (1993) concluded that 'the evidence from meta-analysis indicates that psychological, educational, and behavioral treatments studied by meta-analysts generally have positive effects' (p. 1198). Similar and consistent results showing that psychological treatments were superior to control conditions have been obtained in numerous reviews focusing on specific disorders and specific treatment settings, such as small group treatment (Burlingame *et al.*, 2004). In addition, reviews of outcome studies support the cost-effectiveness of psychotherapy (Chiles *et al.*, 1999; Gabbard *et al.*, 1997) and show that treatment effects are maintained for several years after treatment (Stanton and Shadish, 1997). It is important to note that a small number of patients (5–10%) get worse during psychotherapeutic treatments (*deterioration effect*) (Mohr, 1995).

On the way to reaching this favorable position, outcome research has passed several important milestones, characterized by increased methodological sophistication. Outcome measurement has been differentiated by the specific goals of treatments and standardized measures have been developed for quality assurance, including *core batteries* targeted on specific issues (Strupp *et al.*, 1997). Starting in the 1970s, the development of approaches to determine and test individual changes and their clinical meaning became increasingly important. One of these is the determination of the *social validity* of individual outcome. Social validity is based upon social comparisons, i.e., the evaluation of changes related to a normal reference group, or on subjective evaluation 'by gathering data about clients by individuals who are likely to have contact with the client or are in a position of expertise' (Kazdin, 1998, p. 387). In addition, several statistical methods have been developed to determine the clinical significance of treatment interventions. *Clinical significance* is usually based upon the stringent definition that (1) treated clients make statistically reliable improvements as a result of treatment, and (2) treated clients are empirically indistinguishable from 'normal' peers following their treatment (Jacobson et al., 1999; Kendall et al., 1999; Lambert and Ogles, 2004).

Comparative outcomes of psychological treatments

As well as investigating the general efficacy of psychotherapy, outcome research has focused on the relative effectiveness between treatments. Different treatment modes such as psychodynamic, behavioral, cognitive, or humanistic approaches have been tested in comparative studies. Reviews of comparative studies can be divided into several phases (Lambert and Ogles, in press). Many older reviews reached the startling conclusion that the outcomes of alternative psychotherapies are equivalent. The *equivalence paradox* (Stiles et al., 1986) points to the puzzle that the outcomes of varied psychotherapies appear more-or-less equivalently positive even though their treatment techniques are very different (Luborsky et al., 1975; Lipsey and Wilson, 1993; Lambert and Bergin, 1994; Norcross, 1995). The evidence is often summarized as the Dodo verdict: '*Everybody has won, and all must have prizes*' (Carroll, 1946, p. 28; original work published 1865; italics in original). The Dodo verdict may be an overstatement (Beutler, 1991; Chambless, 2002); there are exceptions, e.g., *in vivo* exposure for phobias and other anxiety disorders has consistently been found more effective than other behavioral procedures (Emmelkamp, 1994); and ultimately no two psychological procedures have exactly equivalent effects, i.e., the null hypothesis is never really true (Meehl, 1978). Nevertheless, the substantial degree of outcome equivalence relative to the technical diversity of treatments has long puzzled observers (Rosenzweig, 1936; Stiles et al., 1986; Luborsky et al., 2002).

Meta-analytic reviews conducted in the 1980s and 1990s generally showed an appreciable advantage for cognitive-behavioral treatment models over psychodynamic, process-oriented and interpersonal therapies (Svartberg and Stiles, 1991; Grawe et al., 1993).

On the other hand, several meta-analyses have shown that comparative studies yield equivalent results, when factors such as investigator allegiance and case severity are controlled (Wampold et al., 1997; Luborsky et al., 1999; Wampold, 2001). In view of this some investigators (e.g., Shoham and Rohrbaugh, 1999) have come to the conclusion that 'the Dodo Bird verdict has been fortified by the allegiance effect bias'.

With the increasing development of outcome research, interest has shifted from testing specific psychotherapeutic theories to teasing out the relative contribution of specific components of various treatments. Such component analyses or *dismantling studies* have been advocated as an important alternative to the usual comparative treatment approach (Borkovec, 1993). Neo Dodo-bird proponents such as Ahn and Wampold (2001) summarized dismantling studies from an 18-year period in a meta-analysis of component analyses and found that these studies reveal 'little evidence that specific ingredients are necessary to produce psychotherapeutic change' p. 126 (Wampold, 2001). From a similar ideological position, Lambert and Ogles (2004) stress this finding as an argument against the identification of *empirically supported therapies* as 'decades of research have not resulted in support for one superior treatment or set of techniques for specific disorders'.

It should, however, be noted that across the range of disorders in which a specific therapy has been shown to be effective, cognitive-behavioral therapies consistently show the greatest versatility and efficacy. Against drawing hasty conclusions from this, however, stands the aphorism that 'absence of evidence does not denote evidence of absence'. In other words, psychodynamic and systemic therapies may well be effective in a range of disorders, but the inclination of their supporters, logistical difficulties, and expense of mounting appropriate trials mean that the results are currently not to hand.

Specific questions in outcome research

Besides the general question of 'how efficacious is (what kind of) psychotherapy?' outcome research has dealt with a variety of more specific problems such as the dosage that is necessary to reach positive outcomes. In addition, outcome research has been increasingly linked with questions of specific and nonspecific ingredients of psychotherapeutic interventions and the amount of variance that can be explained by these factors.

How much psychotherapy is necessary?

In a classical meta-analysis of 2431 patients in psychotherapy in studies published over a period of three decades, Howard, Kopta, Krause, and Orlinsky (Howard et al., 1986) concluded that the relationship between the number of sessions ('dosage') and client improvement 'took the form of a positive relationship characterized by a negatively accelerated curve; that is, the more psychotherapy, the greater the probability of improvement, with diminishing returns at higher doses' (Kopta et al., 1994, p. 1009). This study also clearly supported the view that treatment produces benefits that surpass spontaneous remission rates.

Following this classical dose-effectiveness study, several other investigations were carried out to answer the question: How much therapy would be enough? In summarizing these studies, Lambert and Ogles (2004) conclude: 'Research suggests that a sizeable portion of patients reliably improve after 10 sessions and that 75% of patients will meet more rigorous criteria for success after about 50 sessions of treatment. Limiting treatment sessions to less than 20 will mean that about 50% of the patients will not achieve a substantial benefit from therapy'.

As it is generally the case in outcome research, dose-effectiveness functions reveal differential responses to treatment depending on the level of measurement: Howard et al. (1993) reported an attempt to support empirically the phase model of psychotherapeutic change that has been originally conceptualized by Frank (1973b). This model postulates that the process of psychological restitution reverses the order of development of psychopathology, i.e., failure of functioning in different areas, the development of psychological symptoms and the failure of the individual coping strategies resulting in demoralization. According to the phase model, therapeutic change should first occur in a restitution of well-being (*remoralization*), followed by a relief of symptoms (*remediation*), and finally result in an improvement of functioning (*rehabilitation*). Although the empirical studies related to this model are still equivocal, it is evident that different aspects of functioning respond differentially to treatment; psychological symptoms respond faster than personality and interpersonal aspects of functioning. It is obvious that results like this are of considerable importance in the discussion of the usefulness of long-term psychotherapy such as psychoanalysis or some forms of psychodynamic treatment.

The placebo problem in psychotherapy research

An important obstacle in the way of explaining specific psychotherapeutic effects is the placebo problem. In pharmacological research, placebos should not contain the curative substance. It is evident that ubiquitous psychological factors play an important role in the placebo phenomenon. These factors include the instillation of hope, a decrease in demoralization, the experience of self-efficacy, and the belief in the manageability of a problem. In contrast to pharmacological research, these factors are supposed to play an active role in patient improvement and are known as *common curative factors* in psychotherapy (Frank, 1973a; Strauss and Wittmann, 1999).

There is a long tradition of studies in psychotherapy research studies dealing with the relative benefit of therapies when compared with placebo controls. Recent meta-analyses show that the efficacy of specific treatments is superior to both no treatment and placebo treatments (Lipsey and Wilson, 1993). Grissom (1996) concludes on the basis of a meta-analysis that the 'results are consistent with the view that the ranking for therapeutic success is generally therapy, placebo, and control (do nothing or wait)' p. 979. In Grissom's analysis, the 'probability of superiority' was 0.70 for the therapy versus control comparison, 0.66 for the therapy versus placebo comparison and 0.62 for the placebo versus control comparison, with the latter indicating that placebo conditions that usually emphasize nonspecific or common therapeutic factors such as therapist warmth, attention, or expectations for change contribute to positive outcome, although the effects of these factors are smaller than those of specific psychotherapy.

Common factors and treatment outcome

What are the common factors?

One possible resolution to the equivalence paradox runs as follows: yes, psychotherapies differ in their theories and techniques, but these factors are not the important ones. There are many features that all psychotherapies have in common, and some of these common factors may be responsible for different treatments' equivalent effectiveness—most famously, Rogers's (1957) 'necessary and sufficient conditions,' which included genuineness, unconditional positive regard, and accurate empathy. Process research on common factors has looked at: (1) therapist-provided common factors, including the Rogerian conditions, warm involvement with the patient, and the communication of a new perspective on the patient's person and situation, (2) patient-provided common factors, such as patient self-disclosure (Stiles, 1995) and experiencing (Klein et al., 1986); and (3) the therapeutic alliance or the interaction between the therapist and the patient (Horvath and Bedi, 2002).

Thus one possible explanation for the general finding of only relatively small differences between treatments with respect to several outcome criteria is the assumption that different treatment modalities are characterized by *common curative factors* that are active ingredients of all particular schools (although sometimes not an explicit part of the formal change theory) and that these common factors go beyond those that might be important in explaining the placebo phenomenon.

Meanwhile, there is ample evidence for the relationship of common factors and improvement and even some evidence that common factors are superior to unique factors in explaining the variance of treatment outcome (Castonguay et al., 1996). In their recent review, Lambert and Ogles (2004) group common factors into three categories: *support factors*, such as catharsis, therapeutic alliance, therapist warmth, respect, and empathy; *learning factors*, such as insight, corrective emotional experiences, or assimilating problematic experiences; and *action factors*, such as mastery, reality testing, or behavioral regulation.

These common factors 'loom large as mediators of treatment outcome' (Lambert and Ogles, 2004), but are not sufficient to explain fully psychotherapeutic change. Other sources of variance such as unique interventions, patient and therapist related variables and their interaction have equally to be considered as factors that explain therapeutic improvement. The determination of the influence of such factors is a crucial issue in psychotherapeutic process research.

It is worth noting that an emphasis on common factors does not necessarily contradict the overall finding of the general superiority of CBT over other modalities, especially in specific disorders. It is possible the CBT is simply more efficient in marshalling the key common factors in its training and delivery. This kind of conclusions, emerging from the research literature is an example of the way in which research can help illuminate pressing clinical and training issues.

What we know about process

The aims of psychotherapy process research can be conveyed as a series of questions: What happens in psychotherapy? How do therapies differ? How do patients act and think differently as a result of therapy? What are the common factors across different therapies? Which are the effective ingredients? What happens as patients improve?

Much of this section is drawn from a chapter by Stiles et al. (1999), to which readers are referred for elaboration and further references concerning this material.

What happens in psychotherapy?

Treatment process research is characterized by a profusion of measures. Researchers have developed thousands of categories and scales, and they have organized these into hundreds of measuring instruments and systems of classification (for some compilations of examples, see Kiesler, 1973; Greenberg and Pinsof, 1986; Beck and Lewis, 2000). So many systems of process classification have been developed that there is even a literature on meta-classification—that is, classification of classifications (Russell and Stiles, 1979; Greenberg, 1986; Russell and Staszewski, 1988; Elliott, 1991; Elliott and Anderson, 1994; Lambert and Hill, 1994). Table 38.2 lists some meta-classificatory principles—ways in which process categories and measures differ.

As an illustration, consider the Working Alliance Inventory, patient form (WAI; Horvath and Greenberg, 1989), in which patients rate their agreement with 36 statements about their relationship with their therapist. It yields three scores reflecting the quality of the Bond, Agreement about Tasks, and Agreement about Goals. In terms of the characteristics listed in Table 38.1, the WAI uses the patient's perspective. Its target is the dyad. The scoring unit is usually the session or a sequence of sessions. It refers to all communication channels. It is a rating measure that is evaluative. It is based on the respondent's personal experience, accessed directly. It uses a pragmatic strategy. It is applicable to treatment of any theoretical orientation and has been used mainly in adult individual therapy, though versions have been developed for other modalities (as well as for therapist and observer perspectives).

Why are there so many measures? We think that informed researchers develop new measures because the old measures have failed to answer their questions or because they are interested in some previously unassessed aspect. Thus, although it may be tempting to advocate arbitrary standardization, this is probably not in the long-term interest of the field.

Do therapies differ?

Process research has led the way in trying to unravel the equivalence paradox. To assess differences in treatment processes, investigators have applied process measures to contrasting treatments or conditions and compared the results. They have repeatedly identified systematic differences in therapists' techniques across different orientations (Strupp, 1957; Stiles, 1979; DeRubeis et al., 1982; Elliott et al., 1987; Stiles et al., 1988; Hill et al., 1992; Startup and Shapiro, 1993). The empirically demonstrated process differences have generally been consistent with the theoretical differences between treatments.

Treatment differences are also important in comparative research. To ensure treatment integrity in clinical trials comparing different treatments, researchers have tried to standardize the treatments using detailed treatment manuals (DeRubeis et al., 1982; Luborsky et al., 1982). This step has led researchers to assess therapists' *adherence* to therapeutic protocols. The logic is that if treatments are to be compared, they must be delivered according to protocol. If an adherence check were to show that the therapists were not following the manual, the treatment was not being delivered correctly and the clinical trial could not be interpreted. For example, Hill et al. (1992) tested therapists' adherence to their respective treatment approaches in the National Institute of Mental Health Treatment of Depression Collaborative Research Program (TDCRP; Elkin, 1994) using a 96-item rating scale, which discriminated between the three different treatments very well. Therapists used more techniques consistent with their respective treatment modality, and fewer techniques appropriate to the other treatments.

Are there systematic differences among patients?

The frequent implicit assumption that all patients with the same diagnosed disorder compose a homogeneous group is certainly false. People differ in all sorts of ways that may be manifested in the therapeutic process. These differences affect the ways patients are treated (Hardy et al., 1998). Process researchers have applied their measures to assess ways in which patients are internally consistent (e.g., self-similar from session to session) but different from other patients. For example, computer-based analyses of the text of psychotherapy sessions have demonstrated consistent patient differences in

Table 38.2 Ways in which process categories and measures differ (after Stiles *et al.*, 1999)

Characteristic	Distinctions or examples
Perspective	*Viewpoint used*: therapist, patient, external observers, or judges
Target person(s)	*Examples*: therapist, patient, dyad, family, group
Size of the scoring unit	*Examples*: single words or gestures; phrases, clauses, sentences, speaking turns, topic episodes, timed intervals of various durations, whole sessions, phases of treatment, whole treatments, series of treatments *Distinctions*: Kiesler (1973) distinguished the *scoring unit* (the material to which the measure is directly applied) from the *contextual unit* (the material that coders or raters are told to consider when assigning the score, which may be considerably larger) and from the *summarizing unit* (the material over which scores are aggregated)
Communication channel	*Examples*: verbal, paralinguistic, kinesic
Measure format	*Examples*: coding, rating, verbal description, Q-sort, questionnaire *Distinctions*: Coding refers to classifications into nominal categories. Rating refers to placement on an (at least) ordinal scale
Evaluative vs descriptive	*Evaluations* require some judgment of quality or competence *Descriptions* concern objective characteristics
Verbal category	*Distinctions*: among the verbal coding measures, *content categories* deal with semantic meaning; *speech act categories* concern what is done when someone says something; *paralinguistic measures* concern behaviors that are not verbal but accompany speech (hesitations, dysfluencies, emphasis, tonal qualities)
Data format	*Materials studied*: transcripts, session notes, audiotape, videotape, current experience, postsession recall, long-term recall
Access strategy	*How observed*: direct observation, self-report, tape-assisted recall
Level of inference	*Distinctions*: in the *classical strategy*, only observable behavior is coded or rated by judges. In the *pragmatic strategy*, the coders or raters make inferences about the speaker's thoughts, feelings, intentions, or motivations based on the observed behavior
Theoretical orientation	*Examples*: psychoanalytic, experiential, cognitive, behavioral, interpersonal
Treatment modality	*Examples*: individual adult, child, family, group therapy

the frequencies of particular words, phrases, or categories in verbatim transcripts of sessions (Hölzer *et al.*, 1996).

Trying to capture the uniqueness of the individual, while at the same time yielding reproducible categorical data is a central task for psychotherapy researchers, especially those in the psychodynamic orientation. The Core Conflictual Relationship Theme method (Luborsky, 1976; Luborsky and Crits-Christoph, 1990) has been developed to assess treatment-relevant transference themes shown by patient narratives in psychotherapy; these commonly focus on interactions with other people in the patient's life, including the therapist (Barber *et al.*, 1995). The Structural Analysis of Social Behavior (Benjamin, 1996; Henry, 1996) uses a complex circumplex coding scheme, in which three underlying dimensions (dominance, affiliation, and individuation) are used to describe patients' interactions with self and others; this approach has been used to distinguish between good and poor outcomes of brief psychodynamic therapy (Henry *et al.*, 1986). In the CBT tradition, researchers interested in the psychotherapy of depression have emphasized such components of patient cognitive processes as causal attributions and depressive schemata—specific knowledge structures that contain undesirable biases, which are a target of interventions (Beck *et al.*, 1979).

Which are the effective ingredients?

Much process research has been driven by a search for the curative factors in psychotherapy. However, from a psychodynamic perspective the results of this search have been oddly disappointing. For example, Orlinsky *et al.* (1994) concluded that there was evidence for differential effectiveness of some therapeutic operations, including interpretation (along with paradoxical intention and experiential confrontation). A review of psychodynamic approaches in the same volume by Henry *et al.* (1994), however, concluded that 'transference interpretations do not elicit differentially greater affective response or necessarily increase depth of experiencing when compared with nontransference interpretations or other interventions' (p. 475). It may be noted that transference interpretations are not equivalent to interpretations, but insofar as the former are a subset of the latter, the contrasting conclusions were striking.

Yeaton and Sechrest (1981) urged therapists and investigators to attend to the strength, integrity, and effectiveness of treatment. Effective treatments, they argued, should contain large amounts of helpful change ingredients (strength) and should be delivered in a pure manner (integrity). If the theory underlying the treatment is correct, then delivering interventions with strength and integrity should be effective in producing patient change. This view of process-outcome relations has been called the *drug metaphor* (Stiles and Shapiro, 1989, 1994). However, the reasoning may be misleading (Stiles, 1988; Stiles *et al.*, 1998).

The *drug metaphor* logic assumes that the cause-effect relations of process and outcome variables run in a single direction (i.e., that process variables cause outcome variables). However, this reasoning neglects therapists' and patients' appropriate *responsiveness*—the tendency of both therapist and patients to make appropriate adjustments in their behavior as a result of ongoing changes in their own and each other's requirements (Stiles *et al.*, 1998). In human interaction, participants are responsive to each other's behavior on time scales that range down to a few tens of milliseconds, and for this reason, linear statistical descriptions of process-outcome relations can fail to reflect the value of a psychotherapy process component (Stiles, 1988).

Dismantling studies, at first glance, seem to offer a way around the responsiveness problem. They employ experimental methods to identify which components of a treatment package are responsible for facilitating change. Two or more treatment groups that vary in only one or a few of the treatment's techniques are compared. One group typically receives a complete treatment, whereas other groups receive only a portion of the treatment (Nezu and Perri, 1989). Dismantling studies represent a valuable tool, but interpreting them requires caution. They assume that components are self-contained modules that can be added and removed independently, which may not be the case in human interaction.

What happens as patients improve?

The difficulties in establishing linear links between process and outcome have encouraged interest in more descriptive studies—including qualitative studies—of what has been called the *process of outcome* or *change process* research. Researchers have tried to study sessions or episodes in which it appears that change is occurring and to describe what they believe to be good therapeutic process.

The *events paradigm* (Rice and Greenberg, 1984) focuses on the intensive analysis of significant events in psychotherapy—recurring categories of events that have a common structure and are important for change. Brief passages sharing some specified common feature are collected and examined using microanalytic techniques and close attention to the context. *Task analysis* is a method for studying a particular type of significant event in therapy (a task) and describing the process of change. Rice and Saperia (1984) illustrated task analysis with their description of a *problematic reaction point* (PRP) as a significant event in therapy. The marker of a PRP is a statement by the patient of finding his or her own behavior as problematic (e.g., 'I overreacted but I don't know why; it was unlike me'). The therapist's task at a PRP is systematic evocative unfolding (Rice, 1974). The therapist directs the patient to reenter the scene of the original stimulus situation vividly and to explore his or her own understanding of the situation at the time of the problematic reaction. The therapist tries to get the patient to focus on either the stimulus or their inner reaction, but not on both at the same time. According to Rice and Saperia (1984), a marker of a PRP followed by therapist use of systematic evocative unfolding led to a resolution more frequently than if the therapist responded with empathic caring.

Qualitative approaches bearing such names as *discourse analysis* (Madill and Barkham, 1997), *grounded theory* (Rennie *et al.*, 1988), *consensual qualitative research* (Hill *et al.*, 1997), and *assimilation analysis* (Stiles and Angus, 2001), have offered a nonlinear approach that seeks to describe the therapeutic more discursively and thoroughly. Typically, these approaches study only one or a few cases at a time, but in far more detail than traditional hypothesis-testing process research. The intended yield of such studies is a richly descriptive understanding of particular processes rather than a specific generalizable finding based on a large sample of different cases.

The goal of a qualitative, descriptive study is often to elaborate a theory rather than to test a particular consequence. For example, the goal of task analysis is often explained as the development of a model of psychotherapeutic change. This gives qualitative studies a greater openness to new information, but their conclusions are correspondingly more tentative than those of hypothesis testing research (Stiles, 1993).

Implementation of evidence into clinical practice

Clinical effectiveness is only one dimension in planning psychotherapy services. In addition, services need to meet the criteria of being *comprehensive, co-ordinated and user-friendly, safe, and cost-effective* (Parry, 1996). Research evidence is at the center of the drive by governments and health strategists in many countries to base practice on robust evidence. Optimally, clinicians would routinely and systematically review the research literature and come to conclusions about best practice. This, of course, is a mammoth task. Fortunately commissioned and individually generated reviews fill the gap. In the UK, the Cochrane database is open to all. The database uses a hierarchy of evidence with RCTs at its pinnacle.

Another source of summary information is to be found in the aptly named *What works for whom?* (Roth and Fonagy, 1996). Concentrating largely on RCTs, the authors review the evidence for benefit in different diagnostic groups, predominantly Axis I. Each chapter ends with a summary and implications for service delivery and future research. When, as now, RCTs are not fully representative of the range of therapies or types of presentation in clinical practice, it has to be recognized, as already stated, that absence of evidence is not evidence of ineffectiveness. Furthermore as previously noted, there is considerable problem in extrapolating from efficacy studies to clinic practice.

In the USA, there has been a move to favor *empirically supported therapies* [see *Special section of psychotherapy research* (1998, Vol. 8., pp. 115–70)

for a critique]. This has the advantage of concentrating the minds of therapists, patients and those responsible for paying for a treatment, but it also has a down side. Concentrating on brand names may overemphasize the difference between approaches and risks fossilizing the field when there is still much innovation to come. As the person of the therapist and their allegiance contributes significantly to outcome, it has been, not entirely with tongue in cheek, suggested that we should speak of *empirically supported therapists* (Wampold, 2001).

Empirical research evidence from RCTs tells us what can be achieved under optimal conditions. The evidence is complementary to clinical judgment. For this reason, we welcome the 'Guideline' subtitle to the useful Department of Health report on treatment choice in psychological therapies and counseling (Parry, 2001).

Research (can) tells us what to do: audit tells us if we are doing it right (R. Smith, 1992). Audit is the systematic review of the delivery of health care in order to identify deficiencies so that they can be remedied (Crombie *et al.*, 1993). Audit measures performance against standards. It is part of the process of ensuring that evidence-based practice is delivered in practice. Each audit cycle of observing current practice, setting standards of care, comparing practice with the standards, and implementing change initiates the next pass through the cycle (Fonagy and Higgitt, 1989; Aveline and Watson, 2000).

A new paradigm of *practice-based evidence* is well established (Margison *et al.*, 2000). Inferences are drawn from naturalistic unselected clinical populations. The samples may be large, particularly when services pool routinely collected data through locally organized practice research networks (PTNs). Typically, the clinic work is with complex cases where therapist competence may be more important then therapy adherence. Here the clinician comes out of the planning and research shadows and is a stakeholder in the form of the service and its delivery. Routine monitoring of outcome is an essential component with performance feedback to the clinicians and the service as a whole. This facilitates *quality management* by charting the expected and actual course of patients in the service with various conditions. *Benchmarks* allow one service to compare and review outcomes with other similar services. Several reliable, relevant, and sensitive psychometric systems for routine use have been developed of which one of the most promising is CORE (Evans *et al.*, 2002).

Once an individual's dose-response curve has been determined, predictions can be made about likely outcome (Lueger *et al.*, 2001). This is the *patient-focused* outcome paradigm. There is good evidence that outcome can be enhanced by *signaling* to clinicians that the clinical course of a particular patient is problematic. Typically, a traffic-light metaphor is used: red signaling clinically significant deterioration, yellow being a lesser alert, and green indicating that the therapy is on its expected beneficial course. Clinical decision making is enhanced and there is an opportunity for timely corrective action (Kordy *et al.*, 2001; Lambert *et al.*, 2001).

Evidence, audit, and quality management are essential complements to clinical judgment (and supervision) in maintaining good practice. The appendix offers guidance on the critical questions in evaluating research studies.

Future directions

Neuroscience is making huge strides in understanding how the brain functions. Static models of localized function are being replaced by that of an integrated collaborative whole brain, which reacts plastically to new experience, modeling that new experience through new, ever-changing arrangements of synapse. The importance of pattern recognition and preconscious processing is coming to the fore (Pally, 1997a,b; Gabbard, 2000). The convergence with basic science offers a rich opportunity for collaborative research as the explanations offered by neuroscience come close to the level of observed process in clinical work.

Another process from the opposite end of the spectrum, namely the user-perspective, is also likely to be highly influential in research design and focus. Users will help determine outcome criteria and shape the form of therapies by voicing their experience of what is helpful and what outcomes they particularly value. Self-help therapies are appearing, especially in primary health care.

Naturalistic effectiveness studies will help translate the lessons of efficacy studies into practice. Instead of pure models of therapy, which often feature for pragmatic reasons in RCTs, there is great scope for the evolution and testing of more complex therapy models, spanning both Axis I and II disorders, and resulting in optimal integration and better principles for their eclectic application. This will have implications for training that we predict will emphasize selection based on the personal qualities shown by effective therapists, the best use of the common therapeutic factors, and the application of phase-specific integrated therapies. *Stepped care* provides an interesting model of repeated review and deployment of different interventions as the patient progresses through a course of health care. The value of these new approaches will need to be tested in a new round of comparative and hermeneutic studies.

Now that there are many established symptom measures, there is a great need to develop useable relationship measures, which address the interpersonal and the interactive intersubjectivity that exists between people and is central to psychotherapy practice (Hobson, 2003). More work needs to be done on the optimal duration, frequency, and techniques for both brief and long-term therapy. Finally, cultural and sociological aspects of psychotherapy need to be investigated to see what is novel and valuable and how approaches may have to be modified to do well in local contexts.

Conclusions

Research is one way of knowing the world. Methods that facilitate precision in application and communication are applied to questions of clinical import; the precision helps colleagues understand what was done, assess its significance, and replicate the study. In short, research is part of discovery. Inevitably, the findings or, even, the process of doing the research raises unexpected questions. Taking new insights forward requires flexibility in attitude and assumptions. The results can benefit clinical practice, especially if the design is practice close and involves clinicians from the outset (Hardy, 1995). Worthwhile research is possible at all levels of complexity of investigation but generally needs team work and funding. The path from clinical insight to 'laboratory' studies to clinic is satisfying but long.

Recommended texts

Lambert, M. J., ed. (2003). *Handbook of psychotherapy and behavior change*. New York: Wiley.

Parry, G. and Watts, F. N., ed. (1996). *Behavioural and mental health research: a handbook of skills and methods*. Hove: Lawrence Erlbaum Associates.

Barker, C., *et al.* (1994). *Research methods in clinical and counselling psychology*. New York: Wiley.

Holloway, I. (1997). *Basic concepts for qualitative research*. Oxford: Blackwell.

Murphy, E., *et al.* (1998). *Qualitative research methods in health technology assessment: a review of the literature*. Southampton: Health Technology Assessment, NHS R&D HTA Programme: 276.

References

Ahn, H. and Wampold, B. E. (2001). Where or where are the specific ingredients? A meta-analysis of component studies in counseling and psychotherapy. *Journal of Counseling Psychology*, **48**, 251–7.

Altman, D. G. (1998). Confidence intervals for the number needed to treat. *British Medical Journal*, **317**, 1309–12.

Ambühl, H. and Strauss, B. (1999). *Therapieziele*. Göttingen: Hogrefe.

Aveline, M. (1999). The advantages of formulation over categorical diagnosis in explorative psychotherapy and psychodynamic management. *European Journal of Psychotherapy, Counselling and Health*, **2**, 199–216.

Aveline, M. (in press). Clinical case studies: their place in evidence-based practice. *Psycho-dynamic Practice*.

Aveline, M. and Watson, J. (2000). Making a success of your psychotherapy service: the contribution of clinical audit. In: C. J. Mace, B. Roberts, and S. Morey, ed. *Evidence in the psychological therapies*, pp. 199–210. London: Routledge.

Aveline, M., Shapiro, D. A., Parry, G., and Freeman, C. (1995). Building research foundations for psychotherapy. In: D. A. Shapiro, ed. *Research foundations for psychotherapy practice*. Chichester: John Wiley and Sons.

Barber, J. P., Luborsky, L., Crits-Christoph, P., and Diguer, L. (1995). A comparision of core conflictual relationship themes before psychotherapy and during early sessions. *Journal of Consulting and Clinical Psychology*, **63**, 145–8.

Barkham, M. (2002). Methods, outcomes and processes in the psychological therapies across four successive research generations. In: W. Dryden, ed. *Handbook of individual therapy*, pp. 372–433. London: Sage.

Beck, A. P. and Lewis, C. M., ed. (2000). *The process of group psychotherapy: Systems for analyzing change*. Washington, DC: APA Books.

Beck, A. T., Rush, A. J., Shaw, B. F., and Emery, G. (1979). *Cognitive therapy of depression*. New York: Wiley.

Benjamin, L. S. (1996). *Interpersonal diagnosis and treatment of personality disorders*. New York: Guilford Press.

Beutler, L. E. (1991). Have all won and must all have prizes? Revisiting Luborsky et al.'s verdict. *Journal of Consulting and Clinical Psychology*, **59**, 226–32.

Bond, T. (2004). British Association for Counselling and Psychotherapy, p. 12. Rugby.

Bond, T., Ashcroft, R., Casemore, R., Jamieson, A., and Lendrum, S. (2002). Ethical Framework for Good Practice in Counselling and Psychotherapy. British Association for Counselling and Psychotherapy, p. 16. Rugby.

Borkovec, T. D. (1993). Between-group therapy outcome research: Design and methodology. In: L. S. Onken, J. D. Blaine, and J. J. Boren, ed. *Behavioral treatments for drug abuse and dependence*. Rockville, MD: National Institute on Drug Abuse, pp. 249–90.

Burlingame, G. M., Strauss, B., and MacKenzie, K. R. (2004). Small group treatment: evidence for effectiveness and mechanisms of change. In: W. Lambert, ed. *Handbook of psychotherapy and behavior change*, pp. 647–96. New York: Wiley.

Carroll, L. (1865/1946). *Alice's adventures in wonderland*. New York: Random House.

Castonguay, L. G., Goldfried, M. R., Wiser, S., Raue, P. J., and Hayes, A. H. (1996). Predicting outcome in cognitive therapy for depression: A comparison of unique and common factors. *Journal of Consulting and Clinical Psychology*, **64**, 497–504.

Chambless, D. L. (2002). Beware the Dodo Bird: The dangers of overgeneralization. *Clinical Psychology: Science and Practice*, **9**, 13–16.

Chiles, J. A., Lambert, M. J., and Hatch, A. L. (1999). The impact of psychological interventions on medical cost offset: A meta-analytic review. *Clinical Psychology: Science and Practice*, **6**, 204–20.

Cohen, J. (1977). *Statistical power analysis for the behavioural sciences*. Hillsdale, NJ: Erlbaum.

Cook, R. J. and Sackett, D. L. (1995). The number needed to treat: a clinically useful measure of treatment effect. *British Journal of Medicine*, **310**, 452–4.

Cook, T. D. and Campbell, D. T. (1979). *Quasi-experimentation: Design and analysis for field settings*. Boston: Houghton-Mifflin.

Crombie, I. K., Davies, H. T. O., Abraham, S. C. S., and Florey, C. d. V. (1993). *The audit handbook*. Chicester: John Wiley & Sons.

DeRubeis, R., Hollon, S., Evans, M., and Bemis, K. (1982). Can psychotherapies for depression be discriminated? A systematic investigation of cognitive therapy and interpersonal therapy. *Journal of Consulting & Clinical Psychology*, **50**, 744–56.

Elkin, I. (1994). The NIMH Treatment of Depression Collaborative Research Program: where we began and where we are. In: A. E. Bergin and S. L. Garfield, ed. *Handbook of psychotherapy and behavior change*, pp. 114–39. New York: Wiley.

Elliott, R. (1991). Five dimensions of psychotherapy process. *Psychotherapy Research*, **1**, 92–103.

Elliott, R. and Anderson, C. (1994). Simplicity and complexity in psychotherapy research. In: R. L. Russell, ed. *Reassessing psychotherapy research*, pp. 65–113. New York: Guilford Press.

Elliott, R., *et al.* (1987). Primary therapist response modes: Comparision of six rating systems. *Journal of Consulting and Clinical Psychology*, 55, 218–23.

Elliott, R. *et al.* (2004). *Learning emotion-focused therapy*. Washington, DC: American Psychological Association.

Emmelkamp, P. M. G. (1994). Behavior therapy with adults. In: A. E. Bergin and S. L. Garfield, ed. *Handbook of psychotherapy and behavior change*, pp. 379–427. New York: Wiley.

Evans, C., *et al.* (2002). Towards a standardised brief outcome measure: psychometric properties and utility of the CORE-OM. *British Journal of Psychiatry*, 180, 51–60.

Eysenck, H. J. (1952). The effects of psychotherapy: An evaluation. *Journal of Consulting Psychology*, 319–24.

Fenichel, O. (1930). Statistischer Bericht über die therapeutische Tätigkeit 1920–1930. In: S. Radó, O. Fenichel, and C. Müller-Braunschweig, ed. *Zehn Jahre Berliner Psychoanalytisches Institut*, pp. 13–19. Zurich, Switzerland: Institut Psychoanalytischer Verlag.

Fonagy, P., ed. (2001). *An open door review of outcome studies in psychoanalysis*. London: University College of London.

Fonagy, P. and Higgitt, A. (1989). Evaluating the performance of Departments of Psychotherapy. *Psychoanalytic Psychotherapy*, 4, 121–53.

Frank, J. D. (1973a). *Persuasion and healing*. Baltimore, MD: Johns Hopkins University Press.

Frank, J. D. (1973b). Therapeutic factors in psychotherapy. *American Journal of Psychotherapy*, 25, 101–11.

Gabbard, G. O. (2000). A neurobiologically informed perspective on psychotherapy. *British Journal of Psychiatry*, 177, 117–22.

Gabbard, G. O., Lazar, S. G., Hornberger, J., and Spiegel, D. (1997). The economic impact of psychotherapy: A review. *American Journal of Psychiatry*, 154, 147–55.

Glaser, B. G. and Strauss, A. L. (1967). *The discovery of grounded theory*. Chicago, IL: Aldine.

Grawe, K., Bernauer, F., and Donati, R. (1993). *Psychotherapie im Wandel*. Göttingen: Hogrefe.

Greenberg, L. S. (1986). Change process research. *Journal of Consulting and Clinical Psychology*, 54, 4–9.

Greenberg, L. S. and Pinsof, W. M., ed. (1986). *The psychotherapeutic process: A research handbook*. New York: Guilford Press.

Grissom, R. J. (1996). The magical number .7 ± .2: Meta-meta-analysis of the probability of superior outcome in comparisions involving therapy, placebo, and control. *Journal of Consulting & Clinical Psychology*, 64, 973–82.

Haaga, D. A. F. and Stiles, W. B. (2000). Randomized clinical trials in psychotherapy research: Methodology, design, and evaluation. In: C. R. Snyder and R. E. Ingram, ed. *Handbook of psychological change: psychotherapy processes and practices for the 21st century*, pp. 14–39. New York: Wiley.

Hardy, G. E. (1995). Organizational issues: making research happen. In: M. Aveline and D. E. Shapiro, ed. *Research foundations for psychotherapy practice*, pp. 97–116. Chichester: John Wiley and Sons.

Hardy, G. E., Stiles, W. B., Barkham, M., and Startup, M. (1998). Therapist responsiveness to client interpersonal styles during time-limited treatments for depression. *Journal of Consulting & Clinical Psychology*, 66, 304–12.

Henry, W. P. (1996). Structural Analysis of Social Behavior as a common metric for programmatic psychopathology and psychotherapy research. *Journal of Consulting and Clinical Psychology*, 64, 1263–75.

Henry, W. P., Schacht, T. E., and Strupp, H. H. (1986). Structural analysis of social behavior: Application to a study of interpsersonal process in differential psychotherapeutic outcome. *Journal of Consulting and Clinical Psychology*, 54, 27–31.

Henry, W. P., Strupp, H. H., Schacht, T. E., and Gaston, L. (1994). Psychodynamic approaches. In: A. E. Bergin and S. L. Garfield, ed. *Handbook of psychotherapy and behavior change*, pp. 467–508. New York: Wiley.

Hill, C. E., O'Grady, K. E., and Elkin, I. (1992). Applying the Collaborative Study Psychotherapy Rating Scale to rate therapist dherence in cognitive-behavioral

therapy, interpersonal therapy, and clinical management. *Journal of Consulting and Clinical Psychology*, 60, 73–9.

Hill, C. E., Thompson, B. J., and Williams, E. N. (1997). A guide to conducting consensual qualitative research. *The Counseling Psychologist*, 25, 517–72.

Hillman, J. (1983). *Healing fiction*. Barrytown, NY: Station Hill.

Hobson, R. P. (2003). Between ourselves: Psychodynamics and the interpersonal domain. *British Journal of Psychiatry*, 182, 193–5.

Hölzer, M., Mergenthaler, E., Pokorny, D., Kächele, H., and Luborsky, L. (1996). Vocabulary measures for the evaluation of therapy outcome: re-studying transcripts from the Penn Psychotherapy Project. *Psychotherapy Research*, 6, 95–108.

Horvath, A. O. and Bedi, R. P. (2002). The alliance. In: J. C. Norcross, ed. *Psychotherapy relationships that work: Therapist contributions and responsiveness to patients*, pp. 37–69. New York: Oxford University Press.

Horvath, A. O. and Greenberg, L. S. (1989). Development and validation of the Working Alliance Inventory. *Journal of Counseling Psychology*, 36, 223–33.

Howard, K. I., Kopta, S. M., Krause, M.S., and Orlinsky, D. E. (1986). The dose-effect relationship in psychotherapy. *American Psychologist*, 41, 159–64.

Howard, K. I., Lueger, R. J., Maling, M. S., and Martinovich, Z. (1993). A phase model of psychotherapy outcome: Causal mediation of change. *Journal of Consulting and Clinical Psychology*, 61, 678–85.

Jacobson, N. S. and Truax, P. (1991). Clinical significance: A statistical approach to defining meaningful change in psychotherapy research. *Journal of Consulting and Clinical Psychology*, 59, 12–19.

Jacobson, N. S., Roberts, L. J., Berns, S. B., and McGlinchey, J. B. (1999). Methods for defining and determining the clinical significance of treatment effects: Description, application, and alternatives. *Journal of Consulting & Clinical Psychology*, 67, 300–7.

Kächele, H., Kordy, H., Richard, M. and TR-EAT (2001). Therapy amount and outcome in inpatient psychodynamic psychotherapy for eating disorders in Germany. *Psychotherapy Research*, 11, 239–58.

Kazdin, A. E. (1998). *Research design in clinical psychology*. Boston, MA: Allyn & Bacon.

Kendall, P. C., Marrs-Garcia, A., Nath, S. R. and Sheldrick, R. C. (1999). Normative comparisons for the evaluation of clinical significance. *Journal of Consulting & Clinical Psychology*, 67, 285–99.

Kiesler, D. J. (1973). *The process of psychotherapy: Empirical foundations and systems of analysis*. Chicago, IL: Aldine.

Klein, M. H., Mathieu-Coughlan, P., and Kiesler, D. J. (1986). The experiencing scales. In: L. S. Greenberg and W. M. Pinsof, ed. *The psychotherapeutic process: A research handbook*, pp. 21–71. New York: Guilford Press.

Kopta, S. M., Howard, K. I., Lowry, J. L., and Beutler, L. E. (1994). Patterns of symptomatic recovery in psychotherapy. *Journal of Consulting and Clinical Psychology*, 62, 1009–16.

Kordy, H., Hannover, W., and Richard, M. (2001). Computor-assisted feedback-driven quality managment for psychotherapy: The Stuttgart-Heidelberg model. *Journal of Consulting & Clinical Psychology*, 69, 173–83.

Krupnick, J. L., Sotsky, S. M., Elkin, I., Simmens, S., Moyer, J., Watkins, J., and Pilkonis, P. A. (1996). The role of the therapeutic alliance in psychotherapy and pharmacotherapy outcome: Findings in the National Institute of Mental health treatment of depression collaborative research program. *Journal of Consulting and Clinical Psychology*, 64, 532–539.

Lambert, M. J. and Bergin, A. E. (1994). The effectiveness of psychotherapy. In: A. E. Bergin and S. L. Garfield, ed. *Handbook of psychotherapy and behaviour change*, pp. 143–189. New York: John Wiley and Sons.

Lambert, M. J. and Hill, C. E. (1994). Methodological issues in studying psychotherapy process and outcome. In: A. E. Bergin and S. L. Garfield, ed. *Handbook of psychotherapy and behavior change*, pp. 72–113. New York: Wiley.

Lambert, M. J. and Ogles, B. M. (2004). The efficacy and effectiveness of Psychotherapy. In: M. J. Lambert, ed. *Handbook of psychotherapy and behavior change*, pp. 139–93. New York: Wiley.

Lambert, M., Hansen, N. B., and Finch, A. E. (2001). Patient-focussed research: using patient outcome data to enhance treatment effects. *Journal of Consulting & Clinical Psychology*, 69, 159–172.

Lilford, R. J. (2003). Ethics of clinical trials from a bayesian and decision analytic perspective: Whose equipose is it anyway? *British Medical Journal*, 326, 980–1.

Lilford, R. J. and Jackson, J. (1995). Equipose and the ethics of randomization. *Journal of the Royal Society of Medicine*, **88**, 552–9.

Lipsey, M. W. and Wilson, D. B. (1993). The efficacy of psychological, educational, and behavioral treatment: Confirmation from meta-analysis. *American Psychologist*, **48**, 1181–209.

Luborsky, L. (1976). Helping alliances in psychotherapy. In: J. L. Cleghhorn, ed. *Successful psychotherapy*, pp. 92–116. New York: Brunner/Mazel.

Luborsky, L. and Crits-Christoph, P. (1990). *Understanding transference. The core conflictual relationship theme method*, New York: Basic Books.

Luborsky, L., et al. (1999). The researcher's own therapy allegiances: A 'wild card' in comparisions of treatment efficacy. *Clinical Psychology: Science and Practice*, **6**, 95–106.

Luborsky, L., et al. (2002). The Dodo Bird Verdict is alive and well—mostly. *Clinical Psychology: Science and Practice*, **9**, 2–12.

Luborsky, L., Singer, B., and Luborsky, E. (1975). Comparative studies of psychotherapies. Is it true that 'Everyone has won and all must have prizes?' *Archives of General Psychiatry*, **32**, 995–1008.

Luborsky, L., Woody, G. E., McLellan, A. T., O'Brien, C. P., and Rosenzweig, J. (1982). Can independent judges recognize different psychotherapies? An experience with manual-guided therapies. *Journal of Consulting and Clinical Psychology*, **49**, 49–62.

Lueger, R. O. J., et al. (2001). Assessing treatment progress of individual patients using expected treatment response models. *Journal of Consulting & Clinical Psychology*, **69**, 150–8.

Madill, A. and Barkham, M. (1997). Discourse analysis of a theme in one successful case of brief psychodynamic-interpersonal psychotherapy. *Journal of Counseling Psychology*, **44**, 232–44.

Margison, F., et al. (2000). Evidence-based practice and practice-based evidence. *British Journal of Psychiatry*, **177**, 123–30.

McLeod, J. and Lynch, G. (2000). 'This is our life:' Strong evaluation in psychotherapy narrative. *European Journal of Psychotherapy, Counselling, and Health*, **3**, 389–406.

McNeilly, C. L. and Howard, K. I. (1991). The effects of psychotherapy: A re-evaluation based on dosage. *Psychotherapy Research*, **1**, 74–8.

Meehl, P. E. (1978). Theoretical risks and tabular asterisks: Sir Karl, Sir Ronald, and the slow progress of soft psychology. *Journal of Consulting and Clinical Psychology*, **46**, 806–34.

Mohr, D. C. (1995). Negative outcome in psychotherapy: A critical review. *Clinical Psychology: Science and Practice*, **2**, 1–27.

Nezu, A. M. and Perri, M. G. (1989). Social Problem-Solving Therapy for Unipolar Depression: An initial dismantling investigation. *Journal of Consulting and Clinical Psychology*, **57**, 408–13.

Norcross, J. C. (1995). Dispelling the dodo bird verdict and the exclusivity myth in psychotherapy. *Psychotherapy*, **32**, 500–4.

Ogles, M. M., Lunnen, K. M., and Bonesteel, K. (2001). Clinical significance: History, application and practice. *Clinical Psychology Review*, **21**, 421–6.

Orlinsky, D. E. and Russell, R. L. (1994). Tradition and change in psychotherapy: Notes on the fourth generation. In: R. L. Russell, ed. *Reassessing psychotherapy research*, pp. 185–214. New York: Guilford Press.

Orlinsky, D. E., Grawe, K., and Parks, B. K. (1994). Process and outcome in psychotherapy—noch einmal. In: A. E. Bergin and S. L. Garfield, ed. *Handbook of psychotherapy and behavior change*, pp. 270–376. New York: Wiley.

Packer, M. J. and Addison, R. B., ed. (1989a). Evaluating an interpretive account. In: *Entering the circle: Hermeneutic investigation in psychology*, pp. 13–36. Albany, NY: State University of New York Press.

Pally, R. (1997a). II: How the brain actively constructs perceptions. *International Journal of Psycho-Analysis*, **78**, 1021–30.

Pally, R. (1997b). Memory: Brain systems that link past, present and future. *International Journal of Psycho-Analysis*, **78**, 1223–34.

Parry, G. (1996). NHS psychotherapy services in England. A review of strategic policy. Department of Health.

Parry, G. (2001). Treatment Choice in Psychological Therapies and Counselling. Department of Health, London.

Rennie, D. L. (1994a). Clients' accounts of resistance: A qualitative analysis. *Canadian Journal of Counselling*, **28**, 43–57.

Rennie, D. L. (1994b). Clients' deference in psychotherapy. *Journal of Counseling Psychology*, **41**, 427–37.

Rennie, D. L., Phillips, J. R., and Quartaro, G. K. (1988). Grounded theory: A promising approach to conceptualization in psychology? *Canadian Psychology*, **29**, 139–50.

Rhodes, R., Hill, C. E., Thompson, B., and Elliott, R. (1994). A retrospective study of the client perception of misunderstanding of events. *Journal of Counseling Psychology*, **41**, 473–83.

Rice, L. N. (1974). The evocative function of the therapist. In: D. A. Wexler and L. N. Rice, ed. *Innovations in client-centered therapy*, pp. 289–311. New York: Wiley.

Rice, L. N. and Greenberg, L. S., ed. (1984). *Patterns of change*. New York: Guilford Press.

Rice, L. N. and Saperia, E. P. (1984). Task analysis and the resolution of problematic reactions. In: L. N. Rice and L. S. Greenberg, ed. *Patterns of change*, pp. 29–66. New York: Guilford Press.

Rogers, C. R. (1957). The necessary and sufficient conditions of therapeutic personality change. *Journal of Consulting Psychology*, **21**, 95–103.

Rosenzweig, S. (1936). Some implicit common factors in diverse methods psychotherapy. *American Journal of Orthopsychiatry*, **6**, 412–15.

Roth, A. and Fonagy, P. (1996). *What works for whom? A critical review of psychotherapy research*. New York: Guilford Press.

Rudolf, G. (1991). *Die therapeutische Arbeitsbeziehung*. Heidelberg: Springer.

Russell, R. L. and Staszewski, C. (1988). The unit problem: Some systematic distinctions and critical dilemmas for psychotherapy process research. *Psychotherapy*, **25**, 191–200.

Russell, R. L. and Stiles, W. B. (1979). Categories for classifying language in psychotherapy. *Psychological Bulletin*, **86**, 404–19.

Schulte, D. (1995). How therapy success should be assessed. *Psychotherapy Research*, **5**, 281–96.

Seligman, M. E. P. (1995). The effectiveness of psychotherapy: The Consumer Reports study. *American Psychologist*, **50**, 965–74.

Shadish, W. R., et al. (1997). Evidence that therapy works in clinically representative situations. *Journal of Consulting and Clinical Psychology*, **55**, 355–65.

Shapiro, D. A. and Startup, M. (1992). Measuring therapist adherence in exploratory psychotherapy. *Psychotherapy Research*, **2**, 193–203.

Shapiro, D. A., et al. (1995). Decisions, decisions, decisions: determining the effects of treatment method and duration on the outcome of psychotherapy for depression. In: M. Aveline and D. A. Shapiro, ed. *Research foundations for psychotherapy practice* pp. 151–74. Chichester: John Wiley and Sons.

Shoham, V. and Rohrbaugh, M. J. (1999). Beyond allegiance to comparative outcome studies. *Clinical Psychology: Science and Practice*, **6**, 120–3.

Smith, M. L., Glass, G. V., and Miller, T. I. (1980). *The benefits of psychotherapy*. Baltimore, MD: Johns Hopkins University Press.

Smith, R. (1992). Audit and research (editorial). *British Medical Journal*, **305**, 905–6.

Stanton, M. D. and Shadish, W. R. (1997). Outcome, attrition, and family-couples treatment for drug abuse: A meta-analysis and review of the controlled, comparative studies. *Psychological Bulletin*, **122**, 170–91.

Special Section of Psychotherapy Research (1998). **8**, 115–70.

Startup, M. J. and Shapiro, D. A. (1993). Therapist treatment fidelity in Prescriptive vs Exploratory psychotherapy. *British Journal of Clinical Psychology*, **32**, 443–56.

Stiles, W. B. (1979). Verbal response modes and psychotherapeutic technique. *Psychiatry*, **42**, 49–62.

Stiles, W. B. (1988). Psychotherapy process-outcome correlations may be misleading. *Psychotherapy*, **25**, 27–35.

Stiles, W. B. (1993). Quality control in qualitative research. *Clinical Psychology Review*, **13**, 593–618.

Stiles, W. B. (1995). Disclosure as a speech act: Is it psychotherapeutic to disclose? In: J. W. Pennebaker, ed. *Emotion, disclosure, and health*, pp. 71–91. Washington, DC: American Psychological Association

Stiles, W. B. (2003). Qualitative research: Evaluating the process and the product. In: S. P. Llewelyn and P. Kennedy, ed. *Handbook of clinical health psychology* pp. 477–99. London: Wiley.

Stiles, W. B. and Angus, L. (2001). In: J. Frommer and D. L. Rennie, ed. *Qualitative psychotherapy research: Methods and methodology*, pp. 112–27. Lengerich, Germany: Pabst Science Publishers.

Stiles, W. B. and Shapiro, D. A. (1989). Abuse of the drug metaphor in psychotherapy process-outcome research. *Clinical Psychology Review*, **9**, 521–43.

Stiles, W. B. and Shapiro, D. A. (1994). Disabuse of the drug metaphor: Psychotherapy process-outcome correlations. *Journal of Consulting and Clinical Psychology*, **62**, 942–8.

Stiles, W. B., Shapiro, D. A., and Elliott, R. (1986). Are all psychotherapies equivalent? *American Psychologist*, **41**, 165–80.

Stiles, W. B., Shapiro, D. A., and Firth-Cozens, J. A. (1988). Verbal response mode use in contrasting psychotherapies: A within-subjects comparison. *Journal of Consulting and Clinical Psychology*, **56**, 727–33.

Stiles, W. B., Honos-Webb, L., and Surko, M. (1998). Responsiveness in psychotherapy. *Clinical Psychology: Science and Practice*, **5**, 439–58.

Stiles, W. B., Honos-Webb, L., and Knobloch, L. M. (1999). Treatment process research methods. In: P. C. Kendall, J. N. Butcher, and G. N. Holmbeck, ed. *Handbook of research methods in clinical psychology*, pp. 364–402. New York: Wiley.

Strauss, B. and Kächele, H. (1998). The writing on the wall. *Psychotherapy Research*, **8**, 158–70.

Strauss, B. and Wittmann, W. W. (1999). Wie hilft Psychotherapie? In: W. Senf and M. Broda, ed. *Praxis der Psychotherapie*, pp. 734–46. Stuttgart: Thieme.

Strupp, H. H. (1957). A multidimensional comparison of therapists in analytic and client-centered therapy. *Journal of Consulting Psychology*, **21**, 301–8.

Strupp, H. H., Lambert, M. J., and Horowitz, L. M., ed. (1997). *Measuring patient changes in mood, anxiety and personality disorders*. Washington DC: American Psychological Association Press.

Svartberg, M. and Stiles, T. C. (1991). Comparaive effects of short-term psychodynamic psychotherapy: A meta-analysis. *Journal of Consulting and Clinical Psychology*, **59**, 704–14.

Wallerstein, R. S. (1986). *Forty-two lives in treatment: A study of psychoanalysis and psychotherapy*. New York: Guilford Press.

Waltz, J., Addis, M. E., Koerner, K., and Jacobson, N. S. (1993). Testing the integrity of a psychotherapy protocol: Assessment of adherence and competence. *Journal of Consulting and Clinical Psychology*, **61**, 620–30.

Wampold, B. E. (2001). *The great psychotherapy debate: Models, methods, and findings*. Mahwah, NJ: Lawrence Erlbaum Associates, Inc.

Wampold, B. E., *et al.* (1997). A meta-analysis of outcome studies comparing bona fide psychotherapies: Empiricially, 'all must have prizes'. *Psychological Bulletin*, **122**, 203–15.

Woolfolk, R. L., Sass, L. A., and Messer, S. B. (1988). Introduction to hermeneutics. In: S. B. Messer, L. A. Sass, and R. L. Woolfolk, ed. *Hermeneutics and psychological theory: interpretive perspectives on personality, psychotherapy, and psychopathology*, pp. 2–26. New Brunswick, NJ: Rutgers University Press.

Yeaton, W. H. and Sechrest, L. (1981). Critical dimensions in the choice and maintenance of successful treatments: Strength, integrity, and effectiveness. *Journal of Consulting and Clinical Psychology*, **49**, 156–67.

Appendix: how to read a research paper

The research literature is vast and time is limited. Published work varies in quality and significance. How can the busy clinician sift the wheat from the chaff?

General questions

These apply to all studies.

1. What is the study about? What hypotheses are being tested?

2. What is being 'done' between whom and whom? Can you understand the context?

   (a) type, duration, frequency, and setting of intervention. Adequacy of the intervention. Degree of standardization.

   (b) real or quasi-patients, diagnosis (type, homogeneity, comorbidity), severity of disturbance, exclusion and inclusion criteria.

   (c) representative exemplars in quantitative research, informative exemplars in qualitative studies.

   (d) novice or experienced therapists, degree of competence in and commitment to interventions.

3. Are the change measures convincing?

   (a) relevance.

   (b) validity.

   (c) sensitivity.

   (d) reliability.

   (e) multiperson perspective and dimension.

   (f) multi-time point.

   (g) in common usage (allowing comparison with other studies).

4. Is the research ethical?

   (a) informed consent.

Specific questions for quantitative research

1. How well has bias been excluded?

   (a) randomization.

   (b) stratification.

   (c) representiveness.

   (d) blindness.

   (e) independent rators.

   (f) practice distortion.

   (g) practice bias.

2. Is the study powerful enough to yield significant results? What assumptions for clinically significant effects have been made and do you agree with them?

   (a) size of sample and power analysis.

3. Are the results invalidated by attrition? *Intention-to-treat numbers* should be reported.

4. Are the statistics valid?

Specific questions for qualitative research

1. How permeable is the study, i.e., does it show capacity for understanding to be changed by encounters with observations?

2. Validity of an interpretation is always in relation to some person, and criteria for assessing validity depend on whom that person is, e.g., reader, investigator, research participant. Is this explicit?

3. Has sample size and composition been informed by emerging results, e.g.. cases chosen to fill gaps; data gathering continued until new cases appear redundant.

4. Are the methods for gathering and analyzing observations clearly described to the point where you could replicate them?

5. Is permeability enhanced by:

   (a) Engagement with material.

   (b) Grounding.

   (c) Asking 'what,' *not* 'why'.

6. Can you as reader can make adjustments for differing forestructure in the author, e.g., initial theories, relevant personal experience, preconceptions and biases and assess how well the observations permeate the interpretations?

(a) Is there disclosure of investigators' forestructure.

(b) Explication of social and cultural context, e.g., shared assumptions between investigators and participants, relevant cultural values, data-gathering circumstances, meaning of the research to the participants.

(c) Description of investigators' internal processes.

7. Is there convergence across several perspectives and types of validity, i.e., triangulation?

8. In making your own assessment of validity, look for:

(a) Coherence.

(b) Uncovering; self-evidence.

(c) Testimonial validity.

(d) Catalytic validity.

Conclusions for evidence-based practice

1. Is the author's selection of positive findings and interpretation of the results justified by the evidence? Do you agree with them?

2. How representative is the study of your clinical practice (what is being done between whom and whom)?

3. If the results are sufficiently robust, representative, and significant, what are the implications for your practice?

4. What further evidence do you require before changing or confirming practice?

5. What further questions does the study raise?

6. If you change your practice, how are you going to audit the implementation?

39 Psychotherapy and medication

Jerald Kay

Introduction

The treatment of patients with psychotherapy and medication simultaneously is a common practice throughout the world. When a psychiatrist, nurse specialist, or in some countries, a psychologist, initiates and manages both psychotherapy and medications this practice is referred to as integrated treatment (Kay, 2001). If these professionals, or any other physician, is responsible for medication management only and the patient is seen in psychotherapy by another mental health professional, such as a psychologist, psychoanalyst, social worker, nurse specialist, or counselor, this treatment is termed combined, split, or collaborative treatment. Integrated treatment should be distinguished from psychotherapy integration (Norcross and Goldfried 1992). This term describes a movement within the field of psychotherapy to develop treatment modalities that are derived from effective and shared components from many theoretical models.

The rapid explosion in the development of psychopharmacologic agents in the twentieth century has yielded an impressive array of helpful new medications to combat mental illness but it has also seduced many into adopting an unbalanced or unidimensional view of the patient in both health and illness. In the UK, psychotherapy training has only recently become a mandatory part of residency training in psychiatry. In the US, calls for the remedicalization of psychiatry have strongly urged that the psychotherapies be delegated to nonphysician therapists (Lieberman and Rush, 1996; Detre and McDonald, 1997, and for a response, see Kay, 1998). Any devaluation of psychotherapeutic treatments is especially short sighted in light of the exciting research in the neurobiology of psychotherapy that points to the powerful and common effects of these two treatments (Gabbard, 2000; Lehrer and Kay, 2002).

Combined treatment has become increasingly popular and clinicians of all persuasions are obligated to work with the challenges of this treatment approach for the betterment of patient care. This chapter therefore will apprise the reader of the most recent research on this subject and present the clinical indications, challenges, helpful approaches, and interventions in employing concurrent psychotherapy and medication within a single or dual caregiver model.

Advantages of combining psychotherapy and medication

Controversies and benefits

With the introduction of new compounds to treat mental illness during the last half of the twentieth century came some resistance to their use within the psychotherapeutic relationship (Karasu, 1982; Klerman, 1991). Fears were expressed that medication would somehow submerge important feelings and conflicts and therefore impede psychotherapy and/or provide the message that the patient was less rewarding or even too ill for more formal psychotherapeutic interventions. Few psychiatrists, psychoanalysts, and

other clinicians maintain this position any longer. Instead, most mental health professionals, regardless of discipline, maintain that psychotropic medications, in conjunction with psychotherapy, are enormously helpful to patients and can often provide the following benefits to the psychotherapeutic process.

Pharmacotherapy can reduce uncomfortable levels of anxiety and depression allowing the patient greater access, expression, and understanding of feelings.

◆ Medications, through the reduction of acute symptoms, may enhance the patient's self-esteem by decreasing feelings of helplessness, futility, and passivity as well as enhancing the acceptability of treatment.

◆ Medication may increase the safety with the therapeutic relationship permitting more open expression of fantasies, feelings, and fears.

◆ Pharmacotherapy, for some patients, may have a positive placebo effect allowing a more substantial therapeutic alliance and decreasing the stigma of seeking mental health treatment.

◆ Medication, from the viewpoint of ego psychology, may improve autonomous ego functions (concentration and recall for example) that allow the mobilization of greater resources for the therapeutic process.

◆ Improvement from medication. Feelings about medication-related side-effects and pharmacologically unrelated nonspecific medication side-effects (Barsky *et al.*, 2002) often provide invaluable insight into the patient's personality and emotional experience, both conscious and unconscious, and clarify countertransference issues as well, especially in the case of heightened resistance or therapeutic impasse.

◆ As in psychotherapy, can elucidate the patient's self-defeating conflicts about achievement and success.

◆ Medications may not only increase the likelihood, but also the speed and magnitude of the response to psychotherapy.

◆ During times of interruption of treatment, medication can maintain a connection to the treatment relationship.

On the other hand, psychotherapy, when added to an ongoing pharmacotherapy may have the following benefits.

◆ Psychotherapy promotes improved adaptation and coping.

◆ Psychotherapy improves compliance with pharmacotherapy (Paykel, 1995).

◆ Psychotherapy, even in patients with the most severe disorders, decreases the likelihood of recurrence of symptoms (Kay, 2001).

◆ Psychotherapy decreases relapse when medications are discontinued (Wiborg, 1996; Teasdale *et al.*, 2001).

◆ Psychotherapy provides a much broader and more comprehensive inquiry into the patient's condition than is the case with medication monotherapy.

The flexibility of adding an additional treatment modality when the initial intervention is unsuccessful or partially successful is a major advantage in caring for patients and has been called sequential or stepped treatment.

Some authors have suggested a systematically developed plan to add a second treatment from the outset. For example, Pava *et al.* (1994) and Fava (1999) have proposed the treatment of the acute phase of major depression with antidepressant medication and reserved the use of psychotherapy (cognitive-behavioral therapy, CBT) for the continuation phase to prevent relapse and improve the quality of life by treating residual symptoms. They argue that this approach utilizes psychotherapy resources in a more efficient fashion and specifies the unique advantage of each treatment. Much research is needed in explicating the advantages and disadvantages of sequential interventions.

There are also disadvantages in combining medication with psychotherapy. A significant concern is that patients may attribute their improvement to medication rather than to the active steps they have taken within the psychotherapy. In many such cases, the patient wishes to minimize the importance of the psychotherapeutic relationship. There may be fears that the patient will become too reliant on the therapist, will experience erotic feelings toward the therapist, or may be frightened of rejection, to name but a few. The devaluation of the psychotherapy and the idealization of pharmacotherapy, especially at the beginning of treatment, can be seen as an attempt by the patient to defend against painful feelings and thoughts that would undoubtedly require exploration. Similarly, many educators insist that their trainees treat patients initially, where appropriate, without medication so they may gain some conviction about the usefulness of a psychotherapeutic approach. For some students, especially at the start of their training, it is less anxiety provoking to believe that medication can ameliorate all psychic pain thereby alleviating them from the doubts and uncertainties of engaging in this type of intense work.

There is also some limited literature on the potential of medications in overly dampening a patient's discomfort that is necessary for engaging in a psychotherapeutic experience. Marks *et al.* (1993) have noted that combined treatment with benzodiazepines (a class of anxiolytic medications) may adversely affect the outcome for those patients suffering from panic disorder. They noted that, when compared with panic patients receiving psychotherapy alone, those who received medication and psychotherapy demonstrated increased relapse rates. Moreover, patients with panic and other anxiety disorders such as posttraumatic stress disorder must repeatedly reexperience in psychotherapy painful memories or feelings and begin to appreciate that some symptoms are not as fragmenting, catastrophic, or dangerous as initially experienced. Theoretically, if they are overmedicated, however, the necessary process of increasing insight and the ability to provide new understanding of symptoms may be decreased. A more recent study demonstrated that as needed anxiolytic treatment with benzodiazepines and psychotherapy for patients with panic disorder and agoraphobia was associated with poorer outcome compared to group cognitive behavioral therapy alone (Westra *et al.*, 2002).

Strengthening compliance: understanding the meaning of medication

Whether they are aware of it or not, patients ascribe some psychological meaning to the taking of medication. These feelings may be about the agents themselves, about the prescribing and nonprescribing professionals or, as is often the case, both. Table 39.1 summarizes the feelings a patient may have about the medication and the treatment relationship.

Case example: Mrs James, a 33-year-old accountant, sought treatment for depression, which she attributed to her disappointing marriage. Over the previous year, her husband began drinking heavily, missed work often, was verbally abusive, and showed little sexual interest. She endorsed early morning awakening, anhedonia, and frequent crying spells. The psychiatrist suggested that psychodynamic psychotherapy would be helpful in exploring her marital situation and the impact it had made in her life. In light of the patient's significant discomfort, the clinician also offered the patient an antidepressant. Although Mrs James agreed to enter psychotherapy she adamantly refused any medication. The psychiatrist was puzzled by her strong refusal to consider pharmacotherapy but assured the patient that her strong feelings about this subject could be revisited. In the ensuing sessions, the patient described her chaotic and conflicted formative years with her mother who suffered from severe bipolar disorder and frequently required hospitalization. The patient held intensely ambivalent feelings towards her mother and had little contact with her after leaving home at the age of 18. Exploration of these feelings revealed that Mrs James was frightened that she too might have a mood disorder and would become like her mother whom she viewed as alienated, empty, and despondent. If she were to take medication, the patient feared she would end up like her mother. Complicating the medication issue, was her husband's accusation that if she were to take medication, it would become a 'crutch' because she was such a weak and dependent person.

There are a number of ways to inquire about meaning that patients attribute to medication and to those that prescribe them or treat them in psychotherapy. All, however, are predicated upon the clinician's willingness to recognize and explore a patient's expectable ambivalence about the treatment situation. This ambivalence may manifest itself on a continuum from severe suspiciousness to overidealization of one or more components in the treatment plan. For example, the clinician must recognize a patient's delusional thinking about the toxicity of medications as being representative of paranoid feelings about the treatment experience. The precise manner of the patient's thinking therefore, requires exploration to assess patient resiliency and cohesiveness. Patients who ascribe overly positive or unrealistic qualities or powers to medication at the exclusion of acknowledging their self-experience, also must be questioned about their views on their illness. In these situations it often helpful to inquire about previous relationships with healthcare professionals to ascertain the presence of long-standing characterological difficulties with those who are in authority, or in the case of a treatment relationship, requiring a trusting relationship.

As is the case in any psychotherapy, the patient will readily appreciate their professional's discomfort with psychological pain. For example, the practitioner who does not ask about the experience of psychological discomfort but rather focuses exclusively on phenomenology to arrive at a diagnosis, is more likely to consider medication as a monotherapy and the patient will undoubtedly feel on some level that he or she is dismissed. On the other hand, a clinician that fails to recognize the components of a specific disorder whose symptoms are quite treatable may leave the patient with doubt about the minimization of their painful symptoms. Both of these require that the professional observes the patient's response to the clinician and attention to countertransferential issues. Ultimately, regardless of

Table 39.1 Patient's feelings about the psychiatrist (integrated treatment) or prescribing physician and psychotherapist (combined treatment) and about medication

Positive	Negative
Optimism about symptom relief	Minimization or dismissal of patient's problems
Understanding of patient's psychological pain	Discomfort with patient's situation or condition
Caring and safety	Fear of being controlled or it's the easiest thing the doctor can do
Comfort with prescriber's knowledge	Anger/disappointment of not receiving and/or changes in the medication that patient desires
Relief from scientifically based medical decision	Fear of being harmed/poisoned/addicted
Delayed therapeutic onset of medication	Fear that physician is unempathic to patient's level of discomfort
Relief from increases in medication dosage	Concern about new side effects or being viewed as sicker or constitutionally weaker
Gratification from discontinuation of medications	Fear that symptoms will recur

Adapted from Kay (2001, p. 21).

theoretical orientation, clinicians must attend to the distortions that patients bring to the treatment situation. In the case of psychoanalytic psychotherapy, this is termed transference. These phenomena in CBT are called beliefs and automatic thoughts. At the initiation of treatment, for most patients these transferences and beliefs and automatic thoughts are outside of awareness. Moreover, regardless of the patient's level of psychopathology, these issues must be understood and brought to light for treatment to be effective. This is true for the continuum of psychotherapy from predominantly supportive to expressive or insight-oriented modalities.

Because as many as 60% of all patients do not take their medications as prescribed, appreciating the reasons for noncompliance becomes a powerful tool in the therapeutic armamentarium (Baso and Rush, 1996; Ellison and Harney, 2000). A recent comprehensive review of the prevalence of and risk factors for medication nonadherence in patients with schizophrenia noted that nearly 50% of these patients did not take their medications as prescribed (Lacro et al., 2002). Demyttenaere et al. (2001) studied depressed patients treated in primary care settings who dropped out of continuation treatment. They found that nearly 30% of patients stopped treatment because they worried about becoming drug dependent, felt uncomfortable taking medications, or were concerned that they were relying inappropriately on medication to solve their problems. Similarly, a study of 155 depressed patients in primary care revealed that 28% had stopped taking their antidepressants by the first month and 44% had done so by the third month of treatment (Lin et al., 1995). American and Canadian researchers studied why patients may drop out from mental health care (Edlund et al., 2002). This study examined 1200 patients from the US and Ontario, Canada in the early 1990s and found that the dropout rates from treatment were, 19.2% and 16.9% respectively. This difference was not statistically significant despite the fact that mental health insurance is a major problem for US subjects, whereas Canadians have access to unlimited care. Reasons for dropping out of treatment included: belief that mental health treatment is ineffective, embarrassment about seeking help, and being offered only medication or only psychotherapy instead of combined treatment. Only Americans endorsed not having insurance as an important reason for discontinuing treatment. Lastly, respondents who had received combined treatment were less likely than their counterparts offered only monotherapies to leave treatment prematurely.

Noncompliance behaviors are associated with automatic thoughts about the particular medication, about the psychiatrist (or other physician and therapist), about the illness, and about oneself and others (Beck, 2001). Table 39.2 provides a summary of typical beliefs associated with noncompliance.

The unanticipated prevalence of public antimedication beliefs was illustrated in one public opinion poll of approximately 2200 adults in Germany that found that attitudes toward psychotropic medication were much more negative than those associated with cardiac drugs (Benkert et al., 1997). Even in the case of schizophrenia, 76% felt that psychotherapy was the treatment of choice and only 8% advocated medication. As most respondents were not knowledgeable about these medications nor did they know many people with mental disorders, the authors attributed their findings to lack of information and negative reports from the mass media. Similarly, Jorm

et al. (1999), studied the Australian public and mental health professionals regarding the treatment of depression and found that the former frequently believed that antidepressants were potentially addictive and, along with electroconvuslive therapy, considered to be harmful.

It is not surprising therefore, that adherence problems with medications are ubiquitous. Rush (1988) has argued that until proven otherwise, every clinician should assume that noncompliance is present in each patient they treat. There are a number of questions that can be asked of the patient in anticipating medication noncompliance (Beck, 2001). Above all, the clinician must not shy away from exploring particular facets of medication beliefs and behaviors. For example, patients should be asked directly if they believe the medication that is being prescribed will be effective and are they willing to take the medication exactly as instructed. They should be prompted to consider the advantages and disadvantages of following treatment recommendations. Additional questions should attempt to elicit any problems with the purchase of medication and the ability to remember to take the medication at appropriate times. Assessing the impact of family beliefs about taking medication is critical. Patients will not follow medication regimens, especially with psychotropic drugs, when the prevailing belief by influential family members is that these medications are 'crutches' for the weak and dependent or required by those with only the most severe and chronic of mental illnesses. Patients should routinely be asked their fantasies about taking medication. Beck has further advocated that covert rehearsal in which patients are instructed to visualize how and when they would take their medication as well as appreciating any negative feelings about this activity. This technique will provide the basis for interventions that will strengthen compliance behaviors.

There is an unfortunate and simplistic view that is held by many prescribers that arriving at the correct diagnosis and providing the appropriately evidence-based medication guarantees that a patient will improve. The ability of a patient to follow medication plans is strongly predicated upon the establishment of a solid therapeutic alliance. Just as the strongest predictor for a positive psychotherapy outcome is the strength of the therapeutic alliance, it is also the strongest predictor for successful pharmacological outcome (Krupnick et al., 1996). No treatment will succeed without a safe, uncritical, empathic, and educative working relationship. There are additional behavioral techniques that some clinicians find helpful. These include:

- asking the patient to call at regularly scheduled times to assess if adherence is problematic;
- meeting with family members to defuse antimedication beliefs and inviting them to assist the patient in following the medication regimen;
- requesting that the patient complete a written record indicating when they took their prescription;
- the use of written coping cards that the patient carries with him that remind him of his unhelpful automatic thoughts about taking medication (Beck, 2001).

Case example: Ms S is a 24-year-old graduate student who was referred to a psychiatrist for twice-weekly psychoanalytic psychotherapy. Since the age of 13, this patient has experienced three episodes of major depression, the last of which took place approximately 2 years earlier. In each case, she had responded well to antidepressants. She had been euthymic for 2 years while on medication but expressed an interest in psychotherapy to explore her inhibitions with men as well as with the monitoring of her medication. As a child, the patient had grown up in a sexually stimulating and unsafe home. Ms S was a striking woman who became quite anxious when, as frequently was the case, she was the object of inappropriate sexual remarks or rude glaring from men. The patient had never developed a serious relationship with a man, although she had many friendships. The patient acknowledged that because of her beginning work in psychotherapy, she was able to enter into a relationship with a young man.

After a month of intense and rewarding dating, Ms S felt she could no longer resist her boyfriend's wish for a more intimate relationship. Her first and subsequent sexual relations with this boyfriend were unsatisfying and she could not achieve orgasm. She did not speak about these experiences with her psychiatrist initially because she was uncomfortable in discussing sexual topics. Shortly after beginning

Table 39.2 Some typical beliefs associated with noncompliance

Beliefs about medications
Medications don't work
Medications are dangerous
Medications are for 'crazy' people
Medications should be considered only as a last resort
Medications should only be taken when someone is feeling bad/sick

Beliefs about illness
There is no such thing as mental illness
It's terrible to need treatment for a mental illness
Ignoring symptoms will make them go away
Mental illness can't be cured

Modified from J. S. Beck (2001, p. 116).

sexual relations, she became depressed again. After rather persistent exploration of her mood change by her psychiatrist, she finally admitted to discontinuing her medication because she attributed her sexual dysfunction to her antidepressant. A different medication, with less sexual side-effects, was provided and her depression cleared. In her therapy, she came to realize that her fear of discussing intimate matters with her psychiatrist was related to her earlier experiences as a child and adolescent. She worried that to speak about her sexual relationship with her boyfriend, which she found very anxiety and guilt provoking, would overstimulate the psychiatrist with the resultant loss of safety within the therapeutic dyad.

How advantageous is combined treatment?

An important meta-analysis of 13 studies comparing psychodynamic psychotherapy with other types of psychotherapies and combined treatment demonstrated that, although there were no significant differences between types of psychotherapy, combined treatment was clearly more effective than any monotherapy (Luborsky *et al.*, 1993). In reviewing the growing body of evidence that supports the helpfulness of employing medication and psychotherapy in the treatment of psychiatric disorders, there are three points to keep in mind. First, the literature on using psychotherapy and medication, while growing, is limited. Second, not all studies have found that combined treatment is superior to either monotherapy with medication or with psychotherapy in depression except in the case of severe disorders (Hollon *et al.*, 1992; Manning *et al.*, 1992; Wexler and Chicchetti, 1992; Antonuccio, 1995). Third, while this very brief review will focus on randomized controlled trials (RCT), there remains controversy about their generalizability to everyday clinical practice as these studies often have involved homogeneous patient populations who are without comorbid disorders, employ tightly supervised manualized treatments, and fail to report exclusion rates (Westen and Morrison, 2001). Nevertheless it is important for the clinician to have familiarity with recent research supporting the advantages of providing both medication and psychotherapy to patients.

To provide the reader with some appreciation of the evidence for combined treatment, it would be helpful to review selectively a few studies in major depression. There is, however, strong evidence for the helpfulness of combined treatment in patients with schizophrenia (Falloon *et al.*, 1982; Leff *et al.*, 1985; Hogarty *et al.*, 1991, 1997a,b; Kuipers *et al.*, 1998; Tarrier *et al.*, 1998; Sensky *et al.*, 2000; Granholm *et al.*, 2002; McQuaid *et al.*, 2002; McGorry *et al.*, 2002) but only limited data in the treatment of personality disorders (Bateman and Fonagy, 2001), substance abuse (McLellan *et al.*, 1993; Woody *et al.*, 1995; Feeney *et al.*, 2001), eating disorders (Walsh *et al.*, 1997; Ricca *et al.*, 2001), anxiety disorders (Spiegal *et al.*, 1994; Wiborg and Dahl, 1996; Bruce *et al.*, 1999; Barlow *et al.*, 2000; Stein *et al.*, 2000; Whittal *et al.*, 2001; Kampman *et al.*, 2002), and bipolar disorder (Miklowitz *et al.*, 2000; Fava *et al.*, 2001). For an in-depth review of these studies the reader is referred to Kay (2001) and Grech (2002).

An additional word is in order about the treatment of severe mental illness for which clinicians in many countries believe psychotherapy is ineffective. Researchers from the UK have recently made exciting advances in integrating CBT with medication for patients with acute and chronic schizophrenia.

There is mounting evidence that combined therapy with CBT has been noted to:

♦ improve medication compliance

♦ improve hallucinations and delusions among medication-resistant patients

♦ improve recovery from acute psychotic and first episodes

♦ decrease relapse and rehospitalization.

The continuing emphasis on combined interventions has underscored the importance of providing comprehensive psychosocial treatment in treating a severe, chronic, and often disabling disorder, which is arguably the most expensive of mental disorders (Knapp, 1997). Moreover, patients with schizophrenia and their families value psychotherapy as a very helpful intervention (Coursey *et al.*, 1995; Hatfield *et al.*, 1996; Kuipers *et al.*, 1998). In treating psychotic disorders as is true with personality, substance abuse, eating, and many mood disorders, medication as monotherapy produces modest effects only and is rarely as effective as combined treatment. Clinicians should be skeptical of a biomedical orientation that reduces psychiatric and emotional disorders to phenomenology and therefore encourages unidimensional treatment approaches. On the other hand, nonprescribing professionals would be most unwise and shortsighted to dismiss the potential for pharmacotherapy in helping those who seek treatment.

Major depression

Major depression or unipolar nonpsychotic depression has been the most studied disorder in the combined treatment literature. The largest randomized controlled study of depression has supported the advantage of combined therapy over monotherapy. A multicenter study of 681 patients with chronic depression compared treatment with nefazadone and a CBT to patients who received only medication or psychotherapy (Keller *et al.*, 2000). The specific type of psychotherapy provided in this study was the cognitive-behavioral analysis system of psychotherapy (CBASP), which is more directed and structured than interpersonal psychotherapies and differs from CBT by focusing on interpersonal interactions via the use of a social problem-solving algorithm. Those that received combined treatment had an 85% response rate, whereas patients treated with the antidepressant alone and those treated with only psychotherapy had response rates of 55% and 52%, respectively.

A meta-analysis of the treatment of 600 patients from six standardized protocols at the University of Pittsburgh demonstrated that patients with severe depression responded best with respect to shorter time to recovery and outcome when provided combined treatment with interpersonal psychotherapy (IPT) and antidepressant medication. However, for those with mild to moderate depression, psychotherapy alone was as effective as combined treatment (Thase *et al.*, 1997).

Most studies of combined treatment in depression have utilized either CBT or IPT. Burnand *et al.* (2002) treated 74 outpatients with acute major depression with medication alone or combined treatment with psychodynamic psychotherapy. In this RCT, marked improvement was noted in both groups; however, the combined treatment group had less treatment failure, better work adjustment postdischarge, better global functioning, and lower hospitalization rates. Combined treatment with psychodynamic psychotherapy and clomipramine also was associated with both lower direct and indirect costs as measured by lost work days. The cost savings per patient amounted to $2311 in those subjects treated with both psychotherapy and medication. A second RCT study compared a 16-session psychodynamic brief supportive psychotherapy with medication to medication monotherapy in the treatment of major depression (de Jonghe *et al.*, 2001). In this Dutch study, 84 patients receiving only medication were compared with 83 subjects who were treated with combined therapy. The medication protocol provided for patients who experienced poor response or significant side-effects the opportunity for successive trials on three different antidepressants: fluoxetine, amitriptyline, or moclobemide. Nearly one-third of patients refused pharmacotherapy and 13% refused combined treatment. In 6 months, 40% of patients who began with pharmacotherapy stopped their medication while only 22% who were treated with combined therapy did so. At 24 weeks, those who received combined treatment had a mean success rate of 59.2% compared with only 40.7% in the medication only group. The authors of this study noted that patients treated with medication and psychotherapy found their treatment significantly more acceptable, were less likely to drop out of treatment, and more likely to recover.

A number of recent studies have examined the treatment of late life depression. A 3-year RCT study demonstrated that elderly patients with recurrent nonpsychotic major depression were helped most by combining medication and psychotherapy (Reynolds *et al.*, 1999). In this study of nearly 200 patients, for the 107 who responded, combined treatment with nortriptyline and IPT was superior to treatment with either monotherapy. Patients treated with combined therapy had only a 20% recurrence rate.

Those patients who received only medication experienced a 43% recurrence rate and rates of 64% and 90%, respectively, were found in the groups treated only with IPT or only with placebo.

Improvement in social adjustment in the depressed elderly who were treated for 1 year was shown to be greater in patients receiving combined therapy compared with those receiving only IPT or a tricyclic antidepressant, or a placebo (Lenze *et al.*, 2002).

As for younger patients, The Treatment for Adolescents With Depression Study (TADS) is the first major randomized control trial strongly supporting the superiority of combined treatment over either medication or psychotherapy as monotherapies (March, 2004). In this large study in 13 academic centers of 439 teenagers (mean age 14.6 years), subjects were provided with 12 weeks of antidepressant therapy or CBT alone or CBT with antidepressant or placebo. The CBT consisted of 15 sessions and included two parent only sessions as well as three family sessions.

One of the striking findings in the depression literature just reviewed is the significant rate of relapse and recurrence after successful treatment. It is not surprising then, that investigators are now turning their attention to maintaining treatment gains. Segal *et al.* (2002) have reviewed the efficacy of combined, sequential, and crossover psychotherapy and pharmacotherapy in improving outcomes in depression. Sequential treatment involves the augmentation of the initial treatment with a different treatment. Crossover intervention during the maintenance phase of treatment is the selection of a second modality after an adequate response to the first has been achieved to prevent relapse. The helpfulness of sequential treatment was demonstrated in a nonrandomized study of women with recurrent depression who did not respond to IPT but did improve when a tricyclic antidepressant was added (Frank *et al.*, 2000). There was a 79% response rate to sequential treatment compared with 66% of women receiving both psychotherapy and medication from the outset. Unfortunately, there are few well constructed studies examining the use of crossover treatment; however, this practice may be beneficial in preventing relapse and recurrence (Fava *et al.*, 1998). There is one controlled trial of 158 patients that attempted to elucidate how cognitive therapy prevents relapse in residual depression (Teasdale *et al.*, 2001). The authors of this study propose that psychotherapy works by changing the manner in which patients process depression related material and not by changing belief in depressive thought content.

Before leaving the discussion of combined treatment in major depression, one additional comment is in order. The provision of CBT, IPT, or psychodynamic psychotherapy to depressed patients can be a challenging task. Although manualized treatments have been a major advance to psychotherapy research over the last 20 years, assisting patients with chronic mood disorders requires significant training. This point was brought home by the recent RCT from the UK describing the effectiveness of teaching general practitioners how to conduct brief CBT with their depressed patients (King *et al.*, 2002). Eighty-four general physicians were provided with a training package of four half days on CBT. In their treatment of 272 patients, it was clear that the training produced no discernible difference in the physicians' knowledge about depression nor was there any impact on patient outcome. This study invites comparison with a US RCT of the treatment of late life depression in primary care utilizing a model called Improving Mood-Promoting Access to Collaborative Treatment (IMPACT). In this study (Unutzer *et al.*, 2002), 1800 patients from 18 primary care clinics with major depression (17%) dysthymia (30%), or double depression (53%), were assigned in approximate equal numbers to either usual care (with a primary care physician or available mental health services) or the IMPACT intervention. The latter consists of evidence-based components for chronic illness care which included:

- collaboration among generalists, specialists, and patients who have agreed to a common definition of the problem to be treated;
- close attention to the development of a therapeutic alliance;
- personalized treatment plan that included patient preferences;
- proactive follow-up by a depression case manager supervised by a psychiatrist;

- defined use of specialists;
- protocols for stepped care.

At 1 year, patients in the IMPACT arm had more than twice the reduction in symptoms, more satisfaction with their care, less severity of depression, less functional impairment, and greater quality of life than the control group.

General principles of integrated and split treatment

Whether one clinician or two clinicians treat a patient with a mental disorder, there are critical skills, attitudes, and knowledge that are essential. All psychotherapists understand that the establishment of a therapeutic relationship is the single most potent predictor of psychotherapy outcome regardless of modality. However, fewer clinicians appreciate that to treat patients effectively with medication also requires a strong 'pharmacotherapeutic' relationship. In analyzing the National Institute of Mental Health Collaborative Depression Study, which compared different psychotherapies with antidepressant medication, Krupnick *et al.* (1996) found that 21% of the variance in outcome was attributed to therapeutic alliance while only 1% could be ascribed to the specific treatment intervention.

In the US, most malpractice suits in psychiatry arise from failure to intervene appropriately with suicidal patients and adverse drug responses. In the case of split treatment, if a physician sees a patient infrequently but a psychologist or social worker conducts psychotherapy on a regular basis, the nonphysicians must also attend to the side-effects of psychotropic medications, and by virtue of their increased contact with the patient, are more likely to discern untoward medication effects.

Regardless of whether integrated or split treatment is being provided, all clinicians are obligated to obtain a thorough history. Professionals in split treatment relationships should not rely on the collaborator to secure important historical data. As well, all clinicians regardless of type of treatment, are obligated to develop a case formulation that contains an evaluation of the patient's current and past levels of functioning, current life stressors, strengths and weaknesses, diagnostic impression, likely past events that may have disposed to vulnerability, and some appreciation of the specific challenges likely to arise within the therapeutic relationship. The case formulation provides the clinician(s) with hypotheses regarding the timing and nature of the mental illness. From that assessment, regardless of type of treatment, appropriate treatment goals can then be established. Lastly, the requirement for informed consent must be recognized in integrated treatment or collaborative interventions. In the latter case, much more will be said later in this chapter.

The ability to recognize and manage resistance about medication or medication side-effects is required in both models of treatment. The same can be said of compliance to psychotherapy and pharmacotherapy goals. In both types of treatment, clinicians must also understand how patients may frequently abuse or misuse medication. Similarly, it is imperative to address psychological consequences of adverse medication effects. As previously discussed, all patients ascribe certain meanings to medication and the same is true with medication side-effects that require exploration.

In both integrated and split treatment clinicians are required to provide education about the patient's medication regimen. This includes instruction about the acute as well as the maintenance phases of treatment, the latter being instrumental in preventing symptom recurrence, relapse, or rehospitalization.

The ability to discern when patients might require changes in medication is also vital. Frequently, patients experiencing significant psychosocial stressors will require additional medication. On the other hand, it is important to appreciate that despite a patient's request, not all intense stressors require medication changes. Lastly, the development of a termination or discontinuation plan is essential in both types of treatments and will be discussed shortly.

Integrated treatment: advantages, challenges, and principles

Advantages

There are a number of attractive properties in the one clinician model.

First, this approach counters the prevailing conceptual mind-body split that has so dominated modern Western medicine. In psychiatry for example, this is most apparent in the dichotomization of treating patients with pharmacotherapy for 'brain-based disorders' and treating concerns of the mind with psychotherapy. Important neurobiological and neuroimaging research within the last decade has clearly demonstrated the untenability of this position as it is now clear that all mental processes are ultimately products of brain activity (Kandel, 1998, 1999; LeDoux, 2001). In particular, neuronal plasticity (neurogenesis and synaptogenesis) and genetic transduction are central features of learning and memory, which not only determine our knowledge of ourselves and world views, but also how psychotherapy is likely to work (Liggan and Kay, 1999; Lehrer and Kay, 2002). In many ways, this is the most exciting of times because neuroscience has been able to substantiate that psychotherapy can change both brain structure and function. There are a number of comparative studies employing neuroimaging that have illustrated similar effects when patients with obsessive-compulsive disorder or depression are treated with psychotherapy and a second group with medication (L. Baxter et al., 1992; Brody et al., 2001; Martin et al., 2001). Indeed, it may be that these two treatments act on similar pathways (Sacheim, 2001).

Second, the integrated model in many cases allows for closer attention to medication adherence and side-effects. Some have argued that medication noncompliance should be anticipated in all psychiatric patients and vigilance to this issue is a hallmark of successful treatment (Basco and Rush, 1996). It may be easier to appreciate the meaning attached by the patient to medication and medication side-effects (especially sexual side-effects as in the first vignette) in the one clinician model, which does not require the input of a second professional, and for some patients, permits a more secure and safe treatment experience. The same could be said of the ability to understand the meaningfulness of side-effects as they express issues, such as transference, within the therapeutic dyad. Undoubtedly one of the most important qualities of integrated treatment is the likelihood of deeper therapeutic relationships that permit a more in-depth treatment experience through appreciating the subtleties of transference, countertransference, and resistance phenomena.

Third, although it remains to be established, there may be a number of disorders and clinical situations in which the one-person model should at least be considered by psychiatrists who are adept at both the psychotherapeutic and pharmacoptherapeutic models. These include patients with severe medical disorders where a physician may more likely appreciate the interplay between the psychosocial and biological factors, including drug–drug interactions. In addition, perhaps some patients with so-called primitive personality disorders (narcissistic and borderline disorders) who tend to polarize their helping relationships, have a significant propensity for self-harm, and often require hospitalization, can be provided with a more continuous type of care than is possible in the split treatment model. Gunderson and Ridolfi (2001), however, believes strongly that treatment for patients with borderline personality disorder should always have a least two professionals working together to minimize frustration and burnout. He argues that these patients should also receive at least psychotherapy and medication.

There are many psychiatrists who prefer to treat patients with serious disorders, such as schizophrenia and bipolar disorder, in an integrated model. This approach in skilled hands permits closer monitoring not only of symptoms but provides significant opportunities for psychoeducation about the nature of the chronic illness, the importance of medications, and the role of social and family contributions (Gabbard and Kay, 2001).

At least in the US, risk and liability issues are less complicated in an integrated treatment setting. The oversight of a treatment by one professional requires less time, collaboration, and of course paperwork. McBeth (2001)

has elucidated specific risks with the split treatment approach and has noted that seeing greater numbers of patients less frequently carries a greater statistical risk for malpractice suit.

Challenges

The most central challenge in delivering effective integrated treatment is the physician's obligation to master two complicated approaches to the patient. This treatment model requires that a physician be able to integrate the biological with the psychosocial in a moment to moment process. The capacity to 'shift gears' in listening to a patient is a skill that must be mastered for the delivery of effective care. A second challenge in the provision of integrated treatment is the obligation to keep abreast of the burgeoning field of psychopharmacology. It is difficult to underestimate the commitment necessary to stay current not only with new medications but also the increasing awareness of long-term side-effects in some new compounds. Coupled with need to continue to grow in one's psychotherapeutic skills, the responsibility for continuing education is significant.

Some principles of integrated treatment

There are of course many important principles in the provision of medication to all patients. This discussion will be limited, however, to those that will assist the physician in providing integrated treatment (Kay, 2001). The centrality of the therapeutic relationship has been discussed in detail. Some clinicians though believe that arriving at the correct diagnosis guarantees the success of the working alliance. Making the correct diagnosis and providing the most up to date information on medication does not ensure an empathic, nonjudgmental rapport with patients. Without the capacity to establish a safe and secure therapeutic relationship, adherence problems are bound to be more plentiful, including dropouts from treatment. As Frank et al. (1995) have written, a sound philosophy of care should focus on alliance, not compliance.

Along with safety, consistency, and predictability are critical components of the treatment relationship. Technical mistakes and boundary violations are more recognizable when a consistent manner of conducting the psychotherapy has been established. This is also true regarding how the clinician addresses pharmacotherapy issues within an ongoing psychotherapy. Although there is no one correct approach to this issue, the significant element is to establish a routine for such investigation. The examination of when clinicians deviate from their routine is exceptionally helpful in detecting subtle transference or countertransference issues. Some clinicians prefer to address medication concerns at the very beginning of a session, others wait until the end of the session. There are virtues in both methods. In the former case, the clinician will have the entire session to explore the issues surrounding the medication concerns and how it undoubtedly reflects on the therapeutic relationship. The limitation to this approach is that it may artificially set an agenda for a session and derail some of the patients pressing or immediate concerns. Leaving the medication inquiry to the end of a session alleviates the issue of steering the content of the session but may not provide sufficient time to address critical medication-related issues. Still others prefer to address medication-related topics whenever they arise in a psychotherapy session. Regardless of the chosen approach, deviation from the routine will often lead the psychiatrist to question the presence of countertransference. As an example, a beginning psychiatry resident was presenting to his supervisor a challenging and anxiety provoking treatment with a difficult patient. Immediately following the patient's verbalizing her strong sexual feelings for the therapist, he asked her if the medication she had been prescribed was helpful. With the supervisor's assistance, the trainee was able to appreciate that he became anxious about the patient's expression of her erotic longings and switched the subject to medication as an attempt to combat his anxiety.

The potential therapeutic richness of exploring medication side-effects has been discussed. It is imperative that the clinician pay close attention to the patient's questions about side-effects, changes in type and dosage, and to the discontinuation of medication. Often, frequent complaints about improbable side-effects can illustrate a patient's resistance in the psychotherapy. The prescribing of medication for the first time in an ongoing and challenging expressive psychotherapy may signal a growing frustration with a therapeutic impasse.

The termination phase of treatment is often the most overlooked. Novices frequently become overly concerned with the reappearance of symptoms at the very end of psychotherapy. Some attempt to treat this well known phenomenon by increasing or prescribing new medications. Most often, therapists have ambivalent feelings about termination, especially in forced terminations, and can feel conflicted about insufficiently helping their patients. Similarly, a patient's request for additional medication during the termination phase can represent an important entry into the patient's mixed feelings about ending a very meaningful relationship. Lastly, the question of continuing medication and who should monitor this after termination is frequently a challenge and mandates exploration of both the patient's and therapist's feelings.

Advantages, challenges, and principles of providing split treatment

In the US, a number of important issues have led to a significant growth in the practice of split treatment. Many of these issues have already been discussed; however, they include, but are not limited to, the following:

- significant financial incentives for physicians
- diminishing choice for care options under managed care
- inadequate number of psychiatric specialists
- more adequate number of psychologists, social workers, and counselors
- low reimbursement rates for psychiatrists who perform psychotherapy
- the de-emphasis on psychotherapy training among many residency programs
- the growing body of research supporting the efficacy and effectiveness of combined treatment
- the unavailability of insurance coverage for mental health treatment.

Advantages

One advantage frequently cited about the practice of split treatment is that it promotes the use of the unique talents of more than one mental health professional (Balon, 2001) and therefore provides the potential for the patient to receive a more sophisticated and comprehensive treatment experience. Second, many have proposed that it is more cost-effective and affords patients greater access to clinical care. Third, some have argued that more clinical information becomes available for more refined treatments. Fourth, there may be a greater opportunity for patients to be treated by therapists of similar ethnicity to that of the patient. Fifth, there may be greater professional and emotional support for each of the professionals. Sixth, some patients, such as those with severe personality disorders and or histories of overwhelming abuse, establish very intense relationships in treatment and can be enormously taxing to one clinician. The opportunity for sharing treatment responsibility can be protective for the collaborators in terms of decreasing the intensity of feelings on the part of the patient for each. Lastly, there may be an opportunity for collaborators to strengthen their clinical skills through a mutual education process. This is especially true when the result of a collaborative treatment experience provides great insight to the patient's fears and dynamics, thereby presenting a more comprehensive clinical understanding of the patient's plight. On the other hand, the effectiveness of medication has the potential to illustrate some of the biological bases of some disorders for the psychotherapist and demonstrate the usefulness of medication in addressing target symptoms in the areas of impulsivity, affective lability, and cognitive and perceptual limitations.

The collaborative, or two-person model, has other advantages as well. In working with patients with intense transference reactions, these can be somewhat diluted and more easily addressed within the treatment. Similarly, collaborative treatment will decrease a patient's opportunity to spend all or most of the sessions discussing medication at the expense of addressing psychological concerns when integrated treatment is employed.

Challenges

It is not always possible for collaborators to know about each other's qualifications as well as the quality of care routinely provided. Such a situation may leave either or both clinicians anxious about the reliability of the collaborator. This doubt can be readily appreciated by a patient in split treatment and will undoubtedly cause the patient to feel less secure and for some patients, encourage splitting. There are other patients, who as children experienced significant disagreement between their parents. They may, attempt to repeat an important childhood behavior to pacify their parents and diminish conflict when they perceive it between the professionals. This can be accomplished through obsequious behavior or even acting out in an attempt to unite those overseeing the treatment.

A second challenge in the provision of split treatment is the inappropriate prescribing of medication by the physician when he or she is unaware of the process taking place in the psychotherapy (Balon, 2001) or when the prescriber provides medication as a practice routine without careful assessment of the patient's symptoms or feelings about medication. Similarly, a prescriber may insist on medication to dampen the patient's intense feelings in his or her relationship without appreciating the impact on the overall treatment experience. This is often the case for an example, when a physician, without consultation with his collaborator, impulsively begins medication. As well, there may be a wish to provide medication because one collaborator feels they are being ineffective with the patient or cannot tolerate the emotional pain experienced by the patient. If this is the case the patient invariably experiences that one collaborator wishes to become less involved. Also, it may be challenging to collaborate with a prescriber who attempts to treat every symptom experienced by the patient with a different medication because of a lack of an overarching theoretical understanding. This frequently appears as a problem in the treatment of women have been sexually abused because there is a failure by the pharmacotherapist to appreciate that affective lability, perceptual distortions, self-destructive behavior, and hopelessness about life, to mention just a few, are consistent with a traumatic disorder and readily treatable through a psychotherapeutic approach. Other prescribers will give patients multiple medications by rationalizing that they are treating comorbid disorders such as major depression and still others will fail to appreciate the potential for transference reactions to the prescriber in that they are giving the patient something that may be experienced as a significant and highly affect laden gift. Should the medication prove to be ineffective over time, as is often the case in many patients with personality disorders, for example, the physician should not be so quick to ascribe this to drug failure.

A nonprescribing professional my feel it is a violation of their beliefs to request the use of medication. Introducing medication can be experienced as an attack on a theoretical system. When this occurs, the patient is placed in a no-win situation as loyalty to one professional will demand disloyalty to the other.

Despite good intentions, the reality is that effective collaboration takes time and is not accomplished without a strong commitment from both care providers. Another persistent challenge is addressing the propensity for splitting by the patient, especially those with significant character disorders. Most frequently in this situation, one clinician is viewed by the patient as admirable, the other in highly negative terms. When this idealization or de-idealization is expressed in the treatment relationships it can be uncomfortable and difficult to address. Frequently, it may take the form of negativity about one collaborator. That is, some patients will be critical of the physician for only prescribing medication and others will feel similarly about the psychotherapist for not prescribing. Often patients will complain to the nonphysician collaborator that the doctor merely prescribes and is disinterested in any other aspects of the patient's life. Fourth, without consistent and effective collaboration, mental health professionals cannot appreciate that their patient has been providing very different information to each clinician.

Additional challenges are subsumed broadly under legal and ethical tensions. A frequent problem is the failure to establish clear guidelines for the sharing of clinical information between the collaborators. Similarly, the failure to delineate specific responsibilities for each collaborator can be very problematic. For example, who actually decides whether hospitalization is indicated, and if so, who should follow the patient while he or she is hospitalized? Should a diagnostic evaluation be performed by both professionals, or is it sufficient for either to conduct the assessment? Which professional should secure informed consent?

With respect to potential ethical dilemmas, Lazarus (1999) has noted that many psychiatrists are unclear about their supervisory or consultative responsibilities with a nonmedical therapist. In addition, there are inconsistent state licensing laws, the potential for the physician to delegate medical decisions to the collaborator, and the physician being merely a figurehead with responsibility but without the customary contractual safeguards that exist in most doctor–patient relationships. Lazarus also notes that within many managed care organizations in the US, cost containment is the greatest priority. If this is used as the basis for providing split care, then it is possible that the psychiatrist will feel that he or she is providing less than desirable care. This may result in resentment of the collaborator, which may potentially damage the treatment experience for the patient.

Interdisciplinary issues are often an enduring source of tension in collaborative treatments. When split treatment is mandated by a healthcare organization, it may be experienced as a 'shotgun wedding' approach rather than a true collaboration.

Also, competition may be a destructive element in collaborative relationships. Rivalry over inequality in the professional status and reimbursement of physicians may become an unhelpful source of acting out within the psychotherapy. Similarly, some physicians can be quite dismissive of their collaborator's skills and professional backgrounds. At least in the US, communication between the two professionals is rarely done well (Hansen-Grant and Riba, 1995). As a result, one collaborator may not know of a patient's suicidal or homicidal feelings or even when the other professional is out of the office and therefore unavailable to the patient. Some patients will not know whom they should contact if an emergency arises.

In psychoanalytic psychotherapy accepting and understanding transference feelings within the therapeutic dyad is a central, and at times, challenging task. However, this task becomes enormously complicated when there are two clinicians about whom the patient has distinct transference reactions. Consider also that the patient is receiving medication about which he or she may have strong conscious and/or unconscious feelings. To this therapeutic relationship must be added the attendant countertransferences from each of the providers. It is not difficult to imagine that the treatment experience for all participants can become complicated and confusing. The following clinical vignette illustrates nearly every problem (including the failure to ascertain important transference issues and the meaningfulness of medication to the patient) that has been discussed. The frustrating experience for the collaborators, and undoubtedly for the patient as well, can be understood within the context of poorly defined clinical roles, expectations, and professional boundaries.

Ms Jensen is a 27-year-old unmarried secretary who was referred by a recently relocated internist to a social worker for assistance in managing the patient's depression and anxiety. According to her physician, the patient has not responded within the last 6 months to any of the various medications that he has prescribed. She has a long-standing history of depressive episodes beginning as a teenager. The patient has been difficult for the physician as she frequently calls for appointments because of a multiplicity of symptoms and complaints. He is unable to ascertain any significant illness in his patient and all diagnostic tests have proven normal. As the psychotherapist has not worked previously with the referring doctor, she recommends that they meet to discuss the patient before an evaluation for treatment is started. The doctor puts off the therapist saying he is pressed for time in his new practice and would prefer to send a summary of the patient's history. The social worker, not willing to disappoint a new referral source, agrees reluctantly to see Ms Jensen. The patient tells the therapist that her doctor seemed disinterested in her and stated that she was instructed to visit with a mental health professional for counseling. She describes her physician as very controlling and insisting that she take medication. The history indicated that the patient grew up in a household where both her mother and father were very demanding and rigid, always insisting that there was only one way to view life. Ms Jensen acknowledged that she had stopped taking the medications prescribed for her because of side-effects despite the fact that her doctor had reassured her that they would pass after the first week of treatment. She felt he had been dishonest because some side-effects, such as her sexual dysfunction, did not improve. The patient was effusive in her praise for the psychotherapist who clearly was interested in her plight and gave her sufficient time to talk. This was not the case with her internist whom she experienced as somewhat rigid. At the completion of the assessment, the social worker summarized her thoughts about the possible ways in which to proceed and that she would be contacting her internist. She mentioned that the patient should discuss her side-effects with her physician and that perhaps there might be another medication that would be less problematic for her. The social worker tried to contact the referring physician without success to discuss her findings and the appropriateness of psychotherapy in addition to medication. Four days later the psychotherapist received a discouraging phone call from Ms Jensen's doctor who felt he was undercut in his treatment decisions because the patient refused to take any of the medications he wished to prescribe and had nothing but glowing words about her interaction with the therapist. According to the physician, Ms Jensen explained that she was instructed to tell him that psychotherapy was indicated and not medication treatment.

Principles of effective collaborative care: how to communicate effectively and avoid pitfalls

A number of important conclusions can be drawn from this vignette about conducting effective split treatment. First, collaborative treatment cases should be selected carefully and collaborators should meet to discuss the reasons for referral when therapist and physician have never worked together (Rand, 1999). Once a successful working relationship has been established and the clinicians become comfortable with each other, communication then may be via telephone or written reports. Still, at times of crisis, collaborators may need to meet.

The physician or prescriber and therapist must agree on the responsibilities and boundaries of their collaborative work. Is the prescriber being viewed as consultant, equal partner, teacher, or supervisor? Collaborative treatment does not imply that the physician will supervise the treatment provided by the therapist or vice versa. Failure to clarify roles is the source of much confusion and ill will and may have legal implications. This is a particularly important point in the education of psychiatric and primary care residents when they work in medication clinics that employ split treatment. Beginning professionals often lack confidence in their skills and therefore may feel threatened by clinicians who have had different training and are more experienced. Other responsibilities of the collaborators include, but are not limited to agreement on their: frequency of communication, contact with family members where indicated, coverage when one collaborator is out of town, discussion with insurance personnel, and securing of informed consent. This understanding should be documented. As well, the patient must be educated to the characteristics of split treatment by both clinicians regarding their roles as collaborators and the need for constant sharing of treatment information. If splitting becomes prominent resistance in the treatment, collaborators often should meet in person to discuss their united approach to this problem. Physicians have an obligation to educate therapists about why medication is being prescribed as well as possible medication side-effects and how to report them. Therapists should assist the prescriber in identifying conflicts about medication, compliance problems, and the initial presentation of side-effects. In the eventuality of hospitalization, collaborators should be explicit about the level of responsibility and obligations of each. Collaborators must never use the patient to convey information that should be discussed more appropriately with the providers. Sometimes, the request for split treatment with a challenging referral can be a covert wish on the part of one clinician to either terminate or transfer a patient. It is difficult to overestimate the negative impact of such an issue on the patient as well as the collaborative relationship. Similarly, when treatment is to be discontinued, the decision about termination and follow-up (if required) should be jointly made and explained to the patient by each collaborator. In cases where a patient is not be able to establish a therapeutic relationship with one of the collaborators, both have an obligation to support a change in the treatment relationship. A reflection of an effective collaboration is the willingness of both collaborators to identify a therapeutic impasse or plateau and jointly to seek consultation. Lastly, the physician and the psychotherapist should never place each other in legal jeopardy by refusing to see the patient in crisis. At the initiation of each collaborative treatment relationship, therefore, both parties must stipulate about responsibilities in the event of crisis, coverage on vacations and weekends, and how clinical issues such as suicidality and homocidality will be evaluated. However, the physician should never place a therapist in the position of having to make medical decisions.

In the UK, where therapist and psychiatrist or primary care physician are often (but not always) both employees of the National Health Service, regular case conferences including the prescriber, psychotherapist, and care coordinator, and often the patient him/herself and family are an essential component of good mental health care. When patients are hospitalized, it is highly advantageous for members of the hospital treatment team to meet with collaborative treatment professionals. As a corollary, the wisdom of this approach is also helpful in the problems of a treatment impasse with difficult patients in any country. Collaborators should always be open to seek consultation when a treatment is proving to be ineffective, severe symptoms reappear and do not respond to intervention, or when tensions arise in the collaborative relationship.

Some practical issues in using combined treatment

How do nonprescribing clinicians know if medication will be beneficial for their psychotherapy patients?

First and foremost, all clinicians should familiarize themselves with the Diagnostic and Statistical Manual of Mental Disorders IV-TR (DSM-IV) published by the American Psychiatric Association (2000) or in Europe, the ICD-10 or International Classification of Disease and Related Health Problems (1992). Every clinician working with psychiatric patients in any capacity should have an appreciation of the nomenclature of mental disorders and their specific criteria. In addition to helping mental health professionals in their day to day clinical work with eliciting key symptoms and appreciating what diagnostic criteria constitute a particular disorder, these classification systems permit clearer communication from one clinician to another about patients. In the US, the ability to document a diagnosis is required by third party payors such as behavioral healthcare organizations. Moreover, these companies insist that mental health professionals provide a service that is likely to assist a particular patient with a particular psychological problem. Having said this, it is important that all clinicians appreciate the limitations of a categorical approach to understanding mental disorders. These include but are not limited to the following:

◆ each patient with the same diagnosis may not present in the same fashion

◆ each diagnosis may not always be distinguished from others.

This latter point is certainly the case in the classification of personality disorders, which has many clinicians arguing for a dimensional classification scheme. A dimensional model would attempt to quantify the attributes that characterize a patient rather than placing symptoms within a distinct diagnosis. As an example, a patient with borderline personality disorder may also have a number of features common to the diagnosis of narcissistic and histrionic personality disorders. Moreover, at times of maximal stress, some patients with borderline personality disorder may experience short-lived psychotic episodes. In short, providing a DSM-IV diagnosis for

a patient is only one of the important components in developing the biopsychosocial formulation and treatment plan.

The following case example is representative of the issues that should be considered in the treatment of a patient who is depressed in determining whether medication may be of some use in treatment.

Mr Davis is a 38-year-old man who has experienced one previous bout of moderate depression for which he did not seek treatment. He was referred to the social worker by his family physician who could find nothing abnormal on the patient's physical examination and laboratory tests and further acknowledged that his patient was not taking any medication that might account for his depression. His presenting complaints include a sleep disturbance (both difficulty in falling asleep and staying asleep), feeling down in the dumps or blue throughout the day, and difficulty concentrating at work. His recent episode of depression followed a tumultuous separation 3 months earlier in which both partners accused each other of infidelity. Mr Davis completed a Beck Depression Inventory while at the social worker's office and he scored 20. How should the mental health professional proceed?

The clinician must first conduct a comprehensive assessment to elucidate the history of her patient's symptoms and to gain an appreciation for the person behind the emotional disorder.

In her formulation, she then considers those biological, psychological, and social factors that may be contributing to her patient's discomfort. For example, she notes that in addition to his previous episodes of depression, both his mother and brother were hospitalized for severe depression. This may indicate a constitutional predisposition or vulnerability to depression. She also notes the psychological impact of the loss of his wife and the early history of a loss of his father who died when the patient was an adolescent. She also notices the alienation he is now experiencing from the couple's friends. Mr Davis also acknowledges some financial problems and worries that he may lose his job if his performance deteriorates at work. Lastly, his clinician appreciates a strong potential for a working or therapeutic alliance.

The social worker must next establish a working diagnosis. In this case it is obvious that this man is suffering from some type of mood disorder. The social worker has information that the physician could find no medical basis for this depression, which is helpful because it excludes, for example, considerations of brain tumor, endocrine disorder, or a substance-induced disorder. She could discern no other psychopathology, such as a personality disorder, that could complicate this man's depression.

She and her patient decide on a treatment plan and they agree to begin CBT, a psychotherapy with proven efficacy in the treatment of moderate depression. She and Mr Davis meet weekly and the patient adheres to the components of the therapy and completes all assigned homework. Despite a strong therapeutic alliance and the patient's hard work, by week 8, the clinician notes that her patient has only partially responded to the psychotherapy and his symptoms, although less disruptive, nevertheless persist.

The therapist must now consider her options to augment the treatment. She may, for example, meet more often with the patient. The possibility of group psychotherapy is also considered. She may also refer the patient for pharmacotherapy as an adjunct to the psychotherapy work.

This vignette illustrates a number of important steps in conducting this or any other treatment. The clinician should:

◆ take a formal and in-depth history to secure a thorough appreciation of those factors contributing to his illness

◆ develop a formulation to provide a working hypothesis regarding the patient's condition

◆ establish a working diagnosis

◆ appreciate the severity of symptoms

◆ develop a treatment plan

◆ monitor the patient's compliance, his symptomatic and functional status, and response to treatment.

Before presenting the option of medication, the therapist speaks with the referring physician about her observations and the possible helpfulness of combined treatment, and if both clinicians agree, the policies regarding collaboration once medication is started. A thorough discussion with the patient then ensues about the possibility of medications, including highlighting their adjunctive role in treatment, exploring any initial resistance to take medication, encouraging them to ask the physician as much as possible about the medication, the need for the patient to be a collaborator in discussing his responses to the medication with both the social worker and the physician, and the importance of adhering to the medication plan as presented. In the US at least, the patient should sign an informed consent statement that detail the risks and benefits of combined treatment with both clinicians and stipulates that they are free to speak with each regarding the patient's progress in treatment.

Other indications that pharmacotherapy would be helpful for a patient who is treated with psychotherapy alone include the worsening of a patient's disorder, the appearance of a new disorder, and the failure of a patient to respond to the medication currently being prescribed.

When should pharmacotherapy and psychotherapy start at the beginning of treatment?

As a second scenario, let us assume that Mr Davis presented with the following history: three previous episodes of depression, one requiring hospitalization; persistent thoughts of suicide, a weight loss of 12 pounds over a 6-week period without attempting to diet, and a pervasive feeling of hopelessness. On the Beck Depression Inventory he scores 39. In this instance, the social worker would have noted the presence of major depressive episode of significant disruption, safety concerns, and a significant history of depression that required hospitalization. As her patient's depression is severe, he is in significant psychological pain, she is aware that medication, in general, works more quickly than psychotherapy, and of the evidence to support combined treatment in moderately severe to severe depression, she contacts the referring physician and explores his willingness to collaborate with her in Mr Davis's treatment in which psychotherapy and pharmacotherapy will be initiated simultaneously.

When should a therapist consider referral to a psychiatrist for integrated treatment?

It has been discussed previously that many patients who require medication and with severe medical or surgical illnesses may do better with a one-person model. As an example, a panic-disordered patient with severe inflammatory bowel disease may require, among many drugs, very high doses of a corticosteroid. This type of medication has a propensity for producing significant side-effects that often appear to be like other psychiatric disorders. Such patients may become profoundly depressed, manic, or psychotic. A psychiatrist is often able to monitor this patient's treatment more efficiently than might occur in a two-person model. For a surgeon and or gastroenterologist, they may find consulting with another physician to be more conducive to a collaborative situation as well. Also to be considered is the level of anxiety that a nonphysician might experience in treating a medically unstable patient. Of course, some patients who come to a non-medical therapist, may decide that they would prefer seeing only one professional. For some patients who strongly evidence splitting and have demeaned the nonprescribing professional and which does not seem lessened by interpretation, they too may do better in an integrative relationship. A persistently suicidal person may unnerve either collaborator, but there may be times when a psychiatrist who has worked extensively with such patients and who has the opportunity to hospitalize, may treat the patient more efficiently. There are some patients with paranoid disorders requiring medication who threaten litigation consistently and the psychiatrist may be more comfortable with these types of behaviors. Also these patients can only maintain a single treating relationship and will always be a challenge but they may be better contained in an integrated situation. It is important to remember that as yet, data are not available to support any of these assumptions.

How to help patients comply with a medication regimen

It has been noted that medication compliance problems should be anticipated in any treatment relationship be it an integrative or split approach. First and foremost, mental health professionals must understand the characteristics and the natural course of the condition that they are treating. This information must be provided to all patients in treatment. Psychoeducation for the patient, and at times family members or even employers as well, is considered essential to enhancing treatment adherence. For example, some disorders, as in the patient with major depression marked by repeated bouts of his illness, will require lifelong medication. This must be explained to the patient at the initiation of treatment. Often patients who have severe disorders that have been treated effectively in the initial phase will discontinue their medication when feeling better. Some patients, such as those with bipolar disorder, resist taking mood stabilizers because they dislike the dampening of their affect and at times their hyperactivity. These patients not infrequently feel stronger with boundless energy, hypersexuality, and elevated mood.

Patients must be assisted to understand signs of relapse. This is true for the majority of psychiatric disorders. In integrative and split treatment, patients must be educated about the length of time on medication before they experience some relief. This is true for antidepressants, antipsychotics, mood stabilizers, and some anxiolytics. Patients should be warned about discontinuing medication without informing the professional. Many psychotropic medications, if discontinued abruptly, produce rebound effects that patients experience as a worsening of their condition.

Essential to treatment with medication is the appreciation of the occurrence and meaning of side-effects. Nonprescribing professionals with experience generally become familiar with the common side-effects of classes of medication. When in doubt these therapists should routinely consult their collaborator. For common psychotropic medications, the following side-effects are helpful to keep in mind:

◆ Selective serotonin reuptake inhibitor antidepressants (SSRIs) during the first few weeks or treatment or so can produce, among others, headaches, gastroenterological symptoms, sedation, agitation, and sexual dysfunction. With the exception of the latter two, these side-effects will often cease after the first 2 weeks of treatment. Sexual dysfunction occurs in both men and women at significant rates and often lasts as long as patients are on these medications. The therapist can speak with a collaborator about steps to decrease this side-effect. Patients who become severely agitated during the first week of treatment will be instructed by the prescriber to discontinue the medication and an alternate medication may be provided.

◆ Typical antipsychotics, such as chlorpromazine and its relatives or haloperidol, have the potential to cause disturbing side-effects such as abnormal involuntary movements and severe dystonic symptoms such as a very painful stiff neck. In addition, patients who are taking these medications should be observed for a side-effect called tardive dyskinesia that presents as oral facial involuntary movements as this is an irreversible side-effect.

◆ In general, the side-effects of various mood stabilizers used in the treatment of bipolar disorder and to augment severe depression require greater depth of knowledge as these medications differ in their ability to produce specific side-effects.

There a number of rating scales that may assist the psychotherapist in monitoring side-effects. In patients with schizophrenia, for example, abnormal involuntary movements in various parts of the body can be assessed through instruments that do not require extensive training to administer and that can be used repeatedly in monitoring a patient's course. For atypical medications (those prescribed for off label indications) employed in treatment, it is the responsibility of the physician to inform his or her collaborator as well as the patient of side-effects that may occur.

Although every patient ascribes some meaning to their medication, when this meaning interferes with their ability to comply with treatment, this situation demands examination. As discussed earlier in this chapter, patients may hold negative beliefs about their therapist or pharmacotherapist that greatly impede treatment compliance. These beliefs, and specific beliefs about medication, should be anticipated, identified as resistances, and worked through.

Assisting a patient in taking medication can be made easier if clinicians are familiar with certain techniques. Those described by Beck (2001) are illustrative and recommended. Although Beck refers to CBT, her suggestions are helpful to psychotherapy of any theoretical persuasion. To review, she advocates that clinicians identify and address thoughts and beliefs about medication and psychological treatment that frequently interfere with a patient's ability to follow treatment recommendations. In providing any type of psychotherapy, distortions about self, about others, and his or her world view should be appreciated. Direct assessment of likelihood to adhere to treatment is essential. A patient who has failed previous treatments or has not been able to establish a therapeutic alliance should raise concern and requires thorough exploration. Beck suggests that is helpful to ask patients directly if they are likely to follow a medication regimen, whether they believe medication will work, do they have a specific fear about taking a psychotropic medication, would family members be against medication specifically or medication in general, and even if there are transportation or financial difficulties associated with the filling of a prescription. It is often productive to explore if the nonadherence occurs only at certain times. Once a patient's concerns are identified, the clinician in integrated or split treatment situations is obligated to educate and address certain misinformation held by the patient. Beck also notes that frequently in patients with compliance problems that it is facilitating to speak concretely about the advantages and disadvantages of taking medication. Lastly, Beck suggests other formal behavioral techniques may be of some assistance in dealing with noncompliance. These include having the patient accept praise or take credit for complying, visualize their lives if they chose not to comply, using a medication log, and employ coping cards that remind the patient why it is necessary to take the medication and details simultaneously identified resistances.

Unanswered questions

Despite the increasing amount of research on combined treatment, there nevertheless are important issues to be addressed (Kay, 2001).

- For what disorders should psychotherapy precede medication and vice versa?
- For what disorders should combined interventions be implemented from the very beginning of treatment?
- Under what conditions is integrated treatment more advantageous than split treatment?
- For which disorders is it cost effective to provide patients with either integrated or split treatment?
- What factors in integrated and split treatment are critical to improving patient outcome?

Conclusions

There is growing support both from research and clinical practice, about the benefits of combining medication and psychotherapy in the treatment of mental disorders and symptoms. It seems clear that there is much to be gained in helping patients with mental illness by implementing complimentary and comprehensive care, which among other benefits, increases compliance with treatment. This is true for both a one-person model and two-person treatment model. For collaborative treatment to be effective, however, it is essential that communication be consistent, candid, and focused. Perhaps the practice of utilizing psychotherapy and medication will soon put an end to the unproductive tensions created by the anachronistic mind–body split.

References

Antonuccia, J. D. (1995). Psychotherapy for depression: no stronger medicine. *American Psychologist*, **50**, 450–2.

American Psychiatric Association. (2000). *Diagnostic and Statistical Manual of Mental Disorders, Text Revision (DSM-IV-TR)*, 4th edn. Washington, DC: American Psychiatric Association.

Balon, R. (2001). Positive and negative aspects of split treatment. *Psychiatric Annals*, **31**, 598–603.

Barlow, D. H., *et al.* (2000). Cognitive-behavioral therapy, imipramine, or their combination for panic disorder: as randomized controlled trial. *Journal of the American Medical Association*, **283**, 2529–36.

Barsky, A. J., Saintfort, R., Rogers, M. P., and Borus, J. F. (2002). Nonspecific medication side effects and the nocebo phenomenon. *Journal of the American Medical Association*, **287**(5), 622–7.

Basco, M. R. and Rush, A. J. (1996). *Cognitive-behavioral therapy for bipolar disorder*. New York: Guilford Press.

Bateman, A. and Fonagy, P. (2001). Treatment of borderline personality disorder with psychoanalytically oriented partial hospitalization program: an 18-month follow-up. *American Journal of Psychiatry*, **158**, 36–42.

Baxter, K. R., *et al.* (1992). Caudate glucose metabolic rate changes with both drug and behavior therapy for obsessive-compulsive disorder. *Archives of General Psychiatry*, **49**, 681–9.

Baxter, L., *et al.* (1992). Caudate glucose metabolic rate changes with both drug and behavior therapy for obsessive-compulsive disorder. *Archives of General Psychiatry*, **49**, 681–98 [Medline].

Beck, J. S. (2001). A cognitive therapy approach to medication compliance. In: J. Kay, ed. *Integrated psychiatric treatment for psychiatric disorders*, pp. 113–41. Washington, DC: American Psychiatric Press.

Benkert, O., *et al.* (1997). Public opinion on psychotropic drugs: an analysis of the factors influencing acceptance or rejection. *Journal of Nervous and Mental Disease*, **185**(3), 151–8.

Brody, A. L., *et al.* (2001). Regional brain metabolic changes in patients with major depression teated with either paroxetine or interpersonal therapy. *Archives of General Psychiatry*, **58**, 631–40 [Abstract/Free Full Text].

Bruce, T. J., Speigel, D. A., and Hegel, M. T. (1999). Cognitive-behavioral therapy helps prevent relapse and recurrence of panic disorder following alprazolam discontinuation: a long-term follow-up of the Peorian and Dartmouth studies. *Journal of Consulting and Clinical Psychology*, **67**, 151–6.

Burnand, Y., Andreoli, A., Kolatte, E., Venturini, A., and Rosset, N. (2002). Psychodynamic psychotherapy and clomipramine in the treatment of major depression. *Psychiatric Services*, **53**(5), 585–90.

Coursey, R. D., Keller, A. B., and Farrell, E. W. (1995). Individual psychotherapy and persons with serious mental illness: the client's perspective. *Schizophrenia Bulletin*, **21**, 283–301.

Demyttenaere, K., *et al.* (2001). Compliance with antidepressants in a primary care setting, 1: beyond lack of effacacy and adverse events. *Journal of Clinical Psychiatry*, **62**(22), 30–3.

Detre, T. and McDonald, M. C. (1997). Managed care and the future of psychiatry. *Archives of General Psychiatry*, **54**, 201–4 [Medline].

Edlund, M. J., *et al.* (2002). Dropping out of mental health treatment: patterns and predictors among epidemiological survey respondents in the United States and Ontario. *American Journal of Psychiatry*, **159**, 845–51.

Ellison, J. M. and Harney, P. A. (2000). Treatment-resistant depression and the collaborative treatment relationship. *Journal of Psychotherapy and Practice Research*, **9**(1), 7–17.

Falloon, I. R. H., Boyd, J. L., and McGill, C. W. (1982). Family management in the prevention of exacerbations of schizophrenia: a controlled study. *New England Journal of Medicine*, **17**, 1437–40.

Fava, G. (1999). Sequential treatment: a new way of integrating pharmacotherapy and psychotherapy. *Psychotherapy and Psychosomatics*, **68**, 227–9.

Fava, G. A., Rafanelli, C., Grandi, S., Canestrari, R., and Morphy, M. A. (1998). Six-year outcome for cognitive behavioral treatment of residual symptoms in major depression. *American Journal of Psychiatry*, **155**(10), 1443–5.

Fava, G. A., Bartlucci, G., Rafanelli, C., and Mangelli, L. (2001). Cognitive-behavioral management of patients with bipolar disorder who relapsed while on lithium prophylaxis. *Journal of Clinical Psychiatry*, **62**(7), 556–9.

Feeney, G. F., Young, R. M., Connor, J. P., Tucker, J., and McPherson, A. (2001). Outpatient cognitive behavioural therapy programme for alcohol dependence: impact of naltrexone use on outcome. *Australian and New Zealand Journal of Psychiatry*, **35**(4), 443–8.

Frank, E., Kupfer, D. J., and Seigel, L. R. (1995). Alliance not compliance: a philosophy of outpatient care. *Journal of Clinical Psychiatry*, **56**, 11–16, discussion 16–17.

Frank, E., *et al.* (2000). Interpersonal psychotherapy and antidepressant medication: evaluation of a sequential treatment strategy in women with recurrent major depression. *Journal of Clinical Psychiatry*, **61**, 51–7.

Gabbard, G. O. (2000). Combined psychotherapy and pharmacotherapy. In: B. J. Sadock and V. A. Sadock, ed. *Comprehensive textbook of psychiatry*, 7th edn, pp. 2225–34. Baltimore, MD: Lippincott Williams & Wilkins.

Gabbard, G. O. (2000). A neurobiologically informed perspective on psychotherapy. *British Journal of Psychiatry*, **177**, 117–22.

Gabbard, G. O. and Kay, J. (2001). The fate of integrated treatment: whatever happened to the biopsychosocial psychiatrist? *American Journal of Psychiatry*, **158**, 1956–63.

Goldman, W., *et al.* (1998). Outpatient utilization patterns if integrated and split psychotherapy and pharmacotherapy for depression. *Psychiatric Services*, **49**, 477–82.

Granholm, E., McQuaid, J. R., McClure, F. S., Pedrelli, P., and Jeste, D. V. (2002). A randomized controlled pilot study of cognitive behavioral social skills training for older patients with schizophrenia. *Schizophrenia Research*, **53**(1–2), 167–9.

Grech, E. (2002). Psychological interventions for psychosis: a critical review of the current evidence. *The Internet Journal of Mental Health*, **1**(2).

Gunderson, J. G. and Ridolfi, M. E. (2001). Borderline Personality disorder. Suicidality and self-mutilation. *Annals of the New York Academy of Science*, **932**, 61–73 and 73–7.

Hansen-Grant, S. and Riba, M. B. (1995). Contact between psychotherapists and psychiatric residents who provide medication backup. *Psychiatric Services*, **46**(8), 774–7.

Hatfield, A. B., Gearson, J. S., and Coursey, R. D. (1996). Family member's ratings of the use and value of mental health services: results of a national NAMI survey. *Psychiatric Services*, **27**, 825–31.

Hogarty, G. E., *et al.* (1991). The environmental-personal indicators in the course of schizophrenia (EPICS) research group: family psychoeducation, social skills training, and maintenance chemotherapy in the aftercare of treatment of schizophrenia II: two-year effects of a controlled study on relapse and adjustment. *Archives of General Psychiatry*, **48**, 340–7.

Hogarty, G. E., *et al.* (1997a). Three-year trials of personal therapy among schizophrenic patients living with or independent of family, I: description of study and effects on relapse rates. *American Journal of Psychiatry*, **154**, 1504–13 [Abstract/Free Full Text].

Hogarty, G. E., *et al.* (1997b). Three-year trials of personal therapy among schizophrenic patients living with or independent of family, II: effects on adjustment of patients. *American Journal of Psychiatry*, **54**, 1514–24 [Abstract/Free Full Text].

Hollon, S. D., *et al.* (1992). Cognitive therapy and pharmacotherapy for depression: singly and in combination. *Archives of General Psychiatry*, **49**, 774–81.

de Jonge, F., Kool, S., van Aalst, G., Dekker, J., and Peen, J. (2002). Combining psychotherapy and antidepressants in the treatment of depression. *Journal of Affective Disorders*, **64**(2–3), 217–29.

Jorm, A. F., Korten, A. E., Jacomb, P. A., Christensen, H., and Henderson, S. (1999). Attitudes towards people with a mental disorder: a survey of the Australian public and health professionals. *Australian and New Zealand Journal of Psychiatry*, **33**, 77–83.

Kampman, M., Keijsers, G. P., Hoogduin, C. A., and Hendriks, G. J. (2002). A randomized, double-blind, placebo-controlled study of the effects of adjunctive paroxetine in panic disorder patients unsuccessfully treated with cognitive-behavioral therapy alone. *Journal of Clinical Psychiatry*, **63**(9), 772–7.

Kandel, E. R. (1998). A new intellectual framework for psychiatry. *American Journal of Psychiatry*, **155**, 457–69 [Abstract/Free Full Text].

Kandel, E. R. (1999). Biology and the future of psychoanalysis: a new intellectual framework for psychiatry revisited. *American Journal of Psychiatry*, **156**, 505–24 [Abstract/Free Full Text].

Karasu, T. B. (1982). Psychotherapy and pharmacotherapy: toward an integrative model. *American Journal of Psychiatry*, **139**, 1102–13.

Kay, J. (1998). The demise of comprehensive clinical psychiatry. *Archives of General Psychiatry*, **55**(2), 183–4.

Kay, J. (2001). Integrated treatment: an overview. In: J. Kay, ed. *Integrated Treatment for Psychiatric Disorders: Review of Psychiatry*, Vol. 20, pp. 1–29. Washington, DC: American Psychiatric Press.

Keller, M. B., *et al.* (2000). A comparison of nefazodone, the cognitive behavioral-analysis system of psychotherapy, and their combination for the treatment of chronic depression. *New England Journal of Medicine*, **342**, 1462–70 [Abstract/Free Full Text].

King, M., *et al.* (2002). Effectiveness of teaching general practitioners skills in brief cognitive behaviour therapy to treat patients with depression: randomised controlled trial. *British Medical Journal*, **324**, 947.

Klerman, G. L. (1991). Ideological conflicts in integrating pharmacotherapy and psychotherapy. In: B. B. Beitman and G. Klerman, ed. *Integrating pharmacotherapy and psychotherapy*, pp. 3–20. Washington, DC: American Psychiatric Press.

Knapp, M. (1997). Costs of schizophrenia. *British Journal of Psychiatry*, **171**, 509–18.

Krupnick, J. L., *et al.* (1996). The role of therapeutic alliance in psychotherapy and pharmacotherapy outcome: findings in the National Institute of Mental Health Treatment of Depression Collaborative Research Program. *Journal of Consulting and Clinical Psychology*, **64**, 532–9 [CrossRef] [Medline].

Kuipers, E., *et al.* (1998). London-East Anglia randomized controlled trial of cognitive-behavioural therapy for psychoses. *British Journal of Psychiatry*, **173**, 61–8.

Lacro, J. P., Dunn, L. B., Dolder, C. R., Leckband, S. G., and Jeste, D. V. (2002). Prevalence of and risk factors for medication nonadherence in patients with schizophrenia: a comprehensive review of recent literature. *Journal of Clinical Psychiatry*, **63**(10), 892–909.

Lazarus, J. A. (1999). Ethical issues in collaborative or divided treatment. In: M. B. Riba and R. Balon, ed. *Psychopharmacology and psychotherapy: a collaborative approach*, pp. 159–78. Washington, DC: American Psychiatric Press.

LeDoux, J. (2002). Synaptic self: how our brains become who we are. London: Viking Penguin Group.

Leff, J. P., *et al.* (1985). A controlled trial of social intervention in the families of schizophrenic patients: a two-year follow-up and issues in treatment. *British Journal of Psychiatry*, **146**, 594–600.

Lehrer, D. and Kay, J. (2002). Neurobiology. In: M. Hersen and W. Siedge, ed. *Encyclopedia of Psychotherapy*, pp. 207–22. New York: Academic Press.

Lenze, E. J., *et al.* (2002). Combined pharmacotherapy and psychotherapy as maintenance treatment for late-life depression: effects on social adjustment. *American Journal of Psychiatry*, **159**, 466–8.

Lieberman, J. A. and Rush, A. J. (1996). Redefining the role of psychiatry in medicine. *American Journal of Psychiatry*, **153**, 1388–97 [Abstract].

Liggan, D. Y. and Kay, J. (1999). Some neurobiological aspects of psychotherapy: a review. *Journal of Psychotherapy and Practice Research*, **8**, 103–14.

Lin, E. H., *et al.* (1995). The role of the primary care physician in patients' adherence to antidepressant therapy. *Medical Care*, **33**, 67–74.

Luborsky, L., *et al.* (1993). The efficacy of dynamic psychotherapies: is it true that 'everyone has won and all must have prizes'? In N. E. Miller, L. Luborsky, J. P. Barber, and J. P. Docherty, ed. *Psychodynamic treatment research: a handbook for clinical practice*, pp. 497–516. New York: Basic Books.

Manning, D. W., Markowitz, J. C., and Frances, A. J. (1992). A review of combined psychotherapy and pharmacotherapy in the treatment of depression. *Journal of Psychotherapy and Practice Research*, **1**, 103–16.

Marks, I. M., *et al.* (1993). Alprazolam and exposure alone and combined in panic disorder with agoraphobia. A controlled study in London and Toronto. *British Journal of Psychiatry*, **162**, 776–87.

Martin, S. D., Marin, E., Rai, S. S., Richardson, M. A., and Royall, R. (2001). Brain blood flow changes in depressed patients treated with interpersonal psychotherapy or venlafaxine hydrochloride. *Archives of General Psychiatry*, **58**, 641–8 [Abstract/Free Full Text].

McBeth, J. E. (2001). Legal aspects of split treatment: how to audit and manage risk. *Psychiatric Annals*, **31**, 605–10.

McGorry, P. D., *et al.* (2002). Randomized controlled trial of interventions designed to reduce the risk of progression to first-episode psychosis in a clinical sample with subthreshold symptoms. *Archives of General Psychiatry*, **59**(10), 921–8.

McLellan, A. T., *et al.* (1993). The effects of psychosocial services in substance abuse treatment. *Journal of the American Medical Association*, **269**, 1953–9.

McQuaid, J. R., *et al.* (2002). A randomized controlled pilot study of cognitive behavioral social skills training for older patients with schizophrenia (Letter). *Schizophrenia Research*, **53**, 167–9.

Miklowitz, D. J., *et al.* (2000). Family-focused treatment of bipolar disorder: 1-year effects of a psychoeducational program in conjunction with pharmacotherapy. *Biological Psychiatry*, **48**(6), 582–92.

Norcross, J. C. and Goldfried, M. R., ed. (1992). *Handbook of psychotherapy integration*. New York: Basic Books.

Pava, J. A., Fava, M., and Levenson, J. A. (1994). Integrating cognitive therapy and pharmacotherapy in the treatment and prophylaxis of depression: a novel approach: *Psychotherapy and Psychosomatics*, **61**(3–4), 211–19.

Paykel, E. S. (1995). Psychotherapy, medication combinations, and compliance. *Journal of Clinical Psychiatry*, **56**, 24–30.

Rand, E. H. (1999). Guidelines to maximize the process of collaborative care. In: M. B. Riba and R. Balon, ed. *Psychopharmacology and psychotherapy*, pp. 353–80. Washington, DC: American Psychiatric Press.

Reynolds, C. F. III, *et al.* (1999). Nortriptyline and interpersonal psychotherapy as maintenance therapies for recurrent major depression: a randomized controlled trial in patients older than 59 years. *Journal of the American Medical Association*, **281**, 39–45 [CrossRef] [Medline].

Ricca, V., *et al.* (2001). Fluoxetine and fluvoxamine combined with individual cognitive-behaviour therapy in binge eating disorder: a one-year follow-up study. *Psychotherapy and Psychosomatics*, **70**(6), 298–306.

Rush, A. J. (1998). Clinical diagnosis of mood disorders. *Clinical Chemistry*, **34**(5), 813–21.

Sacheim, H. A. (2001). Functional brain circuits in major depression and remission. *Archives of General Psychiatry*, **58**(7), 649–50.

Segal, Z., Vincent, P., and Levitt, A. (2002). Efficacy of combined, sequential and crossover psychotherapy and pharmacotherapy in improving outcomes in depression. *Journal of Psychiatry and Neuroscience*, **27**(4), 281–90.

Sensky, T., *et al.* (2000). A randomized controlled trial of cognitive-behavioral therapy for persistent symptoms in schizophrenia resistant to medication. *Archives of General Psychiatry*, **57**, 165–72.

Spiegel, D. A., Bruce, T. J., Gregg, S. F., and Nuzzarello, A. (1994). Does cognitive behavior therapy assist slow-taper alprazolam discontinuation in panic disorder? *American Journal of Psychiatry*, **151**(6), 876–81.

Stein, M. B., Norton R. G., Walker, J. R., Chartier, M. H., and Graham, R. (2000). Do selective serotonin re-uptake inhibitors enhance the efficacy of very brief cognitive behavioral therapy for panic disorder? A pilot study. *Psychiatry Research*, **94**(3), 191–200.

Tarrier, N., *et al.* (1998). Randomised controlled trial of intensive cognitive behaviour therapy for patients with chronic schizophrenia. *British Medical Journal*, **317**, 303–7.

Teasdale, J. D., *et al.* (2001). How does cognitive therapy prevent relapse in residual depression? Evidence from a controlled trial. *Journal of Consulting and Clinical Psychology*, **69**(3), 347–57.

Thase, M. E., *et al.* (1997). Treatment of Major depression with psychotherapy or psychotherapy-pharmacotherapy combinations. *Archives of General Psychiatry*, **54**, 1009–15. [Medline].

Treatment for Adolescents with Depression Study Team. (2004). Fluoxetine, cognitive-behavioral therapy, and their combination for adolescents with depression: Treatment for Adolescents with Depression Study (TADS) randomized controlled trial. *JAMA*, **292**, 807–20.

Unutzer, J., *et al.* (2002). Collaborative care management of late-life depression in the primary care setting: a randomized controlled trial. *Journal of the American Medical Association*, **288**(22), 2836–45.

Walsh, B. T., *et al.* (1997). Medication and psychotherapy in the treatment of bulimia nervosa. *American Journal of Psychiatry*, **154**, 523–31 [Abstract].

Weston, D. and Morrison, K. (2001). A multidimensional meta-analysis of treatments for depression, panic, and generalized anxiety disorder: an empirical examination of the status of empirically supported therapies. *Journal of Consulting and Clinical Psychology*, **69**(6), 875–99.

Westra, H. A., Stewart, S. H., and Conrad, B. E. (2002). Naturalistic manner of benzodiazepine use and cognitive behavior therapy outcome in panic disorder with agoraphobia. *Journal of Anxiety Disorders*, **16**, 233–46.

Wexler, B. E. and Chicchetti, D. V. (1992). The outpatient treatment of depression: implications of outcome research for clinical practice. *Journal of Nervous and Mental Disease*, **180**, 277–86.

Whittal, M. L., Otto, M. W., and Hong, J. J. (2001). Cognitive-behavior therapy for discontinuation of SSRI treatment of panic disorder: a case series. *Behaviour Research Therapy*, **39**(8), 939–45.

Wiborg, I. M. and Dahl, A. A. (1996). Does brief dynamic psychotherapy reduce the relapse rate of panic disorder? *Archives of General Psychiatry*, **53**, 689–94 [Medline].

Woody, G. E., *et al.* (1995). Psychotherapy in community methadone programs: a validation study. *American Journal of Psychiatry*, **152**, 1302–8.

40 Ethics and psychotherapy

Gwen Adshead

Introduction

The term 'ethics' can be defined in many ways. In the context of mental health care, any discussion about an ethical dilemma involves a special type of dialog; the discourse of 'ought' and 'should' in interpersonal relationships. Thus, when we talk about ethics in psychotherapy, we are talking about how therapists *should* behave in clinical practice with patients, and what the therapist *ought* to do in difficult interpersonal situations with patients and colleagues.

There is arguably a close relationship between ethics and psychotherapy, because just as ethical debate is all about how individuals *should* treat other people, and how we *should* act in relationship to each other, so psychotherapy explores interpersonal relating; how patients *actually* do treat other people, and relate to them. Additionally, all psychotherapeutic processes, regardless of school, utilize the therapeutic relationship between patient and therapist in some way, in order to understand and address the patient's problems.

This chapter is written largely from the perspective of psychoanalytic psychotherapy, with some additional reference to cognitive-behavioral therapy (CBT). But whatever the school of therapy, ethical dilemmas will arise that the therapist will have to reason and think about, and resolve; Tjelveit (1999) suggests that there are at least 14 different types of ethical reasoning that may be used in ethical dilemmas in psychotherapy (Box 40.1).

Box 40.1 Fourteen approaches to ethical reasoning (Tjvelveit, 1999)

- *Casuistry*: emphasize the specific circumstances
- *Classic liberal individualism*: emphasize autonomy and justice as ideals
- *Communitarianism*: emphasizes the interests of society
- *Critical psychology*: challenges psychology's claim to be ethically neutral
- *Feminist ethics*: the ethical character of therapy as gendered
- *Hermeneutics*: emphasizes interpretation, not explanation
- *Narrative*: understanding the right through stories
- *Naturalistic*: putting science and ethics together
- *Pragmatic*: emphasizes practical consequences
- *Radical*: the values of the left should be adopted
- *Rational*: ethics based on reason
- *Religious*: linked with varieties of religious tradition
- *Romantic*: linking ethics with the idea of a natural self
- *Virtue ethics*: understanding the character of the ethical actor.

A key theme here is that ethical dilemmas in psychotherapy have to be resolved, one way or the other; the overarching ethical duty of the therapist is to make the best quality decision that can be made.

Some guidance about the ethical duties of therapists can be found in the codes and guidelines that professional bodies hold to define their professional identity. Further guidance can be found in legal statutes and cases that have examined ethical dilemmas in psychotherapy. In this chapter, I will discuss some important legal cases from both US and English jurisdictions, because these give an indication of how the courts resolve ethical dilemmas. However, these cases should not be understood as legal advice (as the law is always subject to interpretation and review); nor does the law always provide an ethically justifiable source of guidance, as is clear if we remember the impact of both the Nazi and South African race laws.

Legal and professional advice may not provide all the answers, and therapists will still have to do some ethical reasoning for themselves. Specifically, therapists are likely to face dilemmas relating to:

- goals and objectives of therapy
- the boundaries between their different identities
- the social and political frameworks in which they work.

Most of the classical ethical dilemmas can be understood in these three domains.

Goals and objectives of therapy

Informed consent

What are the goals of psychotherapy, and who decides? If we apply the traditional medical ethical principles of beneficence and nonmaleficence, then psychotherapy, like any other medical treatment, should aim to help the patients with their problems, make them feel better and do them no harm. Most psychotherapists pursue this aim by working with patients to increase their capacity for self-reflection, and to help them become more aware of the links between their feelings and actions.

But this is not as simple as it seems. Although CBT can make people feel better in the short term by removing their symptoms, psychodynamic therapies may not do so. For example, patients with histories of exposure to traumatic events (whether in childhood or in adulthood) may want the therapy to take their horrible feelings away. However, psychotherapists do not take patients' feelings and memories away, but try and help them to deal with them better. Both CBT and psychodynamic therapy seek to help regulate conscious negative feelings, and modify distorted and dysfunctional meanings of memories. Although these are perfectly reasonable goals for psychotherapists, they may not be what the patient sees as the goal of therapy. Patients may not accept that the meanings attributed to memory are distorted; they may also be unaware of the extent of their negative feelings, especially guilt, shame, and hatred. In CBT, the patient may want to remove all their negative emotion, while the therapist wants to decrease excess emotion.

There are practical techniques that all therapists employ to address these issues clinically. Ethically, however, there may still be uncertainty or conflict about what the goals of therapy are, and who should set them, which can make the issue of informed consent in psychotherapy particularly complex. The ethical principle that underpins the requirement for consent is respect for autonomy: patients should be free to choose or refuse for themselves what treatment they have. Legally, for consent to be valid it must be given voluntarily, by a patient who is competent to make that decision, and the patient must be adequately informed about what the treatment involves, including any possible negative side-effects. However, it may be difficult for therapists to advise patients exactly to what it is they are consenting. Therapists may not be able to predict what patients will experience during the course of therapy, or what the outcome will be. Should therapists inform patients about unconscious transference enactments (both positive and negative), and get specific consent for this possible 'side-effect'? (Holmes and Lindley, 1989). My own view is that therapists need to warn patients that the p_____t always comfortable, and that many patients f_____ his may not be true for CBT). _____ople do not get better with psy- c_____ ccessful psychotherapy matches the right therapy and right therapist _____ patient, which is why therapists need to develop good quality assessment skills, not just for their own dis- cipline but for others. This means being able to formulate problems in different ways, and think about the ways that this particular patient is most likely to make progress.

Autonomy and consent to therapy

For consent to be valid it must be given by competent patients, who are capable of exercising their autonomy in a way that expresses their values and interests, while giving weight to conflicting values and facts. Although in a general sense, most psychotherapy patients will be competent to make decisions about their own treatment, this may not be true for all. For some it is problems with the exercise of autonomy that have led them to seek therapy; for others, their psychological distress may affect their capacity to make choices about treatment. Obvious examples are those people who have very recently suffered psychological trauma or bereavement, or those who are experiencing psychotic symptoms.

There are other groups of patients who may lack competence to make treatment decisions, such as children, or patients with psychotic disorders or learning disabilities. The problem is usually not a global lack of compet- ence, but rather that patients experience fluctuating levels of capacity, or experience rapid changes in how they make decisions. For example, it is hard to know what to make of a child's refusal to have therapy, which they agreed to only a day before. Can this be understood as an informed choice to refuse treatment? Or is this refusal merely evidence that the work has begun? There are also groups of patients are 'coerced' into therapy, such as children who only agree under pressure from family.

It may also be much harder to know how to think through issues of informed consent for family, marital, or group psychotherapy (Lakin, 1988). Children, or other family members may only 'agree' to thera_____ pressure from others in their emotional network. Although s_____ are an essential part of intimate relationships, they raise dilem_____ nature of 'true' voluntariness. Voluntariness is also an obviou_____ domain of forensic psychotherapy, as some patients may be mandated to have treatment, as an alternative to prison, or participation in therapy is expected as part of their detention. Clinically, most therapists in forensic or penal settings get to grips with this issue as part of the therapy from the start; but it does not sit easily with classical medical ethical accounts of informed consent.

Nonmaleficence: do no harm

Psychotherapists, like any other doctor, are under an obligation to do no harm. The question then is what constitutes 'harm' in psychotherapy. Just as defining benefit can be difficult, because of the need to consider different perspectives and time scales, so too is defining harm. It is probably inevitable that effective psychotherapy will sometimes cause people distress,

at least in the short term. Effective psychotherapy may also have unforeseen effects on patient's lives: an unhappy husband may leave his wife, a child may have to leave his family, and a person may change his/her job. These may constitute benefits in the patient's view, but may be seen as harmful by others. For example, there have been cases where patients who recover memories of abuse in therapy may sever ties with their family, causing dis- tress to all involved. Families have sometimes claimed that the therapist has encouraged the patient in their distressing behavior, or even implanted false memories; either through incompetence, or for ideological purposes. In one case of this kind (Appelbaum and Zoltek-Jick, 1996), the patient did retract her account of their abusive childhood experience, and both she, and her family successfully sued the therapist for negligence.

Confidentiality and consent to disclosure

Clearly, negligence and incompetence are potential risks for all clinicians, and these can (and should) be addressed by training, licensing or registration, and supervision processes. But other types of harm are also possible in therapy, which are not so common in other types of medicine: for example, threats to confidentiality and boundary violations. I will deal with boundary viola- tions in more detail below, but at this point it is relevant to consider the issue of breaches of confidentiality, or the boundary of therapeutic privacy, as a type of harm.

My own view is that the principle of confidentiality may be better under- stood as the *principle of informed consent to disclosure*. Therapists are under an ethical duty to obtain their patient's consent before they disclose details of their psychotherapeutic treatment to anyone; including those close to the patient. Although this is undoubtedly a principle that is respectful of the patient's autonomy, it can be problematic when the patient discloses material, which indicates that someone else is (or has been) at risk of harm from them. Most professional codes and guidelines address this issue, and there is relevant case law (see below). In general psychotherapeutic practice, this is probably a rare event; more commonly dilemmas arise when the therapist perceives that it might be helpful to the patient for others to know that a patient is in therapy, and what has been discussed. Of course, the therapist can seek consent from the patient to disclose, but if the patient refuses consent, then the therapist may still face a dilemma. A nonpsycho- therapeutic example occurs when an HIV-positive patient refuses to tell his or her partner (with whom they are still having a sexual relationship), and refuses to let the clinician inform the partner. In the UK, professionals are advised that it may be justified to breach confidentiality in the face of a competent refusal.

Clinicians may also come under pressure from others (family members or employers) who may contact them to discuss the patient, or to seek infor- mation about the therapy. Again, it may usually be possible for the therapist to seek consent to discuss some agreed upon material with others; ethical problems may arise when the third party asks the therapist not to tell the patient about the contact, usually because it will cause distress to the patient. _____ he therapist may have to balance the patient's claim _____ tiality against a possible harm to them.

____ of patient information for research

Getting consent to any form of disclosure can be intrusive into the process of therapy, and this is a particular issue in relation to research. The ethical dilemma here is about whether therapists can use patient material without consent for teaching and research purposes. Traditionally, this has not been an issue for psychotherapists who have assumed some ownership over their experience in the therapeutic space, and who have presumably also assumed that the breach of confidentiality is justified for the public good that arises from teaching and research. The good consequences justification seems plausible enough; clinical material is essential for teaching trainees, and for research. What is different from 20 years ago is the increased social emphasis on respect for individual patient autonomy, in the form of control and ownership over anything personal, which means that therapists may be unwise to assume that it is ethically unproblematic to use patient material for teaching and research without consent, even if it is disguised.

Although some journals do not require patient's consent to publication of their details, there are others that require that the patient has not only given consent, but has read the article in which their case is mentioned or described. Getting consent after therapy has ended is not necessarily the answer, as this might be just as intrusive or distressing for the patient (Winship, 2002). Then there is the question of content. Do patients have to agre░░░░░░░░░░░░░░░░░░ Can they disagree only with matters of fact, rather than ░░░░░░░░░░░░░░░░░░ extent is the therapist allowed to 'own' his or her own vi░░░░░░░░░░░░░░░░ discuss it without the patient's permission?

The issue is further complicated because the therapist's capacity to have a personal and intimate relationship with the patient is part of the therapeutic process (Klauber, 1986). The therapist makes their mind available to the patient to ass░░░░░░░░░░░░░░░░░░░░░░░░ their own feelings and thought░░░░░░░░░░░░░░░░░░░░░░░ way to do this; and also helps ░░░░░░░░░░░░░░░░░░░░░░░░░ssion. However, generally speakin░░░░░░░░░░░░░░░░░░░░░░ts and feelings *about* the patient *with* the patient (the extent to which she might do this is a matter of technique, reflection, and supervision). It is unlikely that the patient will find it helpful to discover what their therapist thinks about them from simply reading the process notes. My own practice is to make a brief note in the medical record that the session has taken place, and then keep some brief notes of the main themes of the session in a file in my office. The American Psychiatric Association recommends this practice to psychotherapists, and this would be consistent with general advice on good record keeping from the UK Royal College of Psychiatrists. Legal jurisdictions, both in the UK and in the US, do, however, make it theoretically possible for the patient to have access to those notes, unless this access would constitute harm to them or another person. The ethical issue here is that therapists cannot assume that they 'own' the notes of their meetings, and that only their views about the process notes need be consulted.

In CBT, it is common practice for the therapist to record the patient's experiences in therapy (thoughts, feelings, behaviors), in the same way as the patient does in 'homework' assignments. For both therapist and patient, sharing of these records and notes is often therapeutically helpful. What may be problematic is when the patient is recording information that may be misunderstood out of context (for example, in cases of sexual dysfunction, or violence). CBT therapists may also wish to record impressions of the patient and his/her progress that they do not wish the patient to see; and to which the patient may have legal access.

Boundaries in psychotherapy

Perhaps one of the few ethical precepts that all trainees learn at medical school is that the Hippocratic Oath forbids doctors from sexual relationships with their patients. However, there is rarely any accompanying discussion about why, or what this proscription represents. This part of the Oath, however, is perhaps the first recorded acknowledgment that the doctor who is working with a patient as a professional cannot also be that patient's lover; that there is a boundary between the two identities that should not be crossed. Such a boundary applies to all professional carers, and not just physicians.

Boundaries and identities

A boundary then is a construct that defines domains as separate and different. One thinks of the boundary round a cricket pitch, or the stage of the theatre, which must be set out and delineated for the play to happen. In medical ethics, the boundary is between personal and professional identities. The doctor (generally) undertakes not to bring his personal identity into the professional space. This is crucially important in medicine because, unlike other professional spaces, the patient is vulnerable as a result of their illness and disease, and may be less able to protect themselves. Professionals do have additional power that comes with knowledge, and like all power discrepancies, this can be abused. Furthermore, the success of any therapeutic relationship relies on trust; in his vulnerable state, the patient has to rely on the doctor to put the patient's interests first, and not exploit his vulnerability. If the patient cannot trust the doctor to do this, then he will not be able to use the therapeutic relationship to its full extent.

So the boundary between the personal and professional identity of doctors needs to be set and thought about as part of regular clinical practice for all doctors. Good doctors pay attention to the construction and maintenance of ░░░░░░░░░░░░ndaries throughout their working life. But psychiatrists and ░░░░░░░░░░░ have a particular duty to think about these issues because ░░░░░░░░░░░░░er of cogent reasons why boundary setting and maintenance ░░░░░░░░░░░ficant and important in psychiatric and psychotherapeutic relationships. First, psychiatric and psychotherapeutic patients are especially vulnerable insofar as they are mentally distressed. Second, the psychotherapeutic space has to be a particularly private one, to enable the patient to explore the most delicate of feelings, especially those of a potentially shameful nature. As many commentators have noticed, the increase in the numbers of people seeking therapy and counseling mirrors the fall in the number of people who attend a church; another place that used to be associated with private and personal disclosure, and self-examination.

Thirdly, for any psychological therapy to be effective, there has to be a trusting empathic relationship between the therapist and the patient, which promotes intimacy. At both conscious and unconscious levels, patients often reenact, with the therapist, relationships they have had before with other intimates (especially common in patients with personality disorders). It is the intimacy of the therapy that makes it useful, by allowing an examination of these reenactments. However, because human intimacy is powerful, and most psychotherapy patients seek therapy because of problems of intimacy with others, it must be managed safely. Boundary setting and maintenance help to establish a secure space to look at what goes wrong with intimacy, and help to think about different ways of managing interpersonal relating. The patient has to trust that therapists will not exploit that intimacy for their own ends. The therapist has to commit to not doing so; and still balance psychological intimacy with distance in the interests of the therapy (Casement, 1985; Karasu, 1992).

Finally, on the theme of intimacy, all psychotherapists have experience of situations where judicious self-disclosure is immensely helpful to the therapeutic process (Yalom, 1986, 2002). The professional skill then is to know when and how to do this, in a way that takes the therapeutic process forward, and is not exploitative or abusive to the patient. The principle of saying less rather than more is a good one; it is also helpful to develop a few stock phrases that gently re-reroute inquiries about the therapist's personal identity ('This is space for you, not me'; 'I wonder if it's easier to talk about me than you'). Inappropriate self-disclosure is discussed in more detail below, as a type of boundary crossing or violation, which it may be. But there is a real danger that rigidly refusing to ever say anything about oneself has a negative ░░░░░░░░░░░░░░░░░░░░░░░░░acy, and can also be a way for the ░░░░░░░░░░░░░░░░░░░░░░; and powerful role.

░░░░░░░░░░░░░░ings

Gutheil and Gabbard (1993) make a useful distinction between boundary crossings and violations (Box 40.2). For example, if the patient brings a gift to the therapist, this is a *crossing* of the boundary between the personal and the professional identity. The professional identity does not require, and is not entitled to, a gift. The giving of a gift is an indication of the patient's wish to relate more personally to the therapist. If the therapist accepts the gift, they are relating more personally. The balance between their professional and personal identity alters. This may or may not be a bad thing; it may be mutative moment for the patient, or it may simply be the therapist pursuing her own wishes or needs of the moment.

The other point about boundary crossings is that they may or may not be consciously intentionally initiated by either party. A chance meeting outside the therapy session, for example, is still a crossing of the boundary, which will need to be addressed technically in terms of its meaning for the patient. Although the therapist may not have initiated the boundary crossing, there is still an ethically sensitive moment when the therapist's personal

Box 40.2 Boundary crossings and violations

Crossings (may or may not be intended or initiated by either party)

- time keeping: lateness, earliness, alteration, or cancellation of sessions without notice
- self-disclosure (verbal and nonverbal)
- discussions of patient material with others, even with consent
- arguments or jokes with patients
- accidental/unexpected contact outside sessions (common in institutional settings)
- any physical contact

Violations (intended and initiated by the therapist)

- abrupt termination of therapy by therapist without warning
- excessive self-disclosure; especially of therapist's distress or anxiety
- prolonged or repeated angry outbursts with patient
- speaking or responding in ways, which humiliate or demean
- coercive behavior (verbal or nonverbal, including financial)
- financial exploitation
- planned contact outside therapeutic setting
- all physical contact that is prolonged or repeated
- any sexual or erotic contact between therapist and patient
- negligent therapy

Box 40.3 A typical boundary crossing moment: what should the good therapist say?

The patient brings a beautiful wooden bowl for the therapist, saying 'I made this for you at my evening class'. Options:

- 'I'm sorry, I don't accept gifts from patients'
- 'I'm sorry, I don't accept gifts from patients while they are in therapy with me'
- 'It is beautiful, but I don't accept gifts from patients'
- 'It is beautiful, and I appreciate that you wanted to give me something. But you know that I do not accept gifts in therapy, so I wonder why it is . . .'
- 'As a therapist, I've found that accepting gifts from people is also taking something away from them. Perhaps you can keep it for me till our work is over. But I wonder why you felt you wanted to give me something . . .'
- 'Thank you very much'
- 'Thank you very much, you know that I love carved wood'
- 'Thank you very much, it will join the other 57 that you have given me'
- 'Thank you very much . . . should we think about why you bring me these gifts?'

Box 40.4 Self-disclosure by the therapist: what should the good therapist say?

Q (from patient) 'What is your son's name?'

Response options

- Silence
- 'None of your business'
- 'I don't give that sort of information to patients'
- 'I'm sorry, I don't give that sort of information to patients'
- 'I'm sorry, I am not allowed to give that sort of information to patients'
- 'His name is Dan.'
- 'His name is Dan; why do you ask?'
- 'How did you know I had a son?'
- 'Why do you want to know?'
- 'I wonder why you want to know'
- 'I think you are asking me this because . . .'
- 'What do you think it is?'
- 'Do you have any thoughts about why the name is important to you?'
- 'I don't think it would be helpful for me to answer that question'
- 'I will give you an answer; but before I do, I am curious to know why you want to know, and what it means to you'.

and professional identity meet. Self-disclosure is another common area where therapists may say more than they consciously intend to the patient. The fact that it is done unconsciously does not make it any less ethically sensitive.

The first step, in terms of ethical analysis and practice, is to notice that the boundary crossing is happening at all. There may be many ways of responding, and the decision-making process must be both ethical and psychodynamic (Box 40.3). The therapist has to formulate an understanding of what this boundary crossing is about for the patient, in order to match their response. If the boundary crossing is aggressive in nature, then this may indicate that the patient is anxious, and needs a reassuring response. An apparently caring or affectionate type of crossing may indicate that the patient needs reassurance that the therapist can keep the boundaries firmly, and is tough enough to keep to task; this is obviously also the case for challenges to therapeutic authority. As with all ethical dilemmas, the therapist will be helped if they discuss the issue with supervisors and colleagues; they also need to review their technical and communication skills. But the key ethical issue is to notice that the boundary is under pressure and needs attention.

Perhaps the most common example of boundary crossing in therapy is inappropriate self-disclosure by the therapist. Again, the patient often initiates this. I give an example in Box 40.4, together with some ways of responding. Like the ethical dilemma about the gift (and many other ethical dilemmas in medical practice), there has to be a resolution; it must be a good quality one, and it will involve good communication skills. What *is* unprofessional is not to explore whether there is a special meaning of the boundary crossing at this point both for the patient, and the therapist. It cannot be assumed that these types of transaction have no meaning or significance. For those therapists working with very disturbed patients, and those who have previously been exploited in intimate relationships,

supervision is highly advisable, because boundary crossings and violations are so common (Holmes and Lindley, 1989). I would argue that it is ethically unjustifiable for a therapist *not* to obtain supervision for this kind of work, although not all would agree.

Boundary crossings may or may not be harmful. Boundary *violations* are those crossings of the boundary that cause harm to the patient, usually because they involve an exploitation of the power difference and the trust between the therapist and the patient. Physical boundary violations, especially those of a sexual nature, change the relationship between the therapist and patient so profoundly that the therapy is lost. The therapist's mind is no longer available to the patient in the professional way it once was; and this means that the therapy has been harmed.

There are many other types of harm done by sexual boundary violations, particularly. First, the patients most likely to be exploited by their therapists in this way are those who have already been victims of sexual exploitation by previous caregivers; this is often the reason that they sought therapy in the first place (Kluft, 1993). The abuse by the therapist is a reenactment of their prior experience, and they are usually placed in exactly the same position as they were before: they have to keep the relationship secret, in order to protect both the abuser and other family members, and they are made to feel responsible for their therapist's comfort, pleasure, and wrong-doing. Research on the effects of sexual abuse by therapists shows that patients are likely to relapse and deteriorate, especially when the relationship ends (Jehu, 1994).

se their patients have found them udes people who are young, old, female (Gabbard, 1989; Schoener, tedly, as a means of getting a sexual partner; for some it will represent a one-off response to external stress. It is probably safest for therapists to assume that everyone (including themselves) is capable of boundary violations; that no one is immune to the risk. As suggested above, this is why supervision is necessary at times for all therapists, even the most experienced, especially for work with difficult and complex patients.

Boundary violations are not only harmful; they also represent a wrong done to the patient. Boundary violations may therefore have legal repercussions. Therapists may be sued for negligence or malpractice; rarely, they may be subject to criminal charges of assault (Strasburger *et al.*, 1991). In some states in the USA, it is a criminal offense to have a sexual relationship with a patient, even after the therapy is ended. Professional sanctions are also likely: therapists who have sexual relationships with their patients usually have their professional registration or license revoked, in recognition of the fact that they gave up their professional identity when they began a personal relationship with the patient.

What goes wrong with boundaries

There are many reasons why therapists cross or violate the boundary between the personal and the professional domain. As we have seen, boundary crossings are commonplace in any setting where the patient and the therapist are involved in a long-term therapeutic relationship, presumably because it is hard for therapists to exclude their personal identity on an indefinite basis. Thus we should not be surprised to find that boundary crossings are common in long-term residential care. Boundary crossings and violations are also more common in relationships of intimacy combined with a power differential; particularly where that power should be used for therapeutic purposes. There is a similarity between abuse by therapists and abuse by parents (Gabbard, 1989): both are in roles of power involving care, trust, and intimacy over time.

Who-ness and what-ness

Another particular difficulty for boundary setting and maintenance in psychotherapy is that the therapist's personal identity is part of her professional identity; the boundary is opaque and semipermeable, rather than hard and clear. Sarkar (2004) makes a nice distinction between the 'who-ness' of a person and the 'what-ness' of a person, in terms of identity. Thus, for surgeons, it may be possible for *what* you are (a good surgeon) to be different from *who* you are (e.g., a bad man). A group of surgeons will have similar professional identities and practices, regardless of how different their

personal identities are; for example, the fact that they cheat at cards or are dishonest in other ways will not affect how they carry out a splenectomy. To some extent, this is also true for CBT therapists; their personal identity is less interwoven with their professional identity.

However, for the psychodynamic psychotherapist, her who-ness is intimately connected with her what-ness. Her personal identity is part of the professional identity; indeed, the long and expensive psychotherapy trainings are designed to help the trainee explore how their personal identity influences their professional identity. This aspect of training is essential precisely because the boundary between identities in psychotherapy is not always hard and clear. Therefore the therapist must pay constant attention to when, how, and why the boundary is being pushed or crossed; remembering that it is not just the therapist who is doing the pushing or crossing (Joannidis, 2002). In terms of reenactments, the patient also pushes and crosses the border, inviting the therapist to relate more as a personal figure than a professional. Lastly, if one considers that much of the pushing and crossing of boundaries in psychotherapy is done unconsciously as well as consciously, it is clear that boundary setting and maintenance occupies much of the therapist's thinking time.

Absolute prohibitions: 'good fences make good neighbors'

Within general psychotherapeutic practice, there may be different ways of understanding and responding to boundary crossings as ethical dilemmas.

Indeed, they would hardly be dilemmas if the answer were so very clear and obvious. But there are some absolutes in relation to boundary setting and maintenance. Sexual relationships with patients do both harm and wrong to the patient and are therefore unethical. Financial exploitation is not only unethical, it is likely to be illegal. In a recent American case, a therapist was charged with insider dealing when he used information obtained in therapy sessions to make money on the stock market. Any physical touching of a patient needs to be thought about carefully, before and after it happens: although it may be therapeutically justified, it is a significant boundary crossing and should be treated as such. I reiterate that supervision is an ethical necessity; while it cannot prevent boundary violations taking place altogether, it can offer containment for the therapist's feelings as they are stirred up in the psychotherapeutic process.

The other absolute prohibition in terms of boundaries is the prohibition on gossip; specifically, talking about patients and their stories without their consent, and for no therapeutic purpose. The use of the term 'gossip' in this context may seem trivial, but it has been described as a subtle form of social aggression, and it can do enormous harm because information is not contained. Gossip is the antithesis of therapeutic discussions of patients; it is the use of individual's private stories for the gossiper's enjoyment, and the entertainment of others. The pleasure and excitement of having and disclosing secrets about others is very powerful, and very tempting; as can be seen daily in the tabloid press and popular magazines. The principle of confidentiality, as well as being respectful of autonomy and promoting trust, is valuable because it is the patient's strongest defense against gossip.

There are, however, circumstances where the therapist will want to breach confidentiality for purposes that are not to do with their own pleasure or entertainment, or even for the enlightening of others. I want now to turn to violations of the boundary of privacy in the public interest.

Boundaries and confidentiality

There is another test of the boundary between the therapist's different identities, which arises when the patient discloses material that is relevant to the external social and political world in which both parties operate. In these dilemmas, however, it is the therapist's identity as a citizen that is brought into the therapeutic space, and clashes with the professional identity as a therapist. If the patient discloses that they are going to cause harm to another person, the therapist's professional duty not to disclose patient information without consent may clash with their social duty as citizens to contribute to public safety; or at least do nothing to reduce public safety. In ethical terms, the therapist's duty to preserve confidentiality and respect the patient's privacy is challenged by (1) a therapist's duty to the public good and the social realm, and (2) the possible harms that may ensue if nothing is done.

Disclosure when other people are at risk

Traditionally, psychotherapists have privileged their therapeutic duties over their duties as citizens. However, there have been cultural changes over the last 30 years that have changed this position. These changes are reflected in legal cases and rulings that say therapists must honor their duties to society.

The most cited case in the area of psychotherapist disclosure is that of *Tarasoff*. Appelbaum (1984) provides a detailed account and there is a useful review by Herbert and Young (2002). An ethical dilemma arose for a therapist when a patient disclosed in therapy sessions that he was thinking of killing a young woman (Ms Tarasoff). The therapist informed the local university police who interviewed the patient and let him go. The patient never returned to therapy, and several months later, he killed Ms Tarasoff. Her family successfully sued the therapist and his employers, on the grounds that the therapist had a duty to both warn and protect Ms Tarasoff, and he had failed to do either. The court's legal response to the therapist's dilemma was to find that the duty to public safety outweighed the duty to preserve the patient's confidentiality, and that the therapist should disclose information that indicates risk to others, even in the face of patient refusal.

Twenty-seven US states have imposed a duty on psychotherapists to breach confidentiality, when a patient makes an explicit threat to physical harm to an identifiable person; either by warning the intended victim or involving the police. Nine states leave it up to the therapist to decide; 13 have no position at all. The American Psychiatric Association Code of ethics makes it clear that it is sometimes necessary for psychiatrists to breach confidentiality to protect others from 'imminent danger'. Therapists in the USA are also *mandated* to disclose information that indicates risk of abuse to a child.

Therapists in the UK are not so mandated, and there have not (yet) been any comparable cases with that of *Tarasoff*. There have been relevant cases about confidentiality in therapeutic relationships. In *W.v.Egdell*, the court found that a psychiatrist would be justified in breaching patient confidentiality in the public interest, and that he had a duty to do so. In *Palmer. v. Te...* the court found that a psychiatrist would have a duty of care to an identifiable victim, and that therefore the psychiatrist would be justified in breaching confidentiality. The UK General Medical Council (GMC, 2000), which provides professional ethical guidelines for psychiatrists, also supports the argument that confidentiality may be breached in order to prevent harm to others.

None of the English cases *require* the therapist to breach confidentiality in the public interest; nor is there any problem with disclosure of material where the patient has consented. If a therapist is concerned about risk of harm to others, there is no reason why she cannot discuss the risk with the patient, and disclose relevant information with the patient's consent. The ethical dilemma arises when the patient refuses to consent, or the therapist does not wish to ask the patient for their consent, but wishes still to disclose information to third parties.

Finally, the principle of absolute confidentiality to an individual patient is hard to maintain for therapists who work with groups and families. Clearly, the group psychotherapist has multiple duties to the group members, and the ordinary prohibitions on gossip apply. But it may be difficult to balance the conflicting interests of the different members of a group; what should happen if a group member tells the therapist something, but begs the therapist not to tell the rest of the group (Yalom, 1986)? It is usual practice in group therapy to explain to patients that all information is shared with the group from the start, and that the therapist does not keep secrets. Assuming that this is the case, the group therapist will not generally wish to agree to keeping the secret (on good clinical grounds), and will want to challenge the request in various ways. Legally, however, the patients have

control over their own information. Here the dilemma is reversed; it is unethical to practice therapy poorly, and keep the secret, but it is also unethical (and possibly illegal) to fail to respect the patient's wishes. Similar issues arise in family therapy, especially if the therapist discovers in the course of therapy that a child or children have been harmed, and remain at risk of harm. The duty to protect the especially vulnerable may outweigh the therapist's duty to maintain the boundary of confidentiality.

Duties of the therapist

In the current cultural climate, there is a good ethical and legal case for the therapist breaching confidentiality in cases where she perceives that there is a high risk of imminent harm to identifiable others, and where the disclosure may reduce the risk of harm. Some authorities (*W.v.Egdell*) will argue that she has a duty to do so. The social benefit in preventing harm (probably) outweighs the harm and wrong done to the patient.

However, it is important to recognize the powerful counterarguments to this position too; the strongest being that the therapy will be damaged, the patient will be harmed and future patients will be deterred from seeking therapy if therapists disclose patient information to others. The consequences of breaching confidentiality could be worse than not doing so, in the long term. There is also an argument (based on the European Convention of Human Rights) that everyone has a right to a private life, even those with mental illnesses or dangerous thoughts.

On a more psychodynamic note, Gutheil (2001) argues that it is the healthy part of a patient's mind that 'employs' or contracts with the patient, and breaches of confidentiality may still be consistent with respect for that aspect of the therapeutic alliance with the patient. It is also respectful to discuss breaches of confidentiality with the patient, and explain to them what the consequences will be. They do not have to like the consequences, but this does not mean that they cannot be supported. If the patient feels so betrayed that they can no longer continue in therapy, it is still possible for this hurt and betrayal to be acknowledged, and for the therapist to assist the patient in continuing their therapy.

Social and political frameworks

Social and cultural issues in psychotherapy

Just like any other form of medical treatment, psychotherapy is not practiced in a social and legal vacuum. One of the enduring myths of medicine is that practitioners use their skills and knowledge in a value-free way, for no other purpose but the patient's good. However, there is good reason to think that medical diagnosis and treatment are value-laden processes from start to finish, and mental health is no exception (Fulford, 1989). The values of the social groups and cultures to which the therapist and patient belong will infuse the dialogue that takes place in therapy. Tensions may particularly emerge in relation to ethnicity and racial identity, gender of either therapist or patient and religious or political beliefs.

For example, take the concept of personal autonomy. Many writers about the values of therapy argue that development of a sense of self-worth and integrity is a crucial goal for psychotherapy (Holmes and Lindley, 1989; Hinshelwood, 1997). Patients are encouraged to take themselves seriously, and to think of themselves as autonomous agents who can choose for themselves, and should (generally speaking) choose courses of action that will help them to flourish as individuals.

Such a vision is consistent with the values of the Enlightenment, which have dominated European thinking since the seventeenth century (Baumeister, 1987). However, such an individualistic, or indexical, view of the self is not found in every cultural group. Different cultures understand the self as referential, rather than indexical (Landrine, 1992); that is, that the experience of the self, rather than being a single orientation of all one's social interactions, is constructed with reference to relationships with others, and social roles. A common example of this is found in British-born Asian men and women, who may seek therapy when their Western experience and expectations of indexical selfhood can clash badly with their Asian parents' experience and expectations of referential selfhood (depicted most poignantly in the film, *East is East*). It may not be helpful for the therapist to take a view on which position is right for the patient; equally, it may be hard to avoid doing so.

To complicate matters further, we do not always understand the relationship between individual and cultural identities and belief systems; cultural stereotypes may blind the therapist into assumptions about the individual's inner world (Akhtar, 1995; Dalal, 1999). How easy is it to assume, for example, that a patient who i█████████████████████████████ho-analytic framework that su█████████████████████████nly a scientific theory of psych██████████████████████████ of culture-specific beliefs, whic█████████████████████████the values of the therapist and the patient clash, must this always be understood as acting out of transference and countertransference, or can there be a real political and ethical diversity also in the therapeutic encounter? The answer to the latter question is that both processes are operating, and the therapist's job is to keep both perspectives in mind.

Legal frameworks for therapy

The legal framework in which both patient and therapist function is also relevant here. Psychotherapeutic relationships are not outside the law, either civil or criminal. Existing statutes and case law that apply to medical treatments will also apply to therapy. Thus, psychotherapists acquire a legal duty of care when they work with a patient, and that duty requires them to practice in accordance with a reasonable body of medical (psychotherapeutic) opinion. This means that they must exercise reasonable professional skills, make logical treatment decisions, conform to professional ethical guidance where it exists, gain informed consent to treatment, and tell the truth when asked. They also have to abide by the laws of the land; so as described above, psychotherapists in the USA are mandated to report suspected child abuse, even when the information comes from their patient, who may be the abuser. In such circumstances, the therapist may feel a conflict between respect for the law, and the avoidance of harm to children, and concerns that disclosure that lead to harm to the patient.

Are there circumstances where the therapist should break the law out of respect for another ethical principle? One answer might be that the therapist is free to break the law at any time in pursuit of their personal values, but law breaking as a professional duty seems incoherent, when most professions regard respect for the law as a major ethical principle guiding conduct. Having said that, if the therapist is faced with patently unjust laws, she might argue that the pursuit of justice requires her to break the law; this presumably was the case for psychiatrists in Nazi Germany who did not comply with the euthanasia laws for psychiatric patients.

Legal frameworks are an issue for therapists who work with those who have committed crimes, or who may have therapy mandated in some way. For example, forensic psychotherapy cannot claim that it is operating in a nonjudgmental value-free way. The psychotherapist is not free to be non-judgmental about the patient's actions, or to allow the patient to set his or her own goals in therapy (Adshead, 2000, 2002). In institutions set apart for offender patients, therapy that does not look at the offending behavior, or does not seek to help the patient to act differently in the future, is probably not therapy that anyone (including the patient) would think is much use. It may not be enough for the patient to simply be more reflective; as one of my patients said to me, 'I'm still the same person I was when I came here, I'm just more aware of myself'.

Social settings: private and public practice

Forensic psychotherapy is only one example of how the social setting may influence on the psychotherapeutic work. Murray Cox (1976) suggests that all relationships are structured by time, depth, and mutuality, and the social setting affects all three dimensions. The type of hospital one works in, as much as training and personal style, may influence how the clinician allocates time, the depth of the relationship formed with the patient and the

degree of mutuality that is possible. Private practice operates as another type of framework, especially in terms of mutuality and the nature of the contract between therapist and patient. In both the institution and private practice, there is a contract between the therapist and the patient, but the contracts are different.

Private practice is the norm for most psychotherapists in the USA and Europe. However, in other countries, medical psychotherapists may work in a centralized public health system, free at the point of service. In such a system, resources have be managed and allocated; there is not enough for all to have as much as they wish. Choices have to be made about how resources are allocated; and for psychotherapists, this will involve not just the resources allocated to psychotherapy, but how resources are allocated to mental health services in general. Mental health services are generally poorly resourced, and dynamic psychotherapy is often seen as low priority, partly because of a perceived lack of an evidence base.

There is not room here to discuss this debate in detail, which is well described in a published debate by Holmes and Tarrier (Holmes, 2002; Tarrier, 2002). In essence, the ethical debate runs on utilitarian lines: if there are not enough resources to go around, how should we share them out? One way to allocate scarce resources is to give more money for treatments that are shown to be effective, using an agreed form of process for assessing that effectiveness. But what does 'effectiveness' mean in psychotherapy? Is the assessment process able to measure subtle forms of benefit? Where should the views of mental health service users fit in? Perhaps the most important thing to notice is that there is a debate to be had, and its fundamental nature is both political and ethical.

Existing codes and guidelines

Where can a therapist seek advice when facing an ethical dilemma? Nearly all the professional bodies that accredit therapists in both the US and the UK have codes of ethics, or codes of conduct, which provide guidance (examples are given in Box 40.5). For medical psychotherapists, the ethical duties of psychotherapists are the same as other doctors, and are detailed in *Good medical practice* (GMC, 1995). Ethical guidance for psychiatrists is also set out in the World Psychiatric Association Declaration of Madrid (WPA, 1996). Recently, the WPA has also set out ethical guidance in relation to sexual boundary violations (WPA, 2002).

Psychiatric psychotherapists in the UK are also bound by policy documents produced by the Royal College of Psychiatrists; specifically, *Good psychiatric practice* (Royal College of Psychiatrists, 2000a), *Good psychiatric practice: confidentiality* (2000b), and a recent document on working with vulnerable patients (Royal College of Psychiatrists, 2001). Psychiatric psychotherapists in the USA, Canada, Australia, New Zealand, and Russia are guided by the codes of ethics for psychiatrists drawn up by their national professional bodies (Sarkar and Adshead, 2003).

Nonmedical psychotherapists are similarly bound by the codes of conduct and ethical principles held by their training organizations that accredit them. Most psychotherapy training organizations in the UK are members of the UK Council for Psychotherapy, which has its own code of ethics. These training organizations not only have codes of ethics, but also have ethics committees that oversee complaints about therapists' practice, and can take disciplinary action. There are similar organizations in the USA for nonmedical psychotherapists (nurses, social workers, and psychologists); therapists will commonly belong to professional associations, which provide ethical advice to them and to the organizations that license and discipline therapists.

There are many types of personal interaction that are called 'therapy', and there are many people called 'therapists'. The Department of Health guidelines for psychotherapy in England (1996) state that it is 'unethical to offer therapy that is not safe, available, evidence based and efficacious'. There can be problems for patients seeking therapy because it is sometimes difficult to get good advice about the types of therapy on offer, and their indications. It is also still possible for persons to practice as a therapist without

Box 40.5 Examples of codes of practice and codes of ethics for psychotherapists

◆ American Group Psychotherapy Association Guidelines for ethics (2002): http://www.groupsinc.org/group/ethicalguide.html

◆ American Psychiatric Association (2001). *The principles of medical ethics with annotations especially applicable to psychiatry.* Washington, DC: American Psychiatric Press.

◆ American Psychological Association. Ethical Principles of psychologists and Code of Conduct (2002): http://www.apa.org/ethics

◆ British Association of Counsellors and Psychotherapists. Ethical Frameworks for Good Practice in counseling and psychotherapy: http://www.bac.com

◆ British Confederation of Psychotherapy Code of Ethics: http//www.bcp.org

◆ European Association for psychotherapy: Ethical Guidelines (1995): http://www.psychother.com/eap/vode-et.htm

◆ New Zealand Association of Psychotherapists Code of Ethics. http://www.nzap.org.nz

◆ Royal Australian and New Zealand College of Psychiatrists Code of Ethics (1992).

◆ Royal Australian and New Zealand College of Psychiatrists. (1990) Sexual relationships with patients. Ethical Guideline no. 8. RANZCP.

◆ United Kingdom Council for Psychotherapy Ethics guidelines for member organisations; http://www.psychotherapy.org.uk

◆ POPAN (Prevention of Professional Abuse Network). http://www.popan.org.uk

being officially accredited, registered, licensed, or affiliated to a professional body, so that if things go wrong, neither the therapist nor the patient will have anywhere to turn for advice. Support for patients who have been subject to abuse or malpractice by their therapists in the UK is available from POPAN (Prevention of Professional Abuse Network; contact given below); the equivalent organization in the USA is Advocate Web, P. O. Box 202961, Austin, TX 78720.

Conclusions: values in psychotherapy

Changing people's minds is a political act. Psychological change in a person may have moral and political implications for him, which cannot be foreseen. The therapist then has to be thoughtful about maintaining the integrity of the psychotherapeutic process in itself, so that the therapy itself is an ethical process. This raises more interesting questions about the role of virtue in psychotherapy; whether it is possible to be a good therapist and a bad person.

It may be helpful to think about the different classical roots of language here. The Latin word *mores* originally means 'customs' or 'practices', and the Greek word *ethos* means character. Both morality and ethics apply to psychotherapy; we can think of the 'morality' of any therapeutic process, in terms of the goodness of its goals and outcomes, and also the 'ethics' of psychotherapy, in terms of how the therapist maintains and serves the therapeutic process. Alternatively, one may think of the 'morality' of any profession as being expressed in its customs and practices (codes, contracts, etc.) and the 'ethics' of a profession as being a reflection of the values and attitudes that underpin identity (Glover, 2003).

However defined, ethical reasoning will always be integral to psychotherapeutic process. Both ethical reasoning and psychotherapy involve the construction of stories that illuminate something important about our experience of ourselves in relationship to others. If life is a moral adventure (Stone, 1984), then engagement in psychotherapy involves a particular type of adventure or journey with another person (Peck, 1983); a journey that is not necessarily comfortable. It is a process by which both patient and therapist can learn something about their values, beliefs, and perceptions, and develop their capacity for ethical reflection. The term 'reflection' is a reminder that the psychotherapist, like the dramatist, holds a 'mirror up to nature', so that the patient can see 'not his face, but some truth about his face' (Day Lewis, 1947). Courage, truthfulness, and personal honesty are perhaps the most important virtues for the psychotherapist to cultivate in order to practice ethically.

Acknowledgments

I am grateful to following people, who provided comments and advice in the writing of this chapter: the editors, Gary Winship, Adam Jukes and Peter Aylward. I am especially grateful to Sameer Sarkar, MD, who gave me time for reflection, robust feedback and allowed me to use his conception of who-ness and what-ness. The views expressed here are mine alone and do not reflect the views of the Royal College of Psychiatrists Ethics Committee, of which I am the current chair.

References

Adshead, G. (2000). Care or custody: ethical dilemmas in medical ethics. *Journal of Medical Ethics,* **26**, 1–2.

Adshead, G. (2002). A kind of necessity: a forensic psychiatric approach to evil. Spirituality Special Interest Group website: http://www.rcpsych.ac.uk

Akhtar, S. (1995). A third individuation: immigration, identity and the psychoanalytic process. *Journal of the American Psychoanalytic Association,* **13**, 1051–84.

Appelbaum, P. (1994). *Almost a revolution: mental health law and the limits of change.* Oxford: Oxford University Press.

Appelbaum, P. and Zoltek-Jick, R. (1996). Psychotherapists' duties to third parties: Ramona and beyond. *American Journal of Psychiatry,* **153**, 457–65.

Baumeister, R. (1987). How the self became a problem: a psychological review of historical research, **52**, 163–76.

Casement, P. (1985). *On learning from the patient.* London: Routledge.

Cox, M. (1976). *Structuring the therapeutic process: compromise with chaos.* London: Jessica Kingsley Publishers.

Dalal, F. (1999). *Taking the group seriously.* London: Jessica Kingsley Publishers.

Day Lewis, C. (1947). *The poetic image.* London: Jonathan Cape.

Department of Health (1996). *Psychological therapies in England.* London: HMSO.

Fulford, K. W. (1989). *Moral theory and medical practice.* Cambridge: Cambridge University Press.

Gabbard, G. (1989). *Sexual exploitation of professional relations.* Washington, DC: American Psychiatric Press.

General Medical Council (1995). *Good medical practice.* London: GMC.

Glover, J. (2003). *Towards humanism in psychiatry: Lecture one. Identity.* Tanner Lectures. Princeton, NJ: Princeton University.

Gutheil, T. (2001). Moral justification for Tarasoff-type warnings and breach of confidentiality: a clinician's perspective. *Behavioural Science and the Law,* **19**, 345–53.

Gutheil, T. and Gabbard, G. (1993). The concept of boundaries in clinical practice: theoretical and risk management dimensions. *American Journal of Psychiatry,* **150**, 188–96.

Herbert, P. B. and Young, K. A. (2002). Tarasoff at twenty five. *Journal of the American Academy of Law and Psychiatry,* **30**, 275–81.

Holmes, J. (2002). All you need is cognitive behaviour therapy? *British Medical Journal,* **324**, 288–94.

Holmes, J. and Lindley, R. (1989). *The values of psychotherapy.* Oxford: Oxford University Press.

Hinshelwood, R. (1997). *Therapy or coercion? Does psychoanalysis differ from brainwashing?* London: Karnac Books.

Jehu, D. (1994). *Patients as victims: sexual abuse in psychotherapy and counselling.* Chichester: John Wiley.

Joannidis, C. (2002). The other patient. *Psychoanalytic Psychotherapy*, **16**, 227–45.

Karasu, T. B. (1992). *Wisdom in the practice of psychotherapy.* New York: Basic Books.

Klauber, J. (1986). *Difficulties in the analytic encounter.* London: Free Association Books.

Kluft, R. (1993). Basic principles in conducting psychotherapy of multiple personality disorder. In: R. Kluft and C. G. Fine, ed. *Clinical perspectives on multiple personality disorder*, p. 39. Washington DC: American Psychiatric Press.

Lakin, M. (1988). *Ethical issues in the psychotherapies.* Oxford: Oxford University Press.

Lambert, M. J. and Bergin, A. E. (1994). The effectiveness of psychotherapy. In: A. E. Bergin and S. L. Garfield, ed. *Handbook of psychotherapy and behavioural change*, 4th edn, pp. 143–89. New York: Wiley.

Landrine, H. (1992). Clinical implications of cultural differences: the referential and indexical self. *Clinical Psychology Review*, **12**, 401–15.

Peck, S. M. (1983). *The road less travelled.* London: Arrow Books.

Royal College of Psychiatrists (2000a). *Good psychiatric practice.* CR83. London: Royal College of Psychiatrists.

Royal College of Psychiatrists (2000b). *Good psychiatric practice: confidentiality.* CR85. London: Royal College of Psychiatrists.

Royal College of Psychiatrists (2001). *Working with vulnerable patients.* CR101. London: Royal College of Psychiatrists.

Sarkar, S. (2004). Boundary violation and sexual exploitation in Psychiatry and Psychotherapy: a review. *Advances in Psyhiatric Treatment*, **10**, 312–20.

Sarkar, S. and Adshead, G. (2003). Protecting altruism: a call for a code of ethics in British Psychiatry. *British Journal of Psychiatry*, **183**, 95–7.

Schoener, G. (1995). Assessment of professionals who have engaged in boundary violations. *Psychiatric Annals*, **25**, 95–9.

Stone, A. (1984). *Law, psychiatry and morality.* Washington, DC: American Psychiatric Press.

Strasburger, L., Jorgenson, L., and Randles, R. (1991). Criminalisation of therapist-patient sex. *American Journal of Psychiatry*, **148**, 859–63.

Tarrier, N. (2002). Commentary: yes, cognitive behaviour therapy may well be all you need. *British Medical Journal*, **324**, 288–94.

Tjelveit, A. (1999). *Ethics and values in psychotherapy.* London: Routledge.

WPA (1996). *Madrid Declaration on ethical standards for psychiatric practice.* Yokohama: WPA.

WPA (2002). *Additional specific guidelines on psychotherapy.* Yokohama: WPA.

Winship, G. (2002). The ethics of reflective research in the psychodynamic laboratory: closed or open, regulated or free. Unpublished lecture, University of Reading.

Yalom, I. (1986). *Love's executioner and other stories from psychotherapy.* London: Penguin.

Yalom, I. (2002). *The gift of therapy: reflections on being a therapist.* London: Piatkus.

Legal cases

Bolam v. Friern Management Committee [1957] 1 WLR 582

Bolitho v. City and Hackney Health Authority [1997] IV All ER 771

W.v Egdell [1990] A All ER

Jaffe v. Redmond, 518 U.S.1. 1996

Palmer v Tees H.A (1999) Times Law Reports. July 6. Court of Appeal.

Sidaway v Bethlem Royal Hospital Governors [1985] 1 All ER 643

Tarasoff v Regents of the University of California 551 P.2d 334 (Cal 1976)

Internet addresses

www.popan.org.uk

www.advocateweb.org

41 Clinical–legal issues in psychotherapy

Robert I. Simon

Introduction

There are over 450 schools of psychotherapy currently in existence (Simon, 2001, p. 90). New schools continue to emerge. Amidst this diversity, basic clinical–legal principles generally apply to most, if not all, forms of psychotherapy. Psychotherapists need to have a working knowledge and comfort managing clinical–legal issues arising in psychotherapy to avoid maladaptive defensive practices that may interfere with treatment. Moreover, legal issues can often be turned to the benefit of the patient's therapy.

It is said that psychotherapy is an 'impossible task', sometimes complicated by litigation (Simon, 1991). In recent years, negligence claims against psychotherapist have substantially increased. Table 41.1 lists typical malpractice claims filed against psychotherapist.

Confidentiality

Patients have the right and psychotherapists the duty to have spoken or written communications during the course of treatment kept confidential. In the US, there is no legal obligation requiring therapists to provide information, even to law enforcement officials, absent statutory disclosure requirements, or judicial compulsion (Simon, 2001, p. 90).

The therapist's duty to safeguard confidentiality arises from four sources:

1. The ethical codes of the mental health professions.

2. States recognize the right of confidentiality through provisions in professional licensure regulations or in confidentiality and privilege statues.

3. The common law has long recognized an attorney-client privilege. Developing case law has carved out similar protection for psychotherapists, although not as stringent.

4. The right of confidentiality derives from various constitutional guarantees. An explicit constitutional right of privacy does not exist.

In Jaffe v. Redmond (1996), the US Supreme Court ruled that communication between the psychotherapist and patient are confidential. The psychotherapist is not required to disclose them in federal trials. The decision does not, however, apply to state courts where most psychotherapist–patient confidentiality matters take place.

The psychotherapist's duty to maintain confidentiality is not absolute. Circumstances arise where it is both ethical and legal to break confidentiality. In the US, for example, 'The Principles of Medical Ethics with Annotations' especially applicable to Psychiatry (American Psychiatric Association, 2001) states: Psychiatrists at times may find it necessary, in order to protect the patient or the community from imminent danger, to reveal confidential information disclosed by the patient (Section 4, Annotation 8). Patients wave confidentiality in a variety of situations; for example, employment and disability examinations, insurance applications and licenses of various kinds. A limited waiver of confidentiality exists when a patient participates in group therapy. In managed care settings, the therapist should inform the patient about any limitation on maintaining confidentiality. In the US, new federal regulations and existing state statutes mandate disclosure by the therapist in a number of situations (see Table 41.2).

In a number of US jurisdictions, therapists have a legal duty to warn and protect third parties endangered by their patients. The therapist is frequently caught in the conflict between warning and risking a breach of confidentiality suit or keeping silent and risking a suit for failure to warn and protect endangered third parties (Herbert and Young, 2002). As no standard of care exists for the prediction of violence, careful assessment of the risk of violence should inform the therapist's decision whether to breach confidentiality and warn (Simon, 2001, pp. 179–80). Warning by itself, however, is usually insufficient. The duty to protect allows for clinical interventions (e.g., increase frequency of outpatient visits, adjust or add medications, hospitalization) that may obviate the need to breach patient confidentiality.

In the UK, by contrast, there is no *binding* requirement on clinicians to disclose dangerousness. The decision to disclose always is based on the judgment that the responsibility to protect the public outweighs the duty to the patient to protect confidentiality.

Case example: A patient suffering from a personality disorder, with a history of pedophilic offences, and currently living with a divorced woman with two young daughters, disclosed during a psychotherapy session that he experienced the dilemma of standing on the landing and being unsure which bedroom to enter—the mother's or the girls.' The therapist chose not disclose the situation to the social

---

Table 41.1 Typical malpractice claims against psychotherapists

Failure to hospitalize suicidal patient
Boundary violations (sexual and nonsexual)
Mismanagement of transference and counter transference
Therapist-induced memories of sexual abuse
Abandonment
Failure to warn and protect endangered third parties
Failure to collaborate ('split-treatment')
Breach of confidentiality

Table 41.2 Statutory disclosure requirements: some examples

Knowledge or evidence of child abuse

Certification for involuntary hospitalization
Duty to warn and protect endangered third parties (some states)
Commission of a treasonous act (past or present)
Intention to commit a crime
HIV infection*

*Some states require reporting the patient's name. Adapted from Simon (2001, p. 42).

services department immediately, but tried instead to use interpretation to remedy the situation. He suggested that the patient was asking the therapist to help curb his impulses. The therapist linked this with the absence of the patient's father who had been killed in actions during the war, and whose uniform he sometimes donned in order to give himself a sense of power and authority. The therapist suggested that the patient was asking him to help find the authority (the 'uniform') within himself to do the 'right' thing. To the therapist's relief, the patient reported at the next session that he had moved out of the house and did not, in fact, reoffend for a further 13 years.

Clearly, the therapist was taking a great risk in delaying disclosure. The justification for this delay was that by doing so he was facilitating a developmental step which might otherwise have been swept aside by instigating the legal process. This example dates from the 1980s. In today's zero tolerance climate, the therapist might have handled the situation differently. Nevertheless, in the UK, the clinician continues to be accorded the responsibility to make a considered decision whether or not to infringe the right to confidentiality. Statute law (e.g., notification of diseases) determines when the clinician *must* infringe that right; case law when he *may* do so. Most psychotherapy falls under the latter. Each case must be considered on its merits, although the courts would expect that the clinician would discuss any difficult or marginal decision with a colleague, and record accurately the reasons for any course of action (or inaction).

Valid, informed authorization for the release of information provides legal protection for the therapist. State laws and mental health confidentiality statues specify the requirements for valid authorization. Consent for the authorization of release of information should be written, not just verbal. Blanket consent forms should be avoided. Instead, consent should be given for the nature of information released, whether a one time or ongoing release and the specific individual or entity that is authorized to receive this information.

An unauthorized or unwarranted breach of confidentiality can cause a patient great harm. In such situations, the therapist may be held liable for the breach under four legal theories:

- malpractice (breach of confidentiality)
- breach of statutory duty
- invasion of privacy
- breach of implied contract.

Testimonial privilege provides the patient the right to prevent the therapist from disclosing confidential information in a judicial proceeding. Privilege statutes recognize the importance of protecting confidential information revealed by the patient during the course of treatment.

A number of exceptions exist to testimonial privilege. These include involuntary hospitalization, child abuse reporting, court-ordered evaluations, and the patient-litigant exception that occurs when patients place their mental state at issue in litigation. This exception usually arises in malpractice claims, personal injury actions, child custody disputes, workers' compensation cases and will contests.

Therapists often confuse confidentiality with testimonial privilege. Although protected by common or statutory law, maintaining confidentiality is an ethical duty of the therapist with a long and venerable history. Testimonial privilege is established by state statute and belongs to the patient.

Therapists who also act as expert witnesses for their patients risk breaching confidentiality and disrupting treatment. Expert and treater roles do not mix. Once the therapist is on the stand and takes the oath, he or she may be required to answer questions that may reveal embarrassing, damaging information about the patient. Such revelations may not only damage the therapist–patient relationship, but also the patient's legal case. The expert-treater role conflict is discussed in greater depth by Strasburger (1987; Strasburger et al., 1997).

Minors are considered by law to be 18 years of age or younger. However, the general rule is that confidentiality follows the ability to legally consent to treatment (Simon, 2001, pp. 45–7). Young minors, usually defined in mental health confidentiality statutes, require parents or guardians as the legal decision makers. Parents or guardians have a right to know about diagnosis, treatment, and prognosis. Minors may be judged to be mature minors by therapists when they possess sufficient maturity to understand and consent to treatment. Minors may be considered emancipated when they are living away from home or are able to support themselves. Consent of parents is not required in emergencies.

In the US, all states, the District of Columbia, and other federal jurisdictions require healthcare providers, as mandated reporters, to report child abuse. Child abuse laws require the reporting of any physical injuries suspected of being inflicted by other than accidental means or where a child is believed to have been injured by a parent.

Confidentiality in mandated psychotherapy

Psychotherapy that takes place in correctional facilities or court-mandated outpatient treatment settings present challenging confidentiality issues. The therapist in these situations must grapple with the problem of double or triple agentry, otherwise known as conflicting loyalties (Weinstein, 1992). For example, the therapist working in a prison often is confronted with choosing to serve the prisoner-patient, prison officials, or society.

In practice, there is very little confidentiality in a correctional facility (Metzner, J. L., 2002, personal communication). The staff and prisoners usually know who is receiving mental health treatment. However, the content of treatment may or may not remain confidential. Prisoners may be informed about the limitations of confidentiality. Most treatment is behaviorally directed in group settings. Prisoners can be harmed if highly sensitive information is revealed in group therapy and then disseminated among the prison population. When a prisoner-patient's treatment plan is reviewed, many of the prisoner's psychological issues are discussed. There is no guarantee that this information will be kept strictly confidential.

Some prisoners want it explicitly known that they are receiving therapy. Their aim is to create the impression of being 'crazy,' which affords some protection against predatory prisoners who avoid them. Other prisoners seek therapy in order to shorten their length of sentence or gain special favors. The lack of confidentiality in correction facilities harms prisoners who genuinely want treatment. Bifurcating treatment content from administrative oversight, whenever possible, may provide some measure of confidentiality for the prisoner-patient. In correctional facilities, the therapist can talk with anyone, if he or she thinks it is appropriate. Such communications are constrained only by the therapist's good judgment. The prisoner-patient should be informed of all disclosures to third parties.

A number of professional organizations attempt to clarify the separation of forensic and therapeutic roles in prisons through standards and guidelines. Confidentiality issues are also addressed in: 'Standards for Health Services in Prisons' by the National Commission on Correctional Health Care (National Commission on Correctional Health Care, 1999), the 'Ethical Guidelines for the Practice of Forensic Psychiatry' (American Academy of Psychiatry and the Law, 1987), and the 'Principles Governing the Delivery of Psychiatric Services in Lock-Ups, Jails and Prisons' published by the American Psychiatric Association's Task Force on Psychiatric Services in Jails and Prisons (American Academy of Psychiatry and the Law, 1989).

'Forced' treatment may occur as a condition for offenders to be diverted from adjudication or incarceration, such as with sex offenders and juveniles (Melton et al., 1997). The maintenance of confidentiality so essential for successful treatment is observed in the breach. Offenders do not reveal information that might lead to their incarceration.

The therapist must issue reports about the offender's participation and progress in treatment. Again, the therapist should not release highly personal information to parole officers or other supervisory personnel that is irrelevant. The offender should be informed of all disclosures, unless informing would create a threat of harm to the therapist. If a realistic threat of harm exists to the therapist, appropriate officials should be informed and treatment should be terminated.

In the noncriminal context, psychotherapists may become involved in 'forced' treatments when they agree, for example, to treat impaired healthcare professionals. As a means of retaining or reinstituting the professional's license to practice, psychotherapy must be undertaken by approved therapists. Licensure boards try to respect the confidentiality of therapist–patient relationship by requiring general reports of attendance, progress in therapy and suitability to practice. Confidentiality is preserved to the greatest extent possible, unless the patient presents a danger of harm to self or to others. Maintenance of confidentiality in 'forced' treatment of healthcare professionals is not substantially different from the usual therapist–patient relationship.

Good clinical care is facilitated by explaining in 'forced' treatment the limitations of confidentiality and sharing with the patient any information released to the third parties, including family members (Simon, 1992a, pp. 133–4). The therapist as a double agent presents formidable challenges to maintenance of confidentiality and the therapeutic alliance, evoking powerful transference and countertransference challenges (Gabbard and Lester, 1995).

Case example: A mental health professional is required by the licensure board to undergo psychotherapy for sexual misconduct with a patient as a condition for regaining the license to practice. During therapy, the therapist discovers that the patient abuses alcohol and drugs. The patient adamantly objects to the therapist reporting the abuse to the licensure board. The therapist feels caught between her reporting responsibilities to the board and preserving the therapeutic alliance essential to the patient's treatment. The therapist decides to maintain her treatment role and to handle the patient's refusal as a treatment issue. Eventually, the patient acknowledges the destructive personal and professional consequences of polysubstance abuse, he voluntarily enters a detox and rehabilitation program approved by the licensure board.

Informed consent

As psychotherapy is a 'talking' treatment, is informed consent necessary? The answer is yes, because all psychotherapies have risks and benefits that patients need to understand. Few therapists warn patients of the risks of a proposed psychotherapy, although the potential benefits may be emphasized. Untoward transference reactions, mismanagement of transference and countertransference, regressive dependency states, and general worsening of a patient's clinical condition are some of the risks of psychotherapy.

Informed consent is important in psychotherapy. Through increased participation of patient—consumers in treatment decisions, the potential for the use of harmful treatments is lessened. Therapists must be prepared to consider thoughtfully the risks and benefits of any treatment they recommend to patients. Informed consent doctrine provides a basis for legal recovery of compensation for patients who are harmed by failures of therapists to obtain informed consent. Some states that have informed consent statutes declare the failure to obtain informed consent to be negligence (Slovenko, 1989).

In recent years, courts have demonstrated a willingness to compensate patients for nonphysical injuries that arise from psychotherapy. Therapists have an increased risk of liability under informed consent doctrine. The concept of informed consent is being applied increasingly to 'nonmedical' treatment situations. As the scientific study of psychotherapeutic efficacy goes forward, therapists are better able to inform patients about the qualitative and quantitative outcome data of alternative therapies.

Two distinct legal principles form the basis of the informed consent doctrine: the patient's right of self-determination and the therapist's duty as a fiduciary. A fiduciary acts for another person in a capacity of confidence or trust. The therapist has a legal duty to disclose the requisite facts to the patient about his or her condition. The purpose of the informed consent doctrine is twofold: to promote individual autonomy and to facilitate rational decision making (Appelbaum *et al.*, 1987). Although informed consent is a legal requirement, it also has an ethical dimension that respects the patient's autonomy in healthcare decision making. Clinically, it promotes collaboration between therapists and patients (American Psychiatric Association, 1997).

Case example: A patient with a prior history of depression during stressful life situations desires to undertake insight psychotherapy. The therapist informs the prospective patient that insight psychotherapy can be stressful, possibly precipitating a depressive episode potential benefits are also discussed. The prospective patient considers the risks and benefits of insight psychotherapy. She desires to enter therapy, noting that she was able to function during prior depressive episodes without the benefit of treatment. The therapist and patient agree to an extended period of evaluation before a final decision is made to begin psychotherapy.

The essential elements of informed consent are competency, information, and voluntariness. The therapist assesses the patient's healthcare decision-making capacity. Competent informed consent also requires that reasonable information be disclosed to the patient. There is no consistently accepted set of information to disclose for any specific medical or psychiatric disorder or condition. Generally, the following information is provided:

♦ *diagnosis:* description of disorder, condition, or problem

♦ *treatment:* nature and purpose of the proposed treatment

♦ *consequences:* risks and benefits of the proposed treatment

♦ *alternatives:* reasonable alternatives to the proposed treatment, including risks and benefits

♦ *prognosis:* expected but not guaranteed outcome with and without treatment.

An increasing number of courts have adopted the material-risk approach (reasonable-man standard). This standard imposes upon the therapist a duty to disclose all the information that a reasonable patient would need in order to make an informed decision about a procedure or treatment. This approach is more consistent with the ascendance of patient autonomy (Canterbury v. Spence, 1972). In a minority of jurisdictions, a truly patient-oriented standard is used, the so-called 'subjective lay standard' (what a particular patient would want to know). Furrow (1980) proposes the subjective lay standard of informing for psychotherapy because professional opinions about risks and benefits appear to be too uncertain and diverse. Moreover, patients may require quite specific information not ordinarily provided. For example, in a managed care setting, restrictions on psychotherapy visits may require the therapist to inform the patient that more sessions may be needed to treat his or her condition than are provided by insurance coverage. Beahrs and Gutheil (2001) recommend that, as a guiding principle, psychotherapists should convey information to a prospective patient that is material to the particular patient's decision.

Slovenko (1985) quotes Freud who advised against 'lengthy preliminary discussions before the beginning of treatment.' Freud felt that the patient should know of the difficulties and sacrifices of analytic treatment so that the patient would not be deprived 'of any right to say later on that he had been inveigled into a treatment whose extent and implication he did not realize.' Some psychodynamic therapists continue to express concern that sharing detailed psychological information about the assessment or the diagnosis may scuttle the fledgling psychotherapeutic process.

An initial period of evaluation allows the patient time to assess the therapist, the therapist's technique, and the interactional process between therapist and patient. A period of evaluation also allows the therapist time to make a reasonable diagnostic assessment and suitability for psychotherapy before committing to treat the patient. The nature of the patient's difficulties can be described in plain language using descriptive terms that form the basis of diagnostic nosology.

Anticipated benefits of treatment may be discussed as altering maladaptive defenses and resolution of underlying conflict, providing symptomatic relief, or instituting crisis intervention, according to the patient's clinical needs and situation. Obviously, no promises of cure can be made. Therapists who are prone to promising too much to patients should keep in mind Freud's well known comment that the object of psychoanalysis (therapy) is to substitute for neurotic misery ordinary human unhappiness, to temper therapeutic overzealousness. As treatment outcome studies become increasingly available, the findings can be shared with patients.

The risks of psychotherapy are more difficult to define when the evaluation reveals past regressive episodes occurring during a personal crisis. The therapist may want to consider with the patient the possibility of a similar recurrence during the course of psychotherapy. A history of serious psychosomatic illnesses, marked dysfunctional periods, or intense transference reactions toward others should alert the therapist to a possible recurrence of the patient's symptoms in psychotherapy. Previous episodes of regression provide indicia of potential risks to the patient. Although major life changes can occur as the result of psychotherapy, specific events such as divorce or occupational reverses that may seriously stress other family members usually are not foreseeable risks. Unpredictable events that are extremely traumatic may arise at anytime to destabilize a patient.

Prognostic statements should be made with great caution. The expected outcome with and without treatment of a particular mental disorder is extremely difficult, if not impossible, to determine. Many unforeseen life factors and the inherent course of any given mental disorder may determine outcome considerations. Spontaneous remissions are not uncommon. Nevertheless, certain mental conditions such as affective disorders and the schizophrenias have a recurrent, chronic course.

Alternative treatments should be discussed with patients. Although therapists may not be fully competent in using more than a few treatment approaches, they should be up to date in their knowledge of the standard treatments used by competent, ethical therapists. Therapists have an ethical and legal duty to stay abreast of new developments in their field. For example, the phobic patient may be treated by cognitive-behavioral therapy, psychodynamic therapy, medications, group therapy, or by a combination of therapeutic modalities. As more outcome studies become available, therapists will be able to better inform patients about the efficacy of specific treatments.

Many therapists employ a combination of treatment modalities. The therapist who primarily uses dynamic, insight-oriented psychotherapy should be reasonably knowledgeable about the methods, indications and contraindications of behavior therapy, cognitive therapy, medications, and group therapies. In Osheroff v. Chestnut Lodge (1985), the plaintiff claimed that he was inappropriately treated with psychotherapy instead of medication for depression. He alleged that the psychotherapy needlessly extended his hospital stay for many months, causing him emotional, professional, and financial harms. Patients have a right to know about alternative therapies that may be reasonably expected to help their condition. In malpractice cases, allegations of lack of informed consent usually accompany other claims of negligence.

Finally, the patient must be able to voluntarily consent or refuse the proposed treatment or proposed procedure. Coercion must not be used. Subtle differences exist between coercion and persuasion (Malcolm, 1986). Persuasion uses the patient's reasoning ability, while coercion undermines and manipulates the patient's ability to reason.

There are advantages and disadvantages to employing consent forms (Simon, 2001, pp. 82–3). Using forms alone makes obtaining informed consent more of an event than a process. Consent forms can introduce an adversarial tone to the therapist–patient interaction. Documenting the informed consent that occurred verbally with the patient is much more likely to obtain competent informed consent than a robotic 'formed' consent. Although a few states specify by statute that a written consent form be utilized; ordinarily, no legal requirement exists for a written consent form. Informed consent statutes in some states, however, do give written informed consent forms the status of presumptive evidence that competent informed consent was obtained (Simon, 1992, pp. 536–8).

Innovative therapies

Innovative therapies may be indicated when standard treatment methods fail (Simon, 1993). Innovation is very important for the development of new treatments that hold promise for the alleviation of mental suffering. Therapists should be aware of judicial decisions and regulations that govern innovative therapies. Patients must be informed for all foreseeable risks, including less risky, alternative treatments. Informed consent requires telling the patient that the therapy is untried, innovative and has possible unforeseeable risks. Written consent should be obtained for innovative therapies.

Innovative therapies, unless egregious, may fall within the 'respected minority rule' (Reisner and Slobgin, 1990). This rule states that therapists are free to choose from any of the available schools of therapy, even from those that most therapists would not use, provided a respected minority of therapists would employ the same therapies under similar circumstances.

The landmark psychiatric battery case is Hammer v. Rose (1960). Battery results from intentional, nonconsenting physical contact that would be offensive to a reasonable person. Dr John Rosen originated the innovative but controversial therapy—direct analysis—whereby schizophrenic patients were initially bombarded with id-type interpretations. The psychotherapist assumed took the position of an all-powerful parent who would use physical methods to make contact with severely regressed patients. The court stated that the beatings Alice Hammer received over the course of 7 years of treatment with Dr Rosen constituted improper treatment and malpractice.

In Abraham v. Zaslow (1972/1975), a 22-year-old graduate student agreed to undergo an experimental treatment called 'rage reduction' or Z-therapy. This treatment was designed primarily for autistic children. The patient is restrained, tickled, and poked when unsatisfactory answers are given to questions asked by the therapist. Ms Abraham was continually poked and abused for 10–12 hours, suffering extensive bruising and acute renal failure. She was awarded $170 000 in damages.

The United States Department of Health and Human Services (DHHS) (1981) has issued informed consent guidelines for research activities with mentally ill individuals. The DHHS disclosure requirements include: the fact and purposes of the proposed research; reasonably foreseeable risks; reasonably expected benefits; appropriate alternatives; a statement about the maintenance of confidentiality; an explanation about possible compensation if injury occurs in research involving more than minimal risks; information about the process of obtaining answers to pertinent questions; and a statement that participation is voluntary and refusal results in no penalties or loss of benefits.

Malpractice and risk management

To prove malpractice, the plaintiff (e.g., patient, family, or estate) must establish by a preponderance of the evidence (more likely than not) that:

♦ A therapist–patient relationship existed creating a *duty* of care to the patient.
♦ There was a *deviation* from the standard of care.
♦ The patient was *damaged*.
♦ The deviation *directly* caused the damage.

These elements of a malpractice claim are sometimes referred to as the four Ds. All elements must be present to pursue a successful malpractice claim. For example, a patient sues her therapist for going on vacation without having arranged for adequate coverage in his absence. The patient is involved in a serious automobile accident that she blames on being upset over the therapist 'abandonment' of her. Although the therapist deviated from the standard of care in not providing adequate coverage in his absence, he was not found to be the cause of the patient's automobile accident and the patient's injuries. Evidence was presented by the defense that the patient's first time use of cocaine while driving was the *direct* cause.

Establishing a general standard of care for therapists when so many schools of psychotherapy exist is very difficult. Therapists disagree among themselves concerning the indications and effectiveness of the many psychotherapeutic modalities now available.

Malpractice claims in psychotherapy

In recent years, malpractice suits against therapists have increased substantially. Generally, legal liability in psychotherapy cases is based on negligence.

Negligent psychotherapy results from the deviation in the standard of care that harms a patient. Intentional torts play a secondary role in litigation. The intentional torts are assault and battery, false imprisonment, invasion of right of privacy, misrepresentation or fraud, and the intentional infliction of emotional distress.

The most common malpractice suits against therapists claim negligence for suicides, boundary violations, and sexual misconduct.

Suicide

Claims against therapists for suicide attempts generally allege failure to monitor, failure to reasonable assess suicide risk, failure to formulate and implement an appropriate treatment plan, and failure to hospitalize the patient, either voluntarily or involuntarily.

Patients who are at risk for suicide require the therapist to take full charge of the treatment and management of the case. Especially, in 'split treatment arrangements' where the psychiatrist provides medication and the therapist performs the psychotherapy, monitoring and treatment may become fragmented and ineffective for the patient at risk for suicide. Communication and collaboration between treaters are essential for the effective treatment and management of patients. Some patients at risk for suicide may not be suitable to 'split treatment' arrangements.

There is no standard of care for the predication of patient suicides. However, the standard of care does require that therapists perform adequate suicide risk assessments (Simon, 2000). Courts carefully scrutinize suicide cases to determine the reasonableness of the risk assessment process and whether the patient's suicide was foreseeable. Foreseeability is a probabilistic legal term of art, not a scientific construct.

Foreseeability is the reasonable anticipation that harm or injury is likely to result from certain acts or omissions (Black, 1990). Only the risk of suicide can be assessed. Therefore, only the risk of suicide is foreseeable. Foreseeability should not to be confused with predictability for which, as stated above, no professional standard exists. Foreseeability must be distinguished from preventability. In hindsight, a suicide may have been preventable but not foreseeable at the time of assessment. Suicide risk assessments, when properly performed, inform the appropriate treatment, safety, and overall management requirements of the patient. Suicide risk assessment is a process, not an event.

Most patients at risk of suicide are treated as outpatients. As determined by the patient's clinical condition and the level of suicide risk, the patient may be seen more frequently, medication increased or changed and situational adjustments made. If the patient is at high risk for suicide and acutely distressed, hospitalization is usually required. However, a patient at high risk for suicide may continue to be treated as an outpatient, if a solid therapeutic alliance exists and a number of protective factors are present. Clinical judgment is determinative. In managed care settings, only patients with serious psychiatric conditions who are at high risk for harming themselves or others are hospitalized.

Involuntary hospitalization is a critical clinical–legal intervention for severely ill suicidal patients who refuse voluntary hospitalization. Some therapists fear damaging the therapeutic alliance by initiating certification of the patient for involuntary hospitalization. At this point, there may be little or no therapeutic alliance between therapist and patient when a very sick patient is refusing critical care. A battle over hospitalization may also emerge because of a therapist's intense negative countertransference. Inappropriate involuntary hospitalization of the patient may result.

Some therapists worry about being sued for false imprisonment. States have provisions in their commitment statutes that grant therapists immunity from liability, if reasonable judgment and good faith dictates petitioning for involuntary hospitalization. The therapist is much more likely to be sued for failure to involuntarily hospitalize a suicidal patient in critical need of treatment and protection, but who refuses voluntary hospitalization. Good clinical care, not fears of being sued, should direct the therapist's decision about involuntary hospitalization. In outpatient suicide cases, it is difficult for the plaintiff to prevail against the defendant therapist because the latter has much less control over the patient.

Maltsberger and Buie (1974) describe complex therapists' reactions to suicidal patients, such as anger, despair, frustration, and hopelessness. Therapists may experience countertransferential hate toward the suicidal patient because the suicide of a patient is perceived as raising significant doubts about their competence. Abandonment of the patient may occur, substantially increasing the patient's risk for suicide. Negative countertransference is an important clinician factor that may increase the risk of patient suicide. Other clinician factors associated with increased risk for patient suicide include physical and mental impairment, 'burn out,' fatigue, indifference, and placing monetary considerations ahead of patient care (Simon, 2004).

Gabbard and Lester (1995) warn that the therapist may use the psychological defense of reaction formation in an effort to deny hostile feelings toward the suicidal patient. Another countertransference reaction is evident when the therapist assumes the role of the 'good patient' rescuer. The therapist feels responsible for the patient's life instead of maintaining a concerned clinical focus on treatment and management. The patient must take responsibility for his or her life, ultimately making the decision to live or die. Therapists cannot stop patients who are determined to commit suicide. Not surprisingly, the 'love and save' approach ends in futility and despair for the therapist, interferes with clinical judgment, dooms the therapy, and may increase the patient's risk for suicide.

A desperate therapist at an impasse with a suicidal patient may seek legal solutions. The focus shifts from the clinical stalemate to a hoped for legal resolution. Although legal consultation may be useful in certain situations, consultation with a respected colleague is often the best initial step in helping the therapist maintain clinical focus. Lawyers tend to be risk averse, providing competent legal opinions that may not necessarily be appropriate clinical interventions for the patient at risk for suicide. Verbal consultations should be documented. In addition, a written report should be requested from the consultant.

The treatment and management of patients at suicide risk can be one of the most difficult clinical challenges encountered in the therapist's practice. The strong emotional reactions evoked by the suicidal patient must be identified and managed. Most therapists cannot treat more than a few suicidal patients at any given time. The uncertainty of treatment outcome; the potentially devastating personal, professional, and legal consequences for the therapist; the intense anguish of bereft, angry suicide survivors—these and other factors can create anxiety that interferes with effective clinical care. Therapist must realistically gauge their ability to tolerate the inevitable anxieties and vicissitudes encountered in treating patients at risk for suicide (Simon, 1998).

Boundary violations

Under the rubric of negligent psychotherapy, the most common allegations involve sexual and nonsexual boundary violations. The latter usually include business, employment, personal service, or social relationship with patients.

Treatment boundaries are set by the therapist that define and secure the therapist's professional relationship with the patient (Simon, 1992b). Once treatment boundaries are established, boundary issues arise from the patient's testing of treatment boundaries. Dealing with boundary issues is an important part of therapeutic work. Boundary violations, however, usually harm the therapy and the patient. Boundary crossings are less serious departures from boundary maintenance that can be rectified and become grist for the therapeutic mill (Gutheil and Gabbard, 1993).

Effective treatment boundaries define a reasonably fluctuating, neutral, safe place that enables the dynamic psychological interaction between therapist and patient to unfold. Boundary setting depends on the nature of the patient, the type of treatment, the personality, training and clinical experience of the therapist and the interaction style between patient and therapist. An absolutist position regarding treatment boundaries cannot be taken, so long as patients or their treatment is not harmed.

Boundary violations that are precursors to therapist–patient sex occur gradually. Sexual exploitation of patients by therapists has a 'natural history' of progressive personal involvement by the therapist with the patient that is remarkably similar from case to case (Simon, 1989). Gutheil and Simon (1995) posit that during the segment of therapy that occurs 'between the chair and the door,' patients and therapists are more vulnerable to committing boundary crossings and violations. They suggest that inchoate boundary violations first appear during this interval, providing an early warning sign for the therapist. The reader is referred to other works addressing the problem of treatment boundaries (Gabbard, 1989; Epstein, 1994; Pope, 1994).

Boundary violations that harm patients may lead to civil liability, criminal sanctions (sexual exploitation), and professional disciplinary actions. Boundary violations that lead to sexual and nonsexual exploitation of patients are often caused by the therapist's mismanagement of transference and countertransference feelings.

Courts may have difficulty understanding the clinical concepts of transference and countertransference in claims of harm from therapists' boundary violations. This point is well illustrated in the case of Hess v. Frank (1975). The patient alleged that during a regularly scheduled session, "without just cause", the psychiatrist became abusive to the patient. He uttered various words and phrases that the psychiatrist knew or should have known, in his professional capacity, would cause grave mental anguish and be injurious to the mental health of the patient. The alleged abusive statements were uttered during the course of an argument over fees as well as the appointment schedule. The patient sought $100 000 in damages.

The court dismissed the patient's case against the psychiatrist. The court held that the argument was outside of the professional treatment relationship. From a clinician's perspective, however, the court's position that discussions or even arguments about billing somehow exist outside the scope of therapy is a legal fiction. Scheduling and fee matters that arise in the course of therapy are initially treatment issues. The court stated: 'The conduct complained of, however, was not part of the course of treatment and there is no claim or indication that defendant failed to provide medical services in accordance with accepted standards or that he did not exercise requisite skills in the treatment of the plaintiff.' Apparently, the court did not consider the possibility that countertransference was the cause of patient mismanagement by the psychiatrist who, after treating the patient for 8 years, "without just cause", became abusive to the patient.

Attention to early boundary violations can alert the therapist to reestablish appropriate treatment boundaries, obtain consultation, or, if necessary, refer the patient. The rule of abstinence is a basic principle underlying boundary maintenance. It states that the therapist must abstain from using the patient for the therapist's personal gratification. The therapist's main source of pleasure is derived from the professional gratification obtained from the psychotherapeutic process and the satisfaction gained in helping the patient. When the therapist's gratification is derived from a personal rather than a professional relationship with the patient, boundary violations invariably occur. However, some therapists do obtain gratification from the 'personal' aspects of the therapeutic relationship but carefully monitor countertransference problems to avoid any exploitation (personal communication, Glen O. Gabbard, M. D., November 3, 2002). Exploitation of a patient rarely occurs in the absence of other negligent practices and deviations in care.

Readings in the prevention of malpractice in psychotherapy include: recovered memories of sexual abuse (Gutheil and Simon, 1997); abandonment (Simon, 2001, pp. 21–2); split treatment (Meyer and Simon, 1999); breach of confidentiality (Slovenko, 1992); duty to warn and protect endangered third parties (Herbert and Young, 2002).

Conclusions

In psychotherapy, therapists try to help patients to better understand their problems and to learn more adaptive ways of coping. For therapists, understanding and coping with the legal requirements governing psychotherapeutic practice should facilitate the provision of good patient care. A working knowledge of the legal regulation of the mental health professions allows therapists to integrate clinical and legal issues, thereby avoiding unduly defensive practices that can inhibit the therapist's ability to conduct effective psychotherapy. Initially, legal issues should be addressed as treatment issues. Often, legal requirements can be handled in such a way as not to harm treatment and, whenever possible, to beneficially facilitate treatment.

Risk management is a reality of clinical practice. Clinically based risk management is patient centered, supporting the treatment process and the therapeutic alliance. It provides the therapist with a helpful measure of practical comfort. Unduly defensive practices must not be allowed to erode the therapist's affirmative professional, ethical, moral, and legal duty to provide adequate care to the patient. Knowledge and insight into the causes of litigation can help psychotherapists preserve the tranquility and composure so necessary for the practice of psychotherapy.

References

Abraham v. Zaslow (1972/1975). No 245862 Super Ct (Cal June 30, 1972), Affirmed, Cal App (Feb 2, 1975).

American Academy of Psychiatry and the Law. (1987). *Ethical guidelines for the practice of forensic psychiatry* (revised 1989, 1991, and 1995). Bloomfield, CT: American Academy of Psychiatry and the Law.

American Academy of Psychiatry and the Law. (1989). *Report of task force on psychiatric services in jails and prisons*. Washington, DC: American Psychiatric Association.

American Psychiatric Association. (1997). Resource document on principles of informed consent in psychiatry. *Journal of the American Academy of Psychiatry Law*, **25**, 121–5.

American Psychiatric Association. (2001). *The principles of medical ethics with annotations especially applicable to psychiatry*. Washington, DC: American Psychiatric Association.

Appelbaum, P. S., Lidz, C. W., and Meisel, A. (1987). *Informed consent: legal theory and clinical practice*, p. 84. New York: Oxford University Press.

Beahrs, J. O. and Gutheil, T. G. (2001). Informed consent in psychotherapy. *American Journal of Psychiatry*, **158**, 4–10.

Black, H. C. (1990). *Black's Law Dictionary*, 6th edn, p. 649. St Paul, MN: West Publishing.

Canterbury v. Spence, 464 F 2d 772 (DC Cir), Cert denied, Canterbury v. Spence, 409 U. S. 1064 (1972).

Department of Health and Human Services. (1981). Final regulations amending basic HHS policy for the protection of human research subjects. *Federal Register*, 1981L 46L8366–8792.

Epstein, R. S. (1994). *Keeping boundaries*. Washington, DC: American Psychiatric Press.

Furrow, B. R. (1980). *Malpractice in psychotherapy*, pp. 68–70. Lexington, MA: DC Health.

Gabbard, G. O., ed. (1989). *Sexual exploitation in professional relationships*. Washington, DC: American Psychiatric Press.

Gabbard, G. O. and Lester, E. F. (1995). *Boundaries and boundary violations in psychoanalysis*. New York: Basic Books.

Gutheil, T. G. and Gabbard, G. O. (1993). The concept of boundaries in clinical practice: theoretical and risk management dimensions. *American Journal of Psychiatry*, **150**, 188–96.

Gutheil, T. G. and Simon, R. I. (1995). Between the chair and the door: boundary issues in the therapeutic 'transition zone'. *Harvard Review of Psychiatry*, **2**, 336–40.

Gutheil, T. G. and Simon, R. I. (1997). Clinically based risk management principles for recovered memory cases. *Psychiatric Services*, **48**, 1403–7.

Hammer v. Rose, 7NY 2d 376, 165 NE 2d 756, 198 NYS 2d 65 (1960).

Herbert, P. B. and Young, K. A. (2002). Tarasoff at twenty-five. *Journal of the American Academy of Psychiatry Law*, **30**, 175–81.

Hess v. Frank, 47 AD 2d 889, 367 NYS 2d 30 (NY App Div 1975).

Jaffee v. Redmond, ll6 S. Ct. 1923 (1996).

Malcolm, J. G. (1986). Treatment choices and informed consent in psychiatry: implications of the Osheroff case for the profession. *Journal of Psychiatry and Law*, **14**, 9–107.

Maltsberger, T. and Buie, D. H. (1974). Countertransference in the treatment of suicidal patients. *Archives of General Psychiatry*, **30**, 625–33.

Melton, G. B., Petrila, J., Pothress, N. G., and Slobogin, C. (1997). *Psychological evaluations for the courts*, 2nd edn, p. 273. New York: Guilford Press.

Meyer, D. J. and Simon, R. I. (1999). Split treatment: clarity between psychiatrists and psychotherapists. *Psychiatric Annals*, **29** (Part 1) 241–5; (Part 2) 327–32.

National Commission on Correctional Health Care. (1999). *Correctional Mental Healthcare: Standards for health services in prisons*. Chicago, IL: National Services Commission on Correctional Health Care.

Osheroff v. Chestnut Lodge, 490 A 2d 720, 722 (MD App 1985).

Pope, K. S. (1994). *Sexual involvement with therapists: patient assessment, subsequent therapy, forensics*. Washington, DC: American Psychological Association.

President's Commission for the Study of Ethical Problems in Medicine and Biomedical and Behavioral Research. (1982). Making Health Care Decisions: A Report on the Ethical and Legal Implications of Informed Consent in the Patient–Practitioner Relationship, Vol. 1: Report. Washington, DC, Superintendent of Documents, October.

Reisner, R. and Slobgin, C. (1990). *Law and the mental health system*, 2nd edn, p. 75. St Paul: West Publishing.

Simon, R. I. (1989). The natural history of therapist sexual misconduct: identification and prevention. *Psychiatric Annals*, **19**, 104–12.

Simon, R. I., ed. (1991). The practice of psychotherapy: legal liabilities of an 'impossible' profession. In: *American Psychiatric Press Review of Clinical Psychiatry and the Law*, Vol. 2. Washington, DC: American Psychiatric Press.

Simon, R. I. (1992a). *Clinical psychiatry and the law*, 2nd edn. Washington, DC: American Psychiatric Press, Inc.

Simon, R. I. (1992b). Treatment boundary violations: clinical, ethical, and legal considerations. *Bulletin of the American Academy of Psychiatry Law*, **20**, 269–88.

Simon, R. I. (1993). Innovative therapies and legal uncertainty: a survival guide for clinicians. *Psychiatric Annals*, **23**, 473–9.

Simon, R. I. (1998). The suicidal patient. In: L. E. Lifson and R. I. Simon, ed. *The mental health practitioner and the law: a comprehensive handbook*, pp. 166–86. Cambridge, MA: Harvard University Press.

Simon, R. I. (2000). Taking the 'sue' out of suicide: a forensic psychiatrist's perspective. *Psychiatric Annals*, **30**, 399–407.

Simon, R. I. (2001). *Psychiatry and law for clinicians*, 3rd edn, p. 90. Washington, DC: American Psychiatric Publishing, Inc.

Simon, R. I. (2004). *Assessing and managing suicide risk*, p. 89. Washington, DC: American Psychiatric Publishing, Inc.

Slovenko, R. (1981). Forensic psychiatry. In: H. I. Kaplan and J. Sadock, ed. *Comprehensive textbook of psychiatry IV*, Vol. 2, p. 1981. Baltimore, MD: Williams & Wilkins.

Slovenko, R. (1989). Misadventure of psychiatry with the law. *Journal of Psychiatry and the Law*, **17**, 115–56.

Slovenko, R. (1992). *Psychotherapy and confidentiality*, pp. 259–445. Springfield, IL: CC Thomas.

Strasburger, L. H. (1987). 'Crudely, without any finesse': the defendant hears his psychiatric evaluation. *Bulletin of the American Academy of Psychiatry Law*, **15**, 229–33.

Strasburger, L. H., Gutheil, T. G., and Brodsky, A. (1997). On wearing two hats: role conflict in serving as both psychotherapist and expert witness. *American Journal of Psychiatry*, **154**, 448–56.

Weinstein, H. C. (1992). Correctional psychiatry. In: R. I. Simon ed. *Review of clinical psychiatry and the law*, Vol. 3, pp. 193–201. Washington, DC: American Psychiatric Press.

42 Psychotherapy supervision

*James W. Lomax, Linda B. Andrews,
John W. Burruss, and Stirling Moorey*

This chapter explores individual supervision as a unique educational structure for psychotherapy education. Such supervision is of paramount importance in the professional formation of the psychotherapist in particular, but it is also important for all mental health practitioners regardless of whether psychotherapy plays a significant role on their professional lives or not (Mohl *et al.*, 1990). Individual supervision as an extended form of case consultation with a focus on both the patient and consultee is also an extremely important (although apparently underutilized) form of continuing professional education for mental health practitioners. The chapter focuses on individual supervision as an educational element for developing competency in psychodynamic psychotherapy but will also address the pros and cons of individual versus group psychotherapy supervision and the similarities and differences between supervision of the psychodynamic therapies and supervision of cognitive-behavioral therapies (CBT).

The chapter begins with a brief historical review of the concept of individual supervision and what makes individual supervision a unique educational structure (Jacobs *et al.*, 1995; Watkins, 1997). Next we focus on establishing the supervisory alliance, clarifications of goals and objectives for the supervisory relationship, and establishing mutually agreeable measurements of progress in supervision. Of particular importance in psychodynamic psychotherapy is the management of personal revelations in individual supervision. The following section of the chapter will comment upon the vulnerabilities of individual supervision that distinguish it from other types of educational experience. A section defines the various supervisory interventions, including both what the supervisor does and what is at risk for the supervisory enterprise with each intervention.

The relationship of individual supervision to assessment of competency will be explored. In most supervisory relationships there is an evaluation of both the supervisee and the supervisor, which is shared with an external entity, such as an educational program director or faculty evaluation committee. The distinction between feedback and evaluation will be reviewed as it pertains to individual supervision along with comments about how management of the power differential in the supervisory relationship influences the authenticity of evaluations. The final section will focus on the termination of the supervisory relationship with examples of useful and problematic termination processes offered as illustrations.

The concept of individual supervision

While 'supervisory relationships' take place in a wide range of educational and routine work situations, individual supervision was developed as a unique interpersonal structure for the purpose of developing competency in psychoanalysis. This unique interpersonal structure utilizes a deceptively simple form (individual meetings between a supervisor and supervisee for a specified amount of time on a regular and recurring basis) for the interaction of complex and sometimes competing aims and goals. The ongoing goal of the supervisor is the creation of a 'safe enough' environment in which the supervisee reports interactions between a learning therapist and a patient. Such reporting requires painstaking honesty in order to learn to

apply psychotherapeutic principles and ideas to a specific and unique therapeutic dyad for which the learner has primary responsibility. Supervisors are responsible for maintaining not only safety in the supervisory relationship, but also vulnerability. The careful titration of safety and vulnerability allows the supervisee to develop professionally (with an inherent ongoing sense of personal vulnerability) while maintaining self-esteem and is accomplished through the experience of safety in the relationship with the supervisor. Learning about both patients *and* self is the primary goal of supervision for the supervisee. Such learning depends upon the tact, sensitivity, and knowledge of boundaries of the supervisor and also the study, courage, and trust of the supervisee. The educational product of individual supervision is new knowledge, skills, and attitudes on the part of both supervisor and supervisee. Good psychotherapy supervision regularly results in the fresh acquisition of knowledge by both parties. (Successful psychodynamic psychotherapy may be likened to participant observation in the co-creation of a novel. Successful individual supervision is subjectively quite similar.)

There are interprofessional differences in the content of individual supervision based upon both cultural and time differences in supervisory relationships. The education of mental health professionals lends itself to shifts in the content of individual supervision depending on the general professional developmental stage of the trainee. Early in professional education, the content of individual supervision may be weighted towards an in-depth discussion of cases and developing a professional relationship with the patient that can be used to implement specific treatment such as psychotherapy. The goal is predominantly to enrich the understanding of these cases beyond a focus on phenomenological diagnosis and/or pharmacological treatment. However, as the trainee begins didactic and experiential conferences about psychotherapy, the individual supervision moves towards a focus on the ongoing long-term or short-term psychotherapy cases. The structure of individual supervision varies somewhat among the main mental health disciplines. A common structure is for weekly individual meetings of about 1 hour in length each with two to four individual supervisors. Typically, new supervisors are assigned for each academic year in order to give the trainee a greater breadth of exposure. Some programs require longer exposure to a given supervisor. Supervisory assignments should take into account supervisee gender differences. These may be of particular importance for the understanding and management of intense erotic or hostile aggressive attachments of patient to therapist. Specifically, it is useful for supervisees to have supervisors of both genders, a woman supervisor is often especially sensitive to women supervisees encountering erotized negative transference with male patients, etc.

The individual supervisor is responsible for both the education of the mental health professional and the assurance of competent care for the patient. These primary aims of the supervisor may be in conflict or at least shift in balance of emphasis early in the mental health professional's development or at any time when the trainee is having difficulty and the patient is in a state of urgent need (Jacobs *et al.*, 1995). This conflict is not limited to mental health professionals in psychotherapy. Each healthcare specialty has an analogous challenge when learners are included in the care of patients.

While the apparent stakes may seem greater when moment to moment life-threatening procedures are talking place (for example, in cardiovascular or neurosurgical education), the highly personal nature of both psychotherapy and individual supervision intensifies the subjective experience of vulnerability for the learner.

Heinz Kohut's emphasis on the developmental needs of the self dramatically changed not only psychotherapeutic, but also educational cultures with a new emphasis on avoiding shame in processes requiring ongoing revision of the sense of self (Jacobs et al., 1995). Both psychotherapy and individual supervision, when successful, involve disruption of existing ways of thinking and behaving. Thus, psychotherapy education needs a special and specific educational structure to develop psychotherapy skills in the 'translational' arena in which concepts learned in classrooms are utilized in a specific treatment relationship. That unique educational structure is individual supervision.

Establishing the supervisory alliance

The term supervisory alliance is used to describe the special relationship between the supervisor and supervisee. The supervisory alliance needs to be established and reinforced early in the relationship with each supervisee. Establishing the alliance requires specific effort on the part of both the supervisor and the supervisee and begins the new learning for both involved in the supervision relationship.

It is often helpful to begin with the supervisor taking an educational history. If the supervisee educational history in terms of formal education is unknown, that should be where the educational history begins. Specific emphasis should then be placed on the supervisee's previous experiences in individual supervision. Asking what the supervisee learned, what was helpful, what was dull or aversive, produces important information that may or may not predict the outcome of the current supervisory relationship but will certainly inform both parties about the context of their new partnership.

It is helpful for the supervisor to have an understanding of the supervisee's knowledge about psychotherapy, including any personal experience with it. However, this involves a significant boundary issue. The supervisor should convey the importance of privacy and confidentiality in psychotherapeutic relationships. Asking the supervisee 'What do you know about psychotherapy?' gives the supervisee an opportunity to reveal or not to reveal any personal experience with psychotherapy and may provide an opportunity for the supervisor to share his or her resources about what psychotherapy is like. For example, a supervisor who has prepared psychodynamic case formulations, process notes, or videotaped case presentations may share those materials with the supervisee along with an explanation of how it is that such personal and confidential material becomes available for dissemination.

Some supervisor/supervisee pairings are made with no input from the supervisee. If, however, the supervisee has to some degree 'chosen' the supervisor, it is important for both parties to be aware of the supervisee's motivations. Asking how the supervisee decided to choose a supervisor allows an opportunity for shared expectations to develop as well as misunderstandings to emerge. Further questions should discern what the supervisee expects to happen in supervision, what the supervisee expects to learn from it, and what the supervisee expects the supervisor and supervisee to do in order to make learning happen. Such exchanges contribute to developing the elements of a successful alliance. During this history taking, the supervisor should not only receive information from the supervisee, but also actively indicate his or her understanding of the questions asked to clarify what is expected of the supervisee. Specifying that the evaluation process will give the pair an opportunity to appreciate how the progress of their relationship will be assessed and should include a discussion of the evaluation instrument to be used and the timing of evaluations.

Individual supervision in each of the mental health disciplines should allow enough freedom to discuss any pressing matter of the supervisee. However, the supervisor should maintain a clear vision of the task of supervision (psychotherapy education) and prevent unhelpful diversions from the explicit task at hand. Excessive diversions may indicate either a general problem in developing psychotherapeutic competency or a specific problem with a patient being discussed that is either embarrassing or has evoked difficulties for the supervisee. It is helpful for the supervisor to clarify expectations about the supervisory appointments. In educational programs supervision time is 'protected' in the sense that it is a designated part of the educational work week, which takes precedence over anything except acute clinical emergencies. However, it is also 'expected' time for the trainee. Cancellations or requests to reschedule should be thoughtfully mentioned in advance when anticipatable and never promote the idea that supervision (and thereby, psychotherapy) is a casual, informal, or trivial matter.

There is no reason to assume that a junior supervisee in psychiatry, psychology, or social work knows what is supposed to happen in this novel and unique educational experience. Therefore, it is up to the supervisor to clarify the structure and expectations of the supervisee. With the current emphasis in psychiatry on phenomenological diagnosis supported by DSM-IV there is often a tendency for trainees to give rather short shrift to the developmental history or personal narrative of the patient, which is a fundamental importance for constructing a psychotherapeutic treatment plan. Thus, it is common and necessary for the supervisor to emphasize that the resident will be expected to present a developmental history with considerable attention to the patient's early interactions with his or her most significant figures. The idea that such information may be important predictors of psychopathology, current interpersonal relationship difficulties, and the therapeutic relationship itself may come as a new concept to the beginning therapist. This may be true even if that beginning therapist has already started the basic psychotherapy didactic courses of the program.

Some specific considerations of structuring the supervisory situation include the use of audiotape or videotape, the pros and cons of using process notes, and whether the supervisor will personally see the patient for whom the supervisee provides the psychotherapy. Eventually most competent supervisees present cases to their supervisors from memory with relatively few notes. For the senior psychotherapist and trainee or practitioners seeking individual supervision to enrich his or her educational possibilities from a busy clinical practice, process notes may be quite adequate. However, for the therapist-in-training or the postgraduate physician who seeks supervisory consultation because of a stalemate or crisis in a therapeutic relationship, a more thorough and systematic approach to getting started in individual supervision is generally advisable. Specifically during education in psychodynamic psychotherapy or psychoanalysis, constructing a psychodynamic case formulation is a fundamental competency. Specifically within psychiatric education, each second year resident should present several complete psychodynamic case formulations using models such as those found in standard textbooks of psychiatry or psychotherapy (Perry et al., 1987; MacKinnon and Yudofsky, 1991; Stoudemire, 1998; Gabbard, 2000).

Also as part of psychotherapy education it is extremely helpful for the therapist to have experience using process notes. Process notes refer to actual or reconstructed comments by the therapist and patient made throughout the session beginning with the first exchanges in the waiting or consulting room through the departure of the patient from the clinic or consulting room. Note taking during a session will often be seen as a distraction by both the therapist and the patient. This is particularly true with face-to-face therapies, but it may also be true for situations when the patient is lying down on a couch in an effort to increase his or her internal focus. A patient is often preoccupied by what motivates the therapist to write and may well be influenced by the therapist's note taking to the detriment of a focus on what is more salient to the person's difficulties. For the therapist, a focus on getting down exactly what is said might significantly interfere with using the self as an observing instrument in the therapeutic relationship and decrease the therapist's awareness of his or her responses to patient communications (particularly countertransference reactions) that could be of clinical or educational utility. Many trainees find it particularly helpful to reserve 10–15 minutes after the end of the session to reconstruct the sequence of exchanges that took place in the previous treatment session.

With practice, the supervisee is usually able to capture adequately the flow of the communications in a way that makes for useful supervisory discussions.

For many psychotherapy educators, a report on the disconcerting concept of 'lying in supervision' provided a sort of traumatic disillusionment but useful reminder of the need for educational vigilance (Hantoot, 2000). It should come as no surprise that psychotherapists-in-training succumb to the all too human propensity for lying, and the biggest determinant of lying may be to protect the supervisee from disruption of 'narcissistic equilibrium.' A developmental basis for lying may be reawakened by separation and individuation efforts on the part of the student. Supervisors should be aware of the problem, sensitive to the emotional elements of the supervisory relationship, avoiding supervisor complacence, and be educated about their educational challenge.

One way to manage omissions and distortions by the supervisee is some form of recording of the sessions. Of course, audiotape is less intrusive than videotape and does not require as much technical support. The problem with audiotaping and videotaping is that some degree of editing is necessary in order for the supervision to involve more than just observing the sessions. In our experience it is unusual for more than about 15–20 minutes of a therapy session to be adequately discussed in a 50-minute supervisory session. Nonetheless, early in the development of psychotherapeutic competency, it is extremely valuable for a supervisor to have unedited information about the supervisee in action with a patient. Many things will simply go unobserved or unrecognized by even a very good supervisee early their professional development. This is particularly true regarding the way in which the supervisee makes transitions between topics or uses facilitatory language. The difference between 'ok' and a curious nonverbal grunt or simple exclamatory remark, for example, can be quite significant for the patient and the process (Havens, 1978).

The decision of the supervisor to meet personally with the patient being supervised is a significant one. Of course, such an interview will have an effect on the relationship between the supervisee and the patient, but that effect can be positive or negative. Influenced in part by billing requirements, supervisors in some clinics participate in the first 10 or 15 minutes of psychotherapy sessions predominantly conducted by a trainee therapist. While this would be a very poor arrangement for the entire psychotherapy education experience of the trainee, it does provide an interesting and sometimes valuable educational experience early in the development of the psychotherapist. Of course, it greatly informs the supervisor about the patient. It can also help the supervisee to both see what the supervisor would actually do with a particular patient and also (for better and worse) affects the idealization of the supervisor by the supervisee. Even as a limited structure for therapists early in training, this arrangement can be damaging to the establishment of a psychotherapeutic relationship. The physical presence of a designated higher authority can undermine the trust or confidence of any patient and may facilitate unhelpful 'splitting' with devaluation of the junior therapist with borderline or narcissistic patients.

In summary, the goals of the supervisory alliance are to overcome the obstacles to learning, to provide nonjudgmental feedback and evaluation, and to explore anxiety on the part of the supervisee as an impediment to learning—both learning from the patient in psychotherapy and from the supervisor in supervision. In subsequent sections of this chapter, more about managing anxiety of the supervisee will be developed. However, an important basic distinction is that a supervisor explores supervisee anxiety as an impediment to learning not as a consequence of a personal history of conflicts. The latter is the domain of personal therapy, which has analogies to supervision but significant boundary differences.

The management of personal revelations in individual supervision

A detailed focus on the patient being presented in individual supervision is a necessary but not sufficient perspective for developing psychotherapeutic competence. Such a focus would unhelpfully limit the supervisory dialog. The supervisory dialog should include discussions of the therapist's feelings, ideas, and images that produce or inhibit therapeutic activity. Such conversations often begin when either the supervisor or supervisee become aware that the supervisee did not act on available information with a therapeutically appropriate question, confrontation, interpretation, or empathic intervention. Curiosity of either the supervisor or supervisee often leads to recognizing a subjective reluctance of the supervisee, which is helpful to name or identify. Commonly, the supervisee was anxious, irritated, sexually aroused, or had some other thought, feeling, or idea which resulted in the withholding of therapeutic activity. The supervisory goal is to help the supervisee contain such uncomfortable experiences without diminishing awareness of them. The capacity for containment in the therapist is similar to the capacity for equanimity espoused as one desirable capacity of physicians by Osler and others (Osler, 1947). While it is important for both the supervisor and supervisee to keep in mind how unusual it is to have an ongoing relationship in which emotions are discussed without leading to a behavior, good supervision involves mutual exploration of exactly such situations in the service of producing therapeutic competence. The supervisor and supervisee should attempt to relate the emergence of the difficult emotion to the specific provoking event in the therapeutic process. Together the supervisor and supervisee should review potential precipitants in the therapist/patient relationship to determine if a substantive connection between the feelings and precipitant can be established and understood. Sometimes the supervisee will be embarrassed by a curiosity that seems 'voyeuristic' and unusual to pursue in most social contexts. Just as psychoanalysis is a relationship for which there is 'no model in the rest of human experience' (Freud, 1958), supervision shares some of this uniqueness, but the focus is on anxiety, which limits therapeutic activity rather than the history of personal adverse relationships or internal conflicts such as is the focus in psychotherapeutic and psychoanalytic relationships.

Good supervision engenders the development of a therapeutic curiosity to review hypotheses in the supervisory relationship and then independently in psychotherapeutic relationships outside the ones being supervised. This curiosity allows the supervisee to reflect upon the nature of the connection being made between any one reaction to a patient and similar reactions in other psychotherapeutic encounters. It often leads the supervisee to appreciate patterns of therapeutic inhibition, which become clues guiding his or her therapeutic conduct. In a somewhat oversimplified way, the therapist-in-training learns to make accommodations based on self-knowledge about what impedes or enhances therapeutic activity. For many therapists, this curiosity and pattern recognition leads the therapist-in-training to pursue personal therapy. For example, in supervisory discussions about two patients with unexpected negative outcomes, it became clear that the therapist had been reluctant to make an observation about evidence of an emerging erotic transference. The supervisory discussion about the pattern of therapeutic inhibition led the supervisee to seek a consultation that led to a recommendation of personal psychoanalysis.

What is different about individual supervision than other types of teacher–learner relationships is that it makes a very personal self-examination a public matter. Such self-examination is not a part of many other professional exchanges and is actively avoided in some. For example, it will be the unusual physician therapist who has experienced these opportunities for reflection in his or her exchanges with surgical and medical attendings in other specialties.

The principle for the supervisor to keep in mind is that the supervision should focus on examining material relevant to the treatment of patients and be pertinent to the educational needs of the supervisee. The examination is not for the personal needs of the trainee or the supervisor. Such examination requires security and predictability of a secure enough consultative relationship. Supervisory tact and timing also are quite important. Especially early on in supervisory relationships, the supervisor may have an idea about the supervisee that is too far ahead of supervisee's psychological development, self-reflecting capacity, or introspective ability. An important question is whether a particular observation of the supervisor is discussible at this point in time. Sometimes, humor can be helpful, but humor at the expense of the supervisor in a somewhat self-depreciatory tone is preferable to any indication that one is laughing at the dilemmas of the therapist-in-training. At times, it is rather clear that a supervisee would benefit from personal therapy. It is important that a supervisee who brings highly personal material into a supervisory relationship be encouraged to seek personal therapy while clarifying the focus of the individual supervision. Once one gets started talking about things in supervision that belong in personal therapy, it is very hard to extricate oneself gracefully. Helping a supervisee 'wonder' whether anxiety limiting therapeutic activity could be addressed in personal therapy is generally better than telling a supervisee that he or she should seek treatment.

Supervisory interventions: what is done and what is at risk

The supervisor has a wide variety of available interventions ranging from active listening and clarification to role playing to interpretation of parallel process (Doeherman, 1976). Each intervention has a particular use and will be employed differently depending upon specifics of the supervisee, the stage of the two relationships involved, the salience of any current crisis, and the opportunity to deal with enduring themes in either (treatment or supervisory) relationship. Each intervention also has potential for both positive and negative consequences for the supervisee and the educational alliance. This section defines and elaborates some of the fundamental supervisory interventions (Jacobs et al., 1995).

Active learning

Active listening on the part of the supervisor involves simultaneous reception and ordering of information about both the patient being discussed and the supervisee doing the presenting and developing a conceptual model of the relevant clinical and educational issues at hand for both the patient being discussed, the supervisee, and the supervisee/supervisor relationship. A constellation of individual and relational perspectives was recently termed 'The Triadic Match' (Kantrowitz, 2002).

Modeling

Early in psychotherapy learning, the supervisee is especially likely to appreciate modeling of therapy interventions on the part of the supervisor. Such demonstrative teaching can promote identification of the supervisee with the supervisor by providing a vivid example utilizing the greater experience of the supervisor. Such modeling is best done in a somewhat tentative format such as 'I can imagine myself saying . . .' or 'Early in therapy I would be more inclined to say ——, but later ——' (for example, when responding to the question of whether to respond to a direct request for advice on the part of the patient). On the downside, modeling can come across as a constricting directive to the supervisee claiming that there is one 'correct' response. It is helpful to remember that the best answer to the novice therapist question by the supervisee of 'What would you say in this situation?' is 'I don't know.' Of course, this response should be followed by the explanation that individual factors prevent a fixed correct response that is inevitably correct. However, it is also helpful to provide examples of 'one way' of responding to the novice therapist with the caveat that whatever is said or done must be done in the language and style of the supervisee in order to be perceived as authentic on the part of the patient.

Didactic review or instruction

Didactic instruction has a significant place in individual supervision, especially early on in any supervisory relationship. It is important to review diagnostic criteria and how diagnosis relates to psychotherapeutic strategies. Every supervisee needs the opportunity to do case formulations. Each training program should ensure that opportunity is available in a systematic fashion. It is also helpful to discuss identifying and assessing different types of defense mechanisms for the psychodynamic psychotherapies. One purpose of this discussion is to help the supervisee understand that the predominance of certain defenses predicts suitability to different types of psychotherapeutic interventions. Such didactic instruction is an invaluable orientation and also often helps titrate supervisee anxiety thereby building the foundation of the alliance. Supervisors should advise early and whenever patient safety is a question. Explanation, as opposed to directives or pronouncements, is preferable. On the downside, excessive didactic instruction can result in a kind of dogmatism and defensive, mutual laziness for both supervisor and supervisee. The supervisor can bask in an aura of supervisor authority at the expense of learning from his supervisee. Security gained by excessive didactic instruction can come at the expense of growth, change, and the capacity to make useful generalizations.

Socratic questioning

Socratic questioning can facilitate supervisee creativity and learning if it is done in an atmosphere of genuine curiosity and exploration, e.g., an emphasis on 'wondering' together. Such questioning encourages imagination if the supervisor does not have 'the correct answer' too firmly in mind. The downside of such questioning is that it leads to a sort of demeaning interrogation when it devolves into an exercise of 'Guess what I am thinking.' Such interrogation can be especially damaging to the therapeutic alliance if a supervisee is prone to shame and not a good guesser about what the supervisor is thinking.

Encouragement and permission giving

Encouragement and permission are very important elements of the typical supervisory relationship. For the most part, mental health practitioners are individuals with temperaments characterized by reward dependence and persistence. We tend to embark cautiously on new activities while looking for the approval of those in authority or with more experience. Encouragement and permission giving facilitate experimentation. Experimental learning is often impeded when the supervisee is unhelpfully afraid of making a patient angry, sad, sexual aroused, dependent, etc. In this situation, there may be a mutual reluctance on the part of the patient and supervisee to disturb a familiar pattern of adaptation or comfortable defensive posture. Conflicts over voyeurism may lead a supervisee to avoid seeking details where specific information is critical, i.e., the masturbatory fantasies of a patient conflicted about sexual orientation. The goal of encouragement and permission is to provide a therapeutically optimal balance of internal freedom with professional restraint. The downside of encouragement and permission-giving interventions is that they can become a burden or demand to perform. The supervisee needs to be ready (or at least almost ready) to inquire, and the supervisor can judge readiness very imperfectly. Exhortations to ask specific questions on the part of the supervisor are generally ill advised and specifically ill advised when they specify the form or language of the therapeutic interventions.

Clarification and confrontation

Clarifications and confrontations about explicit but unacknowledged aspects of the supervisee's observable attitudes or behaviors are the beginnings of a shift in emphasis in the supervisor/supervisee relationship. Clarification involves summarizing congruencies among supervisee reports of a particular case or cases or inquiring about unreported subjective feelings of the supervisee regarding a patient/supervisee interaction. Confrontations involve highlighting expressed inconsistencies in supervisee comments ('You had established a policy that you would charge the patient for cancellations given without 24-hour notice and yet you volunteered to not charge for the session missed because of a possible thunderstorm'). Such confrontations are important steps in helping the supervisee to understand and contain affects in the patient/therapist relationship. Both understanding and containment are facilitated when supervisee affects become the focus of attention. However, this shift from a focus on the patient to a focus on the supervisee inevitably increases the tension in the supervisory relationship and creates a potential for narcissistic injury on the part of the supervisee. The supervisory relationship is inherently unequal and should not be exploited to force a supervisee to reveal highly personal information about the supervisor's personal history or private mental life. Supervisee readiness to embark on such self-reflection should be considered when the safety of a patient is not at stake.

Supervisory interpretation

Supervisory interpretations include interpretations of feelings, psychodynamic factors, motivations, and defenses. Interpretation of negative affect (embarrassment about one's acting on curiosity, feeling insecure as a therapist when being devalued by a patient, etc.) can both add depth to learning and decrease the tension in the supervisor and supervisee relationship by placing something 'on the table' that had been important but not discussed. Interpretation of a motivation, 'I think you were afraid of making the patient angry.' if correct can often lead to an important discussion of an inhibition to therapeutic action that can be overcome with assistance. Interpretation of a defense by a supervisor ('I wonder if you changed the topic because you were intimidated by the patient's deepening sadness and grief?') can help the supervisee both to self-monitor changes and also begin to explore a potential countertransference problem. However, interpretation of defense generally increases supervisee anxiety and is best done after a workable educational alliance has been established.

Parallel process

A particular form of interpretative activity in supervision is the interpretation of 'parallel process.' This extraordinary event in supervision was first described in the late 60s and refers to the situation in which a conflict in a patient is reproduced by the supervisee in the supervisory relationship (Ekstein and Wallerstein, 1958). In some psychotherapy education programs, students are introduced to the concept of individual supervision, which can include a specific example of parallel process such as the following:

> A second year male resident was discussing a 21-year-old woman patient who became transiently psychotic while watching a movie, *The Exorcist*. While the patient had a somewhat turbulent adolescence, she never had identified psychopathology before experiencing a sudden intense panic attack while watching the scene where the little girl protagonist masturbates with a crucifix. The patient had returned to a fairly stable anxiety symptoms and no psychotic symptoms about 3 months later when she was referred for dynamic psychotherapy. The resident was a competent and thorough man, somewhat obsessionally organized, and had been presenting the patient's twice a week psychotherapy to his admired, competent, and quite attractive supervisor. In the supervisory session in question, the resident was complaining that the patient seemed reluctant to deepen the therapy and, in fact, was resistant and 'acting out' by coming late, offering important personal revelations only at the very end of the session and was generally slowing down the process. Summing up his observations at the end of the supervisory session, he grossed 'It is as if she does one thing or another to test the therapeutic boundary and to block my vision of her inner life.' The supervisor smiled sweetly and said in a measured tone 'I wonder if what she is doing with you is like your placing your overcoat on top of my clock so that I cannot see when supervision is over?' The resident's hot and reddened face suggested that indeed there was a connection. There was not much more discussed about the resident's enactment of a parallel process in that session.
>
> Nonetheless, the resident was emboldened to confront and eventually interpret his patient's acting out. Together, the resident and patient eventually learned why that scene caused her such grief, but the supervisor never made the resident confess how his supervisor's attractiveness influenced his choice of her for supervision.

This reported supervisory session is offered both to illustrate how interpretation of parallel process added a depth to learning that could not have been obtained by reading or lecture and also to confirm that supervision may include embarrassing but useful educational development. It is an example

that with the right supervisee, enough information, and an adequate alliance the interpretation of a parallel process can capture a defense of the supervisee, which was analogous to the patient's obfuscating behavior. The supervisor's comment increased the supervisee's anxiety but the alliance was good enough for it to be a productive anxiety that promoted learning.

Interpretations are the riskiest form of interventions and can become a sort of 'patient making' of the supervisee. In academic settings, this would be making the supervisee the equivalent of an involuntary patient as supervision is a required assignment. As in the example, the supervisor should not make the supervisee confess too much personal material. For one thing, the supervisor usually has a much weaker data base than a therapist. There is also great potential for misuse because of the power imbalance in the relationship. Nevertheless, an interpretation of parallel process often assists in getting something important into the supervisory discussion. The capacity to make such interpretations is considered by some to be a developmental marker of competency of supervisors (Rodenhauser, 1994).

Role playing

Role playing is a form of supervisory interaction that can be a source of considerable learning. It is also rather fun. The supervisor and supervisee can take the part of either the patient or the therapist in the role playing once adequate information about the patient is presented. While playing the part of the patient, the supervisee often achieves a new level of empathic appreciation of the patient. Role playing also provides the opportunity to observe *in vivo* modeling on the part of the supervisor. Additionally, when playing the therapist, the supervisor often is presented with new information about the kinds of problems the patient presents in psychotherapy as the supervisee enacts those problems.

Supervision of cognitive-behavior therapy

Supervision in CBT is considerably more structured than psychodynamic therapy supervision. Most of the CBT writing on supervision comes from practitioners of Beck's cognitive therapy. In cognitive therapy the supervision session echoes the design of a typical therapy session (Newman, 1998), so it includes key elements such as agenda setting, bridge from the previous supervision session, use of capsule summaries and request for feedback from the supervisee (Liese and Beck, 1997). Structuring supervision in this way models skills the therapist will be using in sessions with patients. Supervisees often comment on how this approach helps them structure their own therapy sessions. Applying this format to supervision also encourages the best use of the time available, particularly if the supervision is in a group. Supervisor and therapist(s) decide together at the beginning of the session which patients are to be discussed and what is the key supervision question. A bridge is made between this and the previous session to remind the participants of the context and promote continuity in case management. Another important structural element is the use of summaries and feedback. Therapists always go away having been asked to outline what they have learned from the meeting and how they will apply this in their next session with the patient. Just as in therapy, there is flexibility within this scaffolding allowing supervisor and therapist to follow other paths and renegotiate the agenda if necessary.

As in psychodynamic therapy, there is an expectation that the therapist will take responsibility for his or her own learning experience. Again, this is made more explicit in cognitive therapy. At the beginning of the supervisory relationship, the therapist is asked about his or her previous experience of cognitive therapy and of therapy in general, and encouraged to think about the strengths and weaknesses in their cognitive therapy skills. This helps towards the construction of some specific learning objectives. For instance, in a 6-month supervision placement on a CBT course participants identified two main skills they wished to develop: (1) case conceptualization, and (2) dealing with patients who find it hard to be focused and just want to talk.

The therapists were then asked to consider these overarching goals when bringing a case to supervision, i.e., is there any material that might be relevant to the skill they are trying to develop. Therapists are expected to prepare for supervision by listening to an audiotape of their therapy session and selecting a 10-minute segment that illustrates their supervision question. Novice therapists often frame their question as 'What do I do next?' but with time and practice they can make the questions they ask more precise and focused, e.g., 'How can I devise a behavioral experiment to help this patient test her fear of social situations.' This approach is very different from psychodynamic therapy supervision, which usually asks the therapist to relate an account of the session as a whole.

Supervision can focus on a number of different areas. Padesky (1997) suggests that the session can address skills acquisition, case conceptualization, the client–therapist relationship, therapist reactions, and supervisory processes. There are a number of methods for addressing these including case discussion, videotape, audiotape, live observation, and role play. Case discussion is probably most useful when issues of conceptualization are raised, because it allows for a general consideration of the patient's history and early experiences, target problems, thoughts and beliefs elicited, etc. Although this is the traditional mode of operating in much supervision it may be less helpful in developing skills or looking at the therapeutic relationship. Cognitive therapists routinely audiotape or videotape their sessions. Listening to a tape of a session is invaluable for identifying skills deficits and observing difficulties in the therapeutic relationship. Therapists are initially a little nervous about presenting tapes for supervision. This can be overcome by the supervisor discussing his or her own experience of training and supervision and the universality of these fears. The therapist's automatic thoughts about taping sessions can also be examined. We often work on the assumption that our tapes must be perfect, forgetting that the whole purpose of supervision is to learn new skills. Group supervision can be useful in this respect, because supervisees soon realize that they are all in the same boat. Listening to others' tapes usually demonstrates that they have similar areas where they need to improve.

Role play is used increasingly in CBT supervision, and this again lends itself well to a group setting. Listening to a tape can help the supervisor to identify an area where the supervisee needs to practice skills. Then a role play can be set up. Perhaps the supervisor begins by demonstrating how to use the technique with the supervisee playing the patient. Then the therapist can practice the technique with the supervisor or another trainee as the patient. John was a novice therapist who was having difficulty setting an agenda with one of his patients. The patient wanted to talk about what had happened during the week and would launch into a blow by blow account of every encounter and irritation that had occurred since they last met. This was taking up a good part of the session and preventing them from getting down to much problem-focused work. John role played the patient and the supervisor modeled how to gently interrupt and remind the patient that this was just the beginning of the session—the therapist and patient needed to decide what it would be most helpful to discuss in the following 50 minutes. This worked well. However, when John then took the role of therapist with another group member as the patient, he failed to prevent her from going on and on. Observing the role play allowed the supervisor to see that John was very good at facilitating emotional expression in his patient. He would nod and show an interest and say 'aha' thus encouraging the patient to talk even more. John then practiced giving less facilitating responses at this agenda setting stage and determined to try this out in his next session.

John's difficulty in intervening with his patient proved to be a result of an underlying belief that if he interrupted a patient he would be seen as rude. Once this belief became clear, the therapist asked the other supervisees if they had similar beliefs. They all confessed to ideas such as 'If I stop a patient talking, they will be upset and won't come back' or 'If I interrupt a patient, they will be angry with me.' John felt less alone in his problem, and we were all able to acknowledge how difficult it can be to act in ways that we know are therapeutic but may not seem 'nice.' As a group we then came up with an alternative belief: 'If I interrupt, it will help me and the patient get more out of therapy.' Identifying and testing therapists' beliefs like this can greatly

aid their development as cognitive therapists. Paolo (1998) gives an account of how her own experience of cognitive therapy supervision allowed her to discover her assumption that she had to keep things calm, smooth, and rational so that the patient did not get too emotional. With the help of her supervisor she created alternative beliefs, such as 'I can handle emotional arousal in myself and others. Genuineness involves intentionally attending to the affect of the given moment. The risks are worth taking,' that she was then able to test in subsequent work with her patient.

Discussion of transference and countertransference is obviously one of the main concerns in psychodynamic therapy supervision. While these issues are given less attention in cognitive therapy, they are by no means ignored. As Liese and Beck (1997, p. 119) remark:

> For more complicated patients, especially those with personality disorders, the therapeutic relationship becomes a central focus in therapy as therapists help patients identify and modify distorted thoughts and beliefs about the therapist (and they are helped to generalize this learning to other relationships). Supervisors encourage therapists to pay careful attention to the interpersonal processes that occur during treatment (i.e., transference and countertransference) and to resolve any therapeutic difficulties as directly as possible.

Transference can often be conceptualized as a compensatory interpersonal strategy that the patient uses with the therapist and with other important people in his or her life. For instance, patients who have experienced significant neglect, abandonment, or rejection, their life may develop beliefs that people cannot be trusted and that the best strategy is to not let anyone get close. This may cause problems in the therapeutic alliance when, for instance, the cognitive therapist asks the patient to record automatic thoughts as a homework assignment. Revealing intimate feelings may be too threatening for the patient, and they may respond by failing to do their homework. If the therapist's countertransference feelings are of irritation and frustration, there is a danger that these will be picked up by the patient and perceived as yet more evidence for their belief that no one can be trusted. The supervisor can identify these problems when the therapist reports these difficulties in case discussion, through listening to the tape of the session or through role play. The transference and countertransference thoughts, feelings, and behavior can be located within the cognitive case conceptualization. A number of options for handling the situation are then available (all framed as ways to test the transference hypothesis):

1. The therapist can elicit the patient's negative thoughts about homework and use guided discovery to relate them to the conceptualization.

2. The therapist can use standard techniques to help the patient test the belief that the therapist cannot be trusted.

3. Recording thoughts and feelings can be formulated as a behavioral experiment to test whether or not it is safe to reveal feelings in therapy.

4. Therapist and patient can collaboratively agree that it is too early in the therapy for the patient to reveal these feelings, and try other, less threatening homework.

A good supervisor uses guided discovery as well as direct advice to help the therapist understand and generate strategies. The supervisory relationship, like therapy, is collaborative, so there would be an open discussion of which of these approaches the therapist thinks would work with the patient as well as which feel most comfortable.

Supervision has always been recognized as a vital aspect of training in CBT, but research in this area has lagged behind research into therapy outcome. Much of the research that has been done can be found in the behavioral therapy and learning disability literature (Milne and James, 2000). Reviewers have concluded that the evidence supports systematic interpersonal skills training as more effective than 'traditional' supervision that focuses on case reports and discussion (Lambert and Ogle, 1997; Milne and James, 2000). Some support for this use of structured learning comes from an unexpected source. Binder and Strupp (1997) when reporting the experience of training therapists in their time-limited dynamic psychotherapy recommend the use of tape recording to aid skills development, and teaching 'precise case conceptualizations, anchored in the patient's experience' and giving 'precise communications about concepts, principles and evaluative feedback.' Their research showed that a trainer who used a rather general supervisory style was less effective than one who was much more specific (e.g., stopped the tape and asked specific questions, confronted therapists when they went 'off-model'). The therapist with the more focused approach achieved a group effect size pre-post training of 3.58 for adherence to the model as opposed to 0.46 for the less focused therapist (Henry *et al.*, 1993). There was also a difference in quality of general psychodynamic technique (effect size 1.29 versus 0.24). A small amount of evidence exists in the cognitive therapy literature supporting the effectiveness of supervision. Beck found that the skills learned in a 3-month training were lost after 9 months. However, if the training was followed up by regular supervision, there was a cumulative increase in competence. Similarly, cognitive therapists showed a training effect over the course of supervision in a trial of psychotherapy for substance misuse. Supportive-expressive therapists and drug counselors on the other hand did not.

In summary, supervision in CBT has characteristics in common with psychodynamic therapy (interest in case conceptualization, an assumption that therapists will take personal responsibility for their work, attention to the therapeutic relationship and focus on therapists' beliefs). The main differences are in the style and format of therapy. CBT supervision sessions are structured and focused and utilize a number of methods that are not routinely used in psychodynamic therapy supervision (listening to tapes of session and role play). The field is open for research investigating whether or not these specific supervision techniques facilitate learning in the way that cognitive therapists believe.

Use of supervision to assess competency

Documenting the determination of competency has become increasingly critical in mental health professional education. Therefore, most mental health training programs have revised or are in the process of revising evaluation tools to better assess trainees' competence in multiple modes of psychotherapy. Most training programs are also implementing strategies to make programmatic changes in teaching psychotherapies based on accreditation requirements, program feedback, and/or trainee performance trends as evidenced by trainees' individual evaluations. Individual supervision provides an excellent opportunity to follow trainees' progress in attaining the psychotherapy knowledge, skills, and attitudes consistent with being competent in multiple modes of psychotherapy.

By definition, individual supervision occurs on a regular and recurring basis (usually two supervisors weekly for an entire year during every year of psychiatry residency training). This construct of individual supervision is ideal for assessing competency because therapist trainees' knowledge, skills, and attitudes can be followed, and hopefully directly observed, repeatedly by the same person over an extended period of time. Individual supervision (multiple observations by the same person over an extended period of time) provides useful information that is not available from most other existing standard assessment methods [multiple choice tests, clinical attending evaluations, oral examinations, Objective Structured Clinical Evaluation (OSCE), etc.]. As good assessment is a form of learning and should provide guidance and support to address learning needs (Epstein and Hundert, 2002), individual supervision is designed to accomplish exactly such learning and guidance. Few validated strategies to assess actual clinical practice exist in all of medicine or mental health training. Individual supervision seems to come very close to assessing trainee competency as evidenced in actual clinical practice, at least for the practice of psychotherapy. To enhance further its usefulness in the competency assessment of psychotherapy knowledge and skills, individual supervision should include some form of direct observation. This could include actual contact with patients that the therapist trainee sees for therapy, or videotaped or audiotaped recordings of actual psychotherapy sessions, or less ideally, carefully taken process notes.

To improve interrater reliability among supervisors, standardized rating forms might be helpful for supervisors to use when viewing videotaped or audiotaped psychotherapy sessions of supervisees.

An example of a specific written psychotherapy evaluation tool is included at the end of this chapter (Appendix 42.1). Key elements of this evaluation tool include the following: (1) an expectation and reminder to faculty to provide mid-point feedback to the therapist trainee being evaluated; (2) a space for faculty to indicate information sources used on which to base their evaluation (trainee report, direct observation, videotape or audiotape review, record review, or other); and (3) a Likert scale to evaluate knowledge and skills in five forms of psychotherapy, which is designed to be as effective of an evaluation tool for trainees beginning to learn psychotherapy as for the most experienced trainees. Beginning therapists would be expected to receive evaluations of 1, 2, or 3, depending on their native empathic abilities and previous experiences. More experienced trainees would be expected to receive evaluations of 3, 4, or 5, again depending somewhat on their native empathic skills. Remediation programs (didactic and clinical) would need to be designed to raise the level of competency in any areas of knowledge of skills consistently evaluated as not competent. Programmatic changes (didactic or clinical) would need to be made if many or most trainees were consistently evaluated as not competent or approaching competency in any single knowledge or skill area or for any given type of psychotherapy.

Use of this type of psychotherapy evaluation tool may alter the supervisor–supervisee relationship. The expectation that supervisors evaluate supervisee competency, rather than only providing feedback to help teach the knowledge and skills of psychotherapy, expands the role of individual supervision and 'ups the ante' of the supervisory alliance. In addition to teaching psychotherapy and to assuring that competent patient care is being provided, supervisors will now be expected to assess competency in doing psychotherapy. One might assume that 'assuring competent care' is equivalent to 'assuring trainee competency in doing psychotherapy'. It is the authors' contention that these are, in fact, two different supervisor tasks or responsibilities. Training program directors will likely need to demonstrate that they have structures in place to adequately train supervisors to fulfill all three of their key responsibilities (education, clinical care, and competency assessment). Such structures might include new supervisor training sessions, supervisor workshops or retreats, or systematic evaluation of supervisors.

Evaluation of supervisee and supervisor

Feedback and evaluation are critical components of any educational endeavor; however, they are all too often given only very cursory attention and handled in a haphazard fashion. As an academic mental health professional providing supervision, one is obligated to dedicate sufficient time, reflection, and energy to the process of feedback during the supervisory process so that appropriate behavioral changes can occur in trainees. In this section, the differences between feedback and evaluation will be discussed and some barriers to their effective implementation considered.

Though the terms are often used interchangeably, there are important differences between feedback and evaluation that have earned significant recent attention in academic psychiatry and education in general. Frequently, we as teachers are guilty of utilizing evaluative terms and techniques when feedback would be more in order. Consistency in this separation is much trickier than might first be imagined and requires continuous practice and thoughtful, self-reflection to master.

In short, feedback is intended to be *formative*, while evaluation is *summative* in nature. In this sense, formative relates to an ongoing process of growth and development while summative is defined as a conclusion or final assessment. There are important differences in the manner in which a supervisor provides feedback and evaluation that help to maintain this separation.

Feedback, when used properly, molds and improves behavior in the future by identifying strengths and correcting weaknesses or deficiencies.

To do so, feedback must be exquisitely specific, down to the finest of details. Though this might seem to be 'nit picking' and impossibly tedious, it is only with specificity that desired modifications of behavior can be recognized and internalized effectively. Evaluation provides subjective judgment about behavior that has already happened with a final assessment of the quality of that behavior. Feedback ideally employs neutral statements of observed fact with little use of adjectives, whereas evaluation defines the acceptability and quality of a performance compared with a known or presumed benchmark. Feedback should be provided throughout a learning experience and in innumerable, small aliquots, while evaluations are intended for use after educational experiences have been completed and generally in a single, comprehensive format.

It is probably of value to illustrate some comparative examples of feedback statements compared with evaluation statements.

Feedback: You collected information about the patient's developmental history (*fact*), but I did not hear you discuss the provocative relationship he mentioned with his cousin (*fact*).

Evaluation: Your interview skills are quite good (*judgment*) and you develop solid (*judgment*) rapport with patients, but you do not explore sexuality as much as I would like to see at your level of training (*judgment*).

Feedback: It is important for you to recognize that your strong emotions in this case may arise from the difficult and competitive relationship with your father that (*fact*) you told me you anticipated when you first received the referral.

Evaluation: You have an excellent (*judgment*) grasp of the theoretical basis and implementation of the ideas of transference and countertransference and are beginning to translate them into an appropriately chosen long-term therapy case.

In psychotherapy supervision, as in any educational venture, feedback and evaluation must be bidirectional, with flow of corrective comments from learner to teacher as well as the other way around. As mentioned elsewhere in this chapter, the supervisee's goals and expectations for the supervisory work should be explicit from the beginning and the supervisee must feel free to adjust supervisor behavior to steer continuously toward these ends in a fashion that is tolerable to the trainee. Only in a state of mutual respect, safety, and openness can this give and take occur appropriately. If the process has become too intense or stimulating for the leaner, it must be acceptable for him/her to temper the relationship to a more suitable level. This presents some risk for narcissistic injury on the part of the supervisor, in contrast to the supervisee injuries mentioned previously in this chapter, but the more experienced supervisor will have well-developed resources to manage this challenge.

This last situation, that of a wounded party in the supervisor–supervisee dyad, segues well into a discussion of some potential barriers to effective feedback and evaluation. Paramount among these perhaps is the fear within both teacher and student that feedback will have consequences beyond those that were intended (Ende, 1983). This is most often the fear when one is forced to provide feedback that is critical and negative in nature. Few people enjoy being told of their deficiencies, but most tolerate it with reasonable grace. There is often great fear, however, that even well-intentioned comments have the potential to elicit a powerful, emotional reaction on the part of the person receiving the feedback/evaluation. Anger, defensiveness, hurt, sorrow, self-deprecation, and other difficult responses might manifest in the recipient of feedback, whether or not the information was provided in an untoward manner. Trainees and teachers alike can experience feedback as a comment on personal value or worth, leading to great risk for narcissistic injury. In situations where evaluations play a role in promotion or awards, these emotional reactions can sour the process of fair assessment and lead to detrimental results for faculty or student. Finally, the relationship might be fractured irreparably and the popularity of the supervisor might be diminished. While the extreme among these responses are relatively rare, the fear of these unexpected and unintended outcomes conspires within supervisors and supervisees both to foster collusion to avoid feedback and evaluation altogether. The result then is often a perfunctory and grossly inadequate, 'Great job,' or 'You're doing fine, just fine.'

A second impediment to effective feedback and evaluation is the increasing absence of directly observed behavior within training settings. Mechanisms of observation (videotape, audiotape, process notes, sitting in for a session, etc.) have been discussed for their advantages and drawbacks elsewhere in the chapter. It is important, though, in the context of feedback and evaluation to expand on the necessity of direct observation in providing the all important data that will be used during comment on trainee behavior. Particularly in our very subjective field, it is a must to be aware of the literature on trainee self-assessment of interpersonal skill. A number of studies have (Donnelly *et al.*, 2000; Stewart *et al.*, 2000; Zonia and Stommel, 2000; Tulsky *et al.*, 2001; Davis, 2002; Millis *et al.*, 2002) demonstrated the inability of resident trainees in various specialties to self-assess their own interpersonal skill while confirming attending physicians ability to judge accurately these same interactions with patients, both real and standardized, on identical interpersonal measures. This has tremendous ramifications for the supervisory process, essentially demanding that the supervisor directly observe the psychotherapy in some fashion so as to confirm a supervisee's reports of rapport and therapeutic alliance. Only then can accurate and useful feedback be provided.

Some final barriers to effective feedback and evaluation are the significant amount of time, stamina, and organizational skill required to take advantage of the many opportunities for comment on a supervisee's behavior. It is much easier, and often much more intriguing, to passively allow the very titillating stories encountered in supervisory work to evolve unhindered by pauses to address therapeutic technique, countertransference, and the like. Likewise, it is easier to forego the difficult task of formulating specific and thoughtful individualized feedback for each trainee, not to mention the thoroughness required to complete the lengthy evaluation forms currently required by most psychotherapy training programs. Educational efforts are crippled, though, without accurate, specific, bidirectional feedback and thoughtful evaluation, creating a potent argument for persistence in overcoming the many barriers to their provision. We as clinicians owe this a duty to our patients, specifically those that we manage from afar within the supervisory process.

Termination of supervisory relationship

In a manner somewhat similar but perhaps less pronounced than in psychodynamic psychotherapy, the termination phase of the supervisory relationship presents its own opportunity for new learning. In 'good enough' supervision, the supervisor becomes internalized by the supervisee. In a thoughtful termination, there is some discussion of the terms of future availability for the supervisor in either the same or a different relationship. Separation, like attachment is a powerful motivator and evokes new and often deeper feelings. It is also an important opportunity in which implicitly or explicitly, knowingly or unknowingly, the supervisor provides powerful modeling for the supervisee. It is important to set a specific date for the last supervisory session, which should be determined at least a month in advance. That date should be specific and the termination of supervision should not be minimized. Although previous formal and considerable informal feedback is likely to have taken place, there should be some use of a final supervisory session as a time of mutual evaluation. The supervisor should help the supervisee evaluate what has been learned in this supervision and what needs to be learned in future elements of psychotherapy education. Termination is a good time to review the initial supervisory goals and to specify what were disappointments, any unanticipated positive products, and what contributed to both the disappointments and serendipitous outcomes. It is also important that the supervisor ask for a genuine evaluation. However, as the power differential and administrative reporting line continue to exist, this is often the most difficult challenge. Asking for advice on how to become a better supervisor may be somewhat more productive as will discussions in which the supervisor broaches supervisor limitations that he or she knows about in advance.

Both parties should attend to absences during the time of the identified termination process. Absences will often reflect defensively minimized importance of the separation and the prior supervisory relationship. It is a particularly important time to be vigilant about 'countertransference' type responses both as supervisor and supervisee. Occasionally, the termination phase will produce phenomena analogous to the psychotherapeutic concept of 'acting out' in the form of a crisis or a rationalization for continuing the relationship in some other form.

When discussing disappointments of the supervisory relationship, it is important that both parties recognize that every relationship has its disappointments, but also that some people are more prone to disappointments than others. A particular question is structuring the final supervisory session and whether or not there will be some form of 'gift.' There is frequently a tendency to want to end the supervisory relationship with a celebration of some sort as opposed to a 'typical session.' It is best to avoid extremes. The terms of continuing engagement between supervisor and supervisee are generally more variable than that between patient and therapist. A compromise that is often satisfactory is some sort of informal lunch meeting. If that is done, the more evaluative and feedback portions of the termination phase are best done in advance of the lunch.

The terms of continuing engagement between supervisor and supervisee vary widely. Supervisors have written books on supervision with a supervisee. On the other extreme, there was an unfortunate incident of another prominent analyst omitting to tell a supervisee about a published report of their relationship, which resulted in unhappy feelings and litigation.

Concluding comments

The authors wish to conclude with a reminder that psychotherapy supervision is both art and science and best done when it is experienced as a calling as opposed to an obligation. It is also a source of enormous professional gratification and joy. As is unfortunately the case in psychiatric, psychology, and social work education, this chapter has not given deserved attention to the education of psychotherapy supervisors. It is somewhat beyond the charge of the chapter, but it also reflective of how unevenly our major psychotherapy disciplines prepare senior members for roles as supervisors. Almost all of us support (at least in theory) psychotherapy education for new faculty, more psychotherapy supervision research, and for regular meetings of supervisor faculty to discuss the challenges, joys, and academic perspective on supervision. At a time when medical psychotherapy education takes place in an atmosphere of increasing emphasis on financial accountability and productivity, such valuable and important educational support of supervisors is achieved only with great effort on the part of departmental leadership. We support this effort enthusiastically. The support of competence in supervision will be a major determinant of the future of psychotherapy as a core element of the identity of our professions.

References

Binder, J. L. and Strupp, H. H. (1997). Supervision of psychodynamic psychotherapies. In: C. E. Watkins, ed. *Handbook of psychotherapy supervision*, pp. 44–62. New York: John Wiley & Sons.

Davis, J. D. (2002). Comparison of faculty, peer, self, and nurse assessment of obstetrics and gynecology residents. *Obstetrics and Gynecology*, **99**(4), 647–51.

Doeherman, M. J. G. (1976). Parallel process in supervision and psychotherapy. *Bulletin of the Menninger Clinic*, **40**, 1–104.

Donnelly, M. B., *et al.* (2000). Assessment of residents' interpersonal skills by faculty proctors and standardized patients: a psychometric analysis. *Academic Medicine*, **75**(10, October supplement), S93–8.

Ekstein, R. and Wallerstein, R. S. (1958). *The teaching and learning of psychotherapy*. New York: Basic Books.

Ende, J. (1983). Feedback in clinical medical education. *Journal of American Medical Association*, **250**(6), 777–81.

Epstein, R. M. and Hundert, E. M. (2002). Defining and assessing professional competence, *Journal of American Medical Association*, **287**(2), 226–35.

Freud, S. (1958). Observations on transference love. In: J. Strachey, ed. *The standard edition of the complete psychological works of Sigmund Freud*, Vol. XII, pp. 157–74, London: Hogarth Press.

Gabbard, G. O. (2000). Psychodynamic assessment of the patient. In: *Psychodynamic psychiatry in clinical practice*, pp. 67–88. Washington, DC: American Psychiatric Press.

Hantoot, M. S. (2000). Lying in psychotherapy supervision. *Academic Psychiatry*, **24**(4), 179–87.

Havens, L. (1978). Explorations in the use of language in psychotherapy: simple empathic statements. *Psychiatry*, **41**, 336–45.

Henry, W. P., Schacht, T. E., Strupp, H. H., Butler, S. F., and Binder, J. L. (1993). Effects of training in time-limited dynamic psychotherapy: mediators of therapists' responses to training. *Journal of Consulting and Clinical Psychology*, **61**, 441–7.

Jacobs, D., David, P., and Meyer, D. J. (1995). *The supervisory encounter: a guide for teachers of psychodynamic psychotherapy and psychoanalysis*. New Haven, CT: Yale University Press.

Kantrowitz, J. L. (2002). The triadic match: the interactive effect of supervisor, candidate, and patient. *Journal of the American Psychoanalytic Association*, **50**(3), 939–68.

Lambert, M. J. and Ogles, B. M. (1997). The effectiveness of psychotherapy supervision. In: C. E. Watkins, ed. *Handbook of psychotherapy supervision*, pp. 421–46. New York: John Wiley & Sons.

Liese, B. S. and Beck, J. S. (1997). Cognitive therapy supervision. In: C. E. Watkins, ed. *Handbook of Psychotherapy Supervision*, pp. 114–33. John Wiley & Sons New York.

MacKinnon, R. A. and Yudofsky, S. C. (1991). *Principles of the psychiatric evaluation*, pp. 247–83. Philadelphia: J. P. Lippincott Press.

Millis, S. R., *et al.* (2002). Assessing physicians' interpersonal skills: do patients and physicians see eye-to-eye? *American Journal of Physical Medicine & Rehabilitation*, **81**(12), 946–51.

Milne, D. and James, I. (2000). A systematic review of effective cognitive-behavioral supervision. *British Journal of Clinical Psychology*, **39**, 111–27.

Mohl, P. C., *et al.* (1990). Psychotherapy training for the psychiatrist of the future. *American Journal of Psychiatry*, **147**, 7–13.

Newman, C. (1998). Therapeutic and supervisory relationships in cognitive-behavioral therapies: similarities and differences. *Journal of Cognitive Psychotherapy: An International Quarterly*, **12**, 96–108.

Osler, W. (1947). Aequanimitas. *Aequanimitas: with other addresses to medical students, nurses, and practitioners of medicine*, pp. 3–11. New York: McGraw-Hill.

Padesky, C. (1997) Developing cognitive therapist competency: teaching and supervision models. In: P. M. Salkovskis, ed. *Frontiers of cognitive therapy*, pp. 266–92. New York: Guilford Press.

Paolo, S. B. (1998). Receiving supervision in cognitive therapy: a personal account. *Journal of Cognitive Psychotherapy: an International Quarterly*, **12**, 153–62.

Perry, S., Cooper, A. M., and Michels, R. (1987). The psychodynamic formulation: its purpose, structure, and clinical application. *American Journal of Psychiatry*, **144**(5), 543–50.

Rodenhauser, P. (1994). Toward a multidimensional model for psychotherapy supervision based on developmental stages. *Journal of Psychotherapy Practice and Research*, **3**, 1–15.

Stewart, J., *et al.* (2000). Clarifying the concepts of confidence and competence to produce appropriate self-evaluation measurement scales. *Medical Education*, **34**, 903–9.

Stoudemire, A. (1998). Biopsychosocial assessment and clinical formulation. In: A. Stoudemire, ed. *Clinical psychiatry for medical students*, pp. 70–85. Philadelphia, PA: J. B. Lippincott.

Tulsky, D. S., *et al.* (2001). Rating physician interpersonal skills: do patients and physicians see eye-to-eye? *ACGME website* 2001 Available at http://www.acgme.org/outcome/implement/rsvpTemplate.asp?rsvpID=8 Accessed Jan. 26, 2003.

Watkins, C. E. (1997). Some concluding thoughts about psychotherapy supervision. In: C. E. Watkins, ed. *Handbook of psychotherapy supervision*, pp. 603–16. New York: John Wiley Press.

Zonia, S. C. and Stommel, M. (2000). Interns' self-evaluations compared with their faculty's evaluations. *Academic Medicine*, **75**(7), 742.

Appendix 42.1

BAYLOR COLLEGE OF MEDICINE
PSYCHOTHERAPY SUPERVISION EVALUATION
PGY-II, -III, and -IV

Please provide formal, mid-point feedback and complete the signature blanks below <u>quarterly</u> during the psychotherapy supervision period.

Please complete the entire evaluation form semi-annually (usually December and June) during the supervision period.

Resident_____ Supervisor_____
Dates of Evaluation_____

Quarterly Review (verbal feedback) provided on _____. Resident_____

Supervisor_____

Information source (check all that apply):   Resident Report   Direct Observation   Videotape
     Audiotape   Record review   Other

1	2	3	4	5	N/A
Not competent	Approaching competency	Satisfactorily competent	Highly competent	Exceptionally competent	Not applicable

<u>Instructions</u>: *Using the key above, please indicate level of competency by circling the appropriate number 1-5 below. If the category is not appropriate to PGY level or therapeutic experience please circle N/A.*

I.   FUNDAMENTAL PSYCHOTHERAPY SKILLS

IA. Boundaries

1. Ability to manage therapeutic boundaries, including personal space, handling of   1   2   3   4   5
gifts, confidentiality, etc.
2. Ability to define therapeutic contract with patient, including time, fee setting,   1   2   3   4   5
and collections

IB. Therapeutic Alliance

1. Ability to establish rapport and form a therapeutic alliance   1   2   3   4   5

2. Ability to interact non-judgmentally and empathically   1   2   3   4   5

3. Ability to recognize cultural/religious influence in therapeutic process   1   2   3   4   5

IC. Resistance/Defenses

1. Ability to recognize resistances and deal with them effectively to maintain   1   2   3   4   5
stability of the therapeutic process
2. Ability to describe patient's major defensive organization   1   2   3   4   5

ID. Goals

1. Understands the major theoretical frameworks of psychotherapy   1   2   3   4   5

2. Selects an appropriate theoretical orientation for a specific patient   1   2   3   4   5

3. Assesses the patient's progress in therapy   1   2   3   4   5

4. Manages the termination phase effectively   1   2   3   4   5

1 Not competent	2 Approaching Competency	3 Satisfactorily competent	4 Highly competent	5 Exceptionally competent	N/A Not applicable

II. SUPPORTIVE PSYCHOTHERAPY

1.	Ability to identify defense mechanisms while supporting adaptive defenses	1 2 3 4 5 N/A
2.	Ability to assume an active stance including ego lending and ego building	1 2 3 4 5 N/A
3.	Ability to elicit and appropriately contain affect	1 2 3 4 5 N/A
4.	Ability to employ crisis intervention techniques	1 2 3 4 5 N/A
5.	Ability to utilize stress management techniques	1 2 3 4 5 N/A

III. PSYCHODYNAMIC PSYCHOTHERAPY

1.	Ability to recognize central dynamic issues	1 2 3 4 5 N/A
2.	Ability to conceptualize a psychodynamic formulation	1 2 3 4 5 N/A
3.	Ability to link understanding of the patient's past, present, and transference patterns to thoughts, feelings, and behaviors	1 2 3 4 5 N/A
4.	Ability to recognize and use transference and countertransference in the therapeutic process	1 2 3 4 5 N/A
5.	Ability to clarify, confront, and make interpretations at appropriate times	1 2 3 4 5 N/A

IV. COMBINED PSYCHOTHERAPY AND PSYCHOPHARMACOLOGY

1.	Ability to integrate psychotherapeutic and psychopharmacologic interventions in a mutually beneficial manner, so that neither is neglected	1 2 3 4 5 N/A
2.	Conducts a complete medication assessment within the context of a psychotherapeutic process, while making interpretations and empathic comments	1 2 3 4 5 N/A
3.	Appreciates the potential psychodynamic issues around the prescribing of medications (resistance, compliance, transitional object, etc.)	1 2 3 4 5 N/A
4.	Ability to assess suicidality on an ongoing basis as it relates to the prescribing of potentially dangerous medications	1 2 3 4 5 N/A
5.	Provides education about medications in a manner that complements the psychotherapeutic technique, appreciating the limitations of each treatment modality	1 2 3 4 5 N/A

2

1 Not Competent	2 Approaching competency	3 Satisfactorily competent	4 Highly competent	5 Exceptionally competent	N/A Not applicable

V. COGNITIVE/BEHAVIORAL PSYCHOTHERAPY

1. Ability to set a collaborative agenda for each session, manage time limits, and foster the patient's eventual termination and self-management   1 2 3 4 5 N/A

2. Ability to help the patient recognize automatic thoughts, maladaptive assumptions, and core beliefs/schemas   1 2 3 4 5 N/A

3. Ability to identify and alter cognitive distortions in order to alleviate symptoms   1 2 3 4 5 N/A

4. Ability to help patients develop new, more rational responses to automatic thoughts and core beliefs   1 2 3 4 5 N/A

5. Ability to design and help patients plan and implement behavioral experiments such as activity monitoring with reward paradigms, in vivo exposure, and relaxation   1 2 3 4 5 N/A

VI. BRIEF PSYCHOTHERAPY

1. The resident can recognize a patient with sufficient ego strength and psychological mindedness to pursue brief psychotherapy   1 2 3 4 5 N/A

2. The resident is familiar with the many models and paradigms used in brief psychotherapy, including supportive techniques, dynamic/expressive options, and manualized techniques   1 2 3 4 5 N/A

3. The resident is aware that central to all brief psychotherapies is the concept of focus, not global characterological change   1 2 3 4 5 N/A

4. The resident can work in the markedly accelerated models of time-limited therapy while still maintaining a therapeutic alliance and holding environment   1 2 3 4 5 N/A

5. Ability to work toward effective termination from the outset of treatment   1 2 3 4 5 N/A

COMMENTS:

Semi-annual review   DATE: _____

SIGNATURE: _____   SIGNATURE: _____
                Resident   Supervisor

43 Brief and time-limited psychotherapy

Glenys Parry, Anthony D. Roth, and Ian B. Kerr

Introduction

A major shift has occurred in the last 20 years from delivery of long-term psychotherapy to briefer, time-limited approaches. This is most marked in 'managed care' and public service contexts. There are many reasons for this: there have been immense pressures from healthcare funders for cost-effectiveness and cost containment; innovation and refinement of technique has resulted in more efficient therapy; research trials expediently focus on shorter-term approaches, which then become influential; the conventional psychoanalytic view that 'longer is better' has been increasingly challenged by the evidence; and many therapists have espoused brief approaches because they see intrinsic merit and therapeutic potential in this way of working.

There has also been a sea change in the way different therapeutic paradigms approach treatment length. At one time, conventional wisdom suggested that psychodynamic therapy was invariably a long-term enterprise and cognitive-behavioral therapies (CBT) were briefer. This is no longer the case, with the development of a range of brief psychodynamic therapies (to be discussed in this chapter) and of longer-term behavioral and cognitive therapies. These may extend to 2 years or beyond for personality disorders—such as dialectical behavior therapy (Linehan, 1993) and schema-focused therapy (Young, 1990; Young *et al.*, 2003)—and for psychosis (Perris, 1989; Perris and McGorry, 1999).

'Brief' is a relative term, and the time span of 'brief' therapy can vary between one and about 25 sessions, from a single meeting to a year's work. We make a distinction between very brief therapy (one to five sessions, less than 2 months), brief therapy (six to 16 sessions, 2–6 months), and time-limited therapy (17–30 sessions, 6–9 months), while recognizing that such distinctions are inevitably arbitrary. A common definition of brief therapy is up to 25 sessions in duration (Koss and Butcher, 1986; Messer and Warren, 1995).

However, the majority of therapy delivered falls into this category, either because the therapy offered is short term by design, or because although the therapeutic modality is long term or open-ended, by the 25th session most patients have decided to leave (Garfield, 1994; Hansen *et al.*, 2002).

It also used to be common wisdom that only highly selected client groups were capable of benefiting from brief work, and that these methods were unsuitable for people with more severe and complex mental health problems. Now there are powerful arguments and well-developed methods for offering shorter-term interventions to people with higher levels of distress and impairment. For example, Garfield (1995) challenges the assumption that if people do not respond to short-term therapy, they will benefit from long-term work. Leibovich (1983) argues that many people with borderline personality disorder are best suited to short-term integrative psychotherapy. Winston *et al.* (1991) describe brief therapy for personality disorders, which includes CBT and psychodynamic elements and Ryle (1997) has developed a 24-session version of a brief integrative therapy (CAT) for a range of people with severe and complex psychological difficulties including personality disorders.

We have therefore reached the stage in the history of psychotherapy where brief or time-limited therapy is mainstream practice and it will continue to be the norm for psychotherapeutic work to be conducted briefly and to time limits. In the future, 'brief therapy' as a specific topic may seem odd, and perhaps a separate chapter on 'time unlimited therapy' or 'long-term therapy' will be commissioned for future editions of this volume. Shapiro *et al.* (2003) make the point that the fifth edition of Bergin and Garfield's *Handbook of psychotherapy and behavior change*, a key psychotherapy research text, contains no chapter on brief psychotherapy as most contemporary psychotherapy research concerns treatments planned to be no longer than 25 sessions. They also suggest that currently, only psychodynamic therapists would describe a 25-session treatment as 'brief'.

Having said this, there are some shared assumptions and common factors across a range of diverse approaches that give the concept of 'brief therapy' some coherence. The first section of this chapter reviews these defining features. The second section gives an overview of brief therapies and describes examples. The third section summarizes research evidence on the length of therapy in relation to its effects and its suitability for a range of clients. The fourth section discusses professional attitudes, training, and competence. The chapter ends with a summary of key points and future priorities for practice, training, and research.

Defining features of brief therapies

Common features of brief therapies include working to a time limit, the therapeutic focus, and therapist activity. Taken together they imply a form of therapy that is perhaps better termed *intensive* rather than brief, compared with longer-term methods that could be described as *extensive* (Malan, 1976; Ryle and Kerr, 2002).

Time limits

Therapies that set a time limit all manage the frustrations and disappointments that this can arouse, in both patients and therapists, but they do so in contrasting ways, either to facilitate them or to minimize them. Despite the polar differences between these views, there is little research evidence base for which of these two approaches leads to the best outcomes, for which clients.

The former approach sees the time limit itself as of immense therapeutic significance and potential. James Mann (1978) is the prime exemplar and most eloquent advocate of this view. The time limit of therapy is seen as a profound metaphor for the finiteness of time itself for any individual. It evokes, he argues, the reality of loss and death, but, if faced and endured, is a powerful maturational experience. Mann gives the time factor most attention, but a number of psychodynamic and relational therapies emphasize setting an exact, nonnegotiable time limit, to facilitate the experience of anxiety, disappointment, and anger. Expressing these warded-off emotions, it is argued, within a facilitating therapeutic relationship, leads to their being safely experienced, assimilated, and mastered. These therapies work on the assumption that what was perceived as catastrophic can be transformed into something both manageable and personally empowering.

Other therapies take the opposite line, reducing the significance of the time limit, either by interpreting it very flexibly, by using follow-up appointments, or by making it clear further therapy will be available in the future 'as needed'. For example, Budman and Gurman (1998) argue that there is little empirical evidence that emphasizing termination in therapy leads to better outcomes, and assert that it is therapists rather than patients who have difficulty ending. They do not see therapy as a 'one-shot' operation, instead preferring to conceptualize the therapist as a 'psychological family doctor', available over the life span to respond to different needs in a developmental process. They also emphasize a team approach, with no one therapist being all things to all patients. Cummings (1991) describes a similar practice, remaining available to patients for return visits and intermittent brief therapy. He describes making an explicit commitment to patients. 'I will never abandon you as long as you need me. In return for that, I want you to join me in a partnership to make me obsolete as soon as possible' (Cummings, 1991, p. 40). Despite, or perhaps because of, this contract, he reports that one episode of therapy only lasts between one and 20 sessions.

On the whole it is those therapies rooted in psychodynamic theories that emphasize the time limit and the therapeutic value of the fixed termination, and those rooted in pragmatic eclecticism, and the cognitive-behavioral approaches, which are less concerned with this.

The use of time in brief therapy goes beyond fixing the number of sessions or setting a time limit. It can include varying the length of sessions, the frequency of sessions, and the flexibility with which therapy is delivered. For example, Mann's rigid adherence to the 12-session limit does not preclude considerable flexibility in how they are delivered. Variations to weekly sessions are mentioned, including in one instance weekly 15-minute sessions for 48 weeks. The key issue is that there is no ambiguity or uncertainty about the pattern and duration of the sessions (Mann, 1978). Budman and Gurman (1988) cite Johnson and Gelso's (1980) review of the effectiveness of time limits to argue that there is little empirical justification for traditional weekly sessions, suggesting that after weekly contact to begin the improvement, time alone is required for continued improvement. They favor more intensive work for four to eight visits, then 'spreading out' the sessions, to reduce dependency and enhance self-efficacy. It could be argued that there is an irresolvable tension between the therapist being responsive, adaptable, and pragmatic, and the requirement to provide a consistent, secure framework, which is not colluding with an unreflective enactment of a dysfunctional relationship pattern. Binder et al. (1987) advocate a compromise where strict time limits are replaced by a 'time-limited attitude' with defined but flexible duration of treatment. There is also potential for research to address these questions empirically.

Therapy focus

The therapeutic focus is the second broad factor shared by most, if not all, brief therapies. It can relate to manifest symptoms or a presenting problem. For example, cognitive therapy was originally a brief problem-focused therapy for depression (Beck, 1979). Most brief cognitive and behavioral therapies have a problem focus, such as panic (Salkovskis and Clark, 1991), although longer-term cognitive therapy with a schema focus has also been developed (McGinn and Young, 1996). The focus for interpersonal therapy (IPT) is developed in the early sessions, relating to one of four problem areas: grief, role disputes, role transitions, and interpersonal deficits (Klerman et al., 1984). Psychodynamic, relational and some eclectic therapies often take an intrapsychic or interpersonal focus, a central emotional dilemma or an issue in personal development. Such a focus is referred to in diverse ways; the 'dynamic focus' (Schact et al., 1984), 'core conflictual relationship theme' (Luborsky and Crits-Cristoph, 1998), 'core neurotic conflict' (Wallerstein and Robbins, 1956), 'nuclear conflict'

(Alexander and French, 1946), 'central issue' (Mann and Goldman, 1982), 'interpersonal-developmental-existential focus' (Budman and Gurman, 1988).

Omer (1993) describes how the focus in brief therapy has tended to be either symptom focused or person oriented, and argues for the value to the therapeutic alliance of combining the two into an integrative focus. Ryle's (1990) CAT is a good example of a therapy using an integrative focus that relates symptoms and presenting problems to underlying 'problem procedures' and 'reciprocal role relationships'. This method is also unusual in the degree to which the focus is made explicit through collaborative work on successive drafts of letters and diagrams.

Safran and Muran (2000) describing their brief relational therapy (BRT) warn against a focus on content. Their conviction that the therapist is inevitably embedded in an enactment of relationship patterns makes them wary of early formulation of the central difficulty. Instead they offer a *process* focus, emphasizing the importance of developing mindfulness, the capacity to observe internal processes and actions in relation to other people. A focus on process rather than content is also characteristic of Hobson's (1985) psychodynamic IPT where the development of a shared language for feelings between therapist and client is one of the primary tasks.

Therapist activity

An active therapist is a feature of working in short-term therapy. In the behavioral and cognitive methods, therapists have always been active, irrespective of the length of treatment, in collaboratively setting an agenda for the session, teaching, giving advice, using Socratic questions in guiding discovery, suggesting structured activities and coaching. In the psychoanalytic and some humanistic traditions, the therapist is relatively less active—waiting for the client to speak at the start of the session, refraining from intervening to end a silence, following the patient's (or client's) train of thought and rarely initiating a topic or actively structuring the session. Indeed, in some forms of psychoanalytic work, the therapist is abstinent to the point of appearing personally opaque. In brief psychodynamic therapies, by contrast, the therapist is more active in interpreting the transference, unconscious conflicts and in confronting resistance. Therapists in eclectic, relational, or integrative modes are also active, for example in clarifying and collaboratively exploring the client's material, negotiating treatment goals, structuring sessions, making links between interactions in the therapist–client relationship and past relationship patterns, and possibly setting or discussing between-session tasks.

Range of applicability

The brief therapies also differ widely in the range of difficulties to which they are considered applicable. Groves (1996) is not unusual in terming this 'patient selection', although of course one is not selecting patients who suit the therapy so much as selecting therapy to suit the patients. The different forms of symptom-focused CBT have intrinsic selection criteria, with separate therapy 'packages' developed for panic, depression, health anxieties, obsessive-compulsive disorders, eating disorders, substance abuse, anger management problems, posttraumatic stress disorders (PTSD), and suicide prevention (Salkovskis, 1996; Clark and Fairburn, 1997). Some brief psychodynamic therapies are restrictive, with long lists of exclusion criteria. For example, Sifneos (1972) considers his Short Term Anxiety Provoking Psychotherapy suitable only for people of above average intelligence, who have had at least one meaningful relationship, are able to express emotion in the assessment, have a specific chief complaint, are motivated to work hard, and have realistic expectations of treatment. Messer (2001) described brief dynamic therapists as appropriately avoiding clients who are too severely disturbed to use an insight-oriented approach or those who need more time to work through their problems, but other brief therapists take a more liberal view of suitability. For example, Wolberg (1965, p. 140) states that 'The best strategy, in my opinion, is to assume that every patient, irrespective of diagnosis, will respond to short-term treatment unless he proves himself refractory to it.' Garfield (1995), has only the three criteria that the client be in touch with reality, is experiencing some discomfort, and has made the effort to seek help. Malan (1976) while emphasizing the importance of thorough psychodynamic assessment in predicting suitability for brief intensive therapy, used the patient's response to trial interpretation during assessment as a guiding principle. He was also very aware that despite considerable effort, therapists are unable to predict very accurately who will do well or badly in brief therapy, a point underlined by Binder *et al.* (1987).

The question of who is more likely to benefit from brief or from longer-term therapy is an empirical one. Although there is still inadequate research evidence to inform many practice decisions, findings on the relationship between treatment length and outcome for clients with different levels of disturbance are beginning to have an impact on service planning and delivery. After describing the range of approaches to brief therapy, we review research on these issues.

From this overview of common features of brief therapies from a range of theoretical backgrounds and practice methods, we can discern some general working assumptions for brief therapies.

- This way of working tends to see therapy as catalyst for change in a complex system rather than as a 'one-shot' curative method.
- Therapists aim to maximize the therapeutic alliance and avoid regression.

Other more specific techniques include:

- intensifying therapy processes through use of a strict time limit, to maximize the therapeutic impact of working through anxiety aroused by termination issues, and
- psychoeducation, collaborative empiricism, and skills in self-observation to foster the alliance and avoid regression.

Although brief and time-limited therapies have demonstrated their worth, there are no grounds for complacency. Despite some good results for briefer therapies in randomized trials, relapse rates are high, particularly in depression. There also remains the difficulty of generalizing good results obtained in randomized controlled trials to routine service settings, where outcomes depend on many other factors, including treatment milieu, skills of staff, referral practices, availability, and access. For example, despite growth in evidence-based clinical practice guidelines (Department of Health, 2001; Parry *et al.*, 2003a) service configurations are not delivering the therapies likely to be effective for those who need them. For example, a UK survey showed that in the year 2000 very few people with phobic anxiety were receiving CBT (Office of National Statistics, 2000).

Nor can we assume brief work is a panacea. There are cogent arguments for 'more is better', mainly arising from naturalistic studies of dose–response (Hansen *et al.*, 2002) and from consumer surveys of psychotherapy recipients (Seligman, 1995). The former show that, although there are 'diminishing returns' from longer-term therapy, improvement rates continue to rise up to 2 years. The latter suggests that among individuals who choose to reply to a consumer survey, those who have received longer-term therapy are on the whole more satisfied with their progress and rate their own improvement more highly than those in brief therapy encounters.

There is an argument that a distinction needs to be made between therapies given under private contractual arrangements and those funded by third parties, either in health insurance schemes or public sector provision. In the first case, the individual tries to make an informed judgment on what therapy length and style they will find most beneficial and negotiates this with their chosen therapist. In the second, issues of efficient use of finite resources and equity of access also come into play, at the level of whole-system provision. A balance is inevitably struck between individual benefit and overall benefit at the level of the population served. Unfortunately the types of evidence needed for such policy decisions to be well-informed is thin on the ground, with most trials designed to address clinical questions rather than service ones (Halpern, 1999). The growth in health services research methods in psychotherapy is likely to continue to develop, to provide information on relative costs and effectiveness using pragmatic trial designs with economic evaluation. Brief therapies are potentially cost efficient, although as cost-offset may be most marked for severe presentations,

longer-term therapy too has the potential for cost-effectiveness (Gabbard *et al.*, 1997).

Overview of brief therapies

In describing the various models and modalities in shorter-term and time-limited therapy, there are several possible ways to classify them. Groves (1996) uses the categories of interpretive, existential, cognitive, interpersonal, and eclectic. Within dynamic therapies, Messer and Warren (1995) draw on Greenberg and Mitchell's (1983) distinction between drive/structural and relational approaches. The categories used here are broad—psychodynamic, cognitive/behavioral, relational, eclectic, and very brief—and the boundaries between them are not rigid. (For example, one could categorize aspects of Malan's early work as relational and Ryle's method as cognitive.) We emphasize individual psychotherapy, while acknowledging systemic methods and brief couple, family, and group therapies. The overview describes a broad range of therapies that are brief by design not by default, but inevitably it is not exhaustive—other methods are fully described elsewhere in this volume. Nor shall we attempt to describe the theoretical basis of these different paradigms, which is also better covered in other chapters.

Psychodynamic approaches

Early psychoanalytic therapies were much briefer than their successors— some of Freud's early therapies were very brief indeed, famously no longer than a walk in the woods. Modern brief psychodynamic therapies have their roots in the pioneering work of Ferenczi (1920) and Alexander and French (1946). The latter authors felt that, although psychoanalysts knew 'there is no simple correlation between therapeutic results and the length and intensity of treatment', they clung to a belief that quick therapeutic results could not be genuine. They believed they must be either transitory outcomes due to suggestion or an escape into 'pseudo-health'—a view that many still hold today. In the 1960s, Malan, influenced by Balint, both British psychoanalytic therapists practicing in London, and Sifneos in Boston USA, developed methods for shorter-term psychodynamic therapy. The influence of these methods has been far reaching. The result has been, for selected patients, the widespread application of psychoanalytic principles over 10–25 sessions, where therapists reflect on, clarify, interpret, and confront interpersonal patterns, wishes, conflicts, and defenses (Messer and Warren, 1995; Messer, 2001).

Balint was a psychoanalyst whose considerable innovations were met with some distrust and skepticism from the analytic establishment. His experimental work with shorter-term therapy depended on the idea of establishing a focus for the therapy and working persistently with this, rather than being distracted by other aspects of the patient's difficulties (Balint *et al.*, 1972). While orthodox in his use of structural psychodynamic theory and technique, he was a trailblazer both for developing the focus in shorter-term therapy and the value of psychotherapeutic consultancy to family physicians.

David Malan, a colleague of Balint, developed an influential approach to time-limited therapy he first termed 'radical' and later 'intensive' (Malan, 1963, 1976, 1979). The implication was that for some carefully assessed and selected patients, the time limit of a shorter therapy could accelerate the process of resolution of the central problem, or at least an important aspect of psychopathology. Unlike most, this approach favors a time limit (i.e., an agreed end date) rather than a predetermined number of sessions, to avoid the common difficulty of deciding when or whether sessions missed for any reason will count towards the total. However, an upper limit of sessions was set at 30, although most people were seen in fewer. Malan placed great store by a careful psychodynamic assessment of the patient's family and medical history, past and current relationships, to understand how events precipitating the current difficulty had emotional significance in the light of early experience. The therapist also attends carefully to the quality of the interaction. The assessment allows the therapist to judge whether to attempt a trial interpretation and the patient's response to this is an important factor in deciding whether this form of brief dynamic therapy is likely to be of benefit. The method itself is psychoanalytic, interpreting the transference, linking experience in the therapy relationship with childhood.

Malan described this in terms of two triangles—the 'triangle of conflict' (impulse–anxiety–defense) and the 'triangle of persons' (current relationship–therapist–parent). The 'two triangles' formulation is an economical and clear way for therapists to think about the focal conflict. Holmes (2000) gives the example of someone suffering from agoraphobia defending against anxiety by avoidance and dependency. Underlying this there may be hidden feelings of dissatisfaction and aggression, immediately towards a spouse, and in the past towards a controlling but unaffectionate mother. The therapist makes links between the anxiety, the defense, and the hidden impulse and between past relationships (usually with a parent), current relationships with others and the therapeutic relationship. In such a way, the patient is helped to tolerate anxiety and express hidden feelings, so that the 'triangle of conflict' is no longer enacted in current relationships.

The concept of a therapeutic plan was relatively new when Malan undertook his pioneering work in the 1960s and 1970s. Malan also had a profound commitment to research, at a time when respect for empirical evidence, particularly derived from quantitative methods, was unusual in psychoanalytic circles. From the 1980s, Malan espoused the methods of Davanloo, seeing in them a radical fulfillment of his own work.

Davanloo's (1978, 1990) method relies at heart on an orthodox psychodynamic drive/conflict model, derived from early Freud. He attracted controversy because his method involves pressurizing the patient in a relentless pursuit of any prevarication, vagueness, avoidance, or withdrawal, all seen as signs that important anxieties are being warded off. Repeated confrontation elicits anger, which is interpreted in terms of the 'triangle of persons' (i.e., a transference interpretation). This can lead to the powerful reexperiencing of warded-off anger from the past. Gustafson (1986) remarks on Davanloo's invariable focus on the patient's passivity as a way to deal with anger, noting that 'all interviews of Davanloo discover this passivity' (p. 175). Groves describes his method as Davanloo forcing the frigid patient to *feel* and thus creating mastery experience (Groves, 1996, p. 7).

At the same time as Malan was developing a coherent brief dynamic therapy in London, Peter Sifneos was working independently in Boston to develop short-term anxiety arousing therapy (STAPP) (Sifneos, 1972). He contrasted this approach with anxiety-*suppressive* therapy, which he advocated for severely disturbed patients, for crisis support (up to 2 months), brief therapy (from 2 months to 1 year) or in long-term supportive therapy (Sifneos, 1971). The anxiety arousing therapy could either be offered as a crisis resolution or as a time-limited therapy from 12 to 20 sessions (although sometimes longer, as there is a negotiated ending rather than a fixed time limit). The selection criteria were stringent, to exclude anyone with poor motivation, severe or complex difficulties in relationships, unrealistic expectations of treatment, and diffuse disturbances of identity. (This would exclude many of the patients seen in public sector settings or community clinics.) The therapist worked to establish an early alliance, so that the patient views the therapist as an ally and trusted teacher. The focus is on a circumscribed area of unresolved emotional conflicts, typically in terms of links between early and current Oedipal triangle themes, with repeated clarification using anxiety-provoking questions and confrontation. 'Characterological' problems such as excessive dependency or obsessionality were 'bypassed'; that is, the therapist did not allow them to shift the focus. Sifneos warns against the risks of a countertransference problem where the therapist could unconsciously use the method to 'punish the patient, see the patient suffer, or enjoy a position of superiority' (Sifneos, 1972, p. 114).

Psychodynamic brief therapies, particularly those of Sifneos and Davanloo, could also be seen as a form of behavioral intervention, where controlled exposure to feared emotional states reduces the anxiety associated with them, a concept elaborated by McCulloch *et al.* (2003) in terms of 'affect phobia'.

A structured approach to psychodynamic therapy developed by Luborsky (1984) has been applied in a brief format (Luborsky *et al.*, 1995; Book, 1998). The brief form of 'supportive-expressive' therapy evolved in parallel with research on transference using the core conflictual role theme method (Luborsky and Crits-Cristoph, 1998). This method links repetitive relationship patterns in the patient's past and present, and therapy relationships in terms of central themes. Transcripts of patients' narrative accounts of 'relationship episodes' are coded in terms of the psychodynamic triad of Wishes, Responses from Other, Responses of Self; for example 'I wish to be loved and understood, others tend to dislike and reject me, I respond by feeling anxious and unloved'. In addition to its research uses, the core conflictual role theme method has been developed to guide therapists in their formulation, maintenance of the focus, and choice of interventions for a structured, manualized form of brief psychodynamic psychotherapy over 16 sessions (Book, 1998).

James Mann (1978) was working within a psychoanalytic tradition, but has profoundly influenced the field of brief psychodynamic and relational therapy with his existential method of time-limited psychotherapy. He argues coherently that time is insolubly linked to reality and there is a ubiquitous human yearning to deny time, reality, and death by regaining a lost childhood paradise of timelessness. This is achieved in adulthood by dreams, daydreams, falling in love, drinking, or using drugs, or in mystic states of ecstasy. He describes how brief therapies evoke the horror of the finiteness of time and posits that as soon as the patient learns that the amount of time for help is limited, he or she is subject to magical, timeless, omnipotent fantasies. Dismissive of eclecticism, Mann advocates one or two intake interviews to establish a formulation of the central conflict, linking current suffering to past sources, tracing the 'chronically endured pain'. The focus for therapy is on improving the patient's self-image, but the formulation will differ according to the underlying difficulties. This formulation is given to the patient with a goal for therapy and an explicit offer of 12 sessions—no more, no less. The frequency and length of sessions within that limit seems to have been quite flexible, however. The calendar is consulted and the time for each appointment given, plus the exact date of the last (12th) meeting. He argues for as little ambiguity or evasion as possible about the time limit, and describes a typical course of therapy of early relief and improvement, a middle phase where enthusiasm wanes and ambivalence is felt (in a reenactment of earlier relationship patterns). As the patient moves towards ending, anxiety is evoked of 'separation without resolution from the meaningful, ambivalently experienced person'. In the end phase, affects of sadness, grief, anger, and guilt are intensely experienced and relived in the disappointing ending of therapy. The therapist too feels the pressure to prevaricate and imply that the end is not the end, in order to evade the anxiety of separation without resolution. Mann emphasizes that active management of the termination will allow the patient to internalize the therapist and this time the internalization will be more positive, less anger-laden, less guilt-laden, 'thereby making separation a genuine maturational event'. Any anger is acknowledged as normal and explored more rather than less.

Cognitive and behavioral approaches

Following the development of brief psychodynamic therapies, brief therapies based on behavioral, CBT, and cognitive theories began to appear. These arose from a research-based tradition and over the last 30 years have burgeoned, applied to an every-wider range of difficulties in mental health care, physical health problems, and health promotion. Many authors (see for example, Lovell and Richards, 2000) aggregate all these approaches into a common term—CBT—and in routine practice many therapists are rather eclectic in their choice of method within this broad framework. However, there are important differences between forms of CBT that integrated cognitive concepts into behavior therapy (Breger and McCaugh, 1965; Bandura, 1969; Meichenbaum, 1977) and those springing from the work of Beck, a different tradition of cognitive therapy that was not based on behavior therapy (Beck, 1979; Salkovskis, 1996). Goldfried (2003) argues that the lack of a clear distinction between cognitive therapy and CBT has arisen since CT was erroneously labeled CBT in the NIMH Depression Trial (Elkin, 1994).

Both methods were designedly brief, focusing in the first instance on depression, anxiety disorders, and obsessive-compulsive disorders—all without comorbid personality disorders. Since then the range of mental health problems addressed has grown to include PTSDs, eating disorders, and somatic problems (Salkovskis, 1996; Clark and Fairburn, 1997). Some of the newer applications are not brief, for example, CBT for personality disorders and psychosis (Perris, 1989; Linehan, 1993; Perris and McGorry, 1999).

CBT emphasizes a functional analysis of the problematic behavior or unwanted emotion in terms of antecedents, cognitions, behaviors, and consequences. This formulation then guides the choice of active techniques such as psychoeducation, relaxation, imaginal or *in vivo* exposure, response prevention, cognitive restructuring, and behavioral activation. Cognitive-behavioral therapists tend to emphasize the therapist's role in facilitating new experience and behavior as well as cognitive changes, maintaining clients' awareness of their success experiences and the differences between their present and past functioning (Goldfried and Robins, 1983).

Cognitive therapy based on Beck's cognitive model of emotion (Beck, 1967; Beck *et al.*, 1979) emphasizes that there are always alternative ways of perceiving and appraising any situation. People with mental health problems are trapped in a specific and unhelpful way of perceiving events, because of particular assumptions or beliefs they learned earlier in life. The therapist works collaboratively and empirically, inviting the client to explore whether or not there are alternative ways of appraising their situation, and empowering them to have choices over their response. The fundamental concept is of guided discovery of these alternatives, and support in testing out the consequences of new ways of thinking. Cognitive therapists tend to focus less than cognitive-behavior therapists on the role of behavioral antecedents and consequences including the impact of the patient's behavior on other people (Castonguay *et al.*, 1995).

There is sparse discussion of treatment length in cognitive and cognitive-behavioral literature. Therapy length tends to be fixed (either for research purposes or by the constraints of the service setting) or pragmatically negotiated with the client in routine practice. Typically therapies last between 8 and 20 sessions, although the use of follow-up and 'booster' sessions is common, for example in relapse prevention in depression, and in clinical practice many CB therapists not wishing to terminate therapy abruptly will gradually reduce the frequency of sessions and intensity of treatment. For this reason, some CBTs are in practice long term.

There has been a tendency for CBT interventions to become increasingly complex, although whether or in what circumstances 'multistrand' interventions are more effective than simple ones has not yet been established (Chambless and Gillis, 1998; Tarrier *et al.*, 1999) and some authors express skepticism (Lovell and Richards, 2000). This is probably a specific case of the more general finding of outcome equivalence in direct comparisons of different therapies (Stiles *et al.*, 1986; Lambert and Ogles, 2003).

On the other hand, there has also been a significant drive towards distilling the 'essence' of an effective intervention and finding more efficient ways of delivering it in briefer therapies. Often this is done with the support of written materials for clients to read between sessions. For example, Clark *et al.* (1999) describe a seven session cognitive-behavioral treatment for panic disorder, Wells and Papageorgiou (2001) outline a brief cognitive therapy for social phobia where patients received a mean of 5.5 sessions.

Interpersonal therapy (IPT) (Klerman *et al.*, 1984) was developed by psychiatrists as an adjunct to medication in the treatment of depression, and was brought to international attention through the NIMH collaborative research program. It was based on the interpersonal psychiatry of Harry Stack Sullivan and others, and research findings showing the intense impact of the formation, disruption, and renewal of attachment bonds, and the link between neurosis and deficits in social bonds. Theoretically grounded in social risk factors for depression as an illness, practically the method avoids an intrapsychic emphasis, whether psychodynamic or object relations, and

has been shown to have much in common with CBT in using active techniques to ameliorate present difficulties (Ablon and Jones, 2002).

IPT explores which of four problem areas are salient for a given patient—grief, role disputes, role transitions, or interpersonal deficits. In the early phase, assessment and negotiation of the treatment contract includes review of symptoms, confirmation of the diagnosis and legitimization of the sick role, assessment of interpersonal relationships, and choice of problem area, and medication plan. Within a medical model of depression, there is a psychoeducational emphasis in promoting understanding of the effects of depressive illness, hence reducing self-blame. Therapy continues using specific techniques depending on which of the four foci are agreed. For example, the therapist could aim to facilitate mourning, to identify issues in disputes and alternative actions, could encourage the patient to view role transitions in a positive way, or could work on remediating interpersonal deficits. Therapy is time limited but not constrained to a fixed number of sessions. Typically it lasts between 9 and 12 months.

Problem-solving therapy (PST) is a brief psychological treatment for depression based on cognitive-behavioral principles (D'Zurilla and Goldfried, 1971; Nezu *et al.*, 1989). It has also been used extensively as a form of crisis intervention following deliberate self-harm or attempted suicide (Hawton and Kirk, 1989). Like CBT it is structured, collaborative and focuses on generating solutions to current problems. Problem solving is seen as having five stages: adopting a problem-solving orientation; defining the problem and selecting goals; generating alternative solutions; choosing the best solution; and implementing the best solution and evaluating its effects. Methods used include cognitive modeling, prompting, self-instructions, and reinforcement.

It is usually delivered in about six treatment sessions. PST has been used to train nonspecialist health workers as part of primary care provision in a stepped care model. Meta-analytic review of randomized trials was unable to establish its effectiveness at reducing the repetition of deliberate self-harm (Hawton *et al.*, 1998), although in this population a further meta-analysis of six RCTs in terms depression, hopeless, and improvement in problems, found it effective (Townsend *et al.*, 2001).

Computerized CBT and guided self-help have also been developed as brief therapy approaches to anxiety and depression, particularly to reduce the time spent in therapist contact, so that CBT can become more accessible to the large numbers of individuals who may benefit from it. The principles of 'stepped care' (Katon *et al.*, 1999; Haaga, 2000), suggest that briefer, simpler, and most accessible therapies should first be offered, and more complex, expensive, and effortful therapies only if the patient has not responded to the simpler approach. A research review of self-help interventions in mental health reported that almost all are based on CBT principles, and that computers may best be seen as another way of providing access to self-help materials (Lewis *et al.*, 2003). A systematic review of 16 studies of computerized CBT, of which 11 were randomized controlled trials, suggested that for mild to moderate anxiety and depression, CCBT may be as effective as therapist-led CBT and better than standard care, although the evidence was by no means conclusive (Kalenthaler *et al.*, 2003).

Relational approaches

A third broad grouping of focal brief therapies can be termed 'relational' in that they see mental health difficulties as fundamentally interpersonal and they explicitly link the interpersonal to the intrapsychic in a 'two-person' psychology. Although these approaches have been influenced to a greater or lesser extent by psychoanalytic theory, they all emphasize relational rather than drive or structural aspects (Greenberg and Mitchell, 1983). Some have been influenced by cognitive psychology. These therapies pay close attention to the unfolding process within the psychotherapeutic relationship as a metaphor for, or an enactment of, the patient's problematic and repetitive interpersonal and intrapsychic patterns. They tend to use collaborative methods to guide discovery of these links and are wary of any notion that the therapist can stand aside from 'the transference' in order to interpret it authoritatively.

Time-limited dynamic psychotherapy (TLDP) (Schact *et al.*, 1984; Binder and Strupp, 1991) is a collaborative method that avoids the therapist imposing the focus by 'overtly pushing, manipulating, seducing, coercing, badgering, controlling, extorting or indoctrinating' the patient. The aim is to develop a 'working model' (Peterfreund, 1983) of interpersonal roles into which patients unconsciously cast themselves, the complementary roles into which they cast others, and the maladaptive interaction sequences, self-defeating expectations, and negative self-appraisals that result. The TDLP focus is a structure for interpersonal narratives, describing human actions, embedded in a context of interpersonal transactions, organized in a cyclical maladaptive pattern, that have been both a current and recurrent source of problems in living. The time limit is not rigid, depending on the clarity with which a treatment focus can be established, but a 'time-limited attitude' is maintained (Binder *et al.*, 1987).

Psychodynamic-interpersonal therapy (PIT) (Hobson, 1985) uses the 'here-and-now' relationship as a vehicle for learning about oneself in relation to others. Hobson has a process focus on the therapist and patient collaboratively developing a shared language for feelings. The therapist does not 'interpret' transference, but offers tentative exploratory links, making use of metaphor, and seeking to offer his or her own understanding of the patient's unarticulated emotions in the context of an authentic human relationship. Also known as the 'conversational model' of therapy, because of its emphasis on the therapeutic dialogue, a training manual and other materials have been systematically developed and evaluated in the UK. It has been extensively researched in relation to depression (in both eight-session and 16-session formats) (Shapiro *et al.*, 1984; Shapiro and Firth, 1987), psychosomatic difficulties (Guthrie *et al.*, 1991; Hamilton *et al.*, 2000), with treatment-resistant problems in psychiatric outpatient settings (Guthrie *et al.*, 1999) and as a brief intervention following self-poisoning (Guthrie *et al.*, 2001). For example, Guthrie *et al.* (1999) identified 110 patients with a range of long-standing nonpsychotic disorders who had not responded to psychiatric interventions—an unusual sample both in terms of its mix of diagnoses and selection for their challenge to standard care. Patients were randomized to receive eight sessions of PIT or to continue their usual care from a psychiatrist. There was evidence of significant advantage to the active intervention on some measures, in terms of patients' levels of functioning and in their use of health-service resources in the 6 months following treatment. Cost–benefit analysis suggested that this reduction in demand resulted in a cost-offset for psychotherapy provision.

Brief relational therapy (BRT) is a thoroughgoing relational approach developed in the USA by Jeremy Safran and Christopher Muran (2000), based on a 'dialectical constructivist perspective' (Hoffman, 1998). As with Hobson's method, there is an intense focus on the 'here-and-now' of the psychotherapeutic relationship, where the therapist urges collaborative exploration of both the patient's and the therapist's contributions to the interaction. The therapist is urged to be cautious about making interpretations based on generalized relationship patterns, but to explore the nuances of the patient's experience and the relational meaning of this experience, through unfolding therapeutic 'enactments'. There is extensive use of metacommunication about the meaning of what is happening between the therapist and patient, with disclosure of the countertransference.

The therapist refrains from early case formulation or content focus for the sessions. Safran and Muran argue that as the therapist can never stand outside the interaction to create a formulation that is not shaped by unwitting enactment, such a therapist-derived focus is inimical to a fully relational method. Case formulation only arises from the therapist repeatedly 'disembedding' from whatever interpersonal pattern ('matrix') is being enacted. 'Therapy thus consists of an ongoing cycle of enacting, disembedding and understanding—and this understanding is always partial at best' (Safran and Muran, 2000, p. 178). They acknowledge that the lack of a 'tangible' focus can be a problem for brief therapy, linking to the therapist's anxieties about having something substantial to offer within a limited time. Instead they offer the process focus of mindfulness, modeling a capacity to observe one's internal processes and actions in relationship to other people, and thereby helping the patient develop and generalize this skill. As in cognitive analytic therapy (CAT) ruptures and repairs to the therapeutic

alliance are seen as a particularly effective way to gain awareness of problematic relationship patterns. Links between the therapy relationship and relationship patterns outside therapy are made tentatively, the therapist making an effort to be aware of his or her own motivations.

Cognitive analytic therapy (CAT) is an integrative approach developed in the UK by Anthony Ryle (1990) and further extended both theoretically and clinically by others (Ryle and Kerr, 2002). Ryle aimed to integrate the effective elements of various preceding traditions—not simply at the level of therapeutic technique, but in the underpinning theory of development, personality, and psychopathology. CAT theory is rooted in Kelly's (1955) personal construct theory, cognitive and developmental psychology (stressing in particular the actively intersubjective nature of the human infant; Stern, 1984; Trevarthen and Aitken, 2001) and in psychoanalytic object relations theory. Theoretically it emphasizes repetitive aim-directed sequences of cognition, emotion, behavior and their consequences (called 'procedures'), similar to Goldfried's (2003) 'STAIRCASE' (Situation, Thought, Affect, Intention, Response, Consequence, and Self Evaluation) CBT model. However, CAT theory also draws on object relations theory and Vygotsky's activity theory to assert the pervasively dialogic nature of the human world, where internalized self-other relationship patterns become the basis of reciprocal role procedures governing intrapersonal as well as interpersonal relationships. Procedures, including reciprocal role procedures, are problematic to the extent that aims are not achieved yet the maladaptive sequence is not revised. Over the past decade it has integrated Vygotskian activity theory and the Bakhtinian concept of the dialogic self (Leiman, 1992, 1997). The model has thus come to be underpinned by a radically social concept of self.

CAT, while theoretically and methodologically integrative, is therefore a fundamentally interpersonal and relational therapy. In common with BRT it requires the therapist to reflect collaboratively with the patient what reciprocal roles are being enacted in the therapy relationship, particularly at points where the therapeutic alliance is being threatened (Bennett and Parry, 2003). In contrast to BRT, however, the initial few sessions of CAT are devoted to an extended assessment leading to a jointly agreed reformulation of a patient's story, its personal meaning and the relation to it of the problem procedures they have brought with them. The narrative account is redrafted on the basis of the patient's feedback and is supplemented by a diagrammatic reformulation. Both forms of reformulation are seen from the Vygotskian perspective as psychological 'tools', fostering jointly focused attention and the capacity for self-reflection. The reformulation forms the basis of intervention, which often includes cognitive-behavioral methods of procedural revision.

As in psychodynamic brief therapies there is stress on the therapeutic value of the issues provoked by a fixed termination point. Ending is seen from a CAT perspective to minimize regression and avoid protracted, and usually collusive, dependency. It is also an opportunity to work through the unassimilated issues from earlier losses and to enact new reciprocal role procedures. An example might be the reciprocal role *appropriately withholding* in relation to *manageably deprived* leading to the patient being able to feel vulnerable and to tolerate the painful feelings that the ending can provoke. The ending is formally and symbolically celebrated by the therapist writing a further letter—a 'farewell' letter—to the patient. This acknowledges the achievements of therapy but also anticipates loss and possible grief and anger. The patient is encouraged to write a farewell letter from his or her own perspective.

Although a 16-session format lasting approximately 4 months is used for 'neurotic' difficulties, CAT is one of the better-developed models for working briefly with more severely disturbed patients. Here longer contracts (usually 24 sessions) are offered and sometimes further interventions such as group work or consultation to the community mental health team (Kerr, 1999). The CAT model of borderline personality disorder (Ryle and Marlowe, 1995; Ryle, 1997) describes severe damage and disturbance of the self, characterized by a tendency (apparently secondary to chronic psychological trauma) to dissociate into different 'self states' (each characterized by one reciprocal role procedure). One consequence of this, apart from the tendency to enact extreme and disconnected roles, is a poor ability to reflect upon these states and an impaired capacity for empathy and executive function. The extreme role enactments in borderline personality disorder would include, for example, idealized help seeking, abusive, and vengeful anger (expressed to self or others) or dissociated, numb, 'zombie' states in which serious self-harm may be perpetrated. CAT thus offers a clear theoretical basis for engaging and working with the enactment of poorly integrated and maladaptive reciprocal role procedures, with similarities to that developed independently by Benjamin (2003), but applied within a brief therapy format.

Pragmatic, eclectic therapies

A number of brief therapies draw pragmatically on a range of theories and methods to yield approaches that are eclectic.

Budman and Gurman (1988) describe a method they characterize as 'interpersonal–developmental–existential', which includes a range of issues in the formulation including losses, developmental dysynchronies, interpersonal conflicts, symptoms, and personality dysfunction. The focus is used to open the session, maintain a unity within the session and to close the session, drawing together the material linked to the focus in a brief summary statement. They argue for the flexible use of time on the basis of Johnson and Gelso's (1980) review of the effectiveness of time limits and Howard et al.'s (1986) dose–response findings. They suggest more intensive work for four to eight visits then 'spreading out' the sessions to reduce dependency and enhance self-efficacy. They criticize the traditional analytic view of 'once and for all' therapy and criteria for 'completed' therapy as unrealistic and rigid. Instead, brief therapy is available on an intermittent basis as required when facing different developmental challenges.

Cummings (1991) also argues for brief intermittent therapy throughout the life cycle as a pragmatic approach where theory and techniques from different models are synthesized. He argues that 'termination' is not necessarily difficult or painful and suggests it is therapists rather than patients who have difficulty ending. Instead the therapist makes a commitment to be available to the patient 'as long as you need me—in return I want you to join me in a partnership that makes me obsolete as soon as possible'. This is a model of the therapist as a 'psychological family doctor' providing continuity of care over time. This way of working leads to brief treatment episodes of between one and 20 sessions, spaced flexibly.

Garfield (1989, 1995) describes an eclectic brief therapy model based on maximizing the impact of the 'common factors' identified in therapy research; therapists are engaged in listening, reflection, suggestion, explanation, interpretation, providing information, confrontation, reassurance, homework assignments, modeling and role play, questioning, and cautious self-disclosure. In common with Budman and Gurman and Cummings, he takes a relaxed approach to treatment length, and to selection criteria. Garfield also challenges the assumption that if people do not respond to short-term therapy, they will benefit from long-term work. He seems this as having little empirical justification, as there has been almost no research on long-term therapy.

Winston and Winston (2002) describe a pragmatic eclectic approach, which they term 'integrated', although it does not seem fully integrated at the theoretical level, compared with, for example, CAT. Their case formulation method uses the concept of a continuum between psychological sickness and health, according to 'level of psychopathology, adaptive capacity, self-concept and ability to relate to others' (p. 11). The individual treatment plan depends on the patient's position on this continuum, with cognitive-behavioral methods being used for the 'more impaired' and more psychodynamic, expressive techniques for the 'least impaired'. By this means, a brief intervention can be offered for more severe and complex difficulties, such as borderline disorders (Winston et al., 1991).

Very brief therapy, including crisis intervention and critical incident debriefing

Very brief therapies of up to five sessions have been developed in differing treatment modalities. Öst and colleagues have investigated the impact of single-session interventions, finding that one prolonged session of exposure has an equivalent impact to (an already brief) five sessions for a range of specific phobias: injection (Öst et al., 1992); blood injury (Hellstrom et al., 1996); flying (Öst et al., 1997); and claustrophobia (Öst et al., 2001). As other researcher groups have demonstrated the efficacy of single-session exposure (e.g., Thorpe and Salkovskis, 1997) it does seem that—at least for circumscribed behavioral goals in specific phobias—very brief interventions may be adequate.

A three-session therapy in a 'two plus one' format (Barkham, 1989) was developed in a research context for 'subsyndromal depression' on the basis of the research evidence of dose–response (Howard et al., 1986) and Johnson and Gelso's (1980) review of the effectiveness of time limits. Therapy comprises two sessions 1 week apart followed by a follow-up session 3 months later. Barkham et al. (1992) conducted a pilot study of this approach, with reasonably positive outcomes. In a later larger-scale randomized trial, Barkham et al. (1999) allocated 116 patients to CBT or psychodynamic versions of the 2 + 1 model, either immediately or after a 4-week delay. All patients fell below diagnostic thresholds for depression, but were entered into the trial in three bands of severity—stressed (effectively within normal population limits), subclinical (mildly symptomatic), or low-level depression. Clients at all levels made gains, with some evidence from the delayed-treatment condition that this related to the intervention rather than time-effects. Patients receiving the CBT version obtained greater benefit at 1-year follow-up (Barkham et al., 1999), suggesting that Hobson's PIT method may be less well suited to this very brief format. This model was not developed—or intended—as a therapy in its own right, but as a way of offering a more rapid response to clients, and as a way of testing the appropriateness of further therapy. To that degree these studies offer support for the utility of the model.

Sheard et al. (2000) describe a one- to three-session CAT-derived method to improve the response of psychiatrists to repeated deliberate self-harm in he context of emergency hospital care. Outcome studies are not yet available.

Newman et al. used a four-session CBT intervention for panic disorder, assisted by the use of palmtop computers for self-monitoring and assessment, with similar results to a 12-session treatment.

The clinical method of motivational interviewing (Miller and Rollnick, 1991) has been used as a very brief intervention either alone or in addition to standard treatment, particularly for alcohol and substance misuse problems. It was developed on the basis of a review of 'active ingredients' in effective brief therapy with these client groups, which suggested the importance of giving feedback, promoting personal responsibility for change and self-efficacy, giving straightforward advice, and offering a menu of alternative strategies. The method is nondirective and avoids any confrontation with 'resistance' or 'lack of motivation', instead taking an acceptant and empathic approach to changing motivational states. The aim is to help those reluctant to change problematic behaviors move from the *pre-contemplation* stage, or ambivalent *contemplation* (as understood by Prochaska and DiClemente's, 1984, transtheoretical model of change), to *preparation* where change options can be explored and then *action* and *maintenance* of change. A number of randomized trials have demonstrated its value in these settings, although others have shown it is not invariably effective (Dunn et al., 2001; Miller et al., 2003). A meta-analytic review of randomized trials (Burke et al., 2003) found adaptations of motivational interviewing a promising approach to problems involving alcohol, drugs, dieting, and exercise but that the evidence did not support their efficacy in smoking or HIV-risk behaviors.

Solution-focused brief therapy (SFBP: de Shazer, 1985; Walter and Peller, 1992) developed from brief strategic therapy (Weakland et al., 1974) in work with families and individuals, and is often delivered over four to five sessions. It pays no attention whatsoever to the origin or etiology of problems and instead focuses on helping clients to change problem-maintaining behavior, to define their goals (recognizing that their own definition may or may not be congruent with problems as perceived by professionals), and to generate solutions to difficulties they face. Questions about goals are posed in such a way that the client is able to speak about what the world would be like without their current problems. It is in this sense that the method is solution focused rather than problem solving. The focus is on collaborative identification and amplification of the patient's strengths, with extremely positive feedback and an emphasis on small aspects of meaningful change.

A review by Gingerich and Eisengart (2000) identified 15 controlled studies of this approach, five of which met criteria for methodological adequacy, although only one of these (Sundstrom, 1993) was directly related to mental health issues. Sundstrom contrasted one 90-minute session of solution-focused or problem-focused therapy in 40 mildly depressed college students. At 1 week follow-up scores on the Beck Depression Inventory were reduced, and outcomes were equivalent in both therapy groups. However, the nature and size of the sample and the brevity of follow-up makes it difficult to draw conclusions about the efficacy of this approach. There is in any case a conflict between the philosophy of SFBP and research that estimates efficacy using standardized instruments, as this does not reflect user-defined outcomes (which will inevitably be quite varied). However, as with a number of emergent techniques, in the absence of well-conducted research, we are unable to comment on its effectiveness, or the range of difficulties for which it is appropriate.

There is a wide range of brief interventions aimed at responding to crises (Hobbs, 1984). The theory and practice of crisis intervention developed from the work of pioneers in the 1960s, such as the community psychiatrist Caplan (1961), and the psychoanalytic crisis therapist, Jacobson (1980). A fundamental concept is that during crisis, people are unusually receptive to restructuring their psychological processes, providing a window of opportunity for a brief intervention to have a substantial positive effect. Crisis intervention uses the intense affect associated with the crisis state in order to facilitate constructive change. The personal meaning of the crisis is explored, in terms of both present and past aspects (e.g., a loss event could re-evoke feelings associated with an earlier loss), coping resources, and components of crisis that render these ineffective. The crisis may be formulated in a way that gives individuals or family members a cognitive understanding of what has happened, so that the emotional assimilation of this is facilitated, and new coping resources are mobilized. Crisis intervention is a contractual benefit of most Health Maintenance Organization prepaid plans in the USA (Chiefetz and Salloway, 1985), although Adams (1991), writing of family crisis intervention in the San Diego Kaiser Permanente Medical Care Program, argues that virtually none provide a clear definition of what this means. In the UK, although crisis intervention is linked to home treatment of severe mental illness (Joy et al., 2004) as an alternative to hospital admission, crisis theory, and practice has not been generally characteristic of brief approaches to psychotherapy. Research on the effectiveness of crisis intervention is sparse, with the exceptions of critical incident debriefing after a traumatic event and problem solving following suicide attempts or deliberate self-harm.

Critical incident debriefing was designed as a rapid response to a traumatic event, aiming to reduce vulnerability to developing PTSD or other mental health conditions, and usually delivered in a single session. Although intuitively appealing to many clinicians, it is now clear that single-session debriefing immediately after exposure to a traumatic event is ineffective, and that on the contrary there may be an adverse impact for some individuals (e.g., van Emmerik et al., 2002; Rose et al., 2003). Overall it is clear that single-session interventions cannot be recommended as part of routine practice, and the English Department of Health guideline on treatment choice in psychological therapies (2001) explicitly argues against their use. There is very little evidence about the impact of slightly longer interventions, though Bryant et al. (1999) and André et al. (1997) employed five- and one- to six-session interventions, respectively, with more positive results. This does not imply that individuals in distress should not be offered support, nor does this general conclusion contraindicate more extended psychological intervention at some remove from the initial trauma, if posttraumatic disorder were to develop.

Interventions focused on the management of suicide attempts are reviewed by van der Sande et al. (1997), who identified 15 randomized trials of varying forms of intervention, only some of which would be classified as brief interventions. Two trials considered the impact of a 3-month crisis intervention based on a problem-solving model (Gibbons et al., 1978; Hawton et al., 1987). In total, 480 patients were randomized to receive the intervention or to act as controls; overall the interventions did not lead to a reduction in suicidal behavior. In contrast, four trials employed CBT to focus on broader aspects of current and past functioning and coping mechanisms (Liberman and Eckman, 1981; Salkovskis et al., 1990; Linehan et al., 1993; McLeavey et al., 1994). Although these trials demonstrated a significant reduction in suicide attempts, they were relatively small scale, and (in the context of this chapter), some intervention periods were far from brief (for example, treatment in Linehan et al. took place over 1 year). There is some suggestion from these trials that a focus on background rather than on current problems may be more beneficial for this group of patients.

Research questions and findings

Which brief therapy?

Research into brief therapies falls into several areas. The largest source of information comes from 'mainstream' research into psychological therapy. In research contexts interventions are frequently delivered in the form of manualized packages of short duration—it is a matter of observation that most therapies in research trials last between 12 and 16 weeks. In these cases we are examining the impact of therapies, which their originators may or may not have intended to be brief, but which are nonetheless investigated in this form. While there may be arguments about the appropriateness of examining the impact of therapies not intended for implementation over short time-frames (e.g., some forms of psychodynamic therapy), in the present context it is relevant to ask how therapies perform under conditions where termination is clearly signaled from the outset of therapy. From this perspective (ironically) research trials become a better exemplar of brief therapy than in many clinical contexts, where duration is poorly controlled and much more likely to be dictated by patient attrition than therapist intent.

Evidence for the differential efficacy of different forms of brief therapies remains disappointingly weak. This is usually referred to as the 'dodo bird' conclusion (from *Alice in Wonderland*: 'Everybody has won, and all must have prizes'). Where differences are found, they tend to be small. In 1975, Luborsky et al. drew attention to the apparent equivalence of outcomes across different types of psychotherapy and 27 years later, Luborsky et al. (2002) reexamined the issue in 17 meta-analyses of comparisons of active treatments with each other, drawing a similar conclusion. Lambert and Ogles (2003) reviewed results from comparative, dismantling, and components analysis studies as suggesting the general equivalence of treatments based on different theories and techniques. They believe that these findings argue against the current trend of identifying empirically supported therapies that purport to be uniquely effective and conclude in relation to the differential efficacy question, 'Decades of research have not resulted in support for one superior treatment or set of techniques for specific disorders'.

The verdict of the Dodo bird is controversial, and many do not accept it. Norcross (1995) lists many reasons why he finds the verdict untenable— only a handful of the many therapies have been evaluated; similar symptom reduction does not mean identical outcomes; common factors do not preclude specific effects; studies disregard the person of the psychotherapist (different therapists obtain different improvement rates); almost one-half of studies are underpowered; studies ignore the quality of the therapeutic relationship, 'horse-race' outcome studies are insensitive to differential treatment effects (similar group means mask individual outcome differences and mask interaction effects); and most studies examine psychologically irrelevant treatment variables (e.g., in an *ex post facto* search for correlates between client characteristics and outcomes). He asserts that studies with an aptitude-treatment interaction design and sufficient power on psychologically relevant variables do show differential effects. Beutler (1991, 1995, 2002) also argues that the complexity of determining specific effects has been underestimated and that those who believe in outcome equivalence have largely ignored evidence of specific effects. He contends that the gross labels used to identify manual-driven therapies do not eliminate within-therapy variations, or preserve between-therapy variations. A good example of this is discussed by Ablon and Jones (2002) where the NIMH Treatment of Depression Collaborative Research Program compared two apparently different therapies that actually had many similarities.

In addition, diagnostic homogeneity does not remove important patient differences. As a result, it is vital to consider specific types of interventions (irrespective of therapy type) and specific, nondiagnostic aspects of patients. Examples include therapist directiveness interacting with patient receptivity or resistance, and a focus on symptoms versus a focus on insight differentially benefiting those with internal versus externalizing coping styles (Beutler, 1991). Rounsaville and Carroll (2002) argue that the Dodo bird verdict is based on insufficient attention to patient–treatment matching and the many design constraints on efficacy research that reduce the likelihood of detecting large outcome differences between active treatments.

For these methodological reasons, the degree to which outcome equivalence speaks to common therapeutic processes underpinning effective interventions is not yet clear. Certainly however, champions of specific therapies should be appropriately cautious when advocating one approach over another, especially because contrast of therapies in research trials should ensure that they are of equal credibility and presumed potency in relation to the condition for which they are intended. For example, while one review (Gloaguen et al., 1998) showed apparent superiority of CBT for depression, subsequent reanalysis (Wampold et al., 2002) demonstrated that this effect only stood when 'non bone-fide' therapies were included; once these had been removed from the analysis CBT was equivalent in efficacy to other approaches.

There is a relative hegemony of CBT trials, and while this does not diminish the evidence for the efficacy of these approaches, it limits comment on the relative efficacy of other approaches, as direct comparisons in adequately powered trials are rare. Despite this (and the discussion above), in some areas there is evidence for differential efficacy. Many anxiety disorders are effectively treated by relatively brief behavioral and cognitive-behavioral interventions, and in the absence of strong clinical indicators it would be difficult to justify the first-line use of alternative approaches to these conditions (Department of Health, 2001). The strength of this statement is justified by Schulte et al.'s (1992) trial, which examined treatment outcomes for specific phobias. In effect they contrasted standardized *in vivo* exposure against an individualized treatment where therapists were free to implement any therapeutic approach. The greatest benefit was found with *in vivo* exposure, a fact reinforced by the finding that the patients who benefited from an individualized approach were those who had been given *in vivo* exposure. This result is salutary—specific phobia is a condition with a straightforward treatment approach of known efficacy, and yet at least some clinicians elected to employ alternative and less effective techniques. This raises questions about the relative role of clinical judgment and clinical guidelines (Wilson, 1996; Parry et al., 2003a).

How much therapy is enough?

As noted above, most of the research literature on psychological therapies relates to the impact of therapies delivered in a brief form. Most research is now conducted using a manualized form of therapy, sometimes specifying the sequence of therapy, and sometimes acting as a broader guideline to indicate which types of therapeutic intervention are permissible. On this basis therapies conducted under research conditions represent as tight a test of brief interventions as we are likely to see.

A full review of this literature is beyond the scope of this section (see Roth and Fonagy, 1996, 2005; Lambert and Ogles, 2003), but it is worth noting that overall there is good evidence for efficacy of these interventions across a wide range of mental health conditions. Given the restriction on length of research-based therapies noted above, it is reasonable to conclude that clinically significant change is possible for many conditions after about 16 sessions, and people with more circumscribed problems or milder presentations may benefit from briefer interventions. This does not mean that after 16 sessions all clients can be expected to have achieved stable remission—clinicians need to have a realistic idea of what can be achieved in a relatively brief period.

As an example, outcomes from some major studies of interventions for depression (e.g., Frank et al., 1991; Hollon et al., 1992; Elkin, 1994; Shapiro et al., 1994, 1995) act as a helpful benchmark. At posttherapy about 50% of patients had made significant gain, though over the next year about half of those who improved relapsed. This means that at the end of follow-up, only about one-fourth remained well. It could be argued that this apparently poor result reflects the nature of the disorder—depression is potentially a chronic condition marked by a history or relapse and remission, and expected outcomes need to be set against this context. Recognizing this fact, some researchers have investigated the efficacy of a model of maintenance, showing that additional monthly sessions following short-term intervention significantly reduce relapse rates (e.g., Frank et al., 1991).

It is important to recognize that relapse after brief therapy is not uncommon, though there is variation in the extent to which this occurs, in part related to the condition under examination. For example, relapse appears to be less marked in anxiety disorders (such as phobias, panic, PTSD, and obsessive-compulsive disorder) than in mood disorders, and it also clear that some conditions (for example, eating disorders or generalized anxiety disorder) present particular challenge to clinicians. The degree to which a therapy achieves remission is important, as there is evidence that relapse rates are higher among patients who show residual symptoms at termination (e.g., Jarrett et al., 2001). On this basis, there is sound evidence that clinicians need to consider strategies for managing patients who remain vulnerable at the conclusion of brief episodes of therapy, the most obvious being the planned extension of therapy, or the offer of maintenance sessions.

A second area of research focuses on the incremental impact of adding more sessions in a therapy with no fixed time limit—commonly referred to as 'dose–response' research. Here, therapies as delivered may or may not be brief, but the aim is to determine how brief or how extensive a therapy needs to be to achieve impact. The data analyzed in dose–response research are invariably naturalistic rather than experimental, that is, therapies of different lengths are compared but length of treatment is not manipulated experimentally in a randomized design.

The relationship between the amount of therapy received and subsequent benefit is one that has received considerable attention. As a research question this is entirely appropriate, though the analogy with drug treatment implied by 'dose–response' is unfortunate. Howard et al. (1986) collated data from 15 outcome studies of 2431 patients who had completed therapy. The sample of therapies included in this analysis may not be representative—it included longer-than-typical therapies and did not include cognitive and behavioral therapies. Improvement rates can be examined in therapies of differing lengths. Graphical representation shows this to be a negatively accelerating curve—where the percentage of clients who have shown measurable improvement increases with number of sessions but fewer and fewer reach this criterion as therapy length increases. About half of the patients had improved after eight-session therapy, whereas it took 104 sessions before 90% of patients had improved. People with more severe difficulties (such as personality disorder) respond more slowly to therapeutic intervention (Howard et al., 1993). Replications and further studies have since been undertaken by Kopta et al. (1996), Anderson and Lambert (2001), Lambert, Hansen, and Finch (2001), who on the whole give more conservative estimates of the dose of therapy required for clinically significant improvement.

There is also evidence that the shape of the dose–response curve reflects the fact that different aspects of functioning change at different rates. Barkham et al. (1996) and Kopta et al. (1994) followed the pattern of session-by-session changes in questionnaire item-endorsement; both determined that symptoms changed most quickly, while characterological change was slowest. Though this finding is mathematically isomorphous with Howard et al., (1986) it implies that questions about dose–response are best asked in relation to the type of outcome that is intended. Though it seems obvious to state that more seriously disabled individuals will require more time to recover functioning, the implication is that treatment lengths need closely to reflect treatment aims.

In summarizing dose–response evidence, Lambert and Ogles (2003) state that 'a sizeable portion of patients reliably improve after 10 sessions and [...] 75% of patients will meet more rigorous criteria for success after about 50 sessions of treatment. Limiting treatment sessions to less than 20 will mean that about 50% of patients will not achieve a substantial benefit from therapy (as measured by standard self-report scales)' (p. 156). Hence brief therapy cannot be recommended for all patients, but more than half can be helped substantially in this way. This figure is likely to improve as brief therapy methods are refined and developed.

Another approach is to derive dose–effect relationships for individual patients by analyzing session-by-session change from many thousands of patients, using a standardized metric to follow patterns of change. Two groups of workers have used fairly complex (e.g., Leuger et al., 2001) or relatively simple (e.g., Lambert et al., 2001) assessment systems to produce expected profiles of change for patients based (broadly) on their initial level of psychological distress. The benefit of this approach to the individual clinician is severalfold. It makes it clear that the extent and rate of change for more severely disabled clients will be slower than for the less distressed, and—crucially—quantifies this difference. It also enables clinicians to identify those clients who have already made an appropriate amount of change, with the possibility of more rapid discharge. Further, it signals patients who are deteriorating or whose rate of change is significantly slower than expected.

Lambert et al. (2002) randomized therapists either to receive or not to receive feedback on client progress based on individualized dose–response curves. Clients whose therapists received feedback had somewhat greater rates of improvement, but the more striking result was a significant reduction in the rate of deterioration. In addition, there was evidence that feedback enabled therapists more accurately to tailor the number of sessions to clinical need—those who had improved were more likely to be discharged, and those who required more help were more likely to be retained in therapy.

Consensus about the length of therapy is based on clinical judgment rather than empirical data, though the question of how much therapy is needed to make for clinically significant and lasting change is obviously an important one. A small number of trials address this issue directly, by comparing short and longer forms of the same therapy, delivered as part of the same comparative trial by the same group of clinicians.

Clark et al. (1999) contrasted the impact of 14 sessions of panic control therapy (PCT) against seven sessions, in 43 patients with panic disorder and little or no agoraphobic avoidance. The briefer intervention included self-study modules, which the patient read prior to sessions, and introduced many of the ideas used in sessions. At posttherapy and at 3- and 12-month follow-up, both forms of treatment were of equal efficacy. This study was conducted by a group of senior researchers experienced in using PCT, and it is notable that other researchers obtained poor results using such abbreviated forms of therapy. Black et al. (1993) developed an eight-session form of CBT for panic; though not contrasted against a longer form of the therapy, it was no more effective than placebo medication.

Shapiro et al. (1994) investigated two forms of therapy—CBT and PIT—delivered for either 8 or 16 weeks. The trial design ensured that the 120 patients represented varying levels depression (low, moderate, and high). At the end of the initial phase of treatment there were no differences in efficacy between treatments for those patients with low or moderate levels of depression, but more severely depressed patients appeared to do better with a longer duration of treatment. The pattern of gains at 12-month follow-up (Shapiro et al., 1995) suggested that eight sessions of exploratory therapy appeared to be too few, there was some evidence favoring 16 sessions of CBT, and overall, poorer maintenance of gains was evident in patients with greater levels of initial distress.

Hoglend and Piper (1997) review two independent studies of brief dynamic psychotherapy carried out in Canada, and Oslo, one of which used a fixed time-limit, while the other employed open-ended treatment. Although broad outcomes were similar, post hoc analysis using a measure of the maturity of patient's relationships to others (quality of object relations) suggested that patients high in this quality did equally well with therapy of either duration. However, though low-quality of object relations patients did better with fewer sessions when therapy was time-limited, they did better with more than 35–40 sessions when in open-ended therapy—a result that is hard to interpret, and suggests the potential complexity of dose–response relationships.

Are the effects lasting?

Although the foregoing suggests that there is good evidence for the efficacy of brief therapies, it is reasonable to ask whether their effects are lasting, or indeed are as robust over follow-up as their longer-term counterparts. The most rigorous method for investigating this would be a within-study contrast of shorter and longer versions of the same approach. Here there are too few available studies to draw conclusions, and those reviewed above suggest that there is mixed evidence on this point—for example, and perhaps unsurprisingly, outcomes for depression are more complex than for anxiety. More generally, conclusions about the longer-term outcome from briefer therapies is hampered by a lack of follow-up data, despite a general agreement that posttherapy outcomes may not be the most helpful indicator of therapeutic impact. As an example, a recent meta-analytic review for treatments of depression, panic, and generalized anxiety disorder—all common presentations in clinical practice—noted that comment on outcomes beyond 12 months was severely restricted by a lack of relevant studies and variation in reporting of these outcomes (Westen and Morrison, 2001).

Where findings on follow-up are available, there is reasonable evidence for the stability of gains in relation to some conditions such as panic disorder (e.g., Milrod and Busch, 1996) though it is harder to demonstrate enduring change in conditions characterized by relapse–remission cycles, such as depression, where a common finding at 12-month follow-up is that only around a fourth of those entering a trial of brief therapy remain well (Roth and Fonagy, 2005). This raises an important issue for interpreting follow-up, as without knowing something of the likely trajectory over that time period, expectations of continuing efficacy could be unrealistic.

A rather different issue is raised by outcome studies conducted in the context of primary care, where very brief therapies are offered to individuals whose presentations are less severe, chronic, and complex than might be common in other settings. A common contrast here is to 'treatment-as-usual' (TAU), and a common finding is that though active treatment shows benefit at posttherapy, over a relatively short time those receiving TAU show a similar level of gain. Two examples illustrate this phenomenon. Ward et al. (2000) contrasted treatment as usual from a GP to 12 sessions of nondirective counseling or CBT in 463 patients with mild to moderately depression. Though at 4 months both active treatments showed equivalent and significant advantage to TAU, at 1 year there were no differences in outcome. Parry et al. (2003b) randomized 94 patients with asthma-related anxiety to brief CBT or standard care. At the end of treatment, the CBT group were significantly improved compared with controls on panic fear, depression, locus of control and asthma-related quality of life. Six months later, these differences were no longer significant because the control group had also improved. Results such as these require careful interpretation, as the benefits to the individual of an accelerated rate of change may be highly significant, despite an apparent equity of outcome over time.

Professional attitudes, training, and competence

Despite the evidence that brief therapy is effective for many patients and an efficient use of resources, there is considerable professional resistance to working briefly. Hoyt (1991) summarizes several reasons for this, including:

- beliefs that 'more is better' despite the dearth of evidence justifying the greater expense of open-ended treatment
- the overvaluation of insight and a misassumption that change requires 'deep' examination of an individual's unconscious processes and psychological history

- confusion of the patient's interests with the therapist's, and counter-transference problems—the need to be needed and the difficulties of saying goodbye.

Shapiro *et al.* (2003) redress this view by listing opposing reasons why therapists may wish to terminate therapy prematurely in some cases.

Most practitioners believe that outcomes are as dependent on a therapist's competence and personal qualities as the techniques they practice, but evidence to support or refute this position is difficult to come by. Methodological issues make it hard to disentangle therapists from therapies simply because most research trials are designed to identify the impact of the therapy that is delivered, rather than the therapists who deliver them. Our knowledge about the therapist's contribution to outcome is based on *post hoc* exploration of datasets never intended to yield such information; inevitably the information gleaned is somewhat ambiguous.

There are some studies (e.g., Luborsky *et al.*, 1986; Huppert *et al.*, 2001) that confirm the expectation that different therapists achieve different patterns of outcomes with their patients. However, in the latter trial it was only a small number of 'outlier' therapists who had consistently good or consistently poor outcomes; the majority had mixed results. Although it is not clear why this should be, it is reasonable to assume that at least some of this variability reflects the fact that the therapist's ability to implement an intervention is influenced—for good or ill—by the patient's responsiveness and capacity for engagement. As discussed below, there is good evidence for this proposition.

The benefits of therapist experience and training are also hard to detect, and though there have been a series of meta-analytic reviews of this area, even the most thorough (Stein and Lambert, 1995) fails to show much evidence of a relationship. This negative result may reflect methodological difficulties. For example, it is hard to correct for differential attrition between the patients of novice and experienced therapists, with difficult patients dropping out of treatment with novices and being over-represented in the caseloads of experienced therapists, yielding poorer outcomes (Roth and Parry, 1997).

Nonetheless, the mere possession of experience and professional qualifications does not guarantee that therapy will be implemented well. On this basis it makes more sense to examine what therapists actually do in therapy—specifically their ability to implement a therapy congruent with a treatment protocol (usually referred to as adherence), as well as their capacity to do it competently. The former relates to what was done, and the latter to how well it was done. Although it is easy to conflate these two concepts, research techniques have been developed that attempt (not always successfully) to distinguish them. Although there are some indications that adherence is related to outcome (e.g., DeRubeis and Feeley, 1991), slavish adherence at the expense of the therapeutic alliance can have a negative impact (Henry *et al.*, 1993; Castonguay *et al.*, 1996). Both adherence to a treatment manual and the ability to deviate from or modify standard technique when required are both associated with good outcomes, as compared with poor adherence and rigidity (Frank and Spanier, 1995). Competence in delivery appears to be better related to outcomes than adherence alone (O'Malley *et al.*, 1988; Frank *et al.*, 1991; Barber *et al.*, 1996; Shaw *et al.*, 1999).

Adherence to therapeutic methods and competent delivery are more difficult in the face of patients who are hostile and have negative expectations of therapy (Rounsaville *et al.*, 1981; Foley *et al.*, 1987; O'Malley *et al.*, 1988). The relationship between competence and outcome is also likely to be strongest for therapies with patients who have disturbed patterns of interpersonal relationships, lower aptitude for maintaining a therapeutic alliance, and who are least tolerant of therapist errors. With some exceptions these are the least likely to be offered brief therapy, although a central competence in brief therapy is the ability to maintain the therapeutic alliance, resolve threats to the alliance, and repair ruptures in the alliance (Safran and Muran, 2000; Bennett and Parry, 2003).

Although more suggestive than compelling, there is evidence that conducting therapy to a criterion of competence is important to achieving a good outcome. Effectiveness of brief therapy therefore depends as much

on the skilful undertaking of the intervention by the practitioner as on choosing the most appropriate intervention. In this respect psychotherapists are more like surgeons than like physicians—an appropriate procedure can be harmful to the patient if conducted incompetently.

Many therapists, particularly psychodynamic therapists, often conduct brief therapies having only trained in longer-term or open-ended methods. However, brief therapies are not a compressed or truncated form of long-term work, but have developed theories and techniques to maximize the benefits of a finite time frame. There is a dangerous assumption that competence in long-term work can be easily transferred to brief methods. Levenson and Strupp (1999), on the basis of two large surveys of practitioners and graduate school/internship training directors, contradict this assumption. They conclude that it is critical for psychodynamic therapists to receive continuing in-depth training in brief methods and they make recommendations for improvements in the initial training of psychodynamic therapists.

One specific area where psychodynamic therapists trained in longer-term methods are likely to be less competent in brief therapy is in the use of transference interpretation. There is accumulating evidence that an overemphasis on transference interpretation in brief dynamic therapy has an adverse effect on both the therapeutic alliance and outcome (Piper *et al.*, 1993; Hoglend, 1996; Ogrodniczuk *et al.*, 1999). Hoglend (2003) identifies 11 different studies that report a negative association, but points out that the majority have naturalistic designs, and experimental studies including dismantling studies, are urgently needed. Schaeffer (1998) recognizes that these interventions can cause harm or premature termination of therapy and recommends infrequent and cautious use of such interpretations, including crafting them to meet specific patient characteristics and reflecting presenting problems. Hoglend (2003) also recommends the sparing use of transference interpretations, with a greater focus on interpersonal relationships outside therapy.

Treatment manuals used in successful trials of psychological therapies, although drawn up for a different purpose, can be the basis for acquiring competence in a given intervention. Such manuals are now available for a wide variety of brief psychotherapies (Addis, 1997; Wilson, 1998; Najavits *et al.*, 2000) and teaching programs based on these manuals are increasingly delivered (Calhoun *et al.*, 1998).

Formal measures of therapist competence (Chevron and Rounsaville, 1983) are another potential source of intervention guidance that can help practitioners hone their competence in brief methods. Methods include the assessment of case formulations or psychodynamic interpretations (Silberschatz *et al.*, 1986; Crits-Christoph *et al.*, 1988) and of whole sessions using formal rating scales (Vallis *et al.*, 1986; Young and Beck, 1988; Barber and Crits-Christoph, 1996; Bennett and Parry, 2003).

Chapter summary and priorities for research and practice development

We term one to five sessions 'very brief', six to 16 sessions 'brief', and 17–30 sessions 'time-limited' therapy. Therapies of up to 25 sessions are the modal form of therapy delivery, either by design or by default. In third-party payment healthcare systems, there is pressure towards brief therapies because of the need to contain costs, but they also have intrinsic value. Well-conducted brief therapies are effective in a range of moderate difficulties, such as anxiety disorders and depression. There is a plethora of brief and very brief interventions within a range of therapeutic paradigms. Some of these emphasize the time limit as a vehicle for assimilating warded-off anxieties, others do not impose a rigid time limit, using follow-up sessions, or intermittent episodes of therapy, to attenuate the ending. Methods are continuing to develop to find time-efficient ways to benefit people with more severe and complex mental health problems. Training in longer-term methods does not equip practitioners to deliver brief therapies competently. Training specific to brief modalities is required, particularly in the key area of competence in maintaining the therapeutic alliance. Research trials are needed that are designed to address the impact of therapist factors and treatment length, for example randomized, controlled comparison of treatment lengths is needed in addition to dose–response modeling of naturalistic data. Such trials should be supplemented by patient-focused and practice-based evidence on brief and longer-term therapies in different client groups. The relationships between training, competence, and therapy outcome across a range of therapy types are also priorities for research.

References

Ablon, J. S. and Jones, E. E. (2002). Validity of controlled clinical trials of psychotherapy: findings from the NIMH Treatment of Depression Collaborative Research Program. *American Journal of Psychiatry*, **159**, 775–83.

Adams, J. (1991). Family crisis intervention and psychosocial care for children and adolescents. In: C. S. Austad and W. H. Berman, ed. *Psychotherapy in managed health care: the optimal use of time and resources*, pp. 111–25. Washington, DC: American Psychological Association.

Addis, M. E. (1997). Evaluating the treatment manual as a means of disseminating empirically validated psychotherapies. *Clinical Psychology: Science and Practice*, **4**, 1–11.

Alexander, F. and French, T. M. (1946). *Psychoanalytic therapy: principles and applications*. New York: Ronald Press.

Anderson, E. M. and Lambert, M. J. (2001). A survival analysis of clinically significant change in outpatient psychotherapy. *Journal of Clinical Psychology*, **57**, 875–88.

André, C., Lelord, F., Legeron, P., Reignier, A., and Delattre, A. (1997). Etude contrôlée sur l'efficacité a 6 mois d'une prise en charge precoce de 132 conducteurs d'autobus victimes d'aggression. *Encephale*, **23**, 65–71.

Balint, M., Ornstein, P. H., and Balint, E. (1972). *Focal psychotherapy: an example of applied psychoanalysis*. London: Tavistock Publications.

Bandura, A. (1969). *Principles of behavior modification*. New York: Holt, Rinehart and Winston.

Barber, J. P. and Crits-Christoph, P. (1996). Development of a therapist adherence/competence rating scale for supportive-expressive dynamic psychotherapy: a preliminary report. *Psychotherapy Research*, **6**, 81–94.

Barber, J., Crits-Christoph, P., and Luborsky, L. (1996). Effects of therapist adherence and competence on patient outcome in brief dynamic therapy. *Journal of Consulting and Clinical Psychology*, **64**, 619–22.

Barkham, M. (1989). Brief prescriptive psychotherapy in two-plus-one sessions: initial cases from the clinic. *Behavioral Psychotherapy*, **17**, 161–75.

Barkham, M., Moorey, J., and David, G. (1992). Cognitive behavioural therapy in two-plus-one sessions: a pilot field trial. *Behavioral Psychotherapy*, **20**, 147–54.

Barkham, M., *et al.* (1996). Dose-effect relations in time-limited psychotherapy for depression. *Journal of Consulting and Clinical Psychology*, **64**, 927–35.

Barkham, M., Shapiro, D. A., Hardy, G. E., and Rees, A. (1999). Psychotherapy in two-plus-one sessions: outcomes of a randomised controlled trial of cognitive-behavioral and psychodynamic-interpersonal therapy for subsyndromal depression. *Journal of Consulting and Clinical Psychology*, **67**, 201–11.

Beck, A. T. (1967). *Depression: clinical, experimental and theoretical aspects*. New York: Harper and Row.

Beck, A. T., Rush, A. J., Shaw, B. F., and Emery, G. (1979). *Cognitive Therapy of Depression*. New York: Guilford Press.

Benjamin, L. S. (2003). *Interpersonal reconstructive therapy: promoting change in non-responders*. New York: Guilford Press.

Bennett, D. and Parry, G. (2003). A therapeutic task: resolving reciprocal role enactments that threaten the therapeutic alliance. In: D. Charman, ed. *Processes in brief dynamic psychotherapy: training for effectiveness*. Springfield, IL: Lawrence Erlbaum.

Beutler, L. E. (1991). Have all won and must all have prizes? *Journal of Consulting and Clinical Psychology*, **59**, 226–32.

Beutler, L. E. (1995). The germ theory myth and the myth of outcome heterogeneity. *Psychotherapy*, **32**, 489–94.

Beutler, L. E. (2002). The Dodo Bird is extinct. *Clinical Psychology: Science and Practice*, **9**, 30–4.

Binder, J. L., Henry, W. P., and Strupp, H. H. (1987). An appraisal of selection criteria for dynamic psychotherapies and implications for setting time limits. *Psychiatry*, **50**, 154–66.

Binder, J. L. and Strupp, H. H. (1991). The Vanderbilt approach to time limited dynamic psychotherapy. In: P. Critis-Christoph and J. P. Barber, ed. *Handbook of Short-term Dynamic Psychotherapy*. New York: Basic Books.

Black, D. W., Wesner, R., Bowers, W., and Gabel, J. (1993). A comparison of fluvoxamine, cognitive therapy, and placebo in the treatment of panic disorder. *Archives of General Psychiatry*, **50**, 44–50.

Book, H. E. (1998). *How to practice brief psychodynamic psychotherapy: the core conflictual relationship theme method*. Washington, DC: American Psychological Association.

Breger, L. and McGaugh, J. L. (1965). Critique and reformulation of 'learning-theory' approaches to psychotherapy and neurosis. *Psychological Bulletin*, **63**, 338–58.

Bryant, R. A., Sackville, T., Dang, S. T., Moulds, M., and Guthrie, R. (1999). Treating acute stress disorder: an evaluation of cognitive behavior therapy and supportive counseling techniques. *American Journal of Psychiatry*, **156**, 1780–6.

Budman, S. H. and Gurman, A. S. (1988). *Theory and practice of brief psychotherapy*. New York: Guilford Press.

Burke, B. L., Arkovitz, H., and Menchola, M. (2003). The efficacy of motivational interviewing: a meta-analysis of controlled clinical trials. *Journal of Consulting and Clinical Psychology*, **71**, 843–61.

Calhoun, K. S., Moras, K., Pilkonis, P. A., and Rehm, I. P. (1998). Empirically supported treatments: implications for training. *Journal of Consulting and Clinical Psychology*, **66**, 151–62.

Caplan, G. (1961). *An approach to community mental health*. New York: Grune and Stratton.

Castonguay, L. G., Hayes, A. M., Goldfried, M. R., and DeRubeis, R. J. (1995). The focus of therapist interventions in cognitive therapy for depression. *Cognitive Therapy and Research*, **19**, 485–503.

Castonguay, L. G., Goldfried, M. R., Wiser, S., Raue, P. J., and Hayes, A. M. (1996). Predicting the effect of cognitive therapy for depression: a study of unique and common factors. *Journal of Consulting and Clinical Psychology*, **64**, 497–504.

Chambless, D. L. and Gillis, M. M. (1993). Cognitive therapy of anxiety disorders. *Journal of Consulting and Clinical Psychology*, **61**, 248–60.

Chevron, E. S. and Rounsaville, B. J. (1983). Evaluating the clinical skills of psychotherapists: a comparison of techniques. *Archives of General Psychiatry*, **40**, 1129–32.

Chiefetz, D. I. and Salloway, J. C. (1985). Crisis intervention: interpretation and practice by HMOs. *Medical Care*, **23**, 89–93.

Clark, D. M. and Fairburn, C. G. (1997). *Science and practice of cognitive behaviour therapy*. Oxford: Oxford University Press.

Clark, D. M., Salkovskis, P. M., Hackmann, A., Wells, A., Ludgate, J., and Gelder, M. (1999). Brief cognitive therapy for panic disorder: a randomised controlled trial. *Journal of Consulting and Clinical Psychology*, **67**, 583–9.

Crits-Christoph, P., Cooper, A., and Luborsky, L. (1988). The accuracy of therapists' interpretations and the outcome of dynamic psychotherapy. *Journal of Consulting and Clinical Psychology*, **56**, 490–5.

Cummings, N. A. (1991). Brief intermittent therapy throughout the life cycle. In: C. S. Austad and W. H. Berman, ed. *Psychotherapy in managed health care: the optimal use of time and resources*, pp. 35–45. Washington, DC: American Psychological Association.

Davanloo, H. D. (1978). *Basic principles and techniques in short-term dynamic psychotherapy*. New York: Spectrum.

Davanloo, H. D. (1990). *Selected papers*. New York: Wiley.

Department of Health. (2001). *Treatment choice in psychological therapies and counselling: evidence-based clinical guideline*. London: Department of Health.

DeRubeis, R. J. and Feeley, M. (1991). Determinants of change in cognitive therapy for depression. *Cognitive Therapy and Research*, **14**, 469–82.

Dunn, C., Deroo, L., and Rivara, F. P. (2001). The use of brief interventions adapted from motivational interviewing across behavioral domains: a systematic review. *Addiction*, **96**, 1725–42.

D'Zurilla, T. J. and Goldfried, M. R. (1971). Problem solving and behavior modification. *Journal of Abnormal Psychology*, **78**, 107–26.

Elkin, I. (1994). The NIMH treatment of depression collaborative research program: where we began and where we are. In: A. E. Bergin and S. L. Garfield, ed. *Handbook of psychotherapy and behavior change*, 4th edn. pp. 114–42. New York: Wiley.

Ferenczi, S. (1920). The future development of an active therapy in psychoanalysis. In: J. Suttie, ed. (1950). *Further contributions to the theory and technique of psychoanalysis*. London: Hogarth Press and the Institute of Psychoanalysis.

Foley, S. H., O'Malley, S., Rounsaville, B., Prusoff, B. A., and Weissman, M. M. (1987). The relationship of patient difficulty to therapist performance in interpersonal psychotherapy of depression. *Journal of Affective Disorders*, **12**, 207–17.

Frank, E. and Spanier, C. (1995). Interpersonal psychotherapy for depression: overview, clinical efficacy and future directions. *Clinical Psychology: Science and Practice*, **2**, 349–69.

Frank, E., Kupfer, D. J., Wagner, E. F., McEachrn, A. B., and Comes, C. (1991). Efficacy of interpersonal therapy as a maintenance treatment of recurrent depression. *Archives of General Psychiatry*, **48**, 1053–9.

Gabbard, G. O., Lazar, S. G., Hornberger, J., and Spiegel, D. (1997). The economic impact of psychotherapy: a review. *American Journal of Psychiatry*, **154**, 147–55.

Garfield, S. L. (1989). *The practice of brief psychotherapy*. Elmsford, NJ: Pergamon.

Garfield, S. L. (1994). Client variables. In: A. E. Bergin and S. L. Garfield, ed. *Handbook of psychotherapy and behavior change*, 4th edn. New York: Wiley.

Garfield, S. L. (1995). *Psychotherapy: an eclectic-integrative approach*. New York: Wiley.

Gibbons, J. S., Butler, J., Urwin, P., and Gibbons, J. L. (1978). Evaluation of a social work service for self-poisoning patients. *British Journal of Psychiatry*, **133**, 111–18.

Gingerich, W. J. and Eisengart, S. (2000). Solution focused brief therapy: a review of outcome research. *Family Process*, **39**, 477–98.

Gloaguen, V., Cottraux, J., Cucherat, M., and Blackburn, I. M. (1998). A meta-analysis of the effects of cognitive therapy in depressed patients. *Journal of Affective Disorders*, **49**, 59–72.

Goldfried, M. R. (2003). Cognitive-behavior therapy: reflections on the evolution of a therapeutic orientation. *Cognitive Therapy and Research*, **27**, 53–69.

Goldfried, M. R. and Robins, C. (1983). Self-schema, cognitive bias, and the processing of therapeutic experiences. In: P. C. Kendall, ed. *Advances in cognitive-behavioral research and therapy*, Vol. II, pp. 33–80. New York: Academic Press.

Greenberg, J. and Mitchell, S. A. (1983). *Object relations in psychoanalytic theory*. Cambridge, MA: Harvard University Press.

Groves, J. E. (1996). Four 'essences' of short-term therapy: brevity, focus, activity, selectivity. In: J. E. Groves, ed. *Essential papers on short-term dynamic therapy*, pp. 1–26. New York: New York University Press.

Gustafson, J. (1986). *The complex secret of brief psychotherapy*. New York: Norton.

Guthrie, E., Creed, F., Dawson, D., and Tomenson, B. (1991). A randomised controlled trial of psychotherapy in patients with refractory irritable bowel syndrome. *Gastroenterology*, **100**, 450–7.

Guthrie, E., et al. (1999). Cost-effectiveness of brief psychodynamic-interpersonal therapy in high utilizers of psychiatric services. *Archives of General Psychiatry*, **56**, 519–26.

Guthrie, E., et al. (2001). Randomised controlled trial of brief psychological intervention after deliberate self poisoning. *British Medical Journal*, **323**, 135–8.

Haaga, D. A. (2000). Introduction to special section on stepped care models in psychotherapy. *Journal of Consulting and Clinical Psychology*, **68**, 547–8.

Halpern, J. (1999). Philosophical and ethical considerations in the evaluation of the effectiveness and cost-effectiveness of psychotherapy. In: K. Magruder and N. E. Miller, ed. *The cost effectiveness of psychotherapy: a guide for practitioners, researchers and policymakers*. Cambridge University Press.

Hamilton, J., et al. (2000). A randomized controlled trial of psychotherapy in patients with chronic functional dyspepsia. *Gastroenterology*, **119**, 661–9.

Hansen, N. B., Lambert, M. J., and Forman, E. M. (2002). The psychotherapy dose–response relationship and its implications for treatment delivery services. *Clinical Psychology: Science and Practice*, **9**, 329–43.

Hawton, K. and Kirk, J. (1989). Problem-solving. In: K. Hawton, P. M. Salkovskis, J. Kirk, and D. M. Clark, ed. *Cognitive behaviour therapy for psychiatric problems: a practical guide*, pp. 406–26. Oxford: Oxford University Press.

Hawton, K., McKeown, S., Day, A., Martin, P., O'Connor, M., and Yule, J. (1987). Evaluation of out-patient counselling compared with general practitioner care following overdoses. *Psychological Medicine*, **17**, 751–61.

Hawton, K., et al. (1998). Deliberate self-harm: a systematic review of the efficacy of psychosocial and pharmacological treatments in preventing repetition. *British Medical Journal*, **317**, 441–7.

Hellstrom, K., Fellenius, J., and Öst, L. G. (1996). One versus five sessions of applied tension in the treatment of blood phobia. *Behavior Research and Therapy*, **34**, 101–12.

Henry, W. P., Strupp, H. H., Butler, S. F., Schacht, T. E., and Binder, J. L. (1993). Effects of training in time limited dynamic psychotherapy: changes in therapist behavior. *Journal of Consulting and Clinical Psychology*, **61**, 434–40.

Hobbs, M. (1984). Crisis intervention in theory and practice: a selective review. *British Journal of Medical Psychology*, **57**, 23–34.

Hobson, R. F. (1985). *Forms of feeling: the heart of psychotherapy*. London: Tavistock Publications.

Hoffman, I. Z. (1998). *Ritual and spontaneity in the psychoanalytic process: a dialectical-constructivist view*. Hillsdale, NJ: Analytic Press.

Hoglend, P. (1996). Long-term effects of transference interpretations: comparing results from a quasi-experimental and a naturalistic long-term follow-up study of brief dynamic psychotherapy. *Acta Psychiatrica Scandinavica*, **93**, 205–11.

Hoglend, P. (2003). Long-term effects of brief dynamic psychotherapy. *Psychotherapy Research*, **13**, 271–92.

Hoglend, P. and Piper, W. E. (1997). Treatment length and termination contracts in dynamic psychotherapy: a comparison of findings from two independent studies of brief dynamic psychotherapy. *Nordic Journal of Psychiatry*, **51**, 37–42.

Hollon, S. D., et al. (1992). Cognitive therapy and pharmacotherapy for depression: singly or in combination. *Archives of General Psychiatry*, **49**, 774–81.

Holmes, J. (2000). Object relations, attachment theory, self-psychology, and interpersonal psychoanalysis. In: M. G. Gelder, J. J. López-Ibor Jr, and N. C. Andreasen, ed. *New Oxford textbook of psychiatry*. Oxford: Oxford University Press.

Howard, K. I., Krause, M. S., and Orlinsky, D. E. (1986). The dose-effect relationship in psychotherapy. *American Psychologist*, **41**, 159–64.

Howard, K. I., Lueger, R., Maling, M., and Martinovitch, Z. (1993). A phase model of psychotherapy: causal mediation of outcome. *Journal of Consulting and Clinical Psychology*, **61**, 678–85.

Hoyt, M. F. (1991). Teaching and learning short-term psychotherapy. In: C. S. Austad and W. H. Berman, ed. *Psychotherapy in Managed Health Care: the optimal use of time and resources*, pp. 98–107. Washington, DC: American Psychological Association.

Huppert, J. D., et al. (2001). Therapists, therapist variables, and cognitive behavioral therapy outcome in a multicenter trial for panic disorder. *Journal of Consulting and Clinical Psychology*, **69**, 747–55.

Jacobson, G. F. (1980). Crisis theory. In: G. F. Jacobson, ed. *New directions for mental health services: crisis intervention in the 1980s*. San Francisco, CA: Jossey Bass.

Jarrett, R. B., et al. (2001). Preventing recurrent depression using cognitive therapy with and without a continuation phase: a randomized clinical trial. *Archives of General Psychiatry*, **58**, 381–8.

Johnson, D. H. and Gelso, C. J. (1980). The effectiveness of time limits in counseling and psychotherapy: a critical review. *The Counseling Psychologist*, **9**, 70–83.

Joy, C., Adams, C., and Rice, K. (2004). Crisis intervention for people with severe mental illnesses. Cochrane Database of Systematic Reviews. Oct 18; (4): CD001087.

Kalenthaler, E., Parry, G., and Beverley, C. (2003). Computerised cognitive behaviour therapy: a systematic review. *Behavioural and Cognitive Psychotherapy*, **32**, 31–55.

Katon, W., Von Korff, M., Lin, E., Walker, E., Simon, G., and Bush, T. (1999). Collaborative management to achieve treatment guidelines; impact on depression in primary care. *Journal of American Medical Association*, **273**, 1026–31.

Kelly, G. A. (1955). *The psychology of personal constructs*. New York: Norton.

Kerr, I. B. (1999). Cognitive analytic therapy for borderline personality disorder in the context of a community mental health team: individual and organisational psychodynamic implications. *British Journal of Psychotherapy*, **15**, 425–38.

Klerman, G. L., Weissman, M. M., Rounsaville, B., and Chevron, E. S. (1984). *Interpersonal psychotherapy for depression*. New York: Basic Books.

Kopta, S. M., Howard, K. I., Lowry, J. L., and Beutler, L. E. (1996). Patterns of symptomatic recovery in psychotherapy. *Journal of Consulting and Clinical Psychology*, **62**, 1009–16.

Koss, M. P. and Butcher, J. (1986). Research on brief psychotherapy. In: S. L. Garfield and A. E. Bergin, ed. *Handbook of psychotherapy and behavior change*, 3rd edn, pp. 627–70. New York: Wiley.

Lambert, M. J. and Ogles, B. M. (2003). The efficacy and effectiveness of psychotherapy. In: M. J. Lambert, ed. *Bergin and Garfield's handbook of psychotherapy and behavior change*, 5th edn. New York: Wiley.

Lambert, M. J., et al. (2001). The effects of providing therapists with feedback on patient progress during psychotherapy: are outcomes enhanced? *Psychotherapy Research*, **11**, 49–68.

Lambert, M. J., Hansen, N. B., and Finch, A. E. (2001). Patient-focused research: using patient outcome data to enhance treatment effects. *Journal of Consulting and Clinical Psychology*, **69**, 159–72.

Lambert, M. J., et al. (2002). Enhancing psychotherapy outcomes via providing feedback on client progress: a replication. *Clinical Psychology and Psychotherapy*, **9**, 91–103.

Leibovich, M. A. (1983). Why short term therapy for borderlines? *Psychotherapy and Psychosomatics*, **39**, 1–9.

Leiman, M. (1992). The concept of sign in the work of Vygotsky, Winnicott and Bakhtin: further integration of object relations theory and activity theory. *British Journal of Medical Psychology*, **65**, 209–21.

Leiman, M. (1997). Procedures as dialogical sequences: a revised version of the fundamental concept in cognitive analytic therapy. *British Journal of Medical Psychology*, **70**, 193–207.

Leuger, R. J., et al. (2001). Assessing treatment progress with individualised models of expected response. *Journal of Consulting and Clinical Psychology*, **69**, 150–8.

Levenson, H. and Strupp, H. H. (1999). Recommendations for the future of training in brief dynamic psychotherapy. *Journal of Clinical Psychology*, **55**, 385–91.

Lewis, G., et al. (2003). *Self-help interventions for mental health problems. Report to the Department of Health R&D Programme*. Summary at: www.nimhe.org.uk/expertbriefings

Liberman, R. P. and Eckman, T. (1981). Behavior therapy vs insight-oriented therapy for repeated suicide attempters. *Archives of General Psychiatry*, **38**, 1126–30.

Linehan, M. M. (1993). *Cognitive-behavioural treatment of borderline personality disorder*. New York: Guilford Press.

Linehan, M. M., Heard, H. L., and Armstrong, H. E. (1993). Naturalistic follow-up of a behavioral treatment for chronically parasuicidal borderline patients. *Archives of General Psychiatry*, **50**, 971–4.

Lovell, K. and Richards, D. (2000). Multiple access points and levels of entry (MAPLE): Ensuring choice, accessibility and equity for CBT services. *Behavioural and Cognitive Psychotherapy*, **28**, 379–91.

Luborsky, L. (1984). *Principles of psychoanalytic psychotherapy: a manual for supportive-expressive treatment*. New York: Basic Books.

Luborsky, L. and Crits-Christoph, P. (1998). *Understanding transference: the core conflictual relationship theme method*, 2nd edn. New York: Basic Books.

Luborsky, L., Singer, B., and Luborsky L. (1975). Comparative studies of psychotherapies: is it true that 'everybody has won and all must have prizes'? *Archives of General Psychiatry*, **32**, 995–1008.

Luborsky, L., et al. (1986). Do therapists vary much in their success? Findings from four outcome studies. *American Journal of Orthopsychiatry*, **51**, 501–12.

Luborsky, L., et al. (1995). Supportive-expressive dynamic psychotherapy of depression: a time-limited version. In: *Psychodynamic psychotherapies for psychiatric disorders (Axis I)*, pp. 13–42. New York: Basic Books.

Luborsky, L., et al. (2002). The Dodo Bird verdict is alive and well—mostly. *Clinical Psychology: Science and Practice*, **9**, 2–12.

Malan, D. H. (1963). *A study of brief psychotherapy*. London: Tavistock Publications.

Malan, D. H. (1976). *The frontier of brief psychotherapy*. New York: Plenum.

Malan, D. H. (1979). *Individual psychotherapy and the science of psychodynamics*. London: Butterworths.

Mann, J. (1978). *Time-limited psychotherapy*. Cambridge, MA: Harvard University Press.

Mann, J. and Goldman, R. (1982). *A casebook in time-limited psychotherapy*. New York: McGraw-Hill.

McCullough, L., et al. (2003). *Treating affect phobia: a manual for short-term dynamic psychotherapy*. New York: Guilford Press.

McGinn, L. K. and Young, J. E. (1996). Schema-focused therapy. In: P. M. Salkovskis, ed. *Frontiers of cognitive therapy*, pp. 182–207. New York: Guilford Press.

McLeavey, B. C., Daly, R. J., Ludgate, J. W., and Murray, C. M. (1994). Interpersonal problem-solving skills training in the treatment of self-poisoning patients. *Suicide and Life Threatening Behavior*, **24**, 382–94.

Meichenbaum, D. (1977). *Cognitive behavior modification: an integrative approach*. New York: Plenum.

Messer, S. B. (2001). What makes brief psychodynamic therapy time efficient? *Clinical Psychology: Science and Practice*, **8**, 5–22.

Messer, S. B. and Warren, C. S. (1995). *Models of brief psychotherapy*. New York: Guilford Press.

Miller, W. R. and Rollnick, S. (1991). *Motivational interviewing: preparing people to change addictive behavior*. New York: Guilford Press.

Miller, W. R., Yahne, C. E., and Tonigan, J. S. (2003). Motivational interviewing in drug abuse services: a randomized trial. *Journal of Consulting and Clinical Psychology*, **71**, 754–63.

Najavits, L. M., Weiss, R. G., Shaw, S. R., and Dierberger, A. E. (2000). Psychotherapists' views of treatment manuals. *Professional Psychology: Research and Practice*, **31**, 404–8.

Nezu, A. M., Nezu, C. M., and Perri, M. G. (1989). *Problem-solving therapy for depression: theory, research, and clinical guidelines*. New York: Wiley.

Norcross, J. C. (1995). Dispelling the dodo bird verdict and the exclusivity myth in psychotherapy. *Psychotherapy*, **32**, 500–4.

Office of National Statistics. (2000). Psychiatric morbidity among adults living in private households. National statistics website www.statistics.gov.uk

Ogrodniczuk, J. S., Piper, W. E., Joyce, A. S., and McCallum, M. (1999). Transference interpretations in short-term dynamic psychotherapy. *Journal of Nervous and Mental Disease*, **187**, 571–8.

O'Malley, S. S., et al. (1988). Therapist competence and patient outcome in interpersonal psychotherapy of depression. *Journal of Consulting and Clinical Psychology*, **56**, 496–501.

Omer, H. (1993). The integrative focus: co-ordinating symptom- and person-oriented perspectives in therapy. *American Journal of Psychotherapy*, **47**, 283–95.

Öst, L. G., Brandberg, M., and Alm, T. (1997). One versus five sessions of exposure in the treatment of flying phobia. *Behavior Research and Therapy*, **35**, 987–96.

Öst, L. G., Hellstrom, K., and Kåver, A. (1992). One versus five sessions of exposure in the treatment of injection phobia. *Behavior Therapy*, **23**, 263–82.

Öst, L. G., Alm, T., Brandberg, M., and Breitholtz, E. (2001). One versus five sessions of cognitive therapy in the treatment of claustrophobia. *Behavior Research and Therapy*, **39**, 167–83.

Parry, G., Cape, J., and Pilling, S. (2003a). Clinical practice guidelines in clinical psychology and psychotherapy. *Clinical Psychology and Psychotherapy*.

Parry, G., et al. (2003b). *Clinical and cost effectiveness of a cognitive behavioural intervention for improved self-management in adults with psychological complications of asthma*. Final report on project AM1/06/010 to National Research and Development Programme on Asthma Management. London: Department of Health.

Perris, C. (1989). *Cognitive therapy with schizophrenic patients*. New York: Guilford Press.

Perris, C. and McGorry, P. D. (1999). *Cognitive psychotherapy of psychosis and personality disorder*. New York: Wiley.

Peterfreund, E. (1983). *The process of psychoanalytic therapy. Models and strategies*. Hillsdale, NJ: Lawrence Erlbaum.

Piper, W. E., Joyce, A. S., McCallum, M., and Azim, H. F. (1993). Concentration and correspondence of transference interpretations in short-term psychotherapy. *Journal of Consulting and Clinical Psychology*, **61**, 586–95.

Prochaska, J. O. and DiClemente, C. C. (1984). *The transtheoretical approach: crossing traditional boundaries of therapy*. Homewood, IL: Dow Jones/Irwin.

Rose, S., Bisson, J., and Wessely, S. (2003). *Psychological debriefing for preventing post traumatic stress disorder (PTSD).* (Cochrane Review). The *Cochrane Library*, Issue 2. Oxford: Update Software.

Roth, A. D. and Fonagy, P. (1996). *What works for whom? A critical review of psychotherapy research.* New York: Guilford Press.

Roth, A. D. and Fonagy, P. (2005). *What works for whom? A critical review of psychotherapy research*, 2nd edn. New York: Guilford Press.

Roth, A. D. and Parry, G. (1997). The implications of psychotherapy research for clinical practice and service development: lessons and limitations. *Journal of Mental Health*, **6**, 367–80.

Rounsaville, B. J. and Carroll, K. M. (2002). Commentary on Dodo Bird revisited: why aren't we Dodos yet? *Clinical Psychology: Science and Practice*, **9**, 17–20.

Rounsaville, B. J., Weissman, M. M., and Prusoff, B. A. (1981). Psychotherapy with depressed outpatients: patient and process variables as predictors of outcome. *British Journal of Psychiatry*, **13**, 67–74.

Ryle, A. (1977). *Cognitive analytic therapy and borderline personality disorder: the model and the method.* Chichester: Wiley.

Ryle, A. (1990). *Cognitive analytic therapy: active participation in change.* Chichester: Wiley.

Ryle, A. and Kerr, I. B. (2002). *Introducing cognitive analytic therapy.* Chichester: Wiley.

Ryle, A. and Marlowe, M. J. (1995). Cognitive analytic therapy of borderline personality disorder: theory and practice and the clinical and research uses of the self states sequential diagram. *International Journal of Short-term Psychotherapy*, **10**, 21–34.

Safran, J. D. and Muran, J. C. (2000). *Negotiating the therapeutic alliance: a relational treatment guide.* New York: Guilford Press.

Salkovskis, P. M. (1996). *Frontiers of cognitive therapy.* New York: Guilford Press.

Salkovskis, P. M. and Clark, D. M. (1991). Cognitive therapy for panic disorder. *Journal of Cognitive Psychotherapy*, **5**, 215–26.

Salkovskis, P. M., Atha, C., and Storer, D. (1990). Cognitive-behavioural problem solving in the treatment of patients who repeatedly attempt suicide. A controlled trial. *British Journal of Psychiatry*, **157**, 871–6.

van der Sande, R., Buskens, E., Allart, E., van der Graaf, Y., and van Engeland, H. (1997). Psychosocial intervention following suicide attempt: a systematic review of treatment interventions. *Acta Psychiatrica Scandinavica*, **96**, 43–50.

Schact, T. E., Binder, J. L., and Strupp, H. H. (1984). *Psychotherapy in a new key.* New York: HarperCollins.

Schaeffer, J. A. (1998). Transference and countertransference interpretations: harmful or helpful in short-term dynamic therapy? *American Journal of Psychotherapy*, **52**, 1–17.

Schulte, D., Kuenzel, R., Pepping, G., and Schulte-Bahrenberg, T. (1992). Tailor-made versus standardized therapy of phobic patients. *Advances in Behaviour Research and Therapy*, **14**, 67–92.

Seligman, M. E. P. (1995). The effectiveness of psychotherapy: the Consumer Reports study. *American Psychologist*, **50**, 965–74.

Shapiro, D. A., *et al.* (1994). Effects of treatment duration and severity of depression on the effectiveness of cognitive/behavioral and psychodynamic/interpersonal psychotherapy. *Journal of Consulting and Clinical Psychology*, **62**, 522–34.

Shapiro, D. A., *et al.* (1995). Effects of treatment duration and severity of depression on the maintenance of gains following cognitive behavioral and psychodynamic interpersonal psychotherapy. *Journal of Consulting and Clinical Psychology*, **63**, 378–87.

Shapiro, D. A., *et al.* (2003). Time is of the essence: a selective review of the fall and rise of brief therapy research. *Psychology and Psychotherapy: theory, Research and Practice*, **76**, 211–36.

Shaw B. F., *et al.* (1999). Therapist competence ratings in relation to clinical outcome in cognitive therapy of depression. *Journal of Consulting and Clinical Psychology*, **67**, 837–46.

de Shazer, S. (1985). *Keys to solutions in brief therapy.* New York: W. W. Norton.

Sheard, T., *et al.* (2000). A CAT-derived one to three session intervention for repeated deliberate self-harm: a description of the model and initial experience of trainee psychiatrists in using it. *British Journal of Medical Psychology*, **73**, 179–96.

Sifneos, P. E. (1971). Two different kinds of psychotherapy of short duration. In: H. H. Barton, ed. *Brief therapies*, pp. 82–90. New York: Plenum.

Sifneos, P. E. (1972). *Short-term psychotherapy and emotional crisis.* Cambridge, MA: Harvard University Press.

Silberschatz, G., Fretter, P. B., and Curtis, J. T. (1986). How do interpretations influence the process of psychotherapy? *Journal of Consulting and Clinical Psychology*, **54**, 646–52.

Stern, D. N. (1984). *The interpersonal world of the infant: a view from psychoanalysis and developmental psychology.* New York: Basic Books.

Stein, D. M. and Lambert, M. J. (1984). On the relationship between therapist experience and psychotherapy outcome. *Clinical Psychology Review*, **4**, 127–42.

Stiles, W. B., Shapiro, D. A., and Elliott, R. K. (1986). 'Are all psychotherapies equivalent?' *American Psychologist*, **41**, 165–80.

Sundstrom, S. M. (1993). Single-session psychotherapy for depression: Is it better to focus on problems or solutions? Unpublished doctoral dissertation, Iowa State University, Ames IA.

Tarrier, N., *et al.* (1999). A randomised trial of cognitive therapy and imaginal exposure in the treatment of chronic posttraumatic stress disorder. *Journal of Consulting and Clinical Psychology*, **67**, 13–18.

Thorpe, S. J. and Salkovskis, P. M. (1997). The effect of one-session treatment of spider phobia on attentional bias and beliefs. *British Journal of Clinical Psychology*, **36**, 225–41.

Townsend, E., *et al.* (2001). The efficacy of problem-solving treatments after deliberate self-harm: meta-analysis of randomised controlled trials with respect to depression, hopelessness, and improvement in problems. *Psychological Medicine*, **31**, 979–88.

Trevarthen, C. and Aitken, K. J. (2001). Infant intersubjectivity: research, theory, and clinical applications. *Journal of Child Psychology and Psychiatry*, **42**, 3–48.

Vallis, T. M., Shaw, B. F., and Dobson, K. S. (1986). The cognitive therapy scale: psychometric properties. *Journal of Consulting and Clinical Psychology*, **54**, 381–5.

Van-Emmerik, A. A. P., Kamphuis, J. H., Hulsbosch, A. M., and Emmelkamp, P. M. G. (2002). Single session debriefing after psychological trauma: a meta-analysis. *Lancet*, **360**, 766–71.

Wallerstein, R. S. and Robbins, L. L. (1956). The psychotherapy research project of the Menninger Foundation: rationale, method and sample use IV: Concepts. *Bulletin of the Menninger Clinic*, **20**, 239–62.

Walter, J. L. and Peller, J. E. (1992). *Becoming solution focussed in brief therapy.* New York: Brunner/Mazel.

Wampold, B. E., Minami, T., Baskin, T. W., and Callen-Tierney, S. (2002). A meta-(re)analysis of the effects of cognitive therapy versus 'other therapies' for depression. *Journal of Affective Disorders*, **68**, 159–65.

Ward, E., *et al.* (2000). Randomised controlled trial of non directive counselling, cognitive behaviour therapy, and usual general practitioner care for patients with depression. I: clinical effectiveness. *British Medical Journal*, **321**, 1383–8.

Weakland, J. H., Fisch, R., Watzlawick, P., and Bodin, A. (1974). Brief therapy: focused problem resolution. *Family Process*, **13**, 141–68.

Wells, A. and Papageorgiou, C. (2001). Brief cognitive therapy for social phobia: a case series. *Behavior Research and Therapy*, **39**, 713–20.

Westen, D. and Morrison, K. (2001). A multidimensional meta-analysis of treatments for depression, panic and generalized anxiety disorder: an empirical examination of the status of empirically supported therapies. *Journal of Consulting and Clinical Psychology*, **69**, 875–99.

Wilson, G. (1996). Manual-based treatments: the clinical application of research findings. *Behavior Research and Therapy*, **34**, 295–314.

Wilson, G. T. (1998). Manual-based treatment and clinical practice. *Clinical Psychology: Science and Practice*, **5**, 363–75.

Winston, A. and Winston, B. (2002). *Handbook of integrated short-term psychotherapy.* Washington, DC: American Psychiatric Publishing.

Winston, A., *et al.* (1991). Brief psychotherapy of personality disorders. *Journal of Nervous and Mental Disease*, **179**, 188–93.

Wolberg, L. R. (1965). *Short-term psychotherapy.* New York: Grune and Stratton.

Young, J. E. (1990). *Cognitive Therapy for personality disorders: a schema-focused approach.* Sarasota, FL: Professional Resource Exchange.

Young, J. E., Klosko, J., and Weishaar, M. (2003). *Schema therapy: a practitioner's guide.* New York: Guilford Press.

Index